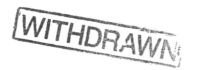

# UROLOGIC NURSING

## Principles and Practice

# UROLOGIC NURSING

## Principles and Practice

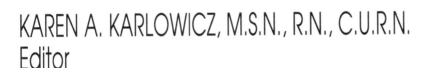

KAREN A. KARLOWICZ, M.S.N., R.N., C.U.R.N.
## Editor
Adjunct Instructor, Old Dominion
University, School of Nursing,
Norfolk, Virginia

**W.B. SAUNDERS COMPANY**
*A Division of Harcourt Brace & Company*
Philadelphia   London   Toronto   Montreal   Sydney   Tokyo

American

Urological

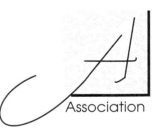

Association

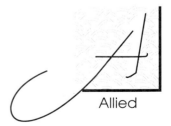

Allied

**W. B. SAUNDERS COMPANY**
*A Division of*
*Harcourt Brace & Company*

The Curtis Center
Independence Square West
Philadelphia, Pennsylvania 19106

## Library of Congress Cataloging-in-Publication Data

Karlowicz, Karen A.

Urologic nursing : principles and practice / Karen A. Karlowicz.

    p.    cm.

Includes index.

ISBN 0–7216–2731–5

1. Urological nursing.    I. American Urological Association
Allied.    II. Title.

[DNLM: 1. Urologic Diseases—nursing.    WY 164 K18a]

RC874.7.K37 1995

610.73′69—dc20

DNLM/DLC                           92–49388

UROLOGIC NURSING: PRINCIPLES AND PRACTICE            ISBN 0–7216–2731–5

Printed in the United States of America.

Last digit is the print number:    9   8   7   6   5   4   3   2   1

To my "boys"—
Gary and Beauregard

KK

**Curriculum Committee of the
American Urological Association Allied**

Karen A. Karlowicz, M.S.N., R.N., C.U.R.N., *Chair*
Christine Hoyler-Grant, M.S.N., R.N., C.P.N.P.
Cindy E. Meredith, M.S.N., R.N.
Janice Robinette, M.A., R.N.
Marsha L. Toner, B.S.N., R.N., C.U.R.N.

# Contributors

**Judith Atkinson-Tighe, R.N.**
Former Unit Manager/Head Nurse, The Hospital for Sick Children, Toronto, Ontario, Canada.
*Pediatric Urologic Oncology*

**Patricia Bates, B.S.N., R.N., C.U.R.N.**
Kaiser Permanente—Urology, Portland, Oregon.
*External Genital Disorders*

**Pamela M. Bilyeu, B.S.N., R.N., C.N.O.R., C.U.R.N.**
Specialty Charge Nurses, St. Vincent Hospital and Health Care Center, Billings, Montana.
*Urologic Instruments*

**Vicki Bowers, B.S.N., R.N.**
Senior Clinical Nurse, Children's Medical-Surgical Center, The Johns Hopkins Hospital, Baltimore, Maryland.
*Bladder Exstrophy and Epispadias*

**Donna F. Brassil, M.A., R.N., C.U.R.N.**
Director of Nursing, Surgical Specialties, New York University Medical Center, New York, New York.
*Sexually Transmitted Diseases*

**Nancy C. Brownlee, B.S.N., R.N.**
Regional Manager, Cook Urological Incorporated, Houston, Texas.
*Urologic Instruments*

**Debra S. Bruton, B.S.N., R.N., C.U.R.N.**
Nurse Clinician II, Cleveland Clinic Foundation, Cleveland, Ohio.
*Urinary Calculi*

**Dorothy A. Calabrese, M.S.N., R.N, C.U.R.N., O.C.N.**
Clinical Nurse Specialist, Urology Oncology, Cleveland Clinic Foundation, Cleveland, Ohio.
*Tumors of the Upper Urinary Tract*

**Susan Carney, B.S.N., R.N.**
Home Health Nurse, Visiting Nurse Services, Columbia Health Center, Seattle, Washington.
*Urinary Tract Obstructions*

viii  *Contributors*

## Carol Einhorn, M.S., R.N., G.N.P., C.U.R.N.
Clinical Nurse Specialist, Urology; Nurse Coordinator, Continence Center/Urodynamics, Northwestern Memorial Hospital, Chicago, Illinois.
*Urinary Calculi*

## Teresa D. Gibbs, B.S.N., R.N., C.U.R.N.
Educator, Nursing Information Systems, The University of Iowa Hospitals and Clinics, Iowa City, Iowa.
*Health Assessment of the Adult Urology Patient*

## Janet A. Giroux, M.S.N., R.N., C.U.R.N.
Research Staff Nurse, Spinal Cord Injury Service, Department of Veterans Affairs Medical Center, Palo Alto, California.
*Urinary Tract Infections in Adults*

## Mikel L. Gray, Ph.D., R.N., C.U.R.N.
UroHealth, Director of Urodynamics, Suburban Medical Center; Adjunct Professor of Nursing, Bellarmine College, Lansing School of Nursing, Louisville, Kentucky.
*Genitourinary Embryology, Anatomy, and Physiology*

## Kathleen F. Hannigan, M.S.N., R.N.
Assistant Professor of Nursing, Union Memorial Hospital School of Nursing, Essex Community College and Anne Arundel Community College; Clinical Nurse Specialist, Johns Hopkins Hospital, Baltimore, Maryland.
*Bladder Exstrophy and Epispadias*

## Christine Hoyler-Grant, M.S.N., R.N., C.P.N.P.
Community Health Nurse, Visiting Nurse Association of Greater Philadelphia, Philadelphia, Pennsylvania; Former Urologic Pediatric Nurse Practitioner affiliated with Joseph Dwoskin, M.D., Buffalo Children's Hospital, Buffalo, New York.
*Health Assessment of the Pediatric Urology Patient*
*Growing Up with a Urologic Disorder: Developmental Considerations*
*Disorders of the External Genitalia in Children*
*Congenital Anomalies That Affect the Kidney, Ureter, and Bladder*

## Karen A. Karlowicz, M.S.N., R.N., C.U.R.N.
Adjunct Instructor, Old Dominion University, School of Nursing, Norfolk, Virginia.
*Perioperative Care of the Urologic Patient*
*Urinary Tract Obstructions*
*Cancer of the Male Genitalia*
*Adult Voiding Dysfunction*
*Radiologic Procedures*
*Information Resources*

## Doris Yukiko Kimura-Van Zant, B.S.N., R.N., C.R.R.N.
Nurse Clinician, Rehabilitation/Urology, Children's Hospital and Medical Center, Seattle, Washington.
*Urinary Tract Infections in Children*

## Angela D. Klimaszewski, M.S.N., R.N., O.C.N.
Former Cancer Research Coordinator, St. Luke Medical Center, Milwaukee, Wisconsin.
*Cancer of the Male Genitalia*

## Karen L. Kushner, B.S.N., R.N.
Head Nurse, Pediatrics, St. Joseph Hospital, Towson, Maryland.
*Bladder Exstrophy and Epispadias*

## Sandra S. La Follette, B.S.N., R.N., C.N.O.R.
Perioperative Clinical Nurse, Center for Health Sciences, University of California, Los Angeles.
*Perioperative Care of the Urologic Patient*

## Catherine-Ann M. Lawrence, M.A., R.N.
Assistant Director, Utilization Management and Quality Improvement; Formerly Nurse Clinician, Pediatrics/Pediatric Genitourinary Service, Montefiore Medical Center—Moses Division, Bronx, New York.
*Pediatric Voiding Disorders*

## Mary Anne Matcham, B.S.N., R.N., C.U.R.N.
Staff Nurse, Cleveland Clinic Foundation, Cleveland, Ohio
*Tumors of the Upper Urinary Tract*

## Cindy E. Meredith, M.S.N., R.N.
Nursing Instructor, University of Michigan, Flint; Urology Nurse Consultant, U.N.C.L.E., Canton, Michigan.
*Urinary Tract Obstructions*
*Erectile Dysfunction*
*Male Infertility*
*Adult Voiding Dysfunction*

## Barbara Montagnino, M.S., R.N.
Clinical Nurse Specialist, Scott Department of Urology, Baylor College of Medicine, Houston, Texas.
*Congenital Anomalies That Affect the Kidney, Ureter, and Bladder*

## Suzanne M. Pear, M.S., R.N., C.I.C., C.U.R.N.
Infection Control Coordinator, Department of Veterans Affairs Medical Center, Tucson, Arizona.
*Urinary Tract Obstructions*

## Lynn M. Reardon, B.S.N., R.N., C.U.R.N.
Former Staff Nurse, Urology, Cleveland Clinic Foundation, Cleveland, Ohio.
*Urinary Calculi*

## Nancy J. Reilly, M.S.N., R.N., C.U.R.N.
Gastrointestinal/Genitourinary Clinical Nurse Specialist, Hospital of the University of Pennsylvania, Philadelphia, Pennsylvania.
*Urinary Tract Obstructions*
*Cancer of the Bladder*
*Genitourinary Trauma*
*Radiologic Procedures*

## Janice Robinette, M.A., R.N.
Laser Education Specialist, Abbott Northwestern Hospital, Laser Center, Minneapolis, Minnesota.
*Information Resources*

### Josette M. Snyder, M.S.N., R.N., C.U.R.N.
Nurse Specialist, Palliative Care, Cleveland Clinic Foundation, Cleveland, Ohio.
*Urinary Calculi*

### Elayne C. Sugar, M.S.N., R.N.
Clinical Specialist in Pediatric Urology, Children's Memorial Hospital, Chicago, Illinois.
*Disorders of the External Genitalia in Children*

### Linda Swibold, B.S.N., R.N., C.U.R.N.
Urology Nurse Clinician, Veterans Administration Medical Center, Tucson, Arizona.
*Urinary Tract Obstructions*

### Kathleen A. Thompson, M.S.N., R.N.C.
Former Nursing Coordinator of the Division of Urology, Children's Hospital, Boston, Massachusetts.
*Problems of Sexual Differentiation and Development*

### Marsha L. Toner, B.S.N., R.N., C.U.R.N.
Nurse Clinician II (Head Nurse), University of Iowa Hospitals and Clinics, Iowa City, Iowa.
*Urinary Tract Obstructions*

### Janet D. Wagner, B.S.N., R.N., C.U.R.N.
Hospital Quality Management Specialist, Veterans Administration Medical Center, Tucson, Arizona.
*Urinary Tract Obstructions*

### Valre W. Welch, M.S.N., R.N, C.P.N.P.
Urology/Nephrology Program Coordinator, Clinical Nurse Specialist, Children's Hospital of the King's Daughters, Norfolk, Virginia.
*Congenital Anomalies That Affect the Kidney, Ureter, and Bladder*

### Julie Wettlaufer, M.S.N., R.N., C.P.N.P.
Family Nurse Practitioner, Children's Hospital of Buffalo, Buffalo, New York.
*Perioperative Care of the Urologic Patient*
*Pediatric Urologic Oncology*

### Angela Williams, B.S.N., R.N., C.U.R.N.
Staff Nurse, Urogynecology, William Beaumont Hospital, Royal Oak, Michigan.
*Urinary Calculi*

# Acknowledgments

Words cannot begin to express my gratitude to the cadre of contributing authors who devoted untold hours to researching, developing, and writing their respective chapters for *Urologic Nursing: Principles and Practice*. I am especially grateful to their families and employers for supporting their involvement in this project. Special recognition and thanks must also be given to Chris Grant, Cindy Meredith, Jan Robinette, and Marsha Toner for their involvement and contributions as members of the Curriculum Committee of the AUAA. Together, our vision and commitment to the creation of an educational resource about the practice of urologic nursing resulted in this publication.

My most sincere appeciation is extended to those who so generously gave their time and expertise as content reviewers for *Urologic Nursing: Principles and Practice*, including: Robert Agee, M.D.; Cheryl Aikey, C.U.R.N.; Leslie Becker, M.D.; Lorraine Carroll, R.N.; Harold A. Fuselier, Jr., M.D.; John P. Gearhart, M.D.; Carolyn Grous, M.S.N., C.N.O.R.; Mertie Jones, B.S.N., M.Ed., C.U.R.N.; M. Gary Karlowicz, M.D.; Gary Kearney, M.D.; Priscilla Krejci, C.U.R.N.; Greg Ott, C.U.T.; Karen Pilkington, R.N.; Carralee Sueppel, B.L.S., R.N., C.U.R.N.; Boyd Winslow, M.D.; and countless other urologic nurses and urologists who served as blind reviewers for the publisher.

Special thanks and recognition are extended to those who provided technical support for this project, including Jerry Bates, for his beautifully prepared medical illustrations; Rochelle Bodner, for her word processing skills and assistance with manuscript preparation; staff of the Moorman Memorial Library of the Eastern Viginia Medical School, for their willingness to assist with literature searches and verification of references; Pam Williams and Nancy Reilly, for their help with the tedious task of proofreading copy; Sue Reilly, Supervising Copy Editor at W. B. Saunders, for her continued understanding and attention to details; and lastly, Dan Ruth, Editor, and the staff at W. B. Saunders Company, for helping to see this project to completion.

I am indebted to the American Urological Association Allied (AUAA) Board of Directors for their financial support, understanding, and patience through what has been the largest project the association has ever undertaken. The membership of the AUAA deserves my thanks, too, for their continued interest in this book and their vote of confidence with the huge number of prepublication orders.

I thank my husband, Gary Karlowicz, for the many sacrifices he made to enable me to undertake the editorial responsibility for this book. I could not have persisted through the many challenges presented by this project without his understanding for my level of commitment and his loving words of encouragement.

Finally, thanks to my unofficial supervisor, Beauregard, who has been a faithful poodle-boy from the day I began working on this book—he never let me forget life's necessities!

KAREN A. KARLOWICZ, *Editor*

# Preface

The practice of urology has become more sophisticated over the past 25 years, and as a result, urologic nursing has become an increasingly important specialty. The urologic nurse is a key member of the health care team whose expertise is essential to the management of acute and chronic urologic problems; the promotion of professional, patient, and public education of urologic issues; and the implementation of urologic nursing research.

## AN ALTERNATIVE APPROACH TO CURRICULUM DEVELOPMENT

*Urologic Nursing: Principles and Practice* was initially planned to be the core curriculum of the American Urological Association Allied (AUAA)—the national organization for urologic nurses and allied health professionals. Like other nursing specialty organizations, the AUAA recognized the necessity and importance of defining that body of knowledge that constitutes the specialty of urologic nursing. We also recognized the critical need for a definitive publication that was written by nurses who are acknowledged as experts in the field of urologic patient care.

Our colleagues in other specialty nursing organizations responded to the task of developing a core curriculum by publishing texts with information presented in an outline format, so designed to aid nurses in preparing for specialty certification examinations. The Curriculum Committee of the AUAA, however, realized that such books were being used for much more than the purpose originally intended. Thus, without conclusive support for the notion that a core curriculum must be written in outline style, we chose to create a comprehensive textbook, complete with detailed discussions, figures, tables, and procedures that would

1. Serve as resource-reference textbook about urologic nursing.
2. Establish a standard of clinical nursing practice in urology.
3. Augment professional nursing education and staff development in urologic nursing practice.
4. Facilitate preparation for specialty certification as a urologic nurse or technician.

## CONTENT AND ORGANIZATION

The scope of this book's content reflects the philosophical belief of the AUAA that urologic nurses, regardless of their area of subspecialty practice, should be knowledgeable about all aspects of urologic nursing care. Thus, *Urologic Nursing: Principles and Practice* addresses urologic diseases and disorders in both the adult and pediatric populations. This comprehensive presentation of information was not only logical but essential, because in many practice settings the urologic nurse cares for persons of all ages, from infancy through older adulthood.

*Urologic Nursing: Principles and Practice* has been developed to focus on the physical and technical aspects of urologic patient care, as well as the urologic patient's developmental, social, psychological, and sexual health needs. The content was planned and organized to include those urologic conditions frequently encountered by most health care providers. However, a considerable effort has been made to present an in-depth discussion of those diseases and disorders that are infrequently discussed in other publications and that may be familiar only to experienced urologic nurses. This information is presented from both the medical and the nursing perspectives to demonstrate the complexities of urologic patient care and to illustrate the necessity for collaboration among health care providers.

Every effort has been made to describe patient care activities without geographic or individual bias. Because of the dearth of published works about urologic nursing care, it was necessary for the authors to draw on their clinical experiences, and that of their colleagues, to present a realistic and accurate view of the care activities and responsibilities of the urologic nurse. Furthermore, the editors and authors have endeavored to present information in a manner that would be applicable to any environment where urologic nursing care is administered. We believe we have succeeded in producing a resource that will be useful to nurses who are practicing in the hospital, as well as those who are working with urologic patients in the clinic or physician's office, home health care program, or long-term care facility. We also believe that this book will be invaluable not only to educators as a supplemental text for medical-surgical and pediatric nursing courses but also to students who yearn for a resource that provides detailed and reliable information about the needs of their assigned patient with a urologic problem.

*Urologic Nursing: Principles and Practice* contains 24 chapters. Chapters 1 through 15 are devoted to the care of the adult with a urologic disease or disorder, whereas Chapters 16 through 24 discuss the urologic nursing care of the child. Each chapter begins with a brief overview of the content contained therein and is followed by a list of study objectives and terms specific to the chapter. At the end of each chapter is a complete list of references. The contributing authors are to be commended for their efforts to include up-to-date clinical and scientific resources. On review of this listing, the reader will no doubt also notice that some references are several years old; these are classic or original papers on a given subject that merit citation in this text. It was the decision of the editors to include such resources to illustrate the rich scientific history of this specialty.

Chapters 1 through 3 contain information that is fundamental to understanding the assessment, treatment, and management of adults with a urologic condition. Included in these introductory chapters are extensive dis-

cussions about the embryology, anatomy, and physiology of the genitourinary system, as well as a comprehensive approach to nursing health assessment and the basics of perioperative nursing care of the adult urology patient. Likewise, Chapters 16 and 17 contain information that is fundamental to the care of the pediatric urology patient. The content of these chapters is devoted to helping the reader develop a basic understanding of the social, psychological, and sexual issues surrounding the growth and development of a child with a urologic condition. In addition, these chapters describe various techniques for the nurse to employ when conducting a thorough assessment of the pediatric urology patient.

Chapters 4 through 15 contain detailed information about specific urologic conditions in adults, including genitourinary obstructions and infections, urinary tract cancers, external genital conditions, sexual and voiding dysfunction, and genitourinary trauma. Chapters 18 through 24 address urologic problems commonly seen in children, including infections; congenital anomalies of the kidney, ureter, bladder, and external genitalia; bladder exstrophy and epispadias; voiding dysfunction; and pediatric urinary tract tumors. In these chapters, information about a specific condition is first presented from the medical perspective and includes discussion about the etiology, pathophysiology, and medical-surgical management of each. A section devoted solely to nursing care then follows and is titled "Approaches to Patient Care."

Material included in the sections on Approaches to Patient Care is organized according to the nursing process, enabling the reader to approach urologic patient care with understanding and in an organized and thoughtful manner. Using the nursing process as the framework for this section required that we carefully analyze urologic nursing care activities related to each disease or disorder and include those tasks or skills unique to the role of the urologic nurse. We have also limited our listing of nursing diagnoses, patient goals, and patient outcomes to those issues that are of the highest priority and that are most specific to the urologic patient. In most instances, North American Nursing Diagnosis Association–approved nursing diagnoses are used to describe commonly identified patient problems, although there are some situations when other terminology has been employed because it was considered descriptive of a particular urologic patient problem. The reader may also find that there is no strict correlation between the number of nursing diagnoses identified and the number of patient goals and patient outcomes listed. Hence, these sections should be approached with the understanding that a single nursing diagnosis could appropriately lead to one or more patient care goals, and one or more expected patient outcomes, depending on the clinical situation.

Anyone familiar with the specialty of urology knows that it is a highly technical field of practice. There are numerous procedural instruments with which the urologic nurse must be familiar, whether he or she is working with urologic patients in a physician's office, clinic, in-patient unit, cystoscopy suite, or operating room. *Urologic Nursing: Principles and Practice* contains three appendices, the first of which is devoted to the topic of urologic instrumentation. Appendix I is without question one of the special features of this book. It was thoughtfully developed to provide urologic nurses with a means for quickly identifying a particular instrument and obtaining basic information about its use. Nearly 100 instruments are catalogued; they are grouped in the appendix with subheadings that indicate their general purpose. Also included in this appendix are examples of setups for common urologic proce-dures and guidelines for the disinfection and sterilization of urologic instruments. Appendix II lists imaging procedures most commonly performed to evaluate urologic diseases and disorders. Appendix III contains a listing of information resources for the urologic allied health care professional.

## FROM PROPOSAL TO PUBLICATION

Eight years have passed since the idea for this project was first discussed and given the green light by the AUAA Board of Directors. Earnest work on this book has been ongoing for nearly 6 years. Development of a urologic textbook of this scope and size proved to be a time-consuming and painstaking process, not only for the authors and editors but also for the AUAA Board of Directors and our publisher, W. B. Saunders Company. Throughout the development of *Urologic Nursing: Principles and Practice,* our sole intent has been to provide the members of the AUAA, and our nursing colleagues, with a quality publication containing the most complete and current information about the practice of urologic nursing. It has been said that good things are worth the wait. We think you will agree with us—*Urologic Nursing: Principles and Practice* was worth the wait!

KAREN A. KARLOWICZ
*for the Curriculum Committee of the AUAA*

# Contents

# PART I

# Introduction to the Adult Urology Patient

# CHAPTER 1

# Genitourinary Embryology, Anatomy, and Physiology

■

*Mikel L. Gray*

## OVERVIEW

The practice of urologic nursing is based on a thorough understanding of the structure and function of the urinary system from the nephron to the urethral meatus. Unlike the nephrologic nurse, however, the urologic nurse concentrates on the transport, storage, and expulsion functions of the end product of renal filtration (urine) rather than its formation. The urologic nurse also applies knowledge of the anatomy, physiology, and embryonic development of the genitourinary system to care for patients with disorders of the genitalia or sexual function.

## BEHAVIORAL OBJECTIVES

After studying this chapter, the reader should be able to

1. Apply knowledge of genitourinary embryology and congenital defects to the care of affected patients.
2. Identify the major structures of the urinary system and their physiologic significance.
3. Synthesize knowledge of the forces of continence into a comprehensive understanding of bladder filling, storage, and emptying functions.
4. Apply knowledge of the hydrodynamics of the urinary system to an understanding of obstructive uropathy.
5. Define the stages of spermiogenesis and their significance to male fertility.

## KEY WORDS

**Antidiuretic hormone**—a hormone produced by the hypothalamus that acts at the distal renal tubule to promote the conservation of water.

**Bowman's capsule**—a membrane that surrounds the glomerulus.

**Calix**—a cuplike cavity that drains urine from the renal parenchyma into the pelvis.

**Cloaca**—a cavity lined with endodermal cells located at the posterior end of the developing fetus; during embryogenesis, it serves as a common passageway for urine and feces.

**Corpus cavernosum**—erectile tissue of the penis.

**Corpus spongiosum**—erectile tissue surrounding the urethra.

**Cortex**—the outer layer of an organ such as the kidney or the adrenal gland.

**Cotransport**—excretion or secretion of a substance along with sodium that accelerates or inhibits its movement.

**Detrusor muscle**—the smooth muscle bundles of the bladder wall.

**Efflux**—the antegrade movement of urine from the upper urinary tracts to the lower urinary tract.

**Erythropoietin**—a hormone secreted by the kidneys that influences the production of erythrocytes (red blood cells) in the bone marrow.

**Follicle-stimulating hormone (FSH)**—a hormone produced in the pituitary gland; in males, FSH stimulates testosterone production.

**Fossa navicularis**—the terminal portion of the urethra located at the glans penis.

**Gerota's fascia**—dense connective tissue encasing the kidney, the superiorly located adrenal gland, and perinephric fat.

**Glomerulus**—a segment of the proximal nephron comprising afferent and efferent arterioles; it is surrounded by Bowman's capsule and filters blood for selective excretion or reabsorption by the kidneys.

**Gubernaculum testis**—a fibrous cord in the fetus extending from the caudad aspect of the testis, through the inguinal canal, and into the scrotum; it guides testicular descent.

**Internal sphincter**—the bladder neck and adjacent smooth muscle; the internal sphincter forms a portion of the urethral sphincter mechanism.

**Isotonic**—having the same osmotic pressure as serum.

**Leydig cell**—a specialized cell located in the seminiferous tubule that produces testosterone.

**Loop of Henle**—a U-shaped tubule composing part of the nephron; it is significant for its thin descending and thick ascending limbs that provide a countercurrent multiplier system affecting the specific gravity of the urine and the internal environment of the body.

**Luteinizing hormone (LH)**—a hormone produced by the pituitary gland; in males, LH contributes to testosterone production.

**Medulla**—the inner layer of an organ such as the kidney or the adrenal gland.

**Mesonephros**—a type of kidney that develops in all vertebrate mammals; it exists only as an embryonic structure in humans.

**Müllerian-inhibiting factor**—a hormone that influences the development of male external genitalia during embryogenesis.

**Nephron**—the functional unit of the kidney; it comprises the glomerulus, the proximal collecting tubule, the loop of Henle, the distal collecting tubule, and the collecting duct.

**Pelvic nerve (plexus)**—originates from spinal roots S2 to S4 and carries primarily parasympathetic innervation to the urinary bladder and the urethra.

**Peristalsis**—a progressive wavelike movement that occurs involuntarily in hollow, tubular viscera of the body; peristalsis transports urine from the renal pelvis to the bladder.

**Pronephros**—a simplistic, primitive form of an excretory organ; in humans, the pronephros exists only as an embryonic structure.

**Pudendal nerve**—the nerve that originates from spinal roots S1 to S3 to provide somatic innervation to the pelvic floor and periurethral musculature.

**Reflux**—the retrograde movement of urine from the lower urinary tract (bladder) into the upper urinary tracts (ureters and renal pelvis).

**Renal parenchyma**—the portion of kidney tissue that contains the nephrons.

**Rhabdosphincter**—series of C-shaped triple-innervated skeletal muscle fibers located in the middle third of the urethra in females and the membranous urethra in males; contributes to the urethral sphincter mechanism.

**Scrotum**—a fibromuscular sac that hangs from the male perineum; it contains the testes.

**Seminiferous tubule**—the functional unit of the testis; the tubule contains spermatogonia and supportive cells for the production of sperm.

**Sertoli cell**—supporting cell of the seminiferous tubules, presumed to nurture maturing spermatids.

**Spermatid**—an immature spermatozoon that is produced by meiotic division of a secondary spermatocyte.

**Spermatocyte**—the precursor to a mature spermatozoon; a *primary spermatocyte* cell arises from a spermatogonia cell in the seminiferous tubule; a *secondary spermatocyte* results from mitotic division of a primary spermatocyte.

**Spermatogonia**—unspecialized germ cells located in the seminiferous tubular wall; they are precursors to spermatozoon.

**Spermatozoon**—mature sperm cell.

**Spermiogenesis**—the process of maturation of a spermatogonia into a mature spermatozoon.

**Starling's forces**—physical factors that govern the rate of ultrafiltration of blood into the glomerulus.

**Testosterone**—an androgenic hormone produced by the testis that affects spermiogenesis and secondary male characteristics.

**Transport maximum**—the maximum concentration (mass) of a solute that can be reabsorbed from the glomerulus.

**Tunica albuginea**—a white, fibrous connective tissue that encases the testis.

**Tunica vaginalis**—the connective tissue membrane surrounding the front and lateral aspects of the testis.

**Tunica vasculosa**—a plexus of vascular structures that provides nourishment for the lobules of the testis.

**Ureterovesical junction**—the union of the ureter and the bladder that is composed of the terminal ureteral segment, the trigone, the adjacent bladder wall, and the ureteral orifice.

**Urethrovesical junction**—the union of the bladder and the urethral orifice.

**Verumontanum**—an elevation on the floor of the prostatic urethra, near the orifices of the ejaculatory ducts.

**Waldeyer's sheath**—the fibromuscular structure that anchors the terminal ureter and the ureterovesical junction to the bladder.

**Wolffian duct**—a duct in the embryo leading from the mesonephros to the cloaca; the vas deferens, epididymis, seminal vesicles, ejaculatory ducts, ureters, and renal pelvis develop from it.

# EMBRYOLOGY

An understanding of the events in the embryonic development of the kidney, the ureters, and the urethrovesical unit is needed to plan the care of children or adults who experience the consequences of congenital anomalies of the urinary system (Table 1–1). The genitourinary system is particularly susceptible to congenital anomalies; these defects may coexist with congenital defects of other organ systems.

## Kidney and Ureter

The embryonic development of the renal parenchyma (the urine-forming tissue of the kidney) is divided into three overlapping phases. The first phase is the development of pronephric tubules, which are the most primitive renal structure in humans. They arise from intermediate mesodermic tissue adjacent to somites 4 to 14 and comprise as many as 10 pairs of rather simple, straight tubules. The pronephros spontaneously degenerates by the fourth week of life as the mesonephric tubules are developing (Tanagho, 1992b).

The second stage of renal development begins with the appearance of the mesonephros around the fourth week of life. Like the pronephros, the mesonephric tubules provide some excretory function for the developing fetus, although the mother still provides the bulk of renal clearance needed to sustain life and the maturation process. The mesonephric tubules also form adjacent to the somites more caudad (nearer the tail) than the pronephros. The mesonephric tubules are more complex than the pronephros in that they contain a more tortuous structure. The mesonephric tubules also contain structures analogous to the nephron of the mature kidney, although they also degenerate around the eighth week of life, before the ascent of the metanephric tubules that will form the kidney in the human infant (Tanagho, 1992b). Following degeneration, the vestigial remnants of the mesonephric tubules contribute to the development of the male genital system (Golimbu, 1981).

The final phase of renal development begins as the metanephric tubules and ureteral bud grow and develop. The metanephric tubules arise before the eighth week of life as the mesonephroi are regressing. They originate as buds arising from the mesonephric duct that joins the cloaca. Simultaneously, the ureteral bud, which originated from the wolffian duct when the fetus was only 0.5 cm long, begins to migrate in a cephalad (toward the head) direction from the sacrum to the retroperitoneal space. During this migration, the metanephric cap continues to grow, and the tubules begin to differentiate into their mature form. While the parenchyma grows and develops, the cephalad bud of the ureteral bud expands to form the renal pelvis.

The renal pelvis pushes into the developing parenchyma to form collecting ducts that will allow urine transport from the upper to the lower urinary tract. As this process occurs, masses of metanephric tissue are formed that lie near the blind end of the newly formed collecting ducts. These masses form a tubular lumen and assume an S-shape. One end merges with the terminal portion of the collecting tubule, forming the distal convoluted tubule, the proximal tubule, and the loop of Henle. The distal portion, in turn, develops into Bowman's capsule and the glomerulus (Pinck, 1981; Tanagho, 1992b).

The ureter ascends and rotates to an approximately 90-degree angle from the kidney. At birth, the kidneys are situated adjacent to the T12 or L1 level in the retroperitoneal space. Each kidney is now rotated so that its convex border faces the spinal column, in contrast with its origin near the sacral spine, with the convex border situated dorsally (Tanagho, 1992b).

## Bladder, Urethra, and Ureterovesical Unit

The bladder, genital system, and rectum are separated into distinctive structures during early embryogenesis. When the fetus is only 0.5 cm long, the primitive gut forms a tail. An ectodermal depression forms under the root of this tail; a thin plane of tissue, the cloaca, separates the proctodeum into the posterior rectal and the anterior urogenital sinuses. The urinary bladder develops from endodermal tissue in the the urogenital sinus (Pinck, 1981). The ventral portion of the urogenital sinus forms the bladder and proximal urethra of males and the bladder and entire urethra of females. Endodermal tissue from the dorsal portion of the urogenital sinus forms the distal urethra in males and the distal vagina and the vestibule in females (Tanagho, 1992b).

The bladder base and the ureterovesical unit have distinct embryonic origins from the bladder and the urethra. The trigone is formed by mesodermal tissue that lies between the com-

TABLE 1–1. Timetable of the Development of the Human Urinary System

| DAYS AFTER OVULATION | EVENTS DURING DEVELOPMENT |
|---|---|
| 18 | Cloacal membrane at caudal end of primitive streak |
| 20 | Para-axial mesoderm and lateral plate mesoderm; tail end of embryo folds to create cloaca |
| 22 | Intermediate mesoderm; pronephric duct present |
| 24 | Nephrotomes of the pronephros disappear; mesonephric ducts and tubules appear |
| 26 | Caudal portions of the wolffian ducts end blindly short of the cloaca |
| 28 | Wolffian duct has fused to the cloaca; ureteral buds appear; septation of cloaca begins |
| 32 | Common excretory ducts dilate and extend into the cloaca; metanephric mesenchyma caps the ureteral buds |
| 33 | Ureteral buds have extended and appear as primitive pelves |
| 37 | Metanephroi are reniform; ureteral bud ampullae divide into cranial and caudal poles |
| 41 | Müllerian ducts appear; cloaca partitioning; genital tubercle prominent; lumen of ureter is discrete |
| 44 | Urogenital sinus separate from rectum; wolffian ducts and ureters drain separately into the urogenital sinus |
| 48 | First nephrons appear; collecting tubules appear; urogenital membrane ruptures |
| 51 | Kidneys in lumbar region; orifices of ureters cranial to those of the wolffian ducts; Müllerian ducts descend adjacent to the mesonephric ducts |
| 52 | Glomeruli appear in the kidney |
| 54 | Müllerian ducts are fused behind the urogenital sinus; Müller's tubercle distinct; testis distinguishable |
| 8 weeks | *Period of the fetus begins* |
| | Primary and secondary urethral grooves |
| 9 weeks | First likelihood of renal function |
| 10 weeks | Genital ducts of opposite sex degenerate |
| 12 weeks | External genitalia become distinctive for sex; male penile urethra forming; urogenital union; apex of bladder separates from allantoic diverticulum; prostate appears; Cowper's glands and Skene's glands appear |
| 13 weeks | Bladder becomes muscularized |
| 14 weeks | Ureter begins to attain submucosal course in bladder |
| 16 weeks | Mesonephros involuted; glandar urethra forms |
| 18 weeks | Ureteropelvic junction apparent |
| 20–40 weeks | Further growth and development complete the urogenital organs |

Adapted from Maizels, M. (1986). Normal development of the urinary tract. In P. C. Walsh, R. G. Gittes, A. C. Perlmutter, & T. A. Stamey (Eds.), *Campbell's urology* (5th ed., p. 1302). Philadelphia: W. B. Saunders. Reprinted by permission.

mon excretory duct and the ureteral bud. During normal development, the ureteral orifices remain within the medial aspects of the trigone in the bladder base; lateral displacement predisposes to reflux or ectopia (Levitt & Weiss, 1985).

## Genital System and Gender Assignment

Determination of genetic sex at the time of fertilization is the first step in gender development. The presence of X and Y chromosomes principally determines the physiologic expression of male and female gender and influences the myriad of other secondary physiologic and psychosocial factors that constitute sexuality (Golimbu, 1981).

During early embryogenesis, the fetus develops genital structures that are influenced by the presence or absence of masculinizing or feminizing hormones. The gonads make their first appearance around the fifth week of life and remain undifferentiated (unidentifiable as male or female) until week 7. At age 7 weeks, a gene on the short arm of the Y chromosome, near the centromere, influences the differentiation of the primitive gonad into testis or ovary (Aaronson, 1992).

If the fetus is male, differentiation of the primordial gonads into functioning testes begins at week 7. Further development of the testes and male external genitalia is influenced by two hormonal substances, müllerian-inhibiting factor and testosterone, produced by the testis as early as the eighth week of life. Under the influence of these substances that act as hormonal and paracrine substances, the wolffian ducts differentiate into epididymis, vas deferens, and seminal vesicles. Testosterone also influences the development of the prostate and the external genitalia with the conversion of testosterone to dihydrotestosterone (Aaronson, 1992).

If the fetus is female, differentiation of the

müllerian ductile system into functioning ovaries occurs later than week 7. It is unclear whether the absence of testosterone and müllerian-inhibiting factor predisposes toward differentiation of the müllerian ducts into female structures or whether feminization is an active response to the estrogens in the fetal environment (Aaronson, 1992) (Fig. 1–1).

## Descent of the Gonads

The testes migrate caudally (toward the tail) early in embryonic development to a retroperitoneal location by the end of the first trimester. The gubernaculum, a fibromuscular band, reaches from the lower aspect of the testis to the subcutaneous tissue of the developing scrotum. Just below the lower aspect of the testis, the peritoneum forms a diverticular structure that reaches the scrotum through the abdominal muscles. The developing testes remain at the abdominal end of this inguinal canal until the seventh month of development, and they migrate into the scrotal sac by the end of the eighth month (Tanagho, 1992b).

The ovaries also undergo early internal descent before becoming attached to the fibromuscular gubernaculum. In females, the portion of the gubernaculum between the ovary and the uterus forms the ovarian ligament, and the portion between the uterus and the labia majora becomes the round ligament of the uterus. The ovaries migrate to the true pelvis to lie behind the fallopian tubes on the superior surface of the urogenital mesentery. This mesentery forms the broad ligament of the uterus (Tanagho, 1992b).

## External Genitalia

The external genitalia can be distinguished as female or male after the first trimester. In males, the genital tubercle elongates and forms the penis. The corpora cavernosa appear in the penile shaft, and the ventral urethral groove tubularizes to form the distal or conduit urethra in males. The scrotal swellings form and fuse, creating the dependent scrotum that will house the testes and distal spermatic cord. In females, the genital tubercle develops into the clitoris at a later stage than does the penis in males. The ventral groove does not tubularize; rather, it differentiates into the labia minora. The genital swellings also remain separate,

forming the labia majora rather than a fused scrotum (Golimbu, 1981).

## KIDNEY

## Anatomy of the Kidney

The kidneys are a pair of brownish-red structures that lie in the retroperitoneal space in the adult human. From their embryonic origins in the sacral region, they have descended and rotated to lie adjacent to the T12 to L2 or L3 levels of the spinal column. Because of the presence of the liver, the right kidney is located slightly lower than the left. Each kidney is situated approximately at a 90-degree angle from the spine. The concave surface of the kidney lies near the spine, and its convex surface is distal. The convex portion of the kidney (renal hilum) is the point at which the renal pelvis, artery, and veins exit the parenchyma (Gray & Dobkin, 1989).

The right and left kidneys are markedly similar in size and shape. Each is surrounded by perirenal fascia and a layer of fat encased by a layer of dense fascia. Gerota's fascia encases the kidney and the superiorly located adrenal gland. Perirenal fascia, fat, and Gerota's fascia, together with the overlying psoas muscle and ribs, form a protective casing for the kidneys that acts as a shock absorber against blunt trauma and shields against penetrating trauma (Gray & Dobkin, 1989; Williams & Warwick, 1980).

The internal architecture of the kidney is appreciated on cross section (Fig. 1–2). Two distinctive regions, the renal pelvis and the parenchyma, are noted. The renal parenchyma is divided into the cortex and the medulla on gross inspection. The medulla is noted as pale, conical pyramids. The pyramids are oriented with the base facing the concave surface of the kidney, and the apex is oriented toward the hilum or the pelvis. Each kidney normally contains 8 to 18 pyramids. They drain into 4 to 13 minor calices that, in turn, drain into two to three major calices that open directly into the pelvis (Gray & Dobkin, 1989; Williams & Warwick, 1980).

The microscopic anatomy of the kidney is centered around the nephron, which is the functional unit of the organ. Each kidney contains approximately 1 million nephrons capable of providing adequate renal function for the body should the contralateral kidney be damaged or rendered nonfunctional. Each nephron

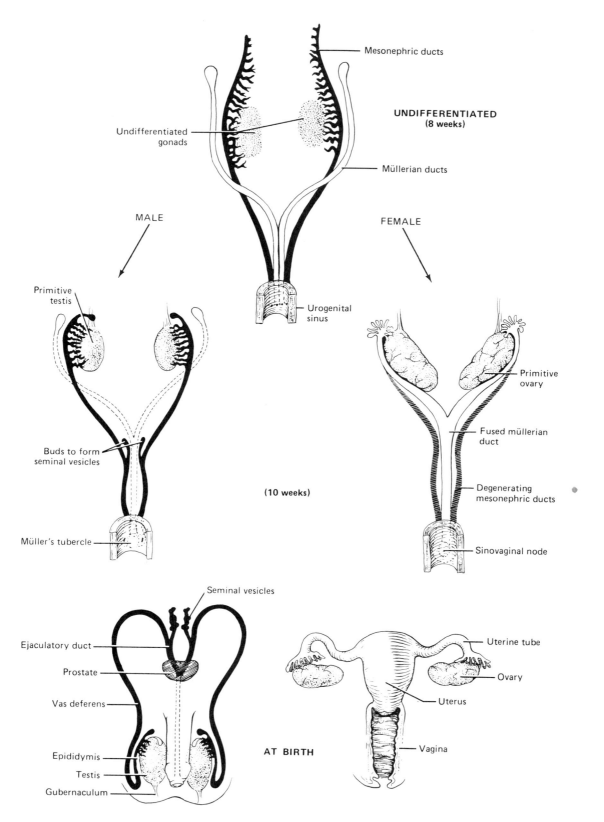

**Mesonephric ducts**

**UNDIFFERENTIATED
(8 weeks)**

Undifferentiated
gonads

Müllerian ducts

MALE

FEMALE

Primitive
testis

Urogenital
sinus

Primitive
ovary

Buds to form
seminal vesicles

(10 weeks)

Fused müllerian
duct

Degenerating
mesonephric ducts

Müller's tubercle

Sinovaginal node

Seminal vesicles

Ejaculatory duct

Prostate

Uterine tube

Vas deferens

Ovary

Uterus

Epididymis

AT BIRTH

Testis

Vagina

Gubernaculum

**FIGURE 1–1** Differentiation of male and female genital systems. (From Tanagho, E. A., & McAninch, J. W. [1992]. Embryology of the genitourinary system. In E. A. Tanagho & J. W. McAninch [Eds.], *Smith's general urology* [13th ed., p. 24]. Norwalk, CT: Appleton & Lange. Reprinted by permission.)

9

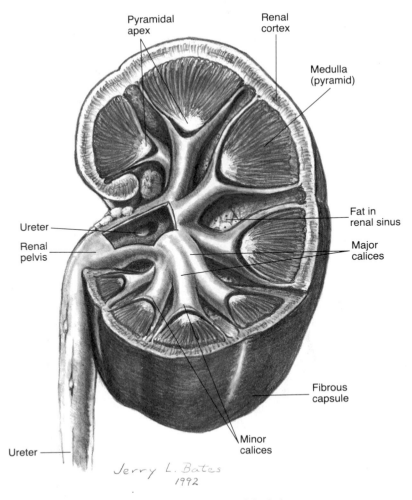

**FIGURE 1–2** Cross section of the kidney.

is composed of a glomerulus containing afferent and efferent arterioles, Bowman's capsule, proximal tubule, loop of Henle, distal tubule, and collecting ducts. The collecting duct empties into the pyramidal apex that leads to a minor calix, a major calix, and the renal pelvis before transport to the lower urinary tract (Brundage, 1992).

Nephrons are structurally divided into superficial, cortical, and juxtamedullary forms. Each nephron is perfused by peritubular capillaries arising from an efferent arteriole. Superficial, cortical, and juxtamedullary nephrons all lie near a network of peritubular capillaries; juxtamedullary nephrons are distinguished by the vasa recta, a series of capillary loops that lies near the loop of Henle. The loop is particularly long in the juxtamedullary nephron (Brundage, 1992).

The parenchymal blood supply arises from the renal arteries that branch at a nearly right angle from the abdominal aorta. In most people, a single artery enters the renal hilum, although two arteries may exist, representing only normal variance. After entering the kidney, the renal artery bifurcates into superior and inferior branches before subdividing into the lobular vessels and, ultimately, into the glomerular capillaries that represent the first step of renal filtration. The renal veins run a course roughly parallel to that of the renal arteries. The major renal veins drain directly into the inferior vena cava; the number of renal veins exiting the hilum typically mirrors the number of renal arteries entering the organ (Gray & Dobkin, 1989; Tanagho, 1992a). Lymphatic drainage from the kidneys collects in the lateral aortic nodes (Redman, 1987).

## Physiology of the Kidney

The excretory functions of the kidney provide homeostasis for the internal environment of the body. This ongoing process impinges on virtually every organ system in the body, including cardiovascular, neurologic, endocrine, and hematologic. The kidney excretes unneeded end products of metabolic function, including creatinine, urea, uric acid, nitrates, and phenol. In addition, the kidney excretes excessive water, sodium, chloride, potassium, and phosphates. The kidney also provides long-term regulation of acid-base balance by selective excretion or reabsorption of hydrogen ions (Guyton, 1991).

### URINE FORMATION AND EXCRETORY FUNCTIONS

The first step in urine formation is the ultrafiltration of urine by the glomerulus (Fig. 1–3). With the exception of periods of intense physiologic distress, each kidney receives approximately 1200 mL of blood per minute; about 125 mL of this blood is filtered through the glomerulus into Bowman's capsule. The rate of ultrafiltration is determined by the influence of (1) Starling's forces; (2) the particularly permeable structure of the glomerular capillary that allows "leakage" of greater amounts of fluid into Bowman's space than do systemic capillaries; (3) the relatively slow rate at which plasma flows into the glomerular capillary; and (4) the total surface area of the glomerular capillaries. These factors favor the movement of fluid and smaller-molecular solutes into Bowman's space while resisting movement of larger proteins or erythrocytes. Once the ultrafiltrate enters the capsule, it is then moved through the tubular system of the nephron and selectively *reabsorbed* (placed back into the systemic circulation) or *secreted* into the urine for disposal from the body (Brundage, 1992; Valtin, 1983).

Most fluid and solutes that enter the glomerular filtrate undergo *reabsorption*. Reabsorption may occur as a result of active or passive mechanisms. Substances are transported from the tubular lumen, through the peritubular interstitium, and back into the peritubular capillaries, returning them to the systemic circulation. Most of the substances that are reabsorbed, such as sodium, bicarbonate, potassium, and water, are essential to internal homeostasis. Many substances are reabsorbed by active (energy-requiring) mechanisms against their osmotic gradient. Because these substances re-

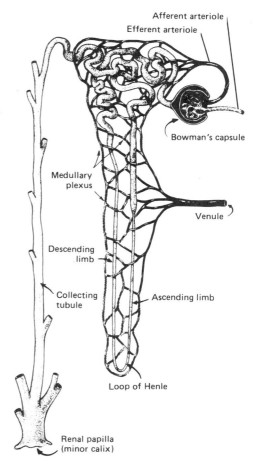

FIGURE 1–3 The nephron, the functional unit of the kidney. (From Tanagho, E. A. [1992]. Anatomy of the genitourinary tract. In E. A. Tanagho & J. W. McAninch [Eds.], *Smith's general urology* [13th ed., p. 5]. Norwalk, CT: Appleton & Lange. Reprinted by permission.)

quire active transport for reabsorption, they are subject to a relatively constant *transport maximum*. Any volume of solute presented to the kidney in a certain period that exceeds this transport maximum is excreted in the urine with its normal osmotic gradient. Certain substances, such as glucose, amino acids, and phosphate, undergo a process called *cotransportation*. Cotransported solutes are influenced by sodium, which acts to accelerate or inhibit their movement from the tubular lumen into the blood stream (Valtin, 1983).

During the course of filtration, a relatively large volume of nearly isosmotic filtrate is converted into a much smaller volume of hyperosmotic filtrate. In the proximal tubule, approximately 87% of the water and solutes, 100% of the glucose, and more than 99% of the amino acids are reabsorbed. Thus, the principal function of the proximal tubule is reabsorbing most of the essential fluids and solutes while resisting the reabsorption of nitrogenous wastes. The proximal tubule employs passive transport (with a substance's osmotic gradient), active transport (requiring energy to move against the substance's osmotic gradient), and cotransport (passively bonded to sodium that is reabsorbed by means of an active transport pathway) (Brundage, 1992; Valtin, 1983). The remaining 13% of the filtrate passes into the loop of Henle and the distal tubule.

The loop of Henle provides a mechanism for the further reabsorption of water that affects the concentration (specific gravity) of the urine produced by the kidney. Through most of the tubular system, active sodium transport results in the passive reabsorption of water across its osmotic gradient. In the loop of Henle, however, a countercurrent multiplier system exists that profoundly influences the concentration of urine (and volume of water reabsorbed by the kidney) with principally or entirely passive reabsorption of the sodium ion. In the juxtamedullary ions with longer loops of Henle and adjacent vasa recta, the hypertonicity of the interstitial fluid may rise dramatically. In the thin, descending limb of the loop of Henle, sodium ions are actively secreted into the interstitial space as water is passively reabsorbed. However, in the thick, ascending limb of the loop, the structure of the tubular cell disallows the reabsorption of water. As a result, the interstitial concentration of sodium near the bottom of the loop of Henle may reach four times that of the blood, causing selective reabsorption of water and concentration of urine (Valtin, 1983).

In the more distal segments of the distal collecting tubule, the permeability of the tubular cells to water is influenced by the antidiuretic hormone. The concentrations of antidiuretic hormone in the nephron also influence the rate of water reabsorption and the specific gravity of the urine. Because of the ability to concentrate urine, the body is able to effectively remove an entire day's worth of metabolic end products and excess solutes in only 500 mL of urine compared with the approximately 2000 mL of fluid required if the urine had remained isotonic (Brundage, 1992).

In addition to the selective reabsorption and excretion of water, solutes, and nitrogenous waste products, the kidneys maintain the internal homeostatic environment of the body by regulation of the hydrogen ion. The concentration of the hydrogen ion is crucial for the main-

tenance of the pH needed for normal functioning. Each day, as a result of normal metabolic processes, the human body produces excess hydrogen ions that must be excreted from the body to prevent the harmful effects of an excessively acidic internal environment. Although the respiratory system, through the expulsion of carbon dioxide, provides short-term regulation of the body's acid-base balance, the kidneys provide long-term maintenance.

The kidneys assist in the regulation of acid-base balance in the body by maintaining adequate serum concentrations of the bicarbonate ion. The store of bicarbonate is provided by reabsorption of virtually 100% of bicarbonate ions filtered into the nephron and by production of additional bicarbonate ions within the tubular cells that are reabsorbed in the blood. In addition to the production of bicarbonate ions, the kidney excretes hydrogen ions by two mechanisms: (1) the excretion of acid into the urine by passive and active transport and (2) the excretion of neutral ammonium salts after ammonium is combined with a hydrogen ion using a nonionic diffusion mechanism (Valtin, 1983).

The renal excretion and reabsorption of potassium ions are also of particular interest to urologic nurses because they are essential cellular functions and because they are directly affected by the use of diuretic drugs. The potassium ion is subjected to bidirectional transport in the course of the proximal and distal tubules. Approximately 80% of potassium excreted in the filtrate is reabsorbed in the proximal tubule and ascending limb of the loop of Henle. In contrast, the distal tubules normally secrete potassium into the urine, except in cases of extreme dietary deprivation, when they actually absorb the substance. Typically, cortical collecting ducts secrete potassium, whereas medullary ducts may reabsorb or secrete ions. The magnitude of secretion of potassium is influenced by three factors: (1) the osmotic gradient of potassium between tubular cells and tubular lumen; (2) the flow rate of water and sodium through the distal tubules and collecting ducts; and (3) the influence of electrical properties of potassium-secreting cells in the tubule (Valtin, 1983). Diuretic medications possess a variety of pharmacologic properties that affect the kidney's ability to reabsorb potassium and its propensity to excrete the substance.

It is particularly important for the urologic nurse to remember that the ultrafiltration and transport of filtrate throughout the nephronic tubules and the subsequent transport of urine from the nephron to the calix and the renal pelvis occur at relatively low pressures. Therefore, it is necessary for the ureters and the urinary bladder to remain at relatively low pressure while the urinary bladder fills with urine. Pathologic states that cause the bladder to fill at abnormally high pressures or that obstruct the transport of urine through the renal pelves and the ureters compromise the kidney's ability to filter, produce, and transport the water, solutes, and nitrogenous waste products that form urine and to maintain normal physiologic homeostasis.

## NONEXCRETORY FUNCTIONS OF THE KIDNEY

The principal nonexcretory functions of the kidney include the maintenance of blood hematocrit levels by regulating the excretion of erythropoietin. The kidney affects blood pressure by regulating the excretion of the endocrine substance renin, and it influences the metabolism of carbohydrates, lipids, plasma proteins, and vitamin D (Guyton, 1991).

The kidney influences systemic blood pressure by several mechanisms, including the excretion or reabsorption of fluid, which profoundly affects circulating plasma volume. The kidneys also affect blood pressure through a set of specialized cells located in or near the glomerulus in the afferent arteriole and the early portion of the distal tubule. These specialized cells secrete a substance called *renin* in response to reduction in blood pressure in the glomerulus, hyponatremia, or ischemia of the renal vascular bed (Guyton, 1991).

Renin is an enzyme that causes the conversion of a hormonal precursor, angiotensinogen, to form angiotensin I. Angiotensin I is converted to angiotensin II by a converting enzyme found in the liver. Angiotensins I and II are powerful vasoconstrictors that produce constriction at the arteriolar level, raising peripheral resistance, which increases systemic blood pressure. Angiotensins II and III (made from the loss of an amino acid) further act to stimulate the release of aldosterone from the adrenal cortex. As a result of aldosterone release, the kidneys retain sodium and water, causing an increase in the circulating blood volume and a further increase in blood pressure (Guyton, 1991).

Renal production of erythropoietin, a hormone that stimulates the production and maturation of red blood cells from the bone marrow, is influenced by hypoxia or anemia. In addition, the substance is produced in response to a reduction in oxygen tension or to renal ischemia. The presence of renal ischemia also stimulates the production of prostaglandins, which act as paracrine substances. Their role in the maintenance of adequate renal perfusion remains unclear (Brundage, 1992).

The kidney also plays a role in the metabolism of vitamin D. Vitamin D is formed in the skin, metabolized in the liver, then metabolized in the kidney to its active, usable form. Vitamin D is produced in response to hypocalcemia or hypophosphatemia. It acts with the parathyroid hormone, parathormone, to increase dietary absorption of calcium and phosphate. In turn, osteoclastic activity is stimulated in the bone that maintains adequate tensile strength in the skeleton. Chronic renal failure frustrates this process, causing excessive mobilization of calcium from the bone and resulting in osteodystrophy (Brundage, 1992).

For a more detailed discussion of the physiology of urine formation and homeostatic renal functions, the reader is referred to a physiology or renal medicine text.

## UPPER URINARY TRACT

The upper and lower urinary tracts comprise the renal pelves, the ureters, and the urethrovesical unit (bladder, urethra, and pelvic floor support structures) (Figs. 1–4 and 1–5).

### Renal Pelvis and Ureter

The renal pelvis and the ureter form a single tube connecting the renal parenchyma and the urethrovesical unit. The renal pelvis is a funnel-shaped structure that originates at the hilum of the kidney and narrows inferomedially to the kidney into the ureter (Tanagho, 1986).

The ureters are narrow, muscular tubes that originate at the lower portion of the renal pelvis and terminate in the bladder wall. Each is 24 to 30 cm long; the left ureter is slightly longer than the right. After exiting the renal pelvis, the ureters pass medially from the kidney along the psoas muscle, course toward the sacroiliac joints, and turn again laterally to pass near the ischium of the bony pelvis. Within the pelvis, they again swing medially to terminate in the trigone located in the bladder base. Three relatively narrow areas are particularly

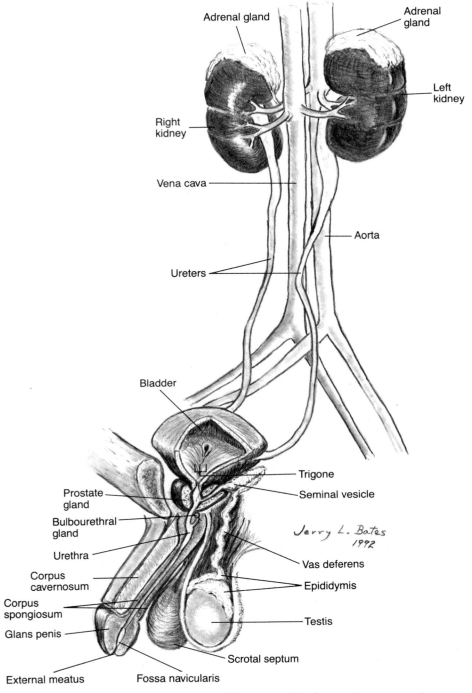

*FIGURE 1–4* Anatomy of the male genitourinary system.

significant because of their propensity to obstruct in the presence of a foreign body, such as calculi. They are the ureteropelvic junction, the ureteral segment near the sacroiliac junction, and the ureterovesical junction (UVJ) (Boyarsky & Labay, 1982; Olsson, 1986).

The renal pelves and the ureters have three histologic layers. The lumen is lined by a tran-

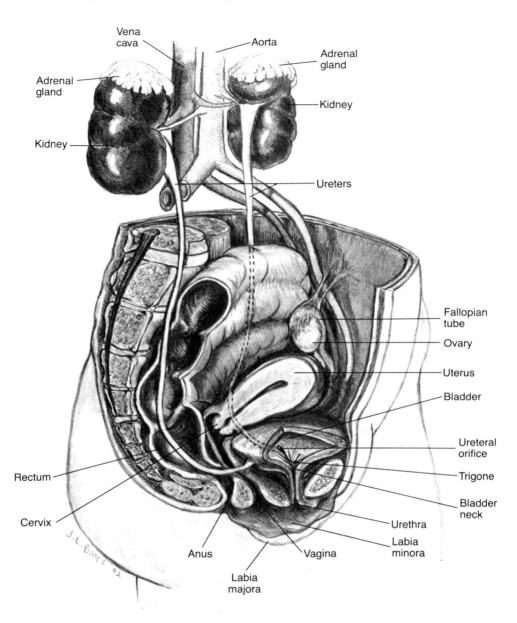

*FIGURE 1–5* Anatomy of the female urinary system.

sitional cell epithelium containing mucus-producing cells. A tunic of smooth muscle lies beneath the epithelial lining. The smooth muscle bundles of the ureter contain relatively small cells that run in longitudinal, circular, helical, or spiral orientations not organized into definite layers (Tanagho, 1981, 1992a). The outer layer of the ureter is an adventitia of connective tissue that encircles the renal pelves and ureters throughout their course and attaches them to the renal hilum and adjacent bladder wall (Williams & Warwick, 1980).

The blood supply of the ureters varies among individuals. Typically, the upper ureter and the renal pelvis may receive blood from branches of the renal, gonadal, or adrenal arteries. The lower or pelvic portion of the ureters receive blood from the common or external iliac artery, the deferential artery in males and the uterine arteries in females, or the obturator artery. Venous drainage parallels the arterial supply (Boyarsky & Labay, 1982).

The primary function of the ureter is the transport of urine from the kidney to the bladder before storage and expulsion from the body. This transport is an active process requiring muscular contraction of the ureteral wall called *peristalsis*. The arrangement and physiology of the smooth muscle bundles in the ureters allow them to propagate contractions caused by neural impulses and mechanical factors, such as mechanical stretching produced when a bolus of urine enters the ureteral lumen (Weiss, 1986).

As urine enters the renal pelvis, pacemaker cells, presumed to exist in the renal calices, are stimulated to propagate a peristaltic wave. The wave originates in the renal pelvis, which pushes the bolus of urine into the ureter. This action forces open the otherwise collapsed ureteral lumen, which reacts by pushing the urine in an antegrade fashion (from the upper toward the lower urinary tract), until it is effluxed into the bladder through the UVJ. Urine travels in response to a pressure gradient; during the resting stage, the intraluminal pressure of the ureter ranges from 2 to 5 cm $H_2O$. A peristaltic wave temporarily raises lumen pressure to 20 to 80 cm $H_2O$, causing the urine to move in a relatively continuous fashion toward the bladder (Ross et al., 1982). The normal ureter is capable of two to six peristaltic waves per minute (Weiss, 1986). Peristaltic waves increase in frequency and amplitude when greater volumes of urine are produced by the kidneys, such as during periods of diuresis, and decrease when less urine is produced.

Ureteral peristalsis also varies in response to neural modulation. Alpha- and beta-adrenergic receptors are found in the ureteral wall. Stimulation of alpha-adrenergic receptors is excitatory to smooth muscle cells, increasing peristalsis, whereas beta-adrenergic stimulation decreases peristalsis by inhibiting smooth muscle tone (Rose & Gillenwater, 1974; Weiss et al., 1978). The effect of cholinergic stimulation on ureteral peristalsis remains less clear; stimulation of cholinergic nerves in the ureteral wall may increase peristalsis directly by stimulation or indirectly by release of catecholamines (Rose & Gillenwater, 1974).

Ureteral peristalsis can be altered by chemical and pharmacologic agents. Predictably, the administration of catecholamines or alpha-adrenergic agonists stimulates peristaltic activity, whereas the administration of a beta-adrenergic agonist or alpha-sympatholytic agent inhibits ureteral tone. The administration of histamines also increases ureteral peristalsis. In contrast, exogenous serotonin, which stimulates peristalsis of the gastrointestinal system,

does not produce any detectable effect on the ureter. Likewise, estrogens, once blamed for ureteral dilatation associated with pregnancy, do not produce clinically apparent effects on ureteral peristalsis. Instead, an increased fluid load and the mechanical aspects of the gravid uterus may produce the dilatation noted in pregnant women (Kiil, 1978).

## Ureterovesical Junction

The UVJ is formed by the intersection of the distal ureter and the bladder wall. The UVJ is of critical importance to urinary system function because it allows *efflux* (antegrade movement) of urine from the kidney to the bladder while it prevents *reflux* (retrograde movement) of urine from the bladder to the upper urinary tract.

In adults, the UVJ contains three distinct components. The *distal* or *intravesical ureter* courses through the bladder wall into the trigone. The *trigone* is a smooth muscle of distinctive embryonic origin compared with the detrusor; it is located in the base of the bladder. The portion of the *bladder wall immediately adjacent to the intravesical ureter* forms the final portion of the UVJ (Tanagho, 1992a).

The distal or intravesical ureter enters the bladder near its base in the lateral aspect of the trigone. It is separated into two components: the intramural ureter is that portion of the tube surrounded by detrusor muscle bundles, and the submucosal ureter lies directly under the bladder mucosa. In the normal person, the intramural ureter is approximately 1.5 cm long, and the submucosal ureter is 0.8 cm long (Tanagho, 1986).

The lower ureter and the bladder are further joined by Waldeyer's sheath. It is a fibromuscular structure that anchors the ureters and the urethrovesical unit. The sheath originates from the wall of the distal ureter just above the bladder surrounding the intramural ureteral segment before fusing with the trigone (Tanagho, 1986; Waldeyer, 1891).

The UVJ functions as a door between the bladder and the upper urinary tracts. The door is designed to allow one-way travel only. During bladder filling, the UVJ remains at a relatively low closure pressure (8–15 cm $H_2O$) to allow an efflux of urine from the ureters to the bladder while preventing a reflux of urine from the bladder to the ureters. This UVJ is easily opened by a bolus of urine pushed into the bladder lumen by a peristaltic contraction generating ureteral pressures of 20 to 80 cm $H_2O$. In contrast, the UVJ must exert considerable active closure pressure over a prolonged period during micturition to prevent urine from escaping from the bladder to the ureters while it is expelled from the urethra.

The UVJ allows efflux while it prevents reflux by active and passive components of its design. The most important passive characteristic of the UVJ is its oblique entry into the lateral aspect of the trigone. An oblique entry angle promotes passive closure during bladder filling. In addition to entry angle, the intravesical ureter relies on a favorable ratio of intramural to submucosal length. Adequate intramural ureteral length promotes passive closure during bladder filling, and it allows effective closure in response to active muscle tone of the trigone and the detrusor muscle. The mechanical characteristics of the bladder wall and the trigone form the third passive characteristic of the UVJ. As the bladder fills, the intravesical pressure rises slightly, stretching the trigone and raising the closure pressure of the UVJ while subtly increasing the acuity of the angle at which the ureter enters the bladder wall (Gray & Dobkin, 1989; Levitt & Weiss, 1985).

In contrast with the passive properties that maintain UVJ closure during bladder filling, active, forceful closure is crucial during micturition, when intravesical pressures rise to 30 to 60 cm $H_2O$ or more and remain at that level for 1 minute or longer. The smooth muscle of the intravesical ureter is arranged differently from the bundles of the upper ureteral segments. Near the ureteral orifice, the smooth muscle bundles are principally longitudinal in orientation, which promotes forceful closure in response to micturition. In addition, the trigone muscle contracts before voiding and remains contracted until several seconds after the detrusor muscle relaxes. This promotes ureteral closure by collapsing the portion of the intramural ureteral wall that courses through its lateral aspect. The smooth muscle bundles of the bladder wall that lie adjacent to the UVJ also contribute to ureteral closure during micturition. Active contraction of detrusor muscle bundles causes stiffening of the bladder wall, further contributing to closure of the intramural ureter (Levitt & Weiss, 1985).

Because of the forceful closure required to maintain UVJ closure during micturition, the efflux of urine from the kidney to the bladder is prevented. Fortunately, this period is relatively brief, and normal urinary transport is reestablished soon after micturition is completed (Gray & Dobkin, 1989).

## LOWER URINARY TRACT

The urethrovesical unit, or lower urinary tract, consists of the urinary bladder, the urethra, and the pelvic floor support structures. It is responsible for the filling and storage of urine before its volitional expulsion from the body by micturition.

### Bladder

The urinary bladder is a hollow, muscular organ that lies in the true pelvis. Its size, shape, and relation to adjacent structures vary with the state of fullness and with age. During infancy, the bladder is found within the abdomen. With growth and maturation, it assumes its position in the true pelvis just before puberty. This change reflects maturation and growth of the bony pelvis rather than a migration of the bladder. The bladder neck retains its location in the midline, just above the symphysis pubis, throughout life, except in cases of pelvic descent or anomaly. In adults, the empty bladder assumes a tetrahedron shape located entirely within the lesser pelvis. As it fills, it assumes a roughly spherical shape, moving upward and anteriorly toward the abdominal cavity at the midline (Sarma, 1969; Williams & Warwick, 1980).

The bladder is characterized by a central hollow area called the *vesicle*, which has two inlets and a single outlet. The inlets are the ureteral orifices of the UVJ, and the outlet is the urethrovesical junction. Five anatomic areas are noted on gross inspection: the bladder neck, base, apex, and superior right and left inferolateral surfaces (Sarma, 1969).

The bladder neck surrounds the urethrovesical junction. Because of its distinctive arrangement of smooth muscle bundles, it forms a portion of the urethral sphincter mechanism sometimes referred to as the *internal sphincter*. In males, the bladder neck is anterior to the rectum and immediately superior to the prostate. In females, the bladder neck sits anterior to the rectum and posterior to the vaginal wall (Williams & Warwick, 1980).

The bladder base is triangular in shape and is defined by the borders of the trigone, which is delineated by the UVJs. In adult males, the base of the bladder lies superior to the seminal vesicles and adjacent to the rectum. Denonvilliers' fascia forms an anatomic border that separates the bladder base and seminal vesicles from the rectum. In adult females, the bladder base lies close to the anterior vaginal wall. At this point, they are anatomically separate structures (Williams & Warwick, 1980).

The apex of the bladder is oriented toward the abdominal wall. When the bladder vesicle is empty, the apex is found in the pelvis. As the bladder fills, it moves anteriorly and superiorly toward the umbilicus. It is connected to the anterior abdominal wall by the urachas. The inferolateral surfaces of the urinary bladder are noted when the vesicle is empty of urine. As the bladder fills, the surfaces become a single, convex area that lies adjacent to the abdominal wall (Sarma, 1969; Williams & Warwick, 1980).

The wall of the bladder is composed of four histologic layers. The outermost layer is an adventitia of connective tissue that provides support and separation from adjacent structures. Immediately beneath the adventitia is a muscular layer composed of smooth muscle bundles collectively called the *detrusor*. The arrangement of these smooth muscle bundles has been described as being in three layers—inner longitudinal, middle circumferential, and outer longitudinal—although a more complex organizational structure consisting of a meshwork of variable orientations is more likely. Interspersed among the smooth bundles is a collagenous framework and autonomic nerve endings. Plentiful cholinergic (muscarinic), occasional adrenergic, and nonadrenergic-noncholinergic nerve receptors are noted (Gosling & Chilton, 1984).

Beneath the smooth muscle tunic is a lamina propria that is loosely attached to the bladder urothelium containing plentiful elastic fibers and areolar tissue. It serves as an interface between urothelium and detrusor muscle throughout the distensible portion of the bladder but is absent beneath the nondistensible bladder base.

Lining the bladder vesicle is a layer of transitional cell epithelium. When the vesicle is empty, the urothelium is six to eight cells deep. As the bladder fills, it progressively stretches and thins to a layer two or three cells deep. The urothelium contains a special membrane that is impermeable to water, preventing reabsorption of urine stored in the bladder (Leeson & Leeson, 1976). It may play a role in protecting the epithelium from the deleterious effects of exposure to urine and may offer clues to understanding the pathophysiology of interstitial cystitis.

Arterial blood is delivered to the bladder by the inferior, superior, and medial vesical arteries that arise from the internal iliac or hypogastric arteries. Smaller branches of the obturator and inferior gluteal arteries may supplement the bladder's blood supply. Venous blood leaves the bladder through Santorini's plexus and a neurovascular sheath near the vesicle ligaments. The venous blood is then directed to the inferior hypogastric vein and the inferior vena cava (Williams & Warwick, 1980).

Lymphatic channels from the bladder drain into the external iliac nodes. Lesser drainage may be provided by hypogastric, common iliac, and lateral sacral chains (Redman, 1987).

## Male Urethra

The urethra is a hollow tube that originates at the bladder neck and terminates at an external meatus. In males, the urethra follows a course from the bladder outlet through the prostate, where it pierces the urogenital diaphragm or pelvic floor muscles before coursing to its termination at the fossa navicularis in the glans penis. It is a conduit for urine or semen, and its posterior segment serves as a sphincter mechanism in preventing urinary leakage during bladder filling and storage. During micturition, the sphincter interacts with the detrusor muscle to determine urinary flow. During ejaculation, the smooth muscle at the bladder neck contracts to prevent retrograde ejaculation of semen into the bladder.

The male urethra is approximately 23 cm long; it is divided into two portions, the anterior and the posterior. The posterior urethra originates at the bladder neck and is composed of a prostatic and a membranous portion. The prostatic urethra is approximately 3 cm long, extending from the bladder neck–prostate apex. It pierces the prostate vertically near its anterior aspect. The prostatic urethra is lined by transitional cell epithelium that forms a mucous membrane. Its posterior floor is raised by the verumontanum that tapers inferiorly and superiorly into the cristae. These folds in the mucous membrane form a depression on the posterior floor known as the *prostatic fossa*. Secretory ducts from the middle lobe of the prostate terminate in the prostatic urethra, contributing to seminal emission during coitus. Smooth muscle bundles that may represent an extension of the bladder neck also are found in the wall of the prostatic urethra (Tanagho, 1986; Williams & Warwick, 1980).

The membranous urethra is 2 to 5 cm long, extending from the prostatic apex to the bulbar urethra. It pierces the area commonly labeled the *urogenital* or *pelvic diaphragm* (Tanagho, 1986). It is lined by a transitional cell epithelial mucous membrane. The membranous urethra is distinguished from the prostatic segment by its proximity to skeletal muscle fibers from the levator ani or urogenital diaphragm. In addition, the membranous urethra contains intrinsic striated and smooth muscle cells that contribute to the urethral sphincter mechanism (Gosling & Chilton, 1984). It is the least distensible segment of the urethra and the most susceptible to stricture (Tanagho, 1986).

The anterior urethra is the segment most distal from the bladder. It tunnels through the corpus spongiosum of the penis and ends at the fossa navicularis of the glans penis. It is approximately 15 cm long. Like the posterior urethra, it is lined by an epithelial mucous membrane that flattens to cuboidal, then squamous cell, configuration by the fossa navicularis. The external meatus of the male urethra forms a vertical slit approximately 8 mm long (Leeson & Leeson, 1976; Williams & Warwick, 1980).

Arterial blood to the urethra is provided by a branch of the pudendal artery, commonly called the *urethral artery*. Venous blood drains by way of the deep penile vein and the pudendal venous plexus (Williams & Warwick, 1980). Lymphatic drainage is provided by the superficial and deep inguinal nodes that drain into the external iliac nodes (Redman, 1987).

## Female Urethra

The female urethra follows a relatively short, straight path that is functionally comparable with that of the posterior segment of the male urethra. In nulliparous women, the urethra is approximately 3.5 to 5.5 cm long. It originates at the bladder outlet and forms a 16-degree angle as it tunnels to the external meatus located immediately superior and midline to the vaginal vestibule.

The female urethra is lined by a layer of columnar-shaped epithelium that forms a mucous membrane. Beneath this membrane is a lamina propria that supports a rich vascular network. The mucosal lining and the submucosal vascular network in the female urethra are influenced by circulating estrogens. The middle third of the female urethra contains specialized striated muscle fibers, whereas longitudinal- and circumferential-oriented smooth muscle bundles are found within the

proximal and middle segments. The lower two thirds of the urethra is anatomically contiguous with the anterior vaginal wall so that the smooth muscle layers become indistinguishable. The meatus is a bud-shaped ellipsoid lined by columnar epithelial cells (Gosling & Chilton, 1984; Tanagho, 1986).

Arterial blood for the female urethra is supplied by branches of the vaginal artery. Venous blood exits the submucosal vascular cushion, draining into the pelvic venous plexus. Lymphatic drainage is primarily by the internal iliac nodes; the external chain may provide additional drainage (Redman, 1987).

## Pelvic Floor Support Structures

The urethrovesical unit maintains its proper anatomic relationships and derives part of its sphincteric function from the supportive structures of the pelvic floor. These structures include the endopelvic fascia, the bony structures of the pelvis, and the pelvic floor musculature.

The pelvic floor musculature is composed of a group of predominantly slow-twitch, striated muscle fibers innervated principally by branches of the pudendal nerve. These fibers originate and insert into the bony pelvis, forming a sling that supports the pelvic viscera, including the urethrovesical unit and the adjacent genital and intestinal organs.

The male membranous segment and the middle portion of the female urethra pass through the pelvic floor musculature. The fibers adjacent to this point are called *periurethral muscle;* they directly affect urethral closure during periods of physical stress through their active tone. The pelvic floor is often called the *levator ani* or the *pelvic diaphragm;* it is further divided into the pubococcygeus (pubis to coccyx) and ischiococcygeus (ischium to coccyx), even though all these muscles act as a single functional unit (Gosling & Chilton, 1984).

As expected, structural differences in the pelvic diaphragm are noted between females and males. In males, a superior portion of the pelvic diaphragm originates at the lateral aspect of the pubic bone. Some fibers sweep around the apex of the prostate to add additional support to its position, whereas others travel under the posterior aspect of the membranous urethra to form the sling of periurethral muscle described previously. The largest portion of fibers from the superior division of the pelvic diaphragm passes behind the rectum and inserts into the rectal wall, forming an anorectal sling and the upper portion of the rectal sphincter. The entire muscle is covered by endopelvic fascia, adding additional support to the urethrovesical unit and the adjacent viscera (Gosling & Chilton, 1984).

The inferior portion of the male pelvic diaphragm also originates at the pubis, caudad to the point of origin for the superior division. The anterior portion forms the puboperineus, which inserts into the perineal body (a fibrous, fat-laden structure located between the membranous urethra and the anorectal junction) and the pubococcygeal portion of the pelvic diaphragm before inserting into the lateral coccyx and the lower sacrum. The more substantial superior portion of the inferior pelvic diaphragm arises from the ischial spine and arcus tendineus to insert into the coccyx and the sacrum. Together, they form a gutter that provides support for the terminal segment of the rectum (Gosling & Chilton, 1984).

The female pelvic floor structures differ from the typical arrangement noted in males. Like the male diaphragm, the female pelvic diaphragm can be divided into superior and inferior segments, although the muscle maintains its functional significance as a single unit. In females, the superior division fibers travel almost exclusively from the lateral aspect of the pubis behind the anorectal junction to insert into the rectal wall and the upper portion of the rectal sphincter.

In addition to the superior portion of the pelvic diaphragm, females also derive support from pubourethral ligaments that correspond to puboprostatic ligaments in males. These structures connect the periosteum of the pubis and the urethra. They are more significant functionally and anatomically in females and may contain muscle fibers that add support for the urethrovesical unit.

The inferior portion of the female pelvic diaphragm is not as substantial as that noted in the male inferior pelvic diaphragm. These relatively sparse muscle fibers play little or no significant role in support of the female urethrovesical unit. Likewise, the female perineal body is considerably smaller than the corresponding male structure and is thought to offer little support to the female lower urinary tract (Gosling & Chilton, 1984).

## Physiology of the Urethrovesical Unit

The goals of motor activity in the urethrovesical unit (bladder and urethra) in humans are to serve as an adequate filling storage compartment for urine and, when an appropriate time arises, to completely evacuate itself. The concept of continence in humans implies a level of control over the urethrovesical unit that allows the person to store urine and remain dry during physical stress for at least 2 hours during waking periods. Continence further implies that the person awakes no more than once during periods of sleep that may span 8 hours or more. Finally, continence requires a complete evacuation of the bladder, which is necessary to prevent excessive frequency of urination and to avoid the adverse effects of urinary stasis. Three forces govern continence in humans: (1) an anatomically intact urinary system, from the renal collecting system to the urethral meatus; (2) a normally functioning neurologic modulatory system, allowing volitional control of micturition; and (3) a competent (watertight) sphincter mechanism.

## INTACT URINARY SYSTEM

An intact urinary system is often assumed when the forces and structures of continence are discussed; however, urinary control relies on the absence of urinary leakage from any extraurethral source. Therefore, the urinary system must contain ureteral orifices that open into the base of the bladder vesicle and a bladder with a single outlet leading to the urethra, and there must be an absence of fistulous or ectopic passages that circumvent the normal sphincter mechanism. Ectopia caused by a congenital defect, fistulas caused by a disease process or trauma, and surgically created urinary diversions all represent interruptions in the structure of the urinary system (Gray, 1990b; Gray & Dougherty, 1987). The resulting extraurethral leakage (incontinence) may occur as a continuous urine loss that may coexist with otherwise normal voiding patterns.

## NEUROMUSCULAR FUNCTION AND THE URETHROVESICAL UNIT

The continent urinary system also relies on input from multiple components of the central and peripheral nervous systems. A stable (normal) bladder may experience small filling contractions but will remain free of contractions of sufficient magnitude to produce leakage or compromise the ability to postpone micturition (Abrams, 1984; Gray et al., 1990). The term *stable bladder* further assumes that the person has reached an age (approximately 4 years) that ensures reasonable maturation of the neurologic structures needed to modulate detrusor control (Kramer, 1986).

Neurologic modulation of bladder control begins in the brain. Multiple portions of the brain contribute to detrusor control; detailed knowledge of their interactions remains elusive. The *detrusor motor area* is located in the frontal lobes of both hemispheres of the cerebral cortex. Fed by the anterior and middle cerebral arteries, the detrusor area has been shown to modulate detrusor contractility in animal models, although its net effect in humans is considered inhibitory (Bhatia & Bradley, 1983).

A separate control center exists for volitional and basal tone of the pelvic floor musculature. This center is located along both sensorimotor cortices near their medial aspects. As is typical of other striated muscles of the body, the pyramidal tracts provide direct neural innervation. This voluntary movement is modulated by components of an extrapyramidal system that include the cerebellum and the basal ganglia (Hald & Bradley, 1983).

The *thalamus* is the relay center for impulses traveling to and from middle and lower brain centers to the cerebral cortex, including the detrusor motor area. Terminal synapses from proprioceptive sensory axons from the detrusor muscle are located in the nonspecific intraluminal nuclei of the thalamus. Unfortunately, the exact location of these pathways remains unclear, and detailed knowledge of the thalamus' role in modulation of lower urinary tract function is not available (Bradley, 1986).

The *limbic system* influences autonomic nervous system modulation of the viscera, including the urinary bladder (Guyton, 1991). Although direct stimulation of the limbic system alters the detrusor reflex (Evardsin & Ursin, 1968), a disease process affecting the limbic system has not been associated with clinically apparent voiding dysfunction in humans (Bradley, 1986).

The *basal ganglia* are a collection of nuclei including the caudate nucleus, putamen, globus pallidus, and substantia nigra (Guyton, 1991). They receive input from multiple neural pathways and affect nervous function as a portion of the extrapyramidal nervous system. The basal ganglia influence striated muscle tone throughout the body, including the pelvic diaphragm, and play a role in detrusor inhibition, which is essential for bladder stability (Lewin et al., 1967).

The *hypothalamus* is a collection of nuclei that regulate the body's internal environment, including neuroendocrine and sexual functions (Guyton, 1991). The role of the hypothalamus in bladder function remains unclear, although it is known that bladder distention produces a discernible effect on neural transmissions to nuclei within this portion of the brain (Stuart et al., 1964).

The *cerebellum* also affects bladder function by its participation in the extrapyramidal system. Like the basal ganglia, it plays a role in the detrusor inhibition that is necessary for bladder stability. In addition, the cerebellum modulates pelvic floor muscle activity affecting the voluntary relaxation of periurethral muscle before micturition (Bradley, 1986).

The *brain stem* has an important role in bladder function. The dorsal aspect of the pons contains two regions that affect detrusor and urethral sphincter function: (1) an "m" region connects parasympathetic fibers that trace their origin to the detrusor muscle and is responsible for initiating the detrusor reflex; and (2) a separate "l" region is responsible for coordinating the pelvic floor striated muscle response and detrusor contractions. Activation of the l region causes inhibition of the pelvic floor muscles (promotion of sphincter relaxation) during detrusor contractions and stimulation of pelvic floor muscle tone during periods of detrusor relaxation and bladder filling (Holstege et al., 1986).

The *spinal cord* affects bladder function through its role as an interface between end organs and the brain. Anatomically separate tracts provide communication between modulatory areas of the brain and the urethrovesical unit.

The reticulospinal tracts of the lateral columns carry messages to and from the brain and the detrusor muscle, whereas the corticospinal tracts communicate with motor units in the pelvic diaphragm (Bradley, 1986). The final central nervous system synapse for both these tracts is located in the lowest portion of the spine, called the *conus medullaris*. Spinal segments S2 to S4 contain pelvic nuclei that travel by way of the pelvic plexus to smooth muscle bundles in the bladder wall, neck, and proximal urethra. Segments S2 to S4 also contain pudendal nuclei that reach the pelvic floor musculature and urethral wall by way of the branches of the pudendal nerve. Stimulation of the pelvic nuclei causes detrusor contraction mediated by the parasympathetic nervous system. Stimulation of the pudendal nerve causes increased tone in the pelvic floor mediated by the somatic system. Interneurons in the spinal cord act under the influence of the pons and provide an inhibitory reflex that ensures coordination between striated muscles of the sphincter and bladder muscle (Bradley, 1986).

In addition to parasympathetic innervation, the spine also provides sympathetic outflow for the urethrovesical unit. Spinal segments T10 to L1 or L2 provide sympathetic outflow to smooth muscle bundles at the bladder neck, the proximal urethra, and the vesicle wall. Stimulation of alpha-excitatory receptors at the bladder neck increases tone and contributes to the urethral closure. Beta-adrenergic receptors in the bladder body inhibit detrusor tone, although their significance in maintaining a stable bladder remains unclear (Bradley, 1986).

Normal filling of the bladder vesicle relies on neural modulation and the vesicoelastic properties of the bladder wall. During periods of bladder filling and storage, the organ must accommodate volumes from 1 to 500 mL or more. Neurologic modulatory centers contribute by inhibiting smooth muscle contraction despite continual distention. Noncontractile, vesicoelastic components of the bladder wall, including the collagenous component of the detrusor muscle and the elastic and connective tissue of the lamina propria and urothelium, also must accommodate expanding volumes to ensure continence.

The vesicoelastic properties of the bladder rely on a marked capacity for distensibility to maintain a relatively low intravesical pressure, except during intermittent periods of physical stress. Mechanically, this relationship is described by Laplace's law, which states that the force exerted against the bladder wall increases during filling in proportion to the increase in radius. This relationship can be stated in mathematical terms:

$$P_{det} = F (pi) / R^2$$

where $P_{det}$ is the pressure exerted by the bladder wall against the vesicle, F is force exerted against the bladder wall, and R is radius. Because the components of the equation—force and radius—tend to increase proportionally, they cancel out each other, and the intravesical filling pressure remains low, allowing passage of large volumes of urine from the upper tracts to the bladder during filling and storage periods (Griffiths, 1984).

In contrast, evacuation of urine during micturition requires neural excitation of smooth muscle bundles in the bladder wall to raise detrusor pressure and increase the force exerted against the urine-filled vesicle. The smooth muscle bundles of the bladder wall receive approximately 1:1 innervation from nerve endings of the pelvic plexus that provide motor innervation needed for contraction. This relatively high proportion of nerves to muscle cells accounts for the volitional control adult humans exert over bladder function, particularly when compared with the lack of control over many other smooth muscle structures, such as the stomach, arterioles, or small or large intestine. Most of these nerve endings release an excitatory neurotransmitter substance called *acetylcholine* in response to parasympathetic stimulation that depolarizes the smooth muscle cell and causes it to contract. Other nerve endings containing norepinephrine are inhibited by acetylcholine release, further encouraging detrusor contraction by blocking inhibitory signals from the sympathetic system. Still other nerve endings in the bladder wall are termed *nonadrenergic-noncholinergic*; they probably contain adenosine triphosphate as their neurotransmitter substance and are believed to contribute directly to detrusor contractility in a manner similar to that of acetylcholine (Dixon & Gosling, 1987).

## Loop Concept and Neurologic Control of Bladder Function

Bradley and associates (1974) conceptualized the neurologic modulation of bladder function as a series of four "loops of innervation." Each loop represents a complete pathway that determines a particular aspect of bladder function based on feedback from the bladder and other modulatory influences of central nervous system structures.

Loop 1 extends from the detrusor motor area in the frontal lobe to the micturition center of the brain stem. It is thought to give rise to social continence in adults. Specifically, loop 1 provides the ability to inhibit micturition in toilet-trained children or adults until an appropriate time and place for urination is found (Bradley et al., 1974).

Loop 2 consists of neural pathways between the brain stem and the micturition center in the sacral spinal cord (segments S2 to S4). Loop 2 is postulated to determine the power and duration of a detrusor contraction (Bradley, 1986; Morrison, 1987a).

Loop 3 consists of the pelvic and pudendal motor neurons and their interneurons. Loop 3 is postulated to play a role in bladder sensations and control of the striated muscle portions of the urethral sphincter mechanism (Bradley et al., 1974).

Loop 4, the final pathway, consists of parts A and B. Loop 4A consists of supraspinal innervation of the pudendal afferents controlling the pelvic floor musculature, including the periurethral muscles. Loop 4A allows humans to volitionally interrupt the urinary stream and voluntarily relax the pelvic floor muscles in preparation for micturition. Loop 4B consists of the segmental (spinal) innervation of the pudendal nerve. Interruption of this loop is believed to cause vesicosphincter dyssynergia or loss of coordination between detrusor and striated sphincter contractions (Bradley, 1986).

## URETHRAL SPHINCTER MECHANISM

The third force that governs continence in humans is the urethral sphincter mechanism. The urethral sphincter is required to perform two significantly different tasks to preserve normal urinary system function. During bladder filling, the sphincter must maintain a watertight seal using both continuous basal tone and some mechanism to compensate for pressure variations produced by physical stress or exertion, such as positional changes, sudden coughing, or prolonged periods of exercise. In contrast, the mechanism must relax during micturition to provide an acceptably low level of resistance to urinary flow needed for efficient evacuation. These functions are performed by a complex physiologic mechanism rather than by the work of any single or pair of muscles.

Urethral closure during bladder filling and storage begins in the presence of a watertight seal formed by the epithelial lining of the organ and the mucosal secretions it produces. The softness of the urethral wall is crucial for effective closure in response to tension from adjacent vascular or muscular structures (Zinner et al., 1980). The concept of urethral mucosal softness is illustrated by the comparison of a drinking straw to a condom. When a straw is held in the hands, the walls remain apart because of their rigidity. If the straw is forced closed, its walls will rapidly return to an open position as soon as the pressure is removed. In contrast, the soft walls of the urethra are more comparable to a condom. Held aloft, the walls of the condom passively appose, that is, rest against each other. In addition, the walls of the condom have relatively little memory; they are easily deformed and have little propensity to

return to a given configuration after this deformation.

The walls of the urethra are even softer than those of a condom. During bladder filling, the horizontal folds of the urethra closely appose each other, contributing to the watertight urethral seal needed for continence. Because of the remarkable softness of the epithelium, these horizontal folds deftly adapt to the introduction of a stiff foreign object such as a tube, disallowing leakage despite obvious deformation.

In addition to the softness of the epithelial lining, the formation of a watertight urethral seal relies on the production of mucosal secretions that raise surface tension and seal the microscopic-sized spaces that remain even after the urethral walls appose during bladder filling. The importance of the deformation properties of the urethral wall and mucosal secretions to the formation of a watertight seal is illustrated by the passage of a catheter through the urethra into the bladder. Urine drains through the tube but not around it. It is the plasticity of the urethral epithelium and mucosal secretions that deforms around the relatively stiff catheter, forming a seal that prevents leakage despite significant deformity in the presence of a foreign object (Staskin et al., 1985; Zinner et al, 1980).

In addition to its ability to form a watertight seal, the sphincter mechanism must also prevent leakage in the presence of physical exertion. When a person changes positions or engages in any form of exercise, the combination of gravity and increased abdominal pressure favors urinary leakage through the urethra. The sphincter mechanism relies on a combination of muscular, vascular, and mechanical properties to protect the person from dribbling urine during these periods of stress.

The lamina propria of the urethra contains a rich vascular network that contributes to urethral tension by two mechanisms. First, it promotes the transmission of pressures from the abdomen to the urethral lumen by serving as a cushion. This mechanism is crucial when the sphincter mechanism responds to a precipitous rise in abdominal pressure caused by a cough or a sneeze. Second, the pressure produced by vascular pulsations contributes to active urethral closure (Staskin et al., 1985).

Smooth muscle bundles in the urethral wall and the bladder neck contribute active tension to augment urethral closure. Muscle bundles arranged in a circular fashion at the bladder neck form an internal sphincter mechanism that contributes to continence in males and females. Smooth muscles extending into the proximal urethra also contribute to closure (Staskin et al., 1985).

Striated muscle fibers found in the urethral wall and in the pelvic diaphragm contribute to the sphincter mechanism with their active tone and their role as a supportive structure for the urethrovesical unit. The striated muscle of the pelvic diaphragm is a mixture of slow- and fast-twitch fibers. Slow-twitch skeletal muscle fibers are particularly suited for sustained periods of tone but are relatively slow to mount a contraction in response to neural stimulation. These fibers contribute to the sphincter mechanism through support of the urethrovesical unit and adjacent structures. Rapid-twitch skeletal muscle fibers, in contrast, fatigue relatively rapidly compared with slow-twitch fibers but quickly contract in response to neural stimulation. They contribute to urethral closure by producing a rapid increase in urethral closure pressure in response to precipitous abdominal pressure increases.

Within the urethral wall, a second set of striated muscle fibers, the rhabdosphincter (Gosling & Chilton, 1984), also contributes to urethral closure. These striated muscle fibers are omega (C)-shaped, with deficient bulk in the posterior aspect of the urethral wall. They receive triple innervation from the somatic, sympathetic, and parasympathetic nervous systems and close the urethra with a circular motion. They are exclusively slow twitch and probably constitute the principal portion of continuous tension produced by the sphincter mechanism (Gosling & Chilton 1984).

The pelvic ligaments interact with the pelvic diaphragm to contribute to urethral closure by maintaining proper anatomic relationships between components of the urethrovesical unit and adjacent structures. The transmission of abdominal pressures to the sphincter mechanism relies on the proper position of the bladder neck and urethra relative to the pelvic bone and adjacent structures. Although the urethra remains in its proper position, pressure transmitted from the abdomen that temporarily increases intravesical pressure also is transmitted to the urethra, maintaining a pressure gradient that favors continence. Descent of the urethra from its proper position disrupts this relationship, so that pressure transmitted from the abdomen to the bladder fails to impact on the sphincter mechanism, causing a disruption of the pressure gradient between these structures that favors leakage. In addition, proper support promotes urethral closure by maintaining the muscular structures of the sphincter in an ideal position for transmission of tension to the urethral lumen. Loss of these relationships, termed *pelvic descent*, may produce stress urinary incontinence, or inability of the sphincter mechanism to maintain closure during periods of physical exertion.

## Sensory Innervation of the Urethrovesical Unit

The sensations of visceral structures in the body, including the urinary bladder and the urethra, are often nonspecific. Unfortunately, their physiologic basis is rather poorly understood by many clinicians, which may cause the significance of sensations of filling, urgency, or pain in the urethrovesical unit to be confused or undervalued.

The presence or absence of two distinctive sensations are of particular significance to the urologic nurse. *Urgency* to micturate and *bladder pain* are associated with a variety of stimuli, including volume, pressure, and inflammation (Morrison, 1987b). Normally, sensations of urgency may be elicited by bladder filling and pressure changes in the vesicle. Among normal subjects, the first sensation of the urgency to void is noted between 90 and 150 mL of filling, whereas sensations of strong urgency or bladder fullness are described at approximately 300 and 600 mL. The sensation of urgency is localized to the urethral meatus or the vaginal vestibule or labia in females and to the penile shaft or point where the urethra courses near the skin just beneath the scrotum in males (Denney-Brown & Robertson, 1933; Gray, 1990). In addition to bladder volume, sensations of urgency may be produced by the presence of unstable detrusor contractions (Gray et al., 1990) and by increases in intravesical pressure, although excessive pressure (higher than 90 cm $H_2O$) produces pain (Morrison, 1987b).

The urethrovesical unit is also capable of distinguishing sensations of warm and cold. These sensations appear to be centered in the urethra. Touching the mucosa of the urethra and trigone produces discomfort described as the burning or stinging sensations associated with inserting a urethral catheter or tugging on the inflated balloon of an indwelling Foley catheter (Morrison, 1987b).

Sensory nerves are located in the bladder wall, the trigone, and the urethra. Impulses from these nerves travel to the central nervous system by way of sympathetic nerves to enter the thoracolumbar spine and by parasympathetic pathways to enter the sacral spine. Sensory nerves from the urethra also reach the spine by way of branches of the pudendal nerve. Hypogastric and pelvic pathways transmit sensations of urgency and pain; pelvic and pudendal pathways transmit sensations of warmth, cold, and urgency (Morrison, 1987b).

The spinal pathways for sensory afferents from the urethrovesical unit are the dorsal, lateral, and, possibly, ventral columns. Dorsal column pathways transmit information concerning touch and pressure in the urethra, whereas the lateral columns transmit sensations concerned with bladder fullness, urgency, dermal sensations from the suprapubic area, and thermal signals from the urethra (Morrison, 1987b).

Unfortunately, the role of supraspinal centers in the modulation and perception of sensations arising from the urethrovesical unit remains unclear. Structures in the brain stem and midbrain (including the thalamus) influence the number and frequency of sensory signals that are transmitted to the cerebral cortex. The precise influence of these areas on the threshold of pain or perceptions of urgency in relation to volume and pressure in the bladder remains uncertain (Morrison, 1987b).

## MALE GENITALIA

The structures of the male genitalia include the penis, scrotum, testis, spermatic cord and its contents, seminal vesicles, ejaculatory ducts, and prostate. Physiologically, the purpose of this organ system is to produce, nourish, and transport mature sperm to the female vagina for reproduction.

### Scrotum

The scrotum is a cutaneous, fibromuscular sac located below the pubis that houses the testes and the lower portion of the spermatic cord. The scrotal skin is thick and rugated and typically contains deeper pigmentation than the surrounding integument. The rugae of the scrotum are formed by dermal fibers separated at a median raphe. Immediately beneath these fibers is the dartos muscle, which is composed of smooth muscle bundles and elastic tissue. The dartos muscle is a continuation of the suspensory ligament of the penis and superficial fascia of the abdominal wall. A reflection of the

dartos muscle creates an incomplete septum between the median ridge and the radix of the penis, forming a cavity in which the testes lie (Williams & Warwick, 1980).

## Testis and Sperm Transport Structures

The testes are a pair of ovoid-shaped organs that lie in the scrotum. They exist under three coverings: the tunica vaginalis, the tunica albuginea, and the tunica vasculosa. The tunica vaginalis is an extension of the peritoneum that forms a fibrous sac around the testis. The tunica albuginea is a white fibrous structure that covers the testis and constitutes a portion of its internal architecture. Its posterior border projects into the testis, forming an incomplete vertical septum called the *mediastinum testis*. The front and lateral aspects of the tunica albuginea project into the testis, dividing it into 200 to 300 lobules containing seminiferous tubules, which are the functional unit of the organ. The tunica vasculosa, or third covering, is a plexus of vascular structures that provides nourishment for each lobule (Williams & Warwick, 1980).

The seminiferous tubule is the functional unit of the testis (Fig. 1–6). Each testicular lobule contains one to three tubules composed of nearly 30 to 60 cm of tortuous tubing that terminates in a relatively short, straight segment called the *canaliculus recti*. The seminiferous tubules constitute approximately 75% of testicu-

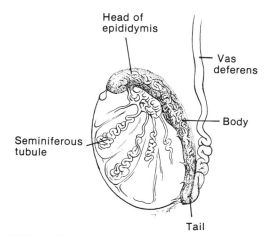

FIGURE 1–6 Testis and epididymis. (From Tanagho, E. A. [1992]. Anatomy of the lower urinary tract. In P. C. Walsh, A. B. Retik, T. A. Stamey, & E. D. Vaughan, Jr. [Eds.], *Campbell's urology* [Vol. 1, 6th ed., p. 59]. Philadelphia: W. B. Saunders. Reprinted by permission.)

lar mass, with a total length of nearly 1 mile (Leeson & Leeson, 1976; Williams & Warwick, 1980).

The seminiferous tubule is composed of four to eight layers of stratified epithelium with an internal lumen. These tubules contain Sertoli cells, spermatogenic germ cells, and an external basement membrane covered by a fibrous tunic. The Sertoli cells are columnar in shape and extend radially from the outer basement membrane toward the central lumen. They are linked in tight junctions that separate the tubule into two identifiable compartments. The outer, or basal, compartment contains more primitive germ cells, whereas the inner, or luminal, compartment houses more mature forms. The precise function of the Sertoli cells remains unclear; they probably provide nourishment for the maturing germ cells and may contribute to the blood-testis barrier. In addition, the Sertoli cells are known to secrete an androgen-binding protein that promotes accumulation of androgen molecules in the immediate area of the germ cell epithelium and the fluid noted throughout the seminiferous tubule (Amelar et al., 1977; Lipshultz et al., 1987).

The germ cell portion of the seminiferous tubular epithelium is composed of continuously maturing germ cells. Spermatogonia, the most primitive form of germ cell, are concentrated at the outer border of the tubule. As they migrate toward the tubular lumen, they undergo maturation to primary, then secondary, spermatocytes before differentiating into spermatids, which are the forerunners of the mature sperm cell (Amelar et al., 1977).

The remaining 25% of the testicular parenchyma is composed of lymphatics, vascular structures, macrophages, and Leydig cells. The Leydig cells are found in small groups of 5 to 20, composing approximately 20% of total parenchymal volume. They affect testicular and systemic function by the secretion of testosterone (Amelar et al., 1977).

The internal spermatic artery provides the bulk of arterial vascularity required for testicular function. The cremasteric and deferential arteries provide supplemental vascularity. The internal spermatic artery branches off from the aorta just below the renal arteries and travels to the testes by way of the spermatic cord. Venous drainage from the testes occurs by way of the internal spermatic vein. The right internal spermatic vein dumps directly into the right inferior vena cava. In contrast, the left internal spermatic vein dumps into the left renal vein following a course that is 8 to 10 cm longer

than the right. Because of its greater vertical length, the left internal spermatic vein must drain against greater hydrostatic pressure than the right, rendering it more susceptible to varicocele (Lipshultz et al., 1987).

Lymphatic drainage from the left testis is provided by the para-aortic and preaortic nodes. Right testicular lymphatics drain into the nodes in the aortocaval zone just below the renal vein (Redman, 1987).

The transportation of sperm from the testes to the urethra requires passage through the epididymis and vas deferens. The sperm interact with secretions from the prostate and seminal vesicles to ensure proper nutrition, support, and maturation of sperm cells before expulsion from the body during ejaculation.

The epididymis is a sausage-shaped structure, approximately 5 cm long, that is attached to the posterolateral aspect of the testis (see Fig. 1–6). It contains a single compartment, which is covered by the tunica vaginalis except on its posterior border, where a fascial reflection forms an epididymal sinus. The single compartment of the epididymis contains a long, tortuous tube with minimal smooth muscle but abundant cilia that transports sperm from the testes to the vas deferens (Williams & Warwick, 1980).

The vas deferens is a firm, cylindrical tube extending from the termination of the epididymis to the ejaculatory duct near the base of the prostate. The initial portion of the vas deferens is tortuous; its latter segment is much straighter. From its origin along the posterior aspect of the testis, the vas deferens travels down to the base of the testis, then curves upward and ascends along the spermatic cord to the bladder base before again descending to the prostatic base. The vas deferens contains a smooth muscle tunic capable of rapidly transporting sperm toward the urethra (Williams & Warwick, 1980).

The smooth muscle action of the vas deferens is moderated by sympathetic fibers from the hypogastric plexus and parasympathetic fibers from the pelvic plexus. The role of the parasympathetic fibers is particularly significant during ejaculation (Lipshultz et al., 1987).

The seminal vesicles are a pair of hollow structures that lie between the posterior bladder and the rectum. Each is 4 cm long, with a pyramidal shape whose apex is oriented laterally and backward from its base. The seminal vesicle is formed by a single tortuous tube from which irregularly diverticular-type structures arise connected by dense fibrous tissue. The diameter of the seminal vesicle tube is approximately 4 mm, with a total length of 10 to 15 cm.

The walls of the seminal vesicles are composed of muscoal epithelium bounded by a muscular tunic and outer areolar covering. The mucosal layer of the vesicles contains numerous goblet-shaped cells and small stellate cells whose significance remains unclear (Lipshultz et al., 1987).

The termination of the sperm transport structures is in the ejaculatory ducts. Beginning in the prostatic base, the ducts are formed by the termination segment of the vas deferens and the seminal vesicles. From their origin in the prostatic base, they travel anteroinferiorly between the right and left median prostatic lobes and past the utricle to terminate in the urethral lumen. The walls of the ejaculatory ducts are relatively thin and have a columnar epithelial inner lining, a muscular tunic, and a fibrous border (Tanagho, 1986).

## Prostate

The prostate contributes to genitourinary function by providing nourishment and volume for the semen before the semen's expulsion from the body during ejaculation. It is a partly glandular, partly fibromuscular organ located immediately beneath the vesicourethral junction. It is pierced by the initial 2 to 3 cm of urethra and terminates at its membranous portion. The prostate has a conical shape that is flattened at its posterior and anterior sides. The organ is approximately 3.4 cm long and 4.4 cm wide, with a maximum depth of 2.6 cm (Tanagho, 1986).

Although no true anatomically separate lobular structure of the prostate exists (Williams & Warwick, 1980), health care professionals divide the gland into several lobes for clinical and surgical purposes. The anterior, subcervical, and right and left lateral intraurethral lobes are felt during endoscopy. The subcervical and right and left lateral lobes are particularly significant when they undergo hyperplasia and produce bladder outlet obstruction. Posterior and median lobes constitute the extraurethral lobes appreciated on digital rectal examination. The posterior lobe is of particular significance because of its propensity to undergo neoplastic changes during later life (Hutch & Rambo, 1978).

The microscopic structure of the prostate is characterized by fibromuscular and glandular components. The fibromuscular capsule surrounds the outer aspect of the organ and extends into the interior organ, including the urethral aspects. The glandular tissue contains numerous follicles that open into a complex system of canals that run from the periphery toward the urethral lumen. The follicles coalesce into 12 to 20 excretory ducts (Hutch & Rambo, 1978).

The arterial blood supply of the prostate is provided by a prostatovesical artery that arises as a branch of the pudendal artery or the superior rectal artery. Venous blood drains into the internal iliac and vesical veins. Lymphatic drainage from the prostate is shared by channels from the posterior urethra. They commonly dump into the internal iliac arteries but may occasionally drain into the external iliac arteries (Redman, 1987).

## Male Reproductive Physiology

Sperm production relies directly on the structures of the genital tract and on neural modulation of smooth muscle bundles that transport sperm to the urethra and into the vaginal vault for reproduction. In addition, spermatogenesis relies on hormonal axes that regulate sperm production and produce the secondary characteristics that differentiate male from female secondary sex characteristics.

The principal hormonal axis affecting spermatogenesis originates in the hypothalamus and terminates at receptor sites in the testicular parenchyma. The hypothalamus begins the cycle by releasing luteinizing hormone-releasing hormone (LHRH), which travels to the median eminence of the adenohypophysis by way of a portal venous system. The pituitary gland then releases luteinizing hormone (LH), which, in turn, leads to release of follicle-stimulating hormone (FSH) (Guyton, 1991).

After their release into the systemic circulation, FSH and LH pass through the vascular supply of the testis, causing production and release of the testicular androgens, primarily testosterone and dihydrotestosterone. LH acts at the Sertoli cell to produce testosterone and stimulate spermatogenesis. FSH plays a more indirect role in the production of testosterone but directly affects the process of sperm production. As blood levels of the gonadal androgens increase, the production of LHRH by the hypothalamus is inhibited, causing an indirect inhibition of FSH and LH production by the pituitary gland. Conversely, as the concentration of circulating androgens decreases below a threshold level, the hypothalamus again produces LHRH, and the cycle begins again (Jenkins et al., 1978).

The process of spermatogenesis begins in the seminiferous tubule. Three phases constitute the portion of the process that occurs within the testis. During phase 1, the primitive spermatogonia enlarge and undergo mitosis to produce primary spermatocytes containing 92 chromosomes. Phase 2 occurs when two consecutive meiotic divisions occur, producing four secondary spermatogonia, each containing 23 chromosomes (haploid number) suitable for union with the ovum. Phase 3 marks the transformation of spermatogonia to spermatozoa (Mann & Lutwak-Mann, 1981).

Maturation of the spermatozoon is slow: 74 days are required to form a mature sperm cell capable of fertilization. The first stage is called the *Golgi phase,* in which small granules of hyaluronidase, proteases, and other substances coalesce into a single acrosomal capsule that attaches to the nuclear membrane at the spot that will form the head of the sperm. During phase 2, a cap is formed around the head of this acrosomal vesicle. The two centrioles of the spermatozoon now begin to move; the proximal centriole assumes a position at the posterior pole of the nucleus, and the distal centriole sprouts a flagellum consisting of two central and nine surrounding pairs of microtubules, thereby forming the tail of the mature sperm.

The third maturational phase is called the *acrosomal stage,* in which the sperm undergoes extensive metamorphosis to assume the appearance of a mature spermatozoon. This stage requires the formation of a mitochondrial sheath around the middle and proximal tail sections needed for sperm motility. The final phase of spermatogenesis is a maturation phase, characterized by shedding of excess cytoplasm with the assistance of the Sertoli cells (Mann & Lutwak-Mann, 1981).

Transport of the spermatozoon from the seminiferous tubule to epididymis occurs by means of the muscular contractions of the tunica muscularis. Although the sperm entering the epididymis appear mature, they are not yet capable of fertilization of the ovum. The epididymis itself plays a role in sperm maturation, accounting for the slow transport time (12 days) through this short segment of the genital tract. Transport through the epididymis allows the sperm cells to gain the potential for motility (forward motion by thrashing of the tail piece), although they become actively motile only after ejaculation. Although the process that causes this change remains unclear, it seems probable that testosterone plays a crucial role (Lipshultz et al., 1987).

After exiting the epididymis, the spermatozoa enter the vas deferens. Transport is then governed by smooth muscle contractions under parasympathetic modulation. During ejaculation, sperm is transported through the vas deferens to the ejaculatory ducts in preparation for expulsion through the urethra. Once in the ejaculatory ducts, the sperm cells are mixed with nutritive secretions provided by the seminal vesicles. In addition to nutritive substances, the vesicles add prostaglandins to the semen, which aids in the sperm's potential for fertilization of an ovum (Lipshultz et al., 1987).

The prostate contributes to male sexual function by adding nutritive secretions to the semen. During ejaculation, the prostatic capsule contracts in synchrony with the vas deferens, secreting a thin, milky fluid containing several substances, including citric acid, calcium acid phosphate, a clotting enzyme, and profibrinolysin. The prostatic fluid is relatively acidic (pH 6.0–6.5), favoring prolonged survival in the acidic environment characteristic of the vaginal mucosa (Lipshultz et al., 1987).

The resulting semen is a mixture of secretions provided by the vas deferens, seminal vesicles, prostate, and posterior urethral glands (principally, the bulbourethral glands). Its pH is approximately 7.5; prostatic secretions give it a milky character, whereas the seminal vesicle secretions provide its characteristically mucoid appearance. A single ejaculate contains from 100 million to 400 million sperm cells. Following expulsion from the body, a weak clotting enzyme in the semen interacts with the profibrinolysin to form a weak coagulum. As this dissolves, the sperm gain their maximal motility as they attempt to penetrate the ovum. Although the spermatozoon may survive several months in the male genital tract, it can survive only 12 to 24 hours in the relatively hostile environment characteristic of the normal female genital tract (Lipshultz et al., 1987).

## Penis

The penis is a cylindrical organ that is attached to the perineum by the suspensory ligament and a reflection of Buck's fascia. The pendulous penis remains visible to the naked eye, and a perineal portion (the radix) lies rooted in the perineum (Redman, 1987). The penile body contains three cylindrical structures composed of erectile tissue. The most inferior is the corpus spongiosum, which also houses the urethra. Immediately superior are paired corpora cavernosa that are capable of significant enlargement when engorged with blood during tumescence. They are surrounded by an extension of the tunica albuginea characterized by two layers. The superficial layer surrounds both corpora cavernosa as a single unit, whereas the deep layer separates the corpora with a fibrous septum with two median grooves. The larger inferior groove houses the corpora spongiosum and pendulous urethra, and the superior smaller groove houses the deep dorsal veins (Williams & Warwick, 1980).

The penile skin is remarkable for its characteristically deep pigmentation and loose connection with underlying fascia allowing expansion during tumescence. At the distal segment, the skin is folded over on itself, forming the foreskin that covers the glans. This fascia contains loose areolar tissue but no fat. A few fibers from the dartos muscle and elements of the suspensory ligament may be present (Williams & Warwick, 1980).

## Physiology of Penile Erection

Advances in understanding of the hemodynamics of penile tumescence have virtually revolutionized clinical wisdom concerning the physiology and pathophysiology of male sexual function. The understanding of erection as a neurovascular event that is modulated by psychogenic and hormonal factors has significantly altered traditional beliefs of erectile physiology and the causes of dysfunction.

The arterial blood supply of the penis arises principally from the pudendal artery, which branches from the internal iliac artery near the sacroiliac joint. The pudendal artery gives rise to the penile artery, which follows only a short course before branching into the dorsal, urethral (spongiosal), deep (cavernous), and bulbar arteries. The dorsal artery enters the penis in the superior groove under Buck's fascia and travels near the dorsal vein and paired dorsal nerves. It is responsible for shunting blood to the cavernous bodies, causing engorgement needed for tumescence. The cavernous or deep artery enters the penis at the hilum along with the cavernosa veins and nerves. It carries blood to the cavernous bodies and communicates with the helicine arteries that empty into sinu-

soidal spaces before venous outflow (Aboseif & Lue, 1988).

The spongiosal and bulbar arteries do not engorge the cavernous bodies during tumescence. The spongiosal or urethral artery supplies the corpus spongiosum, the urethral tissue, and the glans penis. The bulbar artery supplies the Cowper's glands and the proximal urethral bulb (Aboseif & Lue, 1988).

The penis is drained by three sets of veins: deep, superficial, and intermediate. The superficial dorsal vein drains the skin and subcutaneous tissue external to Buck's fascia. The intermediate veins run beneath Buck's fascia but superficial to the tunica albuginea. As many as 15 veins emerge at the glans penis to form a plexus that drains into the dorsal vein, which is the principal intermediate vein. The deep dorsal vein traverses the inferior groove of the tunica albuginea (Aboseif & Lue, 1988).

The act of erection, or tumescence, begins with an inflow of arterial blood caused by a decrease in resistance at the level of the penile arterioles and sinusoids of the cavernous bodies. Resistance to flow is conceptualized by the formula

$$F = P / R$$

where F is flow, P is intra-arterial pressure, and R is resistance. To increase flow, smooth muscle bundles in the arterioles and sinusoids relax, producing greater intraluminal diameter and increased flow. Initially, this increase in flow acts to fill the distensible sinusoids of the cavernosal body with little rise in pressure. Nonetheless, this expansion in volume is limited by the presence of the nondistensible fascial coverings of the corporal bodies. Therefore, after an initial increase in volume, pressure in the cavernous bodies rapidly increases, causing increased penile thickness, size, and rigidity. Ultimately, intracavernosal pressure increases to within 10 to 20 mm Hg of mean arterial pressure (Aboseif & Lue, 1988).

This change in smooth muscle tone at the arteriolar level is mediated by the autonomic nervous system. Although the precise neural mechanisms remain poorly elucidated, an understanding of these relationships is beginning to emerge. It has been assumed that sympathetic-adrenergic nerves that are found throughout the corpora cavernosum smooth muscle favor flaccidity maintained by smooth muscle contraction that produces blood flow sufficient only to meet the nutritional needs of the penile tissue. In contrast, cholinergic receptors that operate under parasympathetic con-

**TABLE 1–2. Phases of Penile Tumescence**

| PHASE | CHARACTERISTICS |
|---|---|
| *Flaccid* | Arterial inflow and venous outflow approximate that of other peripheral tissues; arterial blood gases in corporal bodies are equivalent to those of other tissues |
| *Latent* | Initiation of tumescence begins with smooth muscle relaxation and increased arterial inflow under nervous system influence (psychogenic or reflexogenic); the intracavernous pressure remains near flaccid values, but the volume of blood in cavernous bodies grows, causing elongation of the penis |
| *Tumescent* | Volume of cavernous body reaches point at which the nonelastic components (tunica albuginea and Buck's fascia) limit compliance of system; as a result, intracavernous pressure rapidly increases; penis shows further elongation and increased circumference |
| *Full Erection* | Intracavernous pressure increases to near mean arterial pressure; blood gases in cavernous blood remain comparable to systemic values |
| *Rigid Erection* | As a result of ischiocavernosal muscle contraction, intracavernous pressure briefly exceeds mean arterial pressure, and blood gas values decrease to lower than systemic values. This ischemic phase is short-lived, causing no damage to tissues in the normally functioning system |
| *Detumescent* | Sympathetic tone increases by means of nervous modulation, causing smooth muscle contraction and loss of intracavernous pressure followed by slower loss of volume |

trol were assumed to produce direct relaxation of smooth muscle and increase blood flow needed for tumescence. Recent investigation has not supported this hypothesis. Instead, it has been found that cholinergic nerves *indirectly* facilitate tumescence by inhibiting adrenergic-mediated tone that favors the inflow of blood and by facilitating nonadrenergic-noncholinergic nerves that act directly on smooth muscle to produce relaxation and engorgement of the corporal bodies with blood. The principal neurotransmitter substance contained in nonadrenergic-noncholinergic nerves found in the corporal bodies has not been clearly identified. Several peptides, including substance P, somatostatin, avian pancreatic polypeptide, and neuropeptide Y, have been isolated from nerves in the corporal bodies. Of these neurotransmitters, vasoactive intestinal polypeptide and substance P are the most likely candidates, because only they are known to inhibit smooth muscle tone in corporal vascular tissue (de Tejada et al., 1988).

In addition to neurotransmitter substances, smooth muscle relaxation causing vasodilation of the corporal bodies is modulated by paracrine or endocrine substances, or both. Paracrine substances that are manufactured and released by the endothelium, producing vasodilation, include acetylcholine, adenosine diphosphate and triphosphate, bradykinin, and substance P (de Tejada et al., 1988). Prostaglandin, produced by the cavernosal tissue, also modulates vasodilation. Prostaglandins $E_1$, $E_2$, and $I_2$ are thought to facilitate tumescence by antagonizing adrenergic tone in vascular smooth muscle (de Tejada et al., 1988).

Tumescence in humans also relies on the venous drainage system. Unfortunately, the physiologic mechanisms that govern venous response to tumescence remain unclear. Nonetheless, it is certain that they play a crucial role in the maintenance of an erection necessary for successful intercourse. Three possible explanations for the process of venous occlusion exist. The first relies on active occlusion of venous smooth muscle. A second explanation is that venous occlusion is produced by mechanical means as the engorged corpora crushes the venules that drain it between the sinusoidal wall and rigid, noncompliant tunica albuginea. This mechanical occlusion is further enhanced as the sinusoids occlude the emissary veins during full erection and as the distended tunica albuginea crushes the emissary veins (Aboseif & Lue, 1988). A third potential explanation for venous occlusion during tumescence is a potential role for venous valves in the corporal bodies (Fitzpatrick, 1974, 1975).

Advances in the understanding of the hemodynamic and neurovascular factors that govern tumescence have led to a reorganization of the understanding of the events that cause erections. The six stages of tumescence (Table 1–2) are organized around concepts of *initiation of erection* (mediated by neurally induced smooth muscle relaxation in local arterioles), *filling* with blood (mediated by arteries of the penis), and *maintenance* of erection (storage of blood mediated by venous occlusion mechanisms) (Aboseif & Lue, 1988).

## MODULATORY ROLE OF NERVOUS AND ENDOCRINE SYSTEMS

In addition to understanding erectile function as the result of immediate neurovascular events, it is also important to appreciate the modulatory role played by the endocrine and central nervous systems in the male sexual response. These systems affect the ability to generate an erection and the development of secondary characteristics, libido, and emotional response to sexuality and reproduction.

The central nervous system affects both the immediate mechanism governing erections and the psychogenic response to the complex behaviors that constitute sexuality in human society. The spinal cord is crucial for the initiation of erections, because it is the outflow tract for sympathetic and parasympathetic impulses needed for smooth muscle relaxation and arterial inflow. The brain directly affects the immediate response to erections by responding to continued input necessary for the initiation and maintenance of erections. The psychogenic or brain-mediated erection responds to specific sensory stimulus, producing an erection with the potential for being well sustained compared with the relatively unpredictable and short-lived reflexogenic (spinal cord–mediated) tumescent episode (Gray & Dobkin, 1989).

A number of brain centers contribute to the psychogenic erection. Nuclei in the temporal lobes, cingulate gyrus, gyrus rectus of the cerebral cortex, hypothalamus, hippocampus, and mamillary bodies affect the erectile response experimentally in animals and humans. The hippocampus and cingulate gyrus influence visual stimuli affecting sexual response, whereas the gyrus rectus processes olfactory input (Siroky & Krane, 1983). The complex interactions of the cerebral cortex that shape sexuality from a psychosocial and physiologic perspective are not clearly understood but are known to exert a profound influence on the ability to generate and maintain an erection in a variety of cultural settings.

The hormonal mechanisms that modulate erections are also only partially elucidated. Although it is known that serotonin decreases libido and dopamine stimulates it, their mechanisms of action are not understood. Testosterone also is known to exert an influence on erectile activity. Castration by surgical or medical means is known to result in a gradual decrease in libido and erectile efficiency, although it does not immediately produce adverse effects (Siroky & Krane, 1983; Wagner & Green, 1981).

## SUMMARY

The anatomy and physiology of the genitourinary system are part of the science that un-

derpins the practice of urologic nursing. Detailed knowledge of the physiology of each specific organ system is integrated with a broad base of knowledge of holistic nursing to provide humanistic and technically excellent care of patients with disease or dysfunction of the urinary or genital systems.

## *REFERENCES*

Aaronson, I. (1992). Sexual differentiation and intersexuality. In P. Kelalis, L. R. King, & A. B. Belman (Eds.), *Clinical pediatric urology* (3rd ed.). Philadelphia: W. B. Saunders.

Aboseif, S. R., & Lue, T. F. (1988). Hemodynamics of penile erection. *Urologic Clinics of North America, 15,* 1–7.

Abrams, P. H. (1984). Bladder instability: Concept, clinical causes and treatment. *Scandinavian Journal of Urology and Nephrology, 87* (Supplement), 7–12.

Amelar, R. D., Dubin, L., & Walsh, P. C. (Eds.). (1977). *Male infertility.* Philadelphia: W. B. Saunders.

Bhatia, N. N., & Bradley, W. E. (1983). Neuroanatomy and physiology: Innervation of the lower urinary tract. In S. Raz (Ed.), *Female urology.* Philadelphia: W. B. Saunders.

Boyarsky, S., & Labay, P. (1982). Principles of ureteral physiology. In S. Bergman (Ed.), *The ureter.* New York: Springer-Verlag.

Bradley, W. E. (1986). Physiology of the urinary bladder. In P. C. Walsh, R. F. Gittes, A. D. Perlmutter, & T. A. Stamey (Eds.), *Campbell's urology* (5th ed., pp. 129–185). Philadelphia: W. B. Saunders.

Bradley, W. E., Timm, G. W., & Scott, F. B. (1974). Innervation of detrusor muscle and urethra. *Urologic Clinics of North America, 1,* 3.

Brundage, D. (1992). *Renal disorders.* St. Louis: Mosby-Year Book.

de Tejada, I. S., Goldstein, I., & Krane, R. F. (1988). Local control of penile erections: Nerves, smooth muscle and endothelium. *Urologic Clinics of North America, 15,* 9–16.

Denney-Brown, D., & Robertson, E. G. (1933). On the physiology of micturition. *Brain, 56,* 149–190.

Dixon, J., & Gosling, J. (1987). Structure and innervation in the human bladder. In M. Torrens & J. F. B. Morrison (Eds.), *Physiology of the lower urinary tract.* London: Springer-Verlag.

Evardsin, P., & Ursin, T. (1968). Nervous control of urinary bladder in cats: I. The collecting phase. *Acta Physiologica Scandinavica, 72,* 157.

Fitzpatrick, T. (1974). Venography of the deep dorsal veins and valvular system. *Journal of Urology, 111,* 518.

Fitzpatrick, T. (1975). The corpus cavernosum intercommunicating venous drainage system. *Journal of Urology, 113,* 494.

Golimbu, M. (1981). Embryology of the genital and lower urinary tract. In S. Al-Askari, M. Golimbu, & P. Morales (Eds.), *Essentials of basic sciences in urology.* New York: Grune & Stratton.

Gosling, J. A., & Chilton, C. P. (1984). The anatomy of the bladder, urethra and pelvic floor. In A. R. Mundy, T. P. Stephenson, & A. J. Wein (Eds.), *Urodynamics: Principles, practice and application.* London: Churchill-Livingstone.

Gray, M. L. (1990a). Assessment and investigation of urinary incontinence. In K. Jeter, N. Faller, & C. Norton (Eds.), *Nursing for continence.* Philadelphia: W. B. Saunders.

Gray, M. L. (1990b). Congenital voiding dysfunction in

childhood: Presentation and management. *Journal of Enterostomal Therapy, 17*(2), 47–53.

Gray, M. L., Bennett, J. K., & Green, B. G. (1990). Urodynamic assessment of bladder instability. In *Proceedings: International Continence Society*. Aarhus, Denmark: International Continence Society.

Gray, M. L., & Dobkin, K. (1989). Genitourinary system. In J. M. Thompson, G. K. McFarland, J. E. Hirsch, S. M. Tucker, & A. C. Bowers (Eds.), *Clinical nursing*. St. Louis: Mosby-Year Book.

Gray, M. L., & Dougherty, M.C. (1987). Urinary incontinence: Pathophysiology and treatment. *Journal of Enterostomal Therapy, 14*(4), 152–162.

Griffiths, D. J. (1984). Hydrodynamics and mechanics of the bladder and urethra. In A. R. Mundy, T. P. Stephenson, & A. J. Wein (Eds.), *Urodynamics: Principles, practice and application*. London: Churchill-Livingstone.

Guyton, A. C. (1991). *Textbook of medical physiology* (8th ed.). Philadelphia: W. B. Saunders.

Hald, T., & Bradley, W. E. (1983). *The urinary bladder: Neurology and dynamics*. Baltimore: Williams & Wilkins.

Holstege, G., Griffiths, D. J., Dewall, H., & Dalm, E. (1986). Anatomic and physiologic observations on supraspinal control of bladder and urethral sphincter muscle in the cat. *Journal of Comparative Neurology, 250*, 449–461.

Hutch, J. A., & Rambo, N. O. (1978). A study of the anatomy of the prostate, prostatic urethra and urinary sphincter system. *Journal of Urology, 104*, 443.

Jenkins, A. D., Turner, T. T., & Howards, S. S. (1978). Physiology of the male reproductive system. *Urologic Clinics of North America, 5*, 437.

Kiil, F. (1978). Physiology of renal pelvis and ureter. In J. H. Harrison, R. F. Gittes, A. D. Perlmutter, T. A. Stamey, & P. C. Walsh (Eds.), *Campbell's urology* (4th ed., pp. 55–86). Philadelphia: W. B. Saunders.

Kramer, S. A. (1985). Surgical treatment of urinary incontinence. In P. P. Kelalis, L. R. King, & A. B. Belman (Eds.), *Clinical pediatric urology* (2nd ed., pp. 326–345). Philadelphia: W. B. Saunders.

Leeson, C. R., & Leeson, T. S. (1976). *Histology*. Philadelphia: W. B. Saunders.

Levitt, S. B., & Weiss, R. A. (1985). Vesicoureteral reflux: Natural history, classification and reflux nephropathy. In P. P. Kelalis, L. R. King, & A. B. Belman (Eds.), *Clinical pediatric urology* (2nd ed., pp. 355–419). Philadelphia: W. B. Saunders.

Lewin, R. J., Dillard, G. V., & Porter, R. W. (1967). Extrapyramidal inhibition of the urinary bladder. *Brain Research, 4*, 301.

Lipshultz, L. I., Howards, S. S., & Buch, J. P. (1987). Male infertility. In J. Y. Gillenwater, J. T. Grayhack, S. S. Howards, & J. W. Duckett (Eds.), *Adult and pediatric urology*. Chicago: Year Book.

Mann, R., & Lutwak-Mann, C. (1981). *Male reproductive function and semen*. Berlin: Springer-Verlag.

Morrison, J. F. B. (1987a). Bladder control: Role of higher levels of the central nervous system. In M. Torrens & J. F. B. Morrison (Eds.), *The physiology of the lower urinary tract*. London: Springer-Verlag.

Morrison, J. F. B. (1987b). Sensations arising from the lower urinary tract. In M. Torrens & J. F. B. Morrison (Eds.), *The physiology of the lower urinary tract*. London: Springer-Verlag.

Pinck, B. D. (1981). Embryology of the upper urinary tract. In S. Al-Askari, M. Golimbu, & P. Morales (Eds.), *Essentials of basic sciences in urology*. New York: Grune & Stratton.

Olsson, C. A. (1986). Anatomy of the upper urinary tract. In P. C. Walsh, R. F. Gittes, A. D. Perlmutter, & T. A. Stamey (Eds.), *Campbell's urology* (5th ed.). Philadelphia: W. B. Saunders.

Redman, J. F. (1987). Anatomy of the genitourinary system. In J. Y. Gillenwater, J. T. Grayhack, S. S. Howards, & J. W. Duckett (Eds.), *Adult and pediatric urology*. Chicago: Year Book.

Rose, J. G., & Gillenwater, J. Y. (1974). The effect of adrenergic and cholinergic agents and their blockade on ureteral activity. *Investigative Urology, 11*, 439.

Ross, J. A., Edward, P., & Kirkland, I. S. (1982). *Behavior of the human ureter in health and disease*. Edinburgh: Churchill-Livingstone.

Sarma, K. P. (1969). *Tumors of the urinary bladder*. New York: Appleton-Century-Crofts.

Siroky, M. B., & Krane, R. J. (1983). Neurophysiology of erection. In R. J. Krane, M. B. Siroky, & I. Goldstein (Eds.), *Male sexual dysfunction*. Boston: Little, Brown.

Staskin, D. R., Zimmern, P. E., Hadley, H. R., & Raz, S. (1985). Pathophysiology of stress incontinence. *Clinical Obstetrics and Gynecology, 12*, 357.

Stuart, D. G., Porter, R. W., Adey, W. R., & Kamikawa, Y. (1964). Hypothalamic unit activity: I. Visceral and somatic influences. *Clinical Neurophysiology, 16*, 237.

Tanagho, E. A. (1981). Development of the ureter. In D. R. Smith (Ed.), *General urology* (10th ed.). Los Altos, CA: Lange Medical Publications.

Tanagho, E. A. (1986). Anatomy and surgical approach to the urogenital tract. In P. C. Walsh, R. F. Gittes, A. D. Perlmutter, & T. A. Stamey (Eds.), *Campbell's urology* (5th ed.). Philadelphia: W. B. Saunders.

Tanagho, E. A. (1992a). Anatomy of the genitourinary tract. In E. A. Tanagho & J. W. McAninich (Eds.), *Smith's general urology*. Norwalk, CT: Appleton & Lange.

Tanagho, E. A. (1992b). Embryology of the genitourinary system. In E. A. Tanagho & J. W. McAninich (Eds.), *Smith's general urology*. Norwalk, CT: Appleton & Lange.

Valtin, H. (1983). *Renal function*. Boston: Little, Brown.

Wagner, G., & Green, R. (1981). *Impotence*. New York: Plenum.

Waldeyer, W. (1891). Über die Insel des Gegirns der Anthropoiden. *Korrespondenzblatt der Deutschen Gesselschaft für Anthropologie, Ethnologie abd Urgeschichte, 22*, 110.

Weiss, R. M. (1986). Physiology and pharmacology of the renal pelvis and ureter. In P. C. Walsh, R. F. Gittes, A. D. Perlmutter, & T. A. Stamey (Eds.), *Campbell's urology* (5th ed., pp. 94–128). Philadelphia: W. B. Saunders.

Weiss, R. M., Bassett, A. L., & Hoffman, B. F. (1978). Adrenergic innervation of the ureter. *Investigative Urology, 16*, 123.

Williams, P., & Warwick, R. (1980). *Gray's anatomy*. Philadelphia: W.B. Saunders.

Zinner, N. R., Sterling, A. M., & Ritter, R. C. (1980). Role of inner urethral softness in urinary continence. *Urology, 16*, 115.

# CHAPTER 2

# Health Assessment of the Adult Urology Patient

■

*Teresa D. Gibbs*

## OVERVIEW

Urologic nursing is devoted to the care of patients with disorders of the urinary tract, the adrenal glands, or the male reproductive system. Because approximately 15% of patients who visit a physician have a urologic problem, knowledge about urology is an essential aspect of any nurse's practice (Hanno & Wein, 1987).

Assessment is the first step of the nursing process and is fundamental to nursing practice. A description of assessment is found in *Nursing: A Social Policy Statement*, developed by the American Nurses Association (1980), which states that ``the collection of data about the health status of the client/patient is systematic and continuous. The data are accessible, communicated, and recorded.''

*Systematic* implies that assessment requires a technique that must be learned and practiced to become expert. *Continuous* means ongoing—assessment starts when the nurse first sees the patient and ends when the professional relationship with the patient is terminated. *Accessible, communicated,* and *recorded* signify that if the collected data are not documented, they can serve no purpose for the patient.

This chapter focuses on the general health assessment of the urologic patient—the health history, the physical examination, and the basic laboratory studies.

## BEHAVIORAL OBJECTIVES

After studying this chapter, the reader should be able to

1. List the common signs and symptoms associated with urologic disease.
2. Discuss priority assessments in the physical examination of the urologic patient.
3. Perform urologic assessment using inspection, auscultation, palpation, and percussion.
4. Describe the correct method of urine collection for urinalysis and urine culture.
5. Define normal and abnormal findings in urinalysis.

## KEY WORDS

**Anuria**—a total urine output of less than 100 mL/24 hours.

**Auscultation**—a technique used in physical examination that consists of listening to sounds produced by the body, generally with a stethoscope.

**Azotemia**—an excess of nitrogenous wastes in the blood.

**Bacteriuria**—bacteria in the urine; a bacterial count greater than 100,000/mL in a urine culture usually signifies urinary tract infection, although less than 100,000/ mL may be significant in specially collected specimens.

**Bladder spasms**—sudden, involuntary, intermittent contractions of the bladder.

**Blood urea nitrogen (BUN) determination**—a blood test to monitor renal function that measures the serum concentration of urea, a major end product of protein metabolism that is normally excreted entirely by the kidney.

**Calculus**—a stone found anywhere in the urinary tract.

**Cast**—a clump of material or cells that builds up in the renal tubules and precipitates into the urinary sediment.

**Chyluria**—chyle in the urine (chyle is a product of intestinal digestion normally absorbed into the lymphatic system).

**Colic**—severe pain of sudden onset that may be constant or spasmodic. Renal or ureteral colic is caused by an acute obstruction of the upper urinary tract, hyperperistalsis, and smooth muscle spasms. Renal and ureteral colic are among the worst pain experienced by humans.

**Costovertebral angle (CVA)**—an anatomic landmark on the back that corresponds to the junction of the 12th rib and the lateral border of the sacrospinal muscles.

**Creatinine**—a major end product of muscle metabolism that is excreted by the kidney. The serum creatinine determination is a blood test that measures renal function.

**Dysuria**—painful or difficult urination.

**Eunuchoid features**—physical traits resembling those of a castrated male (due to a deficiency of testosterone), including broad hips, disproportionately long limbs, greater than normal height, lack of facial hair, and poor muscle development.

**Glycosuria**—glucose (sugar) in the urine.

**Grey Turner's sign**—bruising of the skin on the retroperitoneal area, flanks, or upper abdominal quadrants resulting from infiltration of blood into the extraperitoneal tissue. It may be associated with renal trauma.

**Hematuria**—red blood cells in the urine.

**Hemoglobinuria**—hemoglobin in the urine.

**Hypersthenuria**—urine with a specific gravity higher than 1.010 (greater than the specific gravity of plasma filtrate).

**Hyposthenuria**—urine with a specific gravity lower than 1.010 (less than the specific gravity of plasma filtrate).

**Ileus**—intestinal obstruction.

**Inspection**—a technique used in physical examination that involves visually scrutinizing the body to look for relevant details.

**Isosthenuria**—urine with a specific gravity of 1.010 (equal to the plasma filtrate).

**Ketonuria**—ketones (metabolic end products of fat and protein metabolism) in the urine.

**Myoglobinuria**—myoglobin (protein normally found in muscle tissue) in the urine.

**Nocturia**—awakening at night to urinate. Nocturia is considered a disturbance in voiding if it occurs two or more times a night.

**Nycturia**—excreting larger volumes of urine at night than during the day.

**Observation**—a technique used in assessment of the patient that refers to the process of gathering information by using one or more of the senses.

**Oliguria**—total urine output of between 100 and 400 mL/24 hours.

**Palpation**—a technique used in physical examination that involves using touch (the hands and fingers) to feel the physical characteristics of the patient.

**Percussion**—a technique used in physical examination that involves tapping the body surface lightly in a quick, sharp manner to produce a sound.

**Phosphaturia**—phosphate crystals in the urine.

**Pneumaturia**—the excretion of urine containing air or gas.

**Polydipsia**—an excessive thirst persisting for long periods.

**Polyuria**—urinating more than 2000 mL/24 hours.

**Prehn's sign**—a physical assessment finding used to differentiate epididymitis from testicular torsion. When the scrotum is lifted up toward the symphysis, pain due to epididymitis is relieved, but pain due to torsion is worsened.

**Proteinuria**—protein in the urine.

**Pyuria**—white blood cells in the urine.

**Strangury**—frequent, painful urination in small amounts, accompanied by spasms.

**Tenesmus**—ineffectual attempts to urinate accompanied by painful straining.

**Uremia**—a toxic condition that results from severe renal damage, characterized by such signs and symptoms as nausea, vomiting, headache, malaise, pruritus, changes in level of orientation and consciousness, azotemia, and fluid and electrolyte imbalances.

**Urinary incontinence**—the involuntary loss of urine.

**Urinary retention**—an inability to empty the bladder completely when voiding.

## HEALTH HISTORY

The health history is an organized body of historical information provided by the patient describing his or her current state of health. The overall purpose of the health history is to gather data needed to understand the patient's illness and state of health and to formulate the nursing diagnoses. Other purposes include the following:

1. To establish a professional relationship with the patient.
2. To serve as a guide in structuring the physical examination.
3. To help the patient gain insight into his or her own health status by asking questions that suggest relationships that may have been overlooked.
4. To make nursing observations concerning the patient's verbal and nonverbal communication, physical condition, and emotional and behavioral states.

The importance of the health history cannot be stressed enough—it can provide more than 80% of the data gathered in assessment (Ford, 1985).

Skills needed to interview properly and to communicate include knowing how and when to ask the right questions, listening attentively, observing the patient closely, and interpreting the responses objectively and accurately. Taking a urologic history especially requires good communication skills, because many patients are reluctant to discuss genitourinary problems. Because of societal taboos, embarrassment, fear, or anxiety, they may have difficulty talking about genital, sexual, or urinary elimination problems. Another block to communication is the variety of words that exist to describe urinary or sexual functions. Use language the patient understands, avoid medical terminology the patient does not understand, and ask the patient for further explanation if vernacular is used that is unfamiliar.

Begin the interview with broad opening statements or a general question that lets the patient respond in his or her own manner. Examples are "What happened that made you come to the hospital?" and "Tell me about your problem." Follow the patient's lead as much as possible. Encourage the patient to provide details of the history.

It is sometimes necessary to ask direct questions to explore the history. These questions should include information about the onset, duration, and character of any problems. Examples of direct questions to investigate a problem include the following:

1. When did you first notice the problem?
2. How long does the problem last? (Determine if the problem is constant or intermittent and, if it is intermittent, how frequently it occurs and how long it lasts.)
3. Did the problem start gradually or suddenly?
4. What activities were you doing just before the problem started?
5. How does the problem look? smell? feel?
6. Where is the problem located?
7. Does the problem limit your daily activities? If yes, to what extent?
8. What makes the problem(s) worse? better?

Direct questioning is best accomplished and provides the most useful information when certain rules are followed (Bates, 1991), as listed in the following:

1. Begin by asking general questions, and proceed to more specific questions. Using the example of a patient in pain with a kidney stone, first ask for a description of pain— "How does it feel?" Then ask for more specific details—"Please point to where the pain starts"; "Does it stay there or move anywhere else?"
2. Do not ask leading questions, such as "Are you hurting in your back?" It is better to ask, "Where is your pain?" Leading questions limit or bias the information obtained from the patient.
3. Ask questions that require a descriptive response rather than a yes or no answer. For example, "How many times a day do you urinate?" is better than "Do you urinate frequently?" Only limited information can be gathered by yes or no questions.
4. Some patients need more guidance to describe their symptoms. Ask multiple-choice questions to decrease bias. For example, "Do you routinely have a bowel movement every day? every other day? twice a day? something else?"
5. Ask only one question at a time. Let the patient respond to a question before going on to the next one. Asking "Have you ever had pain, burning, frequency, or bleeding with urination?" may be too overwhelming or confusing for the patient to give an accurate response.

At the end of the interview, summarize the information, and say again how the information will be used. Ask the patient if there is anything more he or she wants to discuss. Thank the patient for allowing time and being cooperative, and if appropriate, explain what is expected to happen next.

## Urologic Aspects of the Health History

Following an orderly format when taking a health history ensures that all the significant aspects are covered. The format should be modified to meet the assessment needs of the individual patient, depending on the medical diagnosis, the chief complaint, the physical condition, and the mental and emotional status.

### BACKGROUND INFORMATION

Record the biographic data, such as the patient's name, birth date, marital status, sex, and home address. This information, coupled with the chief complaint and medical diagnosis, provides direction for the rest of the history. Biographic data also include statistical information concerning incidence of disease. Some urologic diseases are more common in certain age groups. For example, prostatic hyperplasia is more common in men older than 45 years of age, and older men should be assessed in more detail concerning changes in voiding pattern. In some instances, incidence of urologic disease is related to sex and race. For example, blacks have a higher incidence of sickle cell disease, which is a cause of priapism. During the physical examination, knowing the patient's age can influence what is viewed as normal versus abnormal. Dry skin, brittle and sparse hair, and pale color may have more clinical significance when observed in a 30-year-old patient with renal failure than in an 80-year-old patient with a kidney stone.

### CHIEF COMPLAINT OR CONCERN

The *chief complaint* is the patient's statement of the reason for consulting a nurse or physician. It usually consists of a quote by the patient regarding the signs or symptoms of a health problem. Generally, the medical diagnosis is not considered a chief complaint. An example of a chief complaint is "I have blood in my urine," whereas the statement "I have bladder cancer" is more a statement of medical diagnosis. However, the medical diagnosis can be used as a chief complaint in the patient who

is examined because of incidental findings on a previous examination. This patient may be asymptomatic and may be seeking health care only because the physician informed him or her of a suspected health problem.

### HISTORY OF THE PRESENT ILLNESS

The next step of the health history is to seek details of the chief complaint. Regardless of the chief complaint, it is standard practice to ask about the most common urologic signs and symptoms—changes in voiding pattern or urine characteristics, systemic manifestations, gastrointestinal (GI) symptoms, and pain.

#### Changes or Disturbances in Voiding

Adults normally void painlessly four to six times a day (about every 3–4 hours). Total daily urine output is usually between 800 and 1800 mL/day, or approximately two thirds of the total fluid intake. People usually void more urine during the day than at night, and the normal bladder capacity is about 400 mL. A change in the voiding pattern is one of the most common reasons patients consult a urologist.

#### Changes in Urine Volume

*Change in urine volume* refers to changes in total daily urine output or in the day-night voiding pattern.

*Anuria,* a total urine output less than 100 mL/day, and *oliguria,* a total urine output between 100 and 400 mL/day, are associated with the following:

1. Prerenal acute renal failure—dehydration, vascular collapse due to septic shock, reduced cardiac output.
2. Vascular renal failure—renal artery embolus, dissecting arterial aneurysms, malignant hypertension.
3. Intrarenal acute renal failure—glomerulonephritis, acute interstitial nephritis, toxic nephritis, acute tubular or cortical necrosis.
4. Postrenal acute renal failure—obstructing renal stone in patients with a solitary kidney, bilateral ureteral obstruction, bladder outlet or urethral obstruction.
5. Chronic renal failure—oliguria may or may not occur, depending on the severity and type of renal disease.

*Polyuria* refers to urinating abnormally large volumes of urine during the entire day. The patient may complain of urinating more frequently and arising at night to urinate because of the larger urine output. Conditions associated with polyuria include the following:

1. Diabetes mellitus.
2. Diabetes insipidus.
3. Psychogenic polydipsia.
4. Chronic renal disease (decreased ability to concentrate urine and reabsorb sodium).
5. Adrenal insufficiency.
6. Diuretic medication.
7. Administration of osmotic diuretics—mannitol, radiographic contrast media, high-protein tube feeding.
8. Ingestion of fluids containing caffeine or alcohol.

*Nycturia* refers to the excretion of larger volumes of urine at night than during the day. To differentiate nycturia from nocturia, ask the patient how much is voided at one time and how many times he or she gets up at night to void. The patient may experience both conditions. Nycturia occurs in older patients who experience dependent edema during the day. At night, the fluid is mobilized and excreted. People who force fluids, drink fluids containing caffeine or alcohol, or take diuretic medications near bedtime may have nycturia.

## Irritative Voiding Symptoms

Irritative voiding symptoms are most often associated with infection, inflammation, or obstruction in the lower urinary tract (bladder, prostate, and urethra). They denote a change in the bladder's ability to fill and store urine but also result when the bladder cannot empty completely.

*Urinary frequency* is urinating more than six times per day or more often than every 3 hours, usually in decreased amounts. Frequency may be the result of a loss of elasticity such that the bladder cannot accommodate or "stretch" to hold normal amounts of urine. Obstruction in the lower urinary tract can cause an overstretching and decompensation of the bladder that results in the inability to empty the bladder completely. The patient has a large amount of residual urine and experiences frequency, because only a portion of the stored urine is voided. The residual urine may also be a source of infection, which could contribute to increased frequency. Extremes of urine pH can cause frequency by irritating the bladder. Nervous tension or anxiety may cause periodic urinary frequency. An extrinsic mass pressing on

the bladder, such as a pelvic tumor and severe constipation, also causes frequency.

*Urgency* is a sudden, strong desire to void. Sometimes the feeling is so acute that it is uncontrollable, causing involuntary urination. The causes of urgency are the same as those for frequency.

*Nocturia* is the number of times a patient awakens during the night to urinate. Nocturia is considered a disturbance in voiding if it occurs two or more times nightly. It is related to the causes of urinary frequency, except that the frequency occurs at night.

Conditions associated with frequency, urgency, and nocturia include the following:

1. Lower urinary tract infection or inflammation of the bladder, prostate, or urethra.
2. Bladder or urethral tumors.
3. Neurogenic bladder disease.
4. Benign prostatic hyperplasia.
5. Bladder outlet or urethral obstruction.
6. Psychogenic disorders—acute spastic bladder reaction related to stress.
7. Foreign body in the lower urinary tract.
8. Fibrotic diseases of the bladder—tuberculosis, interstitial cystitis, schistosomiasis.
9. Radiation therapy or chemotherapy affecting the lower urinary tract.
10. Pregnancy.

*Dysuria*, painful or difficult urination, can manifest in different ways. The patient may complain of a burning sensation at the start of, during, or at the end of urination. The burning may be mild to severe, and it may be located in the distal urethra in men and along the entire urethra in women. It is most often associated with lower urinary tract infection but may be seen with other conditions that cause irritation or inflammation of the bladder or urethra. *Strangury* refers to frequent, painful urination in small amounts, accompanied by spasms. *Tenesmus* refers to ineffectual attempts to void accompanied by painful straining. Strangury and tenesmus are most often associated with severe cases of acute bladder or prostate infection.

## Obstructive Voiding Symptoms

Obstructive voiding symptoms generally denote an inability of the bladder to empty completely. They are related to a lower urinary tract dysfunction causing a blockage of urinary flow and are more commonly found in men.

*Hesitancy* occurs when there is a longer period needed to start urinating voluntarily.

*Straining* refers to the need for an increase in intra-abdominal pressure to start urinating voluntarily. Typically, the patient first notices hesitancy and, as the degree of blockage increases, needs to strain to urinate.

*A sense of residual urine* describes a feeling of incomplete emptying—the patient feels that there is urine still in the bladder right after urination is completed. The patient with this symptom may report double voiding, that is, a repeat trip to the bathroom to urinate again shortly after an initial urination to attempt to empty the bladder.

*Urinary retention* may be of two types. *Acute urinary retention* refers to a sudden inability to void, characterized by increasingly severe suprapubic pain, extreme urgency, and dribbling. *Chronic urinary retention* refers to a long-term residual urine with little pain but accompanying voiding symptoms of hesitancy, straining, and decreased force and caliber of the urinary stream. In more severe cases of chronic urinary retention, there may be significantly more than 1000 mL of urine in the bladder and constant dribbling of urine.

Ask the patient to describe the urinary stream. A normal stream is strong and steady with no dribbling. A *loss of force* and *decrease in size* of stream (force and caliber) describe a urinary stream that is thin (small in diameter), weakened, and slow. *Terminal dribbling* refers to an involuntary dripping or dribbling of urine after the patient has finished urinating. *Interruption of the urinary stream* is a sudden stopping of the stream that can be accompanied by severe pain radiating down the urethra. This symptom suggests the presence of a bladder stone that suddenly blocks the bladder neck during urination. *Bifurcation* or *spraying of the urinary stream* refers to more than one stream or a sprayed stream coming from the urinary meatus, which is most commonly a symptom of a urethral stricture.

Conditions associated with obstructive voiding symptoms include the following:

1. Mechanical obstruction in the lower urinary tract—benign prostatic hyperplasia, cancer of the prostate, urethral stricture.
2. Neurogenic bladder disease.
3. Psychogenic disorders—intermittent periurethral muscle spasm in women, psychogenic urinary retention.
4. Postoperative or postpartum urinary retention.
5. Side effects of medications.

## Urinary Incontinence

Urinary incontinence is an involuntary loss of urine in sufficient amounts or frequency to constitute a social or health problem. If the patient reports incontinence, investigate the problem by including the following questions:

1. Are you able to feel when the bladder is full?
2. Are you aware of losing urine at the time it happens?
3. Do you feel a pressure in the bladder after urinating, a feeling that you did not empty completely?
4. Do you lose urine in large amounts or small amounts?
5. How often does urine leak? Document if it is constant or how many times a day or week, if it is intermittent.
6. Is urinary incontinence a new or a long-standing problem?
7. How do you control urine leakage? Document how many pads or diapers the patient uses a day and how saturated they are, or if the male patient wears a condom catheter or penile clamp.
8. What kind of activity are you doing when the urine leaks? Document if the incontinence is related to physical activity or occurs regardless of activity. Record if the patient is incontinent during sleep or during the daytime or both.

There are several patterns of incontinence, and the patient may exhibit more than one type. An accurate description of the pattern of incontinence is necessary, because nursing interventions differ according to the assessment findings.

*Total incontinence* is characterized by constant dribbling from the bladder. In some instances, the bladder is unable to store urine, but in other instances, the patient is able to store urine in the bladder and void, yet is constantly wet. In the case of the woman with an ectopic ureter or a ureterovaginal fistula, the affected ureter causes a constant dripping, but the unaffected ureter delivers urine to the bladder to be stored and then voided. Conditions that can cause total incontinence include the following:

1. Ectopic ureteral orifice distal to the bladder neck in women.
2. Vesicovaginal or ureterovaginal fistulas from gynecologic surgery or difficult childbirth.
3. Damage to the urethral and bladder neck

sphincters from surgery, trauma, or child-birth.
4. Neurogenic bladder disease.

*Overflow (paradoxic) incontinence* is character-ized by constant dribbling of urine from the urethra. This condition occurs in chronic uri-nary retention, when the bladder has decom-pensated. The bladder stores a fixed amount of urine and cannot empty. Urine entering the bladder over the fixed amount overcomes the resistance pressure of the urinary sphincters, and urine dribbles continuously. Overflow in-continence can occur with lower urinary tract obstructions and neurogenic bladder disease.

*Urge incontinence* is characterized by a sud-den, severe urgency that results in involuntary urination. This state is most commonly associ-ated with severe inflammation or infection of the bladder, often caused by tumors, stones, diverticula, or outlet obstruction. It may also result from nervous tension or anxiety or from neurogenic bladder disease.

*Stress incontinence* is characterized by an in-voluntary loss of urine associated with an in-creased intra-abdominal pressure, such as oc-curs with laughing, coughing, and sneezing. Stress incontinence is most commonly seen with relaxation of the pelvic floor muscles due to childbirth or aging but can be noted in younger nulliparous women. It can also occur after prostate surgery or with neurogenic blad-der disease.

*Functional incontinence* is characterized by a loss of urine control in socially unacceptable situations. The patient voluntarily voids, but at an inappropriate time and place. In most in-stances, the patient fails to recognize the warn-ing signals of a full bladder. Conditions in which functional incontinence may occur in-clude the following:

1. Higher brain level disorders in which neu-rologic impulses fail to be interpreted—Alz-heimer's disease, confused states, closed-head injuries, mental retardation, emotional illness (depression), dementia.
2. Attention-seeking behavior.
3. Physical disability—inability to get to the bathroom, inability to loosen clothing to ur-inate.
4. Environmental factors—lack of clearly marked bathroom, inability to get to the bathroom because of restraints.

(For more detailed information regarding as-sessment of the patient with urinary inconti-nence, refer to Chap. 14.)

## Changes in Urine Characteristics

When assessing changes in urine character-istics, ask the patient to describe the urine color, clarity, and odor.

Changes in urine color can be a result of blood in the urine, ingestion of certain drugs or food, altered hydration states, or certain dis-ease processes (Table 2–1). Red urine does not necessarily indicate blood in the urine. Investi-gate complaints of changes in urine color by asking direct questions, such as when it was first noticed, how long it lasted, if and when it recurred, and if there are any associated symp-toms.

Hematuria, red blood cells in the urine, is a symptom that should never be ignored because it can indicate serious disease. Hematuria can make urine appear shades of pink or red, tea colored, dark brown, or maroon (Table 2–2). Blood clots may or may not be present, and the degree of bleeding is not always an indication of the severity of the disease. Ask the male patient to describe at which point in the uri-nary stream the blood appears. Initial hematu-ria, when the blood appears only at the start of the stream, indicates bleeding from the anterior urethra. Terminal hematuria, in which the blood is noted only at the end of the stream, indicates bleeding from the posterior urethra or bladder neck. Total hematuria, in which the entire stream appears bloody, indicates that the bleeding originates from somewhere above the bladder neck. In female patients, obtain a his-tory of the menstrual pattern to rule out he-maturia due to menstrual contamination. Other causes of hematuria are listed in Table 2–3.

Cloudy urine may be associated with infec-tion or inflammation in the urinary tract but does not necessarily indicate pyuria (white blood cells in the urine). Refer to the section on urinalysis in this chapter for causes of cloudy urine.

Abnormal urine odors can be caused by in-fection or the ingestion of certain drugs or foods. *Pungent, foul, sweet,* and *ammoniacal* are terms often used to describe different odors.

*Pneumaturia* is the passage of air along with urine while voiding. It is usually caused by a fistula between the bowel and bladder due to diverticulosis or cancer of the bowel. An un-common cause is a gas-forming infection in the urinary tract.

## Systemic Manifestations

Fever usually indicates infection somewhere in the urinary tract but does not occur in all

TABLE 2–1. Causes of Urine Color Change

| COLOR | MEDICATION OR DIET | OTHER CAUSES |
|---|---|---|
| Colorless or pale yellow | Diuretics<br>Alcohol | Dilute urine due to diabetes insipidus, diabetes mellitus, overhydration, chronic renal disease, nervousness |
| Bright yellow | Riboflavin (multiple vitamins) | None |
| Dark amber to orange | Phenazopyridine HCl (Pyridium, Azo Gantanol, Azo Gantrisin)<br>Nitrofurantoin (Macrodantin)<br>Sulfasalazine (Azulfidine)<br>Docusate calcium; phenolphthalein (Doxidan) (in alkaline urine)<br>Thiamine (multiple vitamins)<br>Excessive carotene (e.g., carrots) | Concentrated urine due to dehydration or increased metabolic state<br>Urobilinogen<br>Bilirubin |
| Pink to red | Phenothiazines<br>Phenolphthalein (laxatives) (in alkaline urine)<br>Phenytoin (Dilantin)<br>Rifampin<br>Phenolsulfonphthalein (PSP) dye (in alkaline urine)<br>Cascara (in alkaline urine)<br>Senna (X-Prep, Senokot)<br>Beets<br>Blackberries<br>Rhubarb (in alkaline urine) | Hemoglobin<br>Porphyrin<br>Red blood cells<br>Myoglobin<br>Menstrual contamination |
| Brown | Cascara (in acid urine)<br>Metronidazole (Flagyl) (if left standing) | Extremely concentrated urine due to dehydration or increased metabolic state<br>Urobilinogen<br>Porphyrin<br>Bilirubin<br>Red blood cells |
| Blue or green | Triamterene (Dyrenium)<br>Amitriptyline (Elavil)<br>Phenylsalicylate<br>Methylene blue<br>Indigo carmine<br>Vitamin B complex | Bilirubin-biliverdin<br>*Pseudomonas* infection |
| Dark brown to black | Nitrofurantoin (Macrodantin)<br>Iron preparations (if left standing)<br>  Levodopa (if left standing)<br>  Methocarbamol (if left standing)<br>Phenacetin<br>Quinine<br>Cascara (in acid urine)<br>Senna (X-Prep, Senokot)<br>Methyldopa (Aldomet) | Melanin<br>Porphyrin<br>Red blood cells (old blood)<br>Homogentisic acid in alkaptonuria |

cases. Uncomplicated bladder infection and chronic pyelonephritis usually do not cause fever. Fever seen with acute pyelonephritis, prostatitis, or epididymitis may reach 104°F. Fever may also be seen with patients who have renal cell carcinoma or acquired immunodeficiency syndrome (AIDS).

Weight loss may be seen with renal insufficiency, AIDS, or advanced stages of cancer. Malaise may accompany cancer, renal failure, chronic pyelonephritis, or AIDS. Generalized massive edema occurs in patients with nephrotic syndrome. Generalized lymphadenopathy is a feature of AIDS.

## Gastrointestinal Symptoms

GI symptoms may accompany upper urinary tract disorders, such as acute or chronic pyelonephritis, acute or chronic hydronephrosis, staghorn or other obstructing calculi, and cancer. The most frequent complaints are nausea, vomiting, anorexia, diarrhea, and abdominal cramps and distention. In some instances, the GI symptoms may be the only complaint, and these symptoms mimic symptoms of GI diseases such as appendicitis, cholecystitis, and peptic ulcer disease, which leads to some confusion in diagnosis.

**TABLE 2–2. Shades of Red in Urine**

The tendency to describe blood in the urine as "bloody urine" causes concern among clinicians, because it does not accurately communicate the state of the urinary drainage containing varying amounts of blood. The term *bloody urine* should be avoided and a more accurate description rendered so that the clinician can evaluate the situation on the basis of the verbal report. It must be remembered that one drop of blood in a quart of urine is "bloody" urine. Therefore, beginning with the minor states to the major state of blood in the urine, the following descriptions can be made.

| SIGNIFICANCE | DESCRIPTION |
|---|---|
| Minimal clinical | Cranberry-colored urine<br>Rosé wine–colored urine<br>Pale pink urine<br>Light strawberry or Kool Aid–colored urine |
| Minimal to moderate | Cherry red<br>Port wine–colored urine<br>Watermelon-colored urine<br>Coca Cola–colored urine<br>Deep cranberry–colored urine |
| Moderate to severe with unformed clots | Tomato soup–colored urine<br>Port wine–colored urine<br>Tomato paste–type urine<br>Muddy red–colored urine |
| Severe to critical with formed or unformed clots | Thick, ropy, bright red–colored urine |

There are many variations in the types of colors that can be reported, but the description should be of common knowledge to the one who is communicating and the one who is receiving the communication, so that the status of the bleeding process in the urinary tract is understood. When the blood in the urine becomes stagnant, it becomes darker because of oxidation, resulting from deoxygenation; therefore, the darker colors tend to indicate older blood. The brighter and thicker reddish colors result from oxygenation and tend to indicate some degree of active bleeding. The thin reddish colors indicate that blood cells are being actively burst open and the pigment is escaping, coloring the urine. Many times there are clots in the bladder that can color the urine even though there is no active bleeding at the time. The residual clots can cause varying colors in the urine, but usually the darker red colors predominate. The most ominous sign is thick, bright red urine with ill-formed or malformed clots. The more organized clots tend to indicate older or slower bleeding.

Courtesy of Leslie Becker, MD.

GI symptoms occur with urologic disorders for the following reasons (Smith, 1992):

1. The urinary tract and the GI tract have common autonomic and sensory innervations. Afferent stimuli from the renal capsule or smooth muscles of the renal pelvis may cause changes in the smooth muscles of the GI tract by reflex action.
2. The kidneys lie in close proximity to the organs of the GI tract. Inflammation or tumor of the upper urinary tract can extend into the organs of the GI tract. Masses in the upper tract can also displace organs in the GI tract.
3. The peritoneum covers the anterior surfaces of both kidneys. Inflammation of the kidney causes peritoneal inflammation, characterized by involuntary muscle rigidity and rebound tenderness.

In some instances, GI symptoms may be caused by different mechanisms. Extravasation of urine into the abdomen or retroperitoneum can cause chemical irritation of the peritoneum.

An elevated blood urea nitrogen (BUN) level can cause anorexia and nausea.

## Pain

Urologic pain is usually due to distention of one or more parts of the urinary tract. The distention may be caused by inflammation and edema of tissue or by obstruction of urine flow and hydrostatic back pressure on different structures of the urinary tract. The severity of pain is usually a result of the sudden onset rather than the degree of distention.

Determining the presence and severity of pain provides important subjective data. One way to document the severity of pain as accurately as possible is to ask the patient to describe the pain using a scale of 0 to 10, where "0" is the least amount of pain and "10" is the most severe pain.

The different types of renal pain relating to distention can be illustrated using a 0-to-10 pain scale. The patient with a nonfunctioning kidney destroyed by progressive obstruction

## TABLE 2–3. Causes of Hematuria

| RENAL DISORDERS | BLEEDING WITHIN THE URINARY TRACT | SYSTEMIC DISEASE | EXTRAURINARY PATHOLOGIC CHANGES |
|---|---|---|---|
| Glomerulonephritis | Infection and inflammation | Connective tissue disorders | Appendicitis |
| Cancer | Calculus | Systemic lupus erythematosus | Diverticulitis |
| Calculus | Cancer | Acute infections | Tumor of colon, rectum, |
| Infection | Stricture | Scarlet fever | pelvic organs |
| Polycystic disease | Varicose veins | Rheumatic fever | Salpingitis |
| Renal cyst | Prostatic hyperplasia | Subacute bacterial endocarditis | |
| Infarction | Radiation changes | Chronic infection | |
| Hydronephrosis | Cyclophosphamide | Malaria | |
| Renal vein thrombosis | | Tuberculosis | |
| Trauma | | Schistosomiasis | |
| Papillary necrosis | | Hematologic disorders | |
| | | Hemophilia | |
| | | Coagulopathies | |
| | | Sickle cell trait or disease | |
| | | Thrombocytopenic purpura | |
| | | Polycythemia vera | |
| | | Leukemia | |
| | | Dietary deficiency and diseases | |
| | | Drug-induced renal diseases | |
| | | Methicillin | |
| | | Sulfonamides | |
| | | Cantharides | |
| | | Anticoagulants | |
| | | Salicylates | |
| | | Methenamine preparations | |
| | | Hypertension | |
| | | Arteriosclerosis | |

may deny having any pain. At the other end of the scale, the patient with a kidney stone that suddenly obstructs the renal pelvis and causes a mild distention may complain of severe pain (colic), which is 10 on the pain scale. Typical renal pain, a dull, constant pain such as that caused by acute pyelonephritis, which produces sudden edema and distention in the renal capsule, is often described in the middle of the pain scale. These examples show that extensive disease with serious renal damage can occur in the absence of pain.

It is helpful to have the patient point to the location of the pain. The costovertebral angle (CVA) is the point of the back that corresponds to the junction of the 12th rib and the lateral border of the sacrospinal muscle. The iliocostal space is the area between the last rib and the iliac crest on the flank and back. Pain or tenderness in either of these regions suggests a renal or upper ureteral origin.

Two types of pain originate from the genitourinary system: local and referred pain. Local pain is that felt in or around the affected organ. An example is suprapubic discomfort associated with bladder infections. Referred pain originates from the involved organ but is felt at some place other than that organ. Pain asso-ciated with a ureteral stone that is felt in the testis, scrotum, or labia is an example of referred pain. Patients experience referred pain because the genitourinary organs have common sensory nerve supplies with other body organs and structures (Fig. 2–1).

Renal and ureteral colic is one of the most severe types of pain experienced by humans. A frequent cause is when a stone, blood clot, or tissue blocks the urine flow. The ureter and the renal pelvis above the blockage distend from retained urine. This event initiates violent hyperperistalsis and spasms in the smooth muscle, which are an attempt by the kidney to expel the urine past the blockage. Typically, this pain begins suddenly with no apparent reason for the onset. The pain progresses rapidly and in about 30 minutes reaches a plateau. Colic is a continuous or spasmodic, severe, sharp, stabbing pain that can be unbearable. A change in position does not affect renal colic, and the patient is restless. The characteristics of genitourinary pain arising from other sites in the urinary tract are described in Table 2–4.

Bladder spasms are a common complaint of urologic patients. These are spasmodic contractions of bladder muscle, causing pain in the suprapubic or urethral area, that radiate down

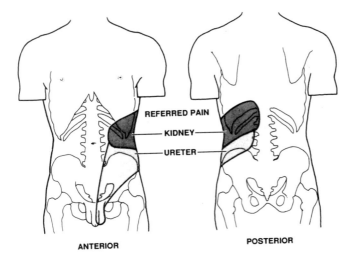

ANTERIOR                POSTERIOR

*FIGURE 2–1* Referred pain from the kidney and ureter. (From Kabalin, J. M. [1992]. Anatomy of the retroperitoneum and kidney. In Walsh, P. C., Retik, A. B., Stamey, T. A., & Vaughan, E. D., Jr. [Eds.], *Campbell's urology* [6th ed., p. 40]. Philadelphia: W. B. Saunders. Reprinted by permission.)

the penis to the meatus in men and to the vulva in women. They may be mild and infrequent or have an acute onset with frequent, sharp pains. The patient usually complains of intermittent, crampy pain or discomfort and often reports an urge to urinate; he or she may occasionally feel the urge to defecate. Bladder spasms are caused by irritation of the bladder wall and are most often caused by a foreign body in the bladder, usually a catheter. Other less common causes include acute inflammation due to severe cystitis, irritation of the bladder and urethra following surgical instrumentation, and vesical irritation due to bladder tumors. It is sometimes difficult to differentiate between the pain caused by bladder spasms and the pain caused by acute overdistention of the bladder. Both begin as spasmodic pain, but the pain from an overdistended bladder typically becomes increasingly severe and constant. Palpating and percussing the bladder and assessing the catheter for patency also provide information to determine the cause of the pain. Leakage of urine around a bladder catheter may be an unreliable indicator, because leakage can occur in patients with a patent catheter if spasms are strong. Accurate assessment is important, because pain from overdistention is relieved by draining the urine from the bladder, whereas bladder spasms are usually relieved by medication.

Pain due to metastasis of a genitourinary tumor may be the first symptom a patient notices. Unfortunately, many tumors of the genitourinary tract do not produce local symptoms and easily recognizable signs in the early stages and become clinically evident only in advanced stages. Low back pain, with radiation to the hips, back, or pelvis, is highly suggestive of metastasis from cancer of the prostate to the pelvis and lumbar spine. Renal cell carcinoma can metastasize to the vertebrae and long bones. Metastatic bladder cancer can also spread to bone. Bone pain arising from sites of metastases is chronic and often difficult to control.

## Abdominal, Flank, or Genital Mass

Patients with renal cell carcinoma, perinephric abscess, polycystic kidneys, or a large hydronephrosis occasionally discover a bulge or fullness in the abdomen or flank as an initial sign. The patient with a large and chronically overdistended bladder may detect a mass in the lower abdomen. The male patient may discover a lump or mass in the genitals during the bath or sexual activity or after trauma to the genitals, or he may find it only after feeling discomfort due to the mass. (See the section on physical examination of the male external genitalia for causes of a mass in the genital area.)

## Abnormal Abdominal or Genital Appearance

Generally, abnormalities in the external anatomy are congenital and are discovered in the pediatric patient, but in some instances the abnormalities are first discovered in the adult as a result of a lack of knowledge about normal anatomy or access to health care. Assess for congenital displacement of the urethral meatus (hypospadias or epispadias) in males and females and an empty scrotum or hemiscrotum (cryptorchidism) in males.

Ascertain for the presence of characteristics of a normal penile erection. The patient with painful curvature of the penis with erection may be exhibiting chordee, a symptom of Peyronie's disease. The condition may be severe enough to interfere with sexual intercourse. Its cause is unknown, and it generally affects middle-aged and older men.

Another condition for which the male patient should be assessed is priapism, which is a sustained, usually painful erection in the absence of sexual desire or excitement. It is a urologic emergency, requiring urgent treatment. Priapism is idiopathic in half of the cases. Other causes include sickle cell disease, leukemia, tumors, trauma, and medication.

Genital lesions may be caused by inflammation, cancerous growths, sexually transmitted diseases, or skin disorders. Ask the patient where the lesion is located and when it was first noticed. Determine if its occurrence can be related to sexual activity.

Urethral discharge is a symptom of urethritis. Ask the patient to describe the color, consistency, and amount of discharge; when the discharge was first noted; and any relation between the onset of discharge and sexual activity. It is most often caused by sexually transmitted disease.

## Sexual and Reproductive Dysfunction

The male patient must be assessed for problems of impotence, an inability to have or sustain an erection long enough for sexual intercourse. It is estimated that about half of the cases of impotence are caused by psychogenic or idiopathic factors. Organic causes of impotence include the following:

1. Vascular disorders—arteriosclerosis, priapism.
2. Surgery—radical prostatectomy or cystectomy, abdominoperineal resection, certain spinal cord or brain surgeries.
3. Neurologic disorders—multiple sclerosis, spinal cord tumors, spina bifida, cerebrovascular accident, Parkinson's or Alzheimer's disease.
4. Endocrine disorders—diabetes mellitus, pituitary tumors, Addison's disease, Cushing's syndrome, hypogonadism.
5. Trauma—spinal cord injury, pelvic fracture, urethral or genital injuries, radiation therapy to the pelvis.
6. Chronic renal failure.
7. Medications—antihypertensives, anticholinergics, phenothiazines, antidepressants, bar-

biturates, sedatives, tranquilizers, antihistamines.

(For more precise guidelines for the assessment of impotence, refer to Chap. 12.)

The male patient must also be evaluated for infertility, the inability to father children. In addition to asking the routine questions in the sexual history, ascertain the patient's understanding of conception. This includes knowing the optimal time (midcycle of the menstruation cycle) and the most effective frequency for intercourse (every 48–72 hours) and avoiding the use of lubricants that could be harmful to sperm (Corriere, 1986). Causative factors in infertility include the following:

1. History of cryptorchidism.
2. History of postpubertal mumps complicated by orchitis.
3. Exposure to pesticides.
4. Excessive heat to the gonads—hot baths or saunas, tight underwear.
5. Retroperitoneal lymph node dissection.
6. Diabetes mellitus.
7. Medications—hormones, nitrofurantoins in high doses, cancer chemotherapeutic agents, phenytoin.
8. Endocrine disorders.
9. Renal failure.
10. Scarring of the bladder neck after transurethral surgery or after Y-V bladder neck plasty for the treatment of primary bladder neck obstruction.
11. Previous vasectomy.

(For further information on the assessment of male infertility, refer to Chap. 13.)

*Hematospermia* is blood in the ejaculate. Its cause is not exactly known but may be related to inflammation or hypertrophy of the seminal vesicles or minor trauma to the seminal vesicles or prostate. It may manifest as a solitary symptom, but in the older man may be related to cancer of the prostate.

## Incidental Findings From a Previous Examination

During a routine physical examination or a diagnostic workup for another health problem, a urologic abnormality may be discovered. The patient, who should be referred to a urologist, may deny any symptoms related to urologic disease. These incidental findings include the following:

1. Suspicious nodule on the prostate found during a rectal examination.

## TABLE 2-4. Characteristics of Genitourinary Pain

| | BLADDER | URETHRAL | TESTICULAR | EPIDIDYMAL | PROSTATIC | RENAL | URETERAL |
|---|---|---|---|---|---|---|---|
| *Location* | Suprapubic area | Male: perineum, along penis to meatus<br>Female: along urethra to meatus | In testicle | In hemiscrotum | Perineum and rectum | Costovertebral angle | Costovertebral angle to flank and lower abdominal quadrant along course of ureter |
| *Radiation* | Low back, urethra, urinary meatus, penis, perineum in female | None | Along spermatic cord into lower abdomen | Groin or lower abdominal quadrant; may reach flank | Low back or testicles | Along subcostal area toward umbilicus, lower abdominal quadrant, groin, testicle | From upper ureter to groin, testis, vulva<br>From mid-ureter to right or left lower abdomen (mimics appendicitis or diverticulitis)<br>From distal ureter to suprapubic area, urethra, penis, scrotal wall |
| *Duration and Intensity* | Dull and continuous with inflammation; may be intense with voiding<br>Onset dull but increases to severe constant pain with acute urinary retention<br>Marked pain when bladder full; relieved by voiding when there is fibrosis or bladder ulceration | Varies in intensity<br>May be severe during and right after voiding | Varies from dull ache to severe pain | Mild to severe | Vague discomfort, feeling of fullness in perineum<br>Mild to moderate back pain | Dull and constant with renal capsular distention<br>Severe, sharp, stabbing colic with sudden distention of collecting system | Severe, sharp, stabbing colic |
| *Associated Symptoms* | Irritative voiding symptoms, possibly urge incontinence with acute inflammation<br>Obstructive voiding symptoms progressing to inability to void, overflow incontinence with acute urinary retention<br>Frequency, nocturia with fibrosis or ulceration of bladder | Irritative voiding symptoms<br>Urethral discharge | Nausea and vomiting with severe pain<br>Scrotal edema | Scrotal edema<br>Urethral discharge<br>Irritative voiding symptoms<br>Pain relieved when scrotum lifted onto symphysis pubis (Prehn's sign) | Pain exacerbated by sitting, riding<br>Suprapubic tenderness<br>Irritative voiding symptoms<br>Varying degrees of obstructive voiding symptoms, possibly acute urinary retention | Unaffected by position<br>Sweating, pallor, shock with colic<br>Gastrointestinal symptoms | Unaffected by position<br>Sweating, pallor, shock<br>Gastrointestinal symptoms<br>Irritative voiding symptoms from distal ureter |

| | Bladder | Urethra | Testis | Epididymis | Prostate | Kidney | Ureter |
|---|---|---|---|---|---|---|---|
| *Mechanism* | Inflammation and infection reduce elasticity of bladder wall; mild stretching of wall causes pain<br>Acute urinary retention results from functional or structural obstruction in lower urinary tract; overdistention causes pain<br>Fibrosis or ulcerations in bladder wall reduces elasticity of wall; filling bladder causes pain | Inflammation and edema in urethra | Infection or inflammation in testis<br>Ischemia in testis<br>Bleeding in testis<br>Rupture of testis | Reflux of infected urine from urethra or prostate to epididymis<br>Lymphatogenous spread of infection to epididymis<br>Sexual transmission of infection<br>Less common: inflammation of epididymis by trauma or reflux of sterile urine into epididymis | Inflammation or infection in prostate | Renal capsular distention due to inflammation or edema<br>Sudden obstruction of urine flow from kidney with distention of collecting system (hydronephrosis) | Sudden obstruction of urine flow in ureter with ureteral distention<br>Edema and inflammation of ureteral orifice with distal ureteral distention |
| *Possible Causes* | Inflammation: cystitis, instrumentation, bladder tumor<br>Acute urinary retention: prostatic hyperplasia with bladder neck obstruction, urethral stricture<br>Fibrosis or ulcerations in bladder wall: interstitial cystitis, tuberculosis | Urethritis<br>Urethral stricture<br>Foreign body in urethra<br>Urethral cancer | Orchitis<br>Torsion of spermatic cord<br>Testicular tumor | Infection or inflammation of epididymis | Acute or chronic prostatitis | Acute pyelonephritis<br>Renal cancer that bleeds into kidney<br>Renal trauma<br>Sudden obstruction due to renal stone or blood clot<br>Obstructed or malpositioned nephrostomy or urethral catheter | Sudden obstruction due to ureteral stone, blood clot, edema<br>Ureteral stricture |

2. Abnormal urinalysis—microhematuria; excessive protein, white blood cells, or casts in the urine.
3. Hypertension—a urologist may be consulted to evaluate renal vascular problems or adrenal disorders as a cause of the hypertension.
4. Mass or lesion in or near the urinary tract discovered on excretory urogram, abdominal or pelvic ultrasound, computed tomography, or magnetic resonance imaging study.
5. Elevated serum creatinine or BUN levels, signs of diminished renal blood flow or renal dysfunction.

## Past History

After investigating the patient's reason for seeking health care, ask about past surgeries, illnesses, and accidents, and obtain a list of current medications and allergies. Collecting data about previous health problems provides information about the patient's present state of health and is used to modify the treatment plan based on individualized health needs.

### HISTORY OF URINARY TRACT PROBLEMS

Many urologic problems are chronic or recurrent. Significant past urinary problems include a history of the following:

1. Urinary tract infection—Determine when any infections started, if they recurred, and how they were treated. Ascending infection from the bladder can cause pyelonephritis, which can be chronic or recurrent and may predispose the patient to renal failure or calculus formation.
2. Urinary incontinence or retention—Ask about its onset and pattern. Determine what treatment was undertaken, especially if the patient had surgical treatment or had to use a catheter.
3. Congenital anomalies—Congenital anomalies occur in the genitourinary tract more often than in any other body system. Examples are hypospadias and exstrophy of the bladder.
4. Surgery or instrumentation of the urinary tract—Surgery may cause problems from trauma or obstruction from edema if it is recent or from scarring if it is remote. Also ask if the patient has a urinary tract diver-

sion. This includes any surgery that alters the urinary tract, or the placement of any urinary catheters. If the patient has a urinary diversion, determine how he or she cares for it, including what kind of equipment is needed, what type of care is given, and how often the care is performed.

5. Urinary stones—Learn how the stone was treated, if the stone passed spontaneously, and if the patient knows the stone's composition. Urinary stones tend to recur, so ask about multiple episodes.
6. Cancer of the urinary tract—Determine what treatment the patient has undergone.
7. Renal disease—Ask about any history of chronic renal failure or insufficiency. If the patient has a history of kidney disease, determine how it was treated. One of the most important points in assessment is to find out if the patient has two functioning kidneys. The patient may have had a prior nephrectomy, for donation or renal disease, or the patient may have been informed by a physician that one kidney is nonfunctioning or congenitally absent. In the presence of a solitary functioning kidney or decreased renal function, treatment may be more conservative to preserve renal function.

### PREVIOUS SURGERIES AND ILLNESSES

A variety of surgical procedures and illnesses affect the genitourinary tract. The following are only a few examples:

1. Cancer of the cervix or prostate may involve metastases that cause urinary obstruction.
2. The patient who has had an ileostomy, colostomy, or jejunoileal bypass may be predisposed to stone formation.
3. Pelvic surgery, such as hysterectomy, can involve accidental trauma to the ureters or bladder.
4. A recent event such as surgery, anesthesia, or any condition that causes shock (e.g., hemorrhage, major trauma, or sepsis) may be a causative factor in acute renal failure.
5. A recent history of significant fluid loss, such as with prolonged fever, diarrhea, and vomiting, may affect the urine output and renal function.
6. A history of external radiation therapy to the pelvis can cause radiation cystitis, ureteral obstruction due to fibrosis, or a fistula in the urinary tract.

## HISTORY OF ACCIDENTS OR TRAUMA

Trauma to the kidney may also involve injury to the renal artery or renal veins. If the patient has a pre-existing renal disease, such as hydronephrosis, tumor, or cystic disease, even a minor trauma can cause extensive renal damage. Trauma to the kidneys results from either of the following categories:

1. *Blunt trauma* accounts for most renal injuries. It may be caused by a direct blow to the abdomen, the flank, the back, or the lower chest by a sudden deceleration, such as occurs in a fall or motor vehicle accident. These may produce contusions (bruises) in the kidney or a laceration due to a fractured rib or vertebra that penetrates renal tissue. The patient most often reports injury from a motor vehicle or an industrial accident, a fall, a fight, or a contact sport.
2. *Penetrating injury* to the kidney can cause a laceration. This type is usually the result of a gunshot or knife wound.

Trauma to the ureter is rare but can occur with pelvic surgery, endoscopic procedures, penetrating wounds, or deceleration accidents in which the ureter can be torn.

Trauma to the bladder is usually secondary to external force. It is often associated with pelvic fracture. Rupture of the bladder may occur in crushing injuries or from a direct blow to the abdomen, such as when a car driver has a full bladder and strikes the steering wheel in an accident. It may also be caused by iatrogenic injury in which the bladder is nicked or torn during surgery or transurethral procedures.

Trauma to the urethra occurs most often in men. It may be associated with pelvic fracture, straddle-type falls, crushing injuries, self-instrumentation, or iatrogenic injury from instrumentation.

For further information on genitourinary trauma, refer to Chapter 15.

## SYSTEMIC DISEASES

When the patient discusses his or her other diseases, be aware of those diseases that can cause urinary problems. The following are examples:

1. Hypertension can cause renal insufficiency, or it may be a symptom of chronic renal failure or renal artery stenosis.
2. Complications of diabetes mellitus include diabetic nephropathy (noted by hypertension, edema, and azotemia) and neurogenic bladder disease.
3. Certain collagen disorders, such as systemic lupus erythematosus, may cause nephritis.
4. Sickle cell anemia and multiple myeloma may cause chronic renal failure.
5. Many diseases predispose to stone formation, including gout, hyperparathyroidism, and Crohn's disease.
6. Cardiac failure, as with congestive heart failure or myocardial infarction, may cause acute or chronic renal failure.

## ALLERGIES

In addition to listing any allergies, document the response in any allergic reaction, because some drug allergy reactions cause a loss of renal function. Be sure to ask about allergies to shellfish, iodine, or radiographic contrast media. Imaging studies using intravascular radiographic contrast media, such as excretory urogram, are commonly performed on urologic patients. These allergies indicate that the studies are contraindicated or must be performed with precautions.

## MEDICATIONS

A list of current medications is an essential part of the health history. By reviewing the pharmacologic history, the patient can confirm or be helped to recall current illnesses. The history also provides insight into causative or contributive factors of the urologic problem and what, if any, treatment is being done currently. For example, a patient may say he takes hydrochlorothiazide but forgot to mention earlier in the interview that he has high blood pressure (BP). Also, always ask why the patient is taking the medication. In this example, hydrochlorothiazide may have been prescribed to prevent calcium stone formation instead of to treat hypertension.

Urologic problems that may be produced by medication include the following:

1. Urinary stone disease—vitamins C and D excess, acetazolamide, chemotherapeutic agents, aspirin, furosemide, mineral supplements.
2. Interstitial nephritis—penicillins, colistin, sulfonamides, phenytoin.
3. Renal papillary necrosis—long-term use of nonsteroidal analgesic and anti-inflammatory drugs.
4. Urinary incontinence—sedative-hypnotics (diazepam), diuretics (furosemide).

5. Urinary retention—anticholinergics (oxybutynin, methantheline), antispasmodics (belladonna and opium suppositories), imipramine, phenothiazines, antihistamines containing phenylpropanolamine or pseudoephedrine.
6. Nephrotoxicity—aminoglycosides (tobramycin, gentamicin, amikacin), cephalosporins, cisplatin, amphotericin B, iodine-containing radiographic contrast media.

Renal implications of drugs should always be assessed. In patients with compromised renal status or decreased renal reserve, such as the elderly, some drugs are contraindicated, whereas others must be given in reduced doses with careful monitoring of the renal function.

Remember to ask about over-the-counter drug use as well. Abuse of drugs such as aspirin, acetaminophen, and laxatives can cause or contribute to renal disease.

## FAMILY HISTORY

Inheritable disorders include polycystic kidneys, familial cystinuria, sickle cell disease, hypertension, and diabetes mellitus. Some other diseases affecting the urinary tract are not inherited but tend to recur in some families. These include urinary stones, urinary tract infections, testicular and prostate cancer, and some congenital anomalies of the urinary tract.

## PSYCHOSOCIAL HISTORY

The psychosocial history examines aspects of personal lifestyle. Ask the patient about his or her occupation and work environment. Is there any exposure to hazardous chemicals or solvents or radiation that could affect fertility? Aniline dyes, known to be bladder cancer carcinogens, are used in the rubber industry and by car mechanics and hairdressers. How does the work environment influence hydration and toileting habits? Some people with limited access to bathroom facilities and water or those with a hectic work schedule develop poor drinking habits (exposing themselves to dehydration) and poor toileting habits (infrequent voiding, which can lead to loss of bladder tone).

Assess the patient's hygiene practices. Too frequent douches and bubble baths may contribute to urinary tract infections in women. Poor personal hygiene can contribute to skin irritations and infections.

Determine the patient's self-image in re-

sponse to illness. Many urologic surgical procedures and chronic diseases alter body image. Has the patient accepted and adapted to bodily changes? Is the patient motivated to be independent in daily activities? What are the expectations for the future? Does the patient feel that he or she receives positive support from family and friends? Has the patient sought support from outside resources?

## SEXUAL HISTORY

A sexual history is obtained as a routine part of the assessment process. Basic screening includes questions about sexual functioning and attempts to identify any sexual concerns or problems. More specific questions must be asked if the diagnosis relates to a sexual problem, such as impotence, infertility, or sexually transmitted disease.

Begin by asking an open-ended question, such as "Tell me about your current sexual activity." If the patient is not sexually active, ask about past sexual experiences and focus on how the patient is meeting his or her sexual needs currently. Determine if the patient is celibate, heterosexual, gay or lesbian, or bisexual. Find out if the patient has one partner or has had several sexual partners in the last year. This necessitates tactfully asking direct questions, in which case a professional, nonjudgmental attitude and good communication skills are essential.

After determining the patient's sexual pattern, ask questions to identify any sexual problems, such as the following:

1. Are you satisfied with your current sexual activity? Is there anything you would like to change?
2. Do you ever have problems getting sexually aroused?
3. Do you have problems achieving or maintaining an erection? If the male has impotence, determine the course or the pattern of impotence and how long it has existed.
4. Have you ever had sexually transmitted disease? How was it treated? For women, any history of vaginal infections or vaginal discharge? For men, any history of urethral discharge?
5. Do you ever experience pain associated with sexual activity? If yes, ask the patient to describe the pain. The patient with Peyronie's disease often complains of penile pain with erections.

Next, ask about the reproductive history. For

women, this includes questions to determine the following:

1. Menstrual history—age of menarche, last menstrual period, regularity of menstruation, pattern of menstrual flow, length of each menstrual period, discomfort or other symptoms associated with menstruation, age of menopause. If the patient is postmenopausal, determine if it was natural or surgically induced and if she takes any hormone replacement.
2. Type of birth control used, if any.
3. Number of pregnancies, live births, abortions, and any complications with pregnancy or delivery—If the patient is premenopausal, ask if she is pregnant or if there is any chance she is pregnant. Always determine this before any radiologic studies or drug administration, to protect the fetus. Pregnancy also has many effects on the urinary tract; renal size increases, and the glomerular filtration rate (GFR) increases. Pregnant women also have an increased risk for pyelonephritis and urinary stones.

For the male reproductive history, ask about the following:

1. Type of birth control used, if any.
2. Number of children he has fathered, if any—If the patient's chief complaint is infertility, ask about this in more detail. What are the ages of the children? Did he father the children with a previous sexual partner? How long have the patient and his current partner been trying to achieve pregnancy?
3. Knowledge and practice of testicular self-examination—If the patient if not informed, schedule a time after the assessment to instruct the patient.

## ACTIVITIES OF DAILY LIVING

Ask the patient if he or she is on a special diet. Prolonged weight-reducing diets with high-protein intake are associated with renal failure. Special renal diets may include restrictions on sodium, potassium, or protein. If the patient has a history of hypertension, ask about salt intake and any use of salt substitutes. Diets that may influence stone formation include those high in calcium (dairy products and milk), purine (meats, fish, and poultry), and oxalate (tea, chocolate, and nuts). Certain foods, such as spicy foods and caffeine, act as bladder irritants in some patients who present with changes in voiding patterns.

Determine how much fluid the patient drinks during an average day. Patients with renal or cardiac disease may need limited fluid intake, whereas patients with urinary stones should have a high fluid intake.

What are the patient's sleep and exercise patterns? Sleep disturbances, such as a reversal of night-day sleep patterns and waking up at night because of muscle cramps in the legs, may be signs of renal failure. Sleep disturbance may also be caused by nocturia. Patients with limited activity or mobility problems are at a higher risk for urinary stasis, retention, or incontinence. If the patient does heavy physical exercise, ask if he or she drinks extra fluids to prevent dehydration.

Obtain a history of the use of tobacco, alcohol, and street drugs. Cigarette smoking has a known association with cancer of the bladder and kidney. Use of marijuana and caffeine contributes to infertility. Alcohol acts as a bladder irritant and may increase voiding problems, and it also contributes to infertility and impotence.

## PHYSICAL EXAMINATION

Physical examination forms the second part of the data base in the patient's assessment. Because information collected during the health history serves as a guide in structuring the physical assessment, the examination should be performed after the health history. The purpose of the physical examination is to detect variations from the normal state by using all the bodily senses and to confirm or rule out suspicious findings detected in the health history.

### Extent of the Physical Examination

The extent of a physical examination depends on many factors. The condition of the patient may influence what is included in the physical examination. The patient who is in severe pain or is critically ill may not tolerate a thorough physical examination. Time is also a factor. The critically ill patient may require immediate treatment, which limits the time to perform in-depth assessments. Every examination must be individualized to meet the needs of the patient and conform to the situation.

The following sections on urologic aspects of physical examination provide detailed infor-

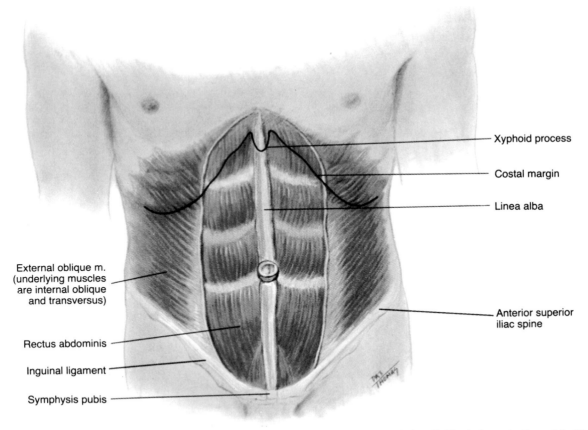

Xyphoid process

Costal margin

Linea alba

External oblique m.
(underlying muscles
are internal oblique
and transversus)

Rectus abdominis

Inguinal ligament

Symphysis pubis

Anterior superior
iliac spine

*FIGURE 2–2* Anatomic landmarks for examination of the abdomen. (From Jarvis, C. [1992]. *Physical examination and health assessment* [p. 586]. Philadelphia: W. B. Saunders. Reprinted by permission.)

mation on the more frequently performed examinations for patients with urologic problems. They do not constitute complete examination. Examination of the respiratory and cardiovascular systems is not discussed but is particularly important. Pulmonary edema and fluid overload that may be a complication of renal disease or postoperative recovery may be discovered during the examination. The condition of the heart and lungs must be determined before any urologic surgery is undertaken. (See Bates, 1991; DeGowin & DeGowin, 1987; or Ford, 1985 for discussion of the examination of the respiratory and cardiovascular systems.)

## Examination of the Abdomen

Examination of the abdomen is carried out to validate any complaints of abdominal, flank, or back pain, or masses or reports of GI problems. In the absence of such complaints, the abdominal assessment evaluates the status of the bowel and the bladder.

Throughout the examination, the use of anatomic landmarks and the division of the abdomen into quadrants is beneficial in documenting the location of findings and in recognizing the location of underlying organs (Fig. 2–2). The four-quadrant method is used more commonly than the nine-section method (Table 2–5).

When assessing the abdomen, an easy way to remember the most common abnormal findings is by the mnemonic of the "six Fs": fat, fluid, feces, flatus, fetus, and fatal (tumor) (DeGowin & DeGowin, 1981).

Inspection, auscultation, percussion, and palpation are all used during the abdominal examination. Auscultation always precedes percussion or palpation, because movement of the abdominal wall can affect peristaltic sounds, causing inaccurate findings.

Position the patient supine with arms at the sides and a small pillow under the head. The knees should be slightly flexed with a pillow under the lower thighs to relax the abdominal muscles. Drape to expose the abdomen fully by

**TABLE 2–5. Organs and Structures in the Four Abdominal Quadrants***

| RIGHT UPPER QUADRANT | LEFT UPPER QUADRANT |
|---|---|
| Liver and gallbladder | Left lobe of liver |
| Pylorus | Spleen |
| Duodenum | Stomach |
| Head of pancreas | Body of pancreas |
| Right adrenal gland | Left adrenal gland |
| Upper lobe of right kidney | Upper lobe of left kidney |
| Hepatic flexure of colon | Splenic flexure of colon |
| Portions of ascending and transverse colon | Portions of transverse and descending colon |
| **RIGHT LOWER QUADRANT** | **LEFT LOWER QUADRANT** |
| Lower pole of right kidney | Lower pole of left kidney |
| Cecum and appendix | Sigmoid colon |
| Portion of ascending colon | Portion of descending colon |
| Bladder (if distended) | Bladder (if distended) |
| Ovary and salpinx | Ovary and salpinx |
| Uterus (if enlarged) | Uterus (if enlarged) |
| Right spermatic cord | Left spermatic cord |
| Right ureter | Left ureter |

**MIDLINE**
Uterus
Bladder

*Loops of small bowel are found in all quadrants.
Adapted from Kozier R. C., and Erb, G. (1987). *Fundamentals of nursing: Concepts, process, and practice* (3rd ed.). Redwood City, CA: Addison-Wesley. Reprinted by permission.

placing a hospital gown or bath towel over the chest and a sheet from the waist to the toes. If the patient has complaints of abdominal pain, note generalized movement during preparation. Patients with peritoneal inflammation tend to lie very still, whereas those with spasms of colicky pain tend to be restless.

## INSPECTION

Inspect the abdomen by looking at it from the patient's side with your head only slightly higher than the abdomen. Using a light source that shines across or lengthwise over the abdomen may assist in detecting shadows or movements. Instruct the patient to relax and breathe normally.

Note the effects of respiration. Watch the abdominal movements through several cycles. On inspiration, the diaphragm normally descends and the upper abdominal wall rises. This is seen especially in men, who tend to do more abdominal breathing. Absence of abdominal wall movement, particularly in men, may be a sign of peritonitis, when the patient tries to hold or splint the diaphragm to decrease abdominal pain. Deep inspiration may reveal enlargement of the liver, gallbladder, or spleen, because these organs move with respirations due to the movement of the diaphragm.

Observe for intestinal movements. Visible movement may be normal if the abdominal wall is thin—a low, wavelike movement may be seen. This is abnormal if visible through a wall of normal thickness, signifying intestinal obstruction. The intestinal movement usually appears as raised ridges in the left upper quadrant that move diagonally downward toward the right. Hyperactive bowel sounds usually accompany this phenomenon.

Note any pulsation. The abdominal wall may pulsate with the heart beat. A normal aortic pulsation is often seen in the epigastric area. An aortic aneurysm or a tortuous aorta may cause a pulsation of greater amplitude.

Inspect the abdomen for asymmetry. Compare the left with the right side and the upper with the lower abdomen. Note the patient's contour, which is a profile inspection from the xiphoid process to the pubis. The contour may be described as flat, scaphoid, or rounded as a normal finding. Masses in the abdomen may be enlarged organs or lymph nodes, or they may be tumors (Fig. 2–3). Examples of asymmetric findings when the left and right sides of the abdomen are compared include an enlarged liver or gallbladder in the right hypochondrium and an enlarged spleen in the left hypochondrium.

A hernia is a protrusion of tissues or organs through a weakening in the abdominal wall. These occur most often in the following areas:

1. Midline—ventral hernia is in the epigas-

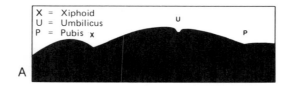

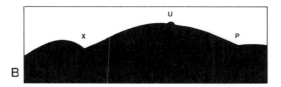

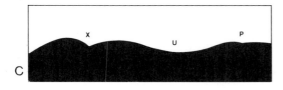

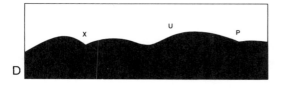

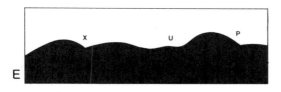

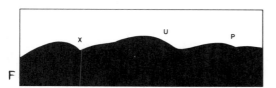

*FIGURE 2–3* Abdominal contours. The profiles show generalized abdominal distention with umbilicus inverted (*A*) or everted (*B*); a scaphoid abdomen (*C*); and distention of the abdominal lower half (*D*), lower third (*E*), and upper half (*F*). (Adapted from DeGowin, E. L., & DeGowin, R. L. [1981]. *Bedside diagnostic examination* [4th ed.]. New York: Macmillan. Reprinted by permission.)

trium; umbilical hernia is usually just above the umbilicus.
2. Surgical scar—incisional hernia.
3. Around a stoma—peristomal hernia.

4. Above or below the inguinal ligament—inguinal hernia.

To check for a hernia in the supine position, instruct the patient to raise the head or cough or strain to increase intra-abdominal pressure. A hernia is usually noted as a bulging mass. Suspected hernias should also be assessed in the standing position. Inspect the skin surface for the following:

1. Scars—they validate the patient's history.
2. Striae ("stretch marks")—silver striae may be seen in postpartum women or when there has been a rapid weight gain in the past. Pinkish-purple striae may be a sign of Cushing's syndrome or a recent stretching of the abdominal wall, as in pregnancy.
3. Dilated veins—these are seen with increased intra-abdominal pressure due to ascites, abdominal tumor, pregnancy, or thrombosis of the vena cava.
4. Pigment changes—bruising around the umbilicus (Cullen's sign) suggests intraperitoneal hemorrhage. Skin changes from recent radiation therapy may include a sunburned appearance in the irradiated area—the ink markings may also still be visible.
5. Lesions or wounds.
6. Stomal openings—document the type of stoma (whether it is a continent diversion or not and what part of the bowel or urinary system it drains) and the appearance of the stoma and its surrounding skin. Note the size of the stoma and its contour and color. Normal stoma size varies according to type, but a very small size may suggest a stomal stenosis. Normal stoma contour is preferably slightly protruding but may be flush with the skin. Prolapsed or retracted stomal contours are abnormal findings. Normal color is pink (like the color of buccal mucosa), whereas abnormal color may be described as blanched, dusky, or necrotic. Peristomal skin should be free of lesions or irritations and have a smooth surface. Skin changes, scars, or an uneven skin surface near the stoma is a potential problem for appliance fit. Document the kind of appliance or other covering used on the stoma.
7. Tubes and catheters—determine the size and type of catheter or tube, what it drains, its patency and positioning, and the appearance of the surrounding skin.
8. Drainage from the umbilicus—a patent urachus may drain urine. Pus may drain from the umbilicus resulting from a urachal cyst or abdominal abscess.

## AUSCULTATION

Immediate auscultation assesses for any flatus or borborygmi. Mediate auscultation is performed to assess peristaltic activity and listen for vascular sounds in the abdomen.

To listen for bowel sounds, use the diaphragm of the stethoscope, and listen in all four quadrants. Describe the sounds in terms of intensity, pitch, frequency, and quality. Document in which quadrant bowel sounds are heard. Normal bowel sounds are auscultated in all four quadrants and can vary greatly in frequency, intensity, and pitch. Assess any accompanying GI symptoms if bowel sounds are abnormal or absent. These include abdominal distention, abdominal cramps or colicky pain, nausea, vomiting, and diarrhea.

Auscultate the abdomen for any bruits, especially if the patient has hypertension. A bruit is an abnormal vascular sound heard over a blood vessel. It is the sound of turbulent blood flow, heard as a low-pitched blowing or swishing sound. A bruit can be heard best during expiration and may be continuous or heard only during systole. Listen for renal bruits by placing the bell of the stethoscope lightly on the skin over the upper abdominal quadrants (Fig. 2–4). A renal bruit can be caused by renal artery stenosis, a large arteriovenous fistula or malformation, or a renal artery aneurysm. Listen for an aortic aneurysm in the midline epigastric area or umbilical area. Cardiac murmurs can be transmitted along the aorta, and these are difficult to distinguish from bruits. If a bruit is heard, deep palpation should not be performed in that area.

## PERCUSSION

Percussion is performed in all four quadrants to define the borders of organs and areas of masses. Tympany usually predominates in the abdomen. A mass in the abdomen may be located when the percussion sounds change from tympanic to dull. In obese abdomens, the percussion sounds may be somewhat dull. Gaseous distention may produce a loud bell-like sound.

Unless the bladder contains more than 150 mL of urine, it cannot be percussed. If the bladder can be percussed, the dome of the bladder wall can be delineated. Start at the midline above the umbilicus and percuss downward. The area where the sound changes from tympanic to dull indicates the level of the bladder.

## PALPATION

Light palpation is always performed before deep palpation. Its purpose is to accomplish the following:

1. Determine muscle tone and resistance.
2. Detect tenderness.
3. Identify superficial organs and masses.
4. Relax the muscles for deep palpation.

To perform light palpation, keep the hand and forearm on a horizontal plane, and use the fat pads of the fingertips with the fingers together. First test the tone of the rectus muscles by gentle pressure with the hand resting against the abdomen. Instruct the patient to breathe deeply with the mouth open. To determine muscle guarding or rigidity, palpate the rectus muscle. If guarding is voluntary, the muscles relax with expiration. If there is involuntary guarding, the muscles remain rigid, which is a sign of peritoneal irritation. Tactile sense is best in the finger pads and most acute when palpation is light. The more forceful the palpation, the less is felt, so use only the amount of pressure necessary. Depress the skin no deeper than 2 cm, and use a light, circular, dipping motion. Move smoothly, and feel in all four quadrants. Be sure to palpate the umbilicus—metastases from intra-abdominal tumors can occur here.

Deep palpation locates abdominal organs and masses and determines the following:

1. Location—document in relation to anatomic landmarks.

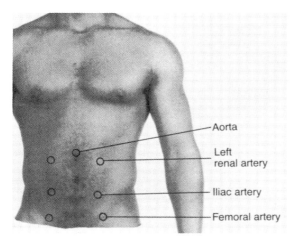

Aorta

Left
renal artery

Iliac artery

Femoral artery

*FIGURE 2–4* Locations for auscultation of renal and abdominal bruits. (From Jarvis, C. [1992]. *Physical examination and health assessment* [p. 600]. Philadelphia: W. B. Saunders. Reprinted by permission.)

2. Size—document in objective terms, such as diameter in centimeters.
3. Contour—smooth, nodular, irregular.
4. Consistency—firm, hard, indurated, soft, cystic.
5. Tenderness—present, absent.
6. Pulsations—present, absent.
7. Mobility—moves with deep inspiration, movable or fixed during palpation.

Deep palpation can be performed in two ways. It can be done by gradually increasing the depth of light palpation, observing the patient's respirations, and palpating deeper with expiration and resting with inspiration. When a maximum depth of about 4 to 5 cm is reached, inspiration brings body organs close to the hand, where they can be felt. The same hand position can be used for deep palpation as for light palpation, but if the patient is obese, bimanual palpation may be more effective. Bimanual deep palpation involves both hands. Place one hand on the patient in the same manner as light palpation. Place the other hand, palm down, on top of it, putting pressure on top of the distal fingers of the bottom hand. The top hand does all the pressing and guides the bottom hand while the fingers of the bottom hand do all the feeling. Palpate in all four quadrants, and identify and describe any masses.

If an area of increased tenderness and rigidity is noted, check for rebound tenderness by firmly and slowly pressing downward over the area of tenderness (or over an adjacent area, if this is too painful). Then quickly withdraw the fingers. If the pain is suddenly worse when the fingers are withdrawn, rebound tenderness, a sign of peritoneal inflammation, is present. This should be done at the end of the examination and should not be performed repeatedly.

The bladder cannot be palpated unless it is moderately distended. Start at the midline at or above the umbilicus and palpate toward the pubis. The distended bladder may be felt as a firm or fluctuant, round, movable mass rising out of the pelvis. In severe distention, the bladder may extend up to the level of the umbilicus. The bladder is usually palpated in the midline, but if a large diverticulum is present, it may extend to the left or the right. In some patients with chronic urinary retention, the bladder wall may be flabby and difficult to palpate, in which case percussion is a more valuable tool.

Normal kidneys may not be palpable because of their location behind other organs or under the ribs and when they are protected by muscles. Men usually have a more fixed kidney position and more resistant muscle tone, making palpation more difficult. Obesity also makes the examination harder to perform. The left kidney is rarely palpable, because it lies 1 to 2 cm higher than the right. The lower pole of the right kidney can sometimes be palpated, but the left kidney cannot usually be palpated unless it is displaced or greatly enlarged. At times, it is also difficult to differentiate the left kidney from the spleen. An enlarged renal mass may indicate hypertrophy (if the other kidney is absent or atrophied), hydronephrosis, cyst, tumor, or polycystic disease. Tumors of the kidney may be smooth or irregular. Ptotic kidneys may be palpated lower in the abdomen or even in the pelvis.

There are two methods of bimanual palpation of the kidney. These procedures explain palpation of the right kidney while standing on the patient's right side as the patient is lying supine. In the first method, place the left hand behind the patient between the rib cage and iliac crest near the CVA to support and elevate the area. Place the right hand below the right costal margin with the fingertips pointing to the left. Press both hands firmly together (deeper than when doing liver palpation). Ask the patient to take a deep breath, and at the peak of inspiration, try to feel the lower pole of the right kidney come down between the fingers of the right hand (Fig. 2–5).

The second method is called the capture technique. Place the hands as before. Ask the patient to take a deep breath. At the peak of inspiration, press the fingers together quickly, exerting slightly more pressure from above than below. Then ask the patient to exhale and stop breathing. Slowly release the pressure of the fingers. If the kidney has been "captured" between the hands, it can be felt as it slips between the fingers back up into place. The patient can usually feel capture and release—normally it does not hurt, but excessive pressure can cause pain.

Deep palpation of the abdomen is contraindicated in any patient with the following:

1. Known history of renal trauma.
2. Polycystic kidneys.
3. Known abdominal aortic aneurysm.
4. Recent kidney transplant.
5. Tender organs.
6. Appendicitis.
7. Known abdominal mass (palpation of a cancerous tumor may cause metastasis).

## Examination of the Back

To examine the back, position the patient in a sitting position with only the back exposed. Stand facing the back, looking down from above.

### INSPECTION

Identify the anatomic landmarks on the back—the CVAs and the iliocostal spaces. Inspect for flank or back bulges. These are most noticeable when the patient sits up and leans slightly forward. The bulging may be caused by a renal tumor or cyst, hydronephrosis, perinephric abscess, or renal trauma. Inspect for bruising of the skin on the retroperitoneal area, flank, or upper abdominal quadrants (Grey Turner's sign). Ecchymosis of this area may be a sign of retroperitoneal bleeding or renal trauma.

Look for any scars. Incisional or percutaneous scars suggest prior renal surgery. Lumbar scarring or disfiguration occurs with meningomyelocele. Scars along the spine suggest a history of spinal surgery that could affect bladder functioning.

Check for edema of the flank and back. Have the patient lie on a rough towel for a few minutes, then look for indentations. Edema may accompany a perinephric abscess. Check also for sacral edema to assess for fluid retention.

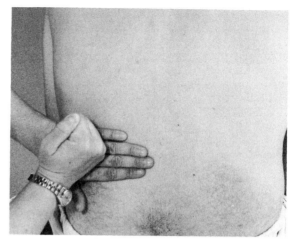

*FIGURE 2–6* Fist percussion over the left costovertebral angle. (Photograph by David Richmond.)

### AUSCULTATION

Place the bell of the stethoscope over each CVA to listen for renal bruits.

### PERCUSSION

Perform fist percussion over each CVA (Fig. 2–6). The patient should perceive a dull thud but no pain. If the patient does complain of pain, it may indicate renal inflammation or tenderness. On the right side, it may also indicate liver or gallbladder inflammation or tenderness. If the patient complains of any pain, be sure to check for any radiation of pain to other areas.

### PALPATION

Finger palpation over the CVA is performed to localize renal pain when percussion would be too painful. Press the fat pads of one or two fingers into the soft tissue of the CVA, and ask the patient to describe any pain. Again, be sure to check for any radiation of pain.

## Examination of the Male External Genitalia

Patients may find physical examination of the genitalia particularly anxiety-producing and embarrassing. Be sure to explain the nature and purpose of this examination, and perform it toward the end of the complete examination. It is important to provide privacy, maintain a

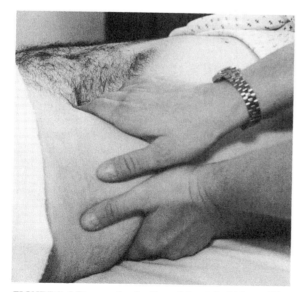

*FIGURE 2–5* Bimanual palpation of the right kidney. (Photograph by David Richmond.)

professional attitude, and perform the examination quickly but thoroughly and gently.

Fully expose the groin and genitalia under adequate lighting. This is best done with the patient standing undressed from the waist down and the examiner sitting in front of the patient. If the patient is unable to assume this position, have him lie supine with a small pillow under the head, the hips externally rotated and knees apart. Use a blanket or sheet to drape the abdomen and chest and another one to drape the thighs to the toes. The examiner should wear gloves for all parts of the examination.

## EXAMINATION OF THE PENIS

Observe the pattern of pubic hair distribution (escutcheon). Normally, hair is thickest over the symphysis pubis and continues over the scrotum and inner thighs. It extends up the lower abdomen in a triangular pattern in most men. Alterations in this pattern suggest an endocrine abnormality. Look at the bases of the pubic hair for any nits or lice. Check the underlying skin for any rash, inflammation, or excoriation. A rash may occur with a fungal infection or contact dermatitis. Excoriation on the pubis or the genitalia may be a sign of lice or scabies.

Note the size of the penis. Document if the penis is unusually small, erect, curved, or generally edematous. The normal size of the penis varies greatly, and it is normally flaccid and without curvature. Certain types of penile prostheses cause a permanent erection. Priapism is a sustained, painful erection in the absence of sexual desire. In priapism, the corpus cavernosa are engorged but the glans and corpus spongiosum are not involved. Curvature of the penis can be caused by scarring or a chordee. A ventral curvature of the penis is associated with epispadias. The penis may appear normal in its flaccid state in those patients who complain of curvature of the penis during erections, a symptom of Peyronie's disease. Penile edema may be noted in the patient on bed rest with dependent edema, or it may be caused by lymphatic or venous obstruction or inflammation. Edema and bruising may also result from trauma, as with a contusion or fracture of the penile shaft or other penile injury.

Inspect the shaft of the penis, looking at the dorsal surface and lifting it toward the abdomen to view the ventral side. Check for any localized edema, discoloration, or visible masses or lesions. Note if the patient has been circumcised. If not, retract the prepuce (foreskin) from the glans. Have the patient do this if possible. Observe the size of the preputial opening. Inspect the glans and inner surface of the prepuce for any discharge, lesions, or inflammation. Note the location of the urethral meatus. Gently squeeze the glans anteroposteriorly between the thumb and index finger to open the meatus and visualize the end of the urethra, inspecting the size of the meatus and any inflammation or discharge from the urethra. Palpate the length of the penis using the thumb and first two fingers on the dorsal, ventral, and lateral sides. Note any masses or areas of induration or tenderness. Replace the prepuce over the glans at the end of the examination to decrease the risk of paraphimosis.

Normally, the penis and prepuce have no lesions or inflammation and are soft to palpation. The preputial orifice should be large enough to move back and forth easily over the glans. The urethral meatus is located at the tip of the glans and has no discharge.

Ulcerations or lesions may be caused by sexually transmitted diseases, other skin diseases, carcinoma of the penis, or other infections. Multiple or secondary infections may be present. If one or more lesions are discovered, describe them in terms of location, size, type (such as vesicle, ulcer, scar, wart, nodule, and erosion), depth (shallow or deeper, with any induration at the base), and color. Note whether the lesion is dry or moist, and describe any drainage.

If the patient complains of urethral discharge, inspect the urethral meatus for discharge before having the patient void. If no discharge is noted, milk the penile shaft from the base to the glans (ask the patient to perform this if he is able). A profuse, thick, yellowish discharge is suggestive of gonococcal infection. Urethral discharge in urethritis from nongonococcal infections is often scanty, thin, and clear or whitish. A bloody discharge may be associated with urethral stricture, trauma, tumor, or foreign body in the urethra. If discharge is present, inspect the edges and visible mucosa of the meatus for inflammation, which often accompanies urethritis. Place a drop of the discharge on a glass slide for microscopic examination, and take a culture if indicated.

After retracting the prepuce, inflammation of the glans (balanitis) or inflammation of the glans and prepuce (balanoposthitis) may cause a foul-smelling discharge. A cheesy, whitish discharge called *smegma* normally may accumulate under the prepuce, but any signs of inflammation or pus indicate poor personal hygiene. Careful inspection of the glans and prepuce is necessary to detect carcinoma of the penis. Most penile cancers appear first in either of these areas and are found almost exclusively in men who were not circumcised in childhood.

Inflammation and infection of the prepuce and glans with resultant scarring can cause phimosis, a narrowing of the orifice of the prepuce. Phimosis can make retraction of the prepuce over the glans difficult or impossible. In severe cases, it can cause obstruction of urinary flow. If the prepuce appears tight over the glans, do not attempt to retract it, because forceful retraction may cause tearing of the fibrotic tissue of the prepuce, or once retracted, paraphimosis may result. Paraphimosis occurs when the prepuce cannot be replaced to its normal position covering the glans. If the prepuce remains in the retracted position, it can restrict venous return in the prepuce and glans, causing edema of those structures. If the restriction is not corrected, the glans can turn color from its normal pink to dusky. Necrosis caused by constriction from the prepuce also may develop.

A meatal stricture is a narrowing of the meatus noted when squeezing the glans. This is usually a congenital anomaly but can be an acquired condition caused by infection or trauma. Congenital malposition of the urethral meatus on the ventral penis is termed *hypospadias*, and congenital malposition of the urethral meatus on the dorsal penis is known as *epispadias*.

A visible swelling on the ventral shaft may be caused by a periurethral abscess, which is usually tender to palpation, or a urethral diverticulum. An induration may be palpable over the site of a urethral stricture or urethral carcinoma. In the patient with acute urethritis, the entire urethra along the ventral shaft may feel indurated. Dense, fibrous plaques palpated near the dorsal midline of the shaft are associated with Peyronie's disease. The dorsal veins of the penis may be visible and palpable if they have varicosities. The superficial dorsal veins and lymph vessels may appear slightly reddened and may be palpable as tender, cordlike strictures on the dorsal shaft near the corona in cases of thrombophlebitis or lymphatic obstruction. A foreign body in the urethra is also usually palpable.

Although not generally considered part of the physical examination, observing the male patient void may sometimes be significant. Such situations include the following:

1. When the patient is unable to provide an adequate history about the character of the urinary stream.
2. When the patient has urethral stricture disease or has recently had urethral surgery.
3. When the patient is suspected of surreptitiously putting blood in the urine sample (men or women). An example of this may be the addicted patient faking kidney stone disease to obtain narcotics, but other patients may do this for secondary gain.

## EXAMINATION OF THE SCROTUM AND GROIN

Lift the penis up toward the symphysis pubis to inspect the anterior surface of the scrotum, and lift the scrotum to inspect its posterior surface. Normally, the scrotal skin is rugated (wrinkled), and small veins may be visible. Spread the rugated surface to assess texture and elasticity. Note any edema, redness, lesions, or cysts. Normal size and color of the scrotum vary. The skin is usually soft and elastic. Generalized scrotal edema may cause the wall to feel thickened and the skin to pit when pressure is applied. The skin may appear smooth and shiny with edema or in the presence of large scrotal masses. Scrotal skin is susceptible to skin diseases that affect other areas of the skin. An uncommon but serious scrotal infection is Fournier's gangrene, a rapidly progressing infection characterized by massive edema and necrosis of the scrotal wall. Sebaceous cysts on the scrotum are common and benign. These are one or more firm, nontender, whitish-yellow nodules approximately 1 cm in diameter. Bruising and edema of the scrotum and perineum may result from bleeding or urinary extravasation after urethral trauma. Atrophy or underdevelopment of the scrotal wall may accompany cryptorchidism. A bifid scrotum, in which the two halves of the scrotum resemble the female labia majora, may be present in cases of severe hypospadias or in intersex.

Palpate the scrotal contents in a systematic manner, attempting to identify the different structures located in the scrotum (Fig. 2-7). If an intrascrotal mass is discovered, attempt to determine if the mass is part of the testis or is separate from it. Any mass found on the testis is assumed to be a testicular tumor until proved otherwise (Corriere, 1986). Note the location, shape, size, and consistency of any masses or indurations. Document any associ-

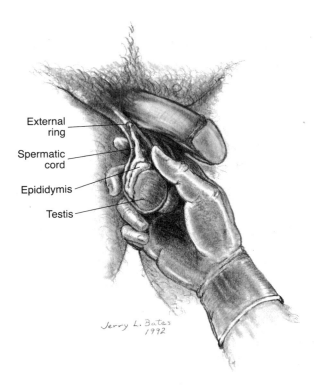

External ring

Spermatic cord

Epididymis

Testis

Jerry L. Bates
1992

*FIGURE 2–7* Palpable structures in the scrotum.

ated signs or symptoms, such as pain or fever (Table 2–6).

Palpate each testis separately. Place each thumb on the anterior surface, and roll the testis between the fingers, feeling its consistency and contour. The testes are egg-shaped structures, located at the base of each hemiscrotum. The normal size is about 2 cm wide and 4 cm long, with the long axis in a vertical position. The left testis usually hangs about 1 cm lower than the right. The testes should feel rubbery with a smooth contour. They are nontender to gentle touch, but pressure on the testes causes a dull ache that radiates to the lower abdomen.

A smaller testis (<3.5 cm long) with a soft or mushy consistency is a sign of atrophy. Absence of the testis from the base of the scrotum may be caused by congenital maldescent (either cryptorchidism or ectopy), congenital absence (which occurs rarely), or an overactive cremasteric reflex, also referred to as *retractile testis*. The retractile testis is pulled to the upper scrotum or near the external inguinal ring with stimulation by cold or excitement. If the testis is not located in the base of the scrotum, palpate the upper scrotum and the area

near the inguinal canal. If the testis is located, attempt to "milk" or gently pull the testis to the base of the scrotum. The maldescended testis cannot be returned to the base of the scrotum, but the retractile testis can be manipulated to the base of the scrotum. If the testis is not palpated in these areas, carefully palpate the inguinal canal, the genitalia, the perineum, and the femoral areas to attempt to locate it.

To palpate the epididymis, use the same hand position as for the testis. The epididymis is a comma-shaped structure extending from the upper to the lower testis, usually near the posterolateral surface of the testis. Normally, it is easily distinguishable from the testis, is nontender to gentle touch, and feels soft and resilient. At the upper pole of the testis is the appendix testis, and near it, on the epididymis, is the appendix epididymis. Both are vestigial organs and typically are not palpable. Occasionally, especially in younger males, these may undergo torsion, a spontaneous twisting. In early torsion the physical examination reveals a painful, pealike mass that appears bluish under the scrotal skin. In later torsion, the entire testicle is edematous.

Next, palpate the spermatic cord with the thumb and forefinger. Palpate from the lower epididymis to the external inguinal ring. Generally the cord is about 3 mm in diameter and feels smooth, round, resilient, and nontender. The different components of the cord can usually be identified. The vas deferens feels cordlike and firm; the blood vessels, nerves, and lymphatics feel threadlike.

If any mass is discovered during examination of the scrotal contents, transillumination should be performed. Darken the room, place the lighted end of a flashlight directly on the posterior scrotal wall behind the mass, and observe the anterior scrotal wall. If the mass contains serous fluid or sperm, the area of the mass will produce a red glow through the anterior scrotal wall. If the mass is solid or contains blood, the mass will appear opaque.

Examination of the groin should be done first with the patient in the supine position as part of the abdominal examination and then repeated with the patient in the standing position as part of the examination of the external genitalia.

First, inspect the inguinal and femoral areas for hernias (Fig. 2–8). Ask the patient to cough or strain, noting any masses. Normally, none are noted. A direct inguinal hernia bulges anteriorly from the inguinal area. An indirect inguinal hernia bulges from the inguinal area,

## TABLE 2–6. Intrascrotal Mass Assessment

| | PHYSICAL EXAMINATION | HISTORY |
|---|---|---|
| **Hydrocele (collection of fluid within tunica vaginalis)** | Size varies; may be large<br>Smooth; soft and cystic or hard<br>Located on anterior surface of testicle or within spermatic cord<br>May not be able to distinguish testis from epididymis<br>Can palpate spermatic cord above mass if spermatic cord not involved; if spermatic cord involved, mass located in upper scrotum<br>Transilluminates | Slow onset<br>Painless<br>Large hydrocele may be uncomfortable and embarrassing<br>If hydrocele secondary to inflammation, onset sudden and mass tender<br>Usually affects men aged 40 yr and older |
| **Hematocele (collection of blood within tunica vaginalis)** | Size and consistency similar to hydrocele<br>Does not transilluminate | History of trauma to genitalia |
| **Spermatocele (mass containing sperm)** | Usually less than 1 cm in diameter; may be large and resemble hydrocele or testicular tumor<br>Firm or cystic<br>Freely movable<br>Palpated above and behind testis; separate from testis<br>Transilluminates | Asymptomatic unless very large |
| **Varicocele (dilatation of veins in spermatic cord)** | Size varies<br>Soft; tortuous; compressible; feels like "bag of worms"<br>Occurs mostly on left side<br>Located above and behind testis; may extend to external inguinal ring<br>May not be palpable in supine position<br>Palpation with patient in standing position doing Valsalva maneuver is best method of detection | Usually nontender; may be painful if inflamed<br>Patient may report infertility<br>If large, patient may report feeling of heaviness or dull ache in scrotum<br>Does not transilluminate |
| **Testicular Tumor (pathologic overgrowth of testicular tissue)** | Size varies<br>Firm to hard mass or nodule on testis<br>Most often located on anterior or lateral surface of testis<br>Usually epididymis and spermatic cord normal<br>Epididymo-orchitis, hydrocele, occasionally hematocele may also be present<br>Does not transilluminate | Usually painless but may be tender<br>Patient may report history of minor genital trauma where mass incidentally discovered<br>Patient may complain of heaviness in testicle<br>Patient may present with metastatic symptoms, e.g., back pain, nonspecific abdominal pain, nausea and vomiting, anorexia, weight loss, cough, dyspnea<br>Most often affects males aged 20–35 yr |
| **Acute Epididymitis (inflammation or infection of epididymis)** | Scrotum enlarged and edematous; overlying skin reddened<br>Early: indurated, swollen epididymis and vas deferens<br>Few hours after onset: hard, swollen mass involving testis and epididymis; unable to distinguish epididymis from testis<br>Affected testis rides low in scrotum<br>Does not transilluminate unless reactive hydrocele present<br>In supine position, pain relieved when scrotum gently lifted onto symphysis pubis (Prehn's sign)<br>Cloudy urine<br>Fever (as high as 40°C); chills<br>Patient may have urethral discharge | Onset usually sudden<br>Pain (usually severe) in scrotum radiating along spermatic cord to lower abdomen<br>Irritative voiding symptoms<br>Usually seen in men 25 yr of age and older<br>May follow episode of physical straining |

*Table continued on following page*

TABLE 2–6. Intrascrotal Mass Assessment *Continued*

| | PHYSICAL EXAMINATION | HISTORY |
|---|---|---|
| **Torsion of the Spermatic Cord (twisting of spermatic cord that compromises blood supply to testicle)** | Scrotal edema; overlying skin reddened<br>Early: may palpate thickening or twisting and shortening of spermatic cord; epididymis may be in anterior position; testis may not be affected<br>Later: thickened spermatic cord; hard swollen mass involving testis and epididymis; unable to distinguish testis from epididymis<br>Affected testis rides high in scrotum<br>Does not transilluminate<br>In supine position, pain increases when scrotum gently lifted onto symphysis pubis (Prehn's sign)<br>May see moderate fever | Onset sudden<br>Severe pain in testicle radiating to lower abdomen, but patient may have little or no pain<br>Often history of previous similar episodes that resolved spontaneously<br>Patient may have nausea and vomiting |
| **Scrotal Hernia (indirect inguinal hernia extending into the scrotum)** | Size varies<br>Feels like soft, thick tube or bulge<br>Extends from external inguinal ring into scrotum; may descend to base of scrotum<br>Descends in front of spermatic cord and testis<br>To differentiate hernia from other masses, grasp neck of scrotum between thumb and first finger to palpate spermatic cord; if mass below fingers, mass is not hernia; if mass palpated at neck of scrotum or above fingers toward inguinal canal, mass may be a hernia<br>Palpation with patient in standing position doing Valsalva maneuver is best method of detection; mass may bulge with Valsalva<br>Auscultation may reveal bowel sounds if bowel in hernia<br>Mass may reduce by gently pressing upward and obliquely lateral with patient supine (do not attempt if patient complains of nausea, vomiting, pain)<br>Does not transilluminate | Usually painless but patient may complain of aching discomfort<br>Nausea, vomiting, or pain in mass suggests trapped obstructed bowel |

but the bulge travels downward toward the scrotum and may enter the scrotum. A femoral hernia bulges anteriorly from below the inguinal area near the skin crease in the groin (Dalton, 1983). With the patient in a supine position, a hernia may be reduced (replaced in the abdominal cavity) by gentle, constant pressure from the fingers. Do not try this if the patient complains of nausea, vomiting, or pain in the area (Bates, 1991).

Palpate the femoral region. The femoral canal lies below the inguinal canal and medial to the femoral blood vessels. Use the femoral pulse as a landmark, and palpate the area about 3 cm medial to the pulse using the middle three finger pads. Normally, the canal is not palpable and has no swelling or tenderness. Swelling or tenderness in this area suggests the possibility of a femoral hernia.

To palpate the inguinal area, use the right hand to palpate the right inguinal area and the left hand to palpate the left inguinal area. Put the index finger on the loose skin of the base of the scrotum. Press upward, invaginating the scrotal skin. Feel for the spermatic cord, and follow its course through the neck of the scrotum until the tip of the finger reaches the triangular-shaped opening of the external inguinal ring. Depending on the size of the external ring, the finger may be able to enter the inguinal canal. With the index finger either at the external inguinal ring or within the ca-

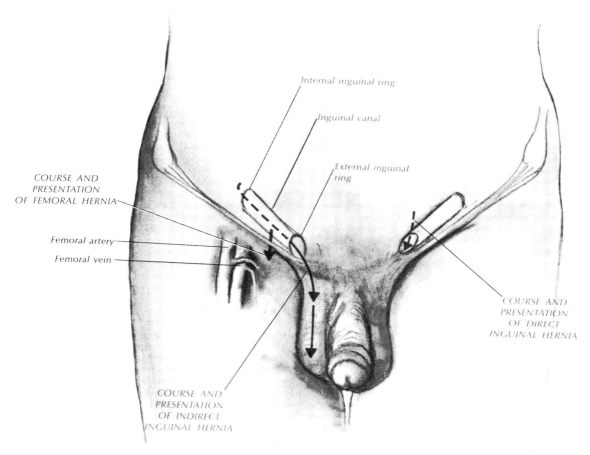

**FIGURE 2–8** Location of inguinal and femoral hernias. (From Bates, B. [1991]. *A guide to physical examination and history taking* [5th ed., p. 382]. Philadelphia: J. B. Lippincott. Reprinted by permission.)

nal, ask the patient to cough or strain (Fig. 2–9). Normally, no pressure should be felt on the fingertip. A small indirect inguinal hernia feels like a pulsation against the fingertip, whereas a larger hernia may feel like a bulging mass (DeGowin & DeGowin, 1981). A direct inguinal hernia feels like a pulsation or mass against the side of the finger pushing outward if the finger is inside the inguinal canal (Bates, 1991).

Palpate the inguinal lymph nodes for any tenderness or enlargement, using the finger pads of the middle three fingers. The superficial inguinal nodes are located parallel to and just below the inguinal ligament. The deep subinguinal nodes lie on either side of the femoral canal and femoral artery (Fig. 2–10) (Jones, 1984). If they are palpable, note the size and consistency. An enlarged node may be indicative of an inflammatory or malignant lesion in the genital or perianal area.

## EXAMINATION OF THE RECTUM AND PROSTATE

With the patient wearing a hospital gown, position him standing bent over an examination table with his elbows on the table to support the weight of the upper body. If the patient is unable to assume this position, have him lie on his side with the legs and knees flexed, pulling the uppermost leg higher toward the chest. Drape the patient with bath blankets or sheets so that only the buttocks are exposed. The knee-chest or lithotomy positions may be alternative choices.

Inspect the perianal region by separating the buttocks with one or both hands. Note any perianal rash, excoriation, ulceration, masses, or inflammation. The skin around the rectum is normally more highly pigmented and coarser than surrounding skin. Ask the patient

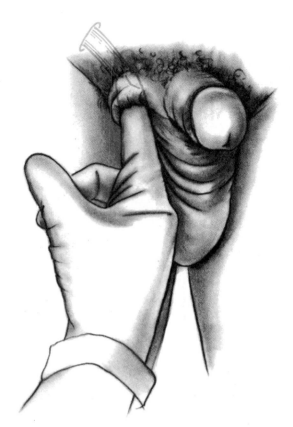

*FIGURE 2–9* Palpation for inguinal hernias. (From Jarvis, C. [1992]. *Physical examination and health assessment* [p. 813]. Philadelphia: W. B. Saunders. Reprinted by permission.)

to bear down, and check for any hemorrhoids or anal fissures. Palpate any abnormal areas, noting any tenderness and the characteristics of any masses. This inspection is particularly important for the homosexual male.

To palpate the rectum and prostate, lubricate the gloved index finger with water-soluble jelly. Explain to the patient that he may feel the urge to move his bowels during the rectal examination and may feel the urge to urinate when the prostate is palpated. Instruct the patient to bear down during insertion of the index finger and to breathe deeply and slowly through his mouth during the examination. Place the finger pad of the index finger over the anus and gently press. As the sphincter relaxes, insert the finger pad and then the tip of the finger, pointing it toward the umbilicus.

Gently insert the finger just past the anal canal, which is about 2.5 to 4 cm long, and position the finger pad against the anterior rectal wall, where the prostate can be palpated. If the finger is inserted too far, the base of the blad-der will be palpated, which is much larger than the prostate. The average prostate is about the size of a walnut and has a heart-shaped configuration, widest at the base of the bladder. It may be felt as a rubbery bulge in the anterior rectal wall with a groove, the median furrow, running down the longitudinal axis. On each side of the prostate lies another groove called the *lateral sulcus*. Palpate the entire prostate between the lateral sulci. The normal consistency is comparable with that of the thenar eminence (the mound of flesh located at the base of the thumb on the palm) when the fist is clenched. The prostate is normally smooth and nontender. Describe any other findings according to size, location, and consistency.

Palpable abnormal findings include the following:

1. A hard nodule or areas of induration that may be associated with cancer of the prostate, chronic infection, or prostatic calculi. The nodule or induration may be located near the surface and raise above the surface or be palpated within the gland (Smith, 1992). The nodule associated with cancer of the prostate can be described as feeling like a knuckle on a clenched fist.
2. A stony-hard consistency that is seen with advanced carcinoma of the prostate.
3. A nontender enlargement that may be associated with benign prostatic hyperplasia (BPH). However, BPH may occur even though the prostate feels normal.
4. A very tender, swollen, firm, indurated prostate that may occur with acute prostatitis.
5. A soft or mushy consistency that may occur with chronic infection and poor drainage or from congestion due to sexual abstinence (Smith, 1992).
6. Areas of bogginess or fluctuation that may be associated with inflammation or abscess.

Slightly above the prostate under the bladder, palpate on either side for the seminal vesicles. The seminal vesicles are normally not palpable, unless they are indurated owing to infection or neoplasm, or distended and cystic owing to sexual abstinence.

Complete the examination by palpating the lateral and posterior walls of the rectum and by noting the amount of stool in the rectum. Note any areas of tenderness, nodules, or induration, and whether a fecal impaction is present. After withdrawing the finger, use a guaiac test for any stool on the glove to assess for occult blood in the stool.

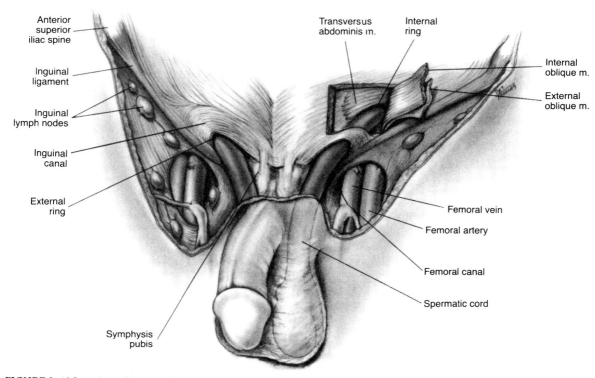

*FIGURE 2–10* Location of inguinal lymph nodes. (From Jarvis, C. [1992]. *Physical examination and health assessment* [p. 800]. Philadelphia: W. B. Saunders. Reprinted by permission.)

## Examination of the Female External Genitalia and the Pelvic Area

If a complete pelvic examination is to be performed, place the patient in the lithotomy position on an examination table with the legs up in stirrups and a small pillow under the head. If a complete examination is not needed, the patient can be placed in bed in the dorsal recumbent position with the knees drawn up and apart and the feet apart. If desired, a bedpan turned upside down and covered with a blanket can be placed under the patient's buttocks (so the flattest part of the bedpan is pushed furthest under the buttocks) to elevate the pelvis and allow better visualization of the genitalia. (Elevate the head of the bed for comfort if a bedpan is used.) The patient is dressed in a hospital gown pulled up to cover the chest and abdomen. A blanket or sheet is placed diagonally over the lower half of the body with two opposite ends wrapped around the legs and feet, another end on the abdomen, and its opposite end draped over the perineum to be lifted to the abdomen during the examination.

A gooseneck lamp provides the best lighting. The examiner is seated at the end of the examination table or, if the patient is in bed, the entire bed should be elevated to a position comfortable for the examiner to stand at the side of the bed. Gloves are worn for all parts of the examination.

First, inspect the mons pubis, the labia majora, and the perineum. Place a hand on the upper inner thigh to prepare the patient for palpation, and explain each step of the examination. Normally, the pubic hair covers the mons pubis and the uppermost inner thighs. Check for any nits or lice at the bases of the pubic hair. Excoriation or rash may be caused by a parasitic infection. If the patient has incontinence, urine contact may have caused skin irritation.

Separate the labia majora, and inspect the labia minora, the clitoris, the urethral meatus, and the introitus. Palpate and describe any lesions noted (such as warts, vesicles, chancre, ulcers, and papules). Lesions can be caused by sexually transmitted diseases, other skin disorders, sebaceous cysts, or cancer of the vulva. An enlarged clitoris and male escutcheon are signs of virilization, which may be seen with adrenogenital syndrome. Labial masses on either side of the posterior vagina may be caused by inflammation of a Bartholin's gland, which is normally not palpable. Palpate the mass by placing the index finger in the vagina and the thumb on the outside over the mass, and feel the swelling between the fingers. Note its size, tenderness, and any discharge.

A reddened, tender nodule at the meatus suggests a urethral caruncle. Eversion and redness of the posterior urethral meatus may be seen with senile urethritis and vaginitis. Inflammation or discharge from the meatus may accompany urethritis or inflammation of Skene's glands, which lie on either side of the urethra and open on the distal urethra just inside the meatus. Palpate the urethra by inserting the index finger into the vagina, and use the finger pad to palpate the urethra through the anterior vaginal wall from the bladder base to the meatus. A localized induration may suggest a tumor. A soft bulging mass may be a urethral diverticulum that, when palpated, may cause a urethral discharge. To detect or express urethral discharge, milk the urethra through the anterior vaginal wall from the base of the bladder to the meatus. Take a sample of the drainage for culture if indicated. Inflamed Skene's or Bartholin's glands may be sites of chronic infection and cause irritative voiding symptoms. Infections of the vagina caused by sexually transmitted diseases or other organisms also can cause urethritis and changes in voiding pattern. With the labia separated, ask the patient to cough or strain, and note any bulging of the vaginal walls. A cystocele is a bulging of the anterior wall due to prolapse of the bladder. A rectocele is a bulging of the posterior vaginal wall due to prolapse of the rectum. A cystocele denotes relaxation of the pelvic muscles and may cause irritative voiding symptoms, stress urinary incontinence, and bladder infection due to residual urine. Coughing or straining may also cause leakage of urine from the meatus due to stress incontinence.

To inspect the vagina and cervix, a speculum is inserted. Choose an appropriate size and type. Warm and lubricate the speculum with warm water. With the index and middle fingers just inside the vagina, press down on the posterior vaginal wall until it relaxes. With the other hand, insert the closed speculum past the finger at a 45-degree angle with more pressure toward the posterior vaginal wall. Hold the blades obliquely to insert them, and use care not to catch any pubic hair or the labia on insertion. Once the speculum is inserted, re-move the fingers and turn the blades to a horizontal position with the handles down, keeping pressure on the posterior vaginal wall. Open the blades and locate the cervix. Once the cervix is in full view, lock the blades open by tightening the thumb screw.

The cervix normally appears smooth and pink. Note any inflammation, erosion, lesions, bleeding, or discharge. These could represent signs of infection or cancer. Obtain any cultures or a Papanicolaou smear if indicated.

Withdraw the speculum slowly while inspecting the vagina. Note any inflammation, lesions, masses, or discharge. After the tips of the blades are withdrawn past the cervix, unlock and close the blades as the speculum is gently removed.

To perform the bimanual examination, lubricate the index and middle fingers with water-soluble jelly and insert them into the vagina. With the other hand, press down on the abdomen about halfway between the umbilicus and the symphysis pubis. Palpate the cervix and uterus for smoothness, size, mobility, and tenderness. Note any tenderness or masses in the anterior vaginal wall or in the area of the bladder. Move the hand on the abdomen to the right lower quadrant to press downward, and move the fingers in the vagina to the right lateral fornix to palpate the right ovary and adnexa. Repeat the procedure for the left ovary. The ovary is normally slightly tender to palpation.

Withdraw the fingers from the vagina, change gloves, and after lubricating the fingers, place the index finger into the vagina and the middle finger into the rectum. Explain to the patient that she may feel as though she needs to have a bowel movement. Repeat the bimanual examination, feeling the area between the cervix and rectum particularly. Finish by examining the rectum, as discussed earlier.

Pain experienced with moving the cervix and palpating the adnexa is associated with acute pelvic inflammatory disease, which is sometimes confused with an acute urinary tract infection. Thickening, or a movable or fixed mass, in the area of the bladder may be noted in advanced cases of bladder cancer. Tumors of the female reproductive system can invade the urinary tract or can extrinsically compress the ureters, causing urinary obstruction.

## Neurologic Examination

Urologic disorders can cause changes in neurologic status. Examples are altered mental states that may accompany renal failure and metastasis from genitourinary cancers to the brain or spine, particularly spinal cord compression from metastatic prostatic cancer. Conversely, urologic disorders can result from neurologic disease or trauma. The major urologic disorders are bladder and sexual dysfunction. Because neurogenic bladder disease is often complicated by upper urinary tract disorders, such as infection, hydronephrosis, and calculi, many urologic patients also have neurologic problems.

The more commonly performed assessment procedures for neurologic examination include determining level of consciousness and orientation and memory span, assessing motor function and sensation, and testing reflexes associated with sacral and lumbar spinal nerves, which are involved in bladder and sexual functioning. Test level of consciousness by determining the least amount of stimulation needed to elicit a response from the patient. Normally, the patient is awake and alert and responds to normal outside stimuli. Abnormal findings include that the patient is

1. Alert only after verbal stimulation (verbal command).
2. Alert only after tactile stimulation (touching or shaking).
3. Alert only after noxious stimulation (pressure on the nail beds, sternal rubbing, pinching the sternocleidomastoid muscle).
4. Not alert, but purposefully responds to noxious stimulation, such as forcing the examiner's hand away.
5. Responds nonpurposefully to noxious stimulation, such as by grimacing, posturing, or changing respiratory rate.
6. Does not respond to noxious stimuli.

Determine the patient's level of orientation to person, place, and time by asking the appropriate questions. Normal response is documented as "oriented × 3." If indicated, also ask the patient to tell his or her name and home address to assess orientation to self.

Assessment of short- and long-term memory is accomplished during the health history when the patient is asked details of his or her recent and past health status. Testing recent history includes asking questions about events occurring within the last 2 days, and past history includes events occurring a week or more earlier. Assessing affect and speech as done with the general survey also provides data about neurologic status.

Check the patient's motor function by testing grip and dexterity of the upper extremities and the gait and strength in the lower extremities. Normal findings are that the patient has equal and strong hand grips, along with fine coordination of all digits; full strength against resistance and a steady gait are expected in the lower extremities.

Test sensation by asking the patient to identify different types of tactile stimulation applied to different parts of the body. Ask the patient to differentiate between light touch, such as gentle stroking with the finger or a wisp of cotton, and pressure, such as gently poking the skin with the wooden end of a cotton-tipped applicator. If indicated, test for pain sensation using a sterile hypodermic needle. Normally, the patient is able to identify the type of stimulation and where the stimulation occurs. This test may be performed in the perianal region when assessing for neurogenic bladder disease.

When testing deep tendon reflexes, the patellar reflex assesses L2, L3, and L4 innervation. Normal response is extension of the leg as the quadriceps muscle contracts. The Achilles tendon reflex assesses S1 and S2 innervation. The normal response is plantar flexion. (See Kozier & Erb, 1991; or King, 1982, for the procedures of testing deep tendon reflexes and abnormal responses.)

During the rectal or pelvic examination, assessment of anal sphincter tone and contraction indicates the level of functioning of the sacral and pelvic nerves. Assess anal sphincter tone with a finger in the rectum. Normally, the rectum closes snugly around the finger. Next, ask the patient to contract the anal sphincter voluntarily and check the response. The bulbocavernosus reflex is elicited by squeezing the glans penis or clitoris when a finger is inserted into the rectum and checking the response of involuntary contraction of the anal sphincter or bulbocavernosus muscles. Hyperactivity or decreased or no response is an abnormal finding (Hanno & Wein, 1987).

## DIAGNOSTIC LABORATORY TESTS

The purposes of diagnostic laboratory testing are the following:

1. Serves as a screening process to detect any problems not uncovered in the history or physical examination.
2. Provides findings that are consistent with

the diagnosis and assessment data or shows significant negative findings.
3. Measures the effectiveness of therapeutic interventions.

Laboratory testing for the urologic patient usually includes examining urine, blood, prostatic fluid, semen, and urethral and vaginal secretions. The laboratory values given are only general guidelines, and values may vary from those used in different laboratories. Also, methods of collection may vary depending on the test required. Always check the laboratory manual specific to the particular work setting.

When collecting specimens to send to a laboratory, the following instructions apply:

1. Follow universal infection control guidelines by wearing gloves when handling any body fluids.
2. Collect the specimen in the proper container. Know if the container must be sterile or if any preservative must be added.
3. Label the specimen container with the patient's name, the type of specimen, the date and time of collection, the patient's identification number, and the physician's name. Note the method of collection for urine specimens. Appropriately label the requisition and the specimens of patients known to have infected body fluids.

## Examination of Urine

Urine testing is one of the most useful assessments for patients with urologic problems. It can provide information about the urinary tract from the kidney to urethral meatus.

### GENERAL GUIDELINES FOR URINE COLLECTION

The timing of a urine collection should always be considered. The following are general guidelines that apply:

1. Random specimens are those collected at any convenient time.
2. A first-voided morning specimen is collected immediately on arising. It is ideal for screening, because it will show the kidney's ability to concentrate; substances that may not be present in a dilute random specimen can also be detected.
3. A "fasting specimen" is collection of the second-voided specimen after a period of fasting. This specimen does not contain any me-

tabolites from eating before the beginning of the fasting period.
4. A 24-hour (timed) specimen is collection of *all* urine during a 24-hour period. Explicit instructions need to be given to the patient. Begin and end the specimen collection period with an empty bladder. This means that the patient will void (or, if necessary, self-catheterize or empty collection device) and discard the urine at the start of the test. Exactly 24 hours later, the patient voids, but adds the voided urine to the specimen collection—this signifies the end of the test. Stress that the patient must save all the urine and restart the test if urine is accidentally discarded.

The method of urine collection varies for different tests as follows:

1. A midstream urine specimen is obtained by having the patient start the stream by voiding in the toilet, collecting about 50 mL of urine in the middle of the stream, and finishing voiding in the toilet.
2. A midstream clean-catch urine specimen decreases contamination from organisms in the urethra of both sexes; the prostate, glans, and prepuce in males; and the vagina and perineum in females. This involves collecting a midstream specimen using precautions to avoid contamination (Procedure 2–1).
3. Multiple-bottle voidings involve collecting individual initial, middle, and terminal parts of the urinary stream to localize the source of bacteria or blood in the urinary tract (Procedure 2–2).
4. Suprapubic aspiration is performed by the physician, who inserts a needle directly into the distended bladder through the lower abdomen above the symphysis pubis and aspirates urine in a syringe. This method avoids any contamination from the urethra, the perineum, or the vagina.
5. A catheterized specimen is obtained by catheterizing the bladder to obtain a urine specimen (Procedures 2–3 and 2–4).
6. Obtaining a urine specimen from a continent urinary reservoir, such as the Kock pouch, is done by catheterizing the stoma, much the same way as bladder catheterization (see Procedures 2–3 and 2–4). This method can also be used for urinary conduit diversions (ileal or colon conduits), but in some settings, nurses are prohibited from catheterizing these stomas if the conduit was created within the past 3 months. Be sure to know the type of stoma—do not catheterize a ure-

**PROCEDURE 2-1**

■

Midstream Clean-Catch Urine Specimen Collection

■ **PURPOSE**

To obtain a voided urine specimen that will be as free of external contaminants as possible.

■ **EQUIPMENT**

Sterile specimen container
Antiseptic towelette or antiseptic-soaked cotton balls
2 aqueous towelettes or water-soaked cotton balls

■ **PROCEDURE**

1. Explain procedure to patient.
2. Wash hands thoroughly.
3. Assemble and prepare equipment.
   a. Open sterile urine specimen container.
   b. Open towelettes.
   c. Prepare area with towelettes.
      (1) Instruct or assist male patient to use one hand to retract the prepuce and expose the urethral meatus. Using the other hand, cleanse the urethral meatus and glans with the antiseptic towelette, starting at the meatus and going outward in a circular motion. Repeat, using the two aqueous towelettes.
      (2) Instruct or assist the female patient to separate the labia minora with one hand. Maintain this position until the specimen is obtained. Using the other hand, cleanse the urethral meatus and vestibule with the antiseptic towelette by wiping toward the rectum with one stroke over the inner surface of the labia minora and over the urethral meatus. Repeat, using the two aqueous towelettes.
4. Collect the sample in the specimen container by having the patient first void into the toilet. Then, with the patient continuing to void, hold the specimen container in "midstream" to interrupt the flow and collect the sample.
5. On the male patient, reposition the prepuce over the glans.
6. Close the specimen container, using care not to touch the inner surface of the lid. Label the specimen as indicated.

---

terostomy. Modifications in the steps of catheterizing a stoma include the following:
a. Remove the covering or stomal appliance before starting the procedure.
b. Prepare the stoma and skin with antiseptic-soaked cotton balls, wiping in a circular motion from the os outward three times.
c. Insert the tip of the catheter through the os until urine returns. In a conduit diversion, the catheter needs to be inserted only about 2 inches; in a continent urinary reservoir, the catheter may have to

be inserted farther. Some physicians recommend that a two-catheter technique be used to obtain urine from a stoma (Fig. 2–11). The technique requires that an outside, larger catheter first be inserted into the stoma. This serves as a protective passage against contamination when the second, smaller catheter is passed through the center of it to collect the urine specimen.
7. The drip method can be used to collect urine from a urinary stoma on the abdomen that continuously drips urine (an ileal or colon

**PROCEDURE 2-2**

■

## Multiple-Bottle Voidings

### ■ PURPOSE

To collect urine specimens from the initial, middle, and terminal parts of the urinary stream to aid in localizing the source of hematuria or urinary tract infection.

### ■ EQUIPMENT

3 sterile specimen containers, separately labeled "initial," "mid," and "terminal"
Aqueous towelette or antiseptic-soaked cotton balls
2 aqueous towelettes or water-soaked cotton balls
Culture materials or material for microscopic examination (smear) if prostatic
   massage is done

### ■ PROCEDURE

1. Explain the procedure to the patient.
2. Wash hands thoroughly.
3. Assemble and prepare equipment.
   a. Open specimen containers.
   b. Open all towelettes on a clean surface.
4. Prepare area with towelettes.
   a. Instruct or assist male patient to use one hand to retract the prepuce and expose the urethral meatus and maintain this position until all specimens are obtained. With the other hand, the patient cleanses the urethral meatus and glans with the antiseptic towelette, starting at the meatus and going outward in a circular motion. Repeat, using the two aqueous towelettes.
   b. With the female patient sitting or leaning far back on the toilet with her legs apart, instruct or assist her to separate the labia minora using one hand and maintain this position until all specimens are obtained. With the other hand, the patient cleanses the urethral meatus and vestibule with the antiseptic towelette by wiping toward the rectum with one stroke over the inner surface of the labia minora and over the urethral meatus. Repeat, using the two aqueous towelettes.
5. Collect the urine specimens.
   a. Instruct the patient to begin voiding into the specimen container labeled "initial." Collect 10–15 mL of urine in this container.
   b. With the patient continuing to void, collect 30–50 mL of urine in the specimen container labeled "mid" during the middle of the urinary stream.
   c. With the patient continuing to void, collect the final 10–15 mL of urine at the end of the urinary stream in the specimen container labeled "terminal."
6. Instruct or assist the male patient to reposition the prepuce over the glans.
7. Close the specimen containers, using care not to touch the inner surface of the lid. Label the specimens with patient's name, identification number, and other data as indicated.

**PROCEDURE 2-2** *Continued*

## Multiple-Bottle Voidings

### ■ PRECAUTIONS, CONSIDERATIONS, AND OBSERVATIONS

1. If multiple-bottle voids are collected on male patients to localize the source of urinary tract infection, the physician may perform prostatic massage after the "mid" urine specimen is collected.
   a. Instruct the patient to stop voiding after the "mid" urine specimen is collected but before he has completely emptied the bladder.
   b. The physician then performs a rectal examination and massages the prostate. If any expressed prostatic secretions are noted at the urethral meatus, obtain them for culture or place them on a glass slide for microscopic examination.
   c. Instruct the patient to resume voiding, and collect the first 10–15 mL of urine in the specimen container labeled "terminal." The prostatic secretions that were expressed into the urethra are washed out and collected in this urine specimen.
2. Multiple-bottle voids in conjunction with prostatic massage are particularly valuable in differentiating urethritis from prostatitis. A significantly higher bacteria count only in the "initial" urine specimen suggests urethritis; in the "terminal" specimen, it suggests prostatitis. Significant bacteria counts in the "mid" specimen indicate infection in the urine itself.
3. If multiple-bottle voids are collected to localize the source of hematuria, significant findings of red blood cells only in the "initial" urine specimen suggest bleeding from the anterior urethra; in the "terminal" specimen, such findings indicate bleeding from the posterior urethra or bladder neck. Significant findings of red blood cells in all specimens indicate that the bleeding originates proximal to the bladder neck (in the bladder, ureters, or kidneys).

---

conduit or a ureterostomy). First, remove the appliance covering the stoma. Place the patient in a prone position leaning on the elbows and knees to keep the abdomen lifted off the bed or examination table. Cleanse the stomal opening with antiseptic-soaked wipes or cotton balls in a circular motion, starting at the os and working outward. Adjust the patient's position so that urine drips directly from the stoma. Hold a urine container a few inches away from the stoma to catch at least 10 mL of urine. Having the patient well hydrated decreases the time involved in collecting this specimen.

8. Collecting urine specimens from a patient with an indwelling catheter should be done without breaking the closed drainage system if at all possible, because opening the system increases the risk of urinary tract infection.
   a. If the catheter is attached to a straight-drainage bag, aspirate urine from the self-sealing port on the drainage tubing.

Position the drainage tubing on the bed so that urine collects at the site of the port or, if necessary, attach a C-clamp below the port on the tubing to collect urine in the drainage tubing. (Clamp the tubing *only* long enough to collect about 10 mL in the tubing.) Cleanse the port with an antiseptic wipe, insert a needle attached to a 10-mL Luer-tip syringe at an oblique angle through the port, and aspirate the urine. Remove the needle from the syringe before emptying the syringe into the specimen container, because forcing urine through a needle breaks up cells in the urine (Corbett, 1987).
   b. If the catheter is not attached to a drainage bag with a self-sealing port, the closed drainage system can be opened. Wearing sterile gloves, cleanse the connection between the catheter and the drainage system, and disconnect the catheter, keeping the ends of the catheter and drainage tubing sterile. Then let the urine

## PROCEDURE 2-3
■
## Catheterization (male) to Obtain a Urine Specimen

### ■ PURPOSE

To obtain a urine specimen directly from the bladder that will be as free of contaminants as possible.

### ■ EQUIPMENT

Sterile disposable catheterization tray
Collection basin
Fenestrated drape
Waterproof underpad
Sterile gloves
6 cotton balls
Forceps
Iodophor cleansing solution
Specimen container
Water-soluble lubricating jelly
Straight catheter, usually a 14 or 16 Fr

### ■ PROCEDURE

1. Explain procedure to the patient.
2. Wash hands thoroughly.
3. Position patient in the dorsal recumbent position with legs extended. Turn down covers below perineum.
4. In a convenient location near the patient, open the catheter tray using aseptic technique.
5. Open appropriate catheter and place on sterile field.
6. Put on sterile gloves.
7. Remove contents of the collection basin, keeping all equipment on the sterile field. Saturate the cotton balls with iodophor solution. Open the lubricating jelly and lubricate the first 18 cm (7 inches) of the catheter, taking care not to obstruct the drainage hole of the catheter. Place the catheter in the collection basin. Remove the lid from the specimen container.
8. Pick up the waterproof underpad by two corners, folding it over gloved hands. Place it below the penis, on the thighs.
9. Pick up the fenestrated drape with your dominant hand. With the other hand, guide the penis through the opening. Consider the nondominant hand contaminated.
10. With contaminated hand, grasp penis firmly, directly behind the glans. Hold penis almost perpendicular to the patient's body (60–90-degree angle). If the penis is not circumcised, retract the prepuce.
11. Use the forceps to pick up a cotton ball saturated with cleansing solution. Cleanse the penis, beginning at the meatus and proceeding 5–7 cm (2–3 inches) down the shaft in a circular motion. Repeat with at least three cotton balls.
12. Move the collection basin close to patient.

## Catheterization (male) to Obtain a Urine Specimen

13. Following the anterior wall, gently insert the catheter into the meatus. Keep the drainage end of the catheter in the collection basin.
    a. Advance the catheter 15–18 cm (6–7 inches) until urine begins to flow. Then advance it another 2.5–5 cm (1–2 inches).
    b. If resistance is felt at the external sphincter (10–12 cm [4–5 inches])
       (1) Encourage the patient to take slow, deep breaths with his mouth open.
       (2) Advance the catheter during deep inspiration.
       (3) Lower the penis level with the body and continue inserting the catheter until urine flows.
    c. If the catheter bends inside the penis or springs back, increase the traction on the penis and gently rotate the catheter. NEVER FORCE THE CATHETER.
    d. If the catheter does not pass after these steps have been taken, stop the procedure and notify the physician.
14. When the urine begins flowing
    a. Hold catheter securely to prevent withdrawal and contamination with reinsertion of the catheter into bladder.
    b. Obtain specimen by allowing at least 30 mL urine to flow from the catheter into the specimen container.
15. Collect the remaining urine in the basin. Withdraw the catheter slowly as urine flow decreases, and remove the catheter when urine stops dripping.
16. Reposition the prepuce over the glans if the patient is not circumcised.
17. Close the specimen container, using care not to touch the inner surface of the lid.
18. Discard equipment and position patient correctly. Label the specimen as indicated.

## ■ PRECAUTIONS, CONSIDERATIONS, AND OBSERVATIONS

1. Contraindications to catheterizing a male patient include
   a. History of urethral stricture.
   b. Observing blood at the urethral meatus, which suggests traumatic injury.
2. To facilitate insertion of the catheter, lubricating jelly in a sterile tube (usually in double-packaged sterile wrap) may be placed into the urethral meatus.
   a. Open the outer strap and place the sterile package of jelly on the sterile field. When preparing equipment with sterile technique, open the package of jelly and pierce the opening of the tube with the cap.
   b. Before inserting the catheter, insert the opening of the lubricant jelly tube into the urethral meatus and squeeze the tube so lubricant flows gently into the urethra.
   c. There may be a sensation of burning in the urethra, but jelly should be allowed to flow until the urethra is full. Gently squeeze the meatus to keep jelly in the urethra.
3. If the catheter is passed and no urine is obtained, reposition the patient or gently apply suprapubic pressure. If urine is still not obtained, remove the catheter and notify the physician.
4. Blood may sometimes be noted in the urine after catheterization. Document this observation and notify the physician.
5. Grasp the penis firmly, because light stimulation could cause an erection. Should an erection occur, stop the procedure and matter-of-factly tell the patient that the catheterization can be done when the erection is gone. Cover the patient and leave him alone for a few minutes. Use a new catheterization set when the procedure is restarted.

## PROCEDURE 2-4
■
## Catheterization (female) to Obtain a Urine Specimen

### ■ PURPOSE

To obtain a urine specimen directly from the bladder that will be as free of contaminants as possible.

### ■ EQUIPMENT

Sterile disposable catheterization tray
Collection basin
Waterproof underpad
Sterile gloves
6 cotton balls
Forceps
Iodophor cleansing solution
Specimen container
Water-soluble lubricating jelly
Straight catheter, usually a 14 or 16 Fr
Proper lighting
Sheet

### ■ PROCEDURE

1. Explain the procedure to the patient.
2. Wash hands thoroughly.
3. Position the patient in the dorsal recumbent position with the knees flexed and feet resting about 2 feet apart. Drape with a sheet.
4. Provide light for good visualization.
5. In a convenient location near the patient, open the catheter tray using aseptic technique.
6. Open the appropriate catheter package and place the catheter on the sterile field.
7. Put on sterile gloves.
8. Remove the contents of the collection basin, keeping all equipment on the sterile field.
9. Pick up the waterproof underpad by two corners, folding the underpad over gloved hands. Place the underpad just under the patient's hips. Pull your hands out, taking care not to touch anything but the center of the sterile underpad to straighten it if needed.
10. Using the nondominant hand, separate the labia minora and maintain this position until catheterization is completed.
11. Use the forceps to pick up a cotton ball saturated with cleansing solution. Cleanse the inner surface of the far labia first by wiping toward the rectum with one stroke. Next, cleanse the inner surface of the near labia and then over the urethral meatus, each with one stroke and a clean cotton ball. Repeat with another three cotton balls.
12. Move the collection basin to the sterile underpad between the patient's legs.

**PROCEDURE 2-4** *Continued*

■
## Catheterization (female) to Obtain a Urine Specimen

13. Gently insert the catheter upward and backward into the meatus. Keep the drainage end of the catheter in the collection basin.
    a. Advance the catheter 8 cm (3 inches) until urine begins to flow. Then advance it another 2.5–5 cm (1–2 inches).
    b. If urine does not flow, slowly rotate the catheter. If urine is still not obtained, reposition the patient or gently apply suprapubic pressure.
    c. If the catheter enters the vagina, leave it in place as a guide when another catheter is inserted into the urethra.
    d. If the catheter passes into the urethra but urine does not return after these steps have been taken, stop the procedure and notify the physician.
14. When urine begins flowing
    a. Release the labia, but continue holding the catheter to prevent withdrawal of the catheter.
    b. Obtain specimen by allowing at least 30 mL of urine to flow from the catheter into the specimen container.
15. Collect the remaining urine in the basin. Withdraw the catheter slowly as urine flow decreases, and remove the catheter when urine stops dripping.
16. Close the specimen container, using care not to touch the inner surface of the lid.
17. Discard equipment and position the patient correctly. Label the specimen as indicated.

---

drip from the catheter into a sterile urine container (do not allow the catheter to touch the container). Reconnect the closed drainage system after the urine is obtained.

c. Send the urine specimen to the laboratory within 30 minutes. Routine urinalysis and urine cultures should be performed on fresh urine. If urine is left at room temperature for longer than 30 minutes, it undergoes changes that alter many test results. For example, there is an increase in the pH and a decrease in the glucose and ketone levels. The number of bacteria multiplies. Red blood cells and casts can disintegrate, especially in dilute alkaline urine. The color and clarity of urine are also affected.

d. If the urine specimen cannot be tested within 30 minutes, it should be preserved. Refrigeration for up to 24 hours is the most common method of preservation. This prevents bacterial growth and does not interfere with the chemical tests. However, refrigeration does increase the specific gravity and can cause precipitation of amorphous phosphates and urates. Many other methods of preserva-

tion involve the use of chemicals, such as formalin, boric acid, toluene, or commercial preservative tablets. None is ideal, because each interferes with some of the tests.

## URINALYSIS

For routine urinalysis, collect a first-voided morning specimen or a random specimen by using the midstream method of collection. Specimens from drainage bags are improper specimens, because the urine is not fresh and may contain contaminants from the drainage bag. Collect urine from the port on the tubing in catheterized patients, and use a drip collection method on patients with stomas. (Obtain a catheterized specimen if the patient is unable to assume the position for a drip collection or has a continent stoma.) Usually, at least 10 mL of urine is required.

### Color

The urine should be examined under good lighting against a white background. Normally, the urine color is yellow, owing to a pigment called *urochrome*. When describing alterations

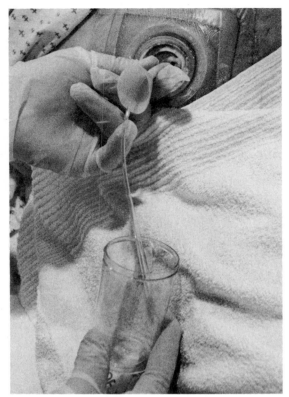

*FIGURE 2–11* Two-catheter technique to access urine from a stoma.

in urine color, use terms that are recognizable to everyone. *Red urine* does not always mean hematuria, but the most common cause of red urine is red blood cells. Many foods, drugs, and diseases can alter urine color (see Table 2–1). Patients with obstructive jaundice excrete bile pigments (bilirubin and biliverdin). In patients taking levodopa or methyldopa, the urine can turn red or red-brown in the toilet bowl if the bowl contains hypochlorite bleach.

## Clarity

The common terminology to report urine appearance is *clear, hazy, slightly cloudy, cloudy, turbid, smoky,* or *milky*. Normally, urine is clear, but clear urine does not always mean "normal" urine. The most common cause of cloudy urine is phosphaturia, a white precipitation of phosphates that occurs in alkaline urine. A pinkish precipitate is caused by precipitation of urates in acidic urine. Cloudy or turbid urine can be caused by white blood cells, red blood cells, bacteria, epithelial cells, colloidal particles, yeast, parasite disease, crystals, or fecal mate-

rial. Mucus can give urine a hazy color. Smoky or milky urine can be caused by prostatic fluid, lipids, blood, chyle, or sperm.

## Odor

Normally, urine is faintly aromatic. Types of abnormal odors include the following:

1. Fecal or sulfurous due to infection with colonic bacilli, for example, *Escherichia coli.*
2. Ammoniacal due to infection with urea-splitting organisms, for example, *Proteus* (urine left at room temperature also smells ammoniacal).
3. Pungent due to eating asparagus.
4. Sweet or fruitlike due to ketonuria.
5. Maple syrup due to maple syrup urine disease, a congenital metabolic disorder.
6. Strongly foul-smelling, usually a sign of infection with gross contamination with pus.

Normal urine produces a slight amount of foam when shaken. Excess foaming with shaking of the specimen is seen when the urine contains bilirubin or large amounts of protein.

## Specific Gravity

The concentration of urine reflects the kidney's ability to regulate fluid balance. Specific gravity measures urine concentration by measuring the density of urine compared with the density of distilled water, which has a density of 1.000 (1 mL distilled water weighs 1 g). The number, size, and weight of solutes in urine determine its density and therefore the specific gravity. Specific gravity can be determined by using a urinometer, refractometer, or other instruments.

The specific gravity of plasma filtrate as it enters the glomerulus is 1.010 (Strasinger, 1989). Urine that has the same specific gravity is *isosthenuric*. Urine that has a specific gravity less than 1.010 is *hyposthenuric* and is usually dilute. Urine with a specific gravity higher than 1.010 is *hypersthenuric* and is generally concentrated. Normally, the specific gravity is inversely proportional to the urine volume; that is, the larger the volume, the lower the specific gravity and vice versa.

Specific gravity can range from 1.003 to 1.035, with most random samples reading between 1.012 and 1.025 (Metheny, 1984). The elderly may have a decreased renal concentrating ability that lowers the upper limits. Values of 1.001 to 1.010 may be caused by fluid volume excess if renal function is normal or by those conditions associated with polyuria (see the section on changes or disturbances in voiding). A false-low value may be obtained when testing refrigerated urine using a urinometer. Values of 1.025 to 1.030 may be due to fluid volume deficit or decreased renal blood flow. A false-high reading may be due to urine temperature higher than 20°C (with urinometer) or the presence of pus, protein, glucose, radiographic contrast media, or dextran in the urine.

When urine contains abnormal constituents, such as albumin and glucose, the specific gravity is increased due to their larger size and weight. This yields a false-positive reading regarding the concentration (the number of solutes). Specific gravity is therefore only a crude indicator of fluid balance and renal concentrating ability in serious conditions. Serum and urine osmolality tests are more accurate in determining the actual dilution or concentration of urine compared with plasma.

A fixed specific gravity, one that remains about 1.010 no matter what the hydration state, indicates that the kidneys have lost the ability to concentrate urine. This is one of the first functions to be lost as a result of renal tubular damage.

## pH

Urinary pH measures the kidney's ability to maintain a normal hydrogen ion concentration in the plasma and extracellular fluid. It can be measured by dipstick or pH paper. Urine pH can range from 4.5 to 8.0 and normally fluctuates throughout the day. The first-voided morning specimen is usually 5.0 to 6.0.

Urine pH may be clinically significant in patients with urinary stone disease. Acidic pH favors formation of uric acid, cystine, and xanthine stones. Alkaline pH favors formation of ammoniomagnesium phosphate stones (struvite). Patients with uric acid stones rarely have a pH higher than 6.5 (uric acid is soluble in alkaline urine). Patients with calcium stones, nephrocalcinosis, or both, may have renal tubular acidosis and be unable to acidify urine at a pH lower than 6.0.

Possible causes of a low urine pH (in the strongly acidic range near 4.5) include the following:

1. Metabolic acidosis.
2. Uncontrolled diabetes mellitus (ketoacidosis).
3. Fever.
4. High-protein diet.

5. Medication use—ammonium chloride, mandelic acid.

Possible causes of high urine pH (in the strongly alkaline range, 7.5 and higher) include the following:

1. Presence of urinary tract infection by urea-splitting bacteria, for example, *Proteus.*
2. Metabolic alkalosis.
3. Hyperaldosteronism.
4. Cushing's syndrome.
5. Medication use—sodium bicarbonate, potassium citrate, thiazide diuretics, acetazolamide.
6. Low-protein diet high in vegetables, diet high in dairy products or citrus fruits.

The presence of glycosuria (glucose in urine) depends on the concentration of glucose in the blood, the GFR, and the degree of renal tubular reabsorption. Normally, only minute amounts of glucose are found in the urine, which are not detected by routine testing methods.

The renal threshold, the blood glucose level at which glucose spills into the urine, is usually around 160 to 180 mg/dL of blood. As the blood glucose level increases, so does the amount of glycosuria. The renal threshold may be lowered in renal disease and pregnancy (the patient may have a blood glucose lower than 160 mg/dL and still have glycosuria). It may be elevated in elderly patients with arteriosclerosis (the patient may have a blood glucose level higher than 180 mg/dL and have little or no glycosuria).

Urinary glucose can be determined by the dipstick or tablet testing method. Usually, the urine specimen is collected before meals and bedtime, and a fasting specimen is preferred in the morning. Many false-negative and false-positive results can occur as a result of interfering substances in urine (Strasinger, 1989; Pagana & Pagana, 1990). Any findings of glycosuria should be reported in terms of percentage.

Possible causes of glycosuria include the following:

1. Diabetes mellitus.
2. Pregnancy.
3. Impaired tubular reabsorptive capacity.
4. Endocrinopathies that may cause hyperglycemia, such as Cushing's syndrome and pheochromocytoma.
5. Administration of nephrotoxic agents.
6. Ingestion of large quantities of carbohydrates.

## Ketones

Ketones are metabolic end products of fat and protein metabolism. When the body does not have sufficient glucose to use for energy, fats are used and ketone excretion increases. Ketonuria (ketones in urine) signifies that the body is using fat as the major source of energy (incomplete carbohydrate metabolism).

Testing can be done using the dipstick or tablet testing method. Specimen collection is the same as for testing glucose. Normally, urine does not contain enough ketones to produce a positive result. Abnormal values are small (20 mg/dL), moderate (30–40 mg/dL), and large (80 mg/dL or higher). Symptomatic ketosis occurs at levels of about 50 mg/dL or higher. Ketones, which are acidic and use up the buffers in the blood stream, can cause a type of metabolic acidosis called *ketoacidosis*.

Causes of ketonuria include the following:

1. Diabetes mellitus.
2. Starvation.
3. Fasting.
4. High-protein diet—weight loss or fad diet, tube feeding high in protein.
5. Pernicious vomiting.

## Protein

Normally, protein is not present in urine, because the glomerular membrane is impermeable to the larger-sized protein molecules. Small amounts of lower-molecular-weight proteins are normally filtered at the glomerulus but are reabsorbed in the proximal tubules. If the glomerular membrane is injured, it becomes more permeable to protein, which seeps out into the glomerular filtrate and into the urine. Tubular dysfunction may result in decreased protein reabsorption.

The dipstick test registers 1+ when there is about 30 mg of protein in the specimen. Less than 30 mg causes a trace reading. Normal values show no more than 10 mg in a random sample. Quantitative protein testing may show as much as 150 mg in a 24-hour urine collection. False-positive readings by dipstick may result from highly alkaline urine, very concentrated urine, or urine containing many white blood cells or vaginal secretions.

Orthostatic or postural proteinuria is an apparently benign condition that occurs only when the patient is in an upright position. Normal levels of protein in the urine are found in specimens obtained before the patient gets out of bed in the morning. This is seen in about 5% of healthy people, usually in adolescent males. Possible causes of proteinuria include the following:

1. Cancer.
2. Severe heart failure.
3. Renal disease—nephrotic syndrome, glomerulonephritis, nephritis, diabetic nephropathy, polycystic kidney disease.
4. Multiple myeloma.
5. Operative trauma.
6. Collagen disease.
7. Fever, heavy exercise, and severe stress may cause transient proteinuria.

## Blood or Hemoglobin

Blood in the urine is in the form of intact red blood cells (hematuria) or hemoglobin, a product of red blood cell destruction (hemoglobinuria). Normally, neither is present in urine. Gross hematuria produces cloudy red urine and may produce clots. Large bulky clots usually implicate the bladder as a source of hematuria; long shoestring- or fishhook-shaped clots suggest bleeding from the upper urinary tract. Microscopic hematuria may produce no visible changes in urine color. Hemoglobinuria produces clear red urine. Intact red blood cells can be seen with a microscope, but free hemoglobin cannot be visualized. Both hematuria and hemoglobinuria are detectable by dipstick.

Hemoglobinuria can be caused by transfusion reactions, hemolytic anemia, severe burns, infections, and strenuous exercise (see Table 2–3 for causes of hematuria).

False-positive results with the dipstick method can be caused by the following:

1. High levels of ascorbic acid in urine.
2. Excessive amounts of urinary nitrite (associated with severe urinary tract infections).
3. Presence of bacterial enzymes, including *E. coli* peroxidase.
4. Contamination of urine with povidone-iodine.
5. Urinary myoglobin.

Urinary myoglobin can produce clear red urine and is associated with conditions of muscle destruction (myoglobin is a protein of muscle tissue). These conditions include muscle trauma, muscle-wasting diseases, prolonged coma, convulsions, and extensive physical exertion.

## MICROSCOPIC EXAMINATION OF URINARY SEDIMENT

Microscopic examination of the urinary sediment is a routine part of urinalysis. Urine is centrifuged in a test tube for 3 to 5 minutes to separate the sediment (which goes to the bottom of the test tube) from the rest of the urine. The urine is poured off, and the sediment is resuspended in a few drops of the urine. One drop of the sediment is placed on a glass slide, covered with a coverslip, and placed under the microscope for low- and high-power examination. Another drop of the sediment can be smeared on a second glass slide for staining.

## White Blood Cells

The normal value for the presence of white blood cells is 0 to 4 per high-power field. Pyuria, white blood cells in the urine, is not an absolute indicator of bacterial infection. Possible causes for increased numbers of white blood cells in the urine include the following:

1. Infection in the urinary tract—acute pyelonephritis, cystitis, urethritis.
2. Renal disease—acute or chronic interstitial nephritis.
3. Urinary stones.

## Red Blood Cells

A normal urinalysis may have 0 to 3 red blood cells per high-power field (see Table 2–3 for causes of hematuria).

## Urinary Casts

Cast formation results from agglutination of cells and the precipitation of protein present in the lumen of the distal tubules and collecting ducts. They are so named because their shape represents a "cast" of the lumen of the kidney tubule. Normally, the urine contains no casts, or a rare hyaline cast may be noted in a high-power field setting. The presence of casts signifies renal disease. Different types of casts result from different disease processes, as follows:

1. Hyaline casts may be of little clinical significance but may be associated with high fever, congestive heart disease, hypertension, eclampsia, diabetic coma, acute glomerulonephritis, collagen diseases, pyelonephritis, or extreme physical exertion.
2. Red blood cell casts suggest disease associated with bleeding within the nephron, such as glomerulonephritis and systemic lupus erythematosus.
3. White blood cell casts indicate a renal par-

enchymal inflammatory process, such as pyelonephritis.
4. Granular casts represent disintegrated epithelial cells, leukocytes, or protein and indicate renal tubular disease, such as chronic renal failure, acute glomerulonephritis, or a collagen disease.
5. Fatty casts may be a sign of a degenerative disease of the kidney, such as nephrosis, glomerulonephritis, or collagen disease.
6. Waxy casts may represent the final stages of degeneration of hyaline casts.
7. Broad casts reflect severe renal dysfunction and may be seen in renal failure that is characterized by an extremely low urine flow.

## Crystals

The presence of crystals is usually not clinically significant except in a few cases. Crystals may be found in patients with urinary stones, but can be found in the urine of healthy people as well. The presence of crystals often occurs in the acute phase of urinary stone disease, and the crystals often accurately reveal the type of stone present. The formation of crystals also varies with the urinary pH. For example, urate crystals can be found in acid urine, and phosphate crystals can be found in alkaline urine. Other crystals that may be noted include the following:

1. Cystine crystals, which are clinically significant because they are found in patients with familial cystinuria.
2. Struvite crystals, which are found in urine that is infected with urea-splitting bacteria.
3. Xanthine crystals, which may appear in patients who produce large amounts of purine or who are taking allopurinol.
4. Uric acid crystals, which may appear in acid urine and may be present in patients with uric acid stones.
5. Oxalate crystals, which are usually seen in acid urine and may be present in patients with oxalate stones.

## Bacteria

The significance of bacteria in the sediment depends on the method used to obtain the urine specimen. Several bacteria from a voided specimen not collected in a midstream clean-catch method from a woman may have little significance. Normally, no bacteria should be noted. If the specimen is properly collected and examined and several bacteria per high-power field are found, urinary tract infection is usually present. The findings of significant bacteriuria should be confirmed by culture.

*Mycobacterium tuberculosis* is identified in concentrated urine sediment by using acid-fast stains. Collect urine for acid-fast bacilli in a first-voided specimen.

## Epithelial Cells

Epithelial cells are derived from the cellular lining of the urinary tract, and small numbers, representing the normal sloughing of old cells, may normally be found in urine. They are an abnormal finding when found in large numbers or in abnormal forms. There are three types, as follows (Strasinger, 1989):

1. Squamous epithelial cells are seen most often and are least important. They originate from the lining of the vagina and the distal urethra in both sexes.
2. Transitional epithelial cells originate from the lining of the renal pelvis, the bladder, and the proximal urethra. The presence of large numbers of transitional cells with abnormal structure suggests cancer in the urinary tract.
3. Renal tubular epithelial cells appear in conditions causing tubular damage or necrosis, such as pyelonephritis, toxic reactions, and viral infections, or as a secondary effect of glomerulonephritis.

## URINE CULTURE

A urine culture estimates the number of bacteria in urine and identifies the exact organism present in the urine. Urine cultures are obtained on patients suspected of having a urinary tract infection and may also be done on patients preoperatively to rule out asymptomatic urinary tract infection.

The culture should be collected before antibiotics are begun. The midstream clean-catch method is used to collect any voided specimens for culture. A catheterized specimen may be ordered if the patient is unable to assume the position for the midstream clean-catch method or if vaginal contamination (either vaginal flora or menstrual blood) occurs with the voided specimen. Rarely, the physician may perform suprapubic aspiration to differentiate urethritis from cystitis in women.

The significance of the number of bacteria depends on the method used to collect the urine and how dilute the urine is. A lower col-

ony count on a catheterized specimen may be more significant, and any bacterial growth on a specimen obtained by suprapubic aspiration is significant. A general, but not absolute, rule is that a bacterial colony count of 10 or more bacteria per milliliter represents a clinical urinary tract infection. Lower counts do not exclude the possibility of an infection, especially if the patient is symptomatic. Cultures with multiple organisms usually signify contamination during collection.

## URINE CYTOLOGIC STUDY

Urine cytologic study (Papanicolaou examination) is done on patients with known or suspected cancer anywhere in the urinary tract. Urine is collected by a voided specimen or by doing bladder washings. Transitional epithelial cells that are present in large numbers or in clumps and that show an abnormal structure (such as large nuclei, multiple nuclei, or an increased ratio of nucleoplasm to cytoplasm) are indicative of cancer affecting the urothelium. Bladder tumors may shed cells more freely than do tumors in the upper urinary tract, and urine cytology is often done as a test for transitional cell carcinoma of the bladder.

# Renal Function Tests

## BLOOD UREA NITROGEN

Normal BUN levels range from 8 to 25 mg/dL. Both the BUN and the serum creatinine levels are obtained by venipuncture. Patients who have elevated BUN levels have *azotemia*, an increase in the nitrogenous wastes in the blood.

Urea is the major end product of protein metabolism and is excreted by the kidneys. Because the kidneys excrete urea, the BUN is used as a test for renal function. Diseased or damaged kidneys cause an elevated BUN because they have impaired ability to excrete urea. Extrarenal factors also influence the BUN level (Table 2–7). Any condition causing low renal blood flow, such as prerenal acute renal failure, dehydration, reduced cardiac output, and early shock, can elevate the BUN even though there is no fixed damage to the renal tubules. Because of the numerous extrarenal influences, BUN as a test for renal function is not as accurate as serum creatinine.

## SERUM CREATININE

Creatinine, a major end product of muscle metabolism, is filtered through the glomeruli and excreted by the kidneys. Daily production of creatinine is fairly constant, and in normal renal function, the creatinine level remains stable, because it is not affected by diet or other factors that affect BUN. (The exception is that serum creatinine may be affected by certain muscle diseases.) The normal levels range from 0.6 to 1.5 mg/dL in men and 0.6 to 1.1 mg/dL in women. The slightly higher normal level for men results from their greater muscle mass.

Because the serum creatinine level is usually unaffected by extrarenal factors, it is an accurate indicator of renal function. It is also a specific test for renal failure. An increase in the serum creatinine level indicates damage to nephrons, the functioning unit of the kidney. In conditions in which there is mild loss of renal function, such as in the early stages of renal insufficiency, the serum creatinine level is not as sensitive to changes in renal function (Table 2–8). In these instances, the creatinine clearance test provides more accurate information.

Renal disorders such as glomerulonephritis, pyelonephritis, acute tubular necrosis, and renal failure due to urinary obstruction cause an elevated serum creatinine level. Nephrotoxicity or hypersensitivity to certain drugs may cause an increase in both the BUN and serum creatinine levels. For this reason, BUN and serum creatinine levels may be measured at specific intervals during drug therapy, especially for aminoglycosides, to monitor for nephrotoxicity.

Because the serum creatinine level is changed only by renal dysfunction, it is not as sensitive an indicator as the BUN level for states of low renal perfusion (prerenal acute renal failure). Comparing the BUN with the creatinine ratio is often done to differentiate between different types of renal failure. The

**TABLE 2–7. Extrarenal Factors That Influence the Blood Urea Nitrogen Level**

Starvation
Sepsis
Fever
Gastrointestinal
   bleeding
Diet very high in protein
Dehydration
Cardiac failure

**TABLE 2–8. Comparison of Serum Creatinine Level With Estimated Loss of Nephron Function**

| CREATININE LEVEL | ESTIMATED LOSS OF NEPHRON FUNCTION |
|---|---|
| Normal creatinine (0.6–1.5 mg/dL) | Up to 50% loss |
| Creatinine level above 1.5 mg/dL | Over 50% nephron function loss |
| Creatinine level of 4.8 mg/dL | As much as 75% nephron function loss |
| Creatinine level about 10 mg/dL | 90% loss of nephron function—end-stage renal disease |

From Corbett, J. V. (1987). *Laboratory tests and diagnostic procedures with nursing diagnoses* (2nd ed., p. 87). Norwalk, CT: Appleton & Lange. Reprinted by permission.

normal ratio is about 10:1. In prerenal acute renal failure, the ratio increases to 20:1 or more.

## CREATININE CLEARANCE

The creatinine clearance test compares the serum creatinine level with the total amount of creatinine excreted in the urine for a specified amount of time. The usual period is 24 hours, but tests can be done over a shorter period. The urine is collected in a 24-hour specimen, and during the test period a serum creatinine level is measured. It is important to keep the patient well hydrated during the test for accuracy. The results may be falsely low if only part of the urine is collected over the timed period or if the serum specimen is not collected at the same time.

The creatinine clearance reflects the GFR (the number of milliliters of filtrate made by the kidneys per minute) and is the most accurate test for renal function without resorting to infusion of exogenous substances, such as inulin and radionuclides. The formula for determining creatinine clearance is (Corbett, 1987)

$$\frac{urine\ creatinine}{creatinine\ in\ serum} \times urine\ volume = creatinine\ clearance\ rate$$

The clearance rate is recorded as milliliters per minute. Additional calculations are done to correct for changes in body surface. Normal values for creatinine clearance in men are 95 to 135 mL/min and 85 to 125 mL/min in women. The values decrease slightly with age, even if no renal disease exists. A minimum creatinine clearance rate of about 10 mL/min is needed to live without dialysis.

A decreased creatinine clearance rate indi-

TABLE 2–9. Nephron Function: Reabsorption-Secretion Sites

| SUBSTANCE | GLOMERULUS | PROXIMAL TUBULE | LOOP OF HENLE | DISTAL TUBULE | COLLECTING DUCT |
|---|---|---|---|---|---|
| Sodium | | Reabsorbed | Reabsorbed | Reabsorbed | Secreted Reabsorbed |
| $K^+$ | | Reabsorbed | Reabsorbed | Reabsorbed Secreted | Reabsorbed Secreted |
| $HCO_3^-$ | | Reabsorbed | | Reabsorbed | |
| $H^+$ | | Reabsorbed Secreted | | Secreted | Reabsorbed Secreted |
| $Cl^-$ | | Reabsorbed | Reabsorbed | Reabsorbed | |
| $NH_3$ | | | | | Secreted Reabsorbed |
| Glucose | Reabsorbed | Reabsorbed | | | |
| $Ca^{2+}$ | | | Reabsorbed | | |
| Amino acids | Reabsorbed | Reabsorbed | | | |
| $H_2O$ | | Reabsorbed | | Reabsorbed | Reabsorbed |
| $PO_4$ | | Reabsorbed | | | |
| Urea | | Reabsorbed | | Reabsorbed | |

cates decreased glomerular function. In the early stages of renal insufficiency, relatively large decreases in clearance are reflected by small changes in serum creatinine levels. As renal failure advances, relatively small changes in clearance result in large changes in the serum creatinine level.

## Blood Studies

(See Appendix I for normal values of frequently ordered blood studies.)

When hemoglobin and hematocrit levels are decreased, it is important to determine whether the decrease is chronic or acute. Levels may be chronically decreased in anemia, which can occur in chronic renal failure, chronic pyelonephritis, and cancer. In chronic renal failure, anemia may become apparent when renal function decreases to a level that is 50% of normal. The major factor is decreased erythropoietin production by damaged nephrons. Levels may be acutely decreased in an acute blood loss, which can occur in renal trauma or severe hematuria. Altered values may also be indicators of fluid imbalance. The hematocrit level may be increased with fluid deficit and decreased with fluid excess. A specific increase in hemoglobin and hematocrit levels may be indicative of a paraneoplastic syndrome associated with renal cell carcinoma.

The red blood cell count is low in some types of anemia and in patients with bone marrow suppression due to chemotherapy or radiation therapy.

The white blood cell count may decrease during chemotherapy or radiation therapy, because these treatments suppress white blood cell production. A complete blood cell count is usually determined at periodic intervals on patients receiving chemotherapy or radiation therapy to monitor for bone marrow suppression. The white blood cell count is elevated with bacterial infection.

### CLOTTING STUDIES

Tests for prothrombin and partial thromboplastin times are routinely done to screen for coagulation disorders, particularly in patients with unexplained hematuria. Many medications can cause elevated or depressed readings. Radiation therapy and chemotherapy suppress platelet production. Purpuric lesions, prolonged bleeding from breaks in the skin, or bleeding from any body orifice is a manifestation of thrombocytopenia, a decreased platelet count. A decrease in the platelet count to $15,000/mm^3$ puts the patient at risk for spontaneous bleeding (Pagana & Pagana, 1990).

### ELECTROLYTES

Patients with renal disorders and other genitourinary diseases may experience alterations in fluid and electrolyte balance. These disturbances may be caused by the inability of the kidneys to maintain fluid and electrolyte balance or may be caused by other disease processes and events that affect renal function.

The fluid and electrolyte reabsorption-secretion sites are identified in Table 2–9. Additional information regarding renal physiology and renal function can be obtained from a nephrology resource.

# Examination of Urethral, Vaginal, and Prostatic Secretions

Examination of urethral, vaginal, and prostatic secretions may be performed when lower urinary tract infection or sexually transmitted disease is suspected. An examination is performed to localize the source of infection and determine the infecting organism. If the male patient complains of urethral discharge or dysuria, if a urethral discharge is observed during physical examination, or if a urethral discharge is expressed after the urethra is milked or stripped from the base of the penis to the urethral meatus, a specimen of the discharge is collected for either culture or microscopic examination (smear). To obtain a smear, a sterile cotton-tipped swab is gently inserted into the urethral meatus to collect the exudate. The swab is then rolled (not rubbed) on a glass slide (Corbett, 1987). If the urethral secretions are copious, a drop of the discharge may be collected directly on a glass slide. A Gram stain of the smear is done to detect the characteristic gram-negative diplococci of *Neisseria gonorrhoeae*, which correctly diagnoses gonorrheal infection in 95% of cases (Halsted & Halsted, 1981, pp. 856–857). Other special preparations of the slide may be done to detect organisms associated with nongonococcal urethritis.

To obtain a culture for *N. gonorrhoeae* in the male patient, the exudate is collected from the urethral meatus in the same manner. Depending on the availability of testing methods, a culture plate at room temperature is directly inoculated, a modified Thayer-Martin medium in a culture bottle is inoculated, or the swab is put in a sterile tube containing a nonnutritive transport medium to be tested in the laboratory (Halsted & Halsted, 1981, pp. 856–857). Other techniques are available to culture organisms for gonorrhea and other infections.

To collect prostatic secretions for culture or smear, the physician may perform prostatic massage. The prostate is located during rectal examination, and the entire posterior surface of the prostate is firmly stroked from its lateral margins toward the midline to express secretions into the urethra (DeGowin & DeGowin, 1981). The urethra is then stripped from the base of the penis to the urethral meatus to collect the secretions on a sterile cotton swab for culture or directly on a glass slide for smear. The glass slide is prepared and examined un-

der high-power field to detect white blood cells and bacteria. Samples for culture are sent to the laboratory to identify any bacterial growth. Prostatic massage is contraindicated in suspected cases of acute prostatitis, because manipulation of the prostate can cause bacteremia and sepsis.

If the urethral discharge or expressed prostatic secretions are scanty, multiple-bottle voids may be done. The secretions are washed out with the urine in different parts of the stream (see Procedure 2–2). The urine is then centrifuged, and the sediment is microscopically examined or cultured to identify infecting organisms.

To obtain a vaginal smear or culture, the patient is placed in the lithotomy position. A sterile cotton-tipped swab is inserted well into the vagina to collect the vaginal discharge or gently scrape the vaginal wall. The labia minora are held far apart, so the swab does not inadvertently touch them. If the test is for gonorrhea, an endocervical specimen is required, which necessitates the insertion of a speculum lubricated with water only (lubricant interferes with the test). Cervical mucus is first wiped away with a dry cotton ball; then a dry sterile cotton-tipped swab is placed into the endocervical canal and left in place for about 30 seconds to absorb the exudate (Corbett, 1987). A smear or culture is performed in the same manner as for urethral discharge. The endocervical smear in women is not as effective in determining the diagnosis of gonorrhea as is the urethral smear in men. Culture of the endocervical exudate is done for definitive diagnosis (Ravel, 1981, pp. 145–147). Tests for other organisms can involve using saline-soaked swabs, special culture media, or special preparation of the smear. For example, testing for *Trichomonas* involves using a saline-soaked swab and a wet-mount glass slide. Always refer to the laboratory's manual for specific instructions on conducting the tests.

To collect a specimen of urethral discharge from a female, a sterile cotton-tipped swab is placed into the urethral meatus to collect the secretions. The urethra can be massaged (by placing a gloved finger into the vagina and milking the urethra from the bladder base to the meatus through the anterior vaginal wall) to increase the amount of urethral secretions.

Oral or anal specimens for culture may also be obtained to test for gonorrhea in persons who engage in oral or anal intercourse.

## Collection of Semen for Analysis

Semen analysis is a routine test for evaluation of infertility. At least two semen analyses are required, at intervals of 2 to 4 weeks, because of normal variations in semen.

Instruct the patient to abstain from ejaculation for 2 to 5 days before the analysis. Prolonged abstinence decreases sperm quality and mobility (Beare et al., 1985). Ejaculation that occurs more often than every 2 days may reduce sperm concentration and semen volume (Shane et al., 1976). Ideally, the specimen is collected in the office or clinic by masturbation. The use of condoms or coitus interruptus (withdrawal) is usually not recommended as the collection method. The powder or lubricants in condoms may be spermicidal, and using a condom during intercourse to collect semen may damage the sperm (Beare et al., 1985). With coitus interruptus, the initial portion of the semen, which contains the highest number of sperm, may be lost (Shane et al., 1976). All the ejaculate is collected in a clean, dry, wide-mouthed container that is free of chemical or soap residue. The specimen is kept at room temperature and transported to the laboratory within 30 minutes of collection. A delay of longer than 1 hour after collection invalidates the testing, so always mark the time the specimen is collected on the container or the requisition. If the patient will be bringing the semen specimen from home, instruct him to wrap the container in a dry towel or washcloth to maintain the temperature of the semen. Stress that the specimen must be delivered to the laboratory within 30 to 60 minutes of collection (Urry, 1986) (see Chap. 13 for specific tests and normal values for semen analysis).

Semen analysis is also performed following a vasectomy to verify sterility. Because the only purpose is to verify the presence or the absence of sperm, testing is much less complex. Specimens are routinely tested starting 2 months postvasectomy and repeated every month until two consecutive monthly specimens are free of sperm (Strasinger, 1989).

## DOCUMENTATION

Documentation of assessment is a written record of what the patient said, what was observed, and what was found during the health history and physical examination. Meticulous care must be taken to ensure that documentation is accurate, concise, and complete. Several guidelines should be followed:

1. Document *all* the assessment data. Documentation may reveal clues or relationships to other professionals later that can lead to better patient care. Also, in a court of law, the medical record is crucial. If the facts are not documented, the implication is that the assessment was not done.
2. Know the standards of nursing care, and document accordingly. For instance, it is standard urologic nursing practice to document the quantity and the characteristics of urine draining from a catheter. These descriptions should be included in the data base.
3. Be sure to document the source of the assessment data. Was the history obtained from the patient or someone else? If it was from someone else, what is that person's relationship to the patient? Some data may be obtained from another source, such as a nursing home referral and medical record from another hospital, and this source should be identified.
4. Document significant negative responses and findings. For example, in a patient admitted with microscopic hematuria, if the dipstick urine shows no blood, that finding should be documented.
5. Do not interpret findings during assessment. An assessment finding can suggest many possible causes, and any interpretation of findings should wait until all data are collected. For example, observing the patient's voided urine to be red with clots is an assessment finding, but documenting it as hematuria is an interpretation of the finding. This may be inaccurate if the patient is a woman who is menstruating.
6. Use correct medical terminology. Avoid general terms like *good*, *poor*, and so forth. "Poor stoma color" provides little information, whereas "stoma dusky red with dark purple area extending from the os to the periphery from 5 to 8 o'clock" tells the reader much more. Use measurements when appropriate—the weight of the dressing or the size of the bruise in centimeters is more precise than "a large amount of drainage" or "a small bruise." Be familiar with the body's landmarks, imaginary lines, and quadrants, and use them in describing location.
7. Document the findings as soon as possible after the assessment.

# REFERENCES

American Nurses' Association. (1980). *Nursing: A social policy statement.* Kansas City: Author.

Bates, B. (1991). *A guide to physical examination* (5th ed.). Philadelphia: J. B. Lippincott.

Beare, P. G., Rahr, V. A., & Ronshausen, C. A. (1985). *Nursing implications of diagnostic tests* (2nd ed.). Philadelphia: J. B. Lippincott.

Corbett J. V. (1987). *Laboratory tests and diagnostic procedures with nursing diagnoses* (2nd ed.). Norwalk, CT: Appleton & Lange.

Corriere, J. N., Jr. (1986). *Essentials of urology.* New York: Churchill Livingstone.

Dalton, J. R. (1983). *Basic clinical urology.* Philadelphia: Harper & Row.

DeGowin, E. L., & DeGowin, R. L. (1981). *Bedside diagnostic examination* (4th ed.). New York: Macmillan.

Halsted, J. A., & Halsted, C. H. (1981). *The laboratory in clinical medicine* (2nd ed.). Philadelphia: W. B. Saunders.

Hanno, P. M., & Wein, A. J. (Eds.). (1987). *Manual of urology.* Norwalk, CT: Appleton-Century-Crofts.

King, R. C. (1983). Refining your assessment techniques. *RN,* February, 43–47.

Kozier, B., & Erb, G. (1991). *Fundamentals of nursing: Concepts, process, and practice* (4th ed.). Redwood City, CA: Addison-Wesley.

Metheny, N. (1984). *Quick reference to fluid balance.* Philadelphia: J. B. Lippincott.

Pagana, K. D., & Pagana, T. J. (1990). *Diagnostic tests and nursing implications* (3rd ed.). St. Louis: C. V. Mosby.

Ravel, R. (1981). *Clinical laboratory medicine.* Chicago: Year Book Medical Publishers.

Shane, J. M., Schiff, I., & Wilson, E. A. (1976). The infertile couple. *Clinical Symposia, 28*(5), 1–40.

Smith, D. R. (1992). *General urology* (13th ed.). Los Altos, CA: Lange Medical.

Strasinger, S. K. (1989). *Urinalysis and body fluids* (2nd ed.). Philadelphia: F. A. Davis.

Urry, R. (1986). Seminal fluid. In C. R. Kjeldsberg & J. A. Knight (Eds.), *Body fluids* (2nd ed.). Chicago: American Society of Clinical Pathologists Press.

# CHAPTER 3

# Perioperative Care of the Urologic Patient

■

*Sandra La Follette, Julie Wettlaufer, and Karen A. Karlowicz*

## OVERVIEW

In recent years, the function of the operating room nurse has expanded from circulating or scrubbing on a case to a more active, involved role—that of the perioperative nurse. Although the terms *operating room nurse* and *perioperative nurse* are used interchangeably, perioperative nursing, as discussed in this chapter, describes a more patient-oriented, personalized form of caregiving.

The perioperative period comprises the time before, during, and after surgery. The *preoperative period* begins when the patient is scheduled for surgery and ends when the induction of anesthesia commences. During this period, the nurse makes contact with the patient (before the surgical procedure) in a home or office visit, in a telephone call, or in the surgical suite. During the preoperative period, the nurse assesses and identifies the patient's needs so that individualized care specific to the planned urologic procedure can be initiated.

The *intraoperative period* begins with the induction of anesthesia and ends when surgery has been completed and patient care is transferred from the operating room nurse to the postanesthesia, intensive care, or primary nurse. During urologic surgery, the perioperative nurse implements the preoperative plan and assists with intraoperative procedures.

The *postoperative period* starts in the recovery room or intensive care unit and ends when the perioperative nurse makes a final or follow-up telephone call or visit with the patient. In this period the perioperative nurse evaluates the effectiveness of the preoperative teaching and intraoperative care.

This chapter focuses on approaches to urologic patient care during the perioperative period for adults and children. Information is organized and presented according to the three time frames within the perioperative period and includes a discussion of common complications of urologic surgical procedures. Most of the chapter is devoted to perioperative care of the urologic patient in the traditional environment of the hospital operating room. However, the impact of ambulatory surgical centers on advances in urologic surgery and the role of the perioperative nurse is also discussed.

## BEHAVIORAL OBJECTIVES

After studying this chapter, the reader should be able to

1. Describe the role of the perioperative nurse.
2. Anticipate questions about urologic surgery a patient or family member might ask the perioperative nurse.
3. Identify possible postoperative complications, including those resulting from patient positioning commonly used during urologic procedures.
4. Establish criteria to evaluate the outcome of the nursing care given by the perioperative nurse to a patient who has undergone urologic surgery.
5. Identify special needs of the pediatric patient undergoing urologic surgery.

## KEY WORDS

**Anesthesia**—an artificially induced insensibility to pain with or without the loss of consciousness.

**Contralateral**—situated on or pertaining to the opposite side.

**Current**—a movement of electricity analogous to the flow of water through a pipe.

**Dispersive electrode**—the accessory that directs current flow from the patient back to the generator; often called the patient plate, return electrode, inactive electrode, ground plate, or ground pad (AORN, 1985).

**Hyponatremia**—a serum sodium level lower than 125 mEq/L.

**Intubation**—the insertion of a tube; as related to surgery, the insertion of a tube into the larynx through the glottis for the administration of anesthetic gases.

**Ipsilateral**—situated on or pertaining to the same side.

**Lithotomy position**—lying on the back with the legs raised and abducted to expose the perineal area.

**Regional anesthetic**—a temporary interruption of sensory nerve conductivity to any region of the body by injection of a local anesthetic.

**Supine position**—lying on the back.

## CARE OF THE UROLOGIC PATIENT IN THE PREOPERATIVE PERIOD

The preoperative period begins when the patient is scheduled for surgery and ends with the induction of anesthesia. Preparation for care begins as soon as the perioperative nurse is aware of the necessity of surgery for the patient.

Initially, the perioperative nurse reviews the patient's record for medical information, including physical examination and diagnostic tests and studies. An interdisciplinary approach involving other members of the health care team facilitates the assessment of the patient's physical status and emotional response to the diagnosis, treatment, and impending surgery. A complete collection of personal data is important in preparation for a preoperative visit or telephone call. However, it is also helpful for the nurse to be familiar with the surgical procedure planned, including special techniques or equipment the urologist may use.

### Preoperative Visit and Teaching

The preoperative visit is an opportunity for the nurse to interview and assess the physical condition of the patient and to familiarize the patient with the operating room environment and routine. This visit also provides a chance for the nurse to teach patient skills that enhance recovery. Ideally, the nurse would meet personally with the patient within a week or two before the planned surgery. However, in the ambulatory surgery setting for urologic procedures, the preoperative contact is often initiated by telephone and continued when the patient is admitted to the ambulatory surgical center the day of surgery.

The role of the urologic nurse and the care activities that occur during the preoperative period are essentially the same as those in other surgical specialties. Nursing care goals are universal and are related to the following:

1. Collection of physiologic data that may be used for comparative purposes during the intraoperative and postoperative periods.
2. Identification of problems requiring nursing intervention throughout the perioperative period.
3. Assessment of the physical preparations for surgery.

4. Determination of the psychological response to and readiness for surgery.
5. Initiation of patient teaching related to the surgical experience.

It is helpful to follow a format that organizes activities and data collection during the preoperative visit (Table 3–1). A variety of forms are available to use in establishing what information should be obtained during assessment.

Throughout the preoperative visit, the nurse decides how much information and teaching the patient and family require. Research findings indicate that well-prepared patients experience less difficulty during anesthesia and have fewer postoperative complications with a shorter postoperative stay than do patients who do not receive preoperative instruction or have the opportunity to discuss their fears and anxieties related to surgery (Gelfant, 1986).

Teaching should begin early in the preoperative period to allow time for patient learning. Preadmission teaching has been shown to be most effective and may be accomplished with a variety of teaching formats. Individual or group instruction, books, pamphlets, and audio-visual presentations all may be employed. The use of a particular teaching strategy depends on the patient's educational level and physical condition, the urologic procedure planned, the date of surgery, and the availability of information. Urologic nurses are fortunate that a variety of patient education materials are widely available, many of which may be used for preoperative teaching. The reader is referred to subsequent chapters for specific preoperative teaching information related to the various surgical procedures employed to treat urologic conditions.

### Preoperative Checklist

To verify preoperative routines and orders, the perioperative nurse must complete a preoperative checklist. Recording of information on this form is initiated before the patient is transported to the operating room. The content and organization of the preoperative checklist vary among facilities; however, all versions include information concerning essential preoperative laboratory results, preoperative preparations undertaken, and safety measures implemented.

## TABLE 3–1. Guidelines for Preoperative Assessment

1. Introduce yourself
2. Identify the purpose of the assessment
   a. To obtain information that will be helpful in planning care in the operating room
   b. To answer questions and concerns about the surgical experience
3. Determine the patient's general knowledge of the intended surgery and the need or desire for additional or supplemental information
4. Explain the routine for the day of surgery
   a. Absence of food or fluid
   b. Premedication
   c. Time to arrive at the hospital
   d. Transportation to operating room (i.e., time and mode)
   e. Location and anticipated length of wait prior to being taken into the operating room
   f. Special skin preparations
5. Familiarize the patient with what he or she will see and experience in the operating room
   a. Operating room lights and table
   b. Accessory equipment
   c. Temperature of the room
   d. Intravenous fluids
   e. Blood pressure cuff
   f. Electrocardiogram monitoring
6. Tell the patient, family, and significant others
   a. Time to arrive at the hospital
   b. Where they should wait during surgery
   c. Restaurant facilities
   d. Anticipated length of time in the operating room and the recovery room
7. Explain the postanesthesia care
   a. Location of PACU
   b. Purpose of the PACU
   c. Routines of postanesthesia care (i.e., vital signs, checking dressings)
   d. Identify anticipated dressings, drains, catheters, packs, casts, traction

8. Discuss any relevant physical problems with the patient to determine the focus of the intraoperative care plan (visual or hearing alterations, joint, or muscle immobility)
9. Formulate a written assessment and individual nursing care plan
   a. Discuss relevant information with the unit nurse
   b. Make an entry on the patient's chart that a preoperative assessment was completed
   c. Formulate a nursing diagnosis, identify expected outcome, and prescribe nursing action
10. Other considerations
   a. Establish an atmosphere of confidence and a climate of acceptance
   b. Give the patient ample opportunity to ask questions or verbalize concerns
   c. Be aware of nonverbal communication
   d. Allow the patient to decide if family or significant others should remain during the interview
   e. Avoid conflict or judgment or instilling false encouragement
   f. Determine the patient's comprehension and use appropriate language; avoid jargon
   g. Write individual care plan after leaving patient's room

PACU, postanesthesia care unit.
From Groah, L. K. (1990). *Operating room nursing: Perioperative practice.* (2nd ed., p. 107). Norwalk, CT: Appleton & Lange. Reprinted by permission.

## CARE OF THE UROLOGIC PATIENT IN THE INTRAOPERATIVE PERIOD

The intraoperative period begins with the induction of anesthesia and ends when patient care is transferred from the operating room nurse to the postanesthesia, intensive care, or primary nurse. During the intraoperative period, the nurse helps maintain a safe environment for the patient by implementing measures to prevent skin breakdown (e.g., from improper positioning) and wound contamination by bacteria or foreign objects. In addition, the nurse is responsible for keeping a record of intraoperative events and providing supplies and assistance to the surgical team.

Nursing care concerns in the intraoperative period of urologic surgery relate to the use of anesthesia, patient positioning, skin preparation, draping, electrical safety, and blood loss. Each of these issues is discussed separately in the following sections.

## Anesthesia

Various types of anesthesia are used during the intraoperative period that cause partial or complete loss of sensation (Table 3–2). General anesthesia, used for extensive procedures (e.g., radical cystectomy), causes a loss of consciousness in the patient and is usually achieved by inhalation agents, intravenous medication, or both. In contrast, regional anesthesia does not cause the patient to lose consciousness because

**TABLE 3–2. Anesthesia Used for Selected Urologic Procedures***

| TYPE OF ANESTHESIA | PROCEDURE | COMMENTS |
|---|---|---|
| Local application | Cystoscopy<br>Urethral dilation<br>Ureteral stent placement | 2% lidocaine jelly is introduced into the urethra with applicator tip affixed to tube or with blunt-tip syringe; penis clamp may be used to help retain anesthetic |
| Intradermal and subcutaneous infiltration | Vasectomy<br>Vasovasotomy<br>Transperineal prostate biopsy | |
| Penile block | Circumcision<br>Penile biopsy<br>Laser ablation of penile lesions | When performed on adult males; also reported to be beneficial in newborns |
| Spinal or epidural block | Endoscopic suspension of vesical neck<br>Transurethral bladder procedures<br>Transurethral prostate procedures<br>Ureteroscopy/stone extraction | Sensory anesthesia to level of T10 required; may need to augment with other anesthetic agents |
| General | All open procedures | |

*This table illustrates the type of anesthesia that may be used for various urologic procedures. It is **not inclusive** of all approaches to anesthesia or all procedures.

the medication is administered by injection into the area to be operated on. This inhibits excitement of the nerve endings and produces a loss of sensation. Local anesthetic agents are administered either topically or by infiltration to block nerve impulses and produce analgesia within tissues in a limited area.

All types of anesthesia require that the nurse be present during administration to assist the patient by offering comfort, explanations when necessary, and reassurance. The nurse may be required to assist the anesthetist by providing equipment and drugs and support in positioning the patient, regulating intravenous fluids, monitoring patient vital signs, and observing the well-being of the patient.

## GENERAL ANESTHESIA

When a patient undergoes general anesthesia, the perioperative nurse should be aware of the stages of anesthesia and the physiologic reaction of the patient during each stage. There are four stages that may evolve, including relaxation, excitement, operative anesthesia, and danger. Each stage dictates the type of action required by the nurse.

The first stage of anesthesia is *relaxation,* when the patient appears sleepy and his or her speech starts to slur. The patient is very sensitive to sounds during this time; therefore, the noise in the room should be minimized. Patient safety is important throughout all stages, necessitating the placement of the safety strap across the patient's thighs just above the knees before induction begins. In the *excitement stage,*

the patient's arms and legs may move involuntarily. The circulating nurse must be available to help restrain the limbs and protect the patient from injury. At the beginning of the *operative anesthesia stage,* the anesthetist lightly touches the patient's eyelid, and if the patient does not respond with a twitching eyelid, then the operation begins. The patient may or may not be intubated at this time, depending on the length of the operation planned. The *danger stage* of anesthesia is not anticipated as part of the usual surgical experience, but as with all emergencies, the perioperative nurse must be prepared to assist in the treatment of cardiac or respiratory arrest.

## REGIONAL ANESTHESIA

In selected urologic procedures, a local anesthetic agent may be administered to produce regional anesthesia. These drugs may be given by spinal or epidural injection, nerve block, infiltration, or topical application. Local anesthetic agents are less expensive than general anesthetic agents, are less restrictive to normal body function, and generally do not cause nausea and vomiting.

This type of anesthesia is used for ambulatory surgery in adults; it may be preferred in the elderly in whom general anesthesia may be contraindicated because of cardiac or pulmonary problems. The use of local anesthetics requires that patients be cooperative and not overly apprehensive about the surgery. For this reason, regional anesthesia is not usually advantageous for young children.

Complications—most often, a toxic reaction to the drug—can occur after the administration of a local anesthetic. The nurse should be alert for signs of emotional excitability, twitching, increased pulse rate, decreased blood pressure, pallor, or respiratory difficulties and be prepared to intervene quickly to restore the patient to normal cardiovascular and respiratory status.

## Positioning for Urologic Procedures

Urologic surgery requires a variety of patient positions to provide adequate exposure of the operative site. Under anesthesia or heavy sedation, all positions are potentially hazardous because the patient cannot voice his or her discomfort. The perioperative nurse who assists in positioning the patient must have an understanding of anatomy and physiology to protect the patient from harmful effects on any part of the body (Table 3–3). The goal of positioning is to maintain unobstructed respiration and circulation. Therefore, the patient needs protection from malalignment or insufficient padding of body parts to avoid numbness, tingling, weakness, or nerve palsy.

Proper patient positioning is required for the following reasons:

1. Optimum exposure of the operative site.
2. Access for the anesthetist to maintain the patient's circulatory and respiratory function.
3. Access for the administration of intravenous solutions.
4. Protection of neuromuscular and skeletal structures.
5. Minimal interference with circulation.
6. Physiologic alignment.
7. Comfort and safety of the patient.
8. Preservation of the patient's dignity (La Follette, 1988).

Most attention is directed toward positioning the surgical patient's extremities and other body parts; however, an anesthetized patient's facial features also should be protected. To protect the cornea, many anesthetists place a small amount of bland ophthalmic ointment in the patient's eyes. If the patient's head is turned to one side, the ear on the underside should be in a natural position and not folded away from the head. If a nasogastric tube has been inserted, careful taping is needed to prevent ala nasi scarring.

There is much for the perioperative nurse to

---

#### TABLE 3–3. Guidelines for Nursing Actions in Positioning All Patients

1. The anesthetized patient is never moved without checking with the anesthesiologist.
2. To prevent damage to the brachial plexus, arms are never abducted beyond 90 degrees.
3. Legs must not be crossed, as this creates pressure on blood vessels and nerves.
4. Body surfaces should not be in contact with one another.
5. Hands and feet should be protected and not allowed to hang off the table.
6. The patient should not be touching any metal part of the table. If the elbow rests on the table edge, ulnar nerve damage may result.
7. Patient exposure is limited to the area required for the surgical procedure.
8. If the patient is conscious, all activities as well as the rationale should be explained.
9. The instrument table, the Mayo stand, or other equipment should not be in contact with the patient's toes or legs.
10. During the surgical procedure, if the Mayo stand, the instrument table, or the operating table is moved, the patient must be checked for pressure points.
11. Movement of the anesthetized patient is done gently and slowly. Turning the patient too quickly may cause circulatory depression.
12. To ensure the patient's safety, adequate numbers of personnel must always be present when positioning the patient. The patient is lifted into position, never pushed or pulled.
13. When moving an anesthetized patient, the anesthesiologist guards the endotracheal tube and protects the patient's head and neck.
14. The position must not obstruct any catheters, tubes, or drains.
15. Team members should be reminded not to lean on the patient.
16. If the surgical procedure is unilateral, the consent form and the x-ray films should be checked and the proper side exposed.
17. If the surgical procedure is on an extremity, such as an amputation, both extremities should be exposed for comparison.
18. All equipment used in positioning patients is padded and terminally disinfected after use.
19. The patient's position is documented as part of the intraoperative nursing notes.

From Groah, L. K. (1990). *Operating room nursing: Perioperative practice* (2nd ed., p. 261). Norwalk, CT: Appleton & Lange. Reprinted by permission.

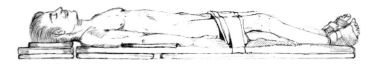

**FIGURE 3–1** Patient in supine position. Note donut at head; elbow pad; padded strap across anterior thighs (2 in. above the knees); egg crate pads for heels; and pillow to knees and calves for slight flexion at 15 degrees. (Drawing by Helen O. Corallo, BSN, RN, CNOR.)

check in ensuring the safety of the patient. A quick head-to-toe visual appraisal after the patient is positioned provides reassurance that the patient's safety needs have been met.

The most common positions used in urologic surgery are described in the following sections.

## SUPINE POSITION

The supine position is used for procedures such as cystectomy, prostatectomy, urethral repairs in males, and kidney transplant. Induction of anesthesia is done with the patient in the supine position (Fig. 3–1); the patient is then repositioned, if necessary, to provide for the optimal surgical approach. The patient's head should be placed on a doughnut or a towel to keep the neck aligned with the spine. Placing a small pillow under the knees makes some patients comfortable and provides slight flexion of the legs, relieving some of the pressure on the spine. Slight separation of the feet gives access to the genitalia and also is a reminder to check the position of the testicles, particularly in older men with copious scrotal skin. Protection of the heels with egg-crate–type padding is required if a long operation is anticipated or if the patient's age or condition warrants extra caution. The safety strap is positioned above the knees, and a blanket is placed between the belt and the patient's skin. Improper placement of the patient's arms

next to the body can cause injury to the median, ulnar, or radial nerve. This problem can occur if the arms are allowed to drape over the side of the operating room bed and come in contact with pressure from the parts of the bed. Postoperative problems may occur if the palm of the hand is turned up and rotated away from the body or if someone from the sterile team inadvertently presses against a unsecured arm. The patient's arms should be on the bed, at the side, palms toward the body, and the fingers should be in a natural position. The properly positioned arms should then be secured with a draw sheet. If the arms are placed on armboards, the nurse should be certain that the armboards are securely attached to the bed and that the arms are not hyperextended to avoid the possibility of a brachial plexus injury. Protective elbow pads may be required, depending on the length of the operation and the age and condition of the patient.

## LITHOTOMY POSITION

The lithotomy position is used for procedures such as urethrovesical suspension, cystoscopy, and perineal prostatectomy. It is often used for urologic surgery in adults (Fig. 3–2). However, because pediatric patients may not "fit" in the standard stirrups, the frog-leg adaptation may be used for this group. The lithotomy position is the position of choice for a

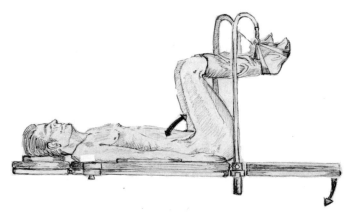

**FIGURE 3–2** Patient in lithotomy position. Note donut at head; elbow pad and padded armboard; candy cane stirrups, pillow cases; angle at hip, not so acute as to impinge on abdomen, lungs, or blood vessels; and buttocks to end of break in table. (Drawing by Helen O. Corallo, BSN, RN, CNOR.)

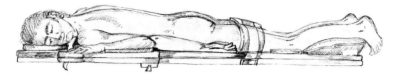

**FIGURE 3–3** Patient in prone position. Note donut at head; double view of arms at side on padded armboard and egg crate; padded safety strap; donut at knees; pillow at shins; and feet and toes free. (Drawing by Helen O. Corallo, BSN, RN, CNOR.)

short procedure like cystoscopy. At other times, it may be used in a quite lengthy surgical operation. Some urologic surgeons use this position for anterior exenteration.

During cystoscopy, the patient's arms may be gently positioned across the chest and held in place by the inverted patient gown. The patient's elbows should be resting on the table and should not be dangling over the side. If the arms are at the sides, extra precautions should be taken to prevent the patient's fingers being pinched in the gap created when the table's bottom is lowered and then raised again after the procedure. Leg warmers or pillow cases are placed on the legs to provide warmth and skin protection and to prevent cross-contamination of the stirrups from one patient to the next. Elastic bandages, antiembolic stockings, or a sequential compression device may be used, if the surgery is lengthy, to help prevent thrombophlebitis postoperatively.

In positioning, the patient's buttocks are placed at the end of the break in the table. Putting the legs in stirrups requires two people raising the legs simultaneously onto or into leg stirrups, which have been placed evenly on the table. Each positioner grabs the sole of a foot in one hand and supports the leg near the knee with the other hand. Both legs are then gently flexed toward the patient's abdomen and placed in stirrup straps (if the "candy cane" type is being used) or onto well-padded knee supports. Unpadded or misplaced stirrups can damage the saphenous and peroneal nerves and predispose the patient to venous thrombosis. Damage to the part of the peroneal nerve located on the outer or lateral aspect of the knee (also called the lateral popliteal nerve) can cause foot drop. Sensory disturbances to the inner aspects of the leg may result from pressure on the femoral and obturator nerves in the groin (Groah, 1990). This complication may result from exaggerated abduction of the legs or from pressure caused by a surgical team member leaning on the patient's leg.

At the end of the procedure, both of the pa-

tient's legs are lifted off the stirrups simultaneously, brought gently toward the chest, and then slowly lowered to the end of the table. In the lithotomy position, blood may pool in the lower body and return too quickly to the legs, if they are lowered to the supine position too rapidly, thus causing a decrease in the patient's blood pressure (Groah, 1990).

## PRONE POSITION

The prone position is used for procedures such as bilateral adrenalectomy and percutaneous nephrolithotomy. Few operations in urology require the prone position, but for those that do, preparation and anticipation are essential in establishing and maintaining this position in a safe manner (Fig. 3–3).

First, the patient is intubated on the gurney, stretcher, or bed on which he or she is brought to the operating room. The endotracheal tube is taped securely in place. Using good body mechanics, at least four people turn and move the patient onto two longitudinally placed chest rolls on the operating room table. This movement is done slowly to allow the patient's cardiovascular system to adjust to the change in position. Rapid turning of the patient can result in hypotension (Groah, 1990). The chest rolls allow for lung expansion and should extend from the shoulder to the iliac crest on either side of the chest (Ricker, 1991). A pillow is placed under the patient's calves, close to the ankles, to prevent pressure on the toes and to avoid hyperextension of the ankles.

The anesthetist should protect the patient's face from pressure, with special attention paid to the downward eye and ear lying on the head support (Tobias, 1980). The head support keeps the neck in line with the rest of the spine. The arms can be placed on armboards or tucked at the patient's side. If the arms are resting on armboards, the elbows should be flexed and padded; the palms of the hands should be facing downward to prevent overextension at the shoulders (Ricker, 1991).

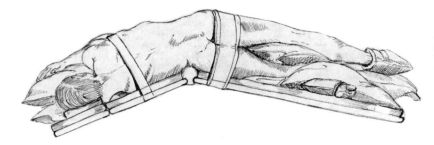

**FIGURE 3–4** Patient in lateral position. Note head on donut; pillows between arms; tape to secure torso; padded safety strap; axillary roll; pillows between legs; heel pads bilaterally; and pillows to dependent legs. (Drawing by Helen O. Corallo, BSN, RN, CNOR.)

A final assessment by the nurse includes checking for any pressure areas that might need extra padding. A blanket should be placed over the lower portion of the body, and the safety strap should be placed above the knees.

## LATERAL POSITION

The lateral position is used for procedures such as nephrectomy, nephrostomy tube insertion, and pyeloplasty. This position is often used for operations on the kidney and upper ureter (Fig. 3–4). The patient is placed on the table with the operative side up and the kidney area above the break in the table. To avoid pressure on the down (contralateral) arm, a small roll is placed just below the axilla, and the arm is placed on an armboard. The up (ipsilateral) arm can be positioned comfortably on a Kraus armrest, pillows, or a double armboard, suspended in a sling hanging from the ether screen, or placed on a padded Mayo stand.

A positioning mattress, which conforms to the patient's contours, padded table braces, sandbags, or body rolls can be used to maintain the patient in the lateral position. The contralateral leg is flexed at the knee, and the top leg is left straight. Pillows are used as padding between the thighs and as support for the top leg.

The kidney rest is raised, and the table is flexed to "open" the area between the 12th rib and the iliac crest. The degree of elevation of the kidney rest depends on the patient's physiologic reaction to this maneuver, because it can create pressure on the area of the inferior vena cava (Ricker, 1991).

## THORACOABDOMINAL POSITION

The thoracoabdominal position is used for procedures such as radical retroperitoneal lymph node dissection, radical nephrectomy, or those done on structures in the retroperitoneum. The abdomen and the peritoneal cavity can also be accessed if necessary. This position is similar to the lateral position, but it does not require rolling the patient completely onto the contralateral side (Fig. 3–5). The chest is rotated to a 30-degree angle in relation to the

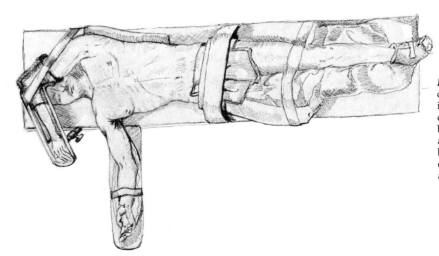

**FIGURE 3–5** Patient in thoracoabdominal position. Note head in alignment with spine; arm on operative side on adjustable board and elbow pad; opposite arm on elbow armboard; pillows between legs; and heel pads bilaterally. (Drawing by Helen O. Corallo, BSN, RN, CNOR.)

operating room table surface. A rolled sheet is tucked under the draw sheet at the patient's ipsilateral flank to help maintain the position. The contralateral leg is bent, and a pillow is placed between the two legs so that the skin surfaces are not in contact and the ipsilateral leg is supported. Heel protectors may be of some benefit. The ipsilateral arm is placed on a padded Kraus armrest, and the other arm is placed in a relaxed position on an armboard. A roll is not needed under the axilla, because the angle of the torso is so slight that there is little pressure on the shoulder (Scardino, 1982).

The patient is held in position at the shoulders, hips, and calves by wide adhesive tape. The genitalia are covered with a towel. A final assessment by the perioperative nurse should include verification that both feet are supported by the operating bed, the contralateral arm is in a natural position on the armboard and not in contact with any metal part from the Kraus armrest, which is supporting the opposite arm, and the patient's neck is aligned with the spine. The lower body may be covered with a light blanket before draping, if desired.

## Skin Preparation

Preparing the patient's skin for an incision requires two steps: the removal of hair and the use of an antimicrobial agent to clean the appropriate area. Some controversy surrounds the first step of skin preparation, including when to shave (the night before the operation, the morning of, or immediately before); how much to shave (just the line of incision or the surrounding area in case the incision has to be extended); and where to shave (in the patient's room, the holding area, or the operating room). According to the 1992 Association of Operating Room Nurses *AORN Standards and Recommended Practice for Perioperative Nursing,* removal of hair should be done only as necessary. In fact, the least amount of shaving done, the better—nonremoval is best. Additionally, the AORN standards suggest that shaving should be done as close to the incision time as possible, in a place that affords privacy and good lighting; the wet shave method is preferred. It is best that shaving be done outside the operating room to prevent hairs from hanging in the air or on the patient's skin and acting as a contaminant to the sterile field.

The object of preoperative skin preparation is to reduce the numbers of microbes on the skin and inhibit their growth, thereby aiding in the prevention of wound infection. The antimicrobial agent used ("prep" solution) is usually the surgeon's choice. There is no proof that one solution is superior to another in preventing wound infection. The perioperative nurse should interview the patient before surgery to determine whether the patient has ever experienced any sensitivity to the prep solution that is used. When scrubbing the incision and the surrounding area, the nurse must be aware that pooling of the solution under the patient could cause skin irritation. This problem can be prevented by using sterile towels to absorb the excess solution. Documentation on the operative record and perioperative nurses notes should include pertinent information concerning the preoperative preparation of the patient's skin.

## Draping

Draping is done to provide a sterile field by separating the microbial-free incisional area from the remainder of the unprepped skin area.

Drapes, as with all materials on the sterile field, should be handled as little as possible to avoid contamination and the possibility of making lint airborne. In urologic procedures, drapes can also be effective in maintaining modesty.

## Electrical Safety

During many urologic procedures, the electrosurgical unit (ESU) is used for cutting and coagulation of body tissues. Protecting the patient from any hazards the ESU may present is a responsibility of the perioperative nurse. Maintenance, inspection, and testing of the ESU are usually provided by the institution's biomedical department, but the nurse should be familiar with basic electrosurgery procedures and the possible consequences of deviating from the manufacturer's user manual.

The ESU functions by delivering an electrical current when it is activated by the operator. The current flows from the machine through the electrical cord and to the active electrode, including the pointed tip, loop (in the case of transurethral resection of the prostate [TURP] or bladder tumor); Bugbee, or roller electrode. The current then travels to patient tissue and eventually back to the machine. The safe mode of return of the current to the machine is through the dispersive electrode (ground pad). The ground pad should be placed on a muscular, hairless, dry part of the patient as close to the area of the incision as possible. Bony prominences and skin folds should be avoided. If the patient is not making good skin contact with the ground pad, the current from the ESU machine may find another mode of ground (through the electrocardiograph electrodes, a place where the patient makes contact with the operating room table, or an instrument that is in contact with the patient). If the current does not return to the machine through a large grounding pad, an electrical burn may result, because excessive heat builds up in a small concentrated area.

## Blood Loss

The circulating nurse helps the anesthetist record blood loss by showing the sponges periodically or weighing them in the case of pediatric surgery or surgery on the critically ill. The scrub nurse should tell the anesthetist when an irrigation solution is used so that the amount can be deducted from the blood and fluid in the suction bottle. Accurate recording of blood loss is important in determining the requirement for timely blood replacement.

## CARE OF THE UROLOGIC PATIENT IN THE POSTOPERATIVE PERIOD

### General Considerations

The postoperative period starts when the patient leaves the operating room and ends the last time the perioperative nurse has contact with the patient. As plans are initiated to transfer the patient from the operating room to the recovery area the perioperative nurse should anticipate the patient's immediate postoperative needs, based on the type of surgery the patient has undergone. These needs may be met by the perioperative nurse or relayed to the postanesthesia or primary care nurse.

On patient transfer, the perioperative nurse reports the type of anesthetic the patient received, how long the operation lasted, the position in which the patient was placed for surgery, and any unusual occurrences during surgery. The location and status of any drains, catheters, lines, or dressings are also reported.

Information such as patient allergies, mobility and hearing limitations, and unusual laboratory, radiographic, or respiratory or cardiac findings should also be conveyed.

Fluid management is critical in the immediate postoperative period. To maintain an accurate record of intake and output measurements, the perioperative nurse should report any urine discarded, any dressing reinforced, or any bagged drainage sites emptied; and the output of closed-suction drainage receptacles, chest drainage systems, and nasogastric tube. The anesthetist formally keeps track of blood loss and reports to the postanesthesia nurse the amount of preoperative and intraoperative fluid therapy received by the patient, including colloid and crystalloid solutions and blood products.

Maintaining the patency of the lines, tubes, drains, and catheters for the regulation of intake and the measurement of output in the postoperative urologic patient is a major responsibility of the postanesthesia nurse. Mucus or blood can clog the tubings and inhibit urine flow. The nurse may find it necessary to milk or gently irrigate a catheter with sterile normal saline. This procedure is done after the tubing has been checked for kinks that may be the cause of the obstruction and after an order from the physician has been obtained. The surgeon should be notified immediately if a tube's patency cannot be re-established. Proper attention and care prevent a catheter from becoming so obstructed that it has to be replaced.

An agitated, restless patient should not be ignored; the complaints may necessitate nursing intervention to relieve pain and discomfort. Bladder spasms are commonly experienced after urologic surgery. Relief may be obtained with the administration of a belladonna and opium suppository (unless contraindicated). Other analgesics, ordered by the physician, may also be required to diminish discomfort at the surgical site.

Complaints about abdominal pain, rigidity, or distention and changes in vital signs should alert the postanesthesia nurse to the possible development of other, more serious postoperative complications. Acute problems such as ileus, thrombophlebitis, pulmonary embolism, shock, transfusion reaction, and dilutional hyponatremia can occur after urologic surgery.

No matter how minor the surgery seems, the danger of postoperative complication is always present. In addition to those complications previously mentioned, infection, hemorrhage, pneumonia, atelectasis, fecal impaction, urinary retention, and even hiccoughs all are possibilities. Shock and dilutional hyponatremia are more common to urologic procedures and are discussed in this chapter. The reader is referred to a medical-surgical nursing text for more information on other problems.

## SHOCK

## Perspective on Disease Entity

**Etiology.** Shock is a condition of acute circulatory failure in which blood flow to vital organs is inadequate and the body is unable to rid itself of waste products. It can occur in response to major insults, such as trauma, hemorrhage, burns, infection, and heart disease. There are different types of shock, depending on its cause.

When shock is caused by fluid or blood loss, it is classified as *hypovolemic shock.* Any surgical procedure involving tissue excision and manipulation causes local trauma and loss of blood and plasma from the circulation, thereby decreasing the circulating blood volume. The urologic surgical patients at highest risk for hypovolemic shock include patients having lymphadenectomy, because of the loss of lymphatic fluid during the removal of lymph nodes. Because the kidney is a highly vascular organ, those patients having a nephrectomy, nephrostomy, or nephrolithotomy are also at risk. Cystectomy, prostatectomy, and urinary diversion all involve excision of a large amount of tissue; the resulting blood and plasma loss during these surgical procedures could predispose a patient to hypovolemia. Considerable bleeding may also occur during TURP and transurethral resection of the bladder.

In some instances, shock develops when bleeding is not recognized and controlled during urologic surgery because of the large amount of irrigating fluid used and the pressure generated by the irrigation. If the pressure of the irrigant is higher than the pressure of the blood in the open vein, the bleeding stops temporarily. Therefore, bleeders may not be recognized, and complete hemostasis may not be achieved. Postoperatively, the severity of bleeding may be difficult to determine if the patient is receiving a continuous bladder irrigation. Having a tumor or undergoing radiation therapy decreases the bladder's healing capacity yet increases the likelihood of bleeding problems.

Shock that is caused by heart failure or poor heart pump function is called *cardiogenic shock.* The heart cannot maintain an adequate cardiac output to meet the body's metabolic demands. This problem results in decreased cardiac output, such as in myocardial infarction, dysrhythmias, tamponade, pulmonary embolism, advanced hypovolemia, and epidural and general anesthesia. Failure of the left ventricle to pump blood into the systemic circulation further contributes to decreased coronary perfusion and decreased oxygen supply to the heart muscle (Canobbio, 1986).

*Vasogenic shock* is characterized by excessive dilatation of blood vessels, loss of vascular tone, and venous pooling that results in decreased venous return and cardiac output. Several conditions cause this type of massive vasodilatation. *Neurogenic shock* occurs when there is an assault or interference to the sympathetic nervous system, which is responsible for vasomotor tone, produced by damage to the spinal cord from disease or trauma or by a pharmacologic block to the nervous system from spinal anesthesia. In contrast an adverse allergic reaction may precipitate the release of histamine, kinins, and prostaglandins to cause vasodilatation. This occurs with *anaphylactic shock* due to an antibody-antigen interaction.

*Septic shock* occurs with an infectious process and is caused by the release of endotoxins into the blood stream. Causative organisms are frequently gram-negative bacteria, including *Escherichia coli, Klebsiella, Enterobacter, Serratia, Pseudomonas,* and *Proteus.* The populations most susceptible are the elderly, the immunosuppressed, patients with indwelling catheters, those with urinary tract infections, and those having gastrointestinal or genitourinary surgery. Urologic patients undergoing manipulative instrumentation procedures, such as TURP or percutaneous catheter placement, are also at risk.

**Pathophysiology.** The physiologic compensation associated with shock is essentially the same for all types, regardless of the cause. Changes that ensue are in response to the imbalance between oxygen demand by the tissues and oxygen delivery by the circulatory system.

During the initial phase of shock, there is stimulation and increased production of epinephrine and norepinephrine. Vasoconstriction occurs in the skin and most visceral organs, whereas vasodilation, increased blood supply, and increased heart rate affect the cardiac and skeletal muscles. Activation of the renin-angiotensin system follows, causing arteriolar vasoconstriction, increased renal tubular reabsorption of sodium and water, increased potassium secretion, and increased aldosterone production, leading to an expansion of the extracellular fluid volume. Eventually, fluid shifts into the capillaries from the interstitial and intracellular spaces so that blood volume and supply to vital organs are improved. These changes represent compensatory mechanisms that allow time for correction of the underlying cause of shock.

If action is not taken, shock progresses, with insufficient tissue perfusion and reduced cardiac output causing further impairment of bodily functions. In response to the decreasing blood flow, the heart's pumping ability becomes compromised, causing a decrease in blood pressure. Oxygen and nutrient delivery to all body tissues diminishes with the further slowing and clotting of blood. Tissues become ischemic, and anaerobic metabolism replaces aerobic metabolism. This leads to acidosis and the conversion of adenosine triphosphate to adenosine diphosphate and adenosine. Damage to the cells occurs and is followed by multisystem organ failure. Shock then becomes irreversible, partly because of the release of myocardial depressant factor by the pancreas. This substance reduces the contractility of the heart and impairs its electrical and mechanical function. By this time, death is likely, even if intervention occurs (DeAngelis, 1985; Huggins, 1990; Osterfield, 1991).

The preceding discussion is intended as a review of the physiologic progression of shock. For a more detailed discussion on this condition, the reader is referred to a medical-surgical or critical care nursing text.

**Medical-Surgical Management.** Treatment for patients in shock is determined partly by the condition that precipitated the shock syndrome. In most types of shock, medical management focuses mainly on replacement and restoration of intravascular volume, followed by the use of drugs to affect vasoactivity.

The fluids used for replacement therapy include (1) blood and blood products, (2) colloid solutions, (3) plasma expanders, (4) isotonic crystalloid solutions, and (5) hypotonic crystalloid solutions. It is unclear which fluids are best for the treatment of shock. Usually, fluid replacement is initiated with an isotonic crystalloid solution, such as lactated Ringer's, which diffuses into the interstitial spaces and buffers acidosis. After the initial volume deficit has been corrected, the use of other fluid replacements may be indicated. For example, whole blood transfusions may be required when hypovolemic shock is the result of excessive blood loss.

In many instances, drug therapy is used to augment fluid replacement to reverse the state of shock. Vasoconstriction is achieved with drugs that stimulate the body's alpha-receptors. The heart's contractility is strengthened and its rate increased with drugs that stimulate beta-receptors. Drugs such as dopamine, norepinephrine, and epinephrine are most often used, because they possess properties that affect both alpha- and beta-receptors. Vasodilating drugs, such as sodium nitroprusside, are given to patients in cardiogenic shock to reduce peripheral resistance; this decreases the work of the heart and increases cardiac output and tissue perfusion. The management of septic shock requires the administration of antibiotics to combat bacterial growth and of steroids to stabilize lysosomal membranes. Patients experiencing anaphylactic shock are also managed with antihistamines and bronchodilators.

Oxygen therapy is begun at the onset of shock and monitored with arterial blood gas measurements and pulse oximetry. Evidence of hypokalemia may necessitate intubation and ventilation.

An intra-aortic balloon is sometimes used to assist circulation in the event of cardiovascular collapse. A catheter with a balloon is inserted into the femoral artery and positioned in the thoracic aorta. The balloon inflates during diastole and deflates during systole to decrease the work of the heart and improve coronary blood flow.

## Approaches to Patient Care

### Assessment

The potential for shock is present in all urologic patients; the degree of the potential varies with the condition of the patient and the type of urologic procedure performed. Nursing assessment, therefore, focuses on the early recognition of symptoms to prevent progression of the shock syndrome.

Initially, it is important to determine whether the patient is at risk for developing shock. As part of the preoperative interview, the nurse should determine whether the patient has a history of intestinal obstruction, diabetes mellitus or insipidus, peritonitis, pancreatitis, cirrhosis, hemothorax, or hemoperitoneum. These problems, along with the prescribed use of diuretics or chronic dehydration, could predispose a patient to hypovolemic shock associated with surgical trauma.

If septic shock is suspected, does the patient have a urinary tract infection that has gone undetected? Are there signs of another infectious process elsewhere in the body? Is the patient receiving immunosuppressant therapy for another condition?

The patient experiencing anaphylactic shock may have received contrast material for diagnostic purposes during a urologic procedure. An allergy to components of the radiographic contrast material, or other drug allergies and blood transfusion reactions, is a predisposing factor.

Any patient who has had anesthesia is at risk for developing neurogenic shock. The nurse should find out what anesthetic agents were used during surgery and their route of administration. When assessing the patient for cardiogenic shock, the nurse should keep in mind that a history of cardiovascular disease, coupled with the stress of a urologic condition or the trauma of urologic surgery, could cause shock. Therefore, the patient should be questioned about a history of myocardial infarction, dysrhythmias, congenital heart disease, myocarditis, congestive heart failure, or aortic aneurysm.

During the physical examination, the nurse should assess the patient for the signs and symptoms common to all types of shock, including hypotension; tachycardia; cool, pale, clammy skin; cyanosis; oliguria or anuria; hypothermia; irritability and anxiety; and lethargy and confusion. In addition to this complex of symptoms, the patient with anaphylaxis may exhibit urticaria, respiratory distress with stridor and wheezing, dysrhythmias, seizures, nausea, vomiting, and diarrhea. Peripheral edema, neck vein distention, and pulmonary congestion may also be evident in patients progressing to cardiogenic shock.

Septic shock evolves from bacteremia. Therefore, the nurse must be alert to subtle signs of an impending problem, such as hyperventilation, hyperthermia, chills, warm and dry skin, vomiting, diarrhea, and altered sensorium. This set of symptoms often precedes those commonly associated with shock.

Finally, the nurse should verify clinical findings by monitoring the results of vital signs, clotting studies, serum electrolytes, blood urea nitrogen, creatinine, glucose, arterial blood gas determinations, and urinalysis and urine culture.

### Nursing Diagnosis

Nursing diagnoses for the patient in shock may include the following:

1. Fluid volume deficit related to
   a. Excessive blood loss.
   b. Shift to and expansion of extracellular fluid volume.
   c. Decompensation of regulatory mechanisms.
2. Altered tissue perfusion related to reduced blood flow.
3. Decreased cardiac output related to alteration in circulation and blood volume.
4. Ineffective breathing pattern related to hypoxia.
5. Alteration in pattern of urinary elimination related to the development of oliguria or anuria.
6. Activity intolerance: lethargy, related to an imbalance between oxygen supply and demand.
7. Anxiety related to a sudden change in health status.

### Plan of Care

Nursing care is directed toward enabling the patient to

1. Restore and maintain circulating blood volume.
2. Maintain adequate ventilation with a clear and patent airway.
3. Re-establish kidney function.
4. Correct electrolyte imbalances.
5. Avoid or reduce anxiety.

### Intervention

Prompt nursing intervention may prevent progression of the shock syndrome and improve the patient's outcome. Fluid replacement is begun at the first signs of any type of shock. When the nature and cause of the shock are determined, fluids are adjusted accordingly. To prevent the complications of peripheral and pulmonary edema, fluids should be administered at a rate that the body can tolerate.

Oxygen therapy is essential for the maintenance of adequate ventilation and the prevention of respiratory problems. It is initiated at the onset of shock and is usually administered by mask or nasal cannula. Frequent turning, with a slight elevation of the head, improves tissue oxygenation and perfusion. Stimulation to cough, postural drainage, chest physiotherapy, and use of a humidifier may be beneficial. In some instances, suctioning may be necessary to keep the airway clear and free of mucus. If breath sounds diminish or arterial blood gas or pulse oximetry determinations suggest hypoxia, be prepared to assist with intubation and artificial ventilation of the patient.

To evaluate the patient's cardiovascular status, continuous electrocardiograph monitoring and frequent blood pressure recordings are required (Huggins, 1990). Various hemodynamic measurements are also employed to determine blood volume and cardiac output.

Urinary output is measured hourly with the insertion of an indwelling catheter required for accurate monitoring. Inadequate renal perfusion accompanied by inadequate arterial pressure is suspected when urinary output is less than 30 mL/h for an adult and 1 mL/kg/h for a child.

It is important to reduce the patient's anxiety to minimize the energy expenditure. Rest is ensured by limiting activities and proper positioning (horizontal with head and feet slightly elevated), and quiet and calm surroundings help decrease the body's demand for oxygen. Frequent neurologic checks should be performed to detect changes in consciousness that may indicate an alteration in cerebral blood flow. Medications to relieve discomfort or chest pain are administered cautiously to prevent further depression of the circulation. Treatments and procedures are clearly and carefully explained in a reassuring manner.

### Patient Outcomes

1. The patient's fluid volume is restored as evidenced by hemodynamic measurements.
2. The patient exhibits no signs of hypoxia as evidenced by the return of normal respiratory rate and rhythm, blood gas measurements within a normal range, and skin color that is pink.
3. The patient's urine output exceeds 30 mL/h.
4. Anxiety is reduced because the patient can express his or her fears and achieve adequate periods of rest.
5. Laboratory analysis of the patient's blood and urine demonstrate stabilization of body chemistry.

## DILUTIONAL HYPONATREMIA

### Perspective on Disease Entity

**Etiology.** Dilutional hyponatremia, otherwise known as TUR syndrome or *water intoxication syndrome*, is a complication that occurs after TURP. It is a problem that results when irrigation fluid is absorbed into the circulatory system. The factors that may predispose a patient to developing intraoperative or postoperative dilutional hyponatremia include the duration of surgery and the amount of tissue resected.

The reader is referred to other texts for discussion of dilutional hyponatremia as the result of an inappropriate secretion of antidiuretic hormone.

**Pathophysiology.** During TURP, venous sinuses are opened as hypertrophied prostate tissue is resected and removed. Depending on the amount of tissue to be excised, these vessels may be exposed to a continuous irrigation of sterile distilled water for a prolonged period. (Normal saline is generally not used as an irrigant in this instance, because it can carry an electrical current and cause injury to the patient.) Open venous sinuses or perforation in the prostatic capsule allows for the absorption of the electrolyte-free irrigant into the circulation, causing chemical imbalances and circulatory overload.

If the patient has received general anesthesia, signs of dilutional hyponatremia may not be readily apparent (Greene, 1986). Therefore, hypertension, an increase in pulse and central venous pressures, or abdominal distention may be the only clue. On the other hand, if regional anesthesia has been used, symptoms such as restlessness, disorientation, dyspnea, nausea, and cyanosis may be observed accompanying bradycardia and a decrease in blood pressure. Hypotension, blindness, loss of consciousness, and seizures may evolve if the hyponatremic state goes undetected and untreated.

**Medical-Surgical Management.** Close observation and aggressive medical management are critical during the first few hours after the onset of hyponatremia to correct fluctuating electrolyte levels. Central venous pressure and blood gas measurements and blood loss and urine output are monitored. Serum electrolyte levels, including osmolality, sodium, and potassium, are measured frequently. A serum sodium level lower than 136 mEq/L, a serum osmolality level lower than 280 mOsm/L, and a decreased hematocrit level indicate water excess. Urine sodium levels may be normal or only slightly increased (>25 mEq/L); urine specific gravity may also be normal (Stark, 1985).

Treatment of dilutional hyponatremia focuses on effecting a net loss of body water. To accomplish this outcome, the intravenous administration of a diuretic, such as furosemide, may be required. An intravenous infusion of a hypertonic (3–5%) saline solution, administered at a rate of 0.1 mg/kg/min, may also be given, although careful consideration is needed before instituting this therapy, because it may cause congestive heart failure in patients at risk (Greene, 1986; Stark, 1985; Thelan, et al., 1990).

## Approaches to Patient Care

### Assessment

The perioperative nurse caring for a patient who has undergone transurethral surgery, such as TURP, must be alert to signs of systemic water intoxication. The patient may complain of a headache or exhibit confusion and lethargy. Abdominal distention, weight gain, nausea, and vomiting may be evident, and seizures may occur. Analysis of laboratory data should reveal a decrease in blood urea nitrogen, hematocrit, and serum osmolality and sodium levels. Urine sodium levels are normal or slightly increased.

Assessment of the patient who may have developed dilutional hyponatremia intraoperatively should also include verification of all fluid intake and output during surgery, including irrigating solutions. The types and concentrations of all fluids used should be noted.

### Nursing Diagnosis

Nursing diagnoses for the patient with dilutional hyponatremia may include the following:

1. Fluid volume excess related to the systemic absorption of an electrolyte-free irrigating solution during surgery.

### Plan of Care

Nursing care is directed toward enabling the patient to

1. Eliminate excess fluid absorbed into the vascular system.
2. Reduce symptoms of hyponatremia.

### Intervention

The nurse caring for the patient with dilutional hyponatremia must maintain accurate intake and output records, because these records are used to calculate fluid replacement and restriction. Seizure precautions should be instituted, and the patient's neurologic status should be checked every 1 or 2 hours. Hemodynamic parameters, including arterial blood, central venous, and pulmonary arterial wedge pressures are measured hourly until the crisis resolves. The patient should be weighed every 12 hours to gauge the degree of fluid retention or loss; this measurement is correlated with laboratory analyses of blood and urine sodium, hematocrit, and serum osmolality.

If the patient is receiving an intravenous infusion of hypertonic saline and exhibits signs of cardiac overload or complains of increased thirst, the infusion should be discontinued immediately. Blood samples should then be collected to check serum electrolyte levels to detect any shift.

Constipation can sometimes be a problem because of the excessive fluid restrictions that may be imposed. If an enema is ordered for bowel evacuation, tap water or hypotonic enemas that permit water absorption through the bowel should be avoided.

### Patient Outcomes

1. The patient's body weight is not increased.
2. The patient's symptoms of hyponatremia have resolved.
3. Electrolyte levels in the patient's blood and urine have returned to normal range.
4. The patient's intake and output measurements reflect a normal state of hydration.

## AMBULATORY CARE

Standards are currently established for ambulatory surgery programs by the Joint Commission on Accreditation of Healthcare Organizations (JCAHO). Two accreditation manuals are available for ambulatory surgery. The first, the *Accreditation Manual for Hospitals* (1989), pertains to facilities that are organized and affiliated with hospitals, even though they may be freestanding. The second manual, the *Accreditation Manual for Ambulatory Health Care* (1989), is written for facilities that are not affiliated with hospitals. With the advent of Diagnosis-Related Groups and other issues of reimbursement, same-day surgery (SDS) centers can provide economical, high-level surgical care.

In reviewing and accrediting ambulatory surgery centers, the JCAHO is particularly interested in four issues: histories and physical examination and operative reports, credentialing and privileging of staff, physician discharge of patients, and quality assurance programs. JCAHO reviews are conducted every 3 years.

With more advanced urologic surgical techniques being perfected and performed on an outpatient basis, visits for SDS are expected to increase. Therefore, it is imperative that the urologic perioperative nurse possess the knowledge necessary to care for the ambulatory urologic patient.

## Preoperative Period

Surgery is a stressful time for patients and their families. The day of surgery is full of unknowns, and that situation breeds fear and anxiety. Dealing with details such as directions to the facility, parking, and the location of the admissions desk can seem like major problems when combined with the stress of surgery. For that reason, it is highly advisable that the patient and responsible support person visit the SDS unit before the actual day of surgery. Gaining familiarity with the details related to physically arriving at the unit can alleviate some anxiety. If the distance from the patient's home to the SDS unit makes the preoperative trip difficult or impossible, the perioperative nurse and the patient are at a disadvantage. In this instance, a preoperative phone call in lieu of a preoperative visit, initiated by the perioperative nurse, may be necessary.

Assuming that the patient and support person can visit the unit before the actual day of surgery, there are some important areas to be covered by the perioperative nurse.

## PATIENT RESPONSIBILITIES

Inform the patient and support person of their responsibilities. Explain the reason for the NPO status and why no jewelry or nail polish is permitted, and encourage them to leave any money or valuables at home. Any skin or bowel preparations the patient must complete before arriving for surgery should be thoroughly explained and demonstrated, if necessary. The preoperative discussion is also an excellent time to review discharge instructions. If special bandages or supplies are needed after surgery, the family will have time to acquire them. The need for a support person to accompany the patient the day of surgery should be emphasized. Registration, paperwork, and financial arrangements can be completed during the preoperative visit.

Because the day of surgery is typically hectic and rushed, and judgment errors can occur more often, it is advantageous for the nurse to assess the patient in a more relaxed environment during the preoperative visit. This visit also gives the perioperative nurse time to develop an individualized plan of care for the patient, so that preparations can be made for any special needs the patient or family may have.

## PATIENT EDUCATION

The SDS unit is set up to accomplish the admission, surgery, and discharge with no overnight stay. Typically, after urologic SDS, the patient is discharged with no professional care provided at home. Education for the patient and support person is imperative to facilitate proper surgical recovery. Problems after

discharge need to be recognized early to prevent disastrous outcomes.

Optimally, the nurse who is working with the patient during surgery should conduct the preoperative visit and patient teaching session. This time can be used to exchange information with the patient and family and to acquaint them with the SDS unit routine. Clear, simple, and concise information should be offered about what will happen to them. The following illustrates how events in the SDS unit can be explained to a male patient:

You and your family will be escorted to the surgical holding area at approximately 10:00 A.M. You will then have to say goodbye to your wife as we wheel you into the operating room. We ask that your wife wait in the surgical waiting room. As soon as your doctor is finished with the surgery, he will contact her either by a visit or by phone. When you get into the operating room, we will help you move onto the operating table. The table has a thin pad on top, and you will notice that the room will feel cool to you. You will see the anesthesia machine, anesthetist, some tables with instruments, the scrub nurse, your surgeon, and myself. I will be there during the entire surgery. The anesthetist will place a needle in your arm for IV fluids and put a blood pressure cuff on your other arm and three heart monitor electrodes on your chest so we can watch everything carefully during your surgery. When you wake up, you will be in the recovery room, and your surgery will be over. You will probably have an oxygen mask over your nose and throat, your throat may feel a little sore, and you will still have your IV. You will also have a catheter into your bladder through your penis. At first you may feel as though you have to go to the bathroom, but after a little while, that urge will pass.

Keep the focus of your explanation on what the *patient* will experience, not the technical aspects of the surgery, unless the patient or support person asks for a specific explanation.

Especially important in urologic nursing is a discussion of sexual activity and what, if any, postoperative changes will be noted or restrictions might be imposed. Patients want to know what to expect, and their physicians often have not discussed sexual activity with them. The nurse should ask the patient if he has any specific questions about postoperative sexual concerns. Permitting and encouraging the patient to raise concerns may reveal any fears or misunderstandings and need for information about sexual activity in the postoperative period.

## Intraoperative Period

The patient depends on the perioperative nurse to be supportive and compassionate. It is helpful to talk to the patient, recognizing that nothing is minor when the patient is lying on a stretcher staring at the ceiling just before surgery.

The patient also depends on the perioperative nurse to be the liaison with the family. It is important to keep the communication between them intact. If surgery is taking longer than expected, let the family know what is happening and why. Was there a technical delay in the operating room? Was the anesthetist late? Was there equipment trouble? The unknown is anxiety producing. If the patient was supposed to be out of surgery by 1:00 P.M. and it is now 3:00 P.M., let the family know what is happening.

## Postoperative Period

General postoperative considerations are the same for all urologic patients. The differentiation between SDS and hospitalized urologic patients has no bearing on postoperative assessment or care.

### DISCHARGE INSTRUCTIONS

Most SDS facilities have a preprinted discharge information sheet for each surgical procedure, because it is important for the patient to have some written material to take home for reference, should a problem arise. Often the family and patient are so anxious to leave the facility that they do not retain information that was discussed verbally.

Discharge instructions should be presented as part of *preoperative* teaching, then reviewed after surgery, just before the patient leaves the SDS facility. Instructions should be specific and direct, including what signs or symptoms are expected and unexpected and what to do if complications arise. The names and telephone numbers of a daytime and a nighttime contact person also should be provided. Any medications prescribed by the health care provider should be reviewed; restrictions, activities, diet and fluids, dressing changes, and follow-up appointments should be included on the discharge form.

Evaluation of the SDS experience should be performed by the perioperative nurse. In most instances, a postoperative telephone call is made to check on the patient's recovery and to find out the patient's impressions of the nursing care provided. A postoperative telephone call or visit is usually done 1 to 7 days after surgery.

## REFERENCES

Association of Operating Room Nurses. (1992). Recommended practices for preoperative skin preparation of patients. *AORN Standards and Recommended Practices for Perioperative Nursing.* Denver, CO: Author.

Canobbio, M. M. (1986). Cardiovascular system. In J. M. Thompson, G. K. McFarland, J. E. Hirsh, S. M. Tucker, & A. C. Bowers (Eds.), *Clinical nursing* (pp. 3–109). St. Louis: C. V. Mosby.

DeAngelis, R. (1985). The cardiovascular system. In J. G. Alspach & S. M. Williams (Eds.), *Core curriculum for critical care nursing* (3rd ed., pp. 101–218). Philadelphia: W. B. Saunders.

Gelfant, B. B. (1986). Minimizing the stress of surgery through patient and family orientation and education. *Point of View, 23,* 9.

Greene, L. F. (1986). Transurethral surgery. In P. C. Walsh, R. F. Gittes, A. D. Perlmutter, & T. A. Stamey (Eds.), *Campbell's urology* (5th ed., pp. 2815–2844). Philadelphia: W. B. Saunders.

Groah, L. K. (1990). *Operating room nursing: Perioperative practice* (2nd ed.). Norwalk, CT: Appleton & Lange.

Huggins, B. (1990). Trauma physiology. *Nursing Clinics of North America, 25*(1), 1–10.

Joint Commission on Accreditation of Healthcare Organizations. (1989a). *Accreditation manual for ambulatory health care.* Chicago: Author.

Joint Commission on Accreditation of Healthcare Organizations. (1989b). *Accreditation manual for hospitals.* Chicago: Author.

La Follette, S. (1988). Perioperative care of the testis tumor patient. *AUAA Journal, 8*(3), 12–18.

Osterfield, G. (1991). Shock. In W. J. Phipps, B. C. Long, N. F. Woods, & V. L. Cassemeyer (Eds.), *Medical-surgical nursing: Concepts and clinical practice* (4th ed., pp. 577–598). St. Louis: Mosby–Year Book.

Ricker, L. E. (1991). Positioning the patient for surgery. In M. H. Meeker & J. C. Rothrock (Eds.), *Alexander's care of the patient in surgery* (9th ed., pp. 103–113). St. Louis: C. V. Mosby.

Scardino, P. T. (1982). Thoracoabdominal retroperitoneal lymphadenectomy for testicular cancer. In E. D. Crawford, D. Borden, & A. Thomas (Eds.), *Genitourinary cancer surgery* (pp. 271–289). Philadelphia: Lea & Febiger.

Stark, J. L. (1985). The renal system. In J. G. Alspach & S. M. Williams (Eds.), *Core curriculum for critical care nursing* (3rd ed., pp. 348–450). Philadelphia: W. B. Saunders.

Thelan, L. A., Davie, J. K., & Urden, L. D. (1990). *Textbook of critical care nursing: Diagnosis and management.* St. Louis: Mosby–Year Book.

Tobias, R. (1980). Circulator, you can help your anesthetist. *Point of View, 17,* 6.

# PART II

# Obstructions and Infections of the Genitourinary Tract

# CHAPTER 4

# Urinary Tract Obstructions

■

*Susan Carney, Karen A. Karlowicz, Cindy Meredith,*
*Suzanne M. Pear, Nancy J. Reilly, Linda Swibold, Marsha L. Toner,*
*and Janet D. Wagner*

## OVERVIEW

The flow of urine may be easily impeded by a blockage anywhere along its path through the urinary system. Pathophysiologic changes resulting from obstruction evolve over time and typically involve those segments of the urinary tract proximal to the obstruction, with the kidney and its structures being protected until all other portions of the system can no longer compensate. All disorders that interfere with the peristaltic movement of urine are considered obstructive and, if undetected, may ultimately lead to hydronephrosis and irreversible damage to renal tissue.

　　Urinary tract obstructions are usually classified in one of four ways, according to (1) the origin (congenital versus acquired), (2) the duration (acute versus chronic), (3) the degree (partial versus complete), or (4) the location (upper urinary tract versus lower urinary tract) (Tanagho, 1992). An obstruction may also be categorized as extrinsic — referring to a source of obstruction outside the urinary tract, or intrinsic — relating to conditions within the urinary tract causing obstruction.

In this chapter, conditions causing obstruction to the urinary tract in the adult patient are described with respect to the location of involvement. Discussions are organized in an anatomic sequence, beginning with the upper urinary tract and progressing to lower urinary tract obstructions. Acute renal failure and postobstructive diuresis, complications that may arise from an obstructive process, are also addressed.

## BEHAVIORAL OBJECTIVES

After studying this chapter, the reader should be able to

1. Classify the types of urinary tract obstruction according to their location and etiology.
2. Identify symptoms of urinary tract obstruction.
3. Discuss complications that may occur as a result of urinary tract obstruction and related nursing activities to prevent or manage those complications.
4. Describe diagnostic tests and procedures for the assessment of urinary tract obstruction and the nursing responsibilities for each.
5. Develop a plan of care for the patient with an upper urinary tract obstruction and for the patient with a lower urinary tract obstruction.

## KEY WORDS

**Antegrade**—moving in a direction of normal flow.

**Bladder neck contracture**—the formation of a fibrous band of tissue at the lower portion of the bladder where it becomes the urethra.

**Compensation**—the correction of an abnormality or the loss of function of an organ by increased functioning of another organ or unimpaired parts of the same organ.

**Contralateral**—used in reference to the kidney on the opposite side.

**Diverticulum**—a blind pouch; in the urinary system, refers to cellules that have pushed their way through the entire bladder wall.

**Extrinsic obstruction**—pressure from outside the urinary tract that causes obstruction within the system.

**Hydroureteronephrosis**—dilatation of the ureter and the pelvis and calices of the kidney caused by an obstruction that prevents urine from passing through the urinary tract.

**Hyponatremia**—decreased sodium concentration in the blood caused by inadequate excretion of water or excessive absorption of fluid into the blood stream, or both.

**Hypertrophy**—increase in volume of a tissue or organ produced by enlargement of existing cells.

**Intrinsic obstruction**—an obstruction due to causes within the urinary tract.

**Natriuresis**—excretion of sodium into the urine.

**Prostatic hyperplasia**—increased development of the glandular and interstitial cellular tissues of the prostate.

**Pyeloplasty**—the revision or surgical reconstruction of the renal pelvis.

**Retrograde**—backward flow.

**Retrograde ejaculation**—the deposit of semen into the bladder instead of expulsion through the urethral meatus; often a consequence of transurethral resection of the prostate.

**Retroperitoneal fibrosis**—a chronic inflammatory process that involves the retroperitoneal tissues over the lower lumbar area.

**Saccule**—a bag or sac of cellules that have forced their way entirely through the muscle of the bladder wall and that may become diverticula.

**Stenosis**—constriction or narrowing of a passage or orifice.

**Stricture**—an abnormal narrowing of a passage, as in the ureter or urethra.

**Trabeculation**—refers to changes in the bladder wall due to the hypertrophy of fibromuscular tissue, causing it to appear thin in some areas and thick in other areas.

**Uremia**—a toxic condition caused by the accumulation of substances in the blood that are ordinarily excreted in the urine.

**Ureteroureterostomy**—the segmental resection of a diseased portion of the ureter and reconstruction in continuity of the two normal segments.

**Urethroplasty**—plastic surgical repair of the urethra.

**Urinary tract obstruction**—a blockage of the flow of urine at any point in the urinary tract from the collecting ducts in the kidney to the urethral meatus.

## THE PROCESS OF OBSTRUCTION

When there is an obstruction within the urinary tract, the effects on the system's structures follow a certain sequence. First, the blockage prevents the antegrade flow of urine, causing urinary stasis behind the obstruction. To compensate, muscle tissues hypertrophy to strengthen their contractions in an effort to propel urine past the obstruction. This creates a back pressure that eventually causes that segment of the urinary tract just above the blockage to dilate to accommodate the stagnated urine. If the obstruction is not relieved, increasing dilation overstretches muscle fibers, thereby decreasing muscle tone and the ability of the affected segment to contract. Because it is unable to maintain its function of elimination, that portion of the urinary tract affected by the obstruction decompensates, allowing increased dilation and thinning and weakening of the atonic muscle wall. With these changes, a back pressure is again created that will be transmitted to the next proximal segment in the urinary tract. This cycle of compensation-decompensation occurs in succession to all segments of the urinary tract above the obstruction until the renal pelvis and calices are reached.

## Effect on the Bladder

The bladder is that portion of the urinary system most immediately affected when there is an obstruction of the lower urinary tract. Incomplete bladder emptying causes stasis of urine and leads to the development of bacterial infections. High intravesical pressures generated to overcome urethral resistance caused by obstruction cause the bladder to become tra-

beculated; diverticula may form in the bladder wall. The build-up of residual urine in the bladder allows stretching of the trigone, causing resistance to urine flowing from the ureter. Hypertrophy of the bladder wall in combination with a continuous residue of urine may further impair the valvelike action of the ureterotrigonal complex, causing urine to reflux into the ureter and inducing a functional obstruction of the ureterovesical junction.

## Effect on the Ureter

Back pressure transmitted from the bladder because of an unrelieved lower urinary tract obstruction eventually causes the ureters to dilate. The term *hydroureter*, which means marked dilation of the ureter, is used to describe this change. In an attempt to push urine toward the bladder, peristaltic action in the ureter increases. The ureter becomes elongated and tortuous, and intraureteral pressure elevates to compensate for the extra workload. In time, the ureter can lose the ability to contract. Extreme dilation can result in the ureter taking on the appearance of a section of bowel.

## Effect on the Kidney

The development of hydronephrosis (distention of the renal pelvis and calices with urine) is the result of pressure on the kidney from obstruction. Hydronephrosis can be bilateral and result from a prolonged and unrelieved obstruction to the lower urinary tract, or it can occur unilaterally with a blockage to either ureter (Fig. 4–1). The extent to which the kidney is affected varies, depending on the location of the obstruction and the degree and duration of back pressure. Generally, the closer the ob-

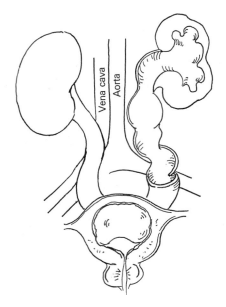

*FIGURE 4–1* Unilateral hydroureter and hydronephrosis.

struction is to the kidney, the greater the impact on renal tissue.

Although the renal pelvis and calices are both affected by obstruction, changes in the musculature of the renal pelvis occur first to decompress and protect the calices. The change is in the form of a compensatory hypertrophy as the renal pelvis tries to force urine past the obstruction (Tanagho, 1992). Increased intrapelvic pressure, in turn, eventually causes the papillae at the end of the calix to become flattened and convex (clubbed). Ischemia and compression atrophy of the parenchyma between the calices also occur. As the pressure from obstruction continues, the tubules become dilated and the cells of the tubules atrophy from ischemia. The glomeruli are the last to show pathologic changes; glomerular filtration and renal plasma flow are decreased, thereby inhibiting the kidney's ability to concentrate and secrete urine. The effects of the distention and destruction of renal tissue that result from hydronephrosis caused by partial obstruction may take months or years to be realized. However, in instances of hydronephrosis associated with complete obstruction, an irreversible loss of function may be evident within 7 days (Kerr, 1954; Klahr et al., 1977; Tanagho, 1992).

Unlike other secreting organs in the body that stop functioning when obstructed, the completely obstructed kidney continues to produce some urine (Tanagho, 1992). However, the amount of urine secreted is reduced, be-

cause there is suppression of renal function with the increased intrarenal pressure. Because it cannot flow down the ureter, urine secreted into the renal pelvis leaves the system in other ways. Pyelovenous reabsorption occurs in the fornix of the minor calix where urine enters the venous system surrounding the base of the calix. Tubular backflow, pyelolymphatic backflow (the most common), and peripelvic extravasation (seen only in acute forms of obstruction) are other methods of reabsorption (Hinman, 1984). As urine leaves the system, there is room for additional urine to be secreted, thus accounting for the changing fluid in the renal pelvis even with complete obstruction.

The greatest and most rapid loss of function due to hydronephrosis occurs when there is unilateral obstruction. By way of compensatory hypertrophy, or counterbalance, the contralateral kidney takes over the work of the affected kidney to maintain renal function as hydronephrosis increases (Hinman, 1984).

Once the function of the contralateral kidney is established, there is little stimulus on the hydronephrotic kidney to continue working (Gillenwater, 1986). In fact, the affected kidney may not resume function even after relief of the obstruction.

## UPPER URINARY TRACT OBSTRUCTIONS

When discussing an obstruction affecting the upper urinary tract, it is important to remember that the ureters assume a critical role in the preservation of renal function. Therefore, obstructions occurring at this level must be recognized quickly so that these narrow tubular structures may remain patent. The ureters lie close to the retroperitoneal musculature, multiple visceral organs, and the vascular tree, progressing down toward the bladder in two graceful curves. Because of their position in the retroperitoneum, the ureters are vulnerable to some of the same pathologic conditions that affect the structures lying adjacent to them (Persky et al., 1986). Extrinsic obstruction includes those conditions causing deviation or compression of the ureters that, in adults, can arise from diseases of the retroperitoneum, vascular lesions, inflammatory conditions of the gastrointestinal tract, or tumors. Acute ureteral obstruction may also be a complication of pregnancy or other benign conditions of the female reproductive system. Intrinsic ureteral obstruction in adults most likely is caused by stricture development, although conditions causing blockage of the ureteropelvic junction (UPJ) or the ureterovesical junction (UVJ) are common.

In this section, the discussion of ureteral stricture disease serves as the basis for understanding all types of upper urinary tract obstruction in adults. Particular attention should be given to the sequence of diagnostic studies employed, for it represents the manner in which most obstructions to the upper urinary tract are assessed; variations in this diagnostic protocol are discussed in the subsequent presentations of other types of obstruction. A complete discussion of the nursing management of the patient with ureteral obstruction (see "Approaches to Patient Care" at the end of this section) also reflects the similarities in diagnosis and treatment.

# Perspective on Disease Entity

## INTRINSIC OBSTRUCTION

## Ureteral Stricture

**Etiology.** A ureteral stricture is an abnormal narrowing of the ureter associated with fibrotic tissue changes. Although stricture formation can occur at any point along the ureter, there are three areas particularly prone to stenosis and stricture development: the UPJ, the midureter (where the ureter crosses the iliac vessels), and the distal ureter above the UVJ (Allen, 1977; Campbell, 1952; Perlmutter et al., 1986).

Narrowing of the ureter can often be attributed to congenital malformation or stenosis. However, a ureteral stricture in an adult is more likely to be an acquired condition, the long-term consequence of another problem. For instance, injuries incurred during an operative procedure, such as that involving instrumentation of the ureter (e.g., ureteroscopy), difficult dissection and excessive handling of the ureter, and the inadvertent ligation or stripping of a ureter, may induce a stricture. Other surgical-related causes of ureteral strictures include the type of incision, the suture material, and the suture method. A failed surgical repair of the ureter may also lead to the development of a stricture.

The passage or presence of a stone can cause localized irritation or pressure necrosis sufficient to lead to stricture formation. Inflammation secondary to renal tuberculosis, retroperitoneal fibrosis, and schistosomiasis may also

induce the development of a ureteral stricture. Other etiologic factors include metastatic tumors, irradiation, and devascularization of a transplanted kidney. Urinary extravasation, infection, and ischemia also make the ureter more susceptible to stricture. Finally, the development of a ureteral stricture may be a complication of traumatic ureteral injury resulting from a penetrating gunshot or knife wound.

**Pathophysiology.** The formation of a ureteral stricture begins with the conversion of fibroblasts to fibrocytes (except in those instances when the stricture is caused by direct permeation of a metastatic tumor). Fibrocytic healing leads to scar formation and increasing constriction of the ureter. Prolonged constriction decreases perfusion of the tissues and inhibits the development of a collateral vascular supply. As the scar increases with age, it becomes less vascular. If the scar is disrupted for any reason, (e.g., ureteral dilatation), it is again replaced by the fibrocytic healing process. Continued reduction of vascular perfusion, along with the build-up of fibrous tissue, ultimately leads to progressive devascularization and an interruption in the flow of urine from the kidney to the bladder (Lang, 1986). An untreated ureteral stricture can eventually lead to hydronephrosis, damage to the renal parenchyma, or both.

**Medical-Surgical Management.** The diagnosis of ureteral stricture is made by a series of radiographic procedures, together with a history and physical examination. These studies serve to verify the presence, the location, and the functional significance of the stricture (Schaeffer and Grayhack, 1986). Initially, ultrasonography may be performed to detect any changes in the ureter and dilatation of the renal pelvis and calices. This study is thought to be a safer and more cost-effective alternative to urography, especially when the patient's symptoms do not clearly indicate an obstruction (Webb, 1990). Despite these benefits, false-positive and false-negative findings are commonly reported, making ultrasonography useful for screening but not diagnostic for ureteral obstruction (Cronan, 1991; Webb, 1990).

For most urologists, the excretory urogram remains the procedure of choice when beginning an evaluation for ureteral stricture. To enhance visualization of the kidney and ureter, delayed films, increased hydration, and drug-induced diuresis may be incorporated into the procedure. Findings of this study allow the urologist to make some general observations concerning the extent of stricture formation, the degree of hydronephrosis, and the effect on the kidney. This is sometimes followed by a computed tomographic scan to further evaluate the hydronephrosis and the viability of the kidney. If there is a suggestion of a poorly functioning or nonfunctioning kidney, radioisotope scanning also is performed.

Definitive diagnosis, however, is usually made by retrograde pyelography, performed cystoscopically, to pinpoint the location of the stricture and inspect the tissue distal to it. At this time, a ureteral biopsy may be obtained to confirm the cause of the ureteral abnormality.

In recent years, the antegrade pyelogram coupled with perfusion (also referred to as the *Whitaker test* or *upper tract urodynamics*) has proved beneficial in demonstrating the degree of obstruction caused by a ureteral stricture. This approach also helps differentiate a ureteral source of obstruction from ureterovesical or intravesical conditions and is especially useful in those instances when symptoms of chronic obstruction persist without other definitive evidence (Cronan, 1991). The procedure requires the percutaneous insertion of one or two needles directly into the renal pelvis of the affected kidney; visual guidance with ultrasonography ensures or confirms the correct location. In addition, an indwelling catheter is inserted into the bladder. Using fluoroscopic monitoring, contrast medium is infused through the needle and into the renal pelvis at a rate of approximately 10 mL/min (Whitaker, 1979). Pressure in the renal pelvis is recorded as the kidney is perfused. When a single needle is used, perfusion and pressure measurements are accomplished through the same line; when two needles are used, the measurement of pressure is independent of that of perfusion. During this time, bladder pressure is also monitored, with bladder filling preferred to continuous drainage in those instances when ureterovesical or intravesical obstruction is suspected. Normally, the difference between renal pelvic pressure and bladder pressure during perfusion is lower than 12 to 15 cm $H_2O$. A pressure differential between 15 and 22 cm $H_2O$ suggests a slight degree of obstruction, whereas pressures higher than 22 cm $H_2O$ suggest moderate obstruction. Severe obstruction is confirmed by a pressure differential higher than 40 cm $H_2O$ (Whitaker, 1979).

The initial management of a ureteral stricture often involves insertion of a ureteral stent or nephrostomy tube to allow for drainage and decompression of the ureter and renal pelvis before surgical correction. Traditionally, strictures at the UPJ are usually corrected by pyeloureteroplasty; a nephrectomy may also be indicated for cases involving extreme hydronephrosis and renal damage. A midureteral stricture often requires excision of the stenotic area followed by ureteroureterostomy (end-to-end anastomosis of the remaining portions of the ureter). Lower ureteral strictures and UVJ strictures may be treated by excision and reimplantation of the ureter into the bladder wall.

Balloon dilation of ureteral strictures is another treatment alternative that has become popular and successful. This procedure is most effective for benign strictures, such as those developed postoperatively and in association with an inflammatory process. Balloon dilatation may be performed with fluoroscopy or under direct vision. Depending on the location of the stricture, angioplastic balloon catheters are passed antegrade through a percutaneous nephrostomy or retrograde through a ureteroscope (Bagley et al., 1985) (Figs. 4–2 and 4–3). The balloon is then inflated, causing dilatation of the strictured portion of the ureter. This is followed by removal of the balloon catheter and insertion of a double-pigtail stent (Bagley et al., 1985). Drainage is maintained for several weeks after the procedure.

Currently, internal ureterotomy via ureterorenoscopy is being used to treat ureteral strictures that result as a complication of surgery. As with other surgical approaches, the success of this endourologic procedure depends on the extent and the duration of the stricture (Thuroff, 1992).

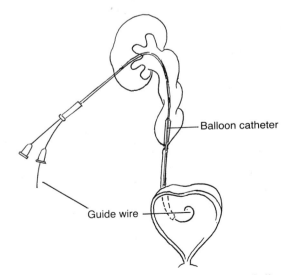

*FIGURE 4–2* Dilation of a ureteral stricture using a balloon passed through a nephrostomy tube.

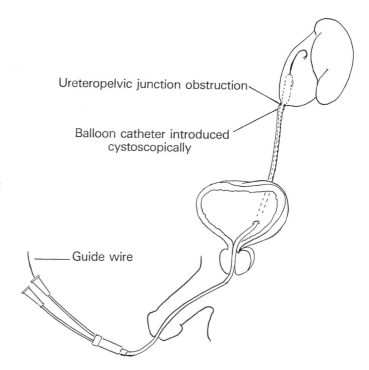

Ureteropelvic junction obstruction

Balloon catheter introduced
cystoscopically

Guide wire

*FIGURE 4–3* Dilation of a ureteral stricture using
a balloon passed cystoscopically.

## Ureteropelvic Junction Obstruction

**Etiology.** In the adult, an obstruction at the UPJ may be a congenital problem that has previously been asymptomatic and therefore unnoticed. However, it is more likely that UPJ obstruction is a condition resulting from inflammation, ischemia, tumors, fibrosis, or calculi. The incidence of UPJ obstruction in adults has not been established; however, evidence suggests that the rate of occurrence is comparable between males and females (Roberts & Slade, 1964).

**Pathophysiology.** Because of the anatomic relationship of the UPJ to the kidney, obstruction at this level is likely to cause a more rapid compromise of renal function than are obstructions in other segments of the ureter (Cronan, 1991). Irreversible renal damage is the most serious consequence of UPJ obstruction. Critical factors that influence the kidney's function at this time include the degree of hydronephrosis, the duration of the obstruction, and the absence or presence of infection. As the obstruction progresses, increased intrarenal pressure, dilatation, atrophy, and ischemia are prevalent throughout the collecting system. Within 7 days of the onset of complete UPJ obstruction, glomerular blood flow and filtration rate may be decreased by as much as 30% in a nonin-

fected kidney and 50% in an infected kidney (Kerr, 1954; Klahr et al., 1977). Symptoms associated with adult-onset UPJ obstruction are initially subtle, yet they worsen with progression of the blockage and increased renal pelvic pressure. The patient may describe a history of chronic, vague back pain that intensifies after an increase in fluid intake. Pyuria and hematuria may also be evident in addition to recurrent urinary tract infections. In some instances, the patient may be hypertensive.

**Medical-Surgical Management.** Once an obstruction at the UPJ has been confirmed, a mechanism for drainage and decompression of the renal pelvis must be implemented before other therapeutic interventions are considered. This is usually achieved with the placement of a percutaneous nephrostomy tube directly into the kidney through the skin on the back flank. Although renal function begins to recover as soon as the UPJ obstruction has been relieved, it may take as long as 6 to 8 weeks for a new level of renal function to be established and the extent of recovery to be realized (Cronan, 1991; Tanagho, 1992). During this interim period, radioisotope scanning and other imaging techniques are used to assess the structures and the function of the contralateral kidney and to determine the amount of useful renal tissue that may be saved in the obstructed kidney.

Surgical correction of a UPJ obstruction in the adult depends on the health status of the patient and the condition of both the obstructed and the contralateral kidneys. The most recent advance in the management of this condition uses endourologic techniques to perform direct-vision internal incision of a stenotic UPJ (Thuroff, 1992). Although there may be advantages to endopyeloplasty, the long-term effects of this approach are unknown. Therefore, most urologists choose to perform a pyeloureteroplasty when there is salvageable renal function in the obstructed kidney. If the obstructed kidney is nonfunctioning, hypoplastic, or dysplastic, a nephrectomy may be required. It is also necessary when the obstruction has caused serious circulatory impairment, stone disease, or infection that threatens to affect an otherwise normal contralateral kidney (Schaeffer and Grayhack, 1986).

See Chapter 20 for additional discussion related to UPJ obstruction in infants and children.

## Ureterovesical Junction Obstruction

The UVJ is that part of the upper urinary tract where the ureters enter the bladder, usually at the proximal border of the trigone area. Those conditions causing obstruction in other segments of the ureter may also affect the UVJ, as do anatomic defects such as ureterocele, bladder diverticula, and obstructive megaureter. The cause of the UVJ obstruction, along with the effect created on the ureter, dictates the course of treatment. In general, UVJ obstruction resulting from infection, tumors, or calculus is first managed medically, with surgical intervention considered on an individual basis. When the obstruction is the result of an anatomic defect, surgical correction is usually indicated. (See other chapters in this text for detailed discussion of those conditions affecting the UVJ.)

## Extrinsic Obstruction

The ureters are normally afforded protection and support by their anatomic positioning in the retroperitoneum. However, it is not uncommon for these conduits between the kidney and the bladder to be displaced, compressed, or blocked as a complication of another disease process occurring in the abdomen or the retroperitoneum. Extensive progression of the underlying condition is usually required before the ureter is affected. Unfortunately, symptoms of secondary ureteral involvement are often overshadowed by the primary disease process and sometimes go unnoticed.

Extrinsic ureteral obstruction may be caused by a variety of disorders. Discovery of the ureteral impairment is usually an incidental finding during diagnostic testing for a retroperitoneal, female reproductive, gastrointestinal, or vascular problem. Although treatment of the primary disease process is usually effective in resolving accompanying ureteral obstruction, urologic intervention, including the insertion of an indwelling ureteral stent, retrograde ureteral catheter, or percutaneous nephrostomy tube is often needed. Table 4–1 lists the most common causes of extrinsic ureteral obstruction and describes each condition's specific effect on the ureter; the usual methods of treatment are also delineated.

## Approaches to Patient Care

### Assessment

The patient with an obstruction to the upper urinary tract may describe a history of chronic, vague back pain. Symptoms such as flank pain, nausea, vomiting, hematuria, and abdominal distention may be exhibited. Generalized malaise, anorexia, weight loss, weakness, and pallor may also be evident if there is an underlying disease process causing extrinsic obstruction. If the right ureter is obstructed, abdominal pain may simulate the pain of appendicitis. In some instances, oliguria or uremia may be the only sign of a blocked ureter, especially in patients with a solitary collecting system. For many patients, though, ureteral obstruction is a silent condition, detected only when radiographic studies are being performed for another problem.

If the involved kidney is enlarged, a palpable flank mass may be detected during the physical examination; a mass in the abdomen, the pelvis, or the rectum may also be detected. Flank tenderness accompanied by fever may be present if an infection exists. Extrinsic conditions compromising peripheral circulation may produce edema in the lower extremities and diminished pulses.

A urinalysis will most likely show microscopic hematuria and pyuria, and urinary cytologic studies may be positive if the obstruction is caused by the growth of malignant tissue. Bacterial cultures confirm the presence of an infectious process, including obstruction as a result of genitourinary tuberculosis. If renal function has been impaired as a result of the obstruction, blood urea nitrogen (BUN) and serum creatinine levels are elevated, and 24-hour creatinine clearance is reduced. Depending on the cause and the extent of the obstruction, alterations in serum electrolyte, hemoglobin, and hematocrit levels and the erythrocyte sedimentation rate may also be noted.

Because the patient suspected of having a ureteral obstruction will undergo multiple radiologic examinations to confirm the diagnosis, the nurse should assess the patient's understanding of and preparation for these procedures. Ask about the patient's previous experiences with radiographic tests—were there any problems or complications? Also inquire about any allergies to radiographic material, iodine, or shellfish and any tendencies to bleed excessively. Because some type of surgical intervention is inevitable for the patient with a ureteral obstruction, it is also important for the urologic nurse to assess the patient's knowledge and understanding of treatment alternatives, preoperative and postoperative routines, recuperation time, and medical follow-up.

### Nursing Diagnosis

Nursing diagnoses for the patient with a ureteral obstruction may include the following:

1. Knowledge deficit related to
   a. Unfamiliarity with the radiologic procedures used to diagnose the presence of a ureteral obstruction.
   b. Unfamiliarity with type of surgical intervention required for treatment of the ureteral obstruction.
2. Anxiety related to
   a. Lack of knowledge regarding the cause of the ureteral obstruction.
   b. Threat to urinary tract function.
   c. Outcome of surgery and postoperative health care needs.
3. Potential for fluid volume deficit related to excessive bleeding after endoscopic instrumentation of the ureter, antegrade perfusion studies, and surgical excision of the strictured or obstructed segment of the ureter.
4. Pain related to tissue trauma and pressure on the renal pelvis caused by hydronephrosis.
5. Potential for infection related to
   a. Stasis of urine caused by ureteral obstruction.
   b. Instrumentation of the upper urinary tract.

6. Potential for impaired tissue integrity related to changes in the renal parenchyma induced by hydronephrosis or upper urinary tract infection.
7. Alteration in pattern of urinary elimination related to the insertion of ureteral stents or a nephrostomy tube for urinary drainage.
8. Self-care deficit related to home maintenance of a percutaneous nephrostomy tube and dressing.

### Plan of Care

Nursing care is planned to enable the patient to

1. Participate cooperatively in diagnostic radiologic procedures to evaluate the obstructed ureter.
2. Prepare for surgery to alleviate ureteral obstruction.
3. Obtain relief from pain and discomfort resulting from hydronephrosis, instrumentation of the ureter, or surgical repair of the obstructed ureteral segment.
4. Prevent problems associated with excessive renal bleeding and urinary tract infection.
5. Maintain the patency of urinary drainage devices to ensure an adequate urinary output.
6. Care for a nephrostomy tube and perform dressing changes in the home setting.

### Intervention

The diagnosis of ureteral obstruction often comes as a surprise to the patient who has been evaluated for another seemingly unrelated condition or who has instead equated chronic back pain with physical exertion and muscle strain. The surprise quickly turns into anxiety on learning of the real or potential threat that ureteral obstruction poses to the function of the kidney. The need for information, support, and reassurance is critical. Initial nursing interventions should therefore be designed to help familiarize the patient with the many radiologic procedures that will likely be performed to verify the location and the severity of the obstruction. Teaching should include a description of the procedure, preparations required, and any special precautions after the procedure (see Appendix III). Bleeding is the most likely, and perhaps the most serious, complication following any radiologic study that requires instrumentation of the ureter and the renal pelvis. Check the patient's vital signs every 15 minutes for up to 1 hour after the completion of a study; decrease the frequency of checks gradually if vital signs remain stable. During the first 24 hours after a study, obtain urine specimens and

*Text continued on page 120*

TABLE 4–1. Common Causes of Extrinsic Ureteral Obstruction

| CATEGORY | SPECIFIC CONDITIONS | CAUSE | EFFECT ON URETER | MEDICAL-SURGICAL TREATMENT |
|---|---|---|---|---|
| **Diseases of the Retroperitoneum** | Retroperitoneal fibrosis | Long-term use of methysergide<br>Retroperitoneal inflammation<br>Radiation therapy<br>Idiopathic | Fibrotic tissue encases the ureter, causing deviation from normal anatomic position; ureter is narrowed and compressed as tissue mass extends | Steroid therapy and ureteral stenting followed by ureterolysis |
| | Retroperitoneal abscess | Renal calculus<br>Renal carbuncle<br>Appendicitis<br>Diverticulitis<br>Enterocolitis (Crohn's disease)<br>Extravasation of infected urine<br>Perinephric abscess | Depending on the size of the abscess, there is displacement of the ureter, kidney, or both, resulting in an alteration in the peristaltic movement of urine toward the bladder | Retroperitoneal drainage and antibiotic therapy essential; irrigation of drain with antibiotic solution may also be performed |
| | Retroperitoneal hematoma | Usually abdominal trauma | Anatomic deviation with varying degrees of obstruction | Surgical evacuation |
| | Retroperitoneal masses | Benign or malignant primary tumors of the retroperitoneum<br>Metastatic tumors spreading most frequently from primary tumors of the cervix, prostate, bladder, or colon (Persky et al., 1986) | Primary tumors most often cause anterior and lateral displacement of ureter and alterations to the kidney that result in distortion to the renal pelvis; obstruction may be partial or complete<br>Metastatic tumors obstruct ureter with direct extension of primary malignant tissue, or with enlargement of retroperitoneal lymph nodes | Depending on the type of tumor, overall effect on the urinary tract, patient's health status, previous treatments, and prognosis, surgical excision and/or urinary diversion—usually with percutaneous nephrostomy—may be done |

**116**

| Conditions of the Female Reproductive System | | | |
|---|---|---|---|
| Pregnancy | | Gravid uterus exerts pressure on the upper urinary tract, causing progressive dilatation of the upper two thirds of the ureter and renal pelvis; elongation and lateral displacement of the ureter, along with tortuosity and kinking at the UPJ, may also occur; urinary stasis results in pyelonephritis | In severe instances, ureteral catheterization and drainage along with antibiotic therapy may be required until pregnancy is completed |
| Benign pelvic masses | Fibroid uterus Cystic ovary | Obstruction usually occurs in that segment where the ureter crosses the iliac vessels; the right ureter is more often affected, with the degree of obstruction related to the size of the pelvic mass | Pelvic laparotomy and excision of the mass |
| Tubo-ovarian abscess | Acute and chronic pelvic inflammatory disease Use of intrauterine device | Blockage occurs at or below the pelvic brim, causing lateral or medial displacement of the ureter; in about 50% of cases, the size of the abscess is sufficient to cause bilateral ureteral obstruction | If patient is of childbearing age, unilateral salpingo-oophorectomy may be considered. However, total abdominal hysterectomy with bilateral salpingo-oophorectomy is recommended |
| Endometriosis | Growth of normal endometrial tissue to an abnormal location outside the uterus | Obstruction to the distal third of the ureter with scarring and inflammation is caused by the development of endometrial adhesions | Total abdominal hysterectomy with oophorectomy and ureterolysis |

*Table continued on following page*

**117**

TABLE 4–1. Common Causes of Extrinsic Ureteral Obstruction *Continued*

| CATEGORY | SPECIFIC CONDITIONS | CAUSE | EFFECT ON URETER | MEDICAL-SURGICAL TREATMENT |
|---|---|---|---|---|
| | Severe uterine prolapse | Weakness of the levator ani muscle | Obstruction could result from stretching and wrapping of uterine vessels around the ureter caused by the herniation of the uterus through the levator ani muscle | Vaginal hysterectomy with vaginoplasty is treatment of choice; a pessary may be used if surgery is contraindicated |
| Diseases of the Gastrointestinal Tract | Enterocolitis (Crohn's disease) | Granulomas form on the mucosa of the distal small intestine and colon, causing thickening of intestinal wall and the formation of scar tissue | Fistulas from the ileum and colon develop, allowing for extension of the inflammatory process into the urinary system, usually causing obstruction to the right distal ureter; retroperitoneal abscess may be a complication | Surgical resection of granulomatous intestinal tissue |
| | Appendicitis | Inflammatory condition of the vermiform appendix | An abscess develops in the appendiceal wall that expands to cause pressure, usually to the right ureter at the pelvic brim | Surgical drainage of abscess with or without appendectomy |
| | Diverticulitis | Diverticula (or sacs) in the muscular wall of the colon fill with colonic contents and become inflamed | Progression of the inflammatory process leads to intestinal perforation and the subsequent development of a retroperitoneal abscess (see retroperitoneal abscess) | Surgical drainage and bowel resection with or without colostomy |

**Vascular Lesions**

| | | | |
|---|---|---|---|
| Abdominal aortic aneurysm | Weakness in the wall of the abdominal aorta, usually below the renal arteries | Depending on the size of the aneurysm, the aortic wall may expand to cause unilateral or bilateral obstruction, usually by displacement of the ureters. In some instances, aortic atherosclerosis leads to inflammation and the development of retroperitoneal scar tissue (see retroperitoneal fibrosis) | Ureteral drainage with resection of the aneurysm; if treatment is for inflammatory aneurysm, ureterolysis and ureteral resection and reanastomosis may also be required |
| Retrocaval ureter | Congenital deformity in which the right ureter passes behind the vena cava | Varying degrees of urethral compression result from the unusual and tortuous position of the ureter in relation to the inferior vena cava | Usually only careful observation of asymptomatic patients is needed; however, surgery may be required if complications occur, such as hydronephrosis or calculus formation, and may involve transection and reanastomosis of the ureter |

inspect for evidence of gross hematuria, encourage an increased fluid intake (if not medically contraindicated), and recommend bed rest. If a procedure required percutaneous puncture of the kidney, examine the puncture site and pressure dressing applied over it for evidence of bleeding (Pagana & Pagana, 1990).

Medical treatment of an upper urinary tract obstruction and the postoperative recovery usually require the placement and maintenance of a percutaneous nephrostomy tube or ureteral stent. Days, weeks, or even months of urinary diversion may be needed, depending on the patient's condition, the severity and the location of the obstruction, and the surgical procedure performed. Because of the length of time often required for recuperation, the nurse caring for the patient with a nephrostomy tube or ureteral stent must ensure that the patient understands the purposes for this alternative form of urinary drainage. Be sure to explain carefully that therapeutic drainage of the ureter and the renal pelvis is essential to the re-establishment of functional renal tissue, the prevention of further renal damage, and the healing of a surgically repaired ureter.

If ureteroureterostomy has been performed, a double-J or "pigtail" type stent is likely to be inserted internally. Usually made of silicone, the stent is a self-retaining device that helps maintain the position and the caliber of the ureter during healing while it prevents extravasation of urine (McAninch, 1992). Nursing care of the patient with an internal stent calls for close observation for signs of urinary tract infection and infection caused by the extravasation of urine into the retroperitoneum. Urinary output should be measured carefully as a way to ascertain the patency of the stent, and urine specimens should be examined for evidence of excessive bleeding. When healing of the ureter is complete, the stent is endoscopically removed through the bladder. Explain to the patient that removal of the stent is usually done on an outpatient basis within 3 to 4 weeks after surgery (McAninch, 1992).

As an adjunct or alternative to ureteral stenting, a percutaneous nephrostomy tube may be inserted intraoperatively for urinary drainage. Placement of a percutaneous nephrostomy tube may also be desired for medical management of obstruction. The procedure can be performed on an inpatient or outpatient basis, although whenever possible, hospitalization is preferred to permit careful observation of the patient during the 24- to 48-hour period after insertion of the tube (Cochran et al., 1991).

Nursing care of the patient after placement of a percutaneous nephrostomy tube includes the following:

1. Maintaining the patency of the tube by preventing kinking or unnecessary tension and positioning the drainage bag below the level of the kidney.
2. Measuring all urinary output, including that from the drainage bag, any that has leaked into the dressing, or any that has been voided.
3. Collecting urine specimens to check for evidence of excessive bleeding; if available, dipstick testing may be used to estimate the amount of blood in the urine.
4. Monitoring laboratory results for hemoglobin and hematocrit levels and bleeding times to detect variations indicative of hemorrhage.
5. Observing the patient for signs of infection, including an elevated temperature, flank pain, cloudy or foul-smelling urine, weakness, and malaise.
6. Collecting urine specimens for culture and sensitivity testing, if infection is suspected.
7. Administering antibiotics, if ordered, for treatment or prevention of infection.
8. Providing analgesics for relief of discomfort caused by skin puncture and insertion of the nephrostomy tube.
9. Encouraging a fluid intake of more than 2000 mL/24 hours, unless medically contraindicated; intravenous fluid replacement may be needed if the patient is unable to tolerate oral fluids.
10. Checking the dressing around the nephrostomy tube, and noting the color and the consistency of any drainage.
11. Inspecting the integrity of the skin around the nephrostomy tube for signs of irritation caused by drainage or moisture.
12. Inspecting the nephrostomy tube for signs of obstruction, including blood clots, sediment, and debris; irrigation of the tube requires an order by the physician and should be performed only by an experienced urologic nurse using 5 to 15 mL of sterile saline (Barr, 1988).
13. Performing nephrostomy tube dressing changes as needed (Procedure 4–1).

Regardless of the setting in which percutaneous nephrostomy tube placement is performed, skilled nursing management, including thorough patient teaching, is needed to prevent complications. Patient instruction begins as soon as the decision for nephrostomy

**PROCEDURE 4-1**

■

Changing a Nephrostomy Tube Dressing

## ■ RATIONALE

A dressing is applied over the nephrostomy tube to protect the skin at the point where the tube is inserted through the skin and into the kidney and to collect any urine or other discharge that may leak from around the tube. A regular schedule for dressing change helps prevent infection and skin irritation.

## ■ FREQUENCY

The nephrostomy tube dressing is changed as needed, depending on the physician's orders and the amount of discharge from around the tube. The procedure may be performed as often as every day, but the minimum frequency is at least once a week.

## ■ TECHNIQUE

In the hospital setting, aseptic technique should be used when changing a nephrostomy tube dressing; in the home setting, this is a clean procedure.

## ■ SUPPLIES

1. Sterile gloves
2. Povidone-iodine solution
3. 4 × 4 gauze sponges (4 packages with 2 per package)
4. 1 roll of tape (1- or 2-inch width)
5. Cotton-tipped applicators
6. Sterile scissors
7. Bedside or urinary leg bag
8. Ureteral connecting tubing

## ■ PROCEDURE

1. Wash hands with soap and water; dry thoroughly.
2. Assemble equipment and arrange sterile field.
3. Pour povidone-iodine solution over two gauze sponges and two cotton-tipped applicators.
4. Carefully, but securely, hold the nephrostomy tube with one hand while removing and discarding the old dressing with the other.
5. Examine the site for signs of redness, swelling, odor, or discharge.
6. Put on sterile gloves.
7. Cleanse the skin around the tube with povidone-iodine–soaked sponges. Wipe in one direction from the insertion site outward, using one sponge for each side (*A*).
8. Remove any crusting from the tube with the cotton-tipped applicators soaked with povidone-iodine.
9. Cut "Y" slits halfway into two gauze sponges.
10. Place the cut gauze sponges around the tube, with the slits in opposing directions (*B*).
11. Roll one 4 × 4 gauze sponge and place it under the tube and over the previously placed gauze sponges to keep the tube from kinking (*C* or *D*).

*Procedure 4–1 continued on following page*

**PROCEDURE 4-1** *Continued*
■
Changing a Nephrostomy Tube Dressing

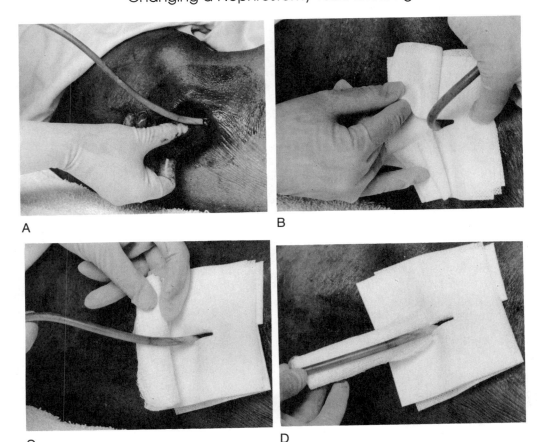

A

B

C

D

12. Place one unsplit gauze sponge over the nephrostomy tube and other sponges, and securely tape the entire dressing to the patient.
13. Wrap one gauze sponge around the tube, approximately 2 inches below the dressing. Then, tape the tube to the patient's skin, allowing for a little slack. This will provide additional stability to the tube, as well as help to maintain its position.
14. If needed, use ureteral connecting tubing to create a link between the nephrostomy tube and drainage bag.
    *Note*: Variations to this procedure may include the use of a hydrocolloidal skin barrier and protective skin film as a base before applying the gauze dressing (Guidos, 1988).

Adapted from guidelines established by the Hospital of the University of Pennsylvania Department of Nursing, Philadelphia, and the University of Iowa Hospital and Clinics Department of Nursing, Iowa City.
Photographs by Susan Leichtman.

tube placement has been made and should include information regarding the preprocedure routine, a description of the procedure itself, and the postprocedure precautions and care. Because long-term management of the tube is often required, guidelines for self-care of the nephrostomy tube and dressing at home must be incorporated into the teaching plan (Procedure 4–2).

**Patient Outcomes**

1. The patient verbalizes an understanding of the radiologic procedures employed to evaluate the obstruction to the upper urinary tract and participates in the completion of those studies needed to confirm the diagnosis.
2. The patient expresses relief of anxiety after receiving information concerning the cause of obstruction, proposed method of treatment, and prognosis for recovery of ureteral and renal function.
3. The patient's urine changes from blood-tinged to clear yellow within 48 hours after instrumentation of the ureter or insertion of a percutaneous nephrostomy tube.
4. The patient's fluid intake is more than 2000 mL/24 hours.
5. The patient's total urinary output is more than 30 mL/h in a 24-hour period.
6. The patient's nephrostomy tube is patent without evidence of kinking, obstruction, or dislodgement.
7. The patient exhibits no signs of urinary tract infection.
8. The patient expresses relief of flank pain after the initiation of comfort measures or the administration of analgesics.
9. The patient's skin around the site of percutaneous nephrostomy tube insertion exhibits no signs of irritation, infection, or breakdown.
10. The patient and caregiver are able to state the signs and symptoms of complications associated with nephrostomy tube drainage.
11. The patient and caregiver demonstrate the procedure to be used at home for changing the nephrostomy tube dressing.

## LOWER URINARY TRACT OBSTRUCTIONS

An obstruction of the lower urinary tract impedes the outflow of urine between the bladder and the urethral meatus. Most types of outlet obstruction are attributed to conditions arising in the urethra that evolve gradually, manifesting with symptoms of slow and difficult urination. Complications associated with incomplete bladder emptying may become evident if the obstructive process continues without treatment. This section reviews the most common causes of lower tract obstruction. Nursing management of the patient with benign prostatic hyperplasia (BPH), bladder neck contracture, urethral diverticula, urethral stricture and meatal stenosis, and urethral obstruction caused by foreign bodies is combined into a single discussion to reflect the similarities in the diagnosis and treatment of all lower urinary tract obstructions.

## Perspective on Disease Entity

### BENIGN PROSTATIC HYPERPLASIA

**Etiology.** Benign enlargement of the prostate gland is a normal physiologic event in aging men. The clinical symptoms caused by this enlargement vary in severity. Many men with significantly enlarged prostates have only mild symptoms of bladder outlet obstruction. Others with minimal enlargement of the prostate are bothered enough by their symptoms to seek medical advice. The process of benign hyperplasia of the prostate is a slow one; in many instances, the lower urinary tract gradually adjusts to the slowly increasing degree of urethral obstruction.

There is no known cause for BPH. All that is known with certainty is that the incidence of BPH increases with age; approximately 75% of men older than 50 years of age will have some symptoms of BPH (Birkhoff, 1983). Much of the epidemiologic data available for BPH refers to the likelihood of surgery for men with BPH: "the probability that a 40-year-old man will undergo prostate surgery if he survives until age 80 will be 30 to 40 per cent for most U.S. men" (Barry, 1990, p 500). Many variables, however, are likely to alter these figures.

Various causal relations have been investigated between factors such as diet, race, religion, and body habitus and the development of BPH. Trends suggest that blacks may have slightly higher occurrence rates than whites, and Asians may have lower rates. Jewish men are more likely to have surgery for BPH, as are nonsmoking men (Barry, 1990). None of these trends is significant enough to validate a causal relation.

**Pathophysiology.** The overall enlargement

## PROCEDURE 4-2
■
## Home Care Instructions for Patients With a Percutaneous Nephrostomy Tube

### ■ GENERAL INFORMATION

1. A percutaneous nephrostomy is the insertion of a catheter or tube through the skin and directly into the kidney that permits urine to be drained into a bag connected to it. The tube is sutured or stitched to the skin to hold it in place.
2. Drink at least eight 8-ounce glasses of water each day.
3. Avoid kinking, twisting, or clamping the nephrostomy tube.
4. Always keep the drainage bag below the waist.
5. During the day, the nephrostomy tube may be connected to a leg bag and concealed under regular clothing. At night, a larger bedside drainage bag must be used.
6. When disconnecting the nephrostomy tube from the drainage system and before reconnecting it, be sure to cleanse the ends of the nephrostomy tube and connecting tube with an alcohol-soaked gauze sponge.

### ■ DRESSING CHANGES

1. The dressing around the nephrostomy should be changed at least once each week or as often as once each day, if needed.
2. Carefully follow the procedure for changing the dressing that was demonstrated by the urologic nurse. [Refer to Procedure 4–1 for specific instructions.]
3. When bathing, place a plastic covering over the dressing to avoid getting it wet.

### ■ CARE OF THE DRAINAGE TUBE AND BAG

1. Clean the drainage tube and bag daily, after each use. To do this:
   a. First, be sure that all urine has been emptied from the tubing and bag.
   b. Wash the tubing and bag in warm, soapy water; allow the entire drainage system (with emptying spout open) to be submerged, filled, and soaked in the wash for 15 minutes. Use a syringe to force soapy water through the tubing for cleansing.
   c. Thoroughly rinse the tubing and bag with warm water to remove the soap.
   d. To disinfect and deodorize the bag, mix a solution consisting of 1 tablespoon of bleach and 2 cups of water. Pour this solution into the bag and rotate it so that all surfaces are rinsed; use the syringe to flush the solution through the tubing, too.
   e. Drain the bleach and water solution from the tubing and bag by way of the emptying spout and rinse the drainage system with warm water again.
   f. Hang to air dry with all ports open.
2. Never leave urine in a drainage bag when the bag is not in use.
3. With proper care, drainage bags may be reused for as long as 4 to 12 weeks.

### ■ WHEN SHOULD THE PHYSICIAN BE NOTIFIED?

1. If the stitches or nephrostomy tube comes out.
2. If there is an excessive leakage of urine from around the tube.
3. If abdominal or back pain, chills, fever higher than 100°F, persistent bloody urine from or around the tube, or cloudy and foul-smelling urine is noted.
4. If there is decreased or no urine output.
5. When it is time for the tube to be changed, usually every 3 months.

Adapted from guidelines prepared by the University of Iowa Hospitals and Clinics Department of Nursing, Iowa City, IA, and Southwest Florida Urologic Associates, Fort Myers, FL.

of the prostate gland that occurs with aging is actually a hyperplastic process—that is, there is an increase in the number of cells in the normal arrangement of tissue. In BPH, this increase in cellular growth causes nodules to develop. This process begins in the transition zone of the prostate or in the inner region adjacent to the urethra (Fig. 4–4). BPH nodules may also arise in the periurethral region (McNeal, 1990). As these nodules enlarge, the surrounding prostatic tissue becomes compressed. If the surrounding tissue responds with elasticity, minimal compression of the urethra will occur. If the capsule has great tensile strength, then obstruction of the lower urinary tract will occur (Hinman, 1986).

Two factors must be present for BPH to occur: aging and the presence of testicular androgens. Rarely does BPH occur in men younger than 40 years of age; it does not occur in men castrated before puberty (McConnell, 1990b). The role of androgens in the development of BPH is further substantiated by the effectiveness of antiandrogen therapy in treating the disease.

The regulation of androgens and estrogens is controlled by pathways involving the hypothalamus and the pituitary gland. The pituitary gland secretes luteinizing hormone, which interacts with receptors on the testicular Leydig cells to increase testosterone production. In the prostate, testosterone diffuses into the tissue and is converted to dihydrotestosterone by an enzyme, 5-alpha-reductase. Ninety percent of total prostatic androgen is in the form of dihy-drotestosterone; androgens from the adrenal gland account for the remaining 10% (McConnell, 1990a, 1990b). The presence of these prostatic androgens seems to be related to both normal and hyperplastic growth of the prostate (Wilson, 1980).

The gradual enlargement of the prostate and narrowing of the urethral lumen affect the ability of the lower urinary tract to perform its normal functions. The urinary bladder must contract with increasing strength and duration to empty against the narrowing urethral lumen. Voiding symptoms often result and are categorized as obstructive or irritative. Obstructive symptoms are those caused by the narrowed lumen of the prostatic urethra. Irritative voiding symptoms are those caused by the effects on the bladder as a result of urethral obstruction, that is, the response of the muscular bladder to the continued pressure at which it must contract (Murphy & Malloy, 1987).

*Silent prostatism* refers to the sudden occurrence of acute urinary retention in men with BPH who claim to be asymptomatic. Even among men who *are* symptomatic, acute retention is a possibility when the prostatic urethra is significantly compressed.

When untreated, BPH can lead to significant urinary tract pathologic conditions. Vesico-ureteral reflux leads to hydroureter and hydronephrosis, eventually compromising renal function. Chronic urinary retention and, subsequently, urinary tract infection and urosepsis are all potential sequelae when the urethral obstruction is severe.

**Medical-Surgical Management.** The diagnosis of BPH can be made using a variety of studies and findings. Several methods can be used to estimate how enlarged the prostate is; however, there is a low correlation between prostate size and severity of symptoms (Christensen & Bruskewitz, 1990). An assessment of the patient's symptoms and the degree to which they bother him is most important in an evaluation for BPH. Symptom scores, such as the Madsen-Iverson system (1983), or 24-hour voiding diaries help determine and quantify this finding.

Most patients being evaluated for BPH undergo a digital rectal examination of the prostate, urinalysis, urinary flow rate, and routine serum blood studies, including a prostate-specific antigen (PSA) determination. Other tests may be indicated depending on the patient's specific symptoms and overall medical condition, including measurement of postvoid residual urine, cystometry or pressure-flow

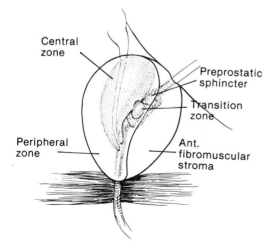

**FIGURE 4–4** Area of the prostate gland where BPH arises (transition zone). (Adapted from McNeal, J. E. [1979]. Prostate cancer. *UICC Technical Report Series, 48,* 24. Reprinted by permission.)

urodynamic studies, prostatic ultrasound, intravenous urography, or cystourethroscopy.

Decisions about treatment options generally depend on the presence or absence of any significant urinary tract pathologic condition and on the severity of the patient's symptoms.

Medical (nonsurgical) management has become an increasingly successful option for patients with mild to moderate symptoms. Several categories of drugs are now recognized for their therapeutic effects, resulting in symptom improvement in those patients with BPH. Those most frequently used are alpha-adrenergic blockers and antiandrogens.

Alpha-adrenergic blocking agents act on the smooth muscle components of the prostate, where alpha$_1$-receptors predominate. When stimulated, the alpha$_1$-receptors cause contraction of the approximately 20% of the prostate gland composed of smooth muscle (Lepor, 1991). Hence, administration of alpha$_1$-blocking agents (or antagonists) results in the opposite reaction, namely, relaxation. The alpha-blockers that have been studied for effectiveness in BPH include phenoxybenzamine (Dibenzyline), prazosin (Minipress), and terazosin (Hytrin). These three drugs are currently approved by the Food and Drug Administration (FDA) for indications other than BPH (Lepor, 1991).

Phenoxybenzamine was among the first of the alpha-blocking drugs to be used for symptoms of BPH. Despite its relative success in improving symptoms, its use has declined because of a questionable carcinogenic effect (Caine, 1990). Prazosin and terazosin are specific alpha$_1$-blockers and are both commonly used for symptoms of BPH. Side effects are usually related to the effects of these agents on alpha-receptors elsewhere in the body and include tachycardia, palpitations, hypotension, fatigue, nasal congestion, and dry mouth. Prazosin has a significant first-dose effect, causing syncopal episodes in many patients after oral administration of the initial dose. Therefore, therapy should always be initiated at night.

Clinical studies on the effectiveness of terazosin in BPH have demonstrated an increase in urinary flow rate, overall improvement in symptom score, and no change in blood pressure in patients who are normotensive (Lepor et al., 1990). Patients taking terazosin are usually dose titrated up to 10 to 20 mg/d. Terazosin has not been used long enough for long-term results to be known (Lepor et al., 1992).

Antiandrogen therapy for BPH has also received much attention. Because the presence of testicular androgens is necessary for BPH to

occur, removing them from the prostatic environment causes BPH to regress (McConnell, 1990a). Most antiandrogen agents, many of which are commonly used in prostate cancer, result in sexual dysfunction because of the interruption of the normal androgen pathway. Obviously, loss of sexual function makes most of these therapies an unattractive option for patients with BPH.

Much attention has surrounded the FDA approval of finasteride (Proscar). Finasteride is a 5-alpha-reductase inhibitor that prevents the conversion of testosterone to dihydrotestosterone within the prostate itself. Circulating testosterone levels are not affected, so sexual dysfunction does not occur as a result of this drug. Clinically, finasteride results in a decrease in prostatic volume and an improvement in urinary flow rate. Long-term data on this drug are needed to determine if finasteride, in fact, alters the natural history of BPH (MK-906 Study Group, 1992).

Combination therapies with alpha$_1$-blockers and antiandrogen drugs are currently being evaluated. One example is the use of flutamide (Eulexin) in combination with finasteride (to block the 10% of circulating androgens from an adrenal source and the 90% from a testicular source). One caution for patients on antiandrogen drugs is that PSA levels may not increase in these patients, even when prostate cancer is present (Lepor et al., 1992). However, the effectiveness of medical treatments for BPH has provided relief of symptoms for many patients without surgery.

Surgical interventions for BPH include transurethral resection of the prostate (TURP), open prostatectomy, transurethral incision of the prostate (TUIP), transurethral laser incision of the prostate (TULIP), visual laser ablation of the prostate (VLAP), balloon dilation, and prostatic stents.

TURP has been the treatment of choice for symptomatic BPH for more than 50 years. TURP is extremely effective in relieving the lower urinary tract obstruction BPH creates, along with the resultant obstructive and irritative voiding symptoms; however, it is an invasive procedure that carries with it certain risks. Some degree of incontinence occurs in 2% to 4% of patients, significant infection in 5% to 10%, bleeding requiring transfusion in 5%, and impotence in 5% to 10% (Lepor et al., 1992). Retrograde ejaculation occurs in as many as 90% of patients after TURP (Murphy & Malloy, 1987).

In recent years, the use of TURP has been

carefully scrutinized by health insurance providers because of the large amounts of money paid out for TURPs. TURP is currently the second most common operation performed in the United States (Graves, 1989). Criteria for selecting patients for surgery for BPH have been established by numerous companies and agencies. It is generally agreed that TURP is the appropriate treatment choice for patients with hydronephrosis (with developing renal failure), acute urinary retention, recurrent urinary tract infections due to stasis, and marked bladder instability with urinary incontinence (Lepor et al., 1992). Patients with extremely large prostates along with the above conditions may require open prostatectomy because of the size of their gland. TURP also remains an option for patients with moderate to severe symptoms who do not respond to other treatment options or who choose the surgery.

TURP is usually performed under regional, spinal, or general anesthesia. A resectoscope is inserted into the urethra, and with continuous irrigation, the prostatic tissue in the periurethral area is gradually resected away and irrigated out of the lower urinary tract (Fig. 4–5). The prostate "chips" are weighed and examined pathologically. A large Foley catheter with a 30-mL balloon is placed to tamponade the surgical area and to drain the bladder. Active

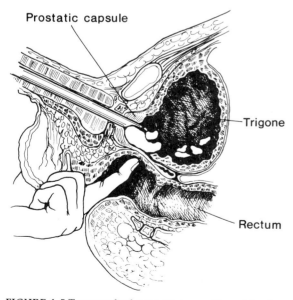

**Prostatic capsule**

**Trigone**

**Rectum**

*FIGURE 4–5* Transurethral prostatectomy. (From Murphy, K., & Malloy, T. R. [1987]. Bladder outlet obstruction. In P. M. Hanno & A. J. Wein [Eds.], *A clinical manual of urology* [p. 229]. Norwalk, CT: Appleton-Century-Crofts. Reprinted by permission.)

bleeding from the vascular prostatic tissue may continue for 24 to 48 hours, requiring continuous or intermittent irrigation to maintain catheter patency.

Open prostatectomy for benign disease is usually carried out using a suprapubic or retropubic approach. The prostatic capsule is opened, and the adenomatous tissue is removed from within. Patients undergoing a suprapubic prostatectomy often require a suprapubic tube in addition to a urethral catheter. Postoperative recovery time after open prostatectomy is significantly longer than after TURP because of the more invasive nature of the procedure.

Late complications after TURP include bladder neck contracture and urethral stricture. Approximately 20% of patients require reoperation (for regrowth of prostatic tissue) 10 years later (Lepor et al., 1992).

Newer procedures designed to be minimally invasive while providing relief of the obstructive symptoms of BPH have evolved in the past decade. Transurethral incision of the prostate (TUIP) has actually been performed for about 20 years but only recently has gained attention in the United States. TUIP involves making incisions in the prostatic tissue to enlarge the lumen of the prostatic urethra and the bladder outlet. Prostate tissue is not resected (Orandi, 1990). TUIP is a treatment option for patients with a small prostate but with bothersome symptoms; usually these are younger or middle-aged patients. TUIP can be performed under local anesthesia in an outpatient setting. In some instances, TUIP has proved to be as successful as TURP in alleviating symptoms for longer periods (Lepor et al., 1992).

TULIP and VLAP are both newer procedures that use laser technology to incise or obliterate prostatic tissue. Long-term results are not yet known.

Balloon dilation of the prostate is a technique that presents an alternative to prostate surgery. It involves inflation of a balloon (under pressure) in the prostatic urethra (Fig. 4–6). The balloon is kept inflated for a period, usually about 15 minutes, then is deflated and removed. Balloon dilation is thought to work by stretching or fracturing the prostatic tissue or by compressing the gland, allowing the prostatic lumen to enlarge (Lepor et al., 1992). Balloon dilation may be performed under local anesthesia in an outpatient setting with minimal complications. A Foley catheter may be left in place for 24 hours to several days.

Relief of symptoms after balloon dilation of

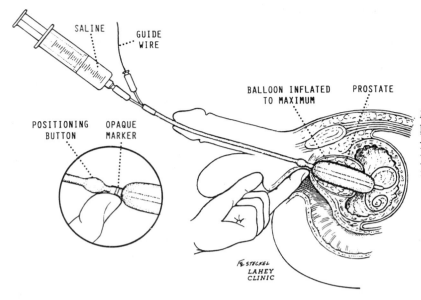

FIGURE 4–6 Balloon dilation of the prostate. (From Dowd, J. B., & Smith, J. J. [1990]. Balloon dilation of the prostate. *Urologic Clinics of North America*, 17[3], 673. Reprinted by permission.)

the prostate is usually immediately apparent (after removal of the catheter), but it tends to be transient. Many patients report that symptoms return within 3 to 42 months (Lepor et al., 1992). Hence, balloon dilation is a treatment option for patients who have not responded to medication (or who choose not to try medication) and for patients who prefer not to undergo invasive intervention. Usually, these are men with mild to moderate symptoms.

Prostatic stents are being used with increasing frequency to open the narrowed lumen of the prostatic urethra. Two types of prostatic stents are currently available: one is a coil, and the other is a tubular mesh made of a biocompatible alloy (Fig. 4–7). The prostatic stent is placed with cystoscopic guidance in the prostatic urethra and expanded to widen the opening; it is then left in place. During a 3- to 6-month period, epithelialization of the stent occurs. The stent is designed to permanently resolve urethral obstruction caused by BPH.

Prostatic stents are relatively new, and no long-term data on their use are available. Initial reports indicate that both symptom scores and flow rates improve after stent placement, although some patients report an increase in irritative symptoms immediately after stent placement (Oesterling, 1991). Patients must be cautioned not to be catheterized through the urethra for any reason for 3 months after stent placement.

Technologies continue to evolve as alternatives to traditional surgery for BPH are sought.

Advances in pharmacologic therapies and localized therapies will doubtless continue.

## BLADDER NECK CONTRACTURE

**Etiology.** Bladder neck contracture is rarely a congenital anatomic variation but rather an iatrogenic abnormality associated with prostatectomy. A contracture may develop after the inadvertent resection or excessive fulguration

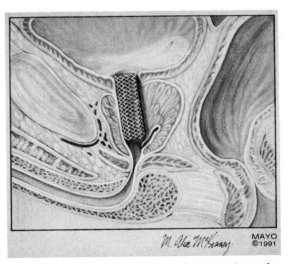

FIGURE 4–7 Intraurethral stent in the prostatic urethra. (From Oesterling, J. E. [1991]. Permanently implanted intraurethral stent may be viable alternative to TURP. *AUA Today*, 4[1], 10, 11. © 1991 Mayo Foundation. Reprinted by permission.)

of smooth muscle tissue at the bladder neck during a transurethral removal of the prostate. It may also occur after radical prostatectomy when reconstruction of the bladder neck, requiring the anastomosis of smooth muscle tissue, is performed. The incidence of bladder neck contracture after the resection of prostatic tissue ranges from 2% to 12% of cases (Bagley et al., 1985; Walsh, 1986).

**Pathophysiology.** During voiding, the bladder neck normally funnels open to permit urine to be evacuated from the bladder. This action may be compromised when bladder neck tissue is resected. A fibrous scar develops in the area disrupted, extending into the lumen of the outlet to cause narrowing and distortion of the bladder neck. The degree of occlusion depends on the extent of tissue growth but may progress to allow only a pinpoint-sized passageway. The bladder compensates for the diminished diameter of the outlet by generating an increased intravesical pressure during bladder emptying. Because the scar tissue is usually dense and relatively immobile, the increased pressure cannot propel urine through the obstructed bladder neck for complete emptying of the vesica. Continued high-pressure voiding against a blocked outlet can eventually lead to bladder wall hypertrophy, trabeculation of the bladder wall, and formation of bladder diverticula.

Symptoms of bladder neck contracture or obstruction are usually noticed several months after prostatectomy (Bagley et al., 1985). Initially, a decrease in the force and the caliber of the stream may be noted, along with hesitancy and postvoid dribbling. If bladder emptying is incomplete, the patient may be experiencing urinary frequency. Stasis of urine in the bladder may precipitate a urinary tract infection, causing the patient to complain of urgency and dysuria.

**Medical-Surgical Management.** The diagnosis of bladder neck contracture may be suspected when passage of a urinary catheter proves difficult. A urinary flow rate study might then be performed to determine if the rate of the urinary stream and the voided amount are decreased and if the voiding time is prolonged. A voiding cystourethrogram (VCUG) may also be obtained to determine the extent of outlet function. A cystourethroscopic examination will confirm the diagnosis of bladder neck contracture, revealing an elevation of the bladder neck above the apex of the trigone, narrowing of the passageway, and tightness of the bladder neck.

A mild bladder neck contracture may be treated with progressive dilation using size-graded sounds or filiforms and followers while the patient is under local or general anesthesia. Bladder neck dilation may also be accomplished by having the patient perform clean intermittent catheterization. This procedure helps maintain a dilated outlet while removing residual urine.

Surgical correction of bladder neck contracture is often favored and may be accomplished by transurethral incision. This usually requires the use of a cold knife blade to make cuts at approximately the 3 and 9 o'clock positions to open up the bladder neck (Bagley et al., 1985). The contracture may also be resected and the remaining tissue injected with steroids to prevent recurrent tissue growth and occlusion (Krongrad & Droller, 1990).

## URETHRAL STRICTURE

**Etiology.** In adults, a urethral stricture is usually an acquired condition commonly occurring in men and infrequently seen in women. The higher incidence of urethral stricture development in men is due to the anatomic structure and length of the urethra.

Most urethral strictures have iatrogenic origins and may be secondary to manipulation of the lower urinary tract during diagnostic procedures and transurethral surgery; they may also be associated with the long-term use of an indwelling urethral catheter. Some reports suggest that as many as 9% of patients who have undergone TURP will later develop urethral strictures (Jorgensen et al., 1986; Krongrad & Droller, 1990). However, traumatic injury to the pelvis or perineum, often caused by crushing accidents, can result in the formation of a urethral stricture in men. Trauma following intercourse, childbirth, or vaginal surgery may be the cause of urethral stricture formation in women. Gonorrhea has historically been the most common cause of infection-induced strictures (Warden & Devine, 1985). In some instances, neoplasms, venereal warts, or urethral polyps are underlying causes of urethral stricture formation.

**Pathophysiology.** An injury to the urethra causes the formation of collagen and fibrous tissue at the area of insult. This leads to a narrowing and loss of elasticity of the passageway that restricts the flow of urine. The scarred tissue may soften as it matures, allowing for improved urine flow. However, repeated infections, attempts at dilation with an instrument too large for the urethra, or high voiding pressures can combine to aggravate the healing tissue, causing a circumferential contraction of the scar that narrows the urethra again and again. The untreated or improperly treated stricture eventually causes sufficient obstruction to dilate the system proximal to the blockage, leading to serious complications.

The male urethra, with its five anatomic segments (prostatic, membranous, bulbous, pendulous, and fossa navicularis), is more prone to stricture formation (Fig. 4–8). Strictures caused by infection and perineal straddle injuries typically affect the bulbous urethra. The membranous or prostatomembranous urethra is the area most likely to develop strictures after pelvic injury. Multiple segments of the urethra may be affected by strictures induced by prolonged catheterization or transurethral instrumentation. In all instances, the severity of a stricture correlates with its cause.

Patients with a urethral stricture exhibit obstructive and irritative voiding symptoms. The most common complaint is prolonged voiding with a thin, weak stream. An intermittent or interrupted stream, double stream, or spraying stream may also be described. Hesitancy, double voiding, postvoid dribbling, a sense of incomplete bladder emptying, dysuria, frequency, nocturia, and urgency or urge incontinence are other complaints typically associated with urethral strictures.

**Medical-Surgical Management.** To confirm the presence of a urethral stricture, the following diagnostic procedures are performed:

1. Urinary flow rate—to measure the length of time required for bladder emptying and the force of the urinary stream; a peak flow rate <10 mL/sec is suggestive of outflow obstruction.

2. Urethral catheterization—to measure the amount of residual urine; an inability to or difficulty in passing a 16 or 18 Fr catheter may suggest a narrowing of the urethra caused by stricture (Bagley et al., 1985).

3. Urine culture—to verify bacterial growth if infection is suspected.

4. Retrograde urethrogram—to demonstrate the location and extent of the stricture.

5. Urethroscopy—for direct visualization and inspection of the stricture to determine the location, the extent, and the degree of urethral scarring.

6. Urethral calibration—done using a bougie à boule to determine the size of the passageway (McAninch, 1992).

A variety of therapies are used to treat urethral strictures. The specific management technique selected depends on the location, the length, and the density of the strictured area. Mechanical dilation of strictures, a nonsurgical approach, is among the oldest and most common therapies employed. A local anesthetic is usually instilled into the urethra before the procedure. Dilation of the stricture is accomplished by inserting a filiform and passing followers of increasingly larger sizes. Van Buren urethral sounds (curved metal rods) may also be used to dilate a strictured urethra; however, these instruments are generally used for strictures that have been previously dilated or for passageways that will readily accept a size 18 sound. The use of smaller sounds for initial dilation of a urethral stricture is not recommended, because they may perforate the urethral mucosa or create false passages (Bagley et al., 1985; McAninch, 1992). Indwelling urethral catheters may also be used to dilate a stricture. This technique requires transurethral insertion of the next larger even-sized catheter every 48

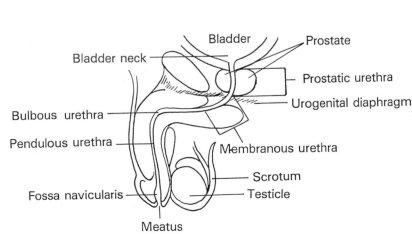

FIGURE 4–8 Male genitourinary system depicting anatomic segments of the urethra.

to 72 hours, until a 20 to 24 Fr tube may be placed with ease. Catheter dilation may be used in combination with dilation by followers or sounds to continue expanding the urethra when larger instruments could not be passed or to maintain a newly dilated passageway (Bagley et al., 1985). Intermittent self-catheterization, if feasible, may accomplish the same objective.

Direct-vision internal urethrotomy represents a surgical approach to the treatment of urethral strictures. The procedure requires the use of a urethrotome to visualize the stricture. A filiform or ureteral catheter is inserted through the strictured segment of the urethra to serve as a guide for incision. The safest and most effective urethral incisions are made at the 12 o'clock or dorsal midline position and extend through the full thickness of the scar to open the lumen of the urethra (Bagley et al., 1985). A 16 or 18 Fr Foley catheter is then placed to minimize bleeding and pain. To prevent recurrence of the stricture after incision, a program of intermittent self-catheterization is recommended.

Surgical reconstruction of the urethra may be necessary when dilation of the stricture is needed more often than every 6 months, when there is recurrence of the stricture after repeated attempts at urethrotomy, or when the strictured area is too large for treatment by dilation or urethrotomy. To refashion the urethra, a urethroplasty is performed as either a one- or two-stage procedure. One-stage urethroplasty requires excision of the stricture and reanastomosis of the urethral ends; a patch tissue graft may or may not be used to secure the anastomosed area. The single-stage urethroplasty is an uncomplicated procedure, preferred by most urologists for its high rate of success (Devine, 1986). The two-stage procedure is reserved for instances of complex or multiple strictures. In the first step, the strictured area is marsupialized to form a pouchlike structure, and a perineal urethrostomy is established. The second step is performed after a 6-month period of healing and involves the recreation of the urethra.

A new treatment alternative for urethral strictures is laser photoradiation. The most favorable results relate to the use of the KTP-532 laser. This is a "frequency-doubled Nd:YAG laser that is passed through a crystal to provide a wavelength of 532 nm" (Malloy & Wein, 1990). Although the KTP-532 laser does not allow for deep penetration of tissue, its ability to precisely cut tissue makes it an effective therapy for urethral strictures. As with other therapeutic approaches, a catheter is required for a period after laser treatment to keep the urethral passage patent.

## URETHRAL DIVERTICULA

**Etiology.** Two types of diverticula are recognized. Primary, or congenital, diverticula are more commonly found in males and result from incomplete development of the urethra with a defect in the ventral wall, a müllerian duct remnant, or an enlarged utricle. Diverticula may also arise from cystic dilatation of Cowper's glands (Bagley et al., 1985). Secondary, or acquired, diverticula are a much more common entity that occurs in both sexes (although this type is more common in females) and is usually caused by infection, instrumentation, or obstruction. In males, for instance, a periurethral or prostate abscess, continued use of an external clamp for urethral compression, frequent instrumentation of the urethra, or prolonged use of an indwelling catheter may induce development of diverticula. In females, diverticula are often associated with severe urethral infection, abscess formation of the periurethral glands, or birth trauma.

**Pathophysiology.** A diverticulum is a blind pouch that forms when muscle fibers become hypertrophied, thereby allowing the protrusion of mucosa. In the urethra, a diverticulum usually has a distinct opening and may take on the appearance of small saccule or globule, or it may look like a separate channel to the bladder (Fig. 4–9). Urine is trapped and collects in the pouch, causing it to expand and obstruct outflow from the bladder. Because the diverticulum has no muscle fibers, it has no expulsive power; accumulated urine stagnates to provide a medium for bacterial growth.

Signs indicative of a urethral diverticulum include a history of chronic urinary tract infection and a palpable perineal mass that empties with compression of the perineum (Bagley et al., 1985). Other clues might be the development of a urethral calculus or difficult catheterization resulting in the discovery of a false passage.

**Medical-Surgical Management.** The presence of a diverticulum is confirmed with urethroscopy. If the protrusion is small and asymptomatic, treatment is generally not required. Otherwise, transurethral drainage and resection of the diverticulum is performed. Postoperatively, suprapubic bladder drainage

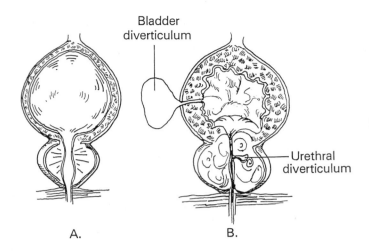

Bladder
diverticulum

Urethral
diverticulum

A.                      B.

*FIGURE 4–9* Comparison of normal bladder *(A)* versus trabeculated bladder with diverticula *(B)*.

may be indicated for a period to prevent further trauma and to allow for healing of the urethra.

## FOREIGN BODIES

**Etiology.** A variety of items of varying sizes and shapes have reportedly been found in the urethra and bladder of men, women, and children. Objects are sometimes inserted in desperation to relieve urinary retention, or they may be introduced during a naive attempt to explore the genitalia. Occasionally, an object has been inserted into the male urethra in the hope of prolonging an erection or in an effort to block the drainage of ejaculate for contraceptive purposes.

The voluntary, unsupervised insertion of an object into one's urethra may be associated with a psychiatric disorder in the adult. Disturbed sexual adjustment, schizophrenia, dementia, or antisocial personality disorders are commonly associated with the performance of such an act; alcohol intoxication may accompany and facilitate urethral insertion. In some instances, the self-insertion of a foreign object may actually be an attempt at mutilation or suicide (Ellison & Dobies, 1984).

**Pathophysiology.** When a foreign object has been inserted into the lower urinary tract, urethritis, cystitis, or both develop and rapidly lead to bacterial infection. If the object has completely blocked the urethra, urinary retention quickly occurs. Prolonged bacterial infection may cause a stone to form on the object; prolonged obstruction eventually leads to hydronephrosis and damage to the kidney.

The patient with a foreign object may describe symptoms such as dysuria, a slow or weak urinary stream, a sense of incomplete bladder emptying, frequency, urgency, and pain. Hematuria or pyuria may also be evident.

**Medical-Surgical Management.** To diagnose the presence of a foreign body in the urethra or bladder, a plain x-ray film of the lower urinary tract is first obtained. If the object is radiopaque or metal, it will be detected. Otherwise, cystourethroscopy should be performed for direct visualization of the object and inspection of the lower tract. Removal of the foreign body is always indicated and may be accomplished during cystourethroscopy. However, suprapubic cystotomy may be required to remove unusually large, long, coiled, or knotted objects. Referral for psychiatric evaluation may be indicated as a secondary measure.

## MEATAL STENOSIS

**Etiology.** Stenosis or stricture of the external urinary meatus can be a congenital condition that, in males, is occasionally associated with hypospadias. In females, the problem may manifest in early childhood as distal urethral stenosis. More likely, however, is the notion that meatal stenosis or stricture is an acquired condition that occurs after inflammation, both specific and nonspecific, after internal or external urethral infections (e.g., balanitis xerotica obliterans), after trauma (e.g., vaginal deliveries), or in association with the use of an indwelling catheter or urethral instrumentation (Devine, 1986). It also may be a late complication of circumcision that occurs because the glans and the meatus are no longer protected by the foreskin, thereby leading to the development of meatitis or meatal ulcer. In newly circumcised infants, diaper irritation may induce the formation of an inflammatory membrane (Kunz, 1986).

**Pathophysiology.** In males, meatal stenosis may appear as a membranous web of tissue that spans the opening of the urethra. In females, the formation of collagenous tissue causes a stenotic ring to form just inside the external urinary meatus.

The problem of meatal stenosis primarily affects the quality and the control of the urinary stream. However, bladder emptying may be compromised when there is extensive blockage. The male patient may complain of difficulty directing his urinary stream to the extent that he must hold the penis downward during voiding to avoid deflecting urine all over the bathroom. Other symptoms that may be described include a fine yet forceful stream, a forked or split stream, a prolonged voiding time, hesitancy, frequency, a sense of incomplete bladder emptying, or terminal hematuria.

**Medical-Surgical Management.** Initially, urethral calibration should be done to determine the size of the meatus. In a child younger than 10 years of age, the tip of an 8 Fr pediatric feeding tube should pass through the meatus without difficulty (McAninch, 1992). In an adult, the urethral meatus should easily accept the tip of a 14 to 18 Fr catheter. If the diameter of the urethral opening is more narrow than this, intervention may be required.

For mild meatal stenosis, dilation with sounds or catheters may be sufficient to expand the opening of the urethra. However, if there is significant obstruction or if the distal urethra is involved, a meatotomy (surgical incision of the meatus) may be performed. Surgical correction is effective in eliminating the problem of meatal stenosis in 95% of cases (Murphy & Malloy, 1987). Regardless of whether meatal stenosis is medically or surgically treated, antibiotic therapy is usually employed to relieve or prevent infection. Routine follow-up and the avoidance of urethral trauma are also important to the long-term effects of treatment.

## Approaches to Patient Care

### Assessment

The patient with a lower urinary tract obstruction may describe a variety of symptoms. Those typically associated with bladder outlet obstruction include hesitancy, a decreased force and caliber of the urinary stream, a slow or prolonged voiding time, double voiding, terminal or postvoid dribble, a sensation of in-

complete bladder emptying, a vague suprapubic discomfort, an interrupted or intermittent urinary stream, and a double or spraying stream. Irritative voiding symptoms such as dysuria, strangury, frequency, urgency, and nocturia are common in persons with a lower tract obstruction and may also be described. Sometimes, the patient may relate findings of blood in the urine.

During the initial collection of data, question the patient about the incidence of any previous urinary tract obstructions, problems with recurrent urinary tract infections, history of sexually transmitted disease, injuries to the pelvis, or prior instrumentation of the urinary tract. In addition, try to ascertain the length of time the patient has been experiencing voiding difficulties.

Depending on the type and extent of lower tract obstruction, physical examination may reveal some of the following findings: palpation of a distended bladder; flank tenderness; palpation of a perineal, penoscrotal, or urethral mass; palpation of a prostate that is (1) enlarged and benign, (2) enlarged, boggy, and tender, or (3) enlarged and hard; difficult passage of a catheter resulting in the discovery of a false passage or a large residual of urine; urethral discharge; cystourethrocele; or perianal or rectal fistulas.

Pertinent laboratory studies include the urinalysis, which may reveal the presence of red blood cells, white blood cells, or pus. A urine culture confirms the presence of bacterial infection; sensitivity studies identify the most effective antibiotic. In some instances, the microscopic examination of prostatic fluid or urethral secretions is performed to look for pathogens. Measurements of BUN, serum creatinine, and serum electrolyte levels may be performed to assess renal function. If carcinoma of the prostate is suspected in a patient with obstruction caused by prostatic enlargement, then the blood levels of prostatic acid phosphatase and PSA should be measured.

Assessment also should include an appraisal of the patient's emotional response to a problem that affects bladder emptying. Inquiry by the nurse may reveal that a patient with a lower urinary tract obstruction is gravely concerned that prostatic enlargement may be due to cancer or that treatment will in some way affect his sexual function. Others may relate feelings of embarrassment over their inability to control the direction of the urinary stream, the inadvertent dribbling of urine, or the length of time and number of visits to the bathroom needed to empty the bladder adequately. For some, discomfort caused by inflammation, infection, or bladder distention may be sufficient to affect their daily routine or job performance, causing unneeded stress and anxiety.

Finally, it is important to determine the patient's knowledge and understanding of his or her urologic condition and the methods that will be employed to confirm and treat an obstruction to the lower tract. The willingness to comply with the treatment plan and recommendations for follow-up care should also be ascertained, because it will impact on nursing care given and the overall therapeutic result.

### Nursing Diagnosis

Nursing diagnoses for the patient with a lower urinary tract obstruction may include the following:

1. Altered pattern of urinary elimination related to
   a. Anatomic obstruction to the lower urinary tract.
   b. Irritative voiding symptoms caused by urinary tract obstruction.
   c. Postoperative placement of an indwelling urethral or suprapubic catheter or the creation of a temporary urethrostomy.
2. Urinary retention related to obstruction to the lower urinary tract caused by prostatic hyperplasia, bladder neck contracture, urethral diverticula, urethral stricture, or the presence of a foreign body in the urethra or meatal stenosis.
3. Pain related to
   a. Bladder spasms.
   b. Bladder distention.
   c. Dysuria.
4. Anxiety related to
   a. Perceived threat to sexual function.
   b. Feelings of embarrassment regarding voiding difficulties.
   c. Effect of voiding disorder on daily routine and job performance.
   d. Fear of prostate cancer.
   e. Ability to be continent after transurethral surgery.
5. Knowledge deficit related to
   a. An unfamiliarity with diagnostic and treatment methods for lower urinary tract obstruction.
   b. Procedure for clean intermittent catheterization for urethral dilation.
   c. Voiding function after removal of catheters.
6. Potential for infection related to
   a. Surgical instrumentation of the lower urinary tract.
   b. Presence of indwelling urethral catheter.
   c. Practice of clean intermittent catheterization for urethral dilation.
7. Potential for fluid volume excess related to postoperative continuous bladder irrigation.
8. Potential for fluid volume deficit related to hemorrhage after transurethral surgery.

### Plan of Care

Nursing care is planned to enable the patient to

1. Verbalize feelings of decreased anxiety after the type of blockage has been confirmed, a treatment plan has been explained, and recovery is assured.
2. Comply with plans for diagnosis, treatment, and long-term management of a condition causing obstruction to the lower urinary tract.
3. Obtain relief from pain and discomfort caused by bladder spasms, bladder distention, and dysuria.
4. Prevent urinary tract infection.
5. Exhibit no signs of an alteration in the volume of bodily fluids.
6. Resume a normal pattern of urinary elimination after intervention for a lower urinary tract obstruction.
7. Achieve complete bladder emptying with each voiding.

### Intervention

The patient with a lower urinary tract obstruction may have been reluctant to seek medical advice for his or her voiding difficulties because of a variety of fears and misconceptions. No doubt, numerous concerns will be expressed, and questions will be asked during the initial evaluation. Nursing intervention involves providing information to the patient (1) to allay the fears regarding the significance and consequences of a bladder outlet obstruction; (2) to prepare for diagnostic procedures that will be performed to assess and confirm the type, the extent, and the location of the obstruction; and (3) to familiarize the patient with postoperative care activities and the routine for follow-up care related to the planned method of treatment for relieving the obstruction.

Postoperative nursing care is directed toward the prevention and recognition of possible complications. Depending on the type of surgical procedure performed, all or some of the following interventions may be used in the care of the patient who has undergone transurethral surgery.

*Catheter Management.* An indwelling urethral catheter is usually inserted intraoperatively after surgical correction of a lower urinary tract obstruction. The catheter provides for drainage of urine from the bladder and serves to support temporarily the surgical site and occlude resected tissue to prevent bleeding. In some instances, a suprapubic catheter is inserted to divert urine when the urethral catheter is intended as a urethral stent. The type and size of catheter used depend on the procedure performed and the preferences of the urologist. Patients who have undergone TURP usually return from surgery with a three-way, 24 to 30 Fr catheter held in place with a 30-mL balloon.

Patency of the Foley catheter is ensured by maintaining a closed drainage system and keeping the drainage bag lower than the bladder level. The patient is also monitored for signs of occlusion, such as suprapubic pain and distention, decreased urine output, severe bladder spasms, and blood clots in the tubing. If clots do threaten to obstruct the catheter and drainage tube, then manual irrigation may be performed as ordered by the physician and as needed to prevent occlusion. If the patient has returned from surgery with a system for continuous bladder irrigation, carefully regulate the rate of infusion to keep the urine pink-tinged. Close monitoring of the amount of irrigant infused and the urine output is essential until the continuous bladder irrigation is terminated—usually within 24 to 48 hours.

*Intake and Output.* A careful record of intake and output is maintained, with hourly measurements recommended while the patient has a continuous bladder irrigation. At the same time, observe the urine color, noting particularly the degree of discoloration caused by bleeding. Also, observe the patient closely for signs of dilutional hyponatremia (water intoxication), such as headache, confusion, lethargy, abdominal distention, weight gain, nausea, vomiting, and seizures. This problem may result from intraoperative bladder irrigation, although it is also likely to occur during the first 24 hours after surgery if continuous bladder irrigation is being maintained. Fluid restriction or replacement should be instituted, as appropriate (see Chap. 3). However, to keep urine dilute, intravenous and oral fluid intake should approximate 1000 mL per 8 hours to induce diuresis, unless medically contraindicated.

*Recognition and Prevention of Infection.* The risk of infection after transurethral surgery is high because of prolonged instrumentation of the urinary tract. Therefore, the patient is observed for signs of bacteremia that may precede the development of septic shock. Observe

for manifestations such as elevated temperature (>101°F), decreased blood pressure (<90/60 mm Hg), increased heart rate (>110 beats per minute), increased respiratory rate (>28 breaths per minute), decreased urinary output, shaking and chills, warm and dry skin, vomiting, and altered consciousness. To minimize the risk of catheter-related infection, maintain a closed drainage system. When manual irrigation of the catheter must be performed, strict aseptic technique is advised. Cleansing of the catheter and urethral meatus performed twice a day and after bowel movements, using soap and water, is also recommended to prevent the ascent of bacteria. Antibiotic medication may be ordered and administered for prophylaxis.

*Pain Management.* Patients who have had transurethral surgery typically experience pain in the form of bladder spasms. The pain is most severe in the 24 to 48 hours after surgery. Although the patient may feel an extraordinary urge to void and at times expel urine from around the catheter, this should be discouraged because bleeding may be induced. Belladonna and opium suppositories may be administered to provide relief from bladder spasms. If they are ineffective in relieving bladder spasms, or if they are contraindicated for the patient (i.e., someone with glaucoma), then lidocaine jelly may be applied to the urethral meatus or a systemic analgesic may be administered.

*Promotion of Voiding.* Catheter drainage is maintained for varying periods, depending on the procedure performed and the practices of the urologist. Indwelling catheters are usually removed on the second or third postoperative day after transurethral resection of the prostate. However, if urethroplasty has been performed, the indwelling catheter will remain in place much longer. The catheter may be irrigated before its removal to evacuate any residual clots. The patient is then encouraged to drink fluids to increase diuresis and to facilitate bladder filling.

Patients should be warned that their first attempt at voiding after surgery may be somewhat difficult and produce sensations of burning and discomfort. An overwhelming fear of pain may cause some patients to avoid urination intentionally. Nonetheless, they must be encouraged to attempt to empty the bladder. If the patient is unable to initiate voiding, suggest measures such as bladder massage, application of heat to the suprapubic area or perineum, running water, and ambulation to help stimulate bladder emptying. Document the time of the first voiding after catheter removal and the volume voided. The frequency and amounts of subsequent attempts at bladder emptying should also be recorded. Notify the physician if the patient is unable to pass urine, voids less than 100 mL of urine with each attempted urination, complains of a persistent urge to void or a feeling of incomplete bladder emptying, has a stream no stronger than a dribble, or exhibits bladder distention. These are indications that the patient has failed the voiding trial and will require recatheterization. Those patients who are unable to void are discharged from the hospital with an indwelling catheter; this occurs in approximately 2.4% of all patients having transurethral surgery (Krongrad & Droller, 1990). Another attempt at catheter removal is usually planned within days and is often done at the time of the patient's postoperative visit to the physician.

*Discharge and Home Care.* In preparation for discharge and home care, the nurse should ensure that the patient has been provided with the necessary instructions and information. Teaching should include the following:

1. Review of the signs and symptoms of urinary tract infection.
2. Review of the signs and symptoms of acute urinary retention.
3. Discussion of measures to promote voiding.
4. Instructions for home maintenance of an indwelling catheter, including catheter and meatal cleansing, emptying of the drainage bag, and daytime use of a leg bag.
5. Instructions on procedure of clean intermittent catheterization for patients who have had urethrotomy (see Chap. 14).
6. Procedure for measurement of intake and output, with emphasis given to maintaining an oral fluid intake of approximately 3000 mL per 24 hours.
7. Recommended use of stool softeners or laxatives for as long as 4 to 6 weeks after surgery to avoid straining with bowel movements.
8. Avoidance of heavy lifting or other strenuous activities for 4 to 6 weeks after surgery.
9. Avoidance of sexual intercourse for 3 to 4 weeks after surgery.
10. Instruction on pelvic muscle exercises to strengthen musculature surrounding the external sphincter for symptoms of urgency, dribbling, or mild incontinence. The patient should be taught to interrupt the urine flow midstream with each void and

to contract pelvic muscles five times each hour during the day (Duffy, 1990).

*Delayed Problems.* For 6 to 8 weeks after transurethral surgery, patients may experience irritative voiding symptoms, such as frequency, urgency, urge incontinence, and dysuria; the urinary stream may also be weak. Patients should be prepared to expect these symptoms, yet be reassured that they are only temporarily bothersome. However, the persistence of irritative voiding symptoms and the recurrence of obstructive voiding symptoms are indications for further evaluation by the physician.

In 2% to 4% of patients, incontinence after transurethral surgery is a persistent problem. Those patients who experience bladder instability before prostatectomy will likely require 6 to 12 months recovery time before regaining continence (Duffy, 1990). They should be counseled about methods to manage postprostatectomy incontinence, including the use of an external catheter connected to a leg bag or an appropriate absorbent product. In some instances, urethral compression devices may prove beneficial when control cannot be achieved by other nonsurgical means. Implantation of an artificial urinary sphincter to control postprostatectomy incontinence is an option only when conservative management has failed and significant amounts of leakage have continued for longer than 12 to 18 months (Duffy, 1990).

Of great concern to many patients are the long-term effects of transurethral surgery on sexual function—especially for those having prostatic resection. Assure the patient that erectile dysfunction is an infrequent complication that occurs in 5% to 10% of cases and only when nerves have been damaged during the resection of prostatic tissue. On the other hand, retrograde ejaculation inevitably occurs in approximately 90% of patients who have had TURP, especially if an extensive resection has been performed or the median lobe of the prostate was involved. Patients need to be assured that the absence of an antegrade ejaculation does not lessen their ability to achieve and maintain an erection or experience orgasm. However, the recovery of semen for insemination may be difficult.

**Patient Outcomes**
1. The patient expresses feelings of reduced anxiety with assurances that the obstruction to the lower urinary tract can be effectively treated without serious side effects.

2. The patient cooperatively participates in diagnostic tests and procedures.

3. The patient verbalizes relief of pain and discomfort caused by dysuria, bladder spasms, or bladder distention.

4. The patient exhibits no signs of urinary tract infection.

5. The patient's fluid and electrolyte status remains stable without signs of hyponatremia.

6. The patient exhibits no signs of excessive bleeding as evidenced by the lessening degree of hematuria.

7. The patient's urinary drainage tube (indwelling catheter or suprapubic tube) remains patent without evidence of occlusion from blood clots.

8. The patient's first attempt at voiding after removal of the urethral catheter yields an output of more than 100 mL, with the patient sensing complete bladder emptying.

9. On discharge, the patient is voiding every 2 to 3 hours, achieving complete bladder emptying, and experiencing only mild irritative voiding symptoms.

10. The patient who is discharged with an indwelling catheter (or suprapubic tube) demonstrates the ability to cleanse the tube and meatus properly and care for the urinary drainage bag.

11. The patient demonstrates the correct procedure for clean intermittent catheterization.

12. The patient verbalizes an understanding of the technique of perineal muscle exercises and the use of devices or absorbent products for temporary management of postprostatectomy incontinence.

13. The patient states relief of anxiety after receiving information regarding sexual function after transurethral surgery.

14. The patient verbalizes an understanding of the need to contact the physician if irritative or obstructive voiding symptoms recur.

15. The patient complies with follow-up visits to the physician.

## COMPLICATIONS OF URINARY TRACT OBSTRUCTION

### Acute Renal Failure

Acute renal failure, as a complication of obstruction to the urinary tract, occurs in approximately 10% of cases (Molitoris & Schrier, 1986). Conditions that contribute to a significant reduction in urine formation include those that create bilateral ureteral obstruction or that involve previously damaged kidneys or a solitary kidney. A urethral blockage, such as prostatic enlargement, starts the cycle of compensation, then decompensation, upward through the urinary tract that eventually leads to impaired kidney function. In rare instances, an extrinsic condition, such as the growth of a tumor, may progress to block both ureters. If only one kidney or its ureter is blocked, acute renal failure is an unlikely consequence, because the contralateral normal kidney is usually able to assume the necessary excretory function of the affected side.

Changes in the kidneys associated with renal failure as a result of obstruction first appear as a transient increase in intratubular pressures, followed by vasoconstriction. With sustained obstruction, inflammation, ischemia, and tubular necrosis may develop. Ultimately, there is a decline in the glomerular filtration rate and tubular function. The degree of change and rapidity of renal deterioration are dependent on the duration and severity of the obstruction (Kaufman & Papper, 1983).

Clinically, the patient exhibits oliguria, with a urine output ranging from 100 to 400 mL per 24 hours over a period of several days. Along with the decrease in urine volume caused by the decrease in the glomerular filtration rate, there is a decrease in the serum creatinine and BUN levels. Variations in serum electrolyte levels are possible, including hyperkalemia, hyponatremia, and acidosis. The acute onset of renal failure may also cause the patient to exhibit a variety of systemic symptoms, such as confusion, lethargy, nausea, vomiting, pulmonary edema, deep and rapid respirations, tachycardia, dysrhythmia, increased blood pressure, and susceptibility to infection.

Although acute renal failure is a serious condition, recovery is possible provided (1) the symptoms of obstruction are recognized and the blockage is quickly relieved and (2) careful fluid management is instituted at the onset of the oliguric phase of acute renal failure (Table 4–2). For some patients, a period of hemodialysis may be needed to retard the development of uremic symptoms and to prevent fluid overload (Walker, 1990). The reader is referred to a nephrology nursing text for further information on the treatment and care of the patient in acute renal failure.

TABLE 4–2. Management of Oliguric Phase of
Acute Renal Failure

**WATER**
Measure fluid intake and *total* fluid output
Reduce fluid intake to 400 mL/day plus measured
losses
Weigh patient daily; if weight increases, reevaluate fluid
intake
Attempt to promote modest but continuing weight loss
(¼–½ lb/day)

**SODIUM**
Place on sodium-free intake
Sodium should be given only to replace measured
sodium losses
Measure sodium content of any urine excreted plus all
other fluids

**POTASSIUM**
Place patient on potassium-free intake
If plasma potassium exceeds 5 mEq/L, place on
regimen of Kayexalate; if this cannot be taken orally,
potassium of 5 m Eq/L is indication for hemodialysis

**ACIDOSIS**
Acidosis should be prevented
Reduce protein intake to minimal levels
Replace sodium as Ringer's lactate or bicarbonate at
earliest signs of acidosis
Provide at least 1,200–1,500 calories/day

**DIALYSIS**
Dialysis should be begun promptly for hyperkalemia,
weight gain, acidosis, BUN >100 mg/dL (>50–60
mg/dL if patient is catabolic)

From Walker, W. G. (1990). Acute renal failure in the
urologic patient. In F. F. Marshall (Ed.), *Urologic complications* (2nd ed.). St. Louis: Mosby-Year Book. Reprinted by
permission.

## Postobstructive Diuresis

After correction of a long-standing obstruction, the patient may experience a period of
profuse urinary output. This response, called
*postobstructive diuresis*, is an acute problem that
is usually mild and self-limiting, but for some
patients it may be severe and life threatening.
The excessive diuresis is due to an inability of
the renal tubules to concentrate and absorb
fluids and electrolytes effectively; it occurs because of tubular atrophy that resulted from
back pressure created by prolonged obstruction (Walker, 1990).

By definition, diuresis is a urine output of
more than 2000 mL in an 8-hour period. However, any increase in urine output after correction of an obstruction may indicate postobstructive diuresis—especially if the output is
more than the volume normally expected
(which in adults can range from 700–2000 mL
per 8 hours).

Postobstructive diuresis is characterized by
polyuria and natriuresis. As the condition progresses, there is a rapid depletion of extracellular fluid volume along with a marked sodium deficit; a state of shock may develop. If
treatment is not quickly initiated, postobstructive diuresis could evolve into a life-threatening situation that may eventually lead to vascular collapse and death.

Management of postobstructive diuresis requires the careful replacement of fluid and sodium (Table 4–3). Parenteral therapy with a
hypotonic solution containing sodium is employed at a rate that will correct for the excessive excretion of urine and alleviate the signs
and symptoms of shock (Walker, 1990). Depending on the severity of the problem, fluid
replacement may be continued for as long as 7
days or more. Although postobstructive diuresis is a reversible condition, full recovery of
normal renal function may not be realized for
several weeks.

TABLE 4–3. Management of Postobstructive
Diuresis

1. Monitor urine output hourly.
2. If urine flow <50 mL/30 min, patient may be managed
with oral fluids and added salts po if there are no other
contraindications to this approach; check blood pressure
every 4 hr.
3. If urine flow 50–100 mL/30 min, obtain sodium and
potassium measurements in urine, as ordered.
   a. Administer intravenous solutions as ordered; use an
   infusion pump to ensure correct rate. (Infusion rate
   usually equals urine output.)
   b. Monitor weight every 12–24 hr.
4. If urine flow >100 mL/30 min
   a. Same as 3a.
   b. Sodium concentration in intravenous fluids may require adjustment, depending on the amount of sodium in urine output.
   c. After 48 hr, reduce infusion rate by 50% and observe
   urine flow and blood pressure carefully.
   d. If urine flow is decreased and blood pressure is stable, continue regimen of progressive reduction.
   e. If urine flow fails to decrease after 2 hr of infusate
   reduction, return to previous infusion rate and repeat.
5. If initially measured urine flow rate >150 mL/30 min,
proceed as outlined in 4 above but wait at least 96 hr
before attempting reduction in infusion rate.
   a. Monitor blood pressure and pulse at least every 30
   min until stability is documented.
   b. Monitor serum electrolytes (particularly potassium,
   sodium, and chloride).
   c. After 96 hr reduce infusion rate by no more than 25%
   and continue to monitor patient very closely.

Adapted from Walker, W. G. (1990). Acute renal failure
in the urologic patient. In F. F. Marshall (Ed.), *Urologic
complications* (2nd ed.). St. Louis: Mosby-Year Book. Reprinted by permission.

## ACKNOWLEDGMENTS

The authors thank Stanley I. Glickman, MD, Chief of Urology, VA Medical Center, Tucson, Arizona, for his professional guidance and Gwen Roske, Medical Media Department, VA Medical Center, Tucson, Arizona, for creating some of the original artwork.

## *REFERENCES*

Allen, T. D. (1977). Discussion. In D. Bergsma & J. W. Duckett, Jr. (Eds.), *Urinary system malformation in children—birth defects: Original article series* (Vol. 13, No. 5, p. 39). New York: Alan R. Liss.

Bagley, D. H., Huffman, J. L., & Lyon, E. S. (1985). *Urologic endoscopy: A manual and atlas.* Boston: Little, Brown.

Barr, J. E. (1988). Standards of care for the patient with a percutaneous nephrostomy tube. *Journal of Enterostomal Therapy, 15*, 147–153.

Barry, M. J. (1990). Epidemiology and natural history of benign prostatic hyperplasia. *Urologic Clinics of North America, 17*(3), 495–507.

Birkhoff, J. D. (1983). Natural history of benign prostatic hypertrophy. In F. Hinman (Ed.), *Benign prostatic hypertrophy.* New York: Springer-Verlag.

Caine, M. (1990). Alpha-adrenergic blockers for BPH. *Urologic Clinics of North America, 17*(3), 641–649.

Campbell, M. (1952). Primary megalo-ureter. *Journal of Urology, 68*, 584.

Christensen, M. M., & Bruskewitz, R. C. (1990). Clinical manifestations of benign prostatic hyperplasia and indications for therapeutic intervention. *Urologic Clinics of North America, 17*(3), 509–516.

Cochran, S. T., Barbaric, Z. L., Lee, J. J., & Kashfian, P. (1991). Percutaneous nephrostomy tube placement: An outpatient procedure? *Radiology, 179*(3), 843–847.

Cronan, J. J. (1991). Contemporary concepts in imaging urinary tract obstruction. *Radiologic Clinics of North America, 29*(3), 527–542.

Devine, C. J. (1986). Surgery of the urethra. In P. C. Walsh, R. F. Gittes, A. D. Perlmutter, & T. A. Stamey (Eds.), *Campbell's urology* (5th ed., pp. 2853–2887). Philadelphia: W. B. Saunders.

Duffy, L. (1990). Male incontinence. In K. Jeter, N. Faller, & C. Norton (Eds.), *Nursing for continence.* Philadelphia: W. B. Saunders.

Ellison, J. M., & Dobies, D. F. (1984). Methamphetamine abuse presenting as dysuria following urethral insertion of tablets. *Annals of Emergency Medicine, 13*(3), 198–200.

Gillenwater, J. Y. (1986). The physiology of urinary obstruction. In P. C. Walsh, R. F. Gittes, A. D. Perlmutter, & T. A. Stamey (Eds.), *Campbell's urology* (Vol. 1). Philadelphia: W. B. Saunders.

Graves, E. J. (1989). Detailed diagnoses and procedures, national hospital discharge survey, 1987. *Vital Health Statistics, 13*(100), 295.

Guidos, B. (1988). Preparing the patient for home care of the percutaneous nephrostomy tube. *Journal of Enterostomal Therapy, 15*, 187–190.

Hinman, F. (1986). Capsular influence on benign prostatic hyperplasia. *Urology, 28*, 347–350.

Hinman, J. R. (1984). Hydronephrosis. In A. R. Kendall & L. Karafin (Eds.), *Practice of surgery: Urology* (Vol. 2, pp. 1–14). Philadelphia: Harper & Row.

Jorgensen, P. E., Weiss, N., & Bruun, E. (1986). Etiology of

urethral stricture following transurethral prostatectomy. *Scandinavian Journal of Urology/Nephrology, 20*, 253–255.

Kaufman, C. E., & Papper, S. (1983). *Review of pathophysiology.* Boston: Little, Brown.

Kerr, W. S. (1954). Effect of complete ureteral obstruction for one week on kidney function. *Journal of Applied Physiology, 6*, 762–772.

Klahr, S., Buerkert, J., & Purkerson, M. L. (1977). The kidney in obstructive uropathy. *Contributions to Nephrology, 7*, 220–249.

Krongrad, A., & Droller, M. J. (1990). Complications of transurethral resection of the prostate. In F. F. Marshall (Ed.), *Urologic complications* (2nd ed.). St. Louis: Mosby-Year Book.

Kunz, H. V. (1986). Circumcision and meatotomy. *Primary Care, 13*(3), 513–525.

Lang, E. K. (1986). Transluminal dilatation of ureteropelvic junction strictures, ureteral strictures and strictures at ureteroneocystostomy sites. *Radiologic Clinics of North America, 24*(4), 601–613.

Lepor, H. (1991). The role of alpha blockade in BPH. *Journal of Andrology, 12*(6), 389–394.

Lepor, H., Brawer, M. K., McConnell, J. D., & Oesterling, J. E. (1992). What will replace TURP? *Contemporary Urology, 4*(2), 30–40.

Lepor, H., Knapp-Maloney, G., & Sunshine, H. (1990). An open label dose titration study evaluating terazosin for the treatment of symptomatic BPH. *Journal of Urology, 144*, 1393–1398.

Madsen, P. O., & Iverson, P. (1983). A point system for selecting operative candidates. In F. Hinman (Ed.), *Benign prostatic hypertrophy.* New York: Springer-Verlag.

Malloy, T., & Wein, A. J. (1990). Complications of lasers in urology. In F. F. Marshall (Ed.), *Urologic complications* (2nd ed.). St. Louis: Mosby-Year Book.

McAninch, J. W. (1992). Injuries to the genitourinary tract. In E. A. Tanagho & J. W. McAninch (Eds.), *Smith's general urology* (13th ed.). Norwalk, CT: Appleton & Lange.

McConnell, J. D. (1990a). Androgen ablation and blockade in the treatment of benign prostatic hyperplasia. *Urologic Clinics of North America, 17*(3), 661–670.

McConnell, J. D. (1990b). Anti-androgen therapy for benign prostatic hyperplasia. In *Monographs in Urology.* West Point, PA: Merck & Co.

McNeal, J. (1990). Pathology of benign prostatic hyperplasia. *Urologic Clinics of North America, 17*(3), 477–486.

MK-906 (Finasteride) Study Group. (1992). One-year experience with finasteride. *Journal of Andrology, 12*(6), 372–375.

Molitoris, B. A., & Schrier M. D. (1986). Etiology, pathogenesis, and management of renal failure. In P. C. Walsh, R. F. Gittes, A. D. Perlmutter, & T. A. Stamey (Eds.), *Campbell's urology* (5th ed.). Philadelphia: W. B. Saunders.

Murphy, K., & Malloy, T. R. (1987). Bladder outlet obstruction. In P. M. Hanno & A. J. Wein (Eds.), *A clinical manual of urology.* Norwalk, CT: Appleton-Century-Crofts.

Oesterling, J. E. (1991). A permanent, epithelializing stent for the treatment of benign prostatic hyperplasia. *Journal of Andrology, 12*(6), 423–428.

Orandi, A. (1990). Transurethral resection versus transurethral incision of the prostate. *Urologic Clinics of North America, 17*(3), 601–612.

Pagana, K. D., & Pagana, T. J. (1990). *Diagnostic testing and nursing implications: A case study approach* (3rd ed.). St. Louis: C. V. Mosby.

Perlmutter, A. D., Retik, A. B., & Bauer, S. B. (1986). Anomalies of the upper urinary tract. In P. C. Walsh, R. F. Gittes, A. D. Perlmutter, & T. A. Stamey (Eds.), *Campbell's urology* (5th ed.). Philadelphia: W. B. Saunders.

Persky, L., Kursh, E. D., Feldman, S., & Resnick, M. I.

(1986). Extrinsic obstruction of the ureter. In P. C. Walsh, R. F. Gittes, A. D. Perlmutter, & T. A. Stamey, (Eds.), *Campbell's urology* (5th ed.). Philadelphia: W. B. Saunders.

Roberts, J. B. M., & Slade, N. (1964). The natural history of primary pelvic hydronephrosis. *British Journal of Surgery, 51*, 759.

Schaeffer, A. J., & Grayhack, J. T. (1986). Surgical management of ureteropelvic junction obstruction. In P. C. Walsh, R. F. Gittes, A. D. Perlmutter, & T. A. Stamey, (Eds.), *Campbell's urology* (5th ed.). Philadelphia: W. B. Saunders.

Tanagho, E. A. (1992). Urinary obstruction and stasis. In E. A. Tanagho & J. W. McAninch (Eds.), *Smith's general urology* (13th ed.). Norwalk, CT: Appleton & Lange.

Thuroff, J. W. (1992). Percutaneous endourology and ureterorendoscopy. In E. A. Tanagho & J. W. McAninch (Eds.), *Smith's general urology* (13th ed.). Norwalk, CT: Appleton & Lange.

Walker, W. G. (1990). Acute renal failure in the urologic patient. In F. F. Marshall (Ed.), *Urologic complications* (2nd ed.). St. Louis: Mosby-Year Book.

Walsh, P. C. (1986). Radical retropubic prostatectomy. In P. C. Walsh, R. F. Gittes, A. D. Perlmutter, & T. A. Stamey (Eds.), *Campbell's urology* (5th ed.). Philadelphia: W. B. Saunders.

Warden S. S., & Devine, C. J. (1985). Urethral stricture disease. In A. R. Kendall & L. Karafin (Eds.), *Practice of surgery: Urology* (Vol. 1). Philadelphia: Harper & Row.

Webb, J. A. (1990). Ultrasonography in the diagnosis of renal obstruction. *British Medical Journal, 301*, 944–946.

Whitaker, R. (1979). Clinical application of upper urinary tract dynamics. *Urology Clinics of North America, 6*(1), 137–141.

Wilson, J. D. (1980). The pathogenesis of benign prostatic hyperplasia. *American Journal of Medicine, 68*, 745.

**CHAPTER 5**

# Urinary Tract Infections in Adults

■

*Janet A. Giroux*

## OVERVIEW OF CHAPTER

Infections and inflammations of the genitourinary tract are among the most common urologic disorders. The occurrence of infections in the urinary tract is second only to respiratory tract infections and continues to be a major source of morbidity in the United States (National Health Survey, 1970–1971). *Urinary tract infection* (UTI) is a broad term that describes microbial colonization of the urine and infection of the urinary tract extending from the kidney to the urinary meatus. Infections of adjacent structures, such as the prostate and epididymis, are included in the definition. According to Kunin (1987), UTIs usually are not isolated events but rather are indications of a more complex situation. Clinical presentation may vary from asymptomatic bacteriuria (colonization of the urine with bacteria but without symptoms) to bacteriuria associated with symptomatic infection of any part of the urinary system.

Infection of the urinary tract can generally be divided into upper and lower tract infections. Upper UTIs may cause parenchymal damage and lead to a decrease in renal function if they are not diagnosed and treated promptly. Populations at risk include women of child-bearing years and elderly men. Lower UTIs encompass a myriad of inflammations, ranging from cystitis to involvement of the reproductive structures. They occur about 10 times more frequently in females than in males of adult age.

Understanding the epidemiology and natural history of UTI is essential for the nurse caring for patients with urologic infections.

This chapter describes the major classification of UTIs, and the routes of infections as well as predisposing factors influencing UTI. After this discussion of fundamentals, specific types of infections and inflammations are presented, along with assessment, diagnostic evaluation, medical-surgical management, and nursing care.

## BEHAVIORAL OBJECTIVES

After studying this chapter, the reader should be able to

1. Discuss common symptoms of upper and lower UTIs.
2. Define the treatment of upper and lower UTIs.
3. Interpret factors involved in the epidemiology of upper and lower UTIs.
4. Formulate specific nursing interventions in caring for patients with upper and lower UTIs.

## KEY WORDS

**Asymptomatic bacteriuria**—the colonization of urine with bacteria in the absence of symptomatology.

**Bacterial adherence**—the interaction between bacteria and uroepithelial cells.

**Bacterial fimbriae (pili)**—nonflagellar, protein appendages that protrude from the bacterial cell surface.

**Bacteriuria**—the presence of bacteria in the urine.

**Pyuria**—the presence of an abnormal amount of pus cells (polymorphonuclear leukocytes) in the urine.

**Significant bacteriuria**—a bacterial colony count greater than or equal to 100,000 ($\geq 10^5$) colony-forming units per mL (cfu per mL) of urine.

## UPPER URINARY TRACT INFECTIONS

### Acute and Chronic Pyelonephritis

PERSPECTIVE ON DISEASE ENTITY

**Etiology.** Pyelonephritis is defined as inflammation of the kidney and renal pelvis (Fig. 5–1). The mode of infection may be (1) hematogenous, (2) local extension from an established cortical focus, or (3) ascending via the ureter from the lower tract. Hematogenous, or blood-borne, transport of bacteria may occur from systemic bacterial infection. Staphylococcal bacteria and systemic candidiasis are often associated with renal infection (Kunin, 1987). In some cases pyelonephritis may be primarily in the kidney itself. Calculi, growth of a neo-

plasm, infection by an acid-fast or staphylococcal organism, and trauma all are possible sources (Lapides, 1976). Vesicoureteral reflux of infected urine and obstruction, which may cause urine to stagnate and thus permit organisms to multiply, are the most common causes of ascending urinary tract infection. Pregnancy, diabetes, analgesic abuse, and polycystic kidney disease are other factors that may predispose to pyelonephritis (Brundage, 1986). Pyelonephritis is seen more frequently in females after urethral catheterization or instrumentation, yet it is uncommon in males free from urinary tract abnormalities. The Enterobacteriaceae organisms, *Escherichia coli*, *Klebsiella*, *Proteus*, *Enterobacter*, *Pseudomonas*, and *Serratia* are commonly cultured from the urine. These organisms are part of the normal fecal flora and generally gain access to the urinary tract through the perineal area. In recent years, re-

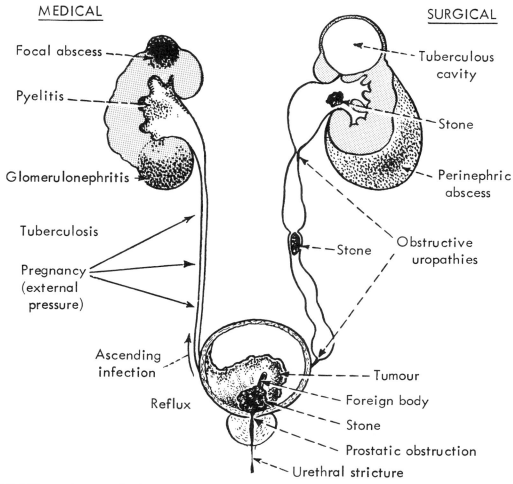

MEDICAL

- Focal abscess
- Pyelitis
- Glomerulonephritis
- Tuberculosis
- Pregnancy (external pressure)
- Ascending infection
- Reflux

SURGICAL

- Tuberculous cavity
- Stone
- Perinephric abscess
- Stone
- Obstructive uropathies
- Tumour
- Foreign body
- Stone
- Prostatic obstruction
- Urethral stricture

*FIGURE 5–1* Sites and causes of urinary tract infection. (From Scott, R., Deane, R. F., & Callander, R. [1982]. *Urology illustrated* [2nd ed., p. 94]. New York: Churchill Livingstone. Reprinted by permission.)

search has shown that most organisms infecting the urinary tract possess bacterial fimbriae, or pili, that allow attachment to squamous and uroepithelial cells. Furthermore, the urinary tract contains receptors for these bacteria to enhance adherence. One host receptor identified for pyelonephritis is the P blood group antigen (Parsons, 1985).

**Pathophysiology.** In the acute phase, the kidneys may be grossly enlarged owing to the inflammatory process. The parenchyma shows fibrosis and scarring, with areas of multiple abscesses. Acute pyelonephritis rarely progresses to renal failure. On the other hand, chronic pyelonephritis causes tissue destruction and small contracted kidneys. Recurrent episodes of acute pyelonephritis usually lead to chronic pyelonephritis, which gradually results in end-stage renal failure.

**Medical-Surgical Management.** Any ureteral obstruction must be ruled out and treated before antibiotic therapy is started, because an obstructed kidney cannot concentrate antibiotics adequately. While awaiting the urine culture report, the standard treatment generally consists of an aminoglycoside along with a synthetic penicillin for broad-spectrum coverage (Roberts, 1986). In acute pyelonephritis, a 10- to 14-day treatment course is the rule. Chronic pyelonephritis, however, may require long-term antibiotic treatment if clinical symptoms remain in spite of a negative urine culture.

## APPROACHES TO PATIENT CARE

### Assessment

In acute pyelonephritis the patient presents with fever, chills, flank pain, and irritative voiding symptoms of dysuria, urgency, and frequency. During the nursing health history interview, the patient is questioned regarding pertinent medical history, that is, diabetes, hypertension, and exposure to substances toxic to renal metabolism. Any previous urologic infections or complications are also ascertained as well as normal voiding habits and perineal hygiene practices. On physical examination, costovertebral tenderness, flank pain, or both are generally present, and the urine is cloudy and foul smelling. Hematuria may be apparent. Urine for culture and sensitivity testing is positive for bacteria, and the urine sediment demonstrates leukocytosis. Chronic pyelonephritis, however, can be clinically silent. It may be diagnosed incidentally during an evaluation for hypertension by an excretory urogram. Renal biopsy is the confirming test but may be unreliable because the infection may be localized and missed by the biopsy puncture. Abnormal laboratory results may include (1) elevated blood urea nitrogen (BUN) and creatinine levels, (2) anemia, (3) acidosis, (4) proteinuria, and (5) poor concentrating ability (urine specific gravity < 1.010).

**Nursing Diagnosis**

The nursing diagnosis for the patient with acute or chronic pyelonephritis may include the following:

1. Potential for alteration in fluid volume excess or deficit related to compromised renal function due to bacterial infection.
2. Knowledge deficit related to the causes, treatment, and prevention of acute or chronic pyelonephritis.
3. Alteration in comfort related to flank pain and dysuria.

**Plan of Care**

Nursing care is directed toward enabling the patient to

1. Maintain a urine output of at least 30 to 40 mL/h.
2. Understand the importance of completing the antibiotic course.
3. Implement measures to prevent recurrent UTI.
4. Understand the causes, signs, and symptoms of pyelonephritis.
5. State relief of symptoms of pyelonephritis.

**Intervention**

There is a potential for alteration in fluid volume excess or deficit caused by inflammation and fibrosis from acute or chronic pyelonephritis. The urine output is maintained at no less

than 30 to 40 mL/h. Oral fluids are encouraged to a level of 2000 to 4000 mL per 24 h, and the patient is encouraged to urinate every 2 or 3 hours. Fluids that may be irritating to the bladder, such as caffeine products and alcohol, are avoided until a clinical response to therapy is verified. The urine is tested for specific gravity, protein, pH, and hematuria at least every 8 hours or more often if abnormalities are noted and until a clinical response to therapy is verified. The patient is assessed for fluid overload by monitoring for the presence of edema (especially in the face, sacrum, and extremities), daily weights, and for any shortness of breath. Vital signs are taken every 8 hours, or more often if indicated. Laboratory values that monitor renal function, such as BUN, serum creatinine, sodium, chloride, and creatinine clearance, are reviewed, and abnormalities are reported. With the administration of prescribed antibiotics, the nurse monitors the patient's response. If the patient is febrile, the temperature is taken at least every 4 hours. Urine cultures are obtained during the course of therapy and at completion.

The patient may lack information related to the causes, treatment, and prevention of acute or chronic pyelonephritis. The nurse must assess what knowledge deficits the patient has and structure an appropriate educational program. Risk factors that might promote the ascending route of infection are reviewed. Does the patient void frequently throughout the day? If not, normal voiding habits that emphasize bladder emptying every 2 or 3 hours and a daily fluid intake of 2000 to 2500 mL are encouraged. Good perineal hygiene practices for women are taught, which emphasize cleansing from front to back, wearing of cotton underpants, and avoidance of tight-fitting jeans. Voiding before and after sexual intercourse is also reinforced for women. Patient education also includes recognizing the signs and symptoms of pyelonephritis, the importance of follow-up urine culture after antibiotic treatment, and the need to seek health care if symptoms recur. The action and any side effects of the prescribed antibiotic are reviewed as well as the need to take the full course even after the symptoms have abated. For the patient with signs of renal failure, the need to continue medical follow-up to control hypertension and monitor renal status is stressed.

During the acute phase, bed rest may be desirable for a few days because of the energy demands of the infectious process and complaints of pain and discomfort; total immobility is not necessary. Frequent voiding is encouraged to empty the bladder, because this can significantly decrease urine bacterial counts and the irritative effect of bacteriuria. Prescribed analgesics, such as aspirin or acetaminophen, are given for complaints of discomfort. The response to these medications is monitored by the nurse. Other comfort measures may include warm, moist soaks and massage to the flank area. If the patient is febrile, tepid sponge baths and fresh, dry linens and bed clothes may be provided as comfort measures.

### Patient Outcomes

1. The patient maintains a normal voiding pattern, averaging 30 to 40 mL/h.
2. The patient can verbalize an understanding of pyelonephritis and describe the signs and symptoms associated with the disease.
3. The patient is aware of the need to seek health care if symptoms recur.
4. The patient expresses an understanding of the rationale for continued antibiotic therapy even when symptoms have resolved.
5. The patient can describe necessary actions to prevent recurrence of infection.
6. The patient reports decrease or relief of pain.

# Papillary Necrosis-Interstitial Nephritis

## PERSPECTIVE ON DISEASE ENTITY

**Etiology.** Renal papillary necrosis is a form of interstitial nephritis in which distal papillae undergo coagulative necrosis and may slough into the urine. This potentially fatal condition is associated with diabetes mellitus, obstructive uropathy, and phenacetin abuse. A compromised circulation may result in an infarct of the papillae. As a result of the infarct, a large slough may pass down the ureter and cause obstruction (Lapides, 1976). Papillary necrosis usually affects both kidneys and involves all the caliceal groups. Papillary necrosis is also known as analgesic neuropathy. The disease appears to be prevalent in Australia and accounts for 20% of terminal renal cases among patients treated with dialysis and transplantation, as compared with 7% in one United States study and 3.1% in Europe. The peculiar geographic distribution is not understood. It commonly affects women between the ages of 40 and 60 years. Emotional factors may play a role in contributing to analgesic abuse (Kunin, 1987). In many instances, the patient is typically depressed, complains of headaches and

abdominal and musculoskeletal disorders, and reports a history of long-term daily ingestion of analgesics. Alcoholism may also be a factor. Other literature reviews show that the habit appears to be largely cultural and related to advertisement of certain agents.

Interstitial nephritis is an inflammation of the interstitial space that has been ascribed to infectious organisms or nonbacterial causes as well as an idiopathic origin. The primary cause is usually nonbacterial and is associated with nephrotoxic agents, including common medications. In addition, chemically induced nephritis has been linked with several agents, including solvents, heavy metals, pesticides, and poisonous mushrooms (Table 5–1).

With chemical-induced nephritis, symptoms usually begin within 15 days of exposure to the chemical. The associated renal failure from interstitial nephritis may be either acute or chronic in onset. An immune response may also cause acute interstitial nephritis (Brundage, 1986).

**Pathophysiology.** The pathogenesis of renal papillary necrosis is thought to be associated with the already precarious blood supply of the papillae being further compromised by the inflammatory reaction to infection often seen in diabetic or obstructive uropathy conditions (Kunin, 1987). The edema and leukocytic infiltrate produces an increase in interstitial pressure that compresses vessels and results in an infarct. In analgesic abuse, a vasculitis or inter-

### TABLE 5–1. Substances Associated with Chemically Induced Nephritis

| CLASSIFICATION | SPECIFIC TYPES |
|---|---|
| Medications | Aspirin |
| | Phenacetin |
| | Penicillins |
| | Sulfonamides |
| | Aminoglycosides |
| | Amphotericin B |
| | Phenytoin |
| | Thiazides |
| | Neomycin |
| Solvents | Carbon tetrachloride |
| | Methanol |
| | Ethylene glycol |
| Heavy metals | Lead |
| | Arsenic |
| | Mercury |
| | Copper |
| | Cadmium |
| | Uranium |
| Other | Pesticides |
| | Poisonous mushrooms |

stitial inflammation may produce a similar reduction in blood supply, leading to an infarct (Lapides, 1976).

In interstitial nephritis, acute inflammation may cause scarring and rapid decline in renal function. As many as 10% to 15% of the cases of acute renal failure may be associated with acute interstitial nephritis (Murray & Goldberg, 1982). The tubular damage is reflected by the kidneys' impaired ability to concentrate urine. Not only is the ability of the glomeruli to filter disrupted, but also the capillary membrane becomes permeable to plasma protein and blood cells.

**Medical-Surgical Management.** Papillary necrosis, particularly that due to phenacetin abuse, is a partially reversible disease. Of prime importance is discontinuing use of the offending analgesic. Affected patients should be cautioned to avoid nonsteroidal anti-inflammatory agents. Those who continue to take even small amounts of analgesics will have progressive deterioration. However, for those patients who stop abusing analgesics, 80% will frequently show an improvement or at least a slowing of deterioration in renal function (Schaeffer & Del Greco, 1986). Fluid intake should be increased to maintain a level of at least 2 L daily. In patients presenting with ureteral obstruction, ureteral catheterization or basket extraction are treatment options. Long-term remission may follow nephrectomy or partial nephrectomy (Schaeffer & Del Greco, 1986). For patients who present with small kidneys, a glomerular filtration rate (GFR) of less than 20 mL/min, hypertension, or persistent proteinuria, the prognosis is poor. Hematuria should be investigated and cytologic studies performed routinely because of the increased incidence of transitional cell carcinoma (Schaeffer & Del Greco, 1986). Careful management of infection, diabetes, and hydration may minimize the progression of decreased GFR and kidney size.

The treatments of interstitial nephritis and papillary necrosis are similar. Discontinuing use of the offending drug, treating infection, and relieving any associated obstruction are necessary steps. If renal function continues to decline, dialysis may be indicated.

## APPROACHES TO PATIENT CARE

### Assessment
The patient with acute papillary necrosis–interstitial nephritis may present with fever, renal and ureteric colic, and symptoms of urinary obstruction. In the chronic type, polyuria, nocturia, hematuria, renal pain, and fatigue may be seen, or, if the disease follows a slow, progressive course, no clinical manifestations may be present. Physical examination may reveal costovertebral tenderness. The patient is questioned regarding pertinent medical history, that is, diabetes, infection, exposure to chemicals, and any past urologic interventions. Analgesic usage is ascertained as well as recent and present medication either prescribed or obtained over the counter. Urine culture may be positive for bacteria, and the urinalysis generally shows pyuria, tubular casts, hematuria, and mild proteinuria. In the presence of either acute or progressive obstruction, BUN and serum creatinine levels are elevated, and the creatinine clearance may be abnormal. Anemia may be present in the chronic type. Serum toxicology screening is performed to possibly yield the source of the nephritis. Excretory urography can demonstrate decreased kidney size, irregular cortical outlines, and scarring of the pelvicaliceal system. With poor renal function, a retrograde pyelogram may be ordered to demonstrate the caliceal changes.

### Nursing Diagnosis
The nursing diagnosis for the patient with papillary necrosis–interstitial nephritis may include the following:

1. Potential for alteration in fluid volume excess or deficit related to impaired renal blood flow caused by acute or chronic inflammation.
2. Knowledge deficit with regard to the causes, treatment, and prevention of papillary necrosis–interstitial nephritis.
3. Potential for alteration in comfort related to renal pain.

### Plan of Care
Nursing care is directed toward enabling the patient to

1. Maintain an adequate urinary output, averaging 30 to 40 mL/h.
2. Understand the nature of papillary necrosis–interstitial nephritis as well as its causes, signs, and symptoms.
3. Comprehend the importance of completing the antibiotic course.
4. Understand the necessity of seeking health care if the symptoms recur.
5. State relief or decrease of symptoms of papillary necrosis–interstitial nephritis.

### Intervention
Nursing intervention for papillary necrosis–interstitial nephritis is aimed at maintaining

adequate urinary output and minimizing renal damage. Intake and output are monitored at least every 8 hours, and fluids adjusted to maintain a urinary output of at least 30 to 40 mL/h. Fluid excess or deficit is also assessed through checking the pulse, respiration, blood pressure, and daily weight; auscultation of the lungs; and observing the neck veins and skin turgor. Laboratory values such as electrolytes, BUN, serum creatinine, and creatinine clearance are monitored, and abnormalities reported.

The nurse assesses the patient's baseline knowledge of the causes, treatment, and prevention of papillary necrosis–interstitial nephritis. If medications or chemical toxins are implicated, the patient is taught the effect that the causative agent has on the genitourinary tract and to avoid further use or exposure. Most important, the patient needs to be aware of those specific medications that might contain phenacetin (i.e., a by-product of acetaminophen [Tylenol]) or phenacetin-containing compounds that could be injurious to the kidney. Stress the fact that some analgesics may contain phenacetin or phenacetin-containing compounds; therefore, caution should be exercised when choosing and using an over-the-counter preparation. Treatment of infection will require that the patient be knowledgeable about the action of the antibiotic, any side effects, and the need to complete the entire course. The importance of a follow-up urine culture after antibiotic treatment and the need to seek health care if symptoms recur should also be emphasized. Because some amount of renal damage may have occurred, the patient is taught about his or her current renal status and the need to continue regular medical follow-up to monitor any progression of renal failure.

**Patient Outcomes**

1. The patient's pulse, respirations, and blood pressure are stable.
2. The patient has adequate urinary output, averaging 30 to 40 mL/h.
3. The patient can verbalize an understanding of papillary necrosis–interstitial nephritis and describe signs and symptoms associated with the disease.
4. The patient is aware of the need to seek health care if symptoms recur.
5. The patient expresses an understanding of the rationale for continuing antibiotic therapy even when symptoms have resolved.
6. The patient is relieved of pain.

# Renal Abscess, Carbuncle, and Perinephric Abscess

## PERSPECTIVE ON DISEASE ENTITY

**Etiology.** Renal abscesses are localized infections confined within the renal cortex. If the abscess becomes extremely large, it is called a *carbuncle.* A renal carbuncle may be confused with a renal tumor. A perinephric abscess, however, extends into the fatty tissue around the kidney and is usually caused by rupture of a renal abscess. Renal and perinephric abscesses are usually spread by the hematogenous route, originating from skin lesions or the respiratory tract. Renal calculi and obstructive uropathy have also been implicated as causes. *Staphylococcus aureus* is a prime offending organism, but enteric gram-negative bacteria are currently being encountered (Kunin, 1987). Multiple renal abscesses can occur in both normal and diseased kidneys.

**Pathophysiology.** An abscess is a circumscribed collection of inflammatory cells that can become necrotic and liquefied (Kunin, 1987). The infection can cause large areas of destruction. Resolution of a renal abscess may leave a scar in the cortex. If the abscess extends into the perinephric space, pus will accumulate, causing local pressure symptoms (Scott et al., 1982). This local pressure can affect the diaphragm, leading to basal atelectasis.

**Medical-Surgical Management.** Renal abscesses may be treated by needle aspiration guided by ultrasound or by surgical drainage. Other treatment modalities include long-term antibiotics and a combination of percutaneous puncture and antibiotic instillation into the abscess cavity (Roberts, 1986). Surgical treatment appears to be the favored choice. Nephrectomy may be required if extensive destruction of the kidney has occurred (Kunin, 1987).

Surgical incision and drainage is generally required for perinephric abscesses along with antibiotic therapy. Reports of successful treatment with antibiotics alone are unusual (Shortliffe & Stamey, 1986). Percutaneous drainage, however, is reported to be contraindicated in large abscess cavities filled with thick purulent fluid (Haaga & Weinstein, 1980).

## APPROACHES TO PATIENT CARE

**Assessment**

The patient with a renal abscess, carbuncle, or perinephric abscess usually appears acutely ill. Fever, unilateral flank or abdominal pain, chills, and dysuria are present, and nausea, vomiting, and hematuria may occur. On physical examination, flank or abdominal tenderness is generally present in patients with renal abscess or carbuncle. But in perinephric abscess, a flank mass can be palpable, and the patient may have abdominal pain with guarding. The patient should be questioned about recent skin infections, cutaneous boils, or a history of kidney stones. Unlike other renal infections, the urine culture may be sterile if the abscess does not communicate with the urinary collecting system. Urinalysis demonstrates pyuria. Leukocytosis is present, and blood cultures may be positive. Radiologic diagnosis shows a renal mass, and caliceal distortion or renal displacement on excretory urography. Sonography and computed tomography may also be helpful in the diagnostic workup. A needle aspiration and culture of the abscess may be done for an analysis of the contents.

### Nursing Diagnosis

The nursing diagnosis for the patient with renal abscess, carbuncle, and perinephric abscess may include the following:

1. Knowledge deficit regarding the causes and treatment of renal abscess, carbuncle, or perinephric abscess.
2. Alteration in comfort related to flank or abdominal pain.
3. Impairment of skin integrity related to surgical drainage or excision of a renal abscess, carbuncle, or perinephric abscess.

### Plan of Care

Nursing care is directed toward enabling the patient to

1. Understand the cause of renal abscess, carbuncle, or perinephric abscess, as well as the treatment options.
2. State relief of or a decrease in the symptoms of flank or abdominal pain.
3. Maintain an infection-free incision.

### Intervention

Nursing care is first directed toward enabling the patient to understand the causes, signs and symptoms, treatment, and prevention of renal abscess, carbuncle, and perinephric abscess. If the patient has a history of skin infections or cutaneous boils, proper hygiene practices are reinforced (if necessary), and the patient is instructed to seek early medical attention when these skin symptoms occur. When antibiotics are the choice of management, the patient is instructed on the action

and side effects of the drug and the need to complete the full course. Warm soaks may be suggested as a means of relieving flank pain if they are not contraindicated. Continued outpatient medical follow-up is stressed, especially if the patient has a history of renal calculi or urinary tract obstruction, which have been implicated in the development of perinephric abscesses. For the patient undergoing surgical incision and drainage of an abscess, preoperative and postoperative instruction is needed to reduce anxiety and speed postoperative recovery.

If drainage of the abscess is required, the nurse assesses the incisional site for signs of infection, the type and amount of drainage from the drain, and the patency of the nephrostomy tube, if one is present, and instructs the patient on self-care of the surgical site. Sterile technique is used during dressing changes, and universal precautions are followed. Antibiotics are administered as prescribed, and patient response is monitored. Vital signs are monitored every 8 hours, or more frequently if the patient is febrile. Discharge teaching is indicated, especially if the patient is sent home with a drain in place. Self-care activities taught during hospitalization are reinforced, as are skin hygiene practices, to avoid skin irritation and the signs and symptoms of incisional infection. Any activity restrictions are reiterated.

### Patient Outcomes

1. The patient can verbalize an understanding of renal abscess, carbuncle, and perinephric abscess, and describe signs and symptoms associated with the condition.
2. The patient is relieved of pain.
3. The patient receiving medical therapy for a renal abscess, carbuncle, or perinephric abscess is aware of the need to seek health care if symptoms recur.
4. The patient expresses an understanding of the rationale for continued antibiotic therapy even when symptoms have resolved.
5. The patient's incision is closed and shows no signs of infections.

# LOWER URINARY TRACT INFECTIONS

## Acute and Chronic Cystitis

### PERSPECTIVE ON DISEASE ENTITY

**Etiology.** Cystitis may occur as part of a generalized UTI, or the infective process may be localized only to the bladder. Bacteria may gain entrance into the bladder by three routes: (1) ascending, the most common; (2) hematogenous; and (3) lymphatic spread. Cystitis may be caused by urine flowing back from the urethra into the bladder (urethrovesical reflux) or by fecal contamination. It may also occur following instrumentation with a catheter or cystoscope. The family of bacteria called Enterobacteriaceae is responsible for approximately 80% of bacterial UTIs, with *E. coli* being the most common offending organism. In young women, *Staphylococcus saprophyticus* is the second most common pathogen isolated. It is widely accepted that bacteria that infect the urinary tract come from normal fecal flora. Susceptibility to recurrent UTI is mainly characterized by an abnormally high number of fecal bacteria on the vaginal and urethral mucosa (Shortliffe & Stamey, 1986). Women are more prone to cystitis than are their male counterparts. Most research, therefore, has been directed toward understanding the natural history of bacteriuria and colonization patterns in the female population.

Studies show that at least 25% of all women develop a UTI at some time in their lives. The incidence of bacteriuria in women, beginning at age 18 years, is reported to be about 4%, with an increase of 1% to 2% during each subsequent decade of life (Stamey, 1980). The short length of the female urethra reduces the distance between the bladder and the external environment, thus making it vulnerable to vaginal and fecal contamination. Numerous studies of female bacteriuria (Elkins & Cox, 1974; Stamey & Sexton, 1975) have shown that colonization of the vaginal introitus and urethra with enterobacteria precedes the onset of cystitis. This risk increases with age, secondary to local estrogen deficiency, incomplete bladder emptying, and chronic medical conditions, such as diabetes mellitus (Luckmann & Sorensen, 1987). The changes in the urinary tract unique to pregnancy are also a factor in female bacteriuria. (UTIs in pregnancy are discussed at length later in the chapter.) Sexual intercourse may play a role in the ascent of organisms from the perineum into the bladder. This appears to be accomplished by urethral manipulation that "milks" the organisms up the urethra into the bladder. Ill-fitting diaphragms have been linked to UTI because of their pressure against the bladder, preventing complete bladder emptying. Vaginal infections secondary to broad-spectrum antibiotic therapy often lead to a UTI owing to the anatomic proximity of the vagina

and bladder (see the section on candidiasis). Factors such as neurogenic bladder and urinary retention provide the bacteria with an environment conducive to proliferation. Other contributing factors include (1) synthetic underwear, (2) pantyhose, (3) tight jeans, (4) feminine hygiene sprays, (5) bubble baths, and (6) sanitary napkins or tampons (Luckmann & Sorensen, 1987).

Most cases of bacteriuria in men occur as a result of a bacterial prostatitis, urethral stricturing, or urinary calculi resulting in urinary retention. Because of the longer length of the male urethra and the antibacterial properties of prostatic secretions, men seldom develop cystitis before the age of 50 years. Contributing factors to UTIs in elderly men are obstructive uropathy, loss of the antibacterial properties of the prostatic secretions, incomplete bladder emptying, and other medical disorders (Luckmann & Sorensen, 1987).

**Pathophysiology.** Bacterial adherence to mucosal cells is a widely accepted prerequisite to colonization and infection of mucosal surfaces including the urinary tract (Eden et al., 1977). The interaction of the mucosal cell and the bacterium is probably dependent on receptors on the mucosal cells and some type of attachment mechanism employed by the bacteria. Several host receptors have been identified, with mannose being linked to cystitis, and the P blood group antigen to pyelonephritis. Bacteria, too, have special types of surface structures that they utilize as adhesions. These bacterial fimbriae, or pili, may be present in large numbers on bacterial cells (Parsons, 1986). Fowler & Stamey (1977 and 1978) showed a possible increased adherence to the cells of cystitis-prone females, suggesting that both host and bacteria play important roles in the adherence process. However, whether this host-bacteria interaction leads to asymptomatic bacteriuria, or tissue invasion causing symptomatic bacteriuria, depends on the intactness of the host defense mechanisms within the urinary tract.

In the normal bladder there is resistance to infection from microorganisms in general. This is due to the bladder's intrinsic defense mechanisms: (1) the bacteriostatic property of urine to most common urinary pathogens, (2) dilution of the bacterial inoculum and effective urine "wash-out factor" with voiding, and (3) an intact bladder mucosal surface (Parsons, 1986). However, structural or functional abnormalities of the urinary tract may interfere with these defense mechanisms and increase the risk of infection. (Many of these abnormalities, such as obstructive components, neurologic lesions, and urinary calculi, are discussed in detail in other chapters.) When an inflammatory process does ensue, it usually involves only the mucosa and submucosa layers.

Chronic cystitis refers to recurrent episodes of cystitis. The women who develop recurrent cystitis differ from normal women in that they tend to carry an increased number of abnormal organisms on their vaginal vestibules, increasing their risk of another UTI. The cause of chronic cystitis in these women appears to be a lack of some form of local defense mechanism, which allows the colonization of bacteria in the vaginal vestibule (Berkow, 1982). With men, chronic bacterial prostatitis is the most common cause of chronic cystitis.

**Medical-Surgical Management.** Medical management is varied yet always directed toward administration of antibiotics specific to the causative organism. Pharmacologic intervention can begin with a broad-spectrum antibiotic while culture reports are pending. The choice of medication may later be narrowed more specifically if necessary. Simple acute bacterial cystitis can generally be treated effectively with single-dose therapy in 80% to 100% of women. Some studies have shown ampicillin, amoxicillin, trimethoprim-sulfamethoxazole, and sulfisoxazole to be effective treatment choices (Buckwold et al., 1982; Rubin et al., 1980). Women should be alerted to the possible complications of vaginal infections when they are placed on broad-spectrum antibiotic regimens. Yogurt or *Lactobacillus* capsules may be used to replace normal vaginal flora and reduce the risk of subsequent infections. Other treatment durations are the typical 7- to 10-day course or the 3-day short-term therapy. A follow-up urine culture after completion of the antibiotic is mandatory. Additional adjuvant therapy may include phenazopyridine hydrochloride (Pyridium) to relieve burning and urgency and acidifying agents, such as ascorbic acid and methenamine mandelate. If the patient has bothersome bladder spasms, propantheline may be prescribed. With chronic recurrent cystitis, long-term antibiotic suppression may be needed for 6 months or up to 24 months. Nitrofurantoin, trimethoprim-sulfamethoxazole, nalidixic acid, cephalexin, and trimethoprim are useful agents for long-term suppression (Shortliffe & Stamey, 1986) and may also be used as a "morning after" medication in women in whom sexual activity is the precipitating factor.

## APPROACHES TO PATIENT CARE

### Assessment

The hallmark symptoms of cystitis are dysuria, frequency, and urgency. Fever, chills, and low back pain may also be present. In chronic cystitis, the symptoms are similar but can be continuous, with mild remissions and frequent exacerbations. On physical examination, the patient may complain of suprapubic or flank tenderness and report hematuria. The urine is cloudy and odorous. During the patient interview, a history of prior UTIs or vaginal infections, the usual pattern of voiding, fluid intake, sexual practices, personal hygiene practices, and contraceptive use are documented. Urine culture generally shows significant bacteria ($>10^5$ cfu per mL); however, symptomatic bacteriuria has been noted with bacterial counts as low as 1000 to 10,000 per mL. Urinalysis is positive for pyuria when there are more than 10 white blood cells (WBCs) per high-power field (HPF). Radiologic diagnosis may include excretory urography, kidney, ureter, and bladder (KUB) urogram, or both to rule out focus of infection.

### Nursing Diagnosis

The nursing diagnosis for the patient with acute or chronic cystitis may include the following:

1. Alteration in the pattern of urinary elimination related to inflammation and irritation of the urinary tract.
2. Knowledge deficit related to the causes, treatment, and prevention of acute or chronic cystitis.
3. Alteration in comfort related to dysuria and suprapubic tenderness.

### Plan of Care

Nursing care is directed toward enabling the patient to

1. State relief of symptoms of acute or chronic cystitis.
2. Understand the importance of completing the antibiotic course.
3. Implement measures to prevent recurrent UTI.
4. Understand the causes, treatment, and prevention of acute or chronic cystitis.

### Intervention

Once appropriate antimicrobial therapy is initiated, the irritative voiding symptoms caused by cystitis are generally relieved. Oral fluids are encouraged, to a level of 2000 to 4000 mL per 24 hours, unless medically contraindicated.

Regular and complete emptying of the bladder is strongly recommended. Fluids that may irritate the bladder, such as alcohol, citrus juices, and caffeine products, should be avoided. To relieve discomfort, analgesics or antispasmodics may be administered. Bed rest, though generally not indicated, may be suggested until the feelings of generalized malaise and fatigue have passed.

Patients with cystitis should be taught to monitor the pH of the urine if they are receiving an acidifying agent. For women, a review of personal hygiene habits and the use of contraceptives is important, especially if these are causative factors. With the older male, the role of the prostate gland as a contributory factor in acute or chronic cystitis is discussed. Other patient education considerations related to the prevention of cystitis are similar to those described in the section on acute or chronic pyelonephritis.

### Patient Outcomes

1. The patient is relieved of pain, urgency, and frequency.
2. The patient resumes a normal voiding pattern.
3. The patient has sterile urine.
4. The patient can verbalize an understanding of acute or chronic cystitis, and describe the signs and symptoms associated with the disease.
5. The patient is aware of the need to seek health care if the symptoms recur.
6. The patient expresses an understanding of the rationale for continued antibiotic therapy even when the symptoms have resolved.
7. The patient can describe techniques to prevent recurrence of infection.

# Abacterial Cystitis, Urethral Syndrome, Interstitial Cystitis, and Radiation Cystitis

## PERSPECTIVE ON DISEASE ENTITY

**Etiology.** There are other forms of cystitis that can produce inflammation of the bladder without a bacterial cause. In the abacterial cystitis syndrome, the signs and symptoms of infection exist, but no bacteria can be cultured in the urine. As a "catch all" phrase, abacterial cystitis seems to include a spectrum of clinical situations from urethral syndrome to interstitial cystitis (Parsons, 1985). Clinically, urethral syndrome is the milder symptom complex in

the spectrum. Urgency and frequency are the characteristic symptoms. These symptoms often resolve spontaneously, but they may persist for an indeterminate amount of time. Women in the child-bearing years are more prone to the syndrome. Even though the cause of urethral syndrome is obscure, certain hypotheses have become popular. These include (1) urethral obstruction (urethral stenosis or glandular enlargement along the urethra), (2) infections, (3) neurogenic causes, and (4) psychogenic mechanisms (Messing, 1986). Bubble baths, perfumed soaps, feminine hygiene sprays, sanitary napkins, and spermicidal jellies have also been implicated as causes (Luckmann & Sorensen, 1987). Schmidt (1985) reports a direct correlation between the high pressure or instability (or both) in the external sphincter, seen urodynamically, and the voiding dysfunction and resultant irritation symptoms. However, a psychogenic etiology concerning women who internalize stress-related tension cannot be negated.

A more severe form of the urgency-frequency syndrome has been termed *interstitial cystitis*. Interstitial cystitis, or Hunner's ulcer, is thought to be a type of local autoimmune phenomenon. However, the etiology is poorly understood. It appears that the combination of defective bladder protective layers and irritative substances in the urine are unsubstantiated. Infections and lymphovascular, neurogenic, endocrinologic, and psychoneurotic causes have also been implicated (Messing, 1986). Both sexes may develop the syndrome, with middle-aged women being affected more commonly. This syndrome is characterized by the triad of chronic, irritative voiding symptoms; sterile, cytologically negative urine; and distinctive cystoscopic findings (Messing, 1986). Symptoms are usually present for 3 to 5 years before the correct diagnosis is made. Unlike bacterial cystitis, micturition does not typically relieve the pain of dysuria. Patients often exhibit despair and frustration in attempting to cope with the chronic and intractable pain of interstitial cystitis. Disruption of family life and work responsibilities is common. Sleep patterns are significantly disturbed because of frequent nocturnal voiding, many times exceeding 12 times a night. Social isolation may occur as a result of the fear of incontinent episodes.

Radiation cystitis may follow accidental exposure to radiation or radiotherapy for pelvic neoplastic disease (Scott et al., 1982). Chemotherapeutic drugs, cyclophosphamide (Cytoxan), and mitomycin may also be etiologic agents. Although the bladder is relatively resistant to radiation, therapeutic doses greater than 60 to 70 Gy during a 6- to 7-week treatment course may result in cystitis (Gray & Broadwell, 1986). The symptoms are similar to those of bacterial cystitis.

**Pathophysiology.** In urethral syndrome, there is no known pathologic entity typical to the condition (Schmidt, 1985). Generally, objective clinical findings are absent, and the diagnosis is made on the basis of exclusion. If there is no evidence for an anatomic, an infectious, an inflammatory, a chemical, or a neurogenic cause of urethral syndrome, then external sphincter spasm of possible psychogenic origin may seem plausible (Messing, 1986).

Interstitial cystitis involves inflammatory infiltration of all four layers of the bladder wall. This leads to ulceration, scarring, and, ultimately, contraction of smooth muscle, causing diminished bladder capacity (Berkow, 1982). White blood cell invasion of the bladder wall is common and consists primarily of lymphocytes. The diagnosis of interstitial cystitis requires cystoscopy. On cystoscopy, diffuse petechial hemorrhages in the bladder mucosa are seen. Hunner's ulcers, red erythematous patches of mucosa that split with bladder distention, may be present (Parsons, 1985).

Radiation cystitis produces inflammatory changes in the bladder wall in the absence of infection. In the acute phase during the course of therapy, bladder mucosa is edematous and congested. There may also be a slight reduction in bladder capacity, but these changes resolve shortly after cessation of therapy. Chronic or late radiation cystitis produces ulcers, fibrosis, vascular stenosis, and a definite diminished capacity (Scott et al., 1982).

**Medical-Surgical Management.** Management of urethral syndrome is varied. Reported treatment options include the use of anticholinergics and urethral dilation (Parsons, 1985). Schmidt (1985) stresses the importance of teaching voiding habits that encourage regular and complete evacuation. Along with this teaching, biofeedback and a combination of skeletal muscle relaxants (diazepam or cyclobenzaprine hydrochloride) and alpha-blockers (prazosin or phenoxybenzamine hydrochloride) seem to be helpful. More recently, neurostimulation has been used in the treatment of urethral syndrome (Schmidt, 1985). This approach appears to fatigue erratic behavior of the striated muscle but will not affect the normal intrinsic sphincter tone. It is important to obtain a 3- to 5-day trial to assess the improvement of patient symptoms before a permanent electrode is implanted.

Treatment of interstitial cystitis can be categorized largely into three groups: (1) surgical, (2) chemotherapeutic, and (3) electromechanical. Surgical options may include transurethral resection and fulguration of the bladder lesions, denervation procedures to manage chronic pain, and bladder substitution or augmentation. Neodymium:yttrium aluminum garnet (Nd:YAG) laser treatments have also been proposed as a palliative option for patients in whom there is proven evidence of interstitial cystitis. Shanberg and Malloy (1987) reported improvement in patient symptoms after the use of Nd:YAG laser photoirradiation therapy. Urinary diversion, a final surgical option, has been used but only when all other treatment modalities have failed (Gray & Broadwell, 1986). In chemotherapeutic treatment, a variety of systemic medications have been tried. The most frequently reported include estrogens, antibiotics, anti-inflammatory agents, antihistamines, vitamins, and analgesics (Messing, 1986). Intravesical agents may consist of silver nitrate, sodium oxychloresene, and dimethyl sulfoxide (Gray & Broadwell, 1986). Electromechanical treatment by hydraulic distention of the bladder is the most traditional therapy. By distending the patient's bladder with an intravesicular balloon, an increase in functional capacity is attempted. The procedure is performed with the patient under anesthesia at controlled pressures, under 30 cm $H_2O$, to avoid potential bladder rupture (Parsons, 1985).

In the acute phase, symptoms of radiation cystitis will usually resolve shortly after cessation of therapy. Bladder distention and, possibly, urinary diversion are treatment options if diminished bladder capacity is a problem. For bleeding symptoms, supplemental iron therapy, transfusion, or both may be indicated. Massive or persistent bleeding may necessitate a cystectomy (Scott et al., 1982).

## APPROACHES TO PATIENT CARE

### Assessment

The presenting symptoms of abacterial cystitis, urethral syndrome, interstitial cystitis, or radiation cystitis mimic those of bacterial cystitis. The patient gives a history of dysuria, frequency, urgency, and nocturia. The pain of interstitial cystitis is typically described as burning and constant. Interruption of a normal sleep pattern is particularly troublesome in interstitial cystitis, and the patient may report frequent nighttime voiding. Hematuria may be present in interstitial and radiation cystitis. Physical examination generally reveals suprapubic or pelvic discomfort. The urethra may be especially tender on examination in urethral syndrome. During history taking, the patient is questioned regarding past history of UTI, recent chemotherapy or radiation exposure, and any personal hygiene and contraceptive practices that might be suspect in causing the symptoms. In contrast to the patient with bacterial cystitis, patients with abacterial cystitis, urethral syndrome, interstitial cystitis, or radiation cystitis have negative urine cultures and urinalysis. Urodynamic evaluation will demonstrate decreased bladder capacity in both radiation and interstitial cystitis. The results of intravenous urography are normal. The diagnosis of interstitial cystitis requires cystoscopy with the patient under anesthesia.

### Nursing Diagnosis

The nursing diagnosis for the patient with abacterial cystitis, urethral syndrome, interstitial cystitis, or radiation cystitis may include the following:

1. Alteration in the pattern of urinary elimination related to inflammation, irritation, and hyperactivity of the urinary tract.
2. Knowledge deficit related to the causes, management, and prevention of abacterial cystitis, urethral syndrome, interstitial cystitis, and radiation cystitis.
3. Alteration in comfort related to dysuria.
4. Potential for ineffective coping mechanisms due to chronicity of interstitial cystitis.

### Plan of Care

Nursing care is directed toward enabling the patient to

1. State relief or reduction of irritative voiding symptoms of abacterial cystitis, urethral syndrome, interstitial cystitis, or radiation cystitis.
2. Understand the rationale behind prescribed treatment modalities.
3. Implement measures to prevent or minimize recurrent episodes of abacterial cystitis, urethral syndrome, interstitial cystitis, or radiation cystitis.
4. Demonstrate effective coping skills related to chronic pain management.

**Intervention.** Many of the nursing care interventions for urinary elimination parallel those of acute or chronic bacterial cystitis. Fluids are encouraged, to 3000 mL per 24 hours, and the patient is instructed to urinate every 2 or 3 hours. In the case of urethral syndrome, proper voiding habits may need to be taught by the nurse. Voluntary tightening and relaxation of the pelvic musculature without the use of the abdominal and gluteal muscles are stressed. Retaining urine in the presence of urgency is encouraged in patients with interstitial cystitis to increase functional bladder capacity. If anticholinergic or antispasmodic medications are ordered, the patient is evaluated for the level of relief of urgency symptoms. Intake and output are monitored every 8 hours, and fluids that are irritating to the bladder are avoided.

It is additionally important, however, to teach the patient's family about the implications of interstitial cystitis and how they may help the affected member cope. Because of the chronicity of the disease and its frequent exacerbations, it is important to keep the patient fully informed regarding each new medication or treatment modality to be used. If surgical intervention is planned, comprehensive preoperative and postoperative teaching pertaining to the specific procedure is done by the nurse.

The patient with abacterial cystitis, urethral syndrome, interstitial cystitis, or radiation cystitis does have to cope with the frustration of an irritative voiding pattern; however, this is usually short-lived. After the offending cause is eliminated, and appropriate intervention instituted, normal voiding habits are generally restored. But in the case of interstitial cystitis, the uncertainty in the diagnosis, the chronic pain, and the long-term effect that it has on the patient's work, social, and personal life can lead to frustration, anger, and feelings of desperation. Many patients are labeled as neurotic and have gone into self-imposed isolation because their bladder symptoms are so severe. The nurse is in a key position to help the patient express these negative feelings and encourage open dialogue with the patient through an understanding and nonjudgmental demeanor. Reassurance should be offered that there are available personnel to assist the patient in developing effective coping mechanisms. Offering information regarding local or national Interstitial Cystitis Association support groups may also be beneficial.

### Patient Outcomes

1. The patient is relieved of pain or reports a decrease in discomfort on voiding.
2. The patient resumes a normal voiding pattern, averaging 30 to 40 mL/h, or the voiding pattern improves.
3. The patient can verbalize an understanding

of abacterial cystitis, urethral syndrome, interstitial cystitis, or radiation cystitis and describe the signs and symptoms associated with the disease.
4. The patient is aware of the need to seek health care if the symptoms recur.
5. The patient expresses an understanding of the rationale for continued medication therapy or the alternative therapies prescribed.
6. The patient is able to cope with feelings of frustration and anger and is aware of support resources.

## Acute Bacterial Prostatitis, Chronic Bacterial Prostatitis, Nonbacterial Prostatitis, and Prostatodynia

### PERSPECTIVE ON DISEASE ENTITY

**Etiology.** There are several types of prostatitis or prostatitis syndromes recognized: (1) acute bacterial, (2) chronic bacterial, (3) nonbacterial, and (4) prostatodynia (Drach et al., 1978). Each has a different cause and clinical presentation. Cultures of prostatic secretions also vary among the different syndromes. Some of the clinical features of the prostatitis syndromes are displayed in Table 5–2.

The bacteria usually responsible for infection in other parts of the urinary tract are the same causative organisms in prostatitis. Most are gram-negative organisms: *Klebsiella*, *Proteus*, *Enterobacter*, and *Pseudomonas*, with *E. coli* being the predominant organism. Gram-positive and gonococcal bacteria may also play a role. Possible routes of infection include (1) the ascending route, (2) reflux of infected urine into prostatic ducts that empty into the posterior urethra, (3) colonization by rectal bacteria, by

direct extension or lymphangial spread, and (4) hematogenous infection (Meares, 1986).

Acute bacterial prostatitis may be precipitated by urethral instrumentation, trauma, an infectious focus elsewhere in the body, bladder outlet obstruction, or prostatic massage in the presence of chronic bacterial prostatitis. An acute episode may be characterized by a sudden onset of fever, chills, general malaise, and urinary retention and will rapidly progress to localized perineal, suprapubic, or back discomfort and irritative voiding symptoms (Gray & Broadwell, 1986). Transient impotency may accompany the attack.

Chronic bacterial prostatitis may follow an inadequately treated episode of acute prostatitis or urethral obstruction or develop insidiously without any prior history of acute prostatitis. This form of prostatitis may be asymptomatic or may demonstrate symptoms similar to those of acute prostatitis. Certain factors have been identified that may predispose to the development of chronic bacterial prostatitis: (1) alcohol excess, (2) perineal trauma, and (3) certain sexual practices (Scott et al., 1982). It is suggested that these factors produce congestion of the prostate, which provides an excellent growth media for bacteria.

Nonbacterial prostatitis is the most common prostatitis syndrome. The etiology of nonbacterial prostatitis is unknown, thus making the condition difficult to treat effectively. This form of prostatitis appears to be either an infectious disease caused by unidentified pathogens or a noninfectious form of inflammation (Meares, 1986). Recent studies have focused on the role of sexually transmitted organisms in the disease. Brunner and colleagues (1983) implicated *Chlamydia* and *Ureaplasma urealyticum* as possible pathogens. Fungi, obligate anaerobic bacteria, *Trichomonas*, and various types of viruses have generally been excluded as etiologic

### TABLE 5–2. Clinical Features of Common Prostatitis Syndromes

| SYNDROME | HISTORY OF CONFIRMED UTI | PROSTATE ABNORMAL ON RECTAL EXAMINATION | EXCESSIVE WBCs IN EPS | POSITIVE CULTURE OF EPS | COMMON CAUSATIVE AGENTS | RESPONSE TO ANTI-MICROBIAL TREATMENT | IMPAIRED URINARY FLOW RATE |
|---|---|---|---|---|---|---|---|
| Acute bacterial prostatitis | Yes | Yes | Yes | Yes | Coliform bacteria | Yes | Yes |
| Chronic bacterial prostatitis | Yes | ± | Yes | Yes | Coliform bacteria | Yes | ± |
| Nonbacterial prostatitis | No | ± | Yes | No | None | Usually no | ± |
| Prostatodynia | No | No | No | No | None | No | Yes |

UTI, urinary tract infection; WBCs, white blood cells; EPS, expressed prostatic secretions.
From Meares, E. M., Jr. (1992). Prostatitis and related disorders. In P. C. Walsh, A. R. Retik, T. A. Stamey, & E. D. Vaughan, Jr. (Eds.), *Campbell's urology* (6th ed., p. 808). Philadelphia: W. B. Saunders. Adapted by permission.

agents of nonbacterial prostatitis (Meares, 1986).

Last, prostatodynia, meaning painful prostate, is the presence of symptoms of prostatitis in the absence of any physical findings. Clinically, it is difficult to distinguish this condition from either chronic or nonbacterial prostatitis. This condition is seen in younger men, aged 25 to 45 years. The etiology is unclear, but several causes have been suggested. Segura et al. (1979) believe that symptoms arise from pelvic floor tension that entails habitual contractions and spasms of the pelvic floor muscles. Psychiatric origins have been proposed by Nilsson et al. (1977). Barbalias et al. (1983) suggest incomplete relaxation of the bladder neck and abnormal narrowing of the urethra at the external urethral sphincter.

**Pathophysiology.** Acute bacterial prostatitis is manifested by marked edema and inflammation of all or part of the prostate gland (Meares, 1986). Small abscesses may occur during the early course of the infection. If these go unchecked, the infection may spread to the periprostatic space, causing urethritis and seminal vesiculitis. Recurrent episodes of acute prostatitis may cause fibrotic tissue to form, which hardens the prostate gland. This fibrosis may initially be confused with carcinoma. The inflammatory reaction in chronic prostatitis is generally less marked and more focal than that in the acute form of the disease.

Objective pathologic findings are difficult in nonbacterial prostatitis and prostatodynia. In nonbacterial prostatitis, the presence of inflammatory cells in the expressed prostatic secretions (EPS) are suspected of causing symptoms. With prostatodynia, there is an absence of any physical findings despite recurrent perineal pain and irritative voiding symptoms.

**Medical-Surgical Management.** Patients with acute bacterial prostatitis usually respond favorably to antibiotic medications, which normally diffuse poorly from plasma into prostatic fluid. It may be that the intense, widespread inflammatory reaction enhances the passage of antibiotic drugs from plasma into the ducts and lobes of the prostate (Meares, 1986). Preferred therapy is trimethoprim-sulfamethoxazole, continued for 30 days, to prevent chronic bacterial prostatitis (Meares, 1986). In a severe case, while awaiting culture and sensitivity results, intravenous gentamicin plus ampicillin is recommended. Urethral instrumentation should be avoided, and vigorous prostatic massage is generally contraindicated. Cases of acute urinary retention are best managed with

suprapubic needle aspiration of the bladder or placement of a punch suprapubic catheter (Meares, 1986).

The distinctive feature of chronic prostatitis is the occurrence of relapsing UTI caused by the same pathogen. Because most antibiotics do not achieve adequate tissue levels in prostatic secretions, organisms persist in prostatic fluid during treatment. Urine may be sterile and symptoms controlled; but as soon as the antibiotic drug is discontinued, infection of the urine and symptoms generally return (Meares, 1986). Trimethoprim-sulfamethoxazole currently has the best cure rates reported. The optimal length of treatment has not been established. Other antibiotics used in chronic prostatitis management include carbenicillin, erythromycin, nitrofurantoin, and tetracycline. For men with chronic prostatitis not cured medically, surgical intervention may be necessary. Transurethral prostatectomy can be a curative procedure if all affected prostatic tissue is removed (Gray & Broadwell, 1986).

Curative therapy for nonbacterial prostatitis is difficult; however, symptomatic relief is possible. It is important to assure the patient that this is not a serious condition and that his sexual ability and fertility should not be affected (Pfau, 1986). If *Chlamydia* is suspected, treatment with tetracycline or erythromycin may prove effective. Normal sexual activity with the use of a condom to protect the partner is encouraged. If spicy foods or alcohol seem to aggravate the symptoms, these items should be eliminated from the diet. Therapeutic prostatic massage has been helpful in some cases. Irritative voiding symptoms may respond to the following: (1) anticholinergic agents (propantheline bromide and oxybutynin chloride) and (2) anti-inflammatory agents, such as indomethacin and ibuprofen (Meares, 1986).

Treatment of prostatodynia with antibiotics is ineffective because patients are not infected. As with nonbacterial prostatitis, therapy goals are to provide patient reassurance and control symptoms (Meares, 1986). Small doses of alpha-adrenergic blockers, such as prazosin, help patients with voiding dysfunction. Diazepam, biofeedback, and hot sitz baths may also alleviate symptoms.

## APPROACHES TO PATIENT CARE

### Assessment
The patient with acute bacterial prostatitis presents with sudden fever, chills, and voiding complaints of dysuria, frequency, urgency, hes-

itancy, nocturia, and possibly acute urinary obstruction. Generalized malaise with low back and perineal pain may also be part of the symptomatic picture. If a rectal examination is performed, the patient will complain of an exquisitely tender prostate gland. The examiner may palpate a swollen, boggy gland that feels warm to the touch, partially or totally firm, and irregular. However, because of the risk of bacteremia, the acutely inflamed prostate gland should not be massaged unless serum levels of an appropriate antibiotic have already been established (Meares, 1986).

Because acute cystitis generally accompanies acute bacterial prostatitis, a urine culture will be diagnostic of the causative organism. A prostatic secretion (EPS) specimen is packed with leukocytes (>10 per HPF), oval fat bodies, and large numbers of the bacterial pathogen. The WBC count will be elevated. Excretory urography may be normal or demonstrate evidence of bladder neck obstruction with elevation of the bladder base.

In chronic bacterial prostatitis, systemic symptoms rarely occur. The patient has varying degrees of irritative voiding symptoms, as described in acute bacterial prostatitis. Perineal discomfort is present and postejaculatory pain, urethral discharge, and hematospermia may occur. Some men may have only recurrent UTIs or asymptomatic bacteriuria. On rectal examination, the gland is usually nontender, but some irregularity or the presence of prostatic calculi may be palpated.

Screening tests include a urine culture and EPS specimen. The urine culture is positive for bacteria, and the EPS reveals excessive numbers of leukocytes and lipid-laden macrophages (oval fat bodies). However, because the same EPS results are also characteristic of nonbacterial prostatitis, the finding is not diagnostic of chronic bacterial prostatitis.

One accurate way of diagnosing chronic bacterial prostatitis is through the 3-4 glass test, also known as the lower tract localization procedure (Shortliffe & Stamey, 1986). These segmental cultures include (1) voided bladder (VB)1 (urethral culture), (2) VB2 (bladder culture), (3) prostatic secretion culture (EPS), and (4) VB3 (voided urine after prostatic massage). The specimens are cultured, and then the quantitative bacterial counts of the four specimens are compared. A diagnosis of prostatitis is made when the bacterial colony counts of the prostatic specimens significantly exceed those of the urethral and bladder specimens.

The patient with nonbacterial prostatitis has symptoms similar to those of chronic bacterial prostatitis. Often postejaculatory pain and discomfort are prominent features. Physical examination may be nonspecific. The patient gives no history of UTIs. The EPS findings parallel those of chronic bacterial prostatitis. The urine culture and sensitivity, however, will be negative. Lower-tract localization fails to reveal any pathogenic organisms.

The predominant symptom of prostatodynia is pelvic pain not necessarily related to voiding. Some patients may complain of symptoms similar to those described in nonbacterial prostatitis, whereas others notice signs of obstructive voiding. These obstructive signs may include hesitancy, weakened stream, and interrupted flow. The patient history is negative for any UTIs. No specific prostate abnormality is palpated on rectal examination. The urine culture and EPS specimen are negative. Urodynamic findings may demonstrate a significant increase in maximum urethral closing pressure and a decrease in peak and average urinary flows (Meares & Barbalias, 1983).

**Nursing Diagnosis**

The nursing diagnosis for the patient with prostatitis or prostatitis syndrome may include the following:

1. Alteration in the pattern of urinary elimination related to inflammation and irritation of the urinary tract and prostate gland.
2. Knowledge deficit related to the causes, treatment, and prevention of acute bacterial prostatitis, chronic bacterial prostatitis, nonbacterial prostatitis, or prostatodynia.
3. Alteration in comfort related to perineal and prostate pain.
4. Anxiety related to sexual concerns and chronicity of condition.

**Plan of Care**

Nursing care is directed toward enabling the patient to

1. Indicate that the symptoms of urinary retention are relieved.
2. Understand the importance of completing the antibiotic course.
3. Implement measures to prevent recurrent UTI.
4. Understand the causes, treatment, and prevention of acute bacterial prostatitis, chronic bacterial prostatitis, nonbacterial prostatitis, or prostatodynia.
5. State that the symptoms of acute bacterial prostatitis, chronic bacterial prostatitis, nonbacterial prostatitis, or prostatodynia are relieved or reduced.

6. Express fears and anxiety related to concerns about sexual function and activity.

### Intervention

Urinary retention is a possible complication in acute bacterial prostatitis owing to local inflammatory response. The nurse monitors the patient's fluid intake and output every 8 hours and assesses the bladder for overdistention. A tympanic sound on percussion is a sign of urinary retention. Frequent voiding is encouraged to decrease irritative symptoms, and fluids are increased to as much as 3000 mL per 24 hours. If a suprapubic catheter is placed to provide for urinary drainage, the nurse assesses the patency and keeps the catheter securely taped to the abdomen or thigh. The patient is taught catheter care if applicable.

Local heat to the perineum by means of sitz baths may be comforting for patients with prostatitis symptoms. Increasing fluid intake and stool softeners aid in preventing discomfort from defecation. Bed rest may be indicated during the acute phase. The nurse administers prescribed antibiotics and analgesics and monitors the patient's response. Vital signs are monitored every 8 hours, or more often if the patient is febrile. For patients with nonbacterial prostatitis or prostatodynia, increased sexual activity may afford some relief of the congested gland. If a sexual partner is not available, masturbation may be offered as an option.

The nurse will be instrumental in helping the patient understand the causes of prostatitis and what preventive and relief measures may be beneficial. Potential risk factors, such as instrumentation and indwelling catheters, are reviewed. If antibiotic therapy is indicated, the patient is instructed in the action of the medication, any side effects, and the importance of completing the full course to prevent episodes of recurrent infection. For those patients with chronic prostatitis, the need for long-term antibiotic compliance is discussed. Dietary instruction includes avoiding any hot or spicy foods that may exacerbate the patient's symptoms and limiting alcohol intake to 2 or 3 ounces per day.

Any infection or condition that affects the reproductive tract can be a source of anxiety for the patient. The patient needs to be reassured that prostatitis does not usually affect fertility or long-term sexual function. Allowing opportunities for the patient to express his fears and frustrations about this chronic and uncomfortable disease is encouraged.

### Patient Outcomes

1. The patient resumes a normal voiding pattern, averaging 30 to 40 mL/h.
2. The patient can verbalize an understanding of acute bacterial prostatitis, chronic bacterial prostatitis, nonbacterial prostatitis, or prostatodynia.
3. The patient is aware of the need to seek health care if symptoms recur.
4. The patient expresses an understanding of prevention factors, relief measures, and the need for continued antibiotic therapy even when symptoms have resolved.
5. The patient is relieved of pain.
6. The patient recognizes that the impact on sexual function is generally transitory.

## Urethritis, Epididymitis, and Orchitis

### PERSPECTIVE ON DISEASE ENTITY

**Etiology.** Urethritis may occur in both men and women. Nongonococcal urethritis (NGU), also called nonspecific urethritis (NSU), will be discussed here as an infection. Urethritis, as a sexually transmitted disease, will be covered in Chapter 7. Epididymitis and orchitis are inflammatory conditions of the male reproductive tract.

The etiology of urethritis includes (1) bacterial infections, (2) sexually transmitted diseases, and (3) chemical irritation secondary to the use of bath powders, spermicidal jellies, and bubble baths (MacGeorge & Bruno, 1986). It is common to have some degree of urethritis in association with bladder or prostatic infection. As an isolated infection, *Chlamydia trachomatis* and *Ureaplasma urealyticum* are the most frequent organisms cultured, with *Mycoplasma* and *Trichomonas vaginalis* less common. The morbidity of clinical infections and the complications of NSU have been reported to be possibly greater than those of gonococcal disease (Berger, 1986). Recurrent or persistent NGU may be due to (1) reinfection with the initial organism (usually from reexposure to the same sexual partner who has not been treated), (2) antibiotic resistance, and (3) idiopathic failure (Berger, 1986).

Epididymitis is the most common of the intrascrotal infections. The route of infection is usually along the vas deferens, from an infection in the urethra or bladder. Pathogens may reach the epididymis from lymphatic pathways, the hematogenous route, or metastatic routes. The etiology of epididymitis is related to bacteria, viruses, parasites, chemicals, or trauma. Generally, epididymitis is divided into three categories: (1) nonspecific, (2) specific, and (3) traumatic. Nonspecific epididymitis encompasses a group of common pathogens that typically gain access to the epididymis via urethral-vasal reflux in the presence of infected urine. Bladder outlet obstruction may be a predisposing factor. Nonspecific epididymitis is also manifested as a complication of certain urologic procedures. Transurethral resection of the prostate and urethral catheterization are cited most frequently (Gray & Broadwell, 1986). Epididymitis is usually unilateral and must be differentiated from testicular torsion, tumor, or trauma (Berger, 1986). In younger men, epididymitis is generally caused by sexually transmitted organisms. On the other hand, in men older than 35 years of age, the cause is generally common urinary pathogens, particularly after instrumentation and prostatectomy or outlet obstruction (Ireton & Berger, 1984).

Orchitis or epididymo-orchitis is the most common complication of epididymitis. Orchitis, infection of the testicle, usually occurs concomitantly with epididymitis, thus the combined name. Infection may reach the testis via (1) the hematogenous route, (2) the lymphatics, or (3) the vas deferens and epididymis. Orchitis may be divided into the following categories: (1) pyogenic, (2) viral, (3) spirochetal, (4) chemical, (5) mycotic, (6) parasitic, and (7) idiopathic (Nickel & Plumb, 1986). In pyogenic orchitis, the usual etiologic agents are common gram-negative pathogens, *Streptococcus* and *Staphylococcus*, all of which may cause UTI as well. The most common cause of suppurative orchitis is epididymitis, complicated UTI, prostatectomy, catheterization, or instrumentation (Nickel & Plumb, 1986). Enlargement of the testis may follow trauma, vas ligation, or surgical manipulation. Chemical substances, such as iodine, thallium, lead, carbon disulfide, and alcohol, have been purported to cause destruction of the seminiferous tubules (Nickel & Plumb, 1986). Orchitis has also been associated with numerous systemic diseases: (1) typhus fever, (2) influenza, (3) leprosy, (4) infectious mononucleosis, (5) filariasis, (6) schistosomiasis, (7) actinomycosis, (8) malaria, (9) endocarditis, and (10) gout, to name just a few (Scott et al., 1982). With these diseases, a specific organism cannot be isolated from the testis. Less frequently, orchitis may be a complication of mumps; however, this is rare before puberty.

**Pathophysiology.** The urethra is a common site of infection in the male urinary tract. The inflammatory response causes irritative voiding symptoms, local tenderness, and usually a urethral discharge. Gram stain reveals abundant polymorphonuclear leukocytes (Kunin, 1987). Urethritis in females may be termed the *pyuria-dysuria syndrome* (Kunin, 1987). The usual offending organism is *Chlamydia,* but many times the etiology is uncertain. Urinary complications of urethritis in men and women are generally uncommon.

Epididymitis occurs most frequently as a result of reflux of urine or some pathogenic entity through the posterior urethra, prostatic ducts, or seminal vesicle (Gray & Broadwell, 1986). In the early phase, epididymitis begins as a type of cellulitis associated with local pain and edema. Following this phase the entire hemiscrotum becomes erythematous and extremely painful. An associated inflammatory hydrocele may be produced in the tunica vaginalis. Late changes may include peritubular fibrosis and occlusion of the epididymis. Sterility is a long-term complication of epididymitis. The pathophysiology of epididymo-orchitis depends on the etiologic cause. In pyogenic orchitis, multiple foci of necrosis are found, with considerable edema and interstitial infiltration of polymorphonuclear cells resulting in ischemia. This process may progress to suppuration involving the entire testis, leading to a testicular abscess (Nickel & Plumb, 1986). Histologic studies in some cases of traumatic orchitis reveal a nonspecific granulomatous reaction to protein. This reaction is prompted by extravasated sperm following an obstruction or traumatic procedure. The tissue reaction comprises giant cells and resembles that of tuberculosis (Nickel & Plumb, 1986). In the myriad of fungal, viral, and parasitic diseases that may cause orchitis, the pathologic process may be the result of the action of bacterial toxins on the testicle (Nickel & Plumb, 1986). Orchitis in any form may result in atrophy, sterility from fibrosis, and destruction of the tubules and ductal system.

**Medical-Surgical Management.** Treatment of urethritis is based on the culture results and appropriate antibiotic. If NGU is diagnosed, a 7-day course of tetracycline or erythromycin is recommended. As part of the management of urethritis, treatment of the patient's sexual partner(s) is imperative.

In a severe episode of epididymitis, hospitalization and treatment with a combination of an aminoglycoside and a synthetic penicillin pending urine culture results might be necessary (Gray & Broadwell, 1986). Less acute cases are generally treated with oral antibiotics. If epididymitis is secondary to a sexually transmitted organism, tetracycline or a related antibiotic is the recommended treatment. All sexual partners should be treated concurrently. On rare occasion, an epididymectomy may be necessary in chronic or tubercular epididymitis.

In the clinical presentation of a painful testis, the possibility of torsion and tumor must be excluded. Treatment of orchitis is aimed at symptomatic relief and specific therapy for the underlying cause. Antibiotic therapy is guided by the urine culture results. Symptomatic relief generally includes scrotal elevation and bed rest. There is some controversy regarding the use of hot compresses on the testis, which may result in destruction of sperm cells (Long & Glazer, 1985). However, there is agreement that cold compresses are beneficial in pain relief. For the presence of a symptomatic hydrocele, aspiration may be required. Gross destruction of the testis, as a complication of orchitis, may necessitate surgical drainage or orchidectomy (Scott et al., 1982).

## APPROACHES TO PATIENT CARE

### Assessment

The patient with urethritis has many of the same symptoms as those seen in cystitis, but, in addition, urethral discharge may be present. Some women, however, may be asymptomatic. Urethral discharge is generally common in men. On physical examination, the patient may complain of local tenderness at the urethral meatus or along the line of the urethra. Physical inspection can reveal a red and swollen urinary meatus. Nursing assessment includes a patient health history. The patient is questioned regarding prior history of UTIs, sexual practices, hygiene health practices (particularly use of bubble baths, perfumed soaps, and feminine hygiene sprays), and contraceptive practices. A Gram stain of the urethral smear will demonstrate an excess of WBCs in the absence of gram-negative diplococci. An endourethral swab may be positive for *C. trachomatis*. If the patient has a concomitant cystitis, the urine culture will be positive.

Epididymitis and orchitis present very similarly. The patient gives a history of acute onset of scrotal swelling, pain, and tenderness. The patient is generally febrile and may complain of nausea and vomiting. In orchitis, the patient may have had a recent viral infection (espe-

cially mumps). Physical examination of the patient with epididymitis reveals a thickened epididymis that is enlarged and very tender. The scrotal skin may be red and warm to the touch. The patient often complains of testicle and lower quadrant abdominal pain on the affected side. A varicocele in the scrotum is a common finding. In orchitis, the involved testis is swollen, tense, and very tender. The scrotal skin may show redness, edema, and evidence of a hydrocele. The nurse documents any recent history of UTI, instrumentation, or surgical procedures on the genitourinary tract. The diagnostic workup for epididymitis and orchitis includes a Gram stain of a urethral smear and an endourethral swab (finding the same as urethritis). Urine culture is positive if there is a bacterial cystitis involved. The WBC count and sedimentation rate are elevated in an acute episode. To rule out torsion of the testis, Doppler ultrasound, a testicular radionuclide scan, or both may be carried out.

### Nursing Diagnosis

The nursing diagnoses for the patient with urethritis, epididymitis, or orchitis may include the following:

1. Alteration in the pattern of urinary elimination related to inflammation and irritation of the lower urinary tract.
2. Alteration in comfort related to the inflammatory response.
3. Knowledge deficit regarding the causes, treatment, and preventive measures for urethritis, epididymitis, or orchitis.
4. Anxiety related to sexual concerns.

### Plan of Care

Nursing care is directed toward enabling the patient to

1. State that the usual pattern of urinary elimination is restored without discomfort.
2. Maintain a urinary output of at least 30 to 40 mL/h.
3. Indicate relief from discomfort.
4. Understand the cause, management, and treatment of urethritis, epididymitis, or orchitis.
5. Understand the importance of completing the antibiotic course.
6. Implement measures to prevent recurrent infection.
7. Express any fears related to concerns about sexual function and activity.

### Intervention

The nursing care interventions related to urinary elimination will be the same as those described for other types of lower tract UTI. Since urinary retention is a possibility, the nurse must monitor the fluid intake and output every 8 hours and assess the bladder for overdistention.

Comfort measures may include application of an ice pack and, in the male, elevation and support of the scrotum by an athletic supporter, folded towel, or Bellevue bridge. If ice is used, the nurse must be aware of the possibility of ice burns and remove the ice pack for short intervals at least every hour. A skin inspection is performed at that time. For the patient with urethritis, a sitz bath may provide local pain relief. Frequent voiding is encouraged to decrease irritative voiding symptoms. The nurse is responsible for administering prescribed antibiotics and analgesics and monitoring patient response. Bed rest may be indicated during the acute phase of epididymitis or orchitis. Vital signs are monitored every 8 hours and more often if the patient is febrile.

The nurse assesses the patient's knowledge of the signs and symptoms, causes, management, and prevention measures associated with urethritis, epididymitis, or orchitis. If spread of infection to a sexual partner or partners is suspected, the nurse discusses with the patient the importance of identifying the sexual contacts so that treatment may be initiated. Treatment of sexual partners is advised whether they are symptomatic or not. Infection control principles are reviewed with the patient as well as safe sex practices, such as the use of condoms and having only one sexual partner. Avoidance of sexual activity is encouraged until treatment of both partners is completed. In the patient with epididymitis or orchitis, strenuous activity is contraindicated until the infection has resolved. As discussed elsewhere, instruction regarding antibiotic therapy is essential to patient compliance.

The nurse needs to be sensitive to the patient's concerns regarding any sexual dysfunction or the spread of infection to sexual partners caused by urethritis, epididymitis, or orchitis. The patient is encouraged to ventilate these concerns to the nurse, who establishes a supportive and nonjudgmental atmosphere. Truthful information needs to be given regarding the need for using a condom and the possibility of sterility in the patient with bilateral epididymitis or orchitis.

**Patient Outcomes**

1. The patient resumes a normal voiding pattern, averaging 30 to 40 mL/h.
2. The patient is relieved of pain.
3. The patient can verbalize an understanding of urethritis, epididymitis, or orchitis and describe the signs and symptoms, causes, and prevention measures associated with the disease.
4. The patient is aware of the need to seek health care if the symptoms recur.
5. The patient expresses an understanding of the rationale for continued antibiotic therapy even when symptoms have resolved.
6. Sexual contacts have been identified and treated if necessary.
7. The patient can verbalize any concerns regarding sexuality and infertility.
8. The patient verbalizes an understanding of safe sex practices.

# PARASITIC AND FUNGAL INFECTIONS

## Schistosomiasis, Filariasis, and Trichomoniasis

### PERSPECTIVE ON DISEASE ENTITY

**Etiology.** Parasitic disease is a major health problem today in developing countries (Lichtenberg & Lehman, 1986). Schistosomiasis, filariasis, and trichomoniasis are infections caused by three species of parasites that regularly affect the urogenital tract. Parasitic infections are frequently related to renal and lower urinary tract disease and are often chronic in nature.

Schistosomiasis is a chronic infection caused by a group of trematode worms; *Schistosoma haematobium* is the organism responsible for invasion of the urinary tract. The disease is endemic in Africa and the Middle East but may occur anywhere in the world. Infection is acquired by exposure to water that harbors the infected snail host. The disease may be asymptomatic or characterized by dysuria, urgency, hematuria, colic, or urinary incontinence (Kunin, 1987). Mortality may result, secondary to renal failure as a complication of obstruction and bacterial infection (Lichtenberg & Lehman, 1986). The incidence of schistosomiasis appears to be higher in males.

Filariasis involves the lymphatic system and is caused by the *Wuchereria bancrofti* parasite. *W. bancrofti* is a human parasite without known animal reservoirs. All lymphatic filarial species are transmitted by mosquitoes. The microfilaria of *W. bancrofti* is endemic in most tropical parts of the world except tropical parts of the United States and Australia (Lichtenberg & Lehman,

1986). Some people infected with filariasis remain asymptomatic, whereas others, who have had repeated and prolonged exposure, develop elephantiasis.

Trichomoniasis is a common cause of vaginitis in women, but it may also be transmitted to men and lead to urethritis and prostatitis. *Trichomonas vaginalis,* a flagellated protozoan, is the only protozoan pathogen found in humans (Lichtenberg & Lehman, 1986). *T. vaginalis* frequently colonizes the vagina and cervix of sexually active women and the anterior urethra of their male sexual partners. Transmission is generally by heterosexual sexual intercourse. The *Trichomonas* organism is viable outside the human body and has been recovered from wet cloths, sponges, and toilet bowls (Halverson & Graham, 1986). The organisms multiply by binary fission, with no intermediary or animal hosts known.

**Pathophysiology.** The disease process in schistosomiasis begins after the infecting organisms penetrate the skin or mucous membranes of the human. The organisms mature in the portal system of the liver, from where they are disseminated (Fig. 5–2).

The chronic disease is caused by persistent infection and granulomatous reaction to the eggs lodged in the bladder wall and ureter. The eggs may protrude into the urinary cavity and be passed into the urine. Chronic infection leads to formation of granulomas, fibrosis, and calcification of the ureter and bladder and may produce obstruction and hydronephrosis (Kunin, 1987). Eggs may be deposited throughout the body and often affect the genital tract and digestive system as well as the central nervous system, resulting in neurologic symptoms. Hemorrhages, ulceration, and diminished bladder capacity are other pathologic changes.

Filariasis exposure begins after a bite from an infected mosquito that affects the lymphatics of the skin. From the skin lymphatics, the worm penetrates the deep lymphatics and then on to lymph nodes, which constitute its natural habitat. The lymphatic channels become obstructed, leading to chyle in the urine and elephantiasis. A granulomatous reaction involving eosinophils, lymphocytes, and giant cells develops around the dead worms, causing the lymphatic channels to swell. Lymphatic varices and calcification may be a feature of the disease. As the lymphatic system in the male genital tract becomes obstructed, scrotal and penile skin swell and become thickened and fibrotic; elephantiasis then becomes apparent. Initially, the lymphatic obstruction may be intermittent, but gradually the edema becomes chronic (Scott et al., 1982).

The pathogenesis of trichomoniasis is still not clearly understood. It is believed that part of the pathology seen in symptomatic trichomoniasis may be due to the effect of bacterial superinfection (Lichtenberg & Lehman, 1986). Part of the host response in this disease may be immunologically determined, because it has been observed that males show more acute urethritis on reinfection during the initial episode. Pathologic lesions are mainly exudate, with reddening of the mucosa, occasional edema, and usually reddish spots, small blisters, or granules. In the uterine cervix, this observation is labeled the "strawberry mucosa" (Lichtenberg & Lehman, 1986). These lesions may be accompanied by extreme tenderness and a burning sensation, especially when they are touched.

**Medical-Surgical Management.** With the advent of less toxic medications, the medical treatment of schistosomiasis has been simplified. Of the three species of *Schistosoma* pathogenic for humans, *Schistosoma haematobium* appears to be the most amenable to treatment. Satisfactory response rates have been seen with metrifonate, hycanthone mesylate, and praziquantel (Lichtenberg & Lehman, 1986). Appropriate treatment should begin at the earliest stage of patient infection, because the reversibility of lesions decreases at later stages. Surgical management is generally confined to treatment of the various urinary complications of schistosomiasis that have not responded to medical therapy. Excision or dilation of the ureter is performed to correct strictures. If at-

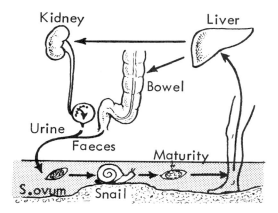

*FIGURE 5–2* Cycle of infection for schistosomiasis. (From Scott, R., Deane, R. F., & Callander, R. [1982]. *Urology illustrated* [2nd ed., p. 190]. New York: Churchill Livingstone. Reprinted by permission.)

tempts to open a ureter fail, a nephrostomy is performed. Surgical correction of bladder lesions can vary from dilation and vesical denervation to urinary shunting and partial cystectomy (Lichtenberg & Lehman, 1986). Prevention, of course, is the most effective type of treatment. Travelers in endemic areas should be warned of the hazards of bathing in potentially infected waters.

The established antifilarial drug is diethylcarbamazine. The drug is useful in the early stage of the disease but has little effect on established pathology in advanced filariasis (Lichtenberg & Lehman, 1986). If there is an element of bacterial lymphatic obstruction, appropriate antibiotic treatment should be instituted. Surgical treatment is aimed at removal of edematous tissue and reconstruction of the scrotum or vulva if necessary. There is a tendency for recurrence after surgery owing to the failure of the lymphatic flow to establish adequate collaterals (Scott et al., 1982).

Metronidazole (Flagyl) is the treatment of choice for trichomoniasis. The medication is contraindicated in pregnancy because of its potential carcinogenicity. Ampicillin is generally prescribed in this case (Kunin, 1987). Both male and female partners should be treated simultaneously to break the cycle of reinfection. Sexual abstinence is advised during the treatment period.

## APPROACHES TO PATIENT CARE

### Assessment

The patient with schistosomiasis may present in either the acute or the inactive phase. The acute phase generally begins 3 to 9 weeks after exposure. The patient complains of hematuria, dysuria, urgency, and slow, painful discharge of urine. In the inactive phase, signs of obstructive uropathy are manifested. Fibrosis causes decreased bladder capacity, and the patient may have severe urgency and incontinence.

On physical examination, colicky flank pain may be present if early obstructive uropathy has occurred. The patient may complain of referred pain in the glans penis or perineal region if there are ulcerations. The nurse continues the assessment by questioning the patient regarding any recent travels to the Middle East or Africa, and any bathing or swimming in potentially infected waters. In moderate to heavy infections, the urine sediment is diagnostic for the presence of eggs. If no eggs are seen, a 24-hour urine collection is necessary. Persistent

proteinuria is common. KUB urogram may reveal calcifications within the urinary tract or in other organs. Evidence of hydroureters, hydronephrosis, ureteral stenosis, and bladder and urethral filling defects (polypoid lesions) may be apparent on excretory urography. Cystourethrography will indicate the presence of vesicoureteral reflux, and cystoscopy will show congestion, ulceration, and cysts.

The male with filariasis presents with swelling and enlargement of the scrotum and penis. Early symptoms may also include fever, redness, and itching or the appearance of a small hydrocele in the affected area. The patient may complain of milky-looking urine. Physical examination demonstrates an enlarged and swollen scrotum and penis. Chyluria may be present. The patient history includes questions regarding travel outside the United States to tropical areas and any known mosquito exposure. Detection of *Wuchereria* microfilariae in a blood smear is diagnostic of filariasis. Any chylous urine or hydrocele fluid is checked for microfilariae. Immunologic tests, such as complement fixation and skin tests, may be useful in suggesting a filarial basis for the lymphedematous state. Lymphangiography can distinguish filariasis from other causes of lymphatic obstruction. KUB urogram may be ordered, but calcified worms are rarely seen.

In trichomoniasis, the patient may complain of dysuria, a painful urethral meatus, and vaginal or urethral discharge that is scanty and frothy. Females may also complain of vulvar itching. Physical examination reveals a reddened and painful urethral meatus. A nursing history includes contact investigation for potentially infected partner(s). A rectal examination in the male can reveal an enlarged and boggy prostate and seminal vesicles. With females, vaginal examination may show a classic "strawberry" cervix from small hemorrhages. Fresh exudate from vaginal, urethral, or vesicoprostatic fluid in which motile trichomonads are seen is diagnostic of trichomoniasis. Trichomonads can also be seen in urine sediment and Papanicolaou (Pap) smears.

### Nursing Diagnosis

The nursing diagnosis for the patient with schistosomiasis, filariasis, or trichomoniasis may include the following:

1. Alteration in the pattern of urinary elimination related to inflammation, irritation, and obstruction of the urinary tract.
2. Knowledge deficit related to the cause, treatment, and prevention of schistosomiasis, filariasis, and trichomoniasis.

3. Alteration in comfort related to dysuria, edema, and flank pain.
4. Alteration in self-concept, disturbance in body image, due to swelling and enlargement of scrotum and penis or vulva.
5. Potential for impairment of skin integrity.
6. Anxiety related to sexual concerns.

### Plan of Care

Nursing care is directed toward enabling the patient to

1. State that the symptoms of schistosomiasis, filariasis, or trichomoniasis are relieved or reduced.
2. Understand the importance of completing the medication course.
3. Implement measures to prevent reinfection.
4. Maintain normal skin integrity.
5. Maintain a healthy self-concept.
6. Express fears and anxiety related to concerns about sexual function and activity.

### Intervention

The nursing care considerations would be the same as those for other types of lower tract UTIs, including the implementation of measures to promote urinary elimination and comfort. Additionally, the nurse is responsible for administering prescribed antiparasitic medications and monitoring patient response.

The excessive swelling and enlargement of the scrotum or vulva can cause potential impairment of skin integrity in patients with filariasis. The lower extremities can also become edematous because of lymphatic obstruction. The nurse should assess the perineal skin areas and other areas of edema at least every 8 hours and should be alert for any signs of skin breakdown. Proper positioning and adequate perineal hygiene are necessary to prevent the complications of ischemia, pressure necrosis, and bacterial colonization.

Because of swelling and enlargement of the scrotum, penis, or vulva, the patient may experience a disturbance in body image that affects self-concept. The nurse should provide a supportive environment and encourage the patient to express any concerns. Sterility issues may not be a factor unless extensive urologic surgery is needed, which might impair sexual or reproductive function. If surgical treatment is planned to reconstruct the scrotum or vulva, the nurse assists the patient and significant other to be active in the preoperative and postoperative plans. A referral to a mental health care professional may be beneficial.

### Patient Outcomes

1. The patient resumes a normal voiding pattern, averaging 30 to 40 mL/h.

2. The patient can verbalize an understanding of schistosomiasis, filariasis, or trichomoniasis and describe the signs and symptoms, causes, treatment, and preventive measures associated with the disease.
3. The patient is aware of the need to seek health care if symptoms recur.
4. The patient expresses an understanding of the rationale for continued antiparasitic therapy even when symptoms have resolved.
5. The patient is relieved of pain.
6. The patient can verbalize concerns regarding disturbance in body image.
7. Skin integrity is maintained.
8. The patient is able to express any fears and anxiety related to sexual concerns
9. Sexual contacts have been identified and treated if necessary.

# Candidiasis and Actinomycosis

## PERSPECTIVES ON DISEASE ENTITY

**Etiology.** Fungi have the ability to invade the urinary tract. The most common of the fungal organisms is *Candida albicans*. *C. albicans* is a yeast fungus that is considered a normal inhabitant of the mouth, vagina, and intestinal canal. It is suppressed by the normal bacterial flora and rarely produces infection unless the usual microbial ecology is altered or the host resistance is decreased (Kunin, 1987). This alteration in the usual microbial ecology is most often influenced by administration of antibiotics. The *Candida* reservoir in the patient's own intestinal tract is the source of infection in most cases of urinary tract candidiasis. The routes of infection are (1) the lymphatics, (2) the hematogenous route, or (3) the ascending route. Glucosuria in diabetes, the use of steroids, and instrumentation of the urinary tract all are predisposing factors in candidiasis (Kunin, 1987). The clinical presentation of urinary tract candidiasis may include (1) asymptomatic candiduria, (2) *Candida* septicemia, (3) *Candida* pyelonephritis, and (4) *Candida* cystitis (Schönebeck, 1986).

Actinomycosis is not commonly seen in the urinary tract. Actinomycosis is an indolent suppurative infection caused by certain anaerobic actinomycetes; *Actinomyces israelii* is the most common pathogen. *Actinomyces* is a genus of nonmotile, non–spore-forming, anaerobic to facultatively anaerobic, gram-positive bacteria.

The disease is seen most often in adults. *Actinomyces* occasionally infects the kidneys or prostate. In the prostate, it causes a chronic prostatitis resembling that seen in tuberculosis of the genitourinary system.

**Pathophysiology.** The body's primary defenses against candidal infections are the presence of normal bacterial flora and the presence of polymorphonuclear neutrophils in the mucosa of the urethra and bladder that have anti-*Candida* effects. Additionally, prostatic fluid is fungicidal, accounting for the low incidence of *Candida* cystitis in males compared with females. Asymptomatic candiduria is always considered pathologic, since fungi are never found in the urine of normal, healthy persons. Generally, asymptomatic candiduria is most often a harmless condition that disappears spontaneously when predisposing factors are eliminated or controlled (i.e., indwelling catheters, antibiotic therapy, or diabetes). However, the condition may also continue for years. *Candida* pyelonephritis occurs in two main forms: (1) multiple abscess formation, primarily in the renal cortex, and (2) diffuse fungal infiltration of the tips of the papillae or along the collecting tubules, sometimes leading to papillary necrosis (Schönebeck, 1986). The first form described usually precedes the second. In *Candida* septicemia, the kidneys appear to be the organ system most frequently involved. Multiple renal abscesses with increased leukocytic reaction, growth of mycelia in the renal tubules, and papillary necrosis are commonly seen (Kunin, 1987). *Candida* cystitis produces bladder mucosal lining changes marked by grayish-white spots that bleed if removed. The cystoscopic findings may resemble tubercular infection of the bladder (Gray & Broadwell, 1986).

One of the main differences between bacterial and fungal infections is the formation of bezoars.

Bezoars, or "fungal balls," occur when the fungi grow long and threadlike, forming pseudomycelia. These threads mingle into small clusters that clump together to form bezoars. Their size may vary from that of a grain of wheat to large enough to fill the bladder. Bezoars may form in the patient with *Candida* pyelonephritis or may be a factor in asymptomatic candiduria. Obstruction from a bezoar may occur in the renal pelvis, ureter, or bladder. The clinical picture can be one of progressive uremia or acute anuria if a bezoar obstructs collecting tubules or the ureters. Small bezoars may pass spontaneously, but large ones may require suprapubic cystotomy for removal (Schönebeck, 1986).

The generalized form of actinomycosis is spread by the hematogenous route and may affect the kidney, ureter, and prostate as well as other organs. All actinomycetes are considered normal bacterial flora of the mouth and gastrointestinal tract in humans. But when actinomycetes are introduced into tissue, they produce chronic, destructive abscesses or granulomas that eventually discharge a viscid pus containing minute, yellowish granules (sulfur granules).

**Medical-Surgical Management.** Amphotericin B, 5-fluorocytosine, or both given intravenously are the drugs of choice in severe candiduria. In the acutely ill patient, an intravenous pyelogram (IVP) should be performed to rule out the possibility of obstruction from bezoars. If the excretory urogram is normal, medical treatment should continue. If obstruction is present, surgical management becomes necessary. In the clinically stable patient, efforts to clear the funguria should be made. Catheters and intravenous lines should be cultured first and then discontinued or replaced. Antibiotics, immunosuppressive medication, and cortisone are discontinued, if possible, and the urine is recultured (Schönebeck, 1986). If candiduria persists, further workup, including IVP, blood cultures, and agglutinin titers, is recommended. Amphotericin B, systemic or by intravesical irrigation, 5-fluorocytosine, or both remain the most effective treatment options (Schönebeck, 1986).

The recommended therapy for milder cases of actinomycosis generally includes oral penicillin or tetracycline (Berkow, 1982). In severe cases, parenteral penicillin G for approximately 6 weeks followed by prolonged therapy with oral penicillin V or tetracycline is recommended (Bennett, 1987).

## APPROACHES TO PATIENT CARE

### Assessment

Asymptomatic candiduria presents without any symptoms and usually resolves spontaneously when predisposing factors are eliminated. Asymptomatic candiduria may develop into a symptomatic infection or give rise to bezoar formation. The urine culture will be positive for *Candida*.

In *Candida* septicemia and pyelonephritis, the patient may be acutely ill and complain of sudden onset of fever, flank pain, or anuria if obstruction from a bezoar has occurred. On physical examination, flank pain is demonstrated on palpation. The urine culture is positive for *Can-*

*dida,* but the blood culture may not be positive in almost half of the patients with disseminated *Candida* infection (Kunin, 1987). If blood cultures are negative, tests to check for the presence of *Candida* metabolites or antigens in the blood or for circulating antibodies to the organism need to be conducted. The enzyme-linked immunosorbent assay (ELISA) technique can detect mannan, a major capsular material in *Candida.* Antibodies can be detected by immunoelectrophoresis, ELISA, or other serologic methods (Kunin, 1987). An IVP may document upper tract changes from obstructive components.

The patient with *Candida* cystitis presents with symptoms similar to those of bacterial cystitis but additionally may complain of air or gas in the urine. However, this symptom is now rare with the improved treatment of diabetes. Physical examination findings were described in the section on acute and chronic cystitis. The urine culture is positive for *Candida.* On KUB urogram, large bezoars may be seen as illuminated, partly radiodense spheres in the bladder region.

Actinomycosis is a slowly progressive disease, and the patient may present with vague symptoms of variable low-grade fever, lethargy, or abdominal or flank pain. If the prostate is affected, a history of chronic prostatitis-type pain may be given. Physical examination may demonstrate flank or abdominal tenderness. The prostatic examination reveals a nodular gland that is rarely tender and generally not enlarged. Diagnosis is based on evidence of *A. israelii* in pus or tissue. The microorganisms appear as tangled masses of branched and unbranched wavy filaments, or as distinctive sulfur granules. These same findings are found in the EPS of a patient with prostatic involvement.

The nursing history for patients with suspected *Candida* infections includes questions on recent catheterization or instrumentation, the use of antibiotics or immunosuppressive medications, and any predisposing conditions, such as diabetes, pregnancy, and prostatic enlargement. Hygiene status is also assessed. The nurse needs to ensure that the urine specimen is not contaminated, especially in women.

**Nursing Diagnosis**
The nursing diagnosis for the patient with candidiasis or actinomycosis may include the following:

1. Alteration in the pattern of urinary elimination related to inflammation and irritation, or obstruction of the urinary tract.

2. Knowledge deficit related to the causes, treatment, and prevention of candidiasis or actinomycosis.
3. Alteration in comfort related to dysuria and flank pain.

**Plan of Care**
Nursing care is directed toward enabling patient to

1. Maintain a urinary output of at least 30 to 40 mL/h.
2. Understand the importance of completing the antibiotic course.
3. Implement measures to prevent reinfection.
4. State that the symptoms of candidiasis or actinomycosis are relieved or reduced.

**Intervention**
The nursing care considerations would be the same as those for other infections of the lower urinary tract. In addition, the patient with candidiasis is instructed to avoid sexual intercourse until antibiotic therapy is completed and follow-up urine cultures are negative. The nurse assists the patient in understanding the importance of identifying any sexual contacts, so appropriate treatment may be instituted if necessary.

**Patient Outcomes**
1. The patient resumes a normal voiding pattern, to average 30 to 40 mL/h.
2. The patient can verbalize an understanding of candidiasis or actinomycosis and describe the signs and symptoms, causes, treatment, and preventive measures associated with the disease.
3. The patient is aware of the need to seek health care if the symptoms recur.
4. The patient expresses an understanding of the rationale for continued antifungal or antibiotic therapy even when symptoms have resolved.
5. Sexual contacts have been identified and treated if necessary.
6. The patient is relieved of pain.

# RELATED PROBLEMS

## Genitourinary Tuberculosis

### PERSPECTIVE ON DISEASE ENTITY

**Etiology.** Infection of the urinary tract due to *Mycobacterium tuberculosis* has become relatively rare in Western countries. However, it still must be considered in patients who present with unexplained persistent hematuria and pyuria, particularly in those who have foci of tuberculosis in other parts of the body (Kunin, 1987). Genitourinary tuberculosis tends to be a late manifestation of a more generalized disease caused by metastatic spread of organisms through the blood stream. As secondary tuberculosis, the disease can occur either by reactivation of an old infection or by reinfection from an active case (Gow, 1986). The kidney and epididymis are the two most common sites where the disease may initially present. However, these sites are usually secondary to a primary focus, such as the lung (Fig. 5–3).

*M. tuberculosis* may infect the kidney, ureter, bladder, testis, epididymis, and rarely the prostate, penis, and urethra. The incidence of genitourinary tuberculosis is more common in men than in women, in a 2:1 ratio (Gow, 1986).

**Pathophysiology.** Renal tuberculosis is a secondary manifestation of the disease and is caused by hematogenous spread of the organism. Once the organism lodges in the kidney, low-grade inflammatory reaction and focal destruction begin, and the characteristic tubercles are seen. If bacilli continue to multiply, the tubercles enlarge to form large cavities containing caseous material. There is destruction of the surrounding parenchymal tissue and dissemi-

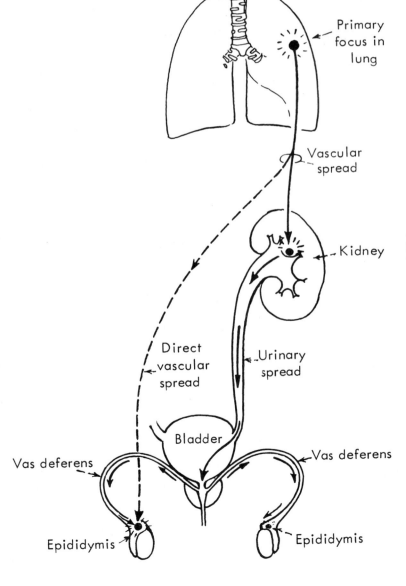

FIGURE 5–3 Tuberculosis of the urinary tract. (From Scott, R., Deane, R. F., & Callander, R. [1982]. *Urology illustrated* [2nd ed., p. 382]. New York: Churchill Livingstone. Reprinted by permission.)

nation of the bacilli down the urinary tract. Renal calcification and hypertension are hazards of renal tuberculosis (Gow, 1986).

Tuberculosis ureteritis is a direct extension of the disease in the kidney. The ureterovesical junction is the most commonly affected site, and stricture formation may result. Strictures may lead to hydronephrosis. Additionally, the infection may cause formation of tubercles and ulcerations of the ureter. Tuberculosis of the bladder is secondary to renal involvement. The lesions usually develop around the ureteric orifice and, as the inflammation progresses, may completely occlude the ureteric opening (Gow, 1986). As the disease continues, inflammation spreads deep into muscle, causing mucosal ulceration and fibrosis that leads to a decrease in functional capacity.

In the testis, tuberculosis is usually secondary to reinfection of the epididymis by the hematogenous route. Rarely, tuberculosis orchitis is seen with no epididymal involvement. It is difficult to differentiate such swelling from a testicular tumor; therefore, exploration is required (Gow, 1986).

Tuberculous foci in the epididymis are the result of hematogenous spread. Clinically, there is enlargement of the epididymis, and a sympathetic hydrocele may form (Scott et al., 1982). In extreme cases, there may be generalized epididymal induration, sinus formation, and even involvement of the testis (Gow, 1986).

Tuberculosis of the prostate, penis, or urethra is rare. Infection of the prostate is through the hematogenous route. Advanced lesions may destroy tissue or lead to a perineal sinus. Penile tuberculosis may be primary from direct infectious contact or secondary from active pulmonary tuberculosis (Gow, 1986). Initially, surface lesions are superficial, but they may progress to a tubercular cavernositis. Last, tuberculosis of the urethra is spread from another focus in the genital tract, such as the epididymis. In the acute phase, urethral discharge and involvement of the epididymis, prostate, and other parts of the urinary system are present. If the disease progresses to the chronic stage, urethral obstruction due to strictures develops.

**Medical-Surgical Management.** Antimicrobial therapy is highly effective in genitourinary tract tuberculosis. Combination therapy is generally prescribed to avoid antimicrobial drug resistance (Scott et al., 1982). The most common combination therapy includes isonicotinic acid hydrazide (isoniazid), ethambutol, and rifampicin. The usual recommended length of treatment is 2 years, but recent literature has sug-

gested that shorter courses of less than 6 months may be equally effective (Gow, 1986). Once treatment has commenced, regular urine screening is necessary during the next 2 years. Generally, tubercle bacilli are absent from the urine after 3 to 6 months of treatment.

Surgical intervention may be required if irreversible changes have occurred in the advanced stage of the disease. In many cases, surgery is combined with short-course medication treatment. Surgical management may include (1) nephrectomy, (2) ureterectomy, (3) epididymectomy, (4) bladder augmentation, and (5) urinary diversion. Reconstructive surgery, to correct tuberculous strictures, is performed most often at the ureterovesical junction, pelviureteric junction, and the middle third of the ureter (Gow, 1986).

## APPROACHES TO PATIENT CARE

### Assessment
The cardinal signs of genitourinary tuberculosis usually include unexplained fever along with painless hematuria and sterile pyuria. The patient may also present with the common irritative voiding symptoms of frequency, dysuria, nocturia, and urgency. Complaints of ureteral colic and renal and suprapubic pain are less common. The patient may give a history of weight loss, fatigue, and anorexia, but these symptoms are generally seen in the later stages of the disease. On physical examination, renal or suprapubic pain may be present on palpation. In males, swelling of the epididymis and evidence of a hydrocele may be seen. The nurse obtains a patient history with particular emphasis on recurrent UTIs not responding to antibiotic treatment, a history of either disease or exposure to the tubercle bacillus, or both. Diagnostic studies generally reveal a sterile urine culture with the presence of pyuria (>20 WBCs per HPF). Secondary bacterial infections, however, are common. Three consecutive early-morning urine specimens are collected and cultured for tubercle bacilli. Blood screening includes an erythrocyte sedimentation rate. This value is usually elevated and needs to be monitored at monthly intervals to assess response to treatment. The general status of renal function is estimated by checking the serum creatinine, BUN, and electrolyte values. A KUB urogram is ordered to evaluate the presence of calculi. Other pathologic changes noted on KUB urogram may include (1) an irregular caliceal pattern, (2) parenchymal damage, (3) hydronephrosis, and (4) a small, contracted

bladder with filling defects. Retrograde pyelography can be diagnostic for strictures at the lower end of the ureter. Ureteric catheterization may be used to obtain urine samples from the kidneys. Cystoscopy reveals patches of inflamed tissue, reddened ureteral orifices, and ulcerations. Poor bladder compliance and limited functional capacity are demonstrated on urodynamic testing.

**Nursing Diagnosis**

The nursing diagnosis for the patient with genitourinary tuberculosis may include the following:

1. Alteration in the pattern of urinary elimination related to inflammation, irritation, and possible obstruction of the urinary tract.
2. Knowledge deficit related to the causes, treatment, prevention, and potential complications of genitourinary tuberculosis.
3. Alteration in comfort related to dysuria, flank pain, or testicular swelling.
4. Alteration in self-concept related to the chronic communicable disease state.

**Plan of Care**

Nursing care is directed toward enabling the patient to

1. Maintain a urinary output averaging 30 to 40 mL/h.
2. Implement measures to prevent reinfection and maintain universal precautions.
3. Understand the importance of completing the entire course of antituberculous medications.
4. State that the symptoms of genitourinary tuberculosis are reduced or relieved.
5. Maintain a healthy self-concept.

**Intervention**

Nursing care for the patient with genitourinary tuberculosis is aimed primarily at helping the patient to understand the effects that the disease has on the urinary tract and its significance as a communicable disease. The method of disease transmission, universal precautions, and the importance of continued compliance with the medical regimen are stressed. The nurse assists the patient in gaining confidence in self-care, because management of the disease is primarily on an outpatient basis. General health measures such as adequate rest, proper nutrition, and good hygiene practices are reviewed with the patient. The use of a scrotal support for genital swelling may be suggested. The importance of continued routine health follow-up is also reinforced. Male patients should be taught to use a protective device (condom)

during sexual intercourse to prevent the transfer of organisms. Patients should abstain from sexual intercourse during the treatment period for penile and urethral tuberculosis. These precautions should be continued until urine cultures are negative. Antituberculous medications are administered as prescribed, and patient response is evaluated. The patient is instructed on the action and side effects of the medication as well as the reasoning behind multiple therapy. If surgical intervention is required, comprehensive preoperative and postoperative instruction is completed.

Because of the social stigma a communicable disease carries, the patient's self-concept may be affected. The nurse is in a prime position to assist the patient in dealing with feelings of social isolation. A supportive and reassuring approach can assist the patient in maintaining a positive self-concept. At the same time, education of the patient, family, and significant other aids in successful adaptation to a chronic long-term illness.

**Patient Outcomes**

1. The patient resumes a normal voiding pattern, averaging 30 to 40 mL/h.
2. The patient can verbalize an understanding of genitourinary tuberculosis and describe the signs and symptoms, causes, treatment, and preventive measures associated with the disease.
3. The patient is aware of the need to seek health care if symptoms recur.
4. The patient expresses an understanding of the rationale for continued antituberculous therapy even when symptoms have resolved.
5. The patient is relieved of pain.
6. The patient is able to maintain a healthy self-concept.

## Genitourinary Fistulas

### PERSPECTIVE ON DISEASE ENTITY

**Etiology.** Genitourinary fistulas are more common in women and constitute one cause of involuntary loss of urine from the urethra or through the vagina. Such fistulas are usually secondary to operative trauma, neoplasms, involvement of the bladder by disease from other organs, and radiation therapy (Scott et al., 1982). Bladder fistulas can extend in almost any direction, to involve (1) uterine, (2) bowel, (3) vaginal, and (4) cutaneous areas. Fistulas involving the vagina and ureter occur most often.

Vesicovaginal fistulas usually develop as a result of gynecologic or obstetric procedures. Pressure necrosis of the bladder by the fetal head in prolonged labor is the most common cause (Turner-Warwick, 1986). Long-term urethral catheterization causes fistula formation at the penile-scrotal junction in men.

**Pathophysiology.** Fistula pathophysiology remains unclear; however, infection and tissue ischemia may be contributing factors (Zimmern et al., 1985).

**Medical-Surgical Management.** In the past, it was common practice to wait 2 to 6 months after a fistula was diagnosed before implementing treatment, to allow tissue around the fistula to mature and become less inflamed and edematous. Today, many urologists advocate prompt repair of vesicovaginal fistula. Conservative management is tried initially. A small fistula may close spontaneously after a Foley catheter is placed for a period of 2 or 3 weeks. If incontinence persists, operative repair is then advised (Zimmern et al., 1985).

The treatment of genitourinary fistula consists of surgical repair either by the transabdominal or the transvaginal route. Any UTI should be treated before the surgery. If feasible, the transvaginal approach is preferred. This procedure avoids a cystotomy, involves minimal blood loss, and consequently results in less postoperative discomfort and a shorter hospitalization (Zimmern et al., 1985). Prophylactic broad-spectrum antibiotic coverage is generally instituted to prevent local tissue infection and avoid breakdown of the repair. Postoperatively, urinary drainage is usually managed by a suprapubic catheter (Turner-Warwick, 1986).

## APPROACHES TO PATIENT CARE

### Assessment

The presenting complaint is incontinence of urine through the urethra or vagina in a patient with vesicovaginal fistula. The incontinence may be total or intermittent if the fistula is small. A watery vaginal discharge accompanied by normal voiding may be the only presenting symptom for fistulas connecting with other areas of the body, such as the bowel. The patient may report abnormal constituents, such as air and fecal material, in the urine. The amount of urinary incontinence varies with the size and location of the fistula. The patient may give a history of recent gynecologic or obstetric surgery. The nurse asks the patient about prior use of urethral catheters, recent radiation treatments, or history of disease in surrounding or-

gans, such as the uterus, cervix, and bowel. The methods used to cope with the incontinence (i.e., pads, plastic pants, or fluid restriction) are also ascertained. If concurrent UTI is present, the patient may complain of dysuria and hematuria. On physical examination, the labia and thighs may be excoriated. Vaginal discharge may also be present. Skin excoriation may be evident on other areas of the body where a urinary tract fistula is suspected. A urine culture and sensitivity rules out any associated UTI. Various diagnostic maneuvers are used to identify small fistulas. The infusion of carbon dioxide into the vagina may induce air bubbles to escape from the fistula tract when the bladder is inspected endoscopically (Zimmern et al., 1985). In the dye test, vaginal packing is placed, and methylene blue is introduced into the bladder by a catheter. If the packing remains dry and only the outer ends become colored, the urethra is the origin of the leakage. The bladder is suspected if the proximal end becomes colored. Last, if the proximal part of the packing becomes wet with unstained urine, the source must be ureteral (Turner-Warwick, 1986). Large vesicovaginal fistulas may be palpated on vaginal examination. With larger fistulas, diagnosis can be made on cystoscopy. A local tissue biopsy is taken if an underlying pathologic condition is suspected. An IVP is ordered to rule out any upper tract pathology. A voiding cystourethrogram is commonly performed to document the extent of the fistula, rule out vesicoureteral reflux, and diagnose a possible associated prolapse of the proximal urethra and bladder neck, which would require additional treatment at the time of the surgical repair (Zimmern et al., 1985).

### Nursing Diagnosis

The nursing diagnosis for the patient with genitourinary fistula may include the following:

1. Knowledge deficit related to the causes and the treatment of genitourinary fistulas.
2. Alteration in the pattern of urinary elimination (loss) due to
   a. Leakage of urine caused by a genitourinary fistula.
   b. Postoperative placement of suprapubic tube.
3. Impairment of skin integrity related to leakage of urine.
4. Potential for infection related to the placement of a suprapubic catheter following surgical repair of a fistula.

5. Alteration in comfort related to surgical repair of a fistula.

**Plan of Care**

Nursing care is directed toward enabling the patient to

1. Understand the medical-surgical management of genitourinary fistula repair.
2. State that the symptoms of incontinence related to genitourinary fistula are relieved.
3. Maintain skin integrity at the site of the fistula tract.
4. Maintain an infection-free suture line and sterile urine.
5. State that the pain relief measures are effective.

**Intervention**

All patients with a genitourinary fistula will inevitably require surgical repair. Nursing interventions are, therefore, directed toward helping the patient understand the course of treatment to prepare for the surgical experience and postoperative recuperation.

Leakage of urine is the most obvious manifestation of a genitourinary fistula. In the interim, before surgery is performed, the nurse should monitor the episodes of incontinence and record each event on the intake and output log. This is especially important when the incontinence is intermittent. If a fistula track is draining elsewhere in the body, attempts should be made to also measure and record that output. Incontinent episodes may excoriate the skin around the vagina, thighs, or other areas of the body where the fistula track drains. Inspect the skin at least every 8 hours. Perineal hygiene with mild soap and water, along with thorough drying, should be performed after each incontinent episode. If a genitourinary fistula track exits at another body site, the drainage is kept away from the skin as much as possible. Dressings are changed when they become wet. For profuse drainage, ostomy skin care products and appliances may be used. By working with the patient to cope with the incontinence while awaiting surgical repair, the nurse can aid the patient in gaining a sense of control over the situation. This will also provide an optimal opportunity to address sexuality issues, which are of greatest concern to female patients who may experience loss of vaginal sensation for several months after surgery.

Postoperatively, the patient is at risk for infection secondary to an abdominal incision and placement of a suprapubic catheter for urinary drainage as well as the manipulation of urethral and vaginal tissue during closure of the fistula. Vital signs should be monitored at least every 8 hours, or more frequently if the patient becomes febrile. Observe for signs of erythema and excessive or odorous drainage. To prevent infection, catheter care is given, and a closed drainage system is maintained; sterile technique is employed for abdominal and perineal dressing changes, and prescribed antibiotics are administered.

During the immediate postoperative period, analgesics may be administered to reduce discomfort. As healing takes place, a heat lamp or warm compresses may provide local pain relief.

Prior to patient discharge, catheter care techniques are reviewed with the patient, as self-care of the suprapubic tube is usually required for several weeks. The procedure for dressing change is also demonstrated and explained. If antibiotics are to be continued at home, instructions about the drug—including side effects and the importance of completing the course—are given. It is also important to advise patients that there is generally a 6-week restriction period on heavy lifting, prolonged standing, and sexual intercourse.

**Patient Outcomes**

1. The patient can verbalize an understanding of genitourinary fistulas and describe the causes and treatment of the condition.
2. Skin integrity is maintained at the site of the fistula tract.
3. The patient resumes a normal voiding pattern, or episodes of incontinence are decreased.
4. The patient is relieved of pain.
5. Incisional area is healing without infection.
6. The patient expresses an understanding of the rationale for continued antibiotic therapy even when dysuria symptoms have resolved.
7. The patient is aware of the need to seek health care if symptoms recur.
8. The patient can verbalize any concerns regarding self-concept.

# Urinary Tract Infection in Pregnancy

## PERSPECTIVE ON DISEASE ENTITY

**Etiology.** Bacteriuria commonly occurs during pregnancy owing to certain anatomic and physiologic alterations that take place during gestation. The rate of cystitis among pregnant women is estimated to be between 4% and 6% (Stamey, 1980). This rate does not differ from that among nonpregnant women. Frequency, however, is increased with parity and age (Kunin, 1987). Recurrent episodes of bacteriuria are common among pregnant women who have positive urine cultures during their initial prenatal examinations (Krieger, 1986). Pregnant women experience a decrease in spontaneous clearing of infection and a higher incidence of acute pyelonephritis. The incidence rate of pyelonephritis is reported to be 2% to 4% in pregnant women (Kunin, 1987). Most cases seem to develop during the third trimester, when hydronephrosis and stasis in the urinary tract are most pronounced.

The complications associated with bacteriuria during pregnancy can affect both mother and fetus. The risk of pyelonephritis has already been addressed. Pregnant women may also develop anemia and toxemia (Krieger, 1986). For the fetus, studies have suggested an association among UTI of pregnancy, prematurity, and neonatal mortality (Naeye, 1979; Sweet, 1977). Whether bacteriuria is asymptomatic or symptomatic when diagnosed, it should be treated to avoid the potential risks of morbidity and mortality.

**Pathophysiology.** The most impressive change in the pregnant woman's urinary tract involves the collecting system. Dilation of the renal calices, pelves, and ureters begins during the first trimester and become markedly increased by the third trimester. Ureteral dilation is more apparent on the right side. Reduced peristaltic activity also accompanies dilation of the upper urinary tract (Krieger, 1986). The muscle-relaxing effects of progesterone, along with mechanical obstruction of the ureters by the enlarging uterus, have been implicated in causing hydroureters (Waltzer, 1981). Other anatomic changes include an increase in ureter length by approximately 1 cm and displacement of the bladder superiorly and anteriorly. Physiologically, there is a transient increase in the GFR and renal plasma flow during pregnancy (Waltzer, 1981). Glomerular filtration may increase by 30% to 50%, and urine protein excretion also increases (Shortliffe & Stamey, 1986). Values considered normal in nonpregnant women may indicate renal insufficiency during pregnancy.

**Medical-Surgical Management.** Management of UTI in pregnancy should be aimed at preventing morbidity and diminishing the rates of prematurity, possible toxemia, and hypertension (Kunin, 1987). Potential injury to the developing fetus and maternal toxicity are prime concerns when choosing the appropriate antimicrobial agent. Maternal expanded fluid volume, fetal distribution of the drug, increased renal blood flow, and increased glomerular filtration will decrease serum drug concentration (Shortliffe & Stamey, 1986). Antibiotics considered safe for use during pregnancy include penicillins, cephalosporins, and those with an erythromycin base.

## APPROACHES TO PATIENT CARE

### Assessment

The assessment for the patient with UTI in pregnancy is the same as that described in the section on acute and chronic cystitis. It should be noted that cystitis may be asymptomatic and diagnosed coincidentally during routine examination. If needed, radiographic studies should be abbreviated to avoid excessive exposure of the fetus to radiation.

### Nursing Diagnosis

The nursing diagnosis for the patient with UTI in pregnancy may include the following:

1. Knowledge deficit related to the causes, treatment, and prevention of UTI in pregnancy.
2. Alteration in comfort related to dysuria or flank pain, or both.
3. Anxiety related to the effect of the UTI on the fetus.
4. Potential for alteration in fluid volume excess related to complications of pregnancy.

### Plan of Care

Nursing care is directed toward enabling the patient to

1. Understand the importance of completing the antibiotic course.
2. Implement measures to prevent recurrent UTI.
3. State that the symptoms of UTI in pregnancy are relieved.
4. Express any concerns related to the effect of UTI on the fetus.
5. Maintain a urinary output averaging 30 to 40 mL/h.

### Intervention

The nursing care considerations would be the same as those described for acute and chronic cystitis. Additionally, the nurse should discuss with the patient the normal changes her body is undergoing during pregnancy and how these might affect the urinary system to cause infection. Naturally, the patient will have concerns about the effect the infection will have on herself and the fetus. By helping her to understand the causes and treatment of UTI, these anxiety feelings may be diminished.

It is probable that an antibiotic will be prescribed; many are considered safe for use during pregnancy. Therefore, the nurse should provide detailed instructions to the patient regarding the dosage and possible side effects. The nurse should advise the patient to be alert to and report any changes in fetal movement while taking the antibiotic. Signs of a change in renal function, such as excessive edema, should also be conveyed. To relieve discomfort, a sitz bath or warm bath may be suggested, if not contraindicated by the obstetrician. Adequate fluid intake, along with regular bladder emptying, should be maintained.

### Patient Outcomes

1. The patient can verbalize an understanding of UTI in pregnancy and describe the signs and symptoms, causes, treatment, and preventive measures.
2. The patient is aware of the need to seek health care if symptoms recur.
3. The patient expresses an understanding of the rationale for continued antibiotic therapy even when the symptoms have resolved.
4. The patient is relieved of pain.
5. The patient can verbalize any fears regarding the effect of UTI on her fetus.
6. The patient resumes a normal voiding pattern averaging 30 to 40 mL/h.

# Urosepsis

## PERSPECTIVE ON DISEASE ENTITY

**Etiology.** The term *urosepsis* implies a gram-negative bacteremia that originates from a genitourinary focus. The urinary tract is reported to be the most frequent site of origin, with the indwelling urinary catheter being the leading cause of nosocomial UTIs (Kreger et al., 1980; Stamm et al., 1977). Catheter-induced infections remain the most frequent problem in hospital infection control. It is reported that approximately 40% of all nosocomial infections are related to the urinary tract, and about 80% of these are preceded by some form of urologic instrumentation (Stamm et al., 1977). The most common offending organism isolated in gram-negative bacteremia is *E. coli*. The prevalence of gram-negative bacteremia in hospitalized

patients is thought to result from (1) bacterial factors, (2) medical practices and procedures, and (3) host factors (Bahnson, 1986).

The prime bacterial factor is the remarkable ability of gram-negative organisms to develop antimicrobial resistance. Drug resistance may be inherent in the microorganism or may be acquired from mutation or genetic exchange (Bahnson, 1986). Medical technology has added devices such as indwelling urethral and venous catheters. However, unless strict aseptic technique is adhered to, these modalities can be of more harm than benefit to patients. Last, older and more medically complex patients along with the increased use of immunosuppression and chemotherapy are responsible for a hospitalized population susceptible to infection (Bahnson, 1986).

**Pathophysiology.** The pathophysiologic mechanisms in urosepsis are complex and not completely understood. The cell wall of gram-negative bacilli is composed of a lipid-carbohydrate complex termed *lipopolysaccharide* (LPS). This complex acts on endotoxin, but its role as the sole initiator of the pathophysiologic changes of septic shock is controversial (Bahnson, 1986). The toxic effects of LPS are believed to be mediated by factors produced by the macrophage system. Endogenous pyrogen (EP) or interleukin-1 is the best defined of these mediators. Table 5–3 lists other postulated mediators of septic shock.

In the acute-response phase of septic shock, the presence of infection causes changes in metabolic, hematologic, and immunologic parameters. Fever is considered the most promi-

**TABLE 5–3. Postulated Mediators of the Pathophysiologic Events in Bacteremia**

Endogenous pyrogen (leukocyte endogenous mediator, interleukin-1)
Catecholamines (epinephrine, norepinephrine)
Serotonin
Histamine
Acetylcholine
Glucocorticoids
Kinins
Complement components (anaphylatoxins)
Coagulation components
Endorphins
Prostaglandins
Lysosomal components
Slow-reacting substance
Macrophage and lymphocyte products
Myocardial depressant factor

From McCabe, W. R., & Treadwell, T. L. (1983). Gram-negative bacteremia. *Monographs in Urology, 4*, 193–214. Reprinted by permission.

nent of these responses and is mediated by EP. It is believed that EP raises the hypothalamic thermal regulatory setpoint, causing vasoconstriction to conserve and generate heat to match the elevated thermal regulatory setpoint (Bahnson, 1986).

Gram-negative bacterial endotoxins appear to activate at least four interacting humoral systems responsible for the pathologic findings and progression to septic shock: (1) activation of complement results in release of C3 and C5, two vasodilating anaphylatoxins enhancing the inflammatory reaction; (2) activation of the coagulation system, causing clotting, tissue ischemia, and necrosis; (3) activation of the plasmin fibrinolytic mechanisms, leading to increased clotting time; and (4) activation of the bradykinin system, which has a role in progression to shock (Grimes, 1986). Characteristic symptoms of early shock may include increased cardiac output, peripheral vasodilation, hyperthermia, increased renal output, and respiratory alkalosis. Progression of the shock syndrome leads to increased peripheral resistance, worsening hypotension, acidosis, and cardiac and renal failure (Grimes, 1986).

**Medical-Surgical Management.** Prompt and aggressive treatment of gram-negative bacteremia is necessary to prevent progression to septic shock. Because bacteremia originating from a urologic focus is most often caused by *E. coli,* members of *Klebsiella, Enterobacter, Serratia,* and *Proteus* genera, as well as *Pseudomonas aeruginosa,* early administration of an antibiotic to which the offending organism is susceptible is of the utmost importance. Therefore, in suspected urosepsis, administration of an antibiotic with the broadest spectrum of activity against the gram-negative bacilli most frequently isolated within that particular hospital is recommended (Bahnson, 1986).

Currently, the use of an aminoglycoside or one of the third-generation cephalosporins (cefotaxime, cefoperazone) provides extended gram-negative coverage pending culture and sensitivity results. A new class of beta-lactam antibiotics (aztreonam) may replace aminoglycosides (amikacin, gentamicin) as the initial drugs of choice in urosepsis. These antibiotics have a wider range of coverage and, in addition, lack the toxicity of aminoglycosides. Once the culture and sensitivity results are obtained, the antibiotic regimen should be changed to the most effective and economical and least toxic agent. The length of antibiotic treatment should be guided by the clinical status of the patient. Generally, treatment should continue until the patient has been afebrile for 3 to 5 days (Bahnson, 1986).

Concurrent treatment of urosepsis includes elimination of the source of infection. In the urologic patient, this might necessitate surgical intervention for obstruction or abscess drainage, or the removal of an infected Foley or intravenous catheter or monitoring device (Bahnson, 1986). Other ancillary treatments are used in the management of septic shock. Administration of large volumes of crystalloid solutions, such as Ringer's lactate or normal saline, are needed to correct the decreased tissue perfusion and hypotension. Either a central venous pressure catheter or a flow-directed pulmonary artery catheter should be inserted (Bahnson, 1986). If fluid replacement fails to correct hypotension, a vasoactive drug should be employed. Patients with hypoxemia or adult respiratory distress syndrome generally require ventilatory assistance. Congestive heart failure is usually managed with digitalis, and other complications of septic shock are treated as the need dictates (Bahnson, 1986).

## APPROACHES TO PATIENT CARE

### Assessment

The patient may report subjective symptoms of fever, shaking, chills, and muscular pain. A history of recent genitourinary instrumentation may be given. The clinical presentation of urosepsis depends on whether the patient is in the early or late stage of shock. In the early stage, the body is attempting to compensate for the hypotension. On physical examination, the respiratory and pulse rates are increased, and the blood pressure may be normal or slightly lowered. The urine output is normal or slightly depressed. The patient's skin may be flushed and warm to the touch. The mental status assessment may reveal variations ranging from alert and restless to confused. The patient may complain of thirst. The symptoms of shock will progress to the later stages if not corrected. Physical examination at this point reveals shallow respirations, decreased blood pressure, and increased tachycardia. Oliguria or anuria may be seen, and the patient's skin is cool and clammy. Signs of edema may be apparent, and the patient's mental status may have deteriorated to lethargic or unconscious.

If urosepsis is suspected, multiple blood cultures for aerobic and anaerobic organisms should be obtained. One or more cultures positive for bacteria are diagnostic of bacteremia. The urine culture and sensitivity is usually positive for bacteria, and the urinalysis shows py- uria. All catheter lines should be cultured as potential sources of infection. The complete blood count shows leukocytosis, and there may be a decrease in platelets. The electrolyte panel demonstrates an elevated BUN and creatinine and hyponatremia and hypochloremia. Coagu- lation studies reveal prolonged partial throm- boplastin time, prothrombin time, thrombocy- topenia, and decreased levels of factors II, V, VII, and VIII (Coleman et al., 1979). Arterial blood gases initially show respiratory alkalosis but then revert to metabolic acidosis. Urine specific gravity is elevated, and creatinine clearance is decreased.

### Nursing Diagnosis

The nursing diagnosis for the patient with urosepsis may include the following:

1. Alteration in the pattern of urinary elimina- tion, oliguria related to diminished renal perfusion.
2. Alteration in body temperature, fever re- lated to acute bacterial infection.
3. Anxiety related to acute illness.
4. Potential for impaired gas exchange related to progression of shock syndrome.

### Plan of Care

Nursing care is directed toward enabling the patient to

1. Maintain a urinary output of at least 30 to 40 mL/h.
2. Maintain an open airway, with adequate pe- ripheral vascular perfusion.
3. Express decreased feelings of anxiety related to acute illness.

### Interventions

One of the nurse's primary goals in caring for the patient with urosepsis is to maintain an adequate urinary output. The nurse monitors the patient's fluid intake and output every 1 or 2 hours in the acute phase. An indwelling uri- nary catheter usually is inserted for purposes of accurate monitoring. Maintenance of patent drainage from the catheter, as well as sterility of the closed urinary system, is essential.

In the initial phase of sepsis, the patient may be febrile. Nursing interventions should in- clude frequent monitoring of the patient's tem- perature and methods of reducing the febrile condition. Prescribed antipyretics are adminis- tered, and patient response is assessed. Tepid water or alcohol baths can assist in lowering body temperature. The patient's room should be maintained between 63 and 68°F to decrease metabolic demands.

Maintaining an open airway for adequate gas exchange is also imperative. Respiratory status is assessed hourly by auscultation of the lungs and by noting the respiratory rate and depth. The nurse should be alert for signs of cyanosis particularly in the patient's nail beds or mucous membranes. Respiratory assistance may be required by means of nasal oxygen or tracheal intubation. Arterial blood gases are drawn as ordered, and abnormalities are re- ported. If the patient is alert, deep breathing and coughing exercises are performed every hour. A semi-Fowler's position may aid in lung expansion.

The patient, if alert, and the family require psychological support during this acute medi- cal crisis. A calm, supportive approach by the nurse assists in reducing the level of anxiety. Simple explanations of care being given and tests ordered can help the patient and family understand what is being done and why. This is crucial to enlisting patient and family coop- eration.

### Patient Outcomes

1. The patient's blood pressure, pulse, and res- piration are stable.
2. The patient is afebrile after antibiotic ther- apy, with the source of bacterial invasion identified.
3. The patient's urinary output is at least 30 mL/h.
4. The patient verbalizes feelings of anxiety concerning the change in or threat to his or her health status.

## REFERENCES

Bahnson, R. R. (1986). Urosepsis. *Urology Clinics of North America, 13,* 627–635.

Barbalias, G. A., Meares, E. M., & Sant, G. R. (1983). Pros- tatodynia: Clinical and urodynamic characteristics. *Jour- nal of Urology, 130,* 514–517.

Bennett, J. E., (1987). Actinomycosis and nocardiosis. In E. Braunwald, K. J. Isselbacher, R. G. Petersdorf, J. D. Wil- son, J. B. Martin, & A. S. Fauci (Eds.), *Harrison's principles of internal medicine* (11th ed., pp. 745–747). New York: McGraw-Hill.

Berger, R. E. (1986). Sexually transmitted disease. In P. C. Walsh, R. F. Gittes, A. D. Perlmutter, & T. A. Stamey (Eds.), *Campbell's urology* (5th ed., pp. 900–945). Philadel- phia: W. B. Saunders.

Berkow, R. (Ed.). (1982). *The Merck manual of diagnosis and therapy* (14th ed.) Rahway, NJ: Merck, Sharp and Dohme Research Laboratories.

Brundage, R. (1986). Renal system. In J. M. Thompson, G. K. McFarland, J. E. Hisch, S. M. Tucker, & A. C. Bowers (Eds.), *Clinical nursing* (pp. 1031–1104). St. Louis: C. V. Mosby.

Brunner, H., Weidner, W., & Schiefer, H. (1983). Studies on

the role of *Ureaplasma urealyticum* and *Mycoplasma hominis* in prostatitis. *Journal of Urology, 147*, 807–812.

Buckwold, F. J., Ludwig P., Godfrey, K. M., et al. (1982). Therapy for acute cystitis in adult women: Randomized comparison of single-dose sulfisoxazole vs. trimethoprim-sulfamethoxazole. *Journal of the American Medical Association, 247*, 1839.

Coleman, R. W., Robboy, S. J., & Minna, J. D. (1979). Disseminated intravascular coagulation: A reappraisal. *Annual Review of Medicine, 30*, 359–374.

Drach, D. W., Fair, W. R., Meares, E. M., & Stamey, T. A. (1978). Classification of benign disease associated with prostate pain: Prostatitis or prostatodynia? *Journal of Urology, 120*, 266.

Eden, C. S., Erickson, B., & Hanson, L. A. (1977). Adhesion of *Escherichia coli* to human uroepithelial cells in vitro. *Infection and Immunity, 18*, 767–771.

Elkins, I. B., & Cox, C. E. (1974). Perineal, vaginal and urethral bacteriology of young women. I. Incidence of gram-negative colonization. *Journal of Urology, 111*, 88–92.

Fowler, J. E., Jr., & Stamey, T. A. (1977). Studies of introital colonization in women with recurrent urinary infections. VII. The role of bacterial adherence. *Journal of Urology, 117*, 472–476.

Fowler, J. E., Jr., & Stamey, T. A. (1978). Studies of introital colonization in women with recurrent urinary infections. X. Adhesive properties of *Escherichia coli* and *Proteus mirabilis*: Lack of correlation within urinary pathogenicity. *Journal of Urology, 120*, 315–318.

Gow, J. G. (1986). Genitourinary tuberculosis. In P. C. Walsh, R. F. Gittes, A. D. Perlmutter, & T. A. Stamey (Eds.), *Campbell's urology* (5th ed., pp. 1037–1069). Philadelphia: W. B. Saunders.

Gray, M., & Broadwell, D. C. (1986). Genitourinary system. In J. M. Thompson, G. K. McFarland, J. E. Hirsch, S. M. Tucker, & A. C. Bowers (Eds.), *Clinical nursing* (pp. 1283–1364). St. Louis: C. V. Mosby.

Grimes, D. E. (1986). Infectious diseases. In J. M. Thompson, G. K. McFarland, J. E. Hirsch, S. M. Tucker, & A. C. Bowers (Eds.), *Clinical nursing* (pp. 1465–1625). St. Louis: C. V. Mosby.

Haaga, J. R., & Weinstein, A. J. (1980). CT-guided percutaneous aspiration and drainage of abscesses. *American Journal of Roentgenology, 135*, 1187.

Halverson, S. G., & Graham, S. K. (1986). Infectious and inflammatory disorders affecting reproductive function. In M. L. Patrick, S. L. Woods, R. F. Craven, J. S. Rokosky, & P. M. Bruno (Eds.), *Medical-surgical nursing: Pathophysiological concepts* (pp. 1499–1523). Philadelphia: J. B. Lippincott.

Ireton, R. C., & Berger, R. E. (1984). Prostatitis and epididymitis. *Urology Clinics of North America, 11*, 83–94.

Kreger, B. E., Craven, D. E., Carding, P. C., & McCabe, W. R. (1980). Gram-negative bacteremia. III. Reassessment of etiology, epidemiology, and ecology in 612 patients. *American Journal of Medicine, 68*, 332–343.

Krieger, J. N. (1986). Complications and treatment of urinary tract infections during pregnancy. *Urology Clinics of North America, 13*, 685–693.

Kunin, C. M. (1987). *Detection, prevention and management of urinary tract infections* (4th ed.). Philadelphia: Lea and Febiger.

Lapides, J. (1976). *Fundamentals of urology*. Philadelphia: W. B. Saunders.

Lichtenberg, F. V., & Lehman, J. S. (1986). Parasitic diseases of the genitourinary system. In P. C. Walsh, R. F. Gittes, A. D. Perlmutter, & T. A. Stamey (Eds.), *Campbell's urology* (5th ed., pp. 983–1024). Philadelphia: W. B. Saunders.

Long, B. C., & Glazer, G. (1985). The patient with reproductive problems. In B. C. Long & W. J. Phipps (Eds.), *Essentials of medical-surgical nursing* (pp. 1044–1084). St. Louis: C. V. Mosby.

Luckmann, J., & Sorensen, K. C. (1987). Assessing people experiencing urinary disorders. In *Medical-surgical nursing: A psychophysiologic approach* (3rd ed., pp. 1157–1219). Philadelphia: W. B. Saunders.

MacGeorge, L. L., & Bruno, P. M. (1986). Renal and urinary infections and inflammatory disorders. In M. L. Patrick, S. L. Woods, R. F. Craven, J. S. Rokosky, & P. M. Bruno (Eds.), *Medical-surgical nursing: Pathophysiological concepts* (pp. 788–797). Philadelphia: J. B. Lippincott.

McCabe, W. R., & Treadwell, T. L. (1983). Gram-negative bacteremia. *Monographs in Urology, 4*, 193–214.

Meares, E. M., Jr. (1986). Prostatitis and related disorders. In P. C. Walsh, R. F. Gittes, A. D. Perlmutter, & T. A. Stamey (Eds.), *Campbell's urology* (5th ed., pp. 868–887). Philadelphia: W. B. Saunders.

Meares, E. M., Jr., & Barbalias, G. A. (1983). Prostatitis: Bacterial, nonbacterial, and prostatodynia. *Seminars in Urology, 1*, 25–40.

Messing, E. M. (1986). Interstitial cystitis and related syndromes. In P. C. Walsh, R. F. Gittes, A. D. Perlmutter, & T. A. Stamey (Eds.), *Campbell's urology* (5th ed., pp. 1070–1093). Philadelphia: W. B. Saunders.

Murray, T. G., & Goldberg, M. (1982). Interstitial renal disease. In W. Flamenbaum & R. J. Hanburger (Eds.), *Nephrology: An approach to the patient with renal disease* (pp. 1127–1139). Philadelphia: J. B. Lippincott.

Naeye, R. L. (1979). Causes of the excessive rates of perinatal mortality and prematurity in pregnancies complicated by maternal urinary tract infections. *New England Journal of Medicine, 300*, 819–823.

*National health survey.* (1970–1971). (DHEW Publication No. 73-1508). Washington, DC: U.S. Government Printing Office.

Nickel, W. R., & Plumb, R. T. (1986). Cutaneous diseases of external genitalia. In P. C. Walsh, R. F. Gittes, A. D. Perlmutter, & T. A. Stamey (Eds.), *Campbell's urology* (5th ed., pp. 956–982). Phildelphia: W. B. Saunders.

Nilsson, I. K., Colleen, S., & Mardh, P. A. (1977). Relationship between psychological and laboratory findings in patients with symptoms of non-acute prostatitis. In D. Danielsson, L. Juhlin, & P. A. Mardh (Eds.), *Genital infections and their complications* (pp. 133–144). Stockholm: Almquist and Wiksell International.

Parsons, C. L. (1985). Urinary tract infections in the female patient. *Urology Clinics of North America, 12*, 355–360.

Parsons, C. L. (1986). Pathogenesis of urinary tract infections: Bacterial adherence, bladder defense mechanisms. *Urology Clinics of North America, 13*, 563–568.

Pfau, A. (1986). Prostatitis: A continuing enigma. *Urology Clinics of North America, 13*, 695–715.

Roberts, J. A. (1986). Pyelonephritis, cortical abscess and perinephric abscess. *Urology Clinics of North America, 13*, 637–645.

Rubin, R. H., Fang, L. S., Jones, S. R., et al. (1980). Single-dose amoxicillin therapy for urinary tract infection. *Journal of the American Medical Association, 244*, 561.

Schaeffer, A. J., & Del Greco, F. (1986). Other renal diseases of urologic significance. In P. C. Walsh, R. F. Gittes, A. D. Perlmutter, & T. A. Stamey (Eds.), *Campbell's urology* (5th ed., pp. 2342–2360). Philadelphia: W. B. Saunders.

Schmidt, R. A. (1985). The urethral syndrome. *Urology Clinics of North America, 12*, 349–354.

Schönebeck, J. (1986). Fungal infections of the urinary tract. In P. C. Walsh, R. F. Gittes, A. D. Perlmutter, & T. A. Stamey (Eds.), *Campbell's urology* (5th ed., pp. 983–1024). Philadelphia: W. B. Saunders.

Scott, R., Deane, R. F., & Callander, R. (1982). *Urology illustrated* (2nd ed.). New York: Churchill Livingstone.

Segura, J. W., Opitz, J. L., & Greene, L. F. (1979). Prostatosis, prostatitis or pelvic floor tension myalgia? *Journal of Urology, 122,* 168–169.

Shanberg, A. M., & Malloy, T. (1987). Treatment of interstitial cystitis with neodymium:YAG laser. *Urology, 29*(4 Suppl.), 31–33.

Shortliffe, L. D., & Stamey, T. A. (1986). In P. C. Walsh, R. F. Gittes, A. D. Perlmutter, & T. A. Stamey (Eds.), *Campbell's urology* (5th ed., pp. 797–830). Philadelphia: W. B. Saunders.

Stamey, T. A. (1980). *Pathogenesis and treatment of urinary tract infections.* Baltimore: Williams & Wilkins.

Stamey, T. A., & Sexton, C. C. (1975). The role of vaginal colonization with Enterobacteriaceae in recurrent urinary infections. *Journal of Urology, 113,* 214–216.

Stamm, W. E., Martin, S. M., & Bennett, J. V. (1977). Epidemiology of nosocomial infections due to gram-negative bacilli: Aspects relevant to development and use of vaccines. *Journal of Infectious Diseases, 136,* 151.

Sweet, R. L. (1977). Bacteriuria and pyelonephritis during pregnancy. *Seminars in Perinatology, 1,* 25–40.

Turner-Warwick, R. (1986). Urinary fistulae in the female. In P. C. Walsh, R. F. Gittes, A. D. Perlmutter, & T. A. Stamey (Eds.), *Campbell's urology* (5th ed., pp. 2718–2738). Philadelphia: W. B. Saunders.

Waltzer, W. C. (1981). The urinary tract in pregnancy. *Journal of Urology, 125,* 271–276.

Zimmern, P. E., Hadley, H. R., Staskin, D. R., & Raz, S. (1985). Genitourinary fistulae: Vaginal approach for repair of vesicovaginal fistulae. *Urology Clinics of North America, 12,* 361–367.

## CHAPTER 6

# Urinary Calculi

◼

*Debra S. Bruton, Carol Einhorn, Lynn M. Reardon,
Josette M. Snyder, Angela Williams*

## OVERVIEW

Within the past 10 years there have been many significant changes related to the care of patients with urinary calculi. New procedures, such as percutaneous ultrasonic pyelolithotomy and extracorporeal shock wave lithotripsy, have resulted in shorter hospital stays, reduced convalescent time, fewer postoperative complications, and less discomfort to the patient. Given these innovations in technology, the nursing care of patients with urinary calculi has expanded from the operating room and the hospital to ambulatory treatment centers and clinics. Regardless of the setting, however, the focus of nursing activity has remained to provide symptomatic relief during the acute phase of an attack, to assess and support patients before and after medical interventions, and to provide patient education to prevent the recurrence of stone formation.

This chapter reviews new procedures available to treat urinary calculi, and it provides a brief description of more traditional treatment options. Nursing care for medical treatments and preoperative and postoperative interventions are discussed. A discussion of the causes, pathophysiology, composition, and complications of urinary stone disease is also included.

## BEHAVIORAL OBJECTIVES

After studying this chapter, the reader should be able to

1. Classify the types and locations of stone formation.
2. Recognize the complications of urinary stone disease and discuss the implications for nursing care.
3. Develop a teaching plan for a patient identified as being at risk for developing calculi.
4. Compare and contrast the medical and surgical treatment of patients with urinary calculi.
5. Formulate a plan of care for patients undergoing surgical intervention for urinary calculi.

## KEY WORDS

**Endourology**—refers to urologic procedures performed with endoscopic instruments, such as nephroscopes, cystoscopes, and ureteroscopes.

**Extracorporeal shock wave lithotripsy**—a noninvasive procedure used for the destruction of calculi. The stone is crushed or exploded by shock waves produced outside the body by a high-voltage spark discharge.

**Litholapaxy**—crushing of a stone in the bladder.

**Lithotomy**—removal of urinary calculi.

**Lithotripsy**—the disintegration or crushing of urinary calculi.

**Matrix**—the organic material in a stone; a derivative of the mucoproteins of urine that may influence urinary calculus formation by permitting chemicals to bind into stone masses.

**Nidus**—the nucleus for the formation of calculi.

**Percutaneous lithotomy (or lithotripsy)**—removal or disintegration of urinary calculi from the renal pelvis or kidney via a tract created from the skin directly into the kidney; various technologies may be employed.

**Plume**—the column of exhaust gases produced during laser surgery.

**Staghorn calculus**—a calculus that grows to fill the renal pelvis and calices; most are ammoniomagnesium phosphate, or struvite, stones.

**Steinstrasse**—the build-up of fragmented stone particles in the ureter, often following extracorporeal shock wave lithotripsy.

**Urinary calculi**—stones occurring in the urinary tract, including the kidney, ureter, bladder, and urethra. They are classified according to their point of origin, location, and composition.

## PERSPECTIVE ON DISEASE ENTITY

### Etiology

#### INCIDENCE AND PREVALENCE

Urinary calculus formation, also known as *stone disease*, is a common medical problem. As many as 2% to 4% of the U.S. population are at risk for forming stones in some portion of the urinary system. Urinary calculus formation is a condition that requires hospitalization for 1 in 1000 people afflicted with the problem each year, yet many other people pass stones spontaneously with only minor symptoms that do not require intervention.

The incidence of urinary calculus formation may be related to geography, climate, season, age, sex, and heredity. In the United States, the incidence of stone disease is highest in the southeast coastal regions, otherwise known as the *stone belt.* However, stone disease is also prevalent in the northwest and arid southwest. Peak occurrence for symptoms of stones is often during the summer months of July, August, and September. Men between 30 and 50 years of age have a 3:1 higher incidence of urinary calculi. Epidemiologic studies suggest that the incidence of urinary calculus formation is highest among people of European and Asian descent yet is extremely low among North American Indians, blacks of African descent, and Israelis. Stone disease can also be found in children. Primary vesical stones are seen in children of the Middle East, India, Indonesia, and parts of China. In the United States, stones found in children are primarily caused by altered metabolic conditions secondary to infection or congenital anomalies and occur following urinary diversion (Schneider, 1986).

## PREDISPOSING FACTORS

The exact cause of calculus formation is not known; however, there are factors that seem to predispose a person to stone formation. Intrinsic factors influencing stone formation include (1) the age, sex, and race of the patient; (2) a family history of stone disease; (3) chronic dehydration, which leads to high urine concentration and a decrease in urinary pH; (4) urinary stasis due to obstruction or immobilization; and (5) metabolic disturbances that increase the concentration of stone-forming solutes in the urine. Extrinsic factors that appear to have some relation to stone formation include (1) geographic and environmental surroundings and climate; (2) water intake and mineral content (e.g., water hardness or softness); (3) diet, specifically an increased ingestion of purines (foods containing uric acid), calcium, and animal proteins; and (4) a sedentary occupation or lifestyle.

Urinary calculi may also be the result of infections. An infection may be the primary cause of a stone, or infection may be a secondary factor, by adding new growth to a preexisting stone. Stones caused by infections are seen primarily in the kidney or the bladder. They are formed by mucoproteins in the urine that collect around the nidus.

## Pathophysiology

### PROCESS OF STONE FORMATION

The process of stone formation is one of crystallization. Crystal growth occurs initially by nucleation, in which crystals gather in clusters to form larger particles. These crystals are thought to form by four different methods: (1) supersaturation, which is an overabundance of solute in the urine (this may be the result of insolubility or a decrease in fluid intake); (2) matrix formation, which is precipitated by mucoproteins binding to form the matrix or mass of a stone; (3) lack of inhibitors or precipitators (the presence or absence of certain protective agents affecting one or more of the processes of crystallization of stone-forming salts); or (4) any combination of these methods (Schneider, 1986). As crystallized particles develop, they may travel through the urinary tract and become lodged at a narrow point that becomes the nidus for the formation of a stone. A crystallized particle may also be deposited and trapped within a fibrous matrix to form the nucleus of a stone.

## TYPES OF URINARY CALCULI

Urinary calculi are classified according to their composition and may be formed of one or more substances. The most prevalent types of stones are calcium, cystine, uric acid, xanthine, and ammoniomagnesium phosphate. Stone analysis reveals that 90% of all calculi contain calcium.

People who are prone to developing stones containing calcium have an abundance of calcium solute in the urine. This condition is called *hypercalciuria* and may be the result of the following conditions:

1. Conditions that cause increased calcium reabsorption from bone and thereby increase calcium in the blood and in the urine, such as bone cancer, immobilization, Cushing's disease, steroids, and primary hyperparathyroidism.
2. A condition called *renal tubular acidosis,* an inability of the kidney to excrete acid, which results in a reabsorption of calcium from bone.
3. Increased absorption of calcium from the intestine as a result of gastric bypass, milk-alkali syndrome, excessive vitamin D ingestion, or a diet high in carbohydrates and proteins.
4. Abnormalities found in the structure of the kidney that may result in hypercalciuria, such as sponge kidney.

Approximately 35% of calcium stone formers have a condition called *idiopathic hypercalciuria.* These patients present with hypercalciuria, but blood studies do not indicate an increased serum calcium level, and no cause is found for the increased urine calcium level.

On analysis, oxalate is commonly found to be a component of many calcium stones. An excess of oxalate in the urine results from the endogenous production of the substance, a diet intake high in green leafy vegetables, and hyperabsorption of oxalates by the body. Primary hyperoxaluria, a rare genetic enzyme deficiency that is characterized by urinary excretion of oxalate, is seldom a cause for calcium-oxalate stone formation.

**Cystine Stones.** Cystine stones, seen most often in children, are caused by a condition known as *cystinuria*. Cystinuria is an inherited defect of the renal tubules that causes the malabsorption or loss of four amino acids (cystine, ornithine, arginine, and lysine). When cystine is excreted into an acidic urine, a favorable environment is created for the precipitation of crystals to form cystine stones.

**Xanthine Stones.** Xanthine stones are caused by xanthinuria, a rare hereditary condition characterized by an excessive excretion of the enzyme xanthine. An acidic urine also forms a favorable environment for xanthine crystals to form into stones. A xanthine calculus is often radiolucent and sometimes is mistaken for a uric acid stone, which always appears radiolucent on x-ray film.

**Uric Acid Stones.** Uric acid stones are caused by urine that is saturated with uric acid, a condition known as *hyperuricosuria*. In this condition, stone formation occurs when the uric acid combines with an acidic and concentrated urine. The administration of uricosuric agents, such as probenecid, and the increased dietary intake of purine may result in hyperuricosuria. Disorders such as primary or secondary gout, lymphoma, and leukemia may also cause hyperuricosuria. Uric acid stones are the only solid calculus considered to be truly radiolucent. They are seen on x-ray film as filling defects.

**Struvite Stones.** Ammoniomagnesium phosphate, or struvite, stones constitute 15% of all calculi. Patients with struvite stones present with alkaline urine and urinary tract infections caused by a urea-splitting organism, such as *Proteus*. Struvite stones are the major cause of staghorn calculus formation. A staghorn calculus is one that grows to occupy the renal pelvis and calices. The struvite stones are difficult to eliminate, because they form a hard shell around a nucleus of bacteria that protects them from antibiotic therapy. Surgical removal of the stone must be complete or the stone may recur.

## COMMON LOCATIONS OF URINARY CALCULI

Urinary calculi can also be classified according to their location in the urinary tract. The kidney is the most frequent site of stone formation; however, calculi may form anywhere in the urinary system. Calculi found positioned in the ureter are usually renal calculi that have migrated by means of peristalsis down through the kidney and into the ureter. A calculus that is 4 to 5 mm in diameter or smaller can easily be passed through the ureter. Stones that are larger than 5 mm are more likely to become trapped in the ureter. The three most common sites of stone obstruction are the ureteropelvic junction; the pelvic brim, where the ureter passes over the iliac vessels; and the ureterovesical junction (Fig. 6–1). Vesical calculi are not unusual in conditions that cause urinary stasis, such as prostatic hypertrophy, bladder diverticula, neurogenic bladder, and cystoceles. Prostate stones form in the tissues or acini of the gland (Drach, 1986).

## SIGNS AND SYMPTOMS OF URINARY CALCULI

The signs and symptoms for all types of stones are essentially the same. A sudden onset of sharp, severe pain is the classic symptom of urinary calculi. Renal calculi cause flank pain on the same side as the affected kidney; this pain may radiate to the groin or genitalia. Ureteral stones cause pain in the flank and abdomen, which may also radiate to the genitalia. Vesical calculi are usually asymptomatic, unless they begin to pass through the urethra, at which time dysuria and genital pain may be experienced.

Gastrointestinal symptoms, such as nausea, vomiting, and paralytic ileus, may be present. When accompanied by severe pain, these symptoms are associated with renal or ureteral colic. Colic is a condition in which the muscular components of the lining of the urinary tract begin to spasm in response to irritation from the calculus. Normal ureteral peristalsis causes movement of the calculus, resulting in tissue trauma and subsequent hematuria. Fever and an elevated white blood cell count may be present if the stone is infected or if there is an infection secondary to a urinary tract obstruction by the calculus. Infections associated with calculi also produce symptoms of urinary frequency, urgency, and dysuria. Patients with a single kidney thought to be obstructed by a

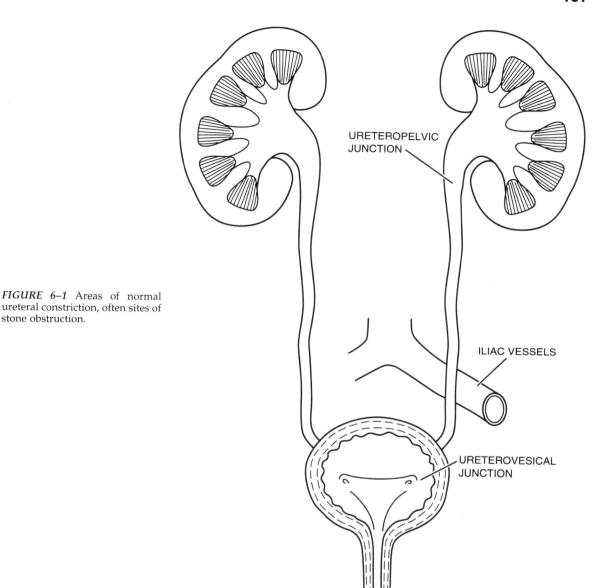

FIGURE 6–1 Areas of normal ureteral constriction, often sites of stone obstruction.

URETEROPELVIC JUNCTION

ILIAC VESSELS

URETEROVESICAL JUNCTION

calculus seem to be anuric because of the blocked flow of urine from the kidney to the bladder.

## COMPLICATIONS OF URINARY CALCULI

The complications of renal and ureteral calculi include (1) an increased risk of infection in the upper urinary tract because of the stasis of urine from obstruction; (2) hydronephrosis due to calculus obstruction of the renal pelvis or ureter; and (3) renal tissue damage from pressure or movement of a calculus (especially staghorn calculus) in either the kidney or the ureter.

Another complication of renal calculi is nephrocalcinosis. This condition occurs when calcium phosphate is precipitated and deposited into the renal tubules, parenchyma, and sometimes the glomeruli. Nephrocalcinosis results in impaired renal function, damage to the kidney due to renal and ureteral calcifications, and chronic kidney infection. Complications of vesical stones include recurrent or chronic bladder infection due to the undetected presence of a calculus in the bladder and to a partial or complete obstruction of the urethra and the bladder neck.

# Medical-Surgical Management

It is estimated that as many as 20% of patients with kidney stones eventually require surgery or other active medical intervention. Therefore, the surgical management of urinary calculi is presented first, to be followed by a discussion on the medical management.

## SURGICAL MANAGEMENT

### Open Procedures

There are several open surgical techniques used to remove urinary calculi. Currently, they are rarely performed unless the patient is not a candidate for newer techniques. These surgical procedures are explained briefly to present a full perspective, whereas the current techniques are explained in more detail. The discussion of open surgical procedures begins with the kidney and progresses down the genitourinary tract.

*Nephrolithotomy* is a surgical procedure that is currently used to remove large staghorn calculi lodged in the renal parenchyma. A surgical incision is made, either by a flank or an abdominal approach, into the kidney, and the stones are extracted in one or more pieces.

*Pyelolithotomy* is a procedure used to remove one or more stones from the renal pelvis. The patient is positioned on his or her side during surgery, and a flank incision is made. The renal pelvis is exposed and incised by one of many different methods, depending on where the stone or stones are located. The stone is then manipulated and removed. After surgery, a transient leakage of urine may occur from the ureter, which was closed in purse-string fashion. Catheters, drains, and stents all may be employed to ensure the patency of the urinary tract, facilitate the passage of any remaining stone fragments, and prevent infection in an effort to promote healing and reduce the chance of stricture formation in the surgically manipulated ureter.

*Nephrectomy* is a surgical procedure in which the entire kidney is removed. The treatment of urinary calculi by partial nephrectomy involves conserving as much renal tissue as possible when progressive infection or diminished renal function secondary to calculi is a health threat.

*Ureterolithotomy* is a surgical procedure used to remove stones lodged in the ureter. A flank approach is made if the stone is in the upper or middle third of the ureter; a supine approach is used for stones in the lower third of the ureter. As with pyelolithotomy, stricture is a common postoperative complication. Therefore, the ureter is closed using a purse-string technique, and careful drainage is required.

*Cystolithotomy* is a suprapubic approach used for the removal of bladder calculi that cannot be removed endoscopically. It is a procedure also employed for uric acid stones, which are usually too hard to be crushed by a lithotrite.

All these procedures usually follow a normal postoperative course of a 7- to 14-day length of stay and as long as 6 weeks' recuperation time. Open surgical procedures for the treatment of urinary calculi produce higher mortality and morbidity rates than do the newer techniques because of their invasiveness. When a flank incision is made for kidney and upper ureteral stones, pneumothorax is a possible complication. Improper positioning for flank incisions may also lead to brachial plexus damage. Another possible complication is ureteral stricture formation due to suture and scar formation. As with any open surgical procedure, pneumonia, infection, bowel obstruction, and hemorrhaging all are possible postoperative complications. Finally, patients with recurrent calculi requiring repeated surgical intervention may form adhesions. Consequently, the risk of serious complications, including kidney damage and renal failure, increases significantly if the patient must undergo a second or other subsequent open procedure.

To learn more about the procedures discussed in this section, the reader is referred to other texts pertaining to urologic surgery. Nursing care is discussed later in this chapter.

### Endourologic Procedures

The second type of surgical intervention began in the early 1980s. Endourologic procedures were refined in this era with the development of semirigid to flexible nephroscopes, cystoscopes, and ureteroscopes and the incorporation of lithotripsy, ultrasound, and laser techniques.

Percutaneous endourologic procedures are indicated in the following situations: for stones larger than 3 cm in diameter, abnormal anatomy of the upper urinary tract, and failure of extracorporeal shock wave lithotripsy (ESWL). Although the advent of ESWL has drastically altered the use of percutaneous extraction, some patients may require repeated procedures or a combination of procedures (Lingeman et al., 1989). (See Table 6–1 for a list of current indications.) The success of percutaneous procedures depends on the patient's understanding of the procedure and its risks, adequate instrumentation, and the skill and experience of the urologist.

*Percutaneous nephrolithotripsy* (PCNL) is a procedure during which upper urinary tract stones are removed through a percutaneous nephrostomy tract. The patient may have the nephrostomy tube placed before the procedure by interventional radiology under local anesthesia or by the urologist at the time of the procedure.

It is important to have the patient positioned properly and under direct fluoroscopic visualization (Fig. 6–2A–C). To place the nephrostomy catheter properly, a guide wire is first inserted; this is a safety mechanism should trauma occur, so that drainage can always be established. A single incision is made in the flank of the affected side with a large-bore needle followed by dilation and insertion of the nephrostomy tube or the nephroscope into the kidney.

There are several methods for removing calculi percutaneously. A stone basket may be used to remove small calculi. Larger stones may be broken up using ultrasonic lithotripsy, laser, or electrolysis techniques. Remaining fragments are removed by a stone basket, mechanical flushing with suction, postoperative chemolysis, or natural passage. After removal of all fragments, the nephroscope is replaced with a nephrostomy tube, which is left in place to assist with drainage.

The benefits of PCNL are reduced length of hospitalization (2–4 days), costs, and recuperation time. There are also complications, because it is an invasive procedure, including the risk of perforation of the kidney, the ureter, and the adjacent organs; urosepsis; obstruction due to stone fragments; and hemorrhage. One of the most common complications is bleeding, sufficient to require transfusion.

Other endoscopic approaches to stone removal are accomplished transurethrally and require the use of the flexible ureteroscope and cystoscope. The primary advantage of this type of procedure, known as *ureteroscopy*, is that it allows maneuvers under direct vision. Indications for the use of ureteroscopy are stones in the lower ureter larger than 4 mm in diameter, obstruction, pain that is intolerable, and fever and chills. Some physicians also remove stones in the middle to upper ureter by this method, depending on their experience.

Care must be taken to prevent proximal stone migration unless ESWL is planned or available. When stones are too large to manipulate through the dilated ureter, they may need to be reduced using lithotripsy (ultrasonic, electrohydraulic, or pulsed laser). With ureteroscopy, stones can also be removed with a basket and forceps.

When ureteroscopy is performed, the patient is given general anesthesia for the procedure and is placed in the lithotomy position. As with the percutaneous extraction, a guide wire is placed to ensure proper drainage. If the patient requires a basketing or lithotripsy procedure, a ureteral catheter is usually left in place for 48 hours. The postoperative complications of ureteroscopy are minimal. If the ureter is perforated, a stent should be left in place to divert drainage. Also, there may be some bleeding, but this is usually not significant.

Bladder stones can be removed through the cystoscope. If they are large, one of two procedures may be performed. *Cystolitholapaxy* is indicated when the stone is soft enough to crush and there is no urethral pathologic condition. An endoscope is inserted into the bladder, the stone is captured in the jaws of the instrument, and then the stone is crushed. *Cystolithotripsy*

**TABLE 6–1. Indications for Removal of Urinary Calculi by PCNL Versus ESWL**

| PCNL | ESWL |
|---|---|
| Cystine calculi, regardless of size | All calculi (except cystine) $\leq 2$ cm |
| Caliceal diverticula | Suspected calcium oxalate dihydrate (low-density) stone $\geq 2$ cm and $\leq 3$ cm |
| Dilated dependent calix | Struvite calculi with nondilated renal collecting system $\geq 2$ cm and $\leq 3$ cm |
| Suspected calcium oxalate monohydrate (radiodense) stones $\geq 2$ cm and $\leq 3$ cm | |
| Struvite calculi $\geq 2$ cm and $\leq 3$ cm | |
| Stones associated with chronic bacteriuria | |
| Dilated renal collecting system | |
| All calculi $\geq 3$ cm | |

Adapted from Lingeman, J., et al. (1989). *Urinary calculi: ESWL, endourology, and medical therapy* (p. 161). Philadelphia: Lea & Febiger. Reproduced with permission.

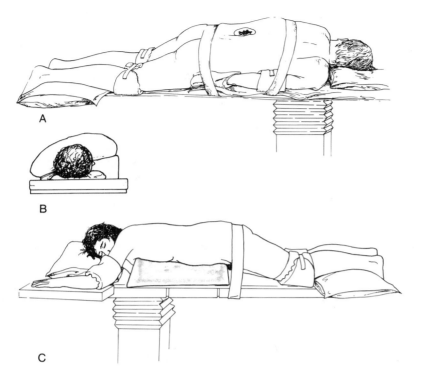

*FIGURE 6–2* Patient position for percutaneous procedures *(A)*. Note that the side to be treated is elevated approximately 30 degrees *(B)* and that all pressure points are carefully padded. The "down" arm should be placed at the patient's side *(A)*, whereas the "up" arm should be placed in an abducted position *(C)*. The patient should be placed far enough down on the table so that movement of the C-arm is not impeded by the center post of the table during imaging of the kidney *(A* and *C)*. *(A* to *C* from J. Lingeman, et al.: *Urinary Calculi: ESWL, Endourology and Medical Therapy.* Philadelphia, Lea & Febiger, 1989. Reproduced with permission.)

may also be performed for the same reason. In this procedure, a lithotriptor is inserted into the bladder, and the bladder is filled with a non-conducting fluid, such as sterile water. An electrode is inserted and comes into contact with the stone; then a high-voltage current disintegrates the stone instantaneously. The fragments are removed through the cystoscope. Usually, there are no complications unless the bladder wall is perforated.

See the section on approaches to patient for nursing care related to endourologic procedures.

## State-of-the-Art Techniques

### Extracorporeal Shock Wave Lithotripsy

Although endourologic procedures have simplified the treatment of urinary calculi, often these procedures are not performed when the newest technology, ESWL, is available. ESWL has revolutionized the treatment of urinary stones because it is noninvasive.

One of the main differences between ESWL and conventional surgery is that the ESWL patient is not 'cured' by the procedure. After he has been treated, he then has to 'cure' himself by passing the stone fragments from his body via the urinary stream (Czarapata, 1988, p. 14).

Most stones that cannot be passed spontaneously are treated with ESWL. There are some limitations with this treatment, so it is important that patients be selected appropriately. Approximately 7% to 10% of stones smaller than 2 cm in diameter need retreatment. Contraindications to ESWL include stones in the lower third of the ureter, cystine stones, and stones contained in diverticula. Patients with stones larger than 3 cm or staghorn calculi may require PCNL in addition to ESWL. Further, in some patients with large stones or in extenuating circumstances, pretreatment stent placement during cystoscopy may be required to minimize possible posttreatment complications and facilitate drainage.

There are several different types of lithotriptors currently available, and future generations of these machines are being continually developed and tested. Their principles are similar, but each works differently; no one machine is best for all patients. The Dornier $HM_3$, the most common machine, is a water bath (Figs. 6–3 and 6–4). Referred to as *shockwave therapy,* the procedure involves the use of high-energy shock waves that are produced extracorporeally, transmitted to the body through the

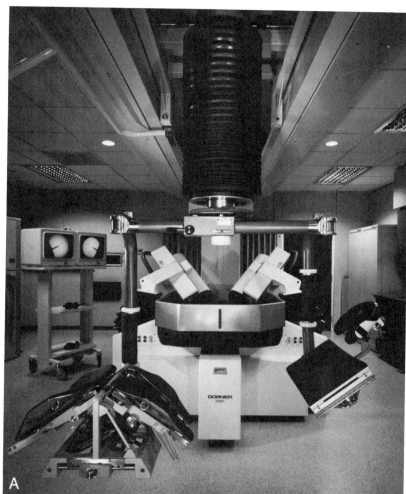

A

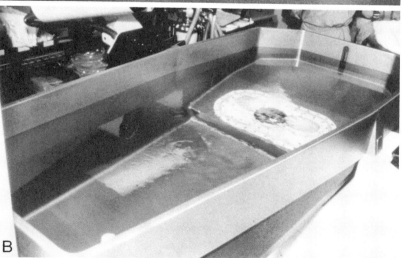

B

***FIGURE 6–3*** *A,* Dornier HM₃ lith-otriptor. (Courtesy of Dornier Medical, Inc., Marietta, GA.) *B,* ESWL water bath.

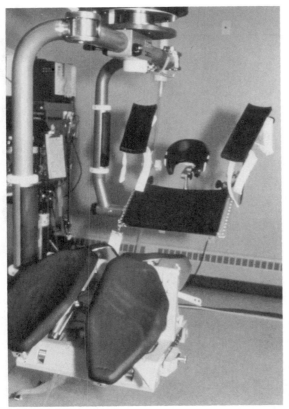

*FIGURE 6–4* Hydraulic lift used to ease patients into water. (Courtesy of Agnes Yost, CURN.)

water, and focused on the stone (Schneider, 1986). Shock waves are produced by a spark from an electrode in the bowl-shaped (or ellipsoid) bottom of the tub. Waves reflect from the ellipsoid and come out at the second focal point in the kidney. This is accomplished by using two fluoroscopy units to position the patient and place the stone within the proper parameters.

Because of the mechanisms of operation and the size of the water bath, there are some patients who are not candidates for ESWL (Table 6–2). If a person does not meet height and weight recommendations, a trial run can be done before anesthesia is administered to ensure an acceptable fit. However, with the new generation of lithotriptors, weight is no longer a consideration because the water bath is eliminated and a flat table with a water cushion is used (Fig. 6–5).

Until recently, persons with pacemakers had been restricted from ESWL procedures, because the lithotriptor is set to be simultaneous with the patient's R waves on an electrocardio-

### TABLE 6–2. Exclusion Criteria for ESWL

Weight exceeding 300 lb (HM$_3$ only)
Height exceeding 6 ft 6 in
Abdominal pacemaker in place
Pregnancy
Poor function of the kidney containing the stone
Very large stones that would cause an overabundance of
    fragmented stone that may lead to obstruction

See Table 6–4 for rejection criteria for patients with pacemakers.

gram and fired during diastole to avoid a possible dysrhythmia. Consequently, it was believed that ESWL might cause direct damage to the pacemaker and that the electrical conductivity from the shock discharge would interfere with the action of the pacemaker.

For patients with pacemakers to be considered for ESWL, they must meet certain criteria (Table 6–3). In addition, many safety measures must be ensured, including the following:

1. Preprocedure and postprocedure monitoring.
2. Ability to reprogram the pacer.
3. Ability to modify the pacer according to ESWL conditions.
4. Ability to trigger ESWL by the patient's QRS complex and not pacemaker stimulus.
5. Ability to evaluate the anatomic placement of the pacemaker in relation to the proposed axis for ESWL.
6. Ability to insert a central venous access catheter capable of holding a pacing lead (McNeave & Mulry, 1989; Weber et al., 1988).

Rejection criteria are also well established (Table 6–4). Needless to say, if patients with pacemakers are to be treated, extensive multi-

### TABLE 6–3. ESWL Requirements for Pacemaker Patients

Patient must have pacemaker for at least 6 months before
    ESWL
Pacemaker must be implanted in the chest area
Only single- or dual-chamber reprogrammable
    pacemakers permitted; manufacturer's representative
    should be notified to assist with reprogramming during
    the ESWL procedure, if necessary
Patient must have cardiology evaluation and clearance
    within 30 days before ESWL treatment; a cardiologist
    should be present during ESWL
A complete history and physical examination, including
    electrocardiogram, should be completed within 30 days
    before the procedure

Adapted from McNeave, C. J., & Mulry, K. (1989). Pacemaker patients as candidates for shock wave lithotripsy. *Urologic Nursing, 9*(5), 17–19. Reprinted by permission.

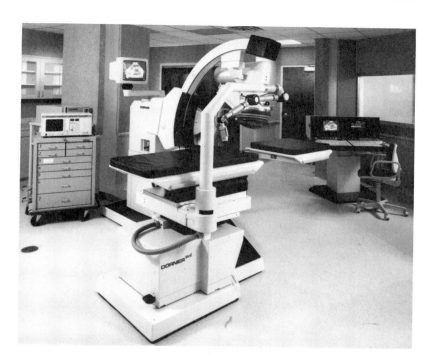

**FIGURE 6–5** Dornier 900 lithotriptor. (Courtesy of Dornier Medical, Inc., Marietta, GA.)

disciplinary planning must be done to ensure patient safety.

The patients who undergo ESWL in the Dornier $HM_3$ usually receive general anesthesia before being placed in the hydraulic lift chair. Anesthesia is necessary because the shocks to the kidney are considerably painful. Further, the patient must not move, once positioned, during treatment so that the stone remains properly aligned. With the use of general anesthesia, breathing is also diminished to prevent a shift in the position or alignment of the stone.

Alternatives to general anesthesia are also employed. If epidural anesthesia is used, the site must be sealed water tight. Cooperative and well-informed patients who have a low

**TABLE 6–4. ESWL Rejection Criteria for Patients with Pacemakers**

Abdominal implant
Motion-sensitive pacer
Temporary pacer
Piezoelectric pacer
Nonprogrammed dual-chamber pacer
History of uncontrolled congestive heart failure
Uncontrolled or newly diagnosed diabetes

See Table 6–2 for exclusion criteria for all candidates for ESWL.

Adapted from McNeave, C. J., & Mulry, K. (1989). Pacemaker patients as candidates for shockwave lithotripsy. *Urologic Nursing, 9*(5), 17–19. Reprinted by permission.

anxiety level may be candidates for intercostal blocks and subcutaneous infiltration of local anesthesia at the site of shock wave entry. Also, some patients with simple stones may do well with intravenous sedation or narcotics (Lingeman et al., 1989). The patient treated with newer machines may need only sedation and a narcotic.

Once sedated or anesthetized, the patient is placed in the hydraulic lift (for the Dornier $HM_3$) and then eased into the tub as far as the clavicles. The entry and exit sites of the shock wave must be below the water level to prevent tissue damage or bruising, although occasional petechiae are seen. In both types of lithotripsy—water and cushion—the patient's affected side is placed over the ellipsoid bowl and the calculus is visualized on two fluoroscopic monitors. The patient is repositioned until the stone is seen at the intersection of both monitors. Once placement is achieved, the shock waves may begin. Depending on the size and type of stone, as many as 500 to 1500 shock waves are delivered over a 30- to 60-minute period; occasionally, as many as 2500 shock waves are needed. The higher the number of shock waves, the greater the possibility of renal damage. The shocks are given in a series of 100, and fluoroscopy is used to view the progress of the dispersal of the calculus and to make sure that the stone is in the proper position.

Once the procedure is finished, the patient is

taken out of the tub or removed from the table and kept in the recovery room until the anesthesia has worn off. The patient is then discharged or taken back to the room and is allowed out of bed immediately, even if an epidural anesthetic has been administered. Ambulation as soon as possible after ESWL promotes the passage of gravel through the urinary system. During this time, the patient's urine is strained for evidence of stone fragments (Fig. 6–6). Pain medication may also be required during this period.

Reduced cost, length of stay, and recuperation time are some of the many benefits of ESWL. Although this mode of therapy is revolutionary, it still has complications, such as stone fragments causing colic or steinstrasse, urosepsis, and perinephric hematoma. Pancreatitis occurs rarely but is still a concern.

Nursing care following ESWL is addressed later in this chapter.

## Laser Treatment

The newest procedure in the treatment of urinary calculi is laser lithotripsy. The term *laser* is an acronym for light amplification by stimulated emission of radiation. There are

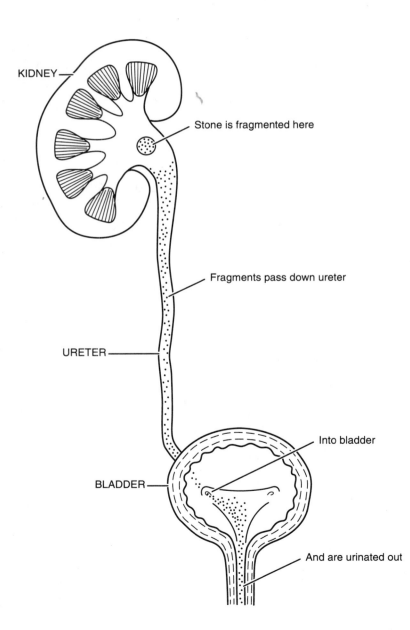

KIDNEY

Stone is fragmented here

Fragments pass down ureter

URETER

Into bladder

BLADDER

And are urinated out

*FIGURE 6–6* Path of stone fragments after disintegration with ESWL or laser.

many types of lasers used for various procedures. One of the main problems encountered with development of the laser was the need to devise a tool for fragmenting kidney stones that did not generate heat sufficient to damage surrounding renal tissue.

Through research, a pulsed dye laser was developed for lithotripsy. This laser works on the principle that as coumarin green dye is exposed to a flash lamp, pulses of green light are emitted. "The concentrated energy emitted from the tip of the laser is absorbed by the stone material, generating a shock wave and creating small stone fragments" (Lingeman et al., 1989, p. 47). There is a maximum absorption of light by the stone but with minimal absorption by hemoglobin and tissues. This mechanism of action is similar to ESWL and electrohydraulic lithotripsy.

The laser is used in conjunction with the flexible or semirigid 9.5 Fr ureteroscope to remove ureteral stones or loosen impacted stones. This procedure requires that water be run continuously through an irrigating channel, as it enhances the fragmentation process. Once the procedure is completed, the fragments are removed.

Patients with impacted stones may need additional therapy with ESWL to fragment the stone completely. For hard stones, a special basket has been designed to encase the stone and allow the laser channel to pass through the middle of the basket. The laser can then be used to make the stone smaller so it can be removed with the basket. On occasion, struvite stones do not respond to laser or ESWL therapy, thereby requiring that stone removal be achieved with other methods. However, the most recent laser technique available permits treatment of all types of stones and uses a 504-nm pulsed dye laser. This laser wavelength offers several advantages over previously used methods, including the use of a smaller ureteroscope; use of a 320-U fiber to deliver laser energy; reduced tissue damage; reduced need for continuous high-flow irrigation throughout the procedure; and the ability to repeatedly deliver laser energy to stone fragments (MacKety, 1990).

While the laser procedure is being performed, adherence to safety precautions is essential. Protective goggles with a yellow filter should be worn over the eyes to prevent retinal damage. Access to the operating room should be restricted during laser intervention. Measures to prevent fire, such as moistening sponges, drapes, and towels, should be employed. Endoscopic equipment should be protected according to the manufacturer's directions to avoid damage when the laser is fired. Finally, masks should be used during the laser procedure, with an adequate system of smoke evacuation available for all procedures that produce plume (Ball, 1990).

The possible complications from laser surgery are the same as those for endourologic procedures. Nursing care is addressed later in this chapter.

## Residual Stones as a Complication of Surgical Intervention

With technologic advances in the treatment of urinary calculi, the complication of residual stones exists. Residual stones can cause two major problems. First, remaining fragments can become acutely dislodged and cause obstruction, with resulting pain and infection. Second, residual stones are believed by some to act as a catalyst for recurrent stone formation.

In most cases, stone formation is secondary to either the supersaturation of stone-forming substances or lack of stone-inhibitor substances; therefore, if residual stones are present and the underlying physiologic or metabolic defects persist, growth of these stones and possibly formation of new calculi may be inevitable (Preminger, 1987, p. 323).

It is interesting to note that for a group of patients with existing stones who received medical therapy, the need for surgery was reduced from 58% to 2%. The incidence of recurrent stone formation is 5% to 21% after open procedures and 8% after endourologic procedures. Early reports with ESWL therapy have suggested a recurrence rate as high as 34% within 3 months after treatment (Preminger, 1987).

Possible causes of residual stones are the improper selection of surgical technique, anatomic abnormalities, stone composition, impatience of the physician, and technical constraints. Two important factors to consider when deciding on a treatment plan are the composition and the location of the stone. For stones that have the potential for obstructing the ureter, an aggressive treatment is indicated. The plan may include the use of chemical dissolution, surgical intervention, or a combination of modalities. If a residual stone does not present problems, then no action is indicated. Consequently, it is important to know what procedures or combination of procedures are appropriate for removing urinary calculi.

## MEDICAL MANAGEMENT

Medical treatment of urinary calculi is initiated only when the patient is suspected of being one who will develop recurrent calculi. The younger the patient, the more likely that stone disease will recur. Stones recur in about 60% of cases; recurrence may be attributed to a patient's disease process or previous surgical interventions. Chronic stone formers include patients with a chronic indwelling urinary catheter, gout, or an ileal conduit.

For patients whose stones are small, the treatment is to observe and wait. The patient should be instructed to alert the physician if he or she experiences any aggravated symptoms (e.g., nausea, vomiting, and hematuria) that indicate that the stone has become larger or is moving. Patients should also be taught to strain all urine to collect stones that may have passed.

Pain relief with oral or intramuscular analgesics may be required if a stone is trying to pass through the urinary system. Exercise may also promote passage of a stone.

All patients who develop calculi should have their stones analyzed for composition, regardless of whether the stone was passed spontaneously or removed through surgical intervention. Once the composition of the stone has been determined, appropriate treatment can be initiated. For patients who chronically form stones, a comprehensive metabolic evaluation should also be performed (Table 6–5). These data, coupled with the results of a stone analysis, will help the health care team develop a plan to prevent the formation of more calculi (Table 6–6).

Regardless of the type of stone, the patient's overall hydrational state is an important common factor. Patients should be encouraged to drink at least 3 L of water a day, unless medically contraindicated. This cleanses the system and prevents supersaturation, which is a causative factor, especially if a patient is prone to dehydration.

In addition to fluids, diet may influence stone formation. Dietary restrictions are specific to the types of stones formed. For instance, a person with calcium stones is encouraged to eat a low-calcium diet that restricts dairy products. An acid-ash diet may be recommended to acidify the urine and increase the solubility of calcium phosphate (Doyle & Reilly, 1985). Oxalate stone formers are encouraged to restrict high-oxalate foods, such as colas, chocolate, and peanuts. Patients who form uric acid

**TABLE 6–5. Metabolic Evaluation of Chronic Stone Formers***

Stone composition analysis
Urinalysis
Urine culture and Gram's stain
Urinary pH × 3 days
Urine spot test for cystine (nitroprusside)
Complete blood count
Serum electrolytes, including blood urea nitrogen, calcium, chloride, creatinine, inorganic phosphate, magnesium, phosphorus, potassium, sodium, and uric acid
Urine acidification test with ammonium chloride
Serum parathyroid hormone
Calcium infusion–calcitonin stimulation test
24-hour urine collection—measurements include urine volume, calcium, phosphorus, uric acid, citrate, and creatinine†

*Any or all of the tests may be done when completing a metabolic evaluation for stone disease.

†Usually, two collections on a random diet are obtained; additional collections may be performed after initiating dietary restrictions specific to the type of stone suspected.

stones are instructed how to select a purine-restricted diet. Foods to avoid in this diet include anchovies, seafood, spinach, poultry, and organ meats, such as liver. Cystine stone formers must eat a diet high in vegetables and exclude animal protein and high-methionine foods, such as fish.

Medications may be used in the treatment of calculi and are prescribed specific to each stone-forming substance. Calcium stone formers may be treated with thiazides to reduce the amount of calcium that is excreted in the urine. Allopurinol may be prescribed to decrease hyperuricosuria. Sodium bicarbonate is used to alkalinize urine in uric acid stone formers. Penicillamine decreases cystine excretion in urine.

In addition to oral medication, stone dissolution may also be performed. Performed as a single procedure or in conjunction with other surgical intervention to ensure removal of all stone fragments, stone dissolution involves inserting a nephrostomy tube on the affected side and administering an irrigation of fluid through the tube to dissolve the calculi. Irrigating solutions are specific for each stone type. Common solutions used are Renacidin and sodium bicarbonate. The results of this treatment take time; therefore, it is not a popular option. Moreover, the medications that may be used for stone dissolution are not approved by the Food and Drug Administration for this route of administration.

Stone dissolution may be used to decrease the size of a stone so it may advance to a posi-

TABLE 6–6. Quick Guide to Kidney Stones

| Type | Characteristics | Possible Causes | Treatment and Prevention |
|---|---|---|---|
| Calcium oxalate or calcium phosphate | White to gray, small, rough, and hard; often form needlelike projections or staghorns | High-calcium intake, hypercalciuria, and sometimes hyperparathyroidism | High fluid intake; decreased calcium and oxalate intake; administration of hydrochlorothiazide diuretics that decrease urinary calcium; removal of parathyroid gland, if necessary; vitamin C, sodium or potassium phosphate, sodium or potassium citrate |
| Struvite (magnesium, ammonium phosphate) | Yellow; crumble easily; staghorn formation common | Infection from urea-splitting organisms | High fluid intake, diet and drugs that decrease urinary pH; administration of antibiotics |
| Cystine | Light yellow to brown, smooth and waxy looking | Cystine amino acid crystals in the urine | High fluid intake; administration of penicillamine and pyridoxine; decreased intake of milk products |
| Uric acid | Yellow to reddish brown, small and hard | High uric acid levels | High fluid intake; administration of alkaline compounds such as allopurinol, sodium citrate, and a mixture of sodium and potassium bicarbonate; diet low in caffeine, theobromine, and other purines |

tion where it can be removed by stone manipulation. When irrigating solution is introduced into the kidney through a nephrostomy tube, intrarenal pressure must be monitored at least every hour. The pressure must be kept lower than 15 cm $H_2O$ to prevent renal damage. It is important to watch the manometer carefully in paraplegic or quadriplegic patients, because they may not sense a pressure increase and could develop autonomic dysreflexia. The irrigation is discontinued if pain, increased renal pressure, and fever above 100.6°F occur. Most institutions develop specific protocols for this type of irrigation.

In conclusion, medical and surgical treatments of stones are effective only if patients follow prescribed plans. Sixty percent of stones recur without proper treatment and can eventually compromise the patient's health status. To prevent other stones from forming, long-term treatment must focus on hydration, diet, medications, and activity.

# APPROACHES TO PATIENT CARE

## Conventional Surgery

### Assessment

The initial nursing assessment is the same for all patients with urinary calculi. First, the nurse should obtain the patient's history of stone disease. Does the patient have another medical problem, such as hyperparathyroidism, gout, or thiazide-treated hypertension, which would predispose him or her to stone disease? At this time, it is important to find out also (1) whether the patient has had a previous incidence of stone formation; (2) what method of treatment was used to remove other calculi; (3) whether the stones have been analyzed, and whether the patient is a chronic stone former; and (4) whether a metabolic evaluation has been done. It is also important to know whether the patient has implemented any measures to prevent stone formation. Because diet and hydration are thought to influence stone disease, a diet history and assessment of fluid intake are also helpful.

Second, a history of the patient's presenting symptoms should be obtained. The onset, quality, and duration of any pain as well as any alleviating factors should be documented. Because pain is the most common symptom that patients with urinary calculi experience, it is important to determine the exact location of that pain. Renal calculi cause flank pain on the same side as the affected kidney, and this pain may radiate to the groin or the genitalia. Ureteral stones cause pain in the flank and abdomen that may also radiate to the genitalia. Ureteral pain, as a result of calculi, is colicky and among the most severe types of pain known. The colic occurs when there is sudden obstruction from a calculus, which then produces hyperperistalsis and spasm of the ureter. In addition to pain, the patient may experience nausea and vomiting. Determine the frequency and duration of these symptoms and whether the patient is dehydrated as a result of them.

An assessment of any chronic illnesses or recent infections is necessary as well as documentation of any allergies, particularly to contrast material (or sensitivity to shellfish). Because patients with infected stones may require antibiotic therapy several days before any planned surgical intervention, be sure to check for any previous adverse reactions or allergies to antibiotics.

Careful monitoring and assessment of all urine for stones or stone fragments are essential. In addition, it is important to note the color, character, and amount of each voiding. Any hematuria should be documented. Hematuria often occurs as a result of tissue trauma incurred from a stone passing through the urinary system. If the patient has a solitary kidney, a calculus that obstructs the ureter may produce symptoms of anuria.

Finally, laboratory values should be obtained and monitored. Tests frequently performed include a urinalysis, urine culture, complete blood count, KP6, and prothrombin and partial thromboplastin times. Results of radiologic procedures, including the kidney, ureter, and bladder (KUB) study and intravenous pyelogram, are also important.

In patients for whom surgery is planned, an in-depth study of respiratory and cardiovascular function is required for pending anesthetic and surgical assault. As with all surgeries, elderly patients and those with chronic medical conditions and disease processes are at increased risk. Additional laboratory data, such as coagulation profile, SMA 20, electrocardiogram, and pulmonary function testing, are needed.

The postoperative assessment of patients who have undergone a surgical intervention for urinary calculi is the same as that of other surgical patients. The postoperative nursing assessment should include an assessment of pain, hydration, hemorrhage, patency of catheters and tubes, the condition of the wound site, mobility, patterns of bowel and bladder elimination, and respiratory status.

In addition, patients who have flank incisions must be monitored for possible pneumothorax. The flank incision is just below the diaphragm, and it is possible to penetrate the pleural cavity. The nurse must monitor for sudden respiratory distress and take immediate action. If the patient already has a chest tube, the output and functioning of the chest drainage system must be monitored for any changes.

**Nursing Diagnosis**

Nursing diagnoses for the patient undergoing conventional surgical intervention for the treatment of urinary calculi may include the following:

1. Alteration in comfort
   a. Pain related to renal or ureteral colic caused by passage of stone or stone fragments.
   b. Pain related to bladder spasms from an indwelling catheter.
   c. Pain resulting from incisional discomfort.
   d. As a result of nausea and vomiting induced by pain.
2. Potential for alteration in urinary elimination related to
   a. Indwelling drainage tubes.
   b. Hematuria.
   c. Obstruction due to stone fragments in the urine.
   d. Dehydration caused by nausea and vomiting.
3. Potential for infection related to
   a. Stasis of urine as a result of urinary tract obstruction caused by calculi.
   b. Disruption in the integrity of the skin caused by a surgical incision.
   c. Insertion of urinary drainage devices.
4. Potential for ineffective breathing related to flank incision.
5. Knowledge deficit related to
   a. Planned surgical intervention.
   b. Discharge planning after conventional surgery for urinary calculi.
   c. The need for medical evaluation to prevent further stone formation.

**Plan of Care**

Nursing care is directed toward enabling the patient to

1. Experience relief from pain and nausea.
2. Maintain adequate hydration and urine output.
3. Maintain the patency of urinary drainage tubes.
4. Remain free from infection.
5. Prevent atelectasis.
6. Verbalize an understanding of planned treatment.
7. Prepare for discharge and follow-up care.

**Interventions**

Analgesics are generously administered preoperatively and postoperatively to relieve the often excruciating pain caused by the presence of a calculus. During the preoperative period, the amount of pain medication required may exceed dosages routinely administered to post-operative patients because of the acute nature of the pain caused by renal or ureteral colic. The analgesia may be administered orally or intramuscularly; epidural catheters or patient-controlled analgesia pumps may also be used. Regardless of the route of administration, the effectiveness of the analgesic and the overall pain management program should be continually evaluated.

Nausea and vomiting often accompany the pain caused by renal calculi. The use of an anti-emetic along with the analgesic is suggested to relieve these symptoms. Adequate hydration is also important to restore any deficit caused by vomiting and to promote the passage of a stone or stone fragments. This result may have to be accomplished with intravenous fluids until the patient is able to tolerate fluids orally. A careful record of intake and output is required to monitor fluid status.

For most conventional types of surgery for removal of a calculus, a urethral catheter is left in place to measure urinary output. In addition, one or more drains may be inserted to promote the drainage of urine and other discharge away from the surgical incision. Such drainage is usually the result of the purse-string closure of the ureter; this type of suture will not be water-tight to prevent stricture formation within the ureter.

Postoperatively, there may be copious amounts of drainage to contend with, and it may be managed in one of two ways: (1) saturated dressings can be frequently changed, approximately every 2 hours, or (2) a urostomy bag may be applied over the drains and connected to a leg bag or nighttime drainage bag. Although a bag is a neat, clean way of containing drainage, it may be difficult to apply and maintain because of the location of the incision. Regardless of the approach taken to contain the drainage, the prime objective is to prevent skin irritation while monitoring the amount of drainage produced.

Measuring output accurately from the drain site and noting the color and odor of the drainage are helpful. Changes should be reported and may require intervention by the physician. Sometimes the drainage persists, because fluid takes the easiest path; a stent may then be necessary for site closure. The drain is usually left in place for 2 or 3 days, then advanced slowly as output decreases, and usually removed by the fifth or sixth day.

As with all surgical procedures, infection is a possible complication. The flank incision site should be observed for redness, swelling, or drainage. Vital signs should be regularly monitored for an increase in body temperature. Changes in the location, intensity, or type of pain may also be indicative of an infectious process. Because infection may also result from the insertion of various urinary drainage devices, urine should be monitored for a cloudy appearance or foul odor—signs of bacterial growth in the urinary tract. Care must also be taken to ensure that drainage systems remain closed and intact; the patency of the system should also be monitored to allow for free drainage of urine. If the patient has a nephrostomy tube, careful dressing change and catheter care at the insertion site minimize the introduction of bacteria.

All surgical patients are at risk for potential pulmonary complications. The patient with a flank incision has a higher incidence of respiratory problems because of the location of the incision. The incision site is in close proximity to the diaphragm, and the chest muscles may have been hyperextended during the surgical procedure. These patients must be reminded to perform deep breathing and coughing exercises at least every 1 or 2 hours for the first 24 to 48 hours and then at least four times a day to ensure good lung expansion and perfusion. If the exercises are not done consistently, the patient is at risk for pneumonia or atelectasis. Patients at risk for developing respiratory complications after surgery for calculi include those who are smokers as well as those whose respiratory system is compromised with chronic obstructive pulmonary disease, asthma, or chronic bronchitis. If these or other conditions exist, the patient may need respiratory therapy to assist in promoting adequate pulmonary toileting.

Preoperative teaching and discharge planning instructions are essential for all surgical patients. As a basis for health care teaching, it is important that the patient understand why conventional surgery was chosen as the treatment alternative for his or her stones. Once this understanding is ensured, the nurse can then proceed to supply the patient with the information necessary to achieve an event-free postoperative recuperation. After discharge, the patient should be cautioned to gradually increase activity and avoid any heavy lifting until healing of the surgical site is complete. Signs of infection, difficulty in voiding, hematuria, or unusual pain should be reported to the physician. Medications should be taken as prescribed, and diet modifications incorporated into daily eating habits. Finally, be sure that the patient understands the importance of follow-up visits to the physician.

**Patient Outcomes**
1. The patient verbalizes an understanding of the treatment alternative selected and the hospital and home courses after surgery.
2. The patient expresses relief from pain.
3. The patient's fluid intake is sufficient to maintain adequate hydration and a urinary output of at least 1000 mL per 24 h.
4. The patient exhibits no signs of infection at the surgical site or as the result of urinary drainage tubes.
5. The patient exhibits no postoperative respiratory difficulties.

# Endourologic Procedures

**Assessment**
The assessment of the patient who is to have an endourologic procedure to remove urinary calculi is the same as that for the patient undergoing conventional surgery. Postprocedure assessment, however, should be specific to the type of endourologic intervention performed. Patients who present with lower tract stones may require intervention with ureteroscopy or cystoscopy. For patients with upper tract stones, the percutaneous route for extraction is preferred.

Hemorrhage, sepsis, and recurrent obstruction from stone fragments are the most frequent problems that occur after an endourologic procedure. Therefore, careful nursing assessment in the first 24 to 48 hours following this type of intervention is essential.

Vital signs should be checked frequently (at least every hour for as long as 4–5 hours following the procedure). Changes such as tachypnea, tachycardia, and hypotension may be suggestive of shock and should be reported immediately. While assessing the vital signs, observe the patient for signs of anxiety or a pale complexion. Note the temperature of the patient's skin, assess skin turgor, observe the percutaneous site for bleeding, and note any increase in pain in the flank area.

Urinary drainage tubes should be observed for a change in urine color that might suggest increased bleeding; the presence or absence of clots should also be noted. Additionally, the patency of the drainage tubes should be ensured. A measurement of urinary output also helps determine whether oliguria, postobstruc-

tive diuresis, or recurrent obstruction has developed.

All patients who undergo percutaneous instrumentation are at risk for extravasation of urine due to the perforation of the kidney's collecting systems. Peritoneal irritation, decreased urinary output, or a change in vital signs may indicate such a problem.

**Nursing Diagnosis**
Nursing diagnoses for the patient undergoing an endourologic procedure for treatment of urinary calculi may include the following:

1. Potential for fluid volume deficit related to
   a. Excessive postprocedure bleeding.
   b. Postobstructive diuresis.
2. Potential for infection related to
   a. Interruption of skin integrity with the establishment of percutaneous access.
   b. Extravasation of urine into peritoneal tissue.
3. Alteration in pattern of urinary elimination related to
   a. Placement of urinary drainage devices.
   b. Recurrent obstruction from stone gravel.
4. Pain related to
   a. Establishment of a percutaneous flank wound.
   b. Extravasation of urine.

**Plan of Care**
Nursing care is directed toward enabling the patient to

1. Avoid dehydration and hypovolemia.
2. Prevent infection.
3. Return to a normal pattern of urinary elimination.
4. Experience relief from pain and discomfort.

**Intervention**
Even though endoscopic removal of calculi is considered to be a minor procedure, a great deal of manipulation is required during the surgery to remove the stone. The stone is often fragmented, making its removal difficult and causing tissue edema and spasm.

The use of urinary catheters and other drainage devices is an integral component of endourologic procedures. For percutaneous extraction, a nephrostomy tube is inserted before the procedure is begun. For other types of endoscopic extraction, stents or catheters are placed after the procedure.

Proper care is necessary for all types of urinary drainage devices. If the patient has a nephrostomy tube, the dressing around the tube should be changed daily. The site is usually cleansed with iodophor or hydrogen peroxide and then redressed by placing a split dressing or two folded 4 × 4s around the tube insertion site. (Refer to Chapter 4 for procedure on changing a nephrostomy tube dressing.) Another 4 × 4 covers the site and is taped in place. In many instances, there is urine leakage from the insertion site because of the dilation of the nephrostomy tract during surgery. Therefore, more frequent dressing changes may be required. If leakage is excessive, a bag may be placed on the site to protect the skin and maintain an accurate record of output.

Following endourologic procedures, it is important to record the amount of urinary output from each device. A sudden increase in urine volume may indicate that the patient is experiencing postobstructive diuresis. If this condition is suspected, closely monitor the vital signs, check the specific gravity and level of albumin in the urine, and analyze the serum electrolyte values. Careful fluid management is essential during this crisis period. Usually, fluid is replaced milliliter for milliliter according to the previous hour's output. (A more detailed discussion of nursing intervention for patients experiencing postobstructive diuresis may be found in Chapters 3 and 4.)

It is possible that the nephrostomy tube may become obstructed with stone fragments. To relieve the obstruction, irrigation of the tube may be needed. In most facilities, the physician is required to perform irrigation procedures. However, irrigation of urinary drainage devices may be performed by the nurse who has expertise in this area. Irrigation must be done using sterile technique. Because the renal pelvis is small and can hold only approximately 5 to 10 mL of fluid, the irrigant must be injected gently and slowly. The irrigation should be discontinued and the physician notified if resistance is met or if the patient complains of pain. The nephrostomy tube is usually left in place for 2 days or longer, depending on the extent of manipulation during the percutaneous extraction. Before the tube's removal, a nephrostogram may be performed to ascertain freedom of stone fragments.

If a ureteral stent has been inserted, it is usually secured in place by attaching it to the urethral catheter. Remember that stents (and nephrostomy tubes) are not retention catheters and must be properly secured. If a stent or other drainage device accidentally falls out, the physician should be notified immediately.

Some patients who have had PCNL require additional therapy, such as chemolysis, to eradicate any remaining stone fragments. The chemolysis is usually accomplished with continuous irrigation to the renal pelvis. A solution of distilled water with an additive formulated for chemical decomposition, such as Renacidin, is used. Magnesium may be added to the solution to reduce any irritating effects on the renal pelvis.

The equipment necessary for chemolysis includes a patent nephrostomy tube with an adapter connected to a drainage system, a central venous pressure manometer, volumetric pump, and irrigating solution. The manometer is set up between the nephrostomy tube and the pump to act as an overflow chamber on the renal pelvis to prevent undue pressure. The pressure should not exceed 15 cm $H_2O$. This is particularly necessary when irrigation is used on paraplegics and quadriplegics, who have no sensation at that level.

The kidney is first irrigated with normal saline to verify the patency of the nephrostomy tube and to determine the patient's ability to tolerate the procedure. Irrigation is begun at 50 mL/h and gradually increased over 4 to 6 hours to 150 mL/h. If the patient has no pain, fever, or increased pressure, the irrigating solution with medication is started. During the irrigation, urine output should be monitored, and the patient observed for changes in body temperature or pain. Encourage the patient to report any other symptoms that may seem unusual. This irrigant is run continuously until all stone fragments are gone. However, if any problems occur, the irrigation should be discontinued immediately. When calculating intake and output measurements be sure to count the irrigating solution as intake, so that the output is reflected accordingly.

Infection is a likely complication of endourologic procedures because of the sometimes excessive manipulation of the urinary tract with various instruments. Therefore, the use of antibiotics before and after the insertion of a nephrostomy tube or the endoscopic procedure is extremely important. Careful observation of the patient for the signs and symptoms of urinary tract infection or septic shock is also imperative.

Patients who have had endoscopic or percutaneous removal of calculi can usually resume their normal activities in 1 or 2 weeks following the procedure. If a nephrostomy tube has been left in place for prolonged drainage of the renal pelvis, self-care needs and care of the tube should be addressed before discharge. Because of the awkward location of the nephrostomy tube, a family member or other caregiver should be enlisted to assist the patient. Other discharge instructions would be similar to those given for patients after conventional surgery.

### Patient Outcomes

1. The patient exhibits no signs of bleeding from the surgical site—the urine is clear, the vital signs are stable, the complexion is pink, and there is no excessive discharge from the surgical site.
2. The patient remains free from urinary tract infection, and the nephrostomy tube and incision sites are free from redness, swelling, and odor.
3. The patient has resumed a normal pattern of urinary elimination, and the nephrostomy tube remains secured with an unobstructed flow of urine.
4. The patient expresses relief from pain.
5. The patient's urinary output is relative to the fluid intake.

# Extracorporeal Shock Wave Lithotripsy

### Assessment

ESWL is different from other surgical treatment modalities in that the calculi are disintegrated but not removed. Patients are usually admitted on the day of the procedure and discharged the same or the next day. Therefore, nursing assessment must be concise and coordinated to deliver all the information needed within a brief period.

The nursing assessment of the patient before ESWL is the same as that for other types of surgical interventions for calculus removal. Additional information that should be obtained includes the patient's height, weight, and cardiac status; the presence or absence of a pacemaker should also be ascertained. If the patient has a history of uncontrolled congestive heart failure or recently diagnosed diabetes, the physician should be alerted, because these conditions may prohibit the patient from undergoing ESWL.

As part of the nursing assessment, determine the patient's understanding of ESWL, including any preparation needed before the procedure. The patient's understanding of care activities after the procedure should also be determined to ensure a safe, uneventful recovery from the treatment.

After the procedure, the patient should be assessed to determine how soon ambulation can be initiated. The patient's ability to tolerate an increased fluid intake should also be assessed. Because fragmented calculi are left to pass through the urinary system, the patient's urine should be checked for signs of hematuria or gravel. Any pain associated with activity or urination should also be noted.

### Nursing Diagnosis

Nursing diagnoses for the patient undergoing ESWL may include the following:

1. Knowledge deficit related to unfamiliarity with the ESWL procedure and course of recovery.
2. Alteration in pattern of urinary elimination related to
   a. Increased fluid intake required to promote passage of disintegrated urinary calculus.
   b. Hematuria due to traumatic passage of calculus fragments.
   c. Upper urinary tract obstruction caused by the development of steinstrasse in the ureter.
3. Pain related to tissue trauma from the ESWL procedure and the passage of stone fragments.

### Plan of Care

Nursing care is directed toward enabling the patient to

1. Verbalize an understanding of the ESWL procedure.
2. Prevent the development of steinstrasse.
3. Resume a normal pattern of urinary elimination without pain or hematuria.
4. Express relief from postprocedure discomfort.

### Intervention

A brief hospital stay with an uneventful recovery period is typical after ESWL. Therefore, nursing interventions are directed toward preventing potential complications and providing educational information in the first 24 to 48 hours after completion of the procedure.

Steinstrasse, the build-up of stone particles in the ureter, is a frequent complication of ESWL. Obstruction may be secondary to the development of steinstrasse. For this reason, an increased fluid intake after ESWL is critical to promoting passage of the stone fragments. When the increased intake is combined with ambulation or postural positioning, patients may find that a greater volume of stone particles is more easily passed (Czarapata, 1988) (Fig. 6–7). If a steinstrasse does occur, stenting or laser lithotripsy may be required to relieve the obstruction (Freeman, 1991).

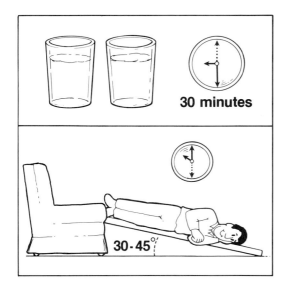 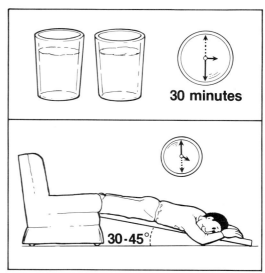

*FIGURE 6–7* Post-ESWL positioning. After the ESWL treatment, the kidney stones are reduced to small particles ranging in size from dust to small gravel. Most of these fragments are passed out of the kidney owing to the normal flushing action of the formation of urine. However, sometimes dust and small fragments settle in the more dependent calices of the kidney. At Georgetown University Hospital, a method was developed which involved drinking fluid and assuming positions to drain those parts of the kidney where fragments seem to become stuck. It has been quite successful in increasing fragment passage in many patients. To perform the positioning procedure the patient should (1) drink two 8-ounce glasses of water; (2) wait 30 minutes (otherwise the patient may experience nausea); (3a) lie on an inclined plane (30–45 degrees), head down, face down for 30 minutes; (3b) lie on an inclined plane (30–45 degrees), head down, affected kidney up; (4) drink another 8-ounce glass of water after getting up. These steps should be followed twice a day, alternating 3a and 3b; and the patient should sleep, whenever possible, with the affected kidney up. (From Czarapata, B. J. R. [1988]. Post-ESWL positioning. *Urologic Nursing, 9*(2), 14–15. Reprinted by permission.)

It is common to have some degree of hematuria after undergoing ESWL. Urinary output should then be monitored closely for changes in color or evidence of blood clots. A careful record of intake and output measurements should also be maintained to detect early signs of a possible obstruction. As is customary with all stone-forming patients, urine should be strained to verify the passage of stone fragments; a sample of the fragmented calculus should also be sent to the laboratory for analysis.

If the patient experiences pain or discomfort, it will most likely be due to tissue trauma in the flank region caused by the repeated shocks delivered to that area for stone disintegration. The flank should be checked for increased bruising; cold compresses may be applied to the area and pain medication administered as needed.

Before discharge from the hospital or lithotripsy center, the patient should be instructed in the signs or symptoms of urinary tract infection and obstruction. The patient should also be taught the procedures for measuring intake and output and for straining urine. Activity may be increased as tolerated, although pa-

tients are typically able to resume their normal routine within days of having the ESWL procedure.

**Patient Outcomes**

1. The patient expresses an understanding of the ESWL procedure and the reasons this treatment alternative was selected.
2. The patient increases his or her fluid intake by approximately 750 to 1000 mL/d.
3. The patient performs postural positioning or some other activity twice a day to promote passage of stone fragments.
4. The patient keeps a record of fluid intake and urinary output measurements.
5. The patient strains all urine to collect fragmented stone.
6. The patient resumes a normal pattern of voiding without evidence of infection, hematuria, or discomfort.

## Laser Therapy

During laser surgery, a flexible ureteroscope or nephroscope is used to gain access to the upper urinary tract. The stone is then fragmented, and the pieces are left to pass spontaneously. Depending on the approach selected, the nursing care of the patient undergoing laser therapy for treatment of urinary calculi is about the same as that for patients having PCNL or ESWL. Hemorrhage, infection, and obstruction resulting from retained fragments all are potential complications. Additionally, perforation of the ureter is a risk because of the manipulation required with instrumentation.

## Nonsurgical Management

Many patients do not require surgery for removal of urinary calculi. Generally, medical management is chosen if

1. There is no obstruction caused by the stone.
2. The stone is smaller than 5 mm in diameter.
3. The stone is moving.
4. The pain is manageable.

Nursing care during this period would be the same as that described for preoperative patients (see section on conventional surgery). The administration of analgesics to control pain as well as antiemetics to control nausea and vomiting is essential as the patient tries to pass the stone spontaneously. As with any urologic condition, a careful record of intake and output measurements should be maintained, and adequate hydration ensured.

## REFERENCES

Ball, K. A. (1990). The basics of laser technology. *Nursing Clinics of North America, 25*(3), 619.

Czarapata, B. J. R. (1988). Post ESWL positioning. *Urologic Nursing, 9*(2), 14–15.

Doyle, J., & Reilly, N. (1985). Genitourinary problems. *RN nursing assessment series 6.* Oradell, NJ: Medical Economics Books.

Drach, G. W. (1986). Urinary lithiasis. In P. C. Walsh, R. F. Gittes, A. D. Perlmutter, & T. A. Stamey (Eds.), *Campbell's urology* (5th ed., pp. 1094–1187). Philadelphia: W. B. Saunders.

Freeman, N. L. (1991). Ureteroscopic laser lithotripsy and extracorporeal shock wave lithotripsy: The advantage of both in a lithotripsy center. *Urologic Nursing, 11*(2), 28–29.

Lingeman, J. E., Smith, L. H., Woods, J. R., & Newman, D. M. (1989). *Urinary calculi: ESWL, endourology and medical therapy.* Philadelphia: Lea & Febiger.

MacKety, C. J. (1990). Lasers in urology. *Nursing Clinics of North America, 25*(3), 697.

McNeave, C. J., & Mulry, K. (1989). Pacemaker patients as candidates for shockwave lithotripsy. *Urologic Nursing, 9*(5), 17–19.

Preminger, G. M. (1987). Management of residual stones. In S. N. Rous (Ed.), *Stone disease: Diagnosis and management* (pp. 323–333). Orlando: Grune & Stratton.

Schneider, H. J. (Ed.). (1985). *Urolithiasis: Etiology, diagnosis.* New York: Springer-Verlag.

Schneider, H. J. (Ed.). (1986). *Urolithiasis: Therapy and prevention.* New York: Springer-Verlag.

Weber, W., et al. (1988). Anesthetic considerations in patients with cardiac pacemaker undergoing extracorporeal shock wave lithotripsy. *Anesthesia and Analgesia, 67*(Suppl. 1), 251.

# CHAPTER 7

# Sexually Transmitted Diseases

■

*Donna F. Brassit*

## OVERVIEW

Society has become startlingly aware of sexually transmitted diseases (STDs) in recent years. The former conception of venereal diseases has now evolved into a classification of STDs. An STD is defined in this chapter as ``any disease in which sexual activity is a significant mode of transmission'' (Krieger, 1984, p. 18). For many of the diseases, there are numerous or more favorable modes of transmission, but they are classified as STDs because they are capable of being transmitted sexually.

The world's attention seems to be focused on acquired immunodeficiency syndrome (AIDS). As health professionals, nurses must not disregard all the other forms of STDs, because their occurrence is increasing. It is difficult to obtain accurate statistical data on the incidence because the Centers for Disease Control and Prevention (CDC) does not require physicians to report all STDs. Aside from that, it is still believed that these diseases are largely under-reported. Greater sexual liberty and changes in behavior such as travel, sexual exploration at an earlier age, the high divorce rate, extramarital affairs, homosexuality, urbanization, the availability of newer birth control methods, and the use of crack cocaine all have contributed to the transmission of STDs.

This chapter explores the transmissibility, evolution, pathophysiology, and treatment for a variety of STDs, based on the CDC's ''Sexually Transmitted Diseases: Treatment Guidelines'' (1989) and *Sexually Transmitted Disease Surveillance, 1990* (1991). The importance of the nurse's role in educating others to prevent the spread of these diseases is emphasized throughout.

## BEHAVIORAL OBJECTIVES

After studying this chapter, the reader should be able to

1. Name at least three factors contributing to the increasing incidence of sexually transmitted diseases.

2. Identify the most common infecting organism in nongonococcal urethritis.

3. Predict the chief complaint of a patient with a protozoan syndrome (trichomoniasis, amebiasis, giardiasis, or cryptosporidiosis).

4. Discuss two serologic antibody tests for human immunodeficiency virus testing.

5. Differentiate between herpes virus hominis types I and II.

6. Create a nursing care plan for a patient who has been diagnosed with *Chlamydia trachomatis* infection.

## KEY WORDS

**Autoinoculation**—secondary infection transmitted from a focus of infection already present in the body.

**Beta-lactamase resistant**—the term used to describe microorganisms that produce the enzyme beta-lactamase and thus have the ability to resist the action of certain types of antibiotics, including penicillin. The enzyme, also called penicillinase, inactivates some forms of penicillin.

**Cryotherapy**—exposing tissues to freezing.

**Culdocentesis**—obtaining material from the retrovaginal cul-de-sac by aspiration or surgical incision through the vaginal wall.

**Curettage**—scraping a cavity.

**Dyspareunia**—painful coitus.

**Electrosurgery**—the division of tissues by high-frequency current applied locally with a hand-held instrument.

**FTA-ABS**—fluorescent treponemal antibody absorption; specific serum test for syphilis.

**Incubation period**—the development, without sign or symptom, of an infection from the time it gains entry until the appearance of the first sign or symptom.

**Inoculation site**—the site of introduction into the body of the causative organism of a disease.

**Kaposi's sarcoma**—an opportunistic neoplasm associated with AIDS; sarcoma that appears as palpable, purplish lesions anywhere on the body that may eventually involve the gastrointestinal tract, the lymph nodes, and the lungs.

**Macules**—small, discolored lesions on the skin, either elevated above or depressed below the skin's surface.

**New York City culture medium**—a selective medium containing vancomycin, colistin, amphotericin B, and trimethoprim used to cultivate *Neisseria gonorrhoeae*. This medium is transparent and allows easy colony identification.

**Papules**—reddened, elevated skin lesions that are solid and well circumscribed.

**Parasite**—an organism that lives within or on a host.

**Self-limiting**—denotes a disease that tends to resolve as a result of its own processes.

**Serology**—the study of serum.

**Serotype**—the subdivision of a species distinguishable from other strains.

**Sterility**—the inability to produce offspring.

**Systemic**—pertaining to the whole body.

**Thayer-Martin culture medium**—a modified chocolate agar containing vancomycin, colistimethate sodium, and nystatin; widely used for cultivation of *Neisseria gonorrhoeae*.

**Tzanck test**—examination of tissue from the lower surface of a vesicular lesion to determine the cell type.

**VDRL**—Venereal Disease Research Laboratory; nonspecific serum test for syphilis.

**Vesicle**—a small, blisterlike elevation containing any type of fluid.

**Viral shedding**—the time in which the virus can be recovered from the lesions.

# PERSPECTIVE ON DISEASE ENTITY

## Bacterial, Chlamydial, and Mycoplasmoid Syndromes

### GONORRHEA

**Etiology.** Gonorrhea is the most commonly reported sexually transmitted disease (STD) in the United States, although the recent trend of incidence has been decreasing from a peak of approximately 1 million cases in the late 1970s to a current level of approximately 700,000. Gonorrhea is a bacterial infection caused by *Neisseria gonorrhoeae*, a gram-negative coccus found in pairs. The organism is most commonly identified by the use of Gram's stain and Thayer-Martin or New York City medium.

Recently, there has been evidence of beta-lactamase–producing *N. gonorrhoeae*, which is resistant to penicillin, and also tetracycline-resistant *N. gonorrhoeae*. If it is suspected that a patient may have penicillinase-producing *N. gonorrhoeae* or tetracycline-resistant *N. gonorrhoeae*, the initial culture should include observation for beta-lactamase production and antibiotic sensitivities.

**Pathophysiology.** Gonorrhea can manifest as an asymptomatic, symptomatic, or complicated infection. Asymptomatic gonorrhea is rare. Symptomatic gonococcal urethritis includes primarily complaints of dysuria and urethral discharge. In males, complications may include epididymitis and proctitis. In females, the primary site is usually the endocervix, and ascending complications involve the fallopian tubes and pelvic peritoneum, causing pelvic inflammatory disease or salpingitis. Many females also develop an abscess of Bartholin's gland.

Anorectal gonorrhea may be evident in homosexual men owing to rectal intercourse or in women secondary to contamination by vaginal secretions. Gonococcal infection of the pharynx is transmitted by fellatio and can cause pharyngitis or tonsillitis. Gonococcal conjunctivitis is rare in adults and usually is caused by autoinoculation or a laboratory accident. Neonatal conjunctivitis is most often caused by *N. gonorrhoeae* and appears within the first week postpartum.

Disseminated gonococcal infection may include arthritis, meningitis, or septicemia. The incubation period for *N. gonorrhoeae* is usually 3 to 5 days.

**Medical-Surgical Management.** Physicians are encouraged to use the 1989 STD treatment guidelines established by the Centers for Disease Control and Prevention (CDC). The recommended regimen for uncomplicated urethral, endocervical, or rectal infection is ceftriaxone 250 mg intramuscularly (IM) once, plus doxycycline 100 mg orally two times a day for 7 days. For patients who cannot take ceftriaxone, the preferred alternative is spectinomycin 2 g IM once, followed by doxycycline.

Sex partners within the past 30 days should be examined, cultured, and treated presumptively.

The CDC recommends re-examination with culture 1 or 2 months after treatment; this strategy detects treatment failures and reinfections. Recurrent infection is usually due to reinfection and indicates a need for improved patient education.

Pharyngeal gonococcal infection should be treated with ceftriaxone 250 mg IM once or ciprofloxacin 500 mg orally once. Because experience with this regimen is limited, patients should be recultured 4 to 7 days after treatment.

Gonococcal ophthalmia should be treated with ceftriaxone 1 g IM once. These patients require ophthalmic assessments and eye irrigations with saline to eliminate discharge.

Disseminated infection that causes arthritis

requires patient hospitalization for treatment with ceftriaxone 1 g IM or intravenously (IV) every 24 hours or ceftizoxime 1 g IV every 8 hours, or cefotaxime 1 g IV every 8 hours. Reliable patients with uncomplicated disease may be discharged 24 to 48 hours after all symptoms resolve and may complete the therapy (for a total of 1 week of antibiotic therapy) with cefuroxime axetil 500 mg twice a day. Meningitis and endocarditis require ceftriaxone 1 to 2 g IV every 12 hours. Most patients with meningitis require therapy for 10 to 14 days, whereas patients with endocarditis require therapy for at least 4 weeks.

## NONGONOCOCCAL URETHRITIS

**Etiology.** *Nongonococcal urethritis* (NGU) is the term applied to evidence of urethritis without the presence of the organism *N. gonorrhoeae*. NGU that occurs soon after treatment of urethral gonorrhea is referred to as postgonococcal urethritis (PGU). There are many organisms that may cause nongonococcal urethritis, but the two most common are *Chlamydia trachomatis* and *Ureaplasma urealyticum*. A small percentage of NGU is caused by *Trichomonas vaginalis* and herpes simplex. NGU is typically diagnosed in males, whereas the equivalent in females, when urethritis is evident without cystitis, is referred to as *urethral syndrome*. NGU is diagnosed by detecting polymorphonuclear leukocytes in the urethral discharge and then performing a Gram's stain to differentiate gonococcal urethritis from NGU.

**Pathophysiology.** The symptoms of urethritis include a mucoid urethral discharge and complaints of burning on urination or an itch at the tip of the urethra. The typical incubation period is 1 to 5 weeks after exposure. Urethritis may be present with balanitis or epididymitis and may involve Reiter's syndrome or urethral strictures.

**Medical-Surgical Management.** The CDC recommends that physicians prescribe doxycycline 100 mg orally twice daily for 7 days or tetracycline 500 mg orally four times daily for 7 days for the patient and any sex partners. If the patient is tetracycline resistant, erythromycin 500 mg four times daily for 7 days may be substituted. Sexual intercourse should not take place during treatment. Posttreatment follow-up is required if any symptoms persist or recur.

## CHLAMYDIAL INFECTION

**Etiology.** *C. trachomatis* is the most prevalent sexually transmitted bacterial pathogen in the United States today. *Chlamydia* is a microorganism that is classified as a bacterium but has qualities of both bacteria and viruses. Like viruses, it grows within the host's cells, and like bacteria, it contains both deoxyribonucleic acid (DNA) and ribonucleic acid (RNA) and divides by binary fission. There are two species of *Chlamydia*. *Chlamydia psittaci* causes infections in birds and can be transmitted to humans, causing pneumonia. *C. trachomatis* infects humans and has subtypes: Types A, B, Ba, and C cause trachoma; types D through K cause STDs, eye infections, and infant pneumonia; and types L1, L2, and L3 are responsible for lymphogranuloma venereum, which is discussed later in the chapter.

The tests available for identifying the organism include culture identification, an enzyme immunoassay, and a direct fluorescent antibody procedure. Although testing for this organism has improved, results are not always accurate. Thus, results of chlamydial tests should be interpreted with caution.

**Pathophysiology.** Chlamydial and gonorrheal infections have similar signs and symptoms and often coexist. Chlamydial infections may be either asymptomatic or symptomatic. The asymptomatic infections that have not been treated have led to the increasing prevalence of chlamydial infection. In men, *C. trachomatis* is the leading cause of NGU (as mentioned previously). It is also a major cause of epididymitis, which could lead to sterility. In women, chlamydial infection may cause vaginal discharge, dysuria, urinary frequency, and soreness, and it may spread, causing endocervicitis and pelvic inflammatory disease. Infants born through an infected vagina may develop conjunctivitis or pneumonia. The incubation period is 7 to 10 days or longer.

**Medical-Surgical Management.** Because *N. gonorrhoeae* frequently coexists with *Chlamydia*, physicians often treat a patient for both organisms, if the test results are positive for *N. gonorrhoeae*. For treatment of *C. trachomatis*, the CDC recommends doxycycline 100 mg orally twice daily for 7 days or tetracycline 500 mg orally four times daily for 7 days. For patients who cannot tolerate tetracycline, erythromycin 500 mg orally four times daily may be substituted. All sexual partners need to be examined for an STD and promptly treated with one of these regimens.

## PELVIC INFLAMMATORY DISEASE

**Etiology.** Pelvic inflammatory disease (PID) denotes an infection of the fallopian tubes and possibly other pelvic structures, such as the ovaries and the peritoneum. The infection originates in the lower genital tract after acquired *N. gonorrhoeae* or *C. trachomatis* infection. During or just after menstruation, the organism ascends the genital tract. Cervicitis leads to endometriosis or salpingitis. Women who have multiple sex partners, use an intrauterine device (IUD), or have an asymptomatic gonococcal or chlamydial infection are the most likely to develop PID.

**Pathophysiology.** Women who have PID most often complain of abdominal pain. They may also present with fever, vaginal discharge, or both. Excessive menstrual bleeding may be caused by endometriosis, and dysuria may be caused by urethritis. Nausea and vomiting usually indicate an inflammation of the bowel. The symptoms differ between gonococcal and nongonococcal PID. In the nongonococcal form, the pain is less severe and is not associated with the menses, whereas in the gonococcal form the pain is most acute and occurs with the menstrual period. PID may lead to pelvic infections, causing perihepatitis or tubo-ovarian abscesses. PID may also lead to tubal scarring or occlusion, thus causing ectopic pregnancies or infertility.

**Medical-Surgical Management.** The signs and symptoms of PID resemble those of appendicitis, endometriosis, ovarian cysts, and ectopic pregnancy. The physician makes the diagnosis of PID based on the signs and symptoms, physical examination, laboratory values, and culdocentesis. The physician obtains cervical cultures for *N. gonorrhoeae* and *C. trachomatis*. Culdocentesis and laparoscopy may also be indicated to examine and obtain specimens to assist in the diagnosis. A pelvic examination usually reveals bilateral lower abdominal pains and adnexal tenderness. The patient may have an elevated white blood cell (WBC) count or sedimentation rate.

The physician is responsible for prescribing antibiotics, monitoring for complications, performing follow-up cultures, and ensuring that the sex partners receive treatment. The patient should be hospitalized if (1) she has peritonitis or is pregnant, (2) surgery for an adnexal mass or ovarian abscess may be required, (3) the diagnosis is uncertain, or (4) she fails to respond to outpatient treatment.

If the patient is treated on an outpatient basis, she must return for follow-up within 48 hours. It is also suggested that any IUD present be removed after antibiotic therapy.

For hospitalized patients, the CDC recommend doxycycline 100 mg IV twice daily plus cefoxitin 2 g IV four times daily for at least 4 days, followed by 100 mg of doxycycline by mouth twice daily to complete 10 to 14 days total, or clindamycin 900 mg IV three times daily plus gentamicin 2 mg/kg IV three times daily for at least 2 days and then doxycycline 100 mg by mouth two times a day for 10 to 14 days total. The outpatient regimen is cefoxitin 2 g IM plus probenecid 1 g orally, or ceftriaxone 250 mg IM followed by doxycycline 100 mg orally twice daily for 10 to 14 days, or tetracycline 500 mg by mouth four times a day for 10 to 14 days. All male sex partners should be treated for uncomplicated gonococcal and chlamydial infections.

## SYPHILIS

**Etiology.** The number of cases of primary and secondary syphilis had been increasing annually in the United States since 1986, but the latest statistics since 1990 indicate that this epidemic has subsided. Syphilis is most frequently transmitted by sexual contact, although it can also be transmitted by kissing someone with lesions on the lips or by contact with a contaminated needle. It is also possible for a fetus to contract the disease through the placenta.

The disease is caused by the spirochete *Treponema pallidum*, a spiral-shaped bacterium that needs the warmth of body temperature to survive.

There are well-defined stages of the progression of the disease. They include primary, secondary, latent, and late or tertiary syphilis.

**Pathophysiology.** The primary stage of syphilis (Fig. 7–1) is characterized by the presence of a chancre at the inoculation site. The

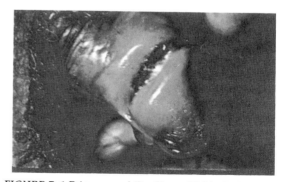

*FIGURE 7–1* Primary syphilis. (From Walsh, P. C., Gittes, R. F., Perlmutter, A. D., & Stamey, T. A. [Eds.]. [1986]. *Campbell's urology* [5th ed., p. 947]. Philadelphia: W. B. Saunders. Reprinted with permission.)

key characteristic to differentiate the chancre from other skin lesions is its painlessness. After exposure, the incubation period is 10 to 90 days. The chancre will appear about 3 weeks after inoculation and disappear in 1 to 6 weeks. Women may present with a chancre evident on the labia, urethra, breasts, axillae, or lips. Men may present with a chancre on any part of the genital area or the lips. Homosexual men may exhibit anal or oral chancres. Nearby lymph node enlargement may occur soon after the chancre appears. If the infection was obtained via a contaminated needle, a chancre will not occur.

Secondary syphilis is a systemic disease in which the spirochetes invade the blood (Fig. 7–2). It begins 6 weeks to 6 months after the onset of primary syphilis. A rash develops that is initially macular and then papular and pustularlike. The rash may be generalized or may present only on the palms or soles. It is accompanied by patient complaints of malaise, sore throat, and a low-grade fever. There is also generalized lymph node enlargement, as in primary syphilis. Secondary syphilis may lead to inflammatory endarteritis, meningeal inflammation, or hepatitis. The rash heals spontaneously in 5 to 12 weeks, although it may recur.

Latent syphilis requires negative results from a spinal tap examination to rule out neurosyphilis. The patient has no symptoms of syphilis at the time. If the latency period is less than 1 year, the disease is infectious. The longer the latent stage, the less possibility of transmission. After 4 years, it is rarely communicable.

Tertiary syphilis is rare today. Lesions progress slowly and involve any organ but are most frequently seen involving the cardiovascular or neurologic system.

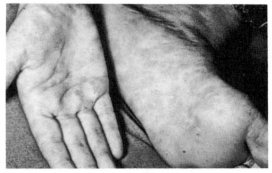

FIGURE 7–2 Secondary syphilis on the palms and soles. (From Walsh, P. C., Gittes, R. F., Perlmutter, A. D., & Stamey, T. A. [Eds.]. [1986]. *Campbell's urology* [5th ed., p. 947]. Philadelphia: W. B. Saunders. Reprinted with permission.)

There are studies taking place hypothesizing that concurrent infection with human immunodeficiency virus (HIV) and syphilis increases the frequency of early neurosyphilis.

**Medical-Surgical Management.** The physician performs a complete physical examination of the patient and then bases the diagnosis on the results of dark-field microscopy and serologic tests that include the venereal disease research laboratory (VDRL), the rapid plasma reagin (RPR), the fluorescent treponemal antibody–absorption (FTA-ABS), and the microhemagglutination–*Treponema pallidum* assay (MHA-TP).

For primary, secondary, and latent syphilis of less than 1 year's duration, the CDC recommend benzathine penicillin G 2.4 million U IM once. If the patient is allergic to penicillin, he or she should receive doxycycline 100 mg twice daily or tetracycline 500 mg four times daily for 2 weeks. For syphilis of more than 1 year's duration, the patient should receive benzathine penicillin G 2.4 million U IM once a week for 3 weeks. Penicillin-allergic patients should be treated with doxycycline 100 mg twice daily or tetracycline 500 mg four times daily for 4 weeks.

For patients with neurosyphilis, the CDC strongly suggest a cerebrospinal fluid examination and recommend aqueous crystalline penicillin G 12 to 24 million U IV daily for 10 to 14 days, or procaine penicillin 2.4 million U IM daily plus probenecid 500 mg orally four times daily, both for 10 to 14 days, followed by benzathine penicillin G 2.4 million U IM weekly for three doses.

Infants with congenital syphilis require aqueous crystalline penicillin G 50,000 U/kg IV every 8 to 12 hours, or procaine penicillin 50,000 U/kg IM daily for 10 to 14 days.

Any form of therapy for syphilis may be followed by an acute febrile reaction, referred to as the *Jarisch-Herxheimer reaction*, and may be accompanied by headache and myalgia. Patients should be informed of this and encouraged to take antipyretics.

## CHANCROID

**Etiology.** Chancroid is caused by a nonmotile gram-negative rod called *Haemophilus ducreyi*. It is commonly seen in tropical countries and causes ulcerative lesions (Fig. 7–3). The term *chancroid* refers to soft chancre. Its importance is enhanced by the knowledge that outside the United States, it has been associated with increased infection rates for HIV. In the

United States, statistics suggest a fivefold increase from early 1980 to the present.

**Pathophysiology.** Most males present with complaints of a penile ulcer or inguinal tenderness. Females usually complain of painful urination, painful defecation, or dyspareunia. The incubation period is between 3 and 10 days. The chancre first appears at the site of inoculation as a tender papule and then becomes an ulcer surrounded by an erythematous reaction. The ulcer may be painful. Some women are unaware of the lesions. Some lesions spread to the thigh via autoinoculation. In women, chancroid may form rectovaginal fistulas.

**Medical-Surgical Management.** The physician performs a complete physical examination of the patient and may obtain cultures and biopsy specimens of the chancre to identify the organism. The physician rules out herpes simplex viral infection, primary syphilis, and lymphogranuloma venereum, because their ulcers resemble chancroid.

According to the CDC, patients and their sex partners should receive erythromycin 500 mg orally four times a day for 7 days or ceftriaxone 250 mg IM once. Alternative regimens include trimethoprim (Bactrim) one double-strength tablet (160/800 mg) by mouth twice daily for 7 days or amoxicillin 500 mg orally plus clavulanic acid 125 mg three times daily for 7 days, or ciprofloxacin 500 mg twice a day for 3 days. One of the alternative regimens is recommended if the initial treatment was not effective. If treatment is successful, ulcers will improve within 7 days after the initiation of therapy. The resolution of lymphadenopathy is slower and may require needle aspiration.

## LYMPHOGRANULOMA VENEREUM

**Etiology.** Lymphogranuloma venereum is one of the STDs caused by serotypes L1, L2, and L3 of *C. trachomatis*. The disease is systemic and chronic and has three stages: primary, secondary, and tertiary. It is most prevalent in Asia (particularly India), Africa, and South America.

**Pathophysiology.** The primary lesion is a small genital papule or herpetiform ulcer that is short-lived and may be accompanied by localized edema. This lesion appears after an incubation period of 3 to 12 days. The most common site in men is the penis or the scrotum; in women, it forms in the urethra or vagina. The lesion will disappear within a few days. Rarely do women realize that there are any lesions at this stage.

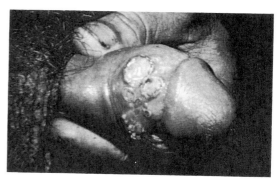

*FIGURE 7–3* Chancroid. (From Walsh, P. C., Gittes, R. F., Perlmutter, A. D., & Stamey, T. A. [Eds.]. [1986]. *Campbell's urology* [5th ed., p. 947]. Philadelphia: W. B. Saunders. Reprinted with permission.)

The secondary stage is manifested by painful, swollen inguinal lymph nodes, and this is usually the first time the patient will seek help. The incubation period may be 10 days to 4 months after acquiring the infection. Because the infection is systemic, the patient may complain of malaise and fever. Complications may include meningitis, hepatitis, pericarditis, pneumonitis, and arthritis.

The tertiary stage involves proctocolitis, perirectal abscesses, rectovaginal fistulas, and rectal strictures. Most patients with the tertiary stage are women or homosexual men. In women, it is caused by anal intercourse or migration of vaginal secretions. In men, it is caused by anal intercourse or lymphatic spread from the urethra.

Lymphogranuloma venereum may be diagnosed using the Frei skin test, the complement-fixation test for *Chlamydia*, the microimmunofluorescence test, or isolation of *C. trachomatis* from a lymph node.

**Medical-Surgical Management.** The physician performs a complete physical examination of the patient to look for any evidence of late-stage disease and may aspirate lymph nodes but not excise them. Surgical intervention may be required for strictures or fistulas. The CDC recommend doxycycline 100 mg orally two times a day for 3 weeks. Alternative regimens include tetracycline 500 mg orally four times a day for 3 weeks, or erythromycin 500 mg orally four times daily for 3 weeks, or sulfisoxazole 500 mg orally four times daily for 3 weeks.

## GRANULOMA INGUINALE

**Etiology.** Granuloma inguinale, also known as *donovanosis*, is caused by *Calymmatobacterium* *granulomatis*, a gram-negative bacillus. The exact mechanisms of infection are controversial, but sexual contact is a mode of transmission.

**Pathophysiology.** The incubation period varies from 1 week to 2 months. The disease begins as a painless, granulomatous lesion that grows to form red granulation tissue. It may involve the genital, inguinal, or anal regions. In males, most lesions form on the penis, whereas in the female, they are evident on the labia. In homosexual males, the lesions are found perianally. If the disease goes untreated, it could progress to destroy the penis or cause an elephantiasis enlargement of the labia.

Granuloma inguinale has often been misdiagnosed as penile carcinoma or secondary syphilis. Biopsy specimens revealing Donovan's bodies, which are blue-staining organisms, aid in the diagnosis.

**Medical-Surgical Management.** A variety of antibiotics are effective against this organism. Most physicians prescribe tetracycline 500 mg orally four times daily. Chloramphenicol 500 mg orally four times daily is also a common regimen. For pregnant women, erythromycin 500 mg orally four times daily is prescribed. Each of these medications is prescribed for 2 to 4 weeks. The lesions will shrink within the first week of therapy and should complete healing within 3 to 5 weeks.

## SHIGELLOSIS

**Etiology.** Shigellosis is a common cause of bacterial dysentery in homosexual men. It is transmitted from person to person via a fecal-oral route. It is caused by the *Shigella* species of enteric bacteria, a non–spore-forming, anaerobic gram-negative rod that is highly infectious.

**Pathophysiology.** After an incubation period of 1 to 7 days, *Shigella* produces a disease of the colon manifested by abdominal cramps, diarrhea, fever, and nausea. The diarrhea may be bloody or mucoid. The disease is confirmed by identification of *Shigella* in a stool specimen.

**Medical-Surgical Management.** The physician prescribes sulfamethoxazole 160 mg orally twice daily for 5 days or ampicillin 500 mg orally four times daily for 5 days. Adequate hydration is also encouraged along with possible electrolyte replacement.

## *CAMPYLOBACTER* ENTERITIS

**Etiology.** *Campylobacter* enteritis is caused by the small, highly motile gram-negative rod *Campylobacter jejuni.* It is likely that active anal-oral sexual activity may contribute to enteritis.

**Pathophysiology.** The patients' first symptoms are fever, malaise, nausea, and headache. They then experience abdominal pain with diarrhea. Blood or mucus may be visible in the stool. The symptoms will subside within 2 or 3 days. The diagnosis is confirmed by microscopic examination of a specimen.

**Medical-Surgical Management.** The physician encourages hydration and a follow-up examination. Symptomatic infection may be treated with erythromycin 500 mg orally four times daily for 7 days.

# Viral Syndromes

## ACQUIRED IMMUNODEFICIENCY SYNDROME

**Etiology.** Acquired immunodeficiency syndrome (AIDS) is an STD caused by HIV. This virus was first identified in humans in 1984. Originally, it was the cause of a benign disease in African green monkeys. HIV destroys T4 lymphocytes, which are helper and regulatory cells essential for immune responses. HIV is a retrovirus whose RNA is transcribed into DNA by an enzyme called *reverse transcriptase.* The viral DNA becomes incorporated into human genetic DNA, thus allowing for replication and A- and ST-cell destruction.

HIV is transmitted through sexual contact and exposure to infected blood or blood components and from mother to neonate. The virus has been isolated from blood, semen, vaginal secretions, saliva, tears, breast milk, cerebrospinal fluid, amniotic fluid, and urine. In August 1977, the CDC mandated universal precautions for all health care workers (see section on assessment).

High-risk groups include homosexual or bisexual men, intravenous drug abusers, transfusion recipients, and hemophiliacs.

**Pathophysiology.** HIV is associated with numerous opportunistic infections. They are called opportunistic because they are seen only in patients who are severely immunodeficient, including those with Kaposi's sarcoma, *Pneumocystis carinii* pneumonia, and other yeast, fungal, bacterial, and parasitic diseases.

In September 1987, the CDC defined three criteria for the diagnosis of AIDS: (1) in the absence of HIV testing, the patient is immunodeficient without cause and has a definite diagnosis of Kaposi's sarcoma or central nervous system lymphoma; (2) the patient is HIV positive and has AIDS dementia complex (ADC), which is HIV encephalopathy, HIV wasting syndrome, tuberculosis, lymphoma, or recurrent bacterial infection; or (3) the patient is HIV negative, although he or she is immunodeficient without cause and has *P. carinii* pneumonia or is immunodeficient with a T-lymphocyte count of fewer than 400 mm$^3$.

In June 1986 the CDC classified HIV infection as follows:

Class I: Acute HIV infection (rash, sore throat, nausea, vomiting, fever within 6–12 weeks of exposure).
Class II: HIV positive, asymptomatic.
Class III: HIV positive; lymphadenopathy evident.
Class IV: HIV disease
- A. Constitutional disease: AIDS-related complex (ARC); 10% weight loss; fever and diarrhea for a month.
- B. Neurologic disease: ADC.
- C. Opportunistic infections: secondary *P. carinii* pneumonia, disseminated histoplasmosis.
- D. Cancers: Kaposi's sarcoma, non-Hodgkin's lymphomas.
- E. Other conditions: clinical symptoms not classified in another group that are associated with HIV.

Note that only class IV is required to be reported to the CDC today.

There are two serologic tests for HIV antibody testing. The first is an enzyme-linked immunosorbent assay (ELISA). This test is not conclusive for AIDS, so if the result is positive, a second test called the *Western blot* is done. If both results are positive, it means that the person has been exposed to HIV and now has the antibody. The time between infection with HIV and the development of AIDS ranges from a few months to more than 10 years.

**Medical-Surgical Management.** The physician manages each patient individually, based on the specific infections the person has acquired and the appropriate treatment. Therapy with zidovudine has been shown to benefit patients with the disease. It suppresses viral replication, thus decreasing the frequency of opportunistic infections, and delays progression of ARC to full-blown AIDS. Serious side effects, usually anemias and cytopenias, are common during therapy. Clinical trials are investigating new drugs or combinations of drugs for persons with different stages of HIV infection.

The research and evidence regarding AIDS are changing rapidly. The continued monitoring of information sources for developments related to this disease is essential.

## GENITAL HERPES SIMPLEX

**Etiology.** Herpes simplex is an infection caused by the virus called herpesvirus hominis, which has two types: The type I strain usually affects the mouth and eyes, whereas type II causes genital lesions. Type I has been found in the genital region, but this is a rare occurrence. This virus is transmitted via a break in the skin or through mucous membranes. The latest statistics indicate a sharp increase in the number of newly diagnosed cases.

**Pathophysiology.** The initial sign of herpes simplex virus is a burning or itch in the affected area. A fluid-filled vesicle is evident and will eventually ulcerate and crust. The patient may exhibit one or many of these lesions. The incubation period is 3 to 12 days, and the lesions last 7 to 21 days. Fever, malaise, edema, and lymphadenopathy may occur. The lesion is infectious until it is totally healed.

After the initial outbreak, the virus may remain dormant or recur. Recurrences are milder, and lesions dissipate more quickly. Some factors responsible for recurrence include exposure to sunlight, emotional stress, hormonal changes, and onset of fever. Diagnosis is made by obtaining a tissue culture of the lesion or a Tzanck test.

Complications of the virus include conjunctivitis, herpes keratitis, and herpes encephalitis. A fetus may also develop herpes in utero or through an infected passage during birth.

**Medical-Surgical Management.** The physician examines the entire body for lesions. According to the CDC, the physician should prescribe acyclovir (Zovirax) 200 mg orally five times daily for 7 to 10 days. Recurrences should be treated with IV acyclovir or a repeat regimen of oral acyclovir. Cool compresses may also provide localized relief. Daily treatment reduces the frequency of occurrences by at least 75% among patients with frequent (more than six per year) recurrences. After 1 year of suppressive therapy (acyclovir 200 mg orally two to five times a day), the medication should be discontinued so the patient's recurrence rate may be reassessed.

## HEPATITIS A

**Etiology.** Hepatitis A is an enteric infection. The hepatitis A virus may be found in contaminated water, shellfish, or blood. It may also be transmitted by oral-anal sexual practices. The virion contains RNA.

**Pathophysiology** The symptoms of hepatitis A, hepatitis B, and hepatitis non-A, non-B are similar, although their incubation periods differ. The incubation period for hepatitis A is approximately 2 to 6 weeks. Generally, the symptoms increase in severity with time. Some people are asymptomatic, whereas others complain of low-grade fever, malaise, headaches, anorexia, nausea, vomiting, and diarrhea. Dark-colored urine and clay-colored stool usually appear prior to jaundice. Jaundice may be evident for 6 weeks, but the disease is not chronic and does not cause severe liver disease. It is contagious during the incubation period and the acute phase of onset. Diagnosis of hepatitis A rests on identification of hepatitis A virus antibodies (anti-HAV) in the serum. The antibodies belong to the IgM class of immunoglobulins, which are replaced after 6 weeks by antibodies of the IgG class. Thus, evidence of anti-HAV of the IgM class indicates a current infection, whereas anti-HAV of the IgG class indicates a past infection.

**Medical-Surgical Management.** In addition to performing a physical examination, the physician obtains serum samples for hepatitis antibodies, liver function tests, and bilirubin. A urine bilirubin measurement also is obtained. The physician may suggest an IM injection of immune globulin, which may decrease the symptoms if given within 2 weeks after exposure. There is no treatment for hepatitis. Rest and good nutrition should be encouraged. Alcohol and hepatotoxic drugs, such as aspirin, acetaminophen, and tetracycline, should be avoided. Patients should be observed for liver failure and encephalopathy and be treated appropriately if they occur.

## HEPATITIS B

**Etiology.** Sexual contact is the most frequently reported mode of transmission of hepatitis B virus in the United States. Hepatitis B is caused by a double-shelled virion containing DNA. It is transmitted via blood or blood products that contain the virus. It is also present in saliva and semen. Sexually, it is transmitted during anorectal intercourse or orogenital contact. Health care workers who are in contact

with blood must abide by their institution's infection control policy to decrease the risk of infection.

**Pathophysiology.** The symptoms of hepatitis B correlate with those previously discussed for hepatitis A. In addition, patients with hepatitis B may complain of a macular-papular skin rash and arthralgia or arthritis. The incubation period is 6 weeks to 6 months. Hepatitis B may lead to cirrhosis. Hepatitis B is diagnosed by the identification of hepatitis B surface antigen ($HB_sAg$) in the serum. It can be found within 60 days after exposure, and if it persists after 6 months, indicates a chronic carrier state. The disease is contagious as long as $HB_sAg$ is present. $HB_sAg$ disappears after the acute illness, and about 3 months later, antibodies to $HB_sAg$ (anti-$HB_s$) appear; these indicate immunity to hepatitis B. Hepatitis B core antigen ($HB_cAg$) and its antibody (anti-$HB_c$) indicate chronic hepatitis. Anti-$HB_c$ is evident during the late acute phase of hepatitis B and is usually lifelong.

**Medical-Surgical Management.** The management is similar to that discussed in the section on hepatitis A. Vaccines are available that are safe and effective for persons at high risk for hepatitis B. The hepatitis B vaccine series requires three inoculations; the vaccine should not be administered in the gluteal or quadriceps muscles. Prophylactic treatment with hepatitis B immune globulin 0.06 mL/kg IM in a single dose should occur in the following situations: sexual contact with a person who has active hepatitis B or sexual contact with a hepatitis B carrier. The injection of immune globulin should be followed by the hepatitis B vaccine series.

## NON-A, NON-B HEPATITIS

**Etiology.** Non-A, non-B (NANB) hepatitis is caused by many NANB viruses. It is transmitted via blood. All donor blood is tested for hepatitis A and hepatitis B, but because there is no screening for NANB hepatitis, most post-transfusion hepatitis is transmitted in this manner. Sexually, it is transmitted during anorectal intercourse or orogenital contact.

**Pathophysiology.** The symptoms of NANB hepatitis correlate to those previously discussed for hepatitis A. The incubation period ranges from 2 weeks to 6 months. NANB hepatitis is diagnosed by ruling out hepatitis A and hepatitis B, cytomegalovirus, and Epstein-Barr virus. The disease may lead to a carrier state, chronic hepatitis, or chronic liver disease.

**Medical-Surgical Management.** The management is similar to that discussed for hepatitis A, including the administration of immune globulin.

## CYTOMEGALOVIRUS

**Etiology.** Cytomegalovirus is one of the herpesviruses that may be transmitted sexually. It is evident in body fluids and is one of the infectious diseases often seen with AIDS. It can be transmitted perinatally from a maternal infection.

**Pathophysiology.** An infant born with cytomegalovirus may have neurologic deficits. Therefore, pregnant women should be told if they have the virus. Patients with AIDS who acquire cytomegalovirus usually manifest pneumonia. Unfortunately, this is fatal, because no effective therapy for the infection is available. The virus can be identified by the complement fixation test or ELISA.

**Medical-Surgical Management.** The physician may prescribe acyclovir, because cytomegalovirus is a herpesvirus.

## CONDYLOMATA ACUMINATA

**Etiology.** Condylomata acuminata are caused by the human papillomaviruses. There are multiple strains of papillomaviruses, but the types associated with this disease are types 6 and 11. They are called genital warts and are sexually transmissible. Statistics from 1990 suggest a sharp increase in the prevalence of this disease.

**Pathophysiology.** The lesions present as soft, fleshy papules. In males, they are found on the penis, and in females, they can be found on the labia, vulva, vagina, or cervix. They can also appear periurethrally and perianally. Complications can lead to hemorrhage or a penile fistula. The literature suggests an association between cervical condylomata and cervical dysplasia. The diagnosis is made with histologic study of a specimen or with a Papanicolaou-stained smear in the instance of a cervical lesion.

**Medical-Surgical Management.** According to the CDC, the therapy for genital, urethral, and perianal warts is cryotherapy or podophyllin 10% in compound tincture of benzoin. Application should be performed by a health care professional to ensure that normal tissue is not affected. It must be washed off thoroughly after 1 to 4 hours. This should take place one or two times a week. Alternative regimens include electrosurgery and surgical removal. The current therapy for vaginal or cervical warts is cryotherapy, trichloroacetic acid, or podophyllin. Anal warts should be treated with cryotherapy, trichloroacetic acid, or surgical removal. Most recently, the $CO_2$ and neodymium:yttrium-aluminum-garnet lasers are being used to treat these lesions.

## MOLLUSCUM CONTAGIOSUM

**Etiology.** Molluscum contagiosum, a viral infection that occurs in children and young adults, has a sexual mode of transmission. It is caused by a poxvirus that carries DNA. The virus attacks epidermal cells.

**Pathophysiology.** The patient presents with a papular lesion that has a dimple. The papules are flesh colored and contain a white secretion. The lesions multiply and are evident in the genital region. The incubation period is between 2 and 6 weeks. The patient usually has no complaints, although some patients report that the lesions are tender or itchy. The disease resolves without treatment within months or years. The diagnosis is made with a biopsy or smear of the lesion.

**Medical-Surgical Management.** The physician performs a complete physical examination of the patient for evidence of other STDs.

# Protozoan Syndromes

## TRICHOMONIASIS

**Etiology.** Trichomoniasis is caused by *T. vaginalis*, a protozoon with flagella that keep it in motion. The disease often coexists with other STDs.

**Pathophysiology.** Most women present with symptoms of watery, odorous vaginal discharges. If the cervix, vagina, or labia are inflamed, there will be complaints of itching, dysuria, and dyspareunia. Most men with the disease are asymptomatic, but some may complain of mucopurulent discharge, dysuria, or urethral irritation. The complications of male trichomoniasis include urethral strictures, epididymitis, and prostatitis. The incubation period varies from 3 to 28 days. The organism is identified by dark-field examination, stained smears, or Papanicolaou smears.

**Medical-Surgical Management.** The physician performs a gynecologic examination that may reveal inflammation of the vulva and the vagina. Vaginal discharge specimens are obtained for examination. The physician may attempt to examine a male's first voided specimen or urethral scraping to identify *T. vaginalis*, although it does not always reveal the organism.

The CDC recommend metronidazole (Flagyl) 2 g orally in a single dose or metronidazole 500 mg orally two times daily for 7 days. Male sex partners of women with trichomoniasis should receive the same regimen and should be examined for coexistent STDs.

## AMEBIASIS

**Etiology.** Amebiasis is caused by *Entamoeba histolytica*, a protozoon. It takes the form of a cyst and a trophozoite. The trophozoite is the stage in the life cycle capable of causing disease. Oral-anal sexual practices lead to the transmission of this parasite. The cyst form contributes to the transmission of the disease.

**Pathophysiology.** *E. histolytica* forms small ulcers within the intestinal mucosa. Intestinal amebiasis includes dysentery, an ameboma, and amebic appendicitis. An ameboma is a mass occurring within the cecum containing lymphocytes, plasma cells, and the organism. Intestinal amebiasis may lead to peritonitis, stricture formation, or hemorrhage. Extraintestinal amebiasis may include involvement of the liver, lung, or spleen.

Many patients are asymptomatic. Others present with complaints of flatulence, abdominal cramping, and irregular bowel habits. Severe cases may reveal bloody diarrhea accompanied by fever.

The laboratory diagnosis is made by examination of stool culture.

**Medical-Surgical Management.** The physician performs a physical examination of the patient. Examination may reveal an enlarged liver due to toxins. A sigmoidoscopy shows mucosal ulcers. For the patient who is symptomatic, the CDC recommend diiodohydroxyquin 650 mg three times daily for 20 days, plus metronidazole 750 mg three times daily for 5 to 10 days.

## GIARDIASIS

**Etiology.** Giardiasis is caused by *Giardia lamblia*, a protozoon with flagella. It presents in two forms: a cyst and a trophozoite. Outbreaks are usually due to ingestion of water contaminated by cyst-passing animals. Some studies indicate a higher incidence of the disease in homosexual men.

**Pathophysiology.** The upper intestinal tract harbors *G. lamblia* and could cause a malabsorption syndrome. Symptoms consist of flatulence, foul-smelling, bulky diarrhea, and abdominal cramping. The disease may be diagnosed by identifying cysts or trophozoites in stool specimens or by intestinal biopsies.

**Medical-Surgical Management.** During the physical examination, the physician observes for evidence of a malabsorption syndrome and may obtain intestinal aspirations. According to the CDC, both asymptomatic and symptomatic patients should be treated with quinacrine (Atabrine) 100 mg orally three times daily for 7 days. An alternative regimen may be metronidazole 250 mg orally three times daily for 7 days.

## CRYPTOSPORIDIOSIS

**Etiology.** Cryptosporidiosis is caused by a protozoan parasite, *Cryptosporidium*. It is known to have caused diarrhea in animals and recently has been identified in humans. It is transmitted via a fecal-oral contamination.

**Pathophysiology.** The patient complains of nausea, vomiting, abdominal cramps, diarrhea, and fever. The incubation period is 1 to 2 weeks. Weight loss may be significant. It is not known how the organism produces diarrhea. The disease is usually self-limiting, but it could be dangerous in immunosuppressed patients if the volume of diarrhea is excessive. The diagnosis may be made by an acid-fast stain of a stool specimen or an intestinal biopsy.

**Medical-Surgical Management.** The physician obtains a thorough history and performs a complete physical examination, noting any evidence of immunosuppression. The patient may require hydration.

## Ectoparasitic Syndromes

### PEDICULOSIS PUBIS

**Etiology.** Pediculosis pubis is caused by *Phthirus pubis*, a pubic or crab louse that is 2 to 3 mm long. Its name comes from its appearance. Four of its six legs have crablike claws used to hold onto pubic or other body hairs. The louse also sucks blood from a cutaneous capillary of the host. The life span of the female louse is 3 to 4 weeks, during which time she can lay three eggs per day. The disease is sexually transmitted, although it can be obtained from contaminated clothing or toilet seats.

**Pathophysiology.** The common symptom of this disease is pruritus in the genital area. The incubation period before pruritus develops is 30 days. The organisms can spread to other hairy body parts, including the thighs, beard, and mustache. Children have involvement of their eyelashes, which is probably the result of close contact with a parent. The parasite can usually be identified with a magnifying glass or, in a difficult case, by placing a hair under a microscope.

**Medical-Surgical Management.** The CDC recommend that physicians prescribe permethrin 1% cream rinse applied to the affected area and washed off after 10 minutes or pyrithrins and piperonyl butoxide applied to the affected area and washed off after 10 minutes, or lindane 1% shampoo applied for 4 minutes and then thoroughly washed off.

Clothing or bed linen that may have been contaminated should be washed and dried on a hot cycle or dry-cleaned.

## SCABIES

**Etiology.** Scabies, or "the itch," is caused by the mite *Sarcoptes scabiei*, a tiny, whitish-brown, eight-legged mite (Fig. 7–4). The female is responsible for the patient's symptoms. It can move at 2.5 cm/min and burrows into the skin, where it lays 10 to 25 eggs before it dies. It is transmitted via direct contact sexually or by handling contaminated clothing.

**Pathophysiology.** The common symptom is itching, which is more pronounced at night. The lesions are tiny papules that may have blood crusts. Sometimes the appearance of the lesions resembles eczema. The burrows are more easily definable. They are short, wavy,

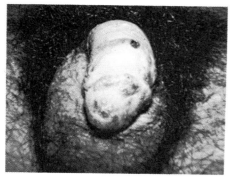

FIGURE 7–4 Scabies. (From Walsh, P. C., Gittes, R. F., Perlmutter, A. D., & Stamey, T. A. [Eds.]. [1986]. *Campbell's urology* [5th ed., p. 966]. Philadelphia: W. B. Saunders. Reprinted with permission.)

gray lines. The lesions are evident on the sides and webs of the fingers, the flexor aspects of the wrists, the extensor portion of the elbows, the axillary folds, the breasts, and the penis. Nodular lesions may form in the axillae or the groin. Scabies is diagnosed by evidence of mites from skin scrapings or by epidermal shave biopsies.

**Medical-Surgical Management.** The physician examines the patient using good lighting to obtain scrapings or biopsy specimens. The CDC recommend that both the patient and any sex partners, or others of close contact, be treated with lindane 1% lotion or cream to the entire body from the neck down and washed off in 8 hours. Alternative regimens include crotamiton 10% applied to the entire body from the neck down nightly for two nights and washed off 24 hours after the second application. The disease is not transmitted after these treatments. All clothing and linen should be washed and dried on hot cycles or dry-cleaned. The patient may be symptomatic for weeks. A single treatment after 1 week may be appropriate if no clinical improvement occurs. The itching may be aided by antipruritic medication.

## STRONGYLOIDIASIS

**Etiology.** Strongyloidiasis is caused by the human roundworm, *Strongyloides stercoralis*. It is transmitted via the oral-anal route.

**Pathophysiology.** The presenting symptom is diarrhea, and the organism is identified in a stool specimen.

**Medical-Surgical Management.** The physician may prescribe thiabendazole 25 mg/kg twice a day for 2 days.

## Fungal Syndromes

### YEAST VAGINITIS

**Etiology.** Yeast vaginitis is most commonly caused by *Candida albicans*. It may also be caused by *Candida tropicalis* or other *Candida* organisms. It may be sexually transmitted. In some, it is also correlated with the use of the birth control pill or the third trimester of pregnancy. It also occurs with the use of antibiotics or steroids. It is highly prevalent in diabetics.

**Pathophysiology.** The common symptom is vulvar pruritus or irritation. It may be accompanied with a scant to moderate amount of white, clumped discharge. The woman is usually symptomatic the week before menstruation. The diagnosis is made based on symptoms, a vaginal pH of less than 4.5, and a direct smear of vaginal discharge.

**Medical-Surgical Management.** According to the CDC guidelines, the physician should prescribe miconazole nitrate (Monistat) 200 mg intravaginally at bedtime for 3 days; clotrimazole (Lotrimin) 200 mg intravaginally at bedtime for 3 days; butoconazole 2% cream 5 g intravaginally at bedtime for 3 days; or terconazole 80-mg suppository or 0.4% cream intravaginally at bedtime for 3 days.

## BALANOPOSTHITIS

**Etiology.** Balanoposthitis is a yeast infection of the uncircumcised penis that may be caused by *Candida* or pyogenic organisms (Fig. 7–5). It may occur in diabetics or men receiving antibiotics, or it may be transmitted sexually.

**Pathophysiology.** The usual symptom is erythema or glazed skin that may be accompanied by edema, desquamation, and encrusting or fissuring of the prepuce. The groin and scrotum are rarely infected. It is diagnosed based on the clinical picture with or without isolation of *Candida* or a pyogenic organism.

**Medical-Surgical Management.** The physician prescribes clotrimazole 1% cream applied twice daily for 7 days, or antibacterial creams. The patient should experience prompt relief, but circumcision may ultimately be necessary.

Table 7–1 is a summary of the recommended regimens for treating STDs.

# APPROACHES TO PATIENT CARE

### Assessment
An accurate diagnosis is necessary to prevent

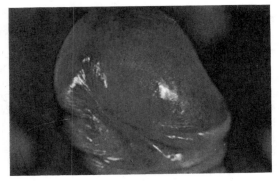

*FIGURE 7–5* Balanitis. (From Walsh, P. C., Gittes, R. F., Perlmutter, A. D., & Stamey, T. A. [Eds.]. [1986]. *Campbell's urology* [5th ed., p. 966]. Philadelphia: W. B. Saunders. Reprinted with permission.)

the numerous complications that may arise from STDs. The assessment phase should take place in a quiet, private environment, and the nurse should maintain a confidential, nonjudgmental, empathetic approach with the patient. A complete assessment should include a complete medical history, sexual history, signs and symptoms, and a physical examination. For females, a menstrual history is necessary to assist in the diagnosis. After obtaining a medical history, the nurse needs to explain to the patient that a sexual history is necessary to assist in diagnosing the problem and understanding how it will affect sexual health.

A sexual history should obtain information regarding the age when the patient first became sexually active; whether the patient is currently sexually active; whether the patient is heterosexual, homosexual, or bisexual; frequency of sexual practices; types of protection used during sexual activity; whether symptoms have affected sexual activity; and whether there are any concerns regarding sexual activity. All these questions should be asked in a nonthreatening, open-ended fashion. The answers to these questions help the nurse decide the diseases to which the patient may be at high risk of exposure, the sites from which cultures should be obtained, and what focus on education the patient needs during the intervention phase.

The physical examination should be thorough, including an inspection of all mucous membrane orifices, the genital area, and the lower abdomen, as well as a complete skin assessment. Be certain that during the physical examination, universal precautions are used (Table 7–2). Because some STDs may be transmitted in modes other than sexual contact, some patients may require additional precautions (Table 7–3). It is recommended that the nurse consult the particular institution's infection control policy to adhere to standards of care. Listed in Table 7–4 is each STD with accompanying symptoms and findings that may be evident on physical examination.

Throughout the assessment phase, the patient's verbal and nonverbal communications assist the nurse in identifying problems related to the patient's disease entity. Be aware of the patient's anxiety level, and decide whether it is sufficient to alter the patient's cooperation in the assessment of the disease. During the sexual history assessment, the nurse should be able to assess the flexibility of the patient to alter the sexual practices. Evidence of any lesion, discharge, or odor found on physical ex-

### TABLE 7–1. Recommended Treatment Regimen for STDs

| DISEASE | RECOMMENDED REGIMEN | ALTERNATE REGIMEN |
|---|---|---|
| Gonorrhea (uncomplicated) | Ceftriaxone + doxycycline | Spectinomycin + doxycycline |
| Gonococcal ophthalmia | Ceftriaxone | |
| Neonatal gonococcal ophthalmia | Ceftriaxone | |
| Disseminated gonococcal infection | Ceftriaxone | Ceftizoxime *or* cefotaxime |
| Nongonococcal urethritis | Doxycycline *or* tetracycline | Erythromycin |
| *Chlamydia trachomatis* infection | Doxycycline *or* tetracycline | Erythromycin |
| Neonatal *Chlamydia* conjunctivitis | Erythromycin | |
| Neonatal *Chlamydia* pneumonia | Erythromycin | |
| Pelvic inflammatory disease | | |
| In-patient | Doxycycline + cefoxitin *or* Clindamycin + gentamicin | |
| Out-patient | Cefoxitin + probenecid + doxycycline *or* Ceftriaxone + doxycycline *or* Cephalosporin + doxycycline | |
| Syphilis | Benzathine penicillin G | Doxycycline *or* tetracycline |
| Neurosyphilis | Aqueous crystalline penicillin G + benzathine penicillin G | Procaine penicillin + probenecid + benzathine penicillin G |
| Neonatal congenital syphilis | Aqueous crystalline penicillin G | Procaine penicillin G |
| Chancroid | Erythromycin *or* ceftriaxone | Sulfamethoxazole-trimethoprim *or* amoxicillin + clavulanic acid |
| Lymphogranuloma venereum | Doxycycline | Tetracycline *or* erythromycin *or* sulfisoxazole |
| Granuloma inguinale | Tetracycline | Chloramphenicol |
| Shigellosis | Sulfamethoxazole-trimethoprim | Ampicillin |
| *Campylobacter* enteritis | Erythromycin | |
| Acquired immunodeficiency syndrome | Zidovudine | |
| Genital herpes simplex | Acyclovir | |
| Hepatitis A | Immune globulin | |
| Hepatitis B | Hepatitis B immune globulin + hepatitis B vaccine series | |
| Non-A, non-B hepatitis | Immune globulin | |
| Cytomegalovirus infection | Acyclovir | |
| Condylomata acuminata | Cryotherapy (liquid nitrogen) | Trichloroacetic acid *or* podophyllin |
| Molluscum contagiosum | None | |
| Trichomoniasis | Metronidazole | |
| Amebiasis | Diiodohydroxyquin + metronidazole | |
| Giardiasis | Quinacrine | Metronidazole |
| Cryptosporidiosis | None | |
| Pediculosis pubis | Permethrin | Pyrethrins + piperonyl butoxide *or* lindane |
| Scabies | Lindane lotion *or* lindane cream | Pyrethrins + piperonyl butoxide *or* crotamiton |
| Strongyloidiasis | Thiabendazole | |
| Yeast vaginitis | Miconazole nitrate *or* clotrimazole | Butoconazole *or* terconazole |
| Balanoposthitis | Clotrimazole | |

amination may trigger a disturbance in self-esteem or body image. This would be noted if, for example, the patient did not want to view the lesion or demonstrated signs of embarrassment. The infected area(s) may also be painful. Therefore, the nurse may perform a pain assessment using a pain scale. The nurse must also elicit the patient's previous coping mechanisms used during stressful situations. The nurse may then employ this information to predict whether these coping mechanisms would be appropriate when the patient is faced with the diagnosis of an STD.

Discharge planning, whether the patient is going to leave the hospital or clinic, must reflect the patient's knowledge of the disease entity, willingness to comply with the treatment modalities, and appropriate coping mecha-

**TABLE 7–2. Universal Precautions**

1. Hands and other skin surfaces should be washed immediately and thoroughly if contaminated with blood or other body fluids.
2. Gloves should be worn for touching blood and other body fluids, mucous membranes, or nonintact skin of all patients; for handling items or surfaces soiled with blood or body fluids; and for performing venipuncture and other vascular access procedures. Gloves should be changed between each patient. Hands should be washed after gloves are removed.
3. Gowns are generally not indicated but should be worn during procedures that are likely to generate splashes of blood or other body fluids.
4. Masks and protective eye wear are generally not indicated but should be worn during procedures that are likely to disperse droplets of blood or other body fluids into the nose, eyes, or mouth.
5. Needles, scalpels, and other sharp instruments should be handled with extreme caution. Needles should not be recapped, purposely bent or broken by hand, removed from disposable syringes, or otherwise manipulated by hand. After use, disposable needles and other sharp items should be placed in puncture-resistant containers for disposal; the containers should be located as close as practical to the area of use. Reusable needles should be placed in a puncture-resistant container for transport to the processing area.
6. Although saliva has not been implicated in HIV transmission, to minimize the need for emergency mouth-to-mouth resuscitation, mouthpieces, resuscitation bags, or other ventilation devices should be available for use where the need for resuscitation is predictable.
7. Health care workers with exudative lesions or weeping dermatitis should refrain from all direct patient care and from handling patient care equipment until the condition resolves.

From Centers for Disease Control. (1987). Recommendations for prevention of HIV transmission in health care setting. *Morbidity and Mortality Weekly Report, 36*(25), 15–18S.

nisms to deal with the diagnosis. Before discharge, the patient's feelings of anxiety, anger, shame, guilt, and fear must be openly discussed, and the patient must be counseled regarding the impact these feelings may have on treatment.

**Nursing Diagnosis**

The nursing diagnoses for the patient with an STD may include the following:

1. Alteration in knowledge related to STD.
2. Altered sexual patterns related to newly gained knowledge of transmission of STDs.
3. Disturbance in body image related to lesions, discharge, odor, or topical medications.
4. Disturbance in self-esteem related to knowledge of an STD diagnosis.
5. Impaired skin integrity related to lesions on or surrounding mucous membranes.

6. Ineffective individual coping related to awareness of the new diagnosis.
7. Alteration in comfort related to painful lesions, lymph nodes, or both.
8. Impaired social interaction related to
   a. Body image changes.
   b. Fear of informing others of the diagnosis.

**Plan of Care**

Nursing care is directed toward enabling the patient to

1. Openly discuss his or her knowledge of newly acquired disease, including its manifestations, mode of transmission, and effects.
2. Reiterate the importance of
   a. Notifying sexual partners.
   b. Refraining from sexual activity during the assessment, diagnosis, and treatment of the disease process.
   c. Using other forms of sexual expression.
3. Verbalize positive feelings regarding sense of well-being.
4. Verbalize anxiety, fear, anger, and other emotions.
5. Discuss the effects of the diagnosis on feelings of self-worth.
6. Verbalize a positive outlook on his or her self-esteem.
7. Demonstrate proper application of prescribed medication.
8. Discuss the basics of good hygiene.
9. Discuss whether it will be difficult to cope with the diagnosis, and if so, how he or she plans to cope.
10. Discuss modes of increasing comfort.
11. Verbalize a plan to participate safely in social activity.

**Interventions**

The diagnosis of an STD can be traumatic to anyone, because it can affect so many aspects of life, such as body image, sexuality, physical changes, comfort, and socialization. It is the nurse's responsibility to address these needs and direct the patient to the optimum level of well-being.

Counseling must take place in an uninterrupted, confidential environment, and the nurse must present all information using a nonthreatening, nonjudgmental approach. The discussion should begin with the patient's specific disease, including its physiology, manifestations, and mode of transmission; how it is diagnosed; and its short- and long-term effects. Eliminate any myths regarding the disease by

## Table 7–3. RECOMMENDED INFECTION CONTROL PRECAUTIONS

| DISEASE | ORGANISM | INFECTION CONTROL PRECAUTIONS |
|---|---|---|
| Gonorrhea | *Neisseria gonorrhoeae* | Universal |
| Gonorrhea | Penicillinase-producing *Neisseria gonorrhoeae* | Universal |
| Nongonococcal urethritis | *Chlamydia trachomatis* *Ureaplasma urealyticum* | Universal |
| Chlamydial infection | *Chlamydia trachomatis* | Drainage/secretion |
| Pelvic inflammatory disease | *Chlamydia trachomatis* *Neisseria gonorrhoeae* | Universal |
| Syphilis | *Treponema pallidum* | Primary: drainage/secretion Secondary: drainage/secretion Latent: universal |
| Chancroid | *Haemophilus ducreyi* | |
| Lymphogranuloma venereum | *Chlamydia trachomatis* | Universal |
| Granuloma inguinale | *Calymmatobacterium granulomatis* | Universal |
| Shigellosis | *Shigella* | Enteric |
| *Campylobacter* enteritis | *Campylobacter jejuni* | Enteric |
| Acquired immunodeficiency syndrome | Human immunodeficiency virus | Universal (may require more if secondary opportunistic infections are present) |
| Genital herpes simplex | Herpesvirus hominis type II | Contact |
| Hepatitis A | Hepatitis A virus | Enteric |
| Hepatitis B | Hepatitis B virus | Universal |
| Non-A, non-B hepatitis | Non-A, non-B virus | Universal |
| Cytomegalovirus infection | Cytomegalovirus | Universal |
| Condylomata acuminata | Papovavirus | Universal |
| Molluscum contagiosum | Poxvirus | Universal |
| Trichomoniasis | *Trichomonas vaginalis* | Universal |
| Amebiasis | *Entamoeba histolytica* | Enteric |
| Giardiasis | *Giardia lamblia* | Enteric |
| Cryptosporidiosis | *Cryptosporidium* | Universal |
| Pediculosis pubis | *Phthirus pubis* | Contact |
| Scabies | *Sarcoptes scabiei* | Contact |
| Strongyloidiasis | *Strongyloides* | Universal |
| Yeast vaginitis | *Candida albicans* | Universal |
| Balanoposthitis | *Candida albicans* | Universal |

Adapted from Garner, J., & Simmons, B. (1983). *CDC guidelines for isolation precautions in hospitals.* Atlanta: Centers for Disease Control.

teaching the patient accurately in lay terms and by providing printed literature to enhance the conversation. It is important to review the signs and symptoms, incubation period, and infectious period of the disease.

Treatment modalities must be defined according to the specific disease. Patient compliance must be emphasized. It must be stressed that the patient does have a certain amount of control over the disease. The medication regimen should focus on the name of the drug, dosage, administration, side effects, and action. The importance of not missing a dose and taking all the prescribed medication, even though symptoms may disappear beforehand, must be emphasized. Along with teaching regarding topical medication administration, a review of basic hygiene must be discussed. Basic hygiene of the lesions should include keeping the sores clean by washing with mild soap and water,

keeping the area dry by possibly using a hair dryer set on low, and wearing loose-fitting cotton undergarments to decrease perspiration.

Often, patients do not understand why their sex partner must be notified. The importance of the disease process, the chance of reinfection, and the prevention of further spread of the disease must be emphasized. Allow the patient and sex partner(s) time to understand the disease itself. Patient confidentiality can also be reinforced at this point. At the same time, the patient must be informed that the infection itself must be reported to the Health Department, as mandated by the CDC. The Health Department will maintain confidentiality.

Sometimes, pain is a problem, especially with lesions. The nurse instructs the patient regarding comfort modalities, such as positioning, activity, and ice application to lesions; if urination is painful, the nurse suggests urinat-

TABLE 7–4. Assessment of Sexually Transmitted Disease

| DISEASE | PATIENT'S COMPLAINTS AND SYMPTOMS | OTHER PHYSICAL EXAMINATION FINDINGS | DIAGNOSTIC STUDY |
|---|---|---|---|
| Gonorrhea | Yellow urethral discharge Urethral itching Burning on urination Reddened, edematous meatus | May have evidence of proctitis, ophthalmitis, pharyngitis | Gram's stain Thayer-Martin medium New York City medium |
| Nongonococcal urethritis | Watery, white or mucoid urethral discharge Slight dysuria Urethra itch | May have ascended to prostate, ejaculatory ducts, seminal vesicles, bladder. Must rule out Reiter's syndrome; assess for conjunctivitis, arthritis, diarrhea | Excess leukocytes; Gram's stain with no gram-negative cocci |
| Chlamydial infection | Male: cloudy urethral discharge; reddened meatus, dysuria Female: dysuria, frequent vaginal discharge | May have epididymitis  May have cervicitis or pelvic inflammatory disease | Enzyme immunoassay test Direct fluorescent antibody Cell culture isolation |
| Pelvic inflammatory disease | Severe abdominal pain | May have vaginal discharge or recent excessive menstrual bleed, indicating endometriosis; pain assessment | Cervical culture; tubal culture CBC count; sedimentation rate Laparoscopy Culdocentesis |
| Syphilis (1st stage) | Chancre | May have localized lymphadenopathy | Examination of serum obtained from a chancre VDRL/RPR, FTA-ABS, MHA-TP |
| Syphilis (2nd stage) | Generalized rash with lymphadenopathy; malaise; sore throat; fever | Check for any invasion of liver or meninges | VDRL/FTA-ABS, RPR/MHA-TP |
| Chancroid | Male: painful ulcer Female: asymptomatic or painful urination | Inguinal tenderness | Smear; culture; biopsy |
| Lymphogranuloma venereum | If early, papule lesions that heal quickly. If later, painful inguinal nodes | May have systemic signs (e.g., fever, arthralgias) | Complement fixation test. Lymph node with a culture of *Chlamydia trachomatis* |
| Granuloma inguinale | Genital papule; granulation of tissue | | Biopsy will reveal Donovan's bodies |
| Shigellosis | Crampy diarrhea, fever | Observe for pus or blood in stool | Direct stool specimen |
| *Campylobacter* enteritis | Diarrhea, fever, malaise Abdominal pain | Observe for pus or blood in stool | Direct stool specimen |
| Acquired immunodeficiency syndrome | Extremely individualized, but usually includes fatigue, fever, recent weight loss, diarrhea | A complete assessment must include observation for opportunistic infections, Kaposi's sarcoma, *Pneumocystis carinii* pneumonia, meningitis, gastrointestinal infection, toxoplasmosis, and others | ELISA Western blot |
| Genital herpes simplex | Vesicles or ulcers | Examine entire body for lesions | Tissue culture Tzanck test |
| Hepatitis | Vary greatly: asymptomatic; fatigue, anorexia, headache, rash, dark-colored urine, clay-colored stool, jaundice, confusion, ascites, and others | Must assess for hepatic failure and encephalopathy | A: anti-HAV IgM in serum B: $HB_sAg$ in serum Check bilirubin levels and liver enzymes |
| Cytomegalovirus infection | Asymptomatic | Assess for signs of other diseases | Complement fixation ELISA |
| Condylomata acuminata | Genital warts | Fistula formation | Histologic scraping, PAP smear |
| Molluscum contagiosum | Papules on external genitalia | May spread to legs or abdomen | Biopsy lesion |

*Table continued on following page*

### TABLE 7–4. Assessment of Sexually Transmitted Disease *Continued*

| DISEASE | PATIENT'S COMPLAINTS AND SYMPTOMS | OTHER PHYSICAL EXAMINATION FINDINGS | DIAGNOSTIC STUDY |
|---|---|---|---|
| Trichomoniasis | Females: watery discharge with foul odor; dyspareunia<br>Males: rarely symptomatic; if so, watery urethral discharge and dysuria | | PAP smear, vaginal pH 7.5 |
| Amebiasis | Bloody diarrhea | | Intestinal biopsy |
| Giardiasis | Abdominal cramping; weight loss; greasy, bulky diarrhea | | Intestinal biopsy |
| Cryptosporidiosis | Nausea, vomiting, fever, abdominal cramps, diarrhea | Assess for excessive stool volume, dehydration | Acid-fast stain of stool<br>Intestinal biopsy |
| Pediculosis pubis | Pruritus | Assess hairy areas of entire body | Microscopic examination of hair follicles |
| Scabies | Itching | Assess for papules or burrows | Microscopic examination of scrapings |
| Strongyloidiasis | Diarrhea | Assess for dehydration | Direct stool specimen |
| Yeast vaginitis | Vulvular pruritus; white, clumpy discharge | Vaginal erythema | Vaginal pH 4.5<br>Direct smear of discharge |
| Balanoposthitis | Penile erythema | Desquamation, crusting, edema, or fissuring of prepuce | Direct isolation |

ing in a bathtub of lukewarm water and then drying well. If the patient seems to have a low tolerance for pain, the nurse may consult a physician regarding the use of mild analgesics or anti-inflammatory agents. The patient and nurse need to evaluate the effectiveness of these interventions.

All patients must be educated regarding safe sex to prevent the spread of the disease, recurrent infections, or both. The patient must refrain from sexual activity during the period of assessment, diagnosis, and treatment, and until a follow-up evaluation indicates a noncontagious state. Alternative affectionate methods of physical expression, such as nongenital massaging and nonerotic hugging, should be suggested until safe sexual activity can be resumed. Safe sex teaching should include the following:

1. Know your partner's sexual history.
2. Limit your own sexual encounters.
3. Practice low-risk sex (Table 7–5).
4. Avoid any exchange of body fluids.
5. Urinate and practice good hygiene before and after sexual contact.
6. Use correctly applied latex condoms and spermicidal cream.
7. Get regular checkups.

If the patient's previous coping mechanisms in dealing with crisis situations did not meet his or her expectations, the nurse may explore new coping mechanisms with the patient that may facilitate adaptation to the present crisis. The nurse may want to teach the patient relaxation or imagery techniques and encourage exercise as useful mechanisms to decrease stress.

It is important for the patient to leave the clinic or hospital with an acceptable self-image. Allow the patient to express his or her emotional response to learning the diagnosis. Allow the patient to ventilate feelings. Explain to the patient that you and your colleagues respect him or her as a person. The patient must be informed of expected body changes that may result from the treatment plan (e.g., le-

### TABLE 7–5. Risk Levels of Sexual Practices

| LOW RISK | MODERATE RISK | HIGH RISK |
|---|---|---|
| Dry kissing<br>Massage (nongenital)<br>Touching, hugging (nongenital)<br>Masturbation with healthy skin<br>Oral sex with a latex condom | Wet kissing<br>Masturbation on broken skin | Oral sex without a latex condom<br>Vaginal intercourse without a latex condom<br>Anal intercourse without a latex condom<br>Fisting (placing a fist into the rectum or vagina)<br>Rimming (oral-anal contact)<br>Watersports (urinating into a mucous membrane) |

sions may weep or crust, depending on the specific disease). Be sure the patient observes the lesions or edematous areas. The actual visualization of them may not be as negative as they may think and will assist in monitoring their progress. Often, these patients require reassurance that they are still worthy of giving and receiving love. Encourage the patient to continue a social life, excluding sexual practices at the present time. Once again, the disease was transmitted sexually; thus, routine asexual activities should not affect the patient. Before the patient leaves, be sure he or she is given ample time to ask any questions. Provide printed literature and a telephone number of the facility. An STD hotline number may also encourage the patient to call for support.

### Patient Outcomes
1. During the discussion of the specific disease, the patient exhibits an understanding of the teaching by
   a. Asking appropriate questions.
   b. Verbally participating in the discussion.
   c. Repeating pertinent information.
2. The patient states a willingness to notify sexual partners of the disease.
3. The patient does not have a recurrence of the disease.
4. The patient expresses a positive body image.
5. The patient expresses a positive self-image that includes coping skills.
6. The patient's skin is free of lesions.
7. The patient states that his or her physical comfort level has improved.
8. The patient verbalizes recent nonsexual social participation.

## REFERENCES

Centers for Disease Control: (1987). Recommendations for prevention of HIV transmission in health care settings. *Morbidity and Mortality Weekly Report, 36*(25), 35–185.

Centers for Disease Control: (1989). Sexually transmitted diseases: Treatment guidelines. *Morbidity and Mortality Weekly Report, 38*(suppl.), 35–385.

Centers for Disease Control: (1991). *Sexually transmitted disease surveillance, 1990.* Atlanta: Author.

Krieger, J. N. (1984). Biology of sexually transmitted diseases. *Urologic Clinics of North America, 11*(1), 18.

# PART III

# Tumors of the Genitourinary Tract

# CHAPTER 8

# Tumors of the Upper Urinary Tract

*Dorothy A. Calabrese and Mary Anne Matcham*

Tumors of the Adrenal Cortex
Tumors of the Adrenal Medulla—
  Pheochromocytoma

Tumors of the Renal Parenchyma
Tumors of the Renal Pelvis and Ureter

## OVERVIEW

The upper urinary tract consists of the adrenal glands, the kidneys, and the ureters. The percentage of cancer deaths from tumors originating in the upper tract is small, only about 2%. These tumors are difficult to detect, and they are not usually noticed until the patient begins to experience symptoms. Cancers of the upper urinary tract are more likely to occur in patients older than 40 years of age, and they are twice as common in men as in women.

Each year about 18,000 new cases of renal cell carcinoma are diagnosed. By comparison, the number of cases of cancer of the ureter and adrenal gland combined is estimated to be fewer than 150 annually. Cancer of the adrenal gland continues to have a high mortality rate.

This chapter describes the tumors occurring in the adrenal gland, the kidney, and the ureters. The complications associated with these tumors and current treatment modalities, as well as implications for nursing care, are discussed.

## BEHAVIORAL OBJECTIVES

After studying this chapter, the reader should be able to

1. Identify the sites and types of tumors of the upper urinary tract, the methods of treatment for each tumor, and possible complications resulting from these tumors.

2. Differentiate the etiology and pathophysiology of renal pelvic versus renal parenchymal tumors.

3. Compare and contrast the signs and symptoms, diagnostic workup, and treatment protocols for renal pelvic and renal parenchymal tumors.

4. Formulate a preoperative and postoperative plan of care for the patient with a diagnosis of renal tumor.

5. Identify nursing diagnoses, nursing interventions, and expected patient outcomes for the patient following surgery for adrenal and ureteral tumors.

## KEY WORDS

**Adrenal tumor**—a benign or malignant tumor of the adrenal gland; the tumor may be unilateral or bilateral, and may involve the cortex (causing adrenogenital syndrome or Cushing's syndrome) or the medulla (pheochromocytoma).

**Cushing's disease (or Cushing's syndrome)**—persistent adrenocortical hypersecretion of cortisol due to either a neoplasm, the excessive secretion of pituitary adrenocorticotropic hormone, or iatrogenic exogenous administration.

**Nephrectomy**—the surgical removal of the kidney. It may be simple (total removal of one kidney), partial (removal of only a portion of the kidney), radical (removal of the kidney and the perinephric fat), or bilateral (removal of both kidneys).

**Nephroureterectomy**—surgical removal of the kidney and ureter.

**Pheochromocytoma**—a tumor of the adrenal medulla that is usually benign. It causes increased secretion of the hormones epinephrine and norepinephrine. Typical symptoms include hypertension, headaches, and palpitations.

**Renal parenchyma**—that portion of the kidney that includes the renal cortex and medulla.

**Renal pelvis**—the main reservoir for the renal collecting system.

**Ureterectomy**—surgical removal of the ureter.

## TUMORS OF THE ADRENAL CORTEX

## Perspective on Disease Entity

### ETIOLOGY

The adrenal cortex makes up 80% of the adrenal gland, yet it is rare to find tumors occurring in this portion of the gland. Tumors found in the adrenal cortex comprise a spectrum of benign and malignant masses, including bilateral adrenal hyperplasia, benign adenoma, adrenal adenocarcinoma, and tumors causing primary hyperaldosteronism.

The incidence of adenocarcinoma of the adrenal cortex is about 2 in 1 million people, and it accounts for less than 0.2% of all cancer deaths combined. No etiologic factors have been identified for this highly malignant tumor. The diagnosis of adrenal cancer usually occurs after regional or distant metastasis; thus, prognosis is often poor. Although adenocarcinoma can be found in all decades of life, the median age at diagnosis is 40 years.

According to Brennan (1982), no data exist regarding the prevalence of benign tumors of the adrenal cortex. However, there are two medical conditions that can develop as a result of benign tumors of the adrenal cortex. The first is primary aldosteronism, or Conn's syndrome, a rare disorder caused by an aldosterone-secreting tumor of the adrenal cortex. It is two or three times more common in females and is most often seen between the ages of 30 and 60. This type of tumor is usually small in size, measuring only about 0.5 to 2 cm (Warner, 1988). The second medical condition that may arise from a mass of the adrenal cortex is Cushing's disease. This is seen more commonly in women and results primarily from a benign adenoma, although malignant-type growths may also cause the disease (Brennan, 1982). The benign adenomas are often slow-growing tumors that may be present for years before diagnosis, whereas the cancerous lesions tend to develop rapidly and metastasize quickly.

Nonfunctioning tumors (tumors that do not cause an increased production of hormones) are more common in males than in females. On the other hand, functioning tumors (those tumors that cause an increase in hormone production) occur more often in females, most of which are usually adrenocortical carcinomas (Warner, 1988). It is the functioning tumors that are responsible for the development of virilism and Cushing's disease.

## PATHOPHYSIOLOGY

Functioning tumors of the adrenal cortex (benign and malignant) can cause an increased production of those hormones normally secreted by the adrenal cortex, including aldosterone, cortisone, and the sex hormones. Usually, there is a predominant increase in one of the hormones. Although these hormones are considered essential to life, the overproduction of any given hormone will produce systemic effects.

An increased production of aldosterone leads to the increased reabsorption of sodium from the distal tubules of the kidney. This results in an increase in circulating blood volume, hypernatremia, and hypokalemia. It can also affect baroreceptors, causing hypotension, as well as carbohydrate intolerance from impaired insulin release secondary to hypokalemia.

The increased production of cortisone and corticosterone, otherwise known as *glucocorticoids*, leads to the symptoms of Cushing's disease. Features associated with Cushing's disease include marked facial roundness or "moon facies," buffalo hump, hirsutism, cutaneous striae, and truncal obesity with thin extremities.

Adrenal tumors can also cause the secretion of excessive quantities of the sex hormones. An increase in the production of androgens causes the following masculinizing effects in women: male pattern baldness, hirsutism, deepening voice, breast atrophy, decreased libido, and oligomenorrhea. The increased production of estrogen causes the following feminizing effects in men: gynecomastia, breast tenderness, testicular atrophy, and decreased libido.

The adrenocortical carcinomas invade locally to involve the retroperitoneum, diaphragm,

kidney, renal vein or vena cava, and pancreas. Metastatic spread commonly involves the regional lymph nodes, liver, lungs, bone, and brain.

Nonfunctioning tumors of the adrenal cortex tend to enlarge and eventually impinge or displace adjacent abdominal organs. The tumor may cause local pain; renal involvement may cause hematuria or infection. In some instances, the effects on adjacent structures will cause the patient to also experience weight loss, weakness, and fever.

## MEDICAL-SURGICAL MANAGEMENT

### Diagnosis

Most tumors of the adrenal glands are associated with hyperfunction. Because these growths are rarely palpable, interventional radiologic procedures, along with various laboratory studies, must be performed to verify the diagnosis. The diagnosis of an adrenocortical tumor is confirmed or disproved based on the results of the following tests.

**Radiologic Procedures**

1. Excretory urogram [or intravenous pyelogram (IVP)] and kidneys, ureters, and bladder (KUB)—done to delineate the tumor and to show displacement of the kidney or other abdominal structures.
2. Computed tomography (CT) scans—used to visualize the adrenal glands; often used as a screening method because the procedure is simple, noninvasive, and capable of detecting tumors smaller than 1 cm in diameter. A negative CT scan does not totally eliminate the possibility of adrenal carcinoma. CT scans of the abdomen and chest are also performed preoperatively if adrenal carcinoma is strongly suspected.
3. Adrenal venography—a less commonly used procedure, yet results can provide the functional location of the tumor causing primary aldosteronism (Conn's syndrome).
4. Angiography—an invasive study that can demonstrate an extensive vascular network and differentiate tumors of the adrenal gland from tumors of the upper pole of the kidney.
5. Nephrotomograms—usually done to support the diagnosis confirmed by other methods.
6. Ultrasound- or CT-guided needle biopsy—reportedly helps establish the diagnosis in more than 80% of cases (Jacobs & Goldin, 1987).

7. Bone scan—used to evaluate for metastatic disease when adrenocortical carcinoma is suspected.

### Laboratory Studies

The results of laboratory tests that specifically assess adrenocortical function are essential to the medical evaluation of a patient suspected of having a tumor of the adrenal cortex. These studies differentiate functioning from nonfunctioning tumors, diagnose adrenal hyperfunction or hypofunction, as well as distinguish among the various causes for adrenal dysfunction. As a general rule, the physician discontinues any medications that may interfere with laboratory results at least 1 week before the tests. This includes birth control pills or estrogens, which may increase renin and angiotensin levels and thus produce a false elevation in aldosterone, as well as diuretics, which decrease blood volume and induce secondary aldosteronism and hypokalemia (Forsham, 1992). Table 8–1 summarizes those laboratory tests used to measure adrenocortical function.

In primary aldosteronism, laboratory findings include a slight increase in the serum sodium level, a decrease in the serum potassium level, an elevated serum bicarbonate level, an increase in serum and urinary aldosterone levels, and an increase in extracellular fluid and blood volume. Additionally, there is a decrease in the plasma renin level. The key to establishing the diagnosis is finding elevated levels of urinary and plasma aldosterone together with unprovoked hypokalemia.

In Cushing's disease, there is an increase in the blood glucose level, as well as the level of glucose in the urine. Twenty-four hour urine collections demonstrate an elevation in 17-ketosteroids and 17-hydroxycorticosteroids if adrenal hyperplasia or adenocarcinoma is present (Forsham, 1992).

## Treatment

Once an adrenal mass has been diagnosed, surgical removal of the tumor is the treatment of choice. Preoperatively, patients receive a soluble preparation of cortisol, which helps main-

**TABLE 8–1. Tests of Adrenocortical Function**

| FUNCTION TEST | PROCEDURE AND PREPARATION | INTERPRETATION |
|---|---|---|
| ACTH stimulation test (various tests available) | Synthetic adrenocorticotropic hormone (ACTH) is given in 500–1000 mL of normal saline at 2 U/24 hr; then 17-OHCS and plasma cortisol levels are measured; alternative way is to infuse 25 units of ACTH over an 8-hr period on 2–3 days and measure 17-OHCS and plasma cortisol levels on these days. | Normally 17-OHCS excretion increases to 25 mg/24 hr, and plasma cortisol increases to 40 µg/100 ml or greater; in patients with secondary adrenal insufficiency, the 17-OHCS rate is 3–20 mg/24 hr, and the cortisol level is 10–40 µg/100 ml. |
| Screening ACTH stimulation test | ACTH, 25 U, is given IM, and plasma cortisol level is measured before and 30 and 60 min after tests. | Normally plasma cortisol increases 7 µg/100 ml. |
| Cortisone suppression test | Twenty-four-hour urine specimen for 17-OHCS is collected for baseline; dexamethasone, 0.5 mg, is given every 6 hr for 2 days; 24-hr urine is collected for these 2 days. | Dexamethasone suppresses pituitary secretion of ACTH and thus steroid levels; normally by second day of dexamethasone, 24-hr urinary level of OHCS should drop more than 50% below baseline. Patients with adrenocortical excess (primary) will not show decrease in 24-hour urine levels; patients with secondary adrenocortical excess will have drop, but less than 50%. |
| Screening suppression test | Dexamethasone, 1 mg, is given at 12 P.M. At 8 A.M. cortisol level is drawn. | Normally cortisol should be less than 5 µg/100 ml. |
| Mineralocorticoid suppression test (various tests are available) | Saline, 500 ml/hr, for 4 hr is infused intravenously. An alternative is that patient is placed on normal sodium diet (100 mEq) or high sodium diet (200 mEq). After patient is in sodium balance, deoxycorticosterone acetate (DOCA) (10 mg q12h) is administered IM for 3–5 days. | Normally saline infusion depresses plasma aldosterone to <8 µg/100 ml if patient has been on a sodium-restricted diet and to <5 µg/100 ml if patient has been on a normal sodium diet. Normal persons on a sodium diet of 100 mEq/day will have a 70% decrease in aldosterone. |

From Phipps, W. J., Long, B. C., Woods, N. F., & Cassmeyer, V. L. (Eds.). (1991). *Medical-surgical nursing: Concepts and clinical practice* (p. 1016). St. Louis: Mosby-Year Book. Reprinted by permission.

tain the balance of sodium and potassium, thereby preventing the occurrence of intraoperative hypotension (Cassmeyer, 1991). If the diagnosis is a benign adenoma or a tumor involving one adrenal gland, a unilateral adrenalectomy is performed, usually through a flank incision. Because there is one remaining adrenal gland that is functioning, hormonal replacement is seldom necessary. If the adrenal tumor has extended into the kidney, a nephrectomy with excision of regional lymph nodes also is performed. The contralateral adrenal gland must be assessed intraoperatively, because approximately 10% of these tumors occur bilaterally. Tumors that involve both adrenal glands require a bilateral adrenalectomy; in this situation, adequate steroid replacement becomes a priority intraoperatively and postoperatively and is a lifelong necessity.

Patients with primary aldosteronism who are not candidates for surgery, those with bilateral disease, and those who may have only mild symptoms of the disease may be treated with 100 to 200 mg/day of spironolactone (Aldactone) to prevent hypertension and hypokalemia. Chemotherapy for those with adrenal adenocarcinoma is used if patients are not candidates for surgery or have metastatic disease. Mitotane (Lysodren), an adrenal cytotoxic agent used to treat functioning and nonfunctioning malignant adrenal tumors, acts to modify the peripheral metabolism of steroids and to suppress the function of the adrenal cortex. Sometimes this therapy causes the tumor to shrink for a brief period. Side effects of mitotane are often quite severe and include nausea, vomiting, diarrhea, extreme lethargy, and headaches. In some instances, patients are treated with a combination of mitotane and 5-fluorouracil, although no single drug or combination of drugs has been proved to be successful in treating this type of tumor.

Adrenocortical carcinoma has a 5-year survival rate of less than 30%. For tumors that are found to be metastatic at the time of diagnosis, the average survival is approximately 8 months (Jacobs & Goldin, 1987; Vaughan & Blumenfeld, 1992).

## Approaches to Patient Care

### Assessment
The variability of clinical presentations makes diagnosis based on symptoms and physical examination difficult and unreliable. The patient may present with vague symptoms that are suggestive of numerous disorders or with symptoms that are fairly indicative of the overproduction of adrenal hormones. Therefore, as part of the nursing assessment, be sure to review the results of pertinent laboratory tests and to correlate those data with information from the health history and physical examination. This will allow you to more accurately determine the patient's state of health.

When completing the health history of the patient with a tumor causing Cushing's disease, ask about a history of fractures (due to osteoporosis), muscle weakness, emotional lability, decreased resistance to infections, hirsutism, amenorrhea, and ecchymosis. Also assess whether or not the patient has noticed any unusual changes in body contour, for example, weight gain or increased fat distribution on the face or trunk of the body. Patients suspected of having a tumor causing primary aldosteronism often describe symptoms such as muscle weakness, nocturia, sustained hypertension, fatigue, visual disturbances, polydipsia, and polyuria (symptoms of diabetes mellitus), paresthesias, and leg cramps.

The most common nonendocrine symptom described by patients with an adrenal tumor is pain, often caused by the displacement, obstruction, or destruction of the kidney. In addition, there may be abdominal distention. Symptoms of advanced malignancy, such as weight loss, anorexia, fever, and sweats, are common because an adrenal tumor is often not diagnosed until metastasis has occurred.

Because pain is often the symptom that precipitates a visit to the physician, the type and management of that pain should be a concern during the initial nursing assessment. Have patients rate the pain on a scale of 1 to 10 (1 being very mild pain and 10 being severe pain). Ask them how this discomfort compares with other types of pain they may have experienced, as well as how they have obtained relief from their discomfort. Once a baseline for the patients has been established, their reaction to various interventions can be more objectively evaluated.

The patient and his or her family may be anxious for many reasons, including unfamiliarity with the diagnosis of adrenal cancer and the disease's prognosis, unusual changes in physical appearance, or a lack of knowledge about possible treatments and their effects. Therefore, the nurse should assess the reasons for the anxiety and the patient's ability to comprehend health information and to participate in decision making regarding the illness, as well as to cooperate with diagnostic tests and selected therapies.

Nursing assessment of the patient with an adrenocortical tumor should also include the measurement of vital signs (particularly blood pressure), weight, 24-hour fluid intake and output, as well as an in-depth neuromuscular examination. A 3-day-recall nutritional history may also provide valuable information regarding the disease process.

**Nursing Diagnosis**

The nursing diagnoses for the patient with an adrenocortical tumor may include the following:

1. Anxiety related to an actual threat to one's personal integrity as a result of the diagnosis of an adrenocortical tumor.
2. Fear related to a lack of knowledge about the disease process, diagnostic testing, and treatment options for an adrenocortical tumor.
3. Pain related to
   a. Obstructed or displaced kidney due to extension of adrenocortical tumor.
   b. Flank incision for adrenalectomy.
4. Body image disturbance related to the systemic effects of an adrenal tumor.
5. Activity intolerance related to the effects of an adrenal tumor.
6. High risk for injury related to physical changes caused by adrenocortical dysfunction.
7. High risk for fluid volume excess or deficit related to adrenocortical dysfunction.

**Plan of Care**

Nursing care is directed toward enabling the patient to

1. Reduce anxiety to cooperate with diagnostic procedures and proposed medical or surgical interventions.
2. Verbalize an understanding of the diagnosis of an adrenocortical tumor and the disease prognosis, as well as expected outcomes for recommended treatments.
3. Obtain relief of discomfort.
4. Demonstrate acceptance of changes in physical appearance.
5. Prevent injury.
6. Maintain fluid balance.

**Interventions**

As with any patient suspected of cancer, the patient with a malignant adrenal tumor requires reassurance and support during the diagnosis and treatment period. The urologic nurse, often viewed as a reliable and dependable member of the health care team, may assist

the patient and family during this time by providing information about the diagnosis and its implications, planned diagnostic studies, medical-surgical interventions, as well as long-term care needs. Additionally, encourage patients to talk about any obvious changes to their physical appearances. Although grief and altered self-concept are feelings often expressed, help the patient to see that the essence of himself or herself as a person has not changed despite the outward appearance.

Preoperative care of the patient undergoing either unilateral or bilateral adrenalectomy for an adrenocortical tumor includes those preparatory activities necessary for any surgical patient. In addition, the nurse should monitor fluid and electrolyte levels, and assist with any corrections to prevent presurgical imbalances. This may involve the administration of intravenous fluids and glucocorticoids. The patient's nutritional intake should also be monitored to ensure that foods consumed contain the necessary vitamins and minerals. Hormonal therapy, if prescribed, should also be maintained.

Patients having adrenalectomy may be admitted to the intensive care unit following surgery, where they are closely monitored for as long as 48 hours. During this postoperative period, blood pressure, pulse, and fluid intake and output are monitored hourly; the blood glucose level is measured every 4 hours; serum electrolytes and body weight are measured daily, or more frequently if needed; and intravenous cortisol is administered for 24 to 48 hours (Cassmeyer, 1991). Other postoperative nursing care activities are summarized in Table 8–2.

The development of an adrenal crisis is a potential risk, especially for persons having bilateral adrenalectomy, because of the depletion of both glucocorticoids and mineralocorticoids. Signs and symptoms of acute adrenal insufficiency to which the urologic nurse should be alert include lethargy, irritability, confusion, hypoglycemia, unusual weakness, anorexia, nausea, vomiting, extreme hypotension, and electrolyte disturbances.

Weakness is a problem that is common after surgery and is brought on by shifts in cortisol levels. Because patients who have undergone adrenalectomy are at great risk for injury, the nurse should assess the environment and eliminate factors that may cause injury. Patients should be instructed to call for assistance when getting out of bed. Maintain the bed in a low position with the side rails raised and the call

## TABLE 8–2. Nursing Care of the Patient Undergoing Adrenal Surgery

**Preoperative**

1. Provide supportive care.
2. Assist patient with usual preoperative care.
3. Maintain nutritional status with a high-protein, prescribed calorie diet with adequate minerals and vitamins.
4. Assist with correction of fluid and electrolyte imbalance.
5. Assist with hormonal therapy as prescribed.
6. Assist with measures used to prevent or treat crises of adrenal hormonal excess or deficit.
7. Administer prescribed intravenous fluids and glucocorticoids before surgery.

**Postoperative**

1. Establish monitoring schedule to detect complications of surgery and
   a. Adrenal crisis.
   b. Blood pressure alterations.
   c. Blood glucose alterations.
   d. Fluid and electrolyte imbalances.
2. Because the patient may have unusual activity intolerance, pace postoperative activities with alternate periods of rest and a gradual increase in self-care.

3. Provide measures to minimize effects of postural hypotension:
   a. Supply Ace bandages or elastic stockings.
   b. Assess effects of posture on blood pressure.
   c. Assist or accompany the patient during ambulation while blood pressure remains labile.
4. Provide measures to decrease risk of infection in the immunosuppressed patient (for instance, strict surgical asepsis, coughing and deep breathing, avoiding contact with persons with upper respiratory infections).
5. Administer cortisol replacement as typically prescribed:
   a. Intravenous route for the first 24 to 48 hours.
   b. Oral route when patient is able to tolerate food by mouth.
6. Administer mineralocorticosteroid (fludrocortisone) replacement, if prescribed; typically prescribed when cortisol replacement is less than 40 to 50 mg/24 hours in the patient with bilateral adrenalectomy.
7. Assist patient and family in learning about required hormonal replacement.
   a. Bilateral adrenalectomy—maintenance dose of cortisol and mineralocorticoids.
   b. Unilateral adrenalectomy—doses of cortisol dependent on degree of suppression of hypothalamic-pituitary-adrenal axis.

From Phipps, W. J., Long, B. C., Woods, N. F., & Cassmeyer, V. L. (Eds.). (1991). *Medical-surgical nursing: Concepts and clinical practice* (p. 1085). St. Louis: Mosby-Year Book. Reprinted by permission.

button readily accessible. It may also be helpful to suggest to the patient ways to conserve energy, such using a bedside commode chair and coordinating similar activities at the same time.

For many patients, cortisol replacement therapy is necessary for a period after discharge from the hospital; patients who have had bilateral adrenalectomy require lifelong treatment. As the nurse preparing the patient for self-care in an environment away from the hospital, be sure that he or she knows the critical nature and effects of the medication, as well as any adverse reactions that may occur. Thoroughly review the dosage schedule, and strongly emphasize the importance of taking the medication according to the regimen prescribed. Patients should also be advised to carry some sort of medical identification on their persons at all times that indicates their need for daily cortisol replacement.

### Patient Outcomes

1. The patient recognizes his or her own anxiety and demonstrates the use of effective coping mechanisms to manage anxiety associated with discovery of the diagnosis of an adrenal tumor.
2. The patient verbalizes an understanding of diagnostic tests and treatment protocols for an adrenocortical tumor.

3. The patient verbalizes improvement of pain following the use of pain medications, or after noninvasive pain relief measures have been implemented.
4. The patient demonstrates acceptance of changes in physical appearance caused by the presence of a functioning adrenal tumor.
5. The patient uses safety measures to prevent injury.
6. The patient avoids fatigue by gradually increasing daily physical activity.
7. The patient's fluid and electrolyte levels remain balanced preoperatively and postoperatively.
8. The patient exhibits physical adjustment to cortisol replacement therapy and verbalizes the importance of compliance and risks of noncompliance with the prescribed drug regimen.

## TUMORS OF THE ADRENAL MEDULLA— PHEOCHROMOCYTOMA

## Perspective on Disease Entity

### ETIOLOGY

Tumors of the adrenal medulla consist of pheochromocytomas, ganglioneuromas, and sympathogoniomas. Pheochromocytomas are the most common of these tumors; the latter two are functionally inactive tumors. The prevalence of tumors occurring in the adrenal medulla is unknown, in part because of their rarity. However, it is estimated that approximately 400 new cases of pheochromocytoma are diagnosed each year (Brennan, 1982).

The exact etiology of pheochromocytoma is also unknown, but a familial tendency suggests a genetic defect (Harris & Dela Roca, 1984). Another theory suggests an autosomal dominant trait (Perkins, 1985). It can occur as an isolated, sporadic tumor or as part of a familial syndrome known as multiple endocrine neoplasia type II (MEN II), which consists of medullary carcinoma of the thyroid, hyperparathyroidism, Cushing's syndrome, and oral mucosal neuromas (Forsham, 1992).

Pheochromocytomas affect all races and both sexes and are most common between the ages of 40 and 60 years. This tumor type can occur in children, in which case it is usually bilateral, multiple, or extra-adrenal. When found in adults, it is usually unilateral and located in the adrenal gland. After surgical removal, there is a 10% to 13% chance of recurrence (Camunas, 1983).

## PATHOPHYSIOLOGY

Pheochromocytomas are usually benign, unilateral, and well-encapsulated tumors. To be considered malignant, metastasis must occur in areas where chromaffin tissue (composed of adrenomedullary-like cells that secrete catecholamines) does not usually occur, such as the bones, lung, liver, and spleen (Jacobs & Goldin, 1987; Perkins, 1985). Pheochromocytomas are often known as the "10% tumor" because 10% are bilateral and 10% are extra-adrenal (Donohue, 1988). Fewer than 5% of pheochromocytomas are truly malignant (Jacobs & Goldin, 1987). These are usually slow-growing tumors with a 5-year survival rate below 50% (Perkins, 1985).

The adrenal medulla produces and stores epinephrine and norepinephrine. These hormones have important metabolic and cardiovascular effects and function according to the "fight-or-flight" response of the body. The adrenal medulla is not essential to life, because the sympathetic nervous system produces a similar response. The sympathetic responses, however, are slower and less extensive.

The presence of a pheochromocytoma causes an increased production of catecholamines. The result is paroxysmal attacks of systolic and diastolic hypertension along with related symptoms, such as headache, increased sweating, flushing, and tachycardia with palpitations, all caused by an excess of epinephrine. Postural hypotension also occurs frequently as a result of the ganglionic blocking of normal pressor pathways by the increase in catecholamines (Forsham, 1992). Following an attack, the patient may experience intense weakness, gastrointestinal disturbances, and emotional irritability.

These attacks seem to occur for any or no apparent reason and may be precipitated by emotional upset, exercise, or straining with a bowel movement. Although pheochromocytomas are rarely palpable, even pressure over the site of the tumor may be sufficient to trigger a hypertensive crisis (Forsham, 1992). The attacks can last for several minutes to as long as several hours, then subside spontaneously. Because these episodes resemble the alarm phase of the stress response, a hypertensive crisis may result (Harris & Dela Roca, 1984).

## MEDICAL-SURGICAL MANAGEMENT

### Diagnosis

The most effective way of establishing the diagnosis of pheochromocytoma is to demonstrate the increased production of urinary catecholamines and vanillylmandelic acid (VMA). The diagnostic accuracy of these measurements alone will detect 95% to 98% of all pheochromocytomas (Donohue, 1988; Forsham, 1992).

A 24-hour urine collection is the test performed to measure excess quantities of metanephrine, normetanephrine, and VMA, all of which are byproducts of epinephrine and norepinephrine. The levels of epinephrine, norepinephrine, and dopamine, the so-called free catecholamines, may also be measured with this same specimen. To obtain a reliable 24-hour urine collection, the physician will order that the patient be restricted from all foods and fluids containing vanilla or aspirin for 2 to 3 days before the start of the collection. All medications, except for diuretics, digitalis, and barbiturates, must also be discontinued (Forsham, 1992; Pagana & Pagana, 1990). Table 8–3 lists the normal levels for VMA and catecholamines when measured from a 24-hour urine specimen. The measurement of plasma catecholamines as a diagnostic indicator of pheochromocytoma is somewhat controversial because

**TABLE 8–3. Twenty-Four Hour Urine Tests for VMA and Catecholamines: Normal Values**

| TEST | NORMAL VALUE |
|---|---|
| VMA | 1–9 mg/24 |
| Epinephrine | <40 μg/24 h |
| Metanephrine | 24–96 μg/24 h |
| Norepinephrine | 10–100 μg/24 h |
| Normetanephrine | 75–375 μg/24 h |

VMA, vanillylmandelic acid.

Data from Forsham, P. H. (1992). Disorders of the adrenal glands. In E. A. Tanagho & J. W. McAninch (Eds.), *Smith's general urology* (13th ed., pp. 495–514). Norwalk, CT: Appleton & Lange; and Pagana, K. D., & Pagana, T. J. (1990). *Diagnostic testing and nursing implications: A case study approach.* St. Louis: C. V. Mosby.

of the highly responsive nature of these substances to stimuli such as stress, activity, and blood loss (Vaughan & Blumenfeld, 1992). Similarly, pharmacologic agents such as glucagon and histamine are rarely used in testing because of the resultant increase in blood pressure.

Once confirmed, the tumor may be localized by excretory urography, ultrasonography, angiography, and computed tomographic (CT) scans. In recent years, magnetic resonance imaging (MRI) has also proved valuable in identifying tumors and defining their anatomic limits (Vaughan & Blumenfeld, 1992).

If a pheochromocytoma outside the adrenal gland is suspected, a wide range of diagnostic tests is used to delineate tumor sites. These tests can include renal, adrenal, and celiac arteriograms; excretory urography; aortogram; and upper gastrointestinal tract series.

## Treatment

Because the tumor is resistant to radiation or chemotherapy, the treatment of choice following diagnosis of a pheochromocytoma is surgical removal (Perkins, 1985). In preparation for surgery, the patient is started on phenoxybenzamine (Dibenzylene) for as long as 3 weeks before hospitalization to control blood pressure and to correct hypovolemia.

The induction of anesthesia and the stress of the surgical procedure are events that can precipitate a hypertensive crisis. Therefore, care must be exercised to maintain the blood pressure at a near normal level to enable the physician to excise the tumor. Often, an intravenous infusion of phentolamine (Regitine), 5 mg in 200 mL of 5% dextrose, is administered intraoperatively to control the patient's blood pressure (Forsham, 1992).

During surgery the tumor is handled as little as possible because excess manipulation can lead to the increased production of catecholamines. Once the adrenal vein has been carefully ligated, the tumor is removed with its capsule intact through a transabdominal or thoracoabdominal incision. After the tumor has been removed, there will naturally be a decrease in blood pressure that may necessitate the administration of a pressor agent to reestablish the patient to a normotensive level (Forsham, 1992).

The usual outcome for the patient is complete remission of the symptoms unless the tumor has metastasized to other sites. To verify that tumor was completely excised, another 24-hour urine collection for VMA is performed on the second or third postoperative day. If an increase in VMA levels persists after surgery, the pheochromocytoma continues to exist elsewhere in the body (Cassmeyer, 1991; Forsham, 1992).

## Approaches to Patient Care

### Assessment
Nursing assessment of the patient suspected of having a pheochromocytoma should consist of identifying those symptoms associated with the paroxysmal elevations of blood pressure. Ask the patient about the following:

Episodes of rapid pulse, chest pain, palpitations, or angina.

Frequency, duration, and severity of headaches.

Neuromuscular changes such as tremors, weakness, extreme nervousness, or attacks of anxiety.

Excessive sweating, heat intolerance, flushing, fevers, or recent weight loss.

Nausea, vomiting, epigastric pain, or other gastrointestinal disturbances.

Episodes of rapid respiration and hyperventilation.

Also inquire about any prescription or over-the-counter medications the patient may be taking, dietary habits, activities that precipitate hypertension, as well as the initial onset, frequency, and duration of the hypertensive events. While completing the nursing health history, take this time to assess the patient's knowledge and understanding of pheochromocytoma, its association with the symptoms he or she is experiencing, and the proposed treatment for the disease. It may be helpful to also determine if the patient is capable of blood pressure self-measurement, or if a family member or friend knows or is willing to learn the procedure.

As part of the physical examination, be sure to include the following:

Measure the patient's blood pressure in the supine, sitting, and standing positions.
Measure the patient's pulse and respiration rates.
Obtain an accurate measurement of the patient's body weight.
Obtain a sample of blood to check for elevations in the serum glucose level.
Perform a thorough neuromuscular examination.

Additionally, the nurse would want to assess the patient's daily fluid intake and output patterns and to review recent laboratory studies for abnormalities in serum electrolyte levels.

**Nursing Diagnosis**

The nursing diagnoses for the patient with pheochromocytoma may include the following:

1. Anxiety related to the perceived threat to one's self caused by the increased production of catecholamines.
2. Activity intolerance related to symptoms associated with paroxysmal hypertension.
3. High risk for injury related to effects of hypertensive episodes, hypovolemia, or postural hypotension.
4. Fear related to a lack of knowledge regarding diagnosis of pheochromocytoma and treatment alternatives.

**Plan of Care**

Nursing care is directed toward enabling the patient to

1. Identify coping mechanisms that will assist in the management of anxiety during hypertensive episodes.
2. Limit physical activity during and after a hypertensive episode to prevent injury.
3. Verbalize an understanding of the diagnosis and treatment for pheochromocytoma to relate psychological comfort.

**Interventions**

The physical and psychological changes that the patient experiences due to the increased production of catecholamines can be frightening. To help the patient cope with these episodes, the nurse should begin by explaining the disease process. Because paroxysmal hypertensive events may occur as a result of physical exertion or stress, suggest that the patient

avoid any seemingly strenuous activity like bending, lifting, or the Valsalva maneuver (Cassmeyer, 1991). Explain that postural hypotension may cause the patient to feel weak and lightheaded, and caution the patient to gradually increase activities after an attack to avoid injury. Ascertain that the patient, or a family member or friend, is able to perform blood pressure self-measurement; this helps monitor the severity and duration of the episodes.

In preparation for surgery, the patient will participate in the 24-hour urine collection to measure VMA and catecholamine levels. Thoroughly explain the procedure for collecting the urine, and inform the patient of dietary or activity restrictions that may be necessary to obtain accurate measurements of epinephrine and norepinephrine levels. Be certain that the collection container has had a preservative added to it; this is usually done by the laboratory and consists of 10 mL of concentrated HCl (Pagana & Pagana, 1990). Other preoperative nursing care activities consist of close monitoring of the patient's blood pressure, neurologic status, serum electrolytes, and fluid intake and output, as well as explaining the surgical procedure and postoperative care activities and needs. When oral alpha-adrenergic blockers are unable to control the patient's blood pressure, the nurse may need to assist with the maintenance of a phentolamine infusion to keep the blood pressure at a safe level (Cassmeyer, 1991).

Postoperative management of the patient who has undergone an adrenalectomy for pheochromocytoma consists of nursing activities common to any surgical patient, in addition to the continued monitoring of blood pressure, neurologic status, and serum electrolyte levels. Intravenous fluids are usually administered to counteract the effects of postoperative hypotension and to prevent fluid volume deficit. In preparation for discharge from the hospital, the nurse should help the patient develop a plan to gradually increase and resume normal physical activity. Discharge teaching should also include counseling regarding diet, blood pressure monitoring, and follow-up visits with the urologist, as well as information about medications, if prescribed.

**Patient Outcomes**

1. The patient recognizes his or her anxiety, and uses effective coping mechanisms to manage anxious episodes.
2. The patient limits preoperative physical activity, then gradually increases activity after surgery to prevent injury.
3. The patient's blood pressure is controlled

preoperatively with medications and returns to a normal level following surgery.

4. The patient's fluid and serum electrolyte levels are stabilized.

5. The patient, family member, or friend is able to demonstrate the proper procedure for blood pressure measurement.

6. The patient verbalizes the importance of continued follow-up with the urologist.

# TUMORS OF THE RENAL PARENCHYMA

## Perspective on Disease Entity

### ETIOLOGY

Approximately 85% of all primary malignant tumors of the renal parenchyma are adenocarcinoma, also known as *renal cell carcinoma* (RCC) (Dreicer & Williams, 1992). This tumor type has also been called *Grawitz's tumor, hypernephroma,* and *clear cell carcinoma.*

The average age at diagnosis for the person with RCC is between 55 and 60 years. There is a 2:1 male to female occurrence. The incidence of frequency is identical between blacks and whites. However, Hispanics develop kidney cancer at a rate one third higher than do whites (Dreicer & Williams, 1992). Genetic influences have been attributed to the development of RCC. Case findings demonstrate that it has occurred in more than one family member (Cohen et al., 1979). RCC has an increased incidence in patients with horseshoe kidneys, polycystic kidney disease, acquired renal cystic disease from chronic renal failure, as well as in those with Von Hippel–Lindau syndrome, an autosomal dominant disease.

Although the cause of RCC is unknown, similar tumors have been produced experimentally with certain agents. Some studies demonstrate a definite correlation between RCC and cigarette smoking. The increased use or abuse of analgesics, particularly those containing phenacetin, is also attributed to the development of RCC. Hormonal influences have been questioned because of the increased number of cases found in males compared with females; exposure to some industrial substances, the excessive use of caffeine products and diuretics, and obesity have also been proposed as risk factors for RCC.

Benign tumors of the kidney, such as adenoma, are usually asymptomatic during a person's life. For this reason, they are commonly found only on autopsy. Despite its classification as a benign tumor, there is really no clinical or histologic difference between renal adenoma and RCC. Thus, the risk of RCC is higher when a renal adenoma is present. It is for this reason that a renal adenoma is commonly treated as an early renal cancer, if it is detected.

### PATHOPHYSIOLOGY

Sudek proposed in 1893 that RCC arises from renal tubular cells (Bennington & Beckwith, 1975). This was confirmed in 1960 when renal adenocarcinoma cells and proximal convoluted tubule cells were compared using an electron microscope. As is now known, RCC originates in the renal cortex, arising from proximal renal tubular epithelium. It expands to compress renal tissue, distorting the contour of the kidney and its collecting systems. As the mass grows, it may spread by direct invasion through the renal capsule and into the perinephric space, creating a bulge that is characteristic of the tumor. Tumors may also spread by direct extension into the renal vein and vena cava.

RCC can occur in the upper or lower pole of either kidney. Most tumors measure approximately 7 to 8 cm in diameter; however, some may grow to fill the entire retroperitoneum or may be of a size to completely occlude vessels. The larger tumors tend to be hemorrhagic and necrotic masses that are dotted with cystic areas or calcifications (Dreicer & Williams, 1992).

Metastatic disease is often present in one third of patients at the time of diagnosis and may occur via the lymphatics or a hematogenous route. The lung is the most common site for distant metastasis; other areas to which the disease is likely to spread include the liver, bone, adjacent regional lymph nodes, adrenal gland, and contralateral kidney.

There are several factors that are used to predict the survival of patients with RCC. The most common and consistent variable is the pathologic stage of the tumor at the time of presentation or surgical intervention (Thrasher & Paulson, 1993). Using either the Robson et al. (1969) or tumor-node-metastasis (TNM) (American Joint Committee on Cancer, 1988) classification, the physician is able to define the anatomic extent of disease to render a prognosis (Tables 8–4 and 8–5). Other factors that are believed to affect survival and, therefore, are closely analyzed include (1) nuclear grade of tumor cells, (2) tumor cell type, (3) histologic

TABLE 8–4. Robson Staging System for Renal Cell
Carcinoma

| STAGE | DESCRIPTION |
|---|---|
| I | Tumor is isolated within the renal capsule |
| II | Tumor extends to the perinephric fat and/or adrenal gland, but within Gerota's fascia |
| IIIA | Growth of tumor extends to the renal vein or vena cava |
| IIIB | Growth of tumor involves regional lymph nodes |
| IIIC | Growth of tumor extends to both vessels and lymph nodes (IIIA + IIIB) |
| IVA | Tumor spreads to adjacent organs (other than ipsilateral adrenal gland) |
| IVB | Distant metastases evident |

or architectural pattern of the tumor, (4) tumor size, and (5) tumor deoxyribonucleic acid content. Demographic variables such as age, race, and sex have been examined for their prognostic significance, but studies have shown that these are not definitive clues to patient survival. Presenting signs and symptoms, although not specific indicators of the chance for survival, often correlate with the stage and grade of the tumor and the presence of advanced disease (Thrasher & Paulson, 1993).

## MEDICAL-SURGICAL MANAGEMENT

### Diagnosis

One method used to confirm the diagnosis of RCC is to analyze the results of various laboratory studies. A urinalysis is usually the first study performed, because as many as 60% of patients presenting with RCC have either gross or microscopic hematuria (Dreicer & Williams, 1992). Anemia is found in 30% of patients with RCC and is probably due to bone marrow depression caused by the tumor-toxic effect (Pritchett et al., 1988). Therefore, a complete blood count (CBC), including hemoglobin, hematocrit, red blood cell count, and erythrocyte sedimentation rate should be performed. Measurement of serum iron and total iron-binding capacity is also indicated, because these values are low in patients with anemia secondary to RCC. The measurement of serum calcium levels may demonstrate hypercalcemia, which is present in about 15% of patients with RCC and is believed to be related to bone metastasis. Along with this, the full complement of serum electrolytes levels should also be measured. Other pertinent laboratory findings might include a prolonged prothrombin time; abnormal

liver function studies, which usually occur when liver metastasis is present; elevated urine lactic dehydrogenase (LDH) levels, which are found in those with malignant renal tumors but are absent in those with benign renal cysts; and elevated levels of renin, believed to be secreted by renal tumor cells and associated with the hypertension experienced by nearly 40% of patients.

Radiologic tests offer a more definitive way to diagnose RCC. Improvement in the quality of equipment and procedures has made it possible for early detection, even in asymptomatic patients. The following is a description of the radiologic procedures that may be used to evaluate suspicious renal lesions.

1. Plain or KUB film—may show enlargement or distortion of the kidney, which may suggest a renal mass.

TABLE 8–5. Tumor Stage of Renal Cell Cancer
Defined by TNM: Current American Joint
Committee on Cancer Recommendations for
Staging

**Primary Tumor (T)**

| | |
|---|---|
| TX | Primary tumor cannot be assessed |
| $T_0$ | No evidence of primary tumor |
| $T_1$ | Tumor ≤2.5 cm in greatest dimension limited to kidney |
| $T_2$ | Tumor >2.5 cm in greatest dimension limited to kidney |
| $T_3$ | Tumor extends into major veins or invades adrenal gland or perinephric tissues but not beyond Gerota's fascia |
| $T_{3a}$ | Tumor invades adrenal gland or perinephric tissues but not beyond Gerota's fascia |
| $T_{3b}$ | Tumor grossly extends to renal vein(s) or vena cava |
| $T_4$ | Tumor extends into adjacent or distant organs |

**Regional Lymph Nodes (N)**

| | |
|---|---|
| NX | Regional lymph nodes cannot be assessed |
| $N_0$ | No regional lymph node metastasis |
| $N_1$ | Metastasis in a single lymph node ≤2 cm in greatest dimension |
| $N_2$ | Metastasis in a single lymph node >2 cm but not >5 cm in greatest dimension, or multiple lymph nodes, none >5 cm in greatest dimension |
| $N_3$ | Metastasis in a lymph node >5 cm in greatest dimension |

**Distant Metastasis (M)**

| | |
|---|---|
| MX | Presence of distant metastasis cannot be assessed |
| $M_0$ | No distant metastasis |
| $M_1$ | Distant metastasis |

From Montie, J. E., Pontes, J. E., & Bukowski, R. M. (1990). *Clinical management of renal cell cancer* (p. 16). Chicago: Year Book. Reprinted with permission of C. V. Mosby.

2. Excretory urogram (or IVP)—may show distortion of the renal collecting system or a filling defect, both of which are characteristic features of a renal mass.
3. Renal ultrasonography—a safe, cost-effective, and noninvasive way to differentiate a renal cyst from a solid tumor.
4. CT scans—widely used to differentiate cystic versus solid masses; used to specify the density of the renal mass; also useful in determining whether or not there is renal vein, vena caval, or lymph node involvement.
5. Arteriography—demonstrates tumor vascularity, including the presence of arteriovenous fistulas; also reveals the extent of the lesion and its blood supply network.
6. Magnetic resonance imaging—used to demonstrate involvement with adjacent tissues, renal vein, vena cava, and lymph nodes to stage renal tumor.
7. Radionuclide isotope scanning—used to determine the presence or absence of metastatic disease associated with RCC.

Percutaneous needle aspiration and biopsy represent another method by which a renal mass may be evaluated. In general, this procedure is performed only when the lesion is believed to be cystic and fluid is needed for cytologic evaluation.

## Treatment

Operative selections for the management of RCC include the following procedures:

Partial nephrectomy—used for patients with bilateral renal tumors or those with a solitary kidney.

Radical nephrectomy—used to treat nonmetastatic RCC; involves the removal of the kidney and Gerota's fascia, proximal ureter, ipsilateral adrenal, and regional lymph nodes (either left para-aortic or right paracaval).

Extended lymphadenectomy—performed as an adjunct to radical nephrectomy; ensures the removal of all lymph nodes that may harbor metastases; if performed on the left side, preaortic, para-aortic, retroaortic, and precaval lymph nodes are removed; if performed on the right side, precaval, paracaval, retrocaval, and preaortic lymph nodes are removed.

In some instances, preoperative renal artery embolization may be used prior to a nephrectomy to reduce blood loss during the operation. It may also be used to palliate pain or hematuria in a patient who is not a candidate for radical nephrectomy. The postinfarction period is often associated with fever, flank pain, and leukocytosis, which lasts for approximately 3 days.

For patients with extension of a tumor thrombus into the vena cava and right atrium, removal of tumor is accomplished with the use of cardiopulmonary bypass and deep hypothermic circulatory arrest. The procedure requires that the surgeon make a thoracoabdominal incision, which extends from the tip of the scapula, across the costal margin, approximately halfway between the umbilicus and xiphoid process of the sternum. Following cannulation of the aorta and right atrium, the patient is connected to the bypass machine, and the process of cooling the body begins. ''Cooling is facilitated by iced saline lavage of the abdominal and chest cavities. When a core temperature of 18° to 20° has been achieved, cardiopulmonary bypass is terminated, and the blood volume is drained into the pump'' (Klein et al., 1991, p. 446). From this point, the surgeon has about 40 to 60 minutes of safe, cold ischemia to complete the dissection. Tumors have been successfully removed from the vena cava, as well as the atria and ventricles of the heart, using this method (Klein et al., 1991; Marshall, 1991). Postoperative complications that may occur following the use of cardiac bypass and hypothermia include hemorrhage, platelet dysfunction, deep vein thrombosis, wound infection, pneumonia, cecal volvulus, pancreatitis, adrenal insufficiency, and acute renal failure (Klein et al., 1991).

Although radiation therapy is controversial in the treatment of RCC, it is used for symptomatic relief of pain from bone metastasis, particularly that which causes spinal cord compression. There are no research findings that show any benefit from preoperative radiation. Postoperative radiation, although it does nothing to prevent distant metastases, can reduce the incidence of local tumor recurrence in patients with gross residual disease. Some of the side effects of radiation therapy are a sunburn-type red patch, nausea, vomiting, diarrhea, and stomach cramps. The side effects experienced by patients differ depending on the area irradiated.

During the past 30 years, as many as 72 cytotoxic drugs have been studied for their therapeutic affect on RCC (Yagoda et al., 1993). Single and combination therapies have been explored, yet none has emerged as an effective treatment for this type of solid tumor. Although studies continue, many researchers are coming to the conclusion that RCCs are not responsive to cytotoxic drugs. "In fact, one must consider the possibility that the few remissions that do occur in renal cancer trials are not attributable to any cytotoxic effect leading directly to cell death but rather to some positive indirect action influencing the patient's immune system" (Yagoda et al., 1993, p. 303).

There is also interest in various hormonal agents as a treatment for RCC. No study to date, however, has proved their efficacy. Progesterone therapy continues as the preferred hormonal treatment for advanced RCC in the absence of other alternatives.

Immunotherapy with bacillus Calmette-Guérin (BCG), infusion of autologous tumor cells, and immune ribonucleic acid has been used for the treatment of RCC. Current protocols, however, are investigating the effectiveness of agents such as interferon (INF)-alpha, INF-beta, INF-gamma, and interleukin-2 (IL-2). These biologic modifiers are given to increase the antitumor responsiveness of the immune system to the growth of tumor cells. Over the years, an average overall response rate of less than 20% for individual preparations has been somewhat disappointing. Nonetheless, there is promising research suggesting the combination of various biologic response modifiers (INF-alpha + IL-2; lymphokine-activated killer [LAK] cells + IL-2; or tumor-infiltrating lymphocytes + LAK + IL-2) may improve outcomes and decrease treatment side effects (deKernion & Belldegrun, 1992; Dreicer & Williams, 1992; Wirth, 1993).

## Approaches to Patient Care

### Assessment

When completing a nursing history on the patient suspected of having RCC, the nurse should inquire specifically about the presence or absence of pain, because it is the most common complaint or symptom in 50% of patients. The type of pain most frequently described is a dull ache in the flank area, which in 40% to 50% of patients is caused by the primary tumor. Severe pain is usually associated with metastatic invasion. Therefore, carefully question the patient about the location and severity of the discomfort. Methods used to relieve the discomfort as well as pain medications that the patient may be taking should be documented.

As part of a nutritional assessment, inquire about any recent changes in the patient's body weight, especially weight loss. The patient's normal weight, approximate number of pounds lost, and the period of time over which the weight loss occurred should be documented. Ask about any food sensitivities, as well as gastrointestinal disturbances such as nausea, vomiting, change in bowel habits, and flatulence.

Hematuria is a frequent complaint among patients with RCC. Therefore, ask the patient to carefully describe the appearance of his or her urine, including when the change from the characteristic clear-yellow color occurred. Most patients will describe gross hematuria, although many are also found to have microscopic blood in the urine. The bleeding is usually painless unless clots are being passed, in which case the patient may relate symptoms suggestive of ureteral colic.

On physical examination, a palpable flank mass may be found in about 50% of patients. Other striking features include edema in the legs and genitalia and dilated surface veins on the abdominal wall. Ascites may be found when there is complex obstruction of the vena cava.

During the initial assessment, the urologic nurse should determine what the patient knows about the diagnosis, prognosis, and treatment plan for RCC. If an experimental treatment protocol is being proposed, determine the patient's understanding, as well as his or her ability and willingness to comply with the program. Because many of these therapies are offered only at major academic medical centers, find out if there are any obstacles to receiving treatment outside of the patient's own community, particularly the availability of reliable transportation and a travel companion. Also discuss any concerns the patient may have regarding the financial responsibilities for hospitalization and treatment, and determine if a consultation with social services may be necessary.

In preparation for discharge and home care, the nurse must begin to consider the following: (1) the extent of the disease and chance for survival; (2) the amount of care that is required postoperatively or following systemic treatments; (3) the availability of a consistent caregiver in the home, as well as other support persons; (4) living environment; and (5) physical or psychological limitations that may affect or impede recovery.

### Nursing Diagnosis

Nursing diagnoses for the patient with renal cell carcinoma may include the following:

1. Anxiety related to perceived threat to physical well-being associated with a diagnosis of malignant disease.
2. Decisional conflict related to a lack of understanding or information about treatment protocols.
3. Pain related to
   a. Compression of kidney by growth of tumor.
   b. Extension of tumor to the renal vein or vena cava or into the retroperitoneum.
   c. Surgical trauma (radical nephrectomy).
   d. Metastatic disease.
4. Alteration in pattern of urinary elimination related to
   a. Presence of hematuria.
   b. Placement of urinary drainage devices after radical nephrectomy.
5. High risk for fluid volume excess (preoperatively) related to extension of the tumor to renal vein and vena cava with subsequent vessel occlusion.
6. High risk for fluid volume deficit (postoperatively) related to hemorrhage.
7. High risk for altered tissue perfusion related to the effects of cardiac bypass and hypothermia.
8. High risk for ineffective breathing patterns related to pain and limited chest expansion due to surgical trauma.
9. High risk for altered health maintenance related to insufficient knowledge about home care needs.

**Plan of Care**

Nursing care is directed toward enabling the patient to

1. Identify methods of coping to reduce anxiety.
2. Verbalize an understanding of the diagnosis and chance for survival from RCC.
3. Make informed decisions about participation in treatment protocols.
4. Verbalize pain relief or improved comfort.
5. Maintain an adequate urine output of at least 30 mL/hr.
6. Avoid problems associated with fluid volume excess or deficit.
7. Maintain adequate tissue perfusion.
8. Sustain adequate respiratory function postoperatively.
9. Prepare for health care needs at home.

**Interventions**

Patients diagnosed with RCC, like most newly diagnosed cancer patients, express feelings of anxiety and fear. Their anxiety may stem from the realization that there is a limited choice of treatment modalities. It may also be due to the fact that he or she might be asked to participate in a clinical trial of an experimental therapy. Often, anxiety is caused by a lack of information or a misunderstanding of information. Find out what the patient knows, clarify fallacies, and provide whatever additional information is necessary for the patient to make an informed decision regarding treatment. It may be beneficial to introduce the patient to another person who has undergone treatment for RCC similar to what he or she has been asked to consider. A referral to the National Kidney Cancer Association for additional information on kidney cancer research or counseling may also be helpful.

Many patients are admitted to the hospital the morning of surgery; they will receive a laxative the day before surgery and will be on a clear liquid diet for 1 to 2 days. If they are admitted to the hospital a day before surgery, preoperative nursing care for the patient undergoing surgery for removal of RCC may include the administration of laxatives or enema; clear liquid diet and antibiotics as part of a bowel preparation program; maintenance of intravenous fluids; and assistance with a body wash and shave, particularly the chest and back areas, according to the institution's operating room policy. In addition, it is important to verify and record if the patient has arranged for dedicated donation or autodonation of blood for use during surgery. Check with the hospital's blood bank to be sure the blood is ready and available immediately prior to the operation.

Patients whose radical nephrectomy was performed using cardiac bypass and hypothermia will be transferred to the intensive care unit following surgery to stay for 24 to 48 hours. Those undergoing a traditional radical nephrectomy usually are returned to their assigned rooms on the acute care unit.

During the immediate postoperative period the nurse is required to manage intravenous fluids and other supports, such as oxygen, cardiac monitors, and patient-controlled analgesia devices for pain management. Vital signs may need to be checked as frequently as every hour for the first 24 hours. On inspection, the nurse should note a large dressing over the surgical incision and the presence of wound drains. There may be some drainage evident from the operative site for 2 to 3 days following surgery, after which time the dressings and drains are usually removed.

Because the patient has one remaining kidney following surgery, it is essential to closely monitor fluid intake and urinary output at least every 8 hours. Discrepancies in fluid balance during the immediate postoperative period may be due to excessive blood loss, poor renal tissue perfusion, or the administration of increased intravenous fluids during surgery. Bladder drainage by means of an indwelling Foley catheter is maintained for several days; the length of time depends on the physician's protocol. In the immediate postoperative period, there may be blood in the urine, but this diminishes and urine returns to the characteristic clear-amber or -yellow color. The physician should be notified if there is an increase in hematuria or the presence of blood clots in the urine. Keep in mind that the presence of a urethral catheter may be a source for entry of bacteria into the lower urinary tract; therefore, monitor vital signs and blood studies for indications of an infection. Prior to catheter removal, a sample of urine should be obtained for culture.

Because of the trauma caused by the flank incision, the patient who has had a radical nephrectomy may exhibit guarded or shallow respirations, and is also at risk for developing a pneumothorax. Most patients express their reluctance to take deep breaths because of the extreme pain experienced when doing so. It is important to explain the rationale for aggressive pulmonary exercises to the patient, and if necessary, initially to adjust the dosage of pain medication to help the patient comply with therapy. Lung sounds should be auscultated each time vital sign measurements are obtained to detect atelectasis or pneumonia; at first, this may be done as frequently as every hour. Be sure to note whether or not the patient has a history of respiratory disease or is a smoker, because this will have an impact on the postoperative respiratory status. The use of an incentive spirometer should be encouraged to assist with coughing and deep-breathing exercises; the patient's goal should be a minimum of 10 deep breaths followed by a cough every hour. To assist with coughing, a pillow splint may be used to support the flank incision. More aggressive therapy may be ordered if needed.

Bowel function resumes in about 3 to 5 days after surgery. Once there are audible bowel sounds and the patient begins to pass gas, oral fluids may be started and the patient's diet should be gradually advanced to solid food. The patient should have a bowel movement within 1 week of surgery; if not, then stool softeners or laxatives may be administered.

Pain medication is switched to oral preparations when the patient is started on a liquid diet. Careful pain assessment must be carried out at regular intervals during this transition period to verify the patient's response to oral pain medications. It may be necessary to initiate noninvasive pain relief methods, such as relaxation techniques, alternative positioning, and distraction. As with any surgical patient, early ambulation is integral to recovery. Complex movements, like getting into and out of bed, will be difficult because of the large flank incision and the trauma to surrounding muscles and tissue. With support from the nurse, however, the patient should be able to get out of bed and walk increasing distances each day.

Assuming there have been no serious postoperative complications, the patient is discharged home approximately 5 to 7 days after surgery. Home care instructions should include the following information:

Avoid heavy lifting and exercises requiring excess exertion (including stair climbing).
Do not drive a car for at least 4 weeks.
Take several short walks each day.
Sponge bathing is recommended; however, showering may be permissible, depending on the type of dressing over the surgical wound, the amount of healing that has occurred, and the physician's protocol.
Increase dietary fiber and fluids to avoid constipation, and maintain adequate urinary output.
Notify the physician or nurse if any of the following symptoms occur: fever, chest pain, respiratory difficulties, abdominal cramps, nausea, vomiting, pain or swelling in the legs, blood in the urine, or wound discharge.
Visit physician for postoperative office visit 2 to 3 weeks after discharge or per physician protocol.

**Patient Outcomes**
1. The patient verbalizes an understanding of the diagnosis and chance for survival from RCC.
2. The patient confirms that anxiety is reduced after receiving information about treatments for RCC.
3. The patient participates in decisions regarding the choice of treatment for RCC.
4. The patient verbalizes an increased level of comfort after measures for pain management have been implemented.
5. The patient has a urine output of at least 30 mL/hr.
6. The patient's urine is clear and free of blood clots.

7. The patient performs pulmonary exercises as instructed.
8. The patient's lungs are clear on auscultation.
9. The patient demonstrates uncomplicated wound healing.
10. The patient walks increasing distances without difficulty.
11. The patient states an understanding of discharge instructions and home care needs.

# TUMORS OF THE RENAL PELVIS AND URETER

## Perspective on Disease Entity

### ETIOLOGY

Malignant tumors of the renal pelvis and ureter account for about 4% to 5% of all genitourinary lesions. Overall, they are two to three times more common in males than females. These tumors are rarely seen in patients younger than 30 years of age; they increase in frequency later in life, being more common in the sixth and seventh decades.

Like renal parenchymal tumors, the etiology of renal pelvic and ureteral tumors is unknown. They are, however, believed to be associated with bladder cancer. It has been estimated that one third of patients with renal pelvic or ureteral tumors will have had, currently have, or will develop other urothelial tumors (Johnson et al., 1984).

Population groups at risk for developing upper urinary tract tumors include

1. Abusers of analgesic compounds, including acetaminophen, aspirin, caffeine, and phenacetin.
2. Workers employed for long periods in rubber, textile, petrochemical, leather, or plastics industries or where exposure to coal, coke, asphalt, and tar are likely.
3. Cigarette smokers.
4. Persons who consume excessive amounts of coffee.
5. Residents of Balkan countries, who tend to develop renal interstitial inflammatory disease (Balkan nephropathy).
6. Persons with chronic bacterial infection of the urinary tract.
7. Patients who were exposed to Thoratrast (thorium dioxide), a contrast material once used for retrograde urography (Carroll, 1992).

### PATHOPHYSIOLOGY

The types of tumors that affect the renal pelvis and ureter include epithelial tumors (transitional cell, squamous cell, adenocarcinoma, and undifferentiated) and mesodermal tumors (sarcomas). Adenocarcinomas and sarcomas are extremely rare, accounting for fewer than 1% of all renal pelvis and ureteral tumors.

Eighty-five percent to 90% of renal pelvis and ureteral tumors are classified as transitional cell carcinoma. Two thirds of these are papillary tumors. Because of the urinary tract's epithelial lining, the transitional cell tumors generally spread throughout the renal pelvis and down the ureter. There may also be invasion to underlying muscle, the lymphatics, and the renal vein. Metastases may occur to the lung, bone, and liver.

Ten percent to 14% of renal pelvis and ureteral tumors are found to be squamous cell carcinoma. This tumor type is associated with chronic irritation and calculus disease. It is unclear, however, whether the inflammation caused by a calculus is a predisposing factor to squamous cell carcinoma or if the presence of squamous cell carcinoma leads to calculus formation (Melamed & Reuter, 1993). Squamous cell carcinoma of the renal pelvis and ureter is highly invasive and malignant. Metastases occur via direct, lymphatic, and blood-borne routes and may be found almost anywhere in the body. Patients with these tumors have a poor life expectancy, usually less than 1 year following diagnosis.

Although tumors affecting the bladder or kidney may also extend to involve the ureter, it is possible for tumors of the ureter to occur independently. Most often, the ureter will be the site of metastasis from adjacent structures, such as the gastrointestinal tract, cervix, breast, lungs, or prostate.

Tumors of the renal pelvis and ureter can cause obstruction of the kidney with subsequent hydroureter and hydronephrosis. Spasms and severe colic-like pain result from the obstruction. Treatment is initially directed toward relief of the hydroureter (and subsequent relief of the pain and spasms) by the insertion of a stent or nephrostomy tube.

As with other genitourinary tumors, the stage of the tumor at the time of diagnosis is directly related to the patient's prognosis. The Grabstald–Cummings system, which is similar to the Jewett–Strong–Marshall system for bladder cancer, is one method for staging renal pelvic and ureteral tumors. Using this method, stage 1 indicates tumors confined to the mucosa; stage 2 indicates tumors involving the submucosa; stage 3 indicates tumors invading the smooth muscle of the ureter, renal pelvis, and renal parenchyma; and stage 4 indicates tumors with lymph node or distant metastases (Catalona, 1992). The other accepted staging method is the TNM system (Table 8–6) established by the American Joint Committee on Cancer–International Union against Cancer (AJC-UICC) (American Joint Committee on Cancer, 1988).

In general, there is a 5-year survival rate of 60% to 90%, or 67 to 91 months, for patients diagnosed with low-stage (1 and 2 or Tis to T1) renal pelvic and ureteral tumors. Compare this with the 5-year survival rate of 0% to 33%, or 13 to 14 months, for patients with higher-stage tumors (Carroll, 1992; Catalona, 1992).

## MEDICAL-SURGICAL MANAGEMENT

### Diagnosis

To confirm the diagnosis of a renal pelvic or ureteral tumor, a urinalysis should first be performed. Possible findings include microscopic hematuria and the presence of bacteria and pus if long-standing obstruction has caused infection. A urine cytologic examination may also be performed and may reveal abnormal cells in the urine. If bleeding has been profuse, a CBC demonstrates anemia.

Radiologic studies and diagnostic procedures used to evaluate patients with renal pelvic or ureteral tumors include the following:

1. Excretory urogram—demonstrates filling defects in the kidney, ureteropelvic stenosis, or hydronephrosis; it is important to distinguish if defects are smooth, round or oval, and radiolucent (suggesting the presence of a stone) versus an irregular outline (suggesting the presence of a tumor).
2. Ultrasound—is a noninvasive procedure that can differentiate a renal pelvis tumor from a calculus or a blood clot.
3. CT scan—most useful to differentiate a tumor from a stone; also identifies nodal or distant metastases.
4. Cystoscopy—permits visualization of the tumor if present in the distal urethra or bladder; useful in identifying bleeding sites.
5. Retrograde ureterography and pyelography—demonstrates the presence of the lesion and defines its distal margins; a retrograde brush biopsy may also be performed

### TABLE 8–6. UICC Staging System for Tumors of Renal Pelvis and Ureter

**T or pT (Primary Tumor)**

| | |
|---|---|
| TX | Primary tumor is occult and cannot be assessed; for example, positive cytology findings in ureteral urine without (or prior to) demonstration of tumor |
| T0 | No evidence of primary tumor |
| Tis | Carcinoma in situ (flat or nonpapillary carcinoma in situ) |
| Ta | Noninvasive papillary carcinoma |
| T1 | Carcinoma involves subepithelial connective tissue |
| T2 | Carcinoma invades muscularis |
| T3 | Carcinoma invades beyond muscularis into periureteric or peripelvic fat. Carcinomas invading into renal parenchyma are also classified T3 in the UICC system* |
| T4 | Carcinoma invades adjacent organs or extends through kidney into perinephric fat |

**N or pN (Regional Lymph Nodes)**

| | |
|---|---|
| NX | Regional lymph nodes cannot be assessed |
| N0 | No regional lymph node metastasis |
| N1 | Metastasis in a single lymph node 2 cm or less in diameter |
| N2 | Metastasis in a single lymph node 2–5 cm in diameter or metastases to multiple lymph nodes, none more than 5 cm in diameter |
| N3 | Metastasis in a lymph node more than 5 cm in diameter |

**M (Distant Metastasis)**

| | |
|---|---|
| MX | Presence of distant metastasis cannot be assessed |
| M0 | No distant metastasis |
| M1 | Distant metastasis |

*See Guinan, P., Vogelzang, N. J., Randazzo, R., et al. (1992). Renal pelvic transitional cell carcinoma: The role of the kidney in tumor–node–metastasis staging. *Cancer, 69*; 1773–1775.
UICC, International Union Against Cancer.
From Melamed, M. R., & Reuter, V. E. (1993). Pathology and staging of urothelial tumors of the kidney and ureter. *Urologic Clinics of North America, 20*(2), 333–347. Reprinted by permission.

at the same time to provide tissue samples for cytologic studies.

6. Ureteroscopy/nephroscopy—allows for direct visualization of renal pelvic and ureteral tumors; during ureteroscopy, ureteral dilatation associated with a coiling of the ureteral catheter at the ureteral defect is believed to indicate cancer of the ureter; endoscopic biopsy forceps may be passed through the ureteroscope to obtain tissue particles from the tumor for analysis.

## Treatment

A nephroureterectomy with excision of the cuff of the bladder and surrounding lymphatic structures is the treatment of choice for renal pelvic tumors and resectable tumors at the proximal end of the ureter. For patients with renal insufficiency, solitary kidney, or bilateral tumors in which preservation of the renal parenchyma is necessary, segmental resection of the ureter with partial pelvic resection or heminephrectomy may be performed (Seaman et al., 1993). This surgical approach is most effective in instances of low-stage disease in which the chance for cure is greater.

A transitional cell cancer at the distal portion of the ureter may dictate an excision of the tumor with reimplantation of the ureter into the bladder (distal ureterectomy with reimplantation). Other surgical options include end-to-end ureteral anastomosis and ureteroneocystostomy. More recently, urologists have employed intraurethral and percutaneous ureteroscopic techniques along with neodymium:YAG laser coagulation for the treatment of renal pelvic and ureteral tumors.

If the patient's prognosis is poor, or if the patient is unable to withstand a major surgical procedure, the insertion of an internal stent or percutaneous nephrostomy may relieve the obstruction caused by the tumor. A urinary diversion may be necessary for severe obstruction.

Theoretically, preparations such as BCG, thiotepa, and mitomycin C should be effective against renal pelvic and ureteral tumors, given the fact that they are histologically similar to transitional cell carcinoma of the bladder. Due to concerns about systemic toxicity, however, the use of topical or instillation therapy has been limited.

Although there are no systemic chemotherapeutic agents proven to be of value in treating malignant renal pelvic and ureteral tumors (Pritchett et al., 1988), chemotherapy is used to treat metastatic lesions found in the lungs, liver, and bone. Radiation therapy is used primarily for symptom control in instances of advanced disease with local extension.

## Approaches to Patient Care

### Assessment

Symptoms of renal pelvic and ureteral tumors are often vague. Sometimes they are present for as long as 2 years before the patient decides to seek treatment, and in other instances they are correlated only when the tumor is an incidental finding on a radiologic test performed for other reasons. Therefore, the nurse must be alert to subtle subjective and objective symptoms that may relate to the presence of an upper urinary tract tumor.

Painless gross hematuria is the most common symptom in patients with renal pelvic and ureteral tumors, occurring in approximately 75% of patients. Bleeding that occurs throughout urination is a further indication of an upper urinary tract disorder (Catalona, 1992).

Flank pain is present in 30% to 50% of patients. A dull ache is usually caused by either obstruction of the ureteropelvic junction or extension of the tumor to the retroperitoneal area. Acute flank pain is often associated with ureteral colic, caused by the passage of blood clots. Be sure to obtain an accurate description of the patient's pain, factors that precipitate the pain, and measures that have helped decrease discomfort. Other complaints that may be elicited during the nursing health history include malaise, anorexia, weight loss, and bone and joint pain.

During the physical examination, the nurse may detect costovertebral tenderness. In 10% to 20% of patients, a flank mass (often a hydronephrotic kidney) may also be palpated. The remaining aspects of the nursing assessment would be the same as have been previously described for RCC.

### Nursing Diagnosis

Nursing diagnoses for the patient with a renal pelvic or ureteral tumor may include the following:

1. Alteration in pattern of urinary elimination related to
   a. Painless gross hematuria.
   b. Placement of a ureteral stent or nephrostomy tube to relieve obstruction.
2. Pain related to
   a. Ureteropelvic obstruction secondary to the presence of a tumor.

b. Ureteral colic caused by the passage of blood clots.
c. Presence of metastatic disease.
d. Surgical trauma.
3. High risk for urinary tract infection related to
a. Stasis of urine caused by obstruction.
b. Placement and long-term management of urinary drainage devices.
4. Fear related to
a. Discovery of a malignant disease affecting the upper urinary tract.
b. Lack of knowledge about treatments, outcomes, and prognosis for renal pelvic or ureteral tumors.
5. Activity intolerance related to the physiologic effects of metastatic disease.

**Plan of Care**

Nursing care is directed toward enabling the patient to

1. Maintain an adequate urine output of at least 30 mL/hr.
2. Avoid urinary tract infection.
3. Experience relief from pain or develop an acceptable method for pain control.
4. Express thoughts and feelings regarding the diagnosis of cancer.
5. Verbalize an understanding of the diagnosis, treatments, outcomes, and prognosis for renal pelvic or ureteral tumors.
6. Tolerate an optimal level of physical activity without fatigue.

**Interventions**

For those patients who are not candidates for surgery, as well as those requiring decompression of the upper urinary tract before surgery, a nephrostomy tube may be inserted. Nursing interventions include monitoring the flow and amount of urine drainage from the tubing and securing the tubing in a manner that prevents kinking. If the urine draining from the nephrostomy tube contains blood clots, the tube may need to be irrigated. This procedure should be performed only with a physician's order, using sterile technique and 5 to 10 mL of sterile saline. The dressing around the nephrostomy should be changed daily or more frequently if wet or soiled (see Procedure 4–2 in Chapter 4).

In some instances, the urologist may choose to place a ureteral stent instead of a nephrostomy tube to facilitate the drainage of urine from the kidney. The internal J-type stent is anchored by coiling one end in the kidney and the other in the bladder. When a Foley catheter has also been inserted, the nurse may find that the stent has been secured alongside the cathe-

ter. If this is the case, carefully observe the urine draining from the stent and report any decreases in output to the physician. Nephrostomy tubes and stents maintained for extended periods must be replaced at regular intervals, at least every 2 to 3 months. Therefore, patients should be advised of the need for regular follow-up appointments.

Preoperative and postoperative nursing care for the patient undergoing a nephroureterectomy is similar to that previously described for simple radical nephrectomy. Guidelines on preoperative and postoperative nursing care for segmental resection of the ureter with partial pelvic resection or heminephrectomy, as well as ureteroscopic approaches to upper urinary tract tumors, are similar to those described for surgical approaches to upper urinary tract obstructions in Chapter 4.

**Patient Outcomes**

1. The patient maintains a urinary output of 30 mL/hr.
2. The patient's urine is clear and free of blood or clots.
3. The patient's nephrostomy tube or ureteral stent remains patent.
4. The patient exhibits no signs or symptoms of urinary tract infection.
5. The patient states that pain is relieved or improved after methods for pain management are implemented.
6. The patient openly expresses his or her thoughts and feelings regarding the diagnosis of renal pelvic or ureteral cancer.
7. The patient verbalizes an understanding of the diagnosis, treatments, outcomes, and prognosis for renal pelvic or ureteral cancer.
8. The patient regains the physical strength that enables him or her to perform daily activities with minimal fatigue.

### ACKNOWLEDGMENT

The authors and editor gratefully acknowledge the reviews and editorial assistance provided by Carol Einhorn, M.S.N., C.U.R.N., G.N.P., and Donna Brassil, M.S.N., C.U.R.N., in completing this chapter.

### *REFERENCES*

American Joint Committee on Cancer. (1988). *Manual for staging of cancer* (3rd ed.). Philadelphia: J. B. Lippincott.
Bennington, J. L., & Beckwith, J. B. (1975). Tumors of the kidney, renal pelvis, and ureter. In fascile 12 of *Atlas of tumor pathology* (2nd series). Washington, DC: Armed Forces Institute of Pathology.

Brennan, M. F. (1982). Cancer of the endocrine system. In V. T. DeVita, S. Hellman, & S. A. Rosenberg (Eds.), *Cancer principles and practices in oncology* (pp. 987–1001). Philadelphia: W. B. Saunders.

Camunas, C. (1983). Pheochromocytoma. *American Journal of Nursing, 83*(6), 887–891.

Carroll, P. R. (1992). Urothelial carcinoma: Cancers of the bladder ureter, and renal pelvis. In E. A. Tanagho & J. W. McAninch (Eds.), *Smith's general urology* (13th ed., pp. 341–358). Norwalk, CT: Appleton & Lange.

Cassmeyer, V. L. (1991). Management of persons with problems of the pituitary, thyroid, parathyroid and adrenal glands. In W. J. Phipps, B. C. Long, N. F. Woods, & V. L. Cassmeyer (Eds.), *Medical-surgical nursing: Concepts and clinical practice* (4th ed., pp. 1021–1090). St. Louis: Mosby-Year Book.

Catalona, W. J. (1992). Urothelial tumors of the urinary tract. In P. C. Walsh, A. B. Retik, T. A. Stamey, & E. D. Vaughan, Jr. (Eds.), *Campbell's urology* (6th ed., pp. 1049–1158). Philadelphia: W. B. Saunders.

Cohen, A. J., Li, F. P., Berg, S., Marchetto, D. J., Tsai, S., Jacobs, S. C., & Brown, R. S. (1979). Hereditary renal cell carcinoma associated with a chromosomal translocation. *New England Journal of Medicine, 301*, 592.

deKernion, J. B., & Belldegrun, A. (1992). Renal tumors. In P. C. Walsh, A. B. Retik, T. A. Stamey, & E. D. Vaughan, Jr. (Eds.), *Campbell's urology* (6th ed., pp. 1053–1093). Philadelphia: W. B. Saunders.

Donohue, J. P. (1988). Diagnosis and management of adrenal tumors. In D. G. Skinner & G. Lieskovsky (Eds.), *Diagnosis and management of genitourinary cancer* (pp. 372–389). Philadelphia: W. B. Saunders.

Dreicer, R., & Williams, R. D. (1992). Renal parenchymal neoplasms. In E. A. Tanagho & J. W. McAninch (Eds.), *Smith's general urology* (13th ed., pp. 359–377). Norwalk, CT: Appleton & Lange.

Forsham, P. H. (1992). Disorders of the adrenal glands. In E. A. Tanagho & J. W. McAninch (Eds.), *Smith's general urology* (13th ed., pp. 495–514). Norwalk, CT: Appleton & Lange.

Harris, R. B., & Dela Roca, R. R. (1984). Pheochromocytoma: A medical review. *Heart and Lung, 13*(1), 73–79.

Jacobs, J. A., & Goldin, N. P. (1987). Disorders of the adrenal gland. In P. M. Hanno & A. J. Wein (Eds.), *A clinical manual of urology* (pp. 481–500). Norwalk, CT: Appleton-Century-Crofts.

Johnson, D. E., Swanson, D. A., & von Eschenbach, A. C. (1984). Tumors of the genitourinary tract. In D. R. Smith (Ed.), *General urology* (pp. 306–404). Los Altos, CA: Lange.

Klein, E. A., Kaye, M. C., & Novick, A. C. (1991). Management of renal cell carcinoma with vena caval thrombi via cardiopulmonary bypass and deep hypothermic circulatory arrest. *Urologic Clinics of North America, 18*(3), 445–447.

Marshall, F. F. (1991). *Operative urology.* Philadelphia: W. B. Saunders.

Melamed, M. R., & Reuter, V. E. (1993). Pathology and staging of urothelial tumors of the kidney and ureter. *Urologic Clinics of North America, 20*(2), 333–347.

Pagana, K. D. & Pagana T. J. (1990). *Diagnostic testing & nursing implications: A case study approach.* St. Louis, MO: C. V. Mosby.

Perkins, M. C. (1985). Would you recognize pheochromocytoma? *Nursing 85, 15*, 64M–64O.

Pritchett, T. R., Lieskovsky, G., & Skinner, D. G. (1988). Clinical manifestations and treatment of renal parenchymal tumors. In D. G. Skinner & G. Lieskovsky (Eds.), *Diagnosis and management of genitourinary cancer* (pp. 337–361). Philadelphia: W. B. Saunders.

Robson, C. J., Churchill, B. M., & Anderson, W. (1969). The results of radical nephrectomy for renal cell carcinoma. *Journal of Urology, 101*, 297.

Seaman, E. K., Slawin, K. M., & Benson, M. C. (1993). Treatment options for upper tract transitional cell carcinoma. *Urologic Clinics of North America, 20*(2), 349–354.

Thrasher, J. B., & Paulson, D. F. (1993). Prognostic factors in renal cancers. *Urologic Clinics of North America, 20*(2), 247–262.

Vaughan E. D., & Blumenfeld, J. D. (1992). The adrenals. In P. C. Walsh, A. B. Retik, T. A. Stamey, & E. D. Vaughan, Jr. (Eds.), *Campbell's urology* (6th ed., pp. 2360–2412). Philadelphia: W. B. Saunders.

Warner, N. E. (1988). Pathology of the adrenal gland. In D. G. Skinner & G. Lieskovsky (Eds.), *Diagnosis and management of genitourinary cancer* (pp. 195–206). Philadelphia: W. B. Saunders.

Wirth, M. P. (1993). Immunotherapy for metastatic renal cell carcinoma. *Urologic Clinics of North America, 20*(2), 283–295.

Yagoda, A., Petrylak, D., & Thompson, S. (1993). Cytotoxic chemotherapy for advanced renal cell carcinoma. *Urologic Clinics of North America, 20*(2), 303–321.

CHAPTER 9

# Cancer of the Bladder

■

*Nancy J. Reilly*

## OVERVIEW

Bladder cancer is the second most commonly occurring genitourinary cancer in adults and the fourth most common cause of cancer deaths among American men older than 75 years of age (Brettschneider & Orihuela, 1990; Catalona, 1991). The incidence of bladder cancer increases with age; it is rarely seen in those younger than 40 years of age and most commonly occurs in people between the ages of 50 and 70 years. Most cases are found to be transitional cell carcinomas, accounting for approximately 95% of all bladder carcinomas in the United States. Squamous cell carcinoma is found in fewer than 3% of cases of bladder cancer, and adenocarcinoma is seen in fewer than 2% (Catalona, 1991).

Much has been discovered in recent years about the clinical course of bladder cancer. Once thought to be a generally progressive carcinoma, it is now believed to be a neoplasm with a wide range of biologic activity. Although some persons diagnosed with bladder cancer are cured or controlled with fairly conservative measures, others are found to have rapidly progressive disease requiring aggressive treatment, usually radical surgery. The past decade has seen great advances in conservative treatment for a form of bladder cancer that once mandated radical surgery: carcinoma in situ (CIS). CIS has been essentially cured in some patients after the intravesical administration of bacille Calmette-Guérin.

Similar advances have been made in techniques for radical surgery in bladder cancer. Although radical cystectomy and ileal conduit urinary diversion remain the gold standard against which other surgeries are measured, continent urinary diversions (both with and without external stomas) are now commonplace. Urologic nurses play a vital role in the rehabilitation of these patients.

This chapter discusses both the clinical pathophysiology of transitional cell carcinoma

**243**

(and other cell-type cancers) of the urinary bladder and the nursing interventions that are crucial to the recovery and rehabilitation of the patient with bladder cancer.

## BEHAVIORAL OBJECTIVES

After studying this chapter, the reader should be able to

1. Determine the factors that differentiate transitional cell carcinomas that may be treated conservatively from those that require radical surgery.

2. Discuss the symptoms most frequently seen in patients with bladder cancer.

3. Describe the staging system for bladder cancer usually used in the United States and its implications for treatment and prognosis.

4. List the chemotherapeutic agents commonly used for the intravesical treatment of bladder cancer, along with their major side effects.

5. Compare the nursing interventions necessary for patients with standard urinary diversions versus continent urinary diversions.

## KEY WORDS

**Bacille Calmette-Guérin (BCG)**—an organism of the strain *Mycobacterium bovis,* originally used as an antituberculosis agent; acts as an antitumor agent when administered intravesically.

**Carcinoma in situ**—a poorly differentiated transitional cell carcinoma, often without any papillary growth; appears as an area of erythema on the bladder wall.

**Continent cutaneous urinary diversion**—a type of urinary diversion in which a pouch constructed of bowel collects urine; an abdominal stoma is periodically catheterized to drain urine from the pouch.

**Dysplasia**—an abnormal cell configuration found in the urothelium; ranges from an increase in the number of normal cells to carcinoma in situ.

**Ileal conduit**—a method of urinary diversion in which a urostomy is created; requires an external collecting device to be worn continuously.

**Intravesical chemotherapy**—the administration of antineoplastic drugs directly into the bladder.

**Intravesical immunotherapy**—the treatment of transitional cell cancer by direct instillation of BCG into the bladder.

**Orthotopic bladder replacement**—a type of urinary diversion in which a pouch constructed of bowel replaces the bladder; performed only on men, who then ''void'' through their urethra after surgery.

**Papillary tumor**—a mushroom-like growth of a transitional cell tumor from the bladder wall; easily seen on cystoscopic examination.

**Radical cystectomy**—the removal of the bladder and adjacent organs along with pelvic lymph nodes—curative surgery for invasive bladder cancer.

**Random bladder biopsies**—the endoscopic sampling of tissue throughout the bladder using biopsy forceps.

**Transitional cell carcinoma**—a type of malignancy that arises from the urothelial lining of the urinary tract.

**Transurethral resection of bladder tumor**—the endoscopic removal of a bladder tumor and surrounding tissue using electrocautery and continuous irrigation.

## PERSPECTIVE ON DISEASE ENTITY

### Etiology

As with most cancers, the exact etiology of bladder cancer remains uncertain. Epidemiologic data have provided much information about factors thought to contribute to the development of bladder cancer. Several of these factors are accompanied by convincing evidence that they may play a causative role in the development of the disease. Etiologic factors associated with transitional cell and squamous cell carcinomas are discussed in this section.

Cigarette smoking is known to increase the risk of developing transitional cell carcinoma in smokers by much as four times that in nonsmokers (Morrison, 1984). This is true for both men and women, although current statistics for bladder cancer indicate that men are three times more likely to develop the disease than are women (Wein & Hanno, 1987). Some authors attribute this difference to a latency period for the onset of the disease in those who smoke. Women generally did not smoke cigarettes with the same frequency as did men until the 1940s and 1950s. These women are only now reaching the age at which bladder cancer usually develops (Armstrong & Doll, 1975; Droller, 1986).

It is thought that the increased concentration of tryptophan metabolites in the urine of cigarette smokers may be the carcinogenic factor that leads to transitional cell carcinoma. Cigarette smoke contains nitrosamines as well as 2-naphthylamine, which is also potentially carcinogenic. However, the same risks do not apply to people who chew tobacco or smoke cigars or pipes (Cole et al., 1971). The risk of developing bladder cancer is significantly reduced over time in those who quit smoking.

Industrial exposure to known carcinogens constitutes a significant risk factor for transitional cell carcinoma. Those people at greatest risk include textile workers, painters, hair-dressers, leather and metal workers, and those employed in the rubber industries (Brettschneider & Orihuela, 1990). All these occupations expose the participants to chemical carcinogens. The latency period of industrial exposure risk may vary from 18 to 45 years (Wein & Hanno, 1987). It has been estimated that one fourth to one third of all cases of bladder cancer are caused by occupational exposure (Catalona, 1991).

The use of artificial sweeteners, caffeine, and the drug phenacetin has been weakly linked with transitional cell carcinoma. Saccharin in extremely high doses caused bladder cancer in rodents and precipitated its removal from the consumer market. Because the dosages of saccharin administered in these studies were extraordinarily high, the clinical relevance of these data in humans is unknown. Coffee drinking was similarly associated with bladder cancer at one time; however, it proved to be impossible to separate caffeine intake from cigarette smoking and the use of artificial sweeteners. Current data suggest only a weak link (if any) between coffee drinking and bladder cancer. Abuse of the analgesic phenacetin was linked with the development of transitional cell carcinoma in several studies published in the late 1960s and early 1970s (Bengtsson et al., 1968). Again, the dosages consumed by the affected patients were extraordinarily high; nonetheless, phenacetin is rarely used today.

Chronic bladder infection and irritation are known to be causative factors in the development of squamous cell carcinoma of the bladder. Usually, those people affected have had indwelling catheters for long periods or have chronic urinary (often bladder) calculi (Catalona, 1991; Droller, 1986). Chronic infection with *Schistosoma haematobium*, the organism responsible for schistosomiasis, has also been found to increase significantly the risk of squamous cell carcinoma of the bladder. In all cases, the period during which squamous cell carcinoma develops is long, and the irritation of the bladder is chronic.

Treatment modalities for pelvic carcinomas have been linked to the later development of bladder carcinomas. Women who have received pelvic radiation for cervical cancer have a twofold to fourfold increased risk of developing transitional cell carcinoma of the bladder. Also, patients treated with cyclophosphamide (Cytoxan) have a nine times greater risk of developing bladder cancer, (Catalona, 1991). The exact mechanism causing bladder cancer in these patients is unknown.

Along with these known risk factors, age and geographic residence contribute to the risk of developing bladder cancer. As mentioned previously, it is unusual for bladder cancer to occur in people younger than 40 years of age. The incidence of the disease is highest in the United States and England. In the United States, those people living in the northern half of the country are at higher risk than are those living in the southern half (Catalona, 1991; Cutler & Young, 1975). Jewish persons are known to have an overall higher incidence than non-Jewish persons. Heredity has not been proved to play a role in the risk of developing bladder cancer (Catalona, 1991).

## Pathophysiology

The urinary bladder is a muscular organ that receives and stores urine excreted from the kidneys by way of the ureters. Its primary functions are to store urine at a low pressure and to contract to empty urine through the urethra. Complex neurologic pathways are responsible for voluntary control of bladder function.

The urinary tract from the renal pelvis to the proximal urethra is lined with specific epithelial cells called the *urothelium.* The urothelium of the normal bladder is composed of three to seven layers of transitional cells (Catalona, 1991). It is these transitional cells that undergo the proliferative changes that begin the disease process in patients with bladder cancer. Beyond the urothelium lie the muscular layers of the bladder, which are then surrounded by perivesical fat. The degree of transitional cell carcinoma invasion is determined by how deeply it has extended into the urothelium (or submucosa) or into or beyond the muscular layer.

Pathologists have identified several types of transitional cell proliferative changes considered to be premalignant. Usually these cellular changes are called *dysplastic* (or *dysplasia*), and this term refers to several types of abnormal cell configurations that range somewhere between normal and carcinoma in situ (CIS) (Brettschneider & Orihuela, 1990). In many instances, urothelial dysplasia is found in patients who are already receiving therapy for bladder tumors. The terms *mild, moderate,* and *severe* are often used to describe the degree of dysplasia. Severe dysplasia may be difficult to distinguish from CIS (Catalona, 1991). *Hyperplasia* refers to an increase in the number of cells present without any premalignant abnormalities.

Pathologically, tumors are graded according to the degree of anaplasia present. The tumor grade assigned to a patient's carcinoma is an important indicator of the aggressiveness of that tumor and the patient's prognosis. Low-grade, or well-differentiated, tumors are usually superficial and not biologically aggressive. High-grade, or poorly differentiated, tumors are usually aggressive and are already invasive. Several different grading systems have been described, and the grading system as defined by the American Joint Commission on Cancer Staging and End Results Reporting is often used. Grade 1 refers to a well-differentiated tumor, and grade 4 represents a poorly differentiated tumor. Whatever grading system is used, the higher the grade, the more malignant the tumor (Brettschneider & Orihuela, 1990). There is a significant correlation between tumor grade and tumor stage and between tumor grade and prognosis (Catalona, 1991).

Transitional cell carcinomas are further described as either CIS (or "flat" CIS) or papillary tumors. Both types arise from transitional cells, and both are capable of resulting in muscle-invasive and, eventually, metastatic disease. CIS tends to be more symptomatic and more rapidly progressive than are papillary tumors. Papillary tumors often respond well to conservative (or local) treatment and may be safely managed in many patients without ever progressing to a life-threatening disease.

CIS is characterized by poorly differentiated transitional cell carcinoma confined to the urothelium. Approximately 11% of patients with superficial papillary tumors are also found to have areas of CIS. Conversely, CIS may occur in the absence of any visible papillary tumors.

CIS may be a biologically aggressive disease; the risk of disease progression ranges from 4% to 8%. Some patients experience a rapid progression to muscle-invasive disease and have a poor prognosis despite aggressive treatment. In other patients diagnosed with CIS, the disease progresses more slowly. Patients with CIS are generally more symptomatic, with irritative voiding symptoms (urgency, frequency, and dysuria) and intermittent gross or microscopic hematuria.

Papillary, or solid, transitional cell carcinomas account for approximately 70% of all bladder cancers. The term *papillary* is usually reserved for superficial lesions that do not extend beyond the mucosa. Papillary tumors are easily seen on cystoscopic examination (whereas CIS may appear as only a reddened or erythematous area). Papillary tumors occur most frequently on the trigone, at the bladder base, and on the lateral bladder walls. Papillary tumors are easily resected transurethrally. The rate of recurrence is approximately 70%; therefore, treatment to prevent recurrence is usually prescribed in the form of intravesical chemotherapy and vigilant repeat cystoscopy. Untreated papillary tumors may eventually progress to muscle-invasive disease. Patients with a history of papillary tumors may additionally develop flat CIS.

Patients with only papillary tumors often do not complain of voiding symptoms but do experience hematuria. For this reason, all patients older than 40 years of age with gross or microscopic hematuria are evaluated for the presence of bladder (or other urothelial) carcinoma.

Bladder cancer metastasizes after it invades through the submucosa and the muscular layer of the bladder wall. Once through the muscle, it gains access to lymphatic channels and the vascular supply. It usually metastasizes first to the pelvic lymph nodes and is often found in the paravesical obturator and the external iliac nodes. Next, it spreads by way of the blood stream to distant sites, including, in order of frequency, the liver, lungs, and bones. Local extension of bladder cancer may affect nearby organs, including the prostate, uterus, vagina, ureters, and rectum (Catalona, 1991).

The likelihood that a patient is initially diagnosed with metastatic disease depends on many factors, including the length of time that has passed between the onset of symptoms and the diagnosis and the grade of that patient's tumor. Patients with metastasis at the time of diagnosis often have a poorly differentiated, high-grade cancer with a high potential for malignancy. Approximately 50% of patients with muscle-invasive disease experience distant or local recurrence within 18 to 24 months of diagnosis. It is far less likely that a patient with a solitary papillary tumor that is low grade and well differentiated will have metastatic disease.

## STAGING

Treatment options for patients diagnosed with cancer of the bladder depend on the staging of their disease. Significant differences exist between treatment for lower-stage disease (stages 0 and A) and treatment for higher stages of bladder cancer. Patients with higher stages of this disease are usually candidates for radical curative surgery, whereas patients diagnosed with lower stages are managed conservatively.

The staging system most commonly used in the United States is the Jewett-Strong-Marshall system (Fig. 9–1). This system describes the stages of bladder cancer from 0 to D. Stages B and D are further divided into B1 and B2, and D1 and D2, respectively.

Stage 0 refers to a tumor that has extended no deeper than the mucosa; stage 0 tumors may be papillary or CIS. Stage A tumors extend through the mucosa to the submucosa. Stage B tumors are muscle invasive and are

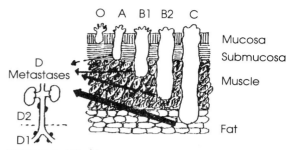

**FIGURE 9–1** Bladder cancer staging: Correlation between local stage of disease and development of metastasis. (Adapted from Brettschneider, N. R., & Orihuela, E. [1990]. Carcinoma of the bladder. *Urologic Nursing, 10*[1], 14–21. Reprinted by permission.)

divided into B1 or B2 lesions, based on the depth of muscle invasion. Stage B1 tumors extend less than halfway through the muscle; stage B2 tumors extend more than halfway. Stage C tumors extend through the muscle and invade the perivesical fat. A diagnosis of stage D disease denotes metastasis. Stage D1 refers to lymph node metastasis; stage D2 refers to distant metastasis.

The TNM staging system, as described by the American Joint Commission on Cancer Staging and End Results Reporting and the International Union Against Cancer (AJC-UICC), is used by some physicians. A comparison between the TNM system and the Jewett-Strong-Marshall system is found in Table 9–1.

Because the management of patients with stage 0 or A disease differs so greatly from the management of stages B to D disease, the remainder of this chapter is divided according to these two subgroups of stages. A discussion of

**TABLE 9–1. Comparison of TNM and Jewett-Marshall-Strong Systems for Staging of Bladder Cancer**

| JEWETT-MARSHALL-STRONG | TNM | |
|---|---|---|
| Stage 0 | T0 | No tumor definitive specimen |
| | TIS | Carcinoma in situ |
| Stage A | T1 | Invasion of lamina propria |
| Stage B1 | T2 | Superficial muscle invasion |
| Stage B2 | T3A | Deep muscle invasion |
| Stage C | T3B | Invasion of perivesical fat |
| Stage D1 | T4A | Invasion of contiguous viscera |
| | N1–3 | Pelvic nodes |
| Stage D2 | M1 | Distant metastases |
| | N4 | Nodes above aortic bifurcation |

From Brettschneider, N. R., & Orihuela, E. (1990) Carcinoma of the bladder. *Urologic Nursing, 10*(1), 14–21. Reprinted by permission.

lower stage disease is followed by a discussion of invasive disease, along with surgical interventions used in the treatment.

# NONINVASIVE BLADDER CANCER (STAGES 0 AND A)

## Medical-Surgical Management

Most bladder cancers determined to be stage 0 or A are transitional cell carcinomas. Pathologically, they may be either papillary or CIS. Papillary transitional cell carcinomas have been managed conservatively for decades with transurethral resection, intravesical chemotherapy, and frequent follow-up cystoscopic examination. Accordingly, much information exists regarding the success of various regimens.

Of significance to the patient is the need for a vigilant follow-up program. Even in the absence of recurrence, patients diagnosed with noninvasive bladder tumors become "permanent patients," requiring (at the least) an annual cystoscopic examination for the rest of their lives. The risk of local recurrence, however, is high, at approximately 70% to 100% over one's lifetime (Brettschneider & Orihuela, 1990).

Conservative management of transitional cell CIS is a development that has occurred in the past two decades. Before the documented success of intravesical immunotherapy with bacille Calmette-Guérin (BCG), a pathologic diagnosis of CIS meant radical surgery. Initial reports of the success of intravesical BCG first appeared in the literature in 1976 (Morales et al., 1976). Since then, BCG has become the standard treatment for the 5% to 10% of all patients with transitional cell carcinoma who present with CIS (Brosman, 1991).

Painless hematuria, either gross or microscopic, occurs in 85% of patients with cancer of the bladder (Wein & Hanno, 1987). Any patient older than 40 years of age who experiences this symptom should be evaluated for the presence of a carcinoma in the bladder or elsewhere in the genitourinary tract. Other symptoms occur less often; frequency, urgency, and dysuria are symptoms associated with bladder irritability, usually an ominous sign of locally advanced disease. Rarely, an asymptomatic patient may be diagnosed with bladder cancer during a urologic workup done for other reasons. Finally, some patients may present with symptoms of metastatic disease.

Most bladder cancers are diagnosed during cystourethroscopy by direct visualization of the tumor. Usually, this initial cystourethroscopy is performed with the patient under local anesthesia in an outpatient setting. When a bladder tumor is found, repeat cystoscopy with transurethral resection and biopsies is then performed under regional or general anesthesia in an inpatient or day surgery setting (Fig. 9–2). A transurethral resection of a bladder tumor (TURBT) allows for both pathologic staging and treatment. Tissue surrounding the area of known tumor is resected in an attempt to remove all areas of malignancy. Many physicians additionally perform random bladder biopsies to evaluate the rest of the bladder.

Treatment of superficial bladder tumors with the neodymium:yttrium-aluminum-garnet (Nd:YAG) laser is an alternative to TURBT for some patients. Rather than removing the tumor, laser therapy destroys it. Some advantages of laser therapy include decreased postoperative bleeding and, in some instances, no need for an indwelling catheter postoperatively. Like TURBT, laser therapy may be performed in an outpatient setting. One disadvantage is that when the tumor is destroyed, specimens cannot be pathologically examined. Random

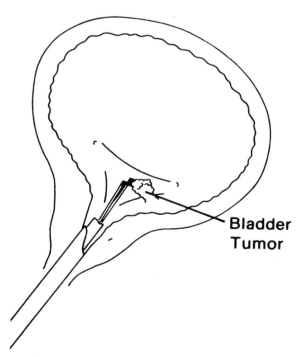

*FIGURE 9–2* Transurethral resection of a bladder tumor. (Illustration courtesy of CIRCON ACMI.)

TABLE 9–2. Agents Used for Intravesical Chemotherapy

| DRUG | MECHANISM OF ACTION | DOSAGE | FREQUENCY | COMMON SIDE EFFECTS |
|---|---|---|---|---|
| Thiotepa | Alkylating agent | 30 mg in 30 mL saline or 60 mg in 60 mL saline | Once a week for 6–8 wk, then monthly | Myelosuppression |
| Mitomycin-C | Antitumor Antibiotic | 40 mg in 40 mL sterile water | Once a week for 8 wk, then monthly | Chemical cystitis Genital skin rashes |
| Doxorubicin (Adriamycin) | Antitumor Antibiotic | 50 mg | Varies from 3 times a week to monthly | Chemical cystitis |

bladder biopsies are performed at the end of the procedure (Malloy & Wein, 1987).

Urinary cytology is an important component of both diagnosis and later monitoring for recurrences. Both conventional microscopic and flow cytometries are used; flow cytometry seems to be preferred because of its improved accuracy in diagnosing CIS and its 80% to 85% sensitivity rate (Catalona, 1991). Saline bladder washings, obtained by barbotage during cystoscopy, are used for flow cytometry. Freshly voided specimens may also be used, although some authors report that bladder washings make better specimens because of tumor cell shedding during barbotage. Specimens of urine that have been stagnant for some time, such as urine voided first in the morning, should not be used for cytologic examination.

Excretory urography (intravenous pyelography [IVP]) is routinely done as part of the diagnostic evaluation for bladder cancer. IVP provides a method of evaluating the upper urinary tract for the presence of other urothelial tumors. It is unusual, but possible, for a bladder tumor to be seen as a filling defect in the bladder on IVP. IVP also plays an important role in the follow-up regimen for superficial bladder tumors, because recurrent transitional cell cancers may arise anywhere in the urothelial lining of the urinary tract.

Once the results of the pathologic examination of the resected tumor and any random biopsy specimens are obtained, along with cytology and IVP results, further treatment options are offered to the patient. The depth of invasion as well as the tumor grade is considered.

The lowest risk scenario is that of a patient with a low-grade, superficial, solitary papillary lesion with a negative cytologic report (Brettschneider & Orihuela, 1990). These patients are treated with TURBT and are then followed, with the usual follow-up regimen involving cystourethroscopy and cytology every 3 months for 1 or 2 years, then every 6 months for 1 or 2 years, then annually. IVP is sched-

uled annually or biannually. Patients at higher risk are those with more than one stage A tumor of a higher grade and those with CIS. Patients with a recurrence are also considered to be at higher risk. These higher risk patients usually receive intravesical chemotherapy or immunotherapy in addition to the previously described follow-up regimen.

Intravesical chemotherapy involves the instillation of one of several chemotherapeutic agents directly into the bladder through a urethral catheter. The three most commonly used agents are described in Table 9–2. Thiotepa probably is the chemotherapeutic agent most often used, primarily because of its proven success in reducing the incidence of tumor recurrence and its relatively low cost. Thiotepa is most effective in patients with low-grade tumors. It is not generally used in patients with higher-grade tumors or CIS. Mitomycin C has yielded complete tumor remissions in 40% of patients, including those with higher-grade tumors (Catalona, 1991). Unfortunately, its extremely high cost may be prohibitive for patients whose insurance does not cover it.

Intravesical immunotherapy with BCG is effective against transitional cell carcinoma of the bladder by a different mechanism of action than the chemotherapeutic drugs. Instead of causing an alteration in the deoxyribonucleic acid structure of tumor cells, "BCG is a biological response modifier which is believed to exert its anti-tumor effect by stimulating various immune responses in the host" (LeBouton, 1990, p. 9). Unlike the chemotherapeutic agents, BCG has proved successful in patients with CIS, as well as in preventing tumor recurrence (Catalona, 1991).

There are five different strains of BCG available, two of which—the Tice and the Connaught strains—are approved by the U.S. Food and Drug Administration for the treatment of CIS of the bladder (Table 9–3). Treatment schedules vary, but most involve at least once-a-week intravesical instillations for as long as 6 weeks. Some authors advocate 12 weekly treat-

**TABLE 9–3. Variations in BCG Preparations**

| STRAIN | CFU/AMPULE | WEIGHT/AMPULE* | EFFECTIVE DOSE |
|---|---|---|---|
| Tice | $2–8 \times 10^8$ | 50 mg | 50 mg |
| Connaught | $8–32 \times 10^8$ | 40 mg | 120 mg† |
| Armand Frappier | $10^7$ per mg | 120 mg | 120 mg |
| Pasteur (France) | $6 \times 10^8$ | 75 mg | 150 mg |

*Approximate wet weight per manufacturer prior to lyophilization.
†Connaught BCG is marketed as TheraCys. Each vial = 27 mg dry weight. The effective dose = 3 vials.
CFU, colony-forming unit.
From LeBouton, J. (1990). Nursing aspects of bacillus Calmette-Guérin immunotherapy for superficial bladder cancer. *Urologic Nursing, 10*(4), 9–13. Reprinted with permission.

ments (Catalona, 1991). Monthly maintenance treatments are usually prescribed for at least 1 year.

The side effects associated with intravesical BCG immunotherapy are significant but usually transient. More than 90% of patients experience symptoms of bladder irritability, frequency, urgency, and dysuria (Lamm et al., 1986). These side effects usually occur shortly after the treatment is given and tend to resolve within a day or two. Most patients seem to tolerate BCG treatments well despite these side effects. Other less frequently occurring side effects include hematuria, fever, malaise, nausea, chills, arthralgia, and pruritus. Granulomatous prostatitis is additionally a frequent side effect following BCG therapy (Catalona, 1991).

The development of a systemic reaction during BCG therapy is a significant complication requiring medical intervention. Patients who develop a fever higher than 100°F that persists for more than 24 hours are considered to have a systemic BCG infection requiring treatment with antituberculosis antibiotics (Brosman et al., 1991; Lamm et al., 1986). The recommended medications and their dosages are isoniazid (INH) 300 mg orally daily and rifampin 600 mg orally daily. Ethambutol 1200 mg orally daily may also be given. The effects of these drugs are not obvious until 3 days after they are started. Cycloserine is given additionally in doses of 250 to 500 mg orally twice daily during the first 3 days when symptoms persist and the risk of fulminating BCG sepsis is high (Brosman et al., 1991).

Most patients with initially diagnosed stage 0 or A transitional cell cancer of the bladder are treated with TURBT, vigilant follow-up, and possible intravesical chemotherapy or immunotherapy. Despite the high rate of recurrence, patients who adhere to this regimen may effectively prevent their disease from progressing.

## Approaches to Patient Care

### Assessment

Nursing assessment of the patient with stage 0 or A bladder cancer may take place in (1) the physician's office or clinic or (2) the hospital when the patient is admitted for transurethral surgery. Obviously, a major difference exists between patients seen in these two settings. When seen in the outpatient setting, the patient may not yet have been diagnosed. Often these patients are being evaluated for painless hematuria, so a nursing assessment must include information about the duration and frequency as well as an approximation of the amount of bleeding, based on the patient's description of the color (intensity) of the blood-tinged urine. Obtain a urine specimen to evaluate for the presence of gross or microscopic hematuria. If available, results of a recent urine culture should be reviewed to check for the presence of bacteria in the urine. Assess the patient for other voiding symptoms, including frequency, urgency, and dysuria, along with the duration of time the patient has experienced them. Information about the patient's exposure to risk factors must be obtained, including a pack-year smoking history and any occupational exposure to known risk factors. Any family history of cancer should be documented. Ascertain any known allergies, especially to shellfish, iodine, or contrast material.

Assess the patient for nonurologic symptoms possibly indicative of progressive disease, including any recent weight loss, gastrointestinal disturbances or changes in bowel habits, or chronic fatigue.

Finally, the nursing assessment must include an evaluation of the anxiety level of the patient as well as his or her significant other. The appearance of blood in the urine may be quite a fearful event, and it may be likely that the patient is well aware he or she will be evaluated for the possibility of cancer. Assess the patient's level of knowledge about what is happening.

When the nursing assessment takes place in the hospital prior to transurethral surgery, all the assessments mentioned earlier should be carried out. The hospitalized patient must also be assessed for factors that may affect the planned surgery, including any history of problems with anesthesia and mobility restrictions or limitations that would prevent the patient from being placed in a lithotomy position. Determine also if there is a history of bleeding disorders or medical conditions requiring anticoagulant therapy or any chronic or acute respiratory disorders.

The preoperative nursing assessment of the patient who will undergo the transurethral surgery should also include an assessment of the patient's knowledge of his or her condition and anxiety level. These patients generally have already been diagnosed and are awaiting the outcome of the upcoming procedure to, in a sense, determine their future. An assessment of the patients' level of understanding about what the transurethral surgery involves and how the biopsy results will affect them is essential in planning nursing care.

### Nursing Diagnosis

The nursing diagnoses for the patient with stage 0 or A bladder cancer may include the following:

1. Altered patterns of urinary elimination related to
   a. Vesical irritation (frequency, urgency, dysuria) due to the presence of a bladder tumor.
   b. Placement of an indwelling urethral catheter (after TURBT or for the instillation of intravesical chemotherapy or immunotherapy).
   c. Bladder irritability from intravesical chemotherapy or immunotherapy.
2. Pain related to
   a. Irritative voiding symptoms.
   b. Urethral irritation caused by placement of indwelling catheter.
   c. Postoperative bladder spasms.
3. Impaired tissue integrity related to
   a. Postoperative bleeding (hematuria) caused by TURBT.
   b. Irritation of the bladder mucosa as a result of intravesical chemotherapy or immunotherapy.
4. Knowledge deficit related to the diagnosis of cancer and proposed treatment plan.

5. Anxiety related to the diagnosis of cancer.
6. Potential for noncompliance with long-term follow-up related to the patient's belief that tumor recurrence is unlikely following initial therapy.

### Plan of Care

Nursing care is directed toward enabling the patient to

1. Increase his or her knowledge about biopsy results, planned interventions, and follow-up regimen.
2. Obtain relief from irritative voiding symptoms.
3. Remain comfortable after transurethral surgery and during intravesical treatment with chemotherapy and immunotherapy.
4. Achieve resolution of postoperative hematuria.
5. Comply with recommendations for long-term follow-up.

### Intervention

Nursing interventions after cystoscopic or transurethral procedures should be directed toward sustaining comfort as well as maintaining the patency of urethral drainage catheters if present. After a diagnostic cystoscopy, the patient may experience dysuria for a short period, primarily as a result of irritation to the urethra that resolves after the first few voidings. When biopsy specimens of the bladder wall have been obtained or when TURBT has been performed, the patient is usually in a day surgery or inpatient setting. Nursing interventions are performed to assist the patient to recover from whatever type of anesthesia was used.

Discomfort related to the presence of the urethral catheter is a common source of pain and bladder spasms after transurethral bladder surgery. Administer analgesic medications, including belladonna and opium suppositories (contraindicated in the patient with glaucoma), to relieve the discomfort.

Patients receiving BCG treatments must be informed about the action and expected side effects of BCG (Procedures 9–1 and 9–2). Most treatment regimens involve weekly visits to the physician's office or clinic. Actual administration of BCG is usually performed by a nurse, after insertion of a urethral catheter. Health professionals who mix and administer BCG should follow safety and handling precautions as advised by the manufacturer (Procedure 9–3). The patients should be instructed to limit their fluid intake and to avoid diuretic medications for several hours preceding the treatment (LeBouton, 1990). Once the BCG is instilled in the bladder, the patient should be

**PROCEDURE 9-1**

■

## Patient Instructions When BCG Bladder Instillations Are Performed

### ■ EXPLANATION

BCG is a solution made of the tubercular bacillus developed in such a way so that it can be used as treatment to prevent recurrences of bladder tumors. This solution is instilled into the bladder using a catheter. This is done in the office once a week for 6 weeks, then once a month for 11 months.

### ■ PREPARING FOR THE INSTILLATION

Before your appointment you will need to limit your fluid intake for 4 hours. Drink only if necessary to take pills or to take a small sip of water. This will allow the medication to remain concentrated in your bladder. This gives better results.

### ■ THE INSTILLATION

When you come to the office, you will be asked to give us a urine specimen and empty your bladder. A catheter will be put into the bladder and the medication put in. The catheter will be removed, and you will be able to go home. You will be able to drive.

Retain the medication for 2 hours.

### ■ EMPTYING THE BLADDER AFTER TREATMENT

1. Urinate in a sitting position for 6 hours after treatment.
2. For these 6 hours, disinfect the urine and toilet bowel with household bleach. Use 2 cups of bleach after each urination and allow it to stand 15 minutes before flushing.
3. Increase fluid intake to "flush" the bladder for several hours after emptying the bladder the first time.

### ■ POSSIBLE SIDE EFFECTS

You will probably experience burning the first time or two after treatment. We will give you medication to help this. If it [the burning] seems unreasonable, please call the office. You may also experience fever, chills, malaise, flu-like symptoms, or increased fatigue. These are usually temporary and may be helped by Tylenol or other over-the-counter pain medicine.

If you experience severe urinary symptoms such as continued burning or pain on urination, urgency, frequency, blood in urine, joint pain, cough, or skin rash, call our office.

### ■ OTHER CONSIDERATIONS

It is best not to be on an antibiotic while on this treatment. This sometimes cannot be helped. Please let us know if another doctor has put you on an antibiotic.

Women should not become pregnant while on this treatment.

If you have any questions, feel free to call our office.

Courtesy of Organon, Inc.

## PROCEDURE 9-2
■
### Tips for Bladder Instillation of Chemotherapy

Bladder instillation is the insertion of fluid, in this case chemotherapeutic drugs, directly into the bladder via a catheter.

Avoid drinking fluids for a minimum of 2 hours prior to bladder instillation; avoid intake of caffeine (in food and drinks) for at least 4 hours prior to instillation.

Void immediately prior to bladder instillation.

Retain solution in bladder for 2 hours; rotate position every 15 to 30 minutes during this period. It may be more comfortable to start the rotation in the prone position to avoid lying on a full bladder. Next, rotate the left side, then back, then right side. Continue rotation schedule until the 2-hour period has elapsed.

Use care while urinating to avoid contaminating genitals or hands with urine. Wash genitals and hands thoroughly after voiding. Rashes on the genitals and palms of the hands are possible side effects due to mitomycin-C.

Report to the physician any discomfort while urinating.

---

Adapted from Taylor, T. K., & Fogleman, J. C. (1993). Patient pointers. *Innovations in Urology Nursing 3*(3), 7. Reprinted by permission.

## PROCEDURE 9-3
■
### Handling BCG—Health Care Worker Safety

### ■ HEALTH CARE WORKER SAFETY

BCG is an active biological, and care should be taken while handling and reconstituting. These instructions apply equally to all types of BCG.

### ■ PPD SKIN TESTING

PPD-negative health care personnel who routinely handle BCG should keep a record of yearly PPD skin testing.

### ■ BCG ACCIDENT INSTRUCTIONS

*Eye splash:* flush affected eye(s) with copious amounts of water for at least 15 minutes while holding the eyelid(s) open; then seek evaluation by a physician.

*Skin exposure/self-inoculation:* in case of skin contact with the drug, exposure of open sores, or finger laceration, thoroughly wash affected area with soap and water and clean wound with alcohol. In case of suspected accidental self-inoculation, PPD skin testing is advised at the time of the accident and 6 weeks later in order to detect skin test conversion. Asymptomatic skin test conversion is equivalent to BCG vaccination and does not require antituberculous medication. Skin test conversion should, however, be evaluated by a physician.

*Note: If finger stick or laceration should develop granulomatous lesion of the skin, treatment may be given with isoniazid (300 mg/day) and continued for 2 weeks after wound has healed.*

*Procedure continued on following page*

**PROCEDURE 9-3** *Continued*

■

Handling BCG—Health Care Worker Safety

### ■ BCG SPILLS

The following recommendations should be followed for proper clean-up of BCG spills:

Use a germicide that passes the A.O.A.C. Tuberculocidal Activity Test (e.g., Sporicidin or household bleach).

Place several layers of disposable towels over spills. Soak towels with germicide solution and allow soaked toweling to sit for at least 10 minutes. Carefully gather all waste materials into a biohazard bag, autoclave or expose to sterilizing conditions, and dispose of properly.

*Note: Report all accidents during the handling of BCG to supervisory personnel.*

### ■ DISPOSAL AND HANDLING OF TICE™ BCG RECONSTITUTING MATERIALS

After completing BCG preparation, wipe down the drug preparation field (safety cabinet) with 70% isopropyl alcohol solution or household bleach using a disposable towel.

Contaminated needles and syringes should be disposed of intact. Place in puncture-proof container. All used materials, including waste BCG drug, should be placed in labeled biohazard containers and disposed of in accordance with federal and state requirements applicable to biohazardous materials.

*Note: Expired BCG should never be used in the clinic. Unopened ampules should be disposed of in accordance with Federal and State requirements applicable to biohazardous materials.*

### ■ DISPOSAL AND HANDLING OF INSTILLATION MATERIALS

All contaminated materials used in the BCG instillation, including the catheter, should be placed in biohazard disposable bags, autoclaved or exposed to sterilizing conditions, and disposed of properly.

Linens and gowns used during an instillation should be placed in isolation bags and handled by the laundry service in routine fashion.

Permanent fixtures, furniture, or other items in the treatment room and bathroom should be scrubbed down with disinfectant in the routine fashion of the urology clinic.

---

Courtesy of Organon, Inc.

---

advised not to void for 1 or 2 hours, depending on the physician's treatment protocol. Patients who are unable to refrain from voiding for this period should be advised to delay bladder emptying for as long as possible.

Irritative and systemic symptoms considered to be side effects of intravesical BCG immunotherapy have been previously described and should be reviewed with the patient, along with the appropriate steps to take if they occur. Instruct patients to increase their fluid intake in the 24 hours following an instillation of BCG

to speed up the resolution of voiding symptoms.

Side effects associated with intravesical chemotherapy are less prevalent but are possible. Patients should be informed about the likelihood of developing decreased white blood cell or platelet counts and advised to avoid contact with other persons known to have contagious illnesses.

Following transurethral bladder biopsies or resection of a bladder tumor (or tumors), an indwelling urethral catheter is usually present.

Monitor the catheter for patency, which is best accomplished through accurate recording of intake and output measurements. Gross hematuria may be present initially but should lessen over time. The color of the patient's urine should be characterized and documented (e.g., "punch-colored," "burgundy-colored"; see Table 2–2 in Chap. 2) every 4 to 8 hours, depending on the severity of the hematuria. Continuous bladder irrigations are rarely used after TURBT, and manual irrigation of an indwelling urethral catheter is similarly discouraged—open blood vessels within the bladder are likely to absorb the irrigant. When necessary because there is an occlusion of the catheter, *gentle* irrigation to restore catheter patency may be performed.

In rare instances, hematuria does not resolve spontaneously and requires the patient to return to the operating room for cauterization of bleeding vessels. Other interventions may be attempted for persistent gross hematuria, including oral administration of aminocaproic acid (Amicar) or intravesical instillation of formalin.

The urethral catheter is removed within 24 hours after surgery or when hematuria is sufficiently resolved. Advise the patient that normal comfortable voiding will resume within several days. Maintaining a high fluid intake (at least eight glasses of water a day) speeds up the resumption of normal voiding.

Patient education is a vital component of nursing interventions for the patient after transurethral surgery. Patients at this stage of their treatment plan are likely to begin a regimen of intravesical therapy. The interpretation of their biopsy results and recommendations for what medication they are to receive intravesically and how often they should receive it are all vital information. Often, the information must be repeated verbally as well as given to the patient in writing owing to the high level of anxiety that accompanies a new diagnosis of cancer.

Patients also must be instructed about their long-term follow-up plan, specifically about the need for repeat cystoscopy at regular intervals and the importance of vigilantly adhering to this schedule. This information should also be provided to the patient in writing.

### Patient Outcomes

1. The patient expresses relief from pain and discomfort after transurethral bladder surgery or during treatment with intravesical chemotherapy or immunotherapy.
2. The patient states that hematuria has re-

solved after surgical interventions; voided urine is clear yellow.
3. The patient's normal voiding function is restored, with the elimination of irritative voiding symptoms.
4. The patient verbalizes an understanding of the prognosis according to biopsy results and asks questions that are appropriate to health teaching.
5. The patient states an intent to comply with treatment regimens and long-term follow-up plans.

# INVASIVE BLADDER CANCER (STAGES B TO D)

## Medical-Surgical Management

The management of invasive bladder cancer has changed significantly in recent years. Given the success of intravesical immunotherapy with BCG, not all patients whose initial diagnosis is stage B bladder cancer must necessarily undergo radical surgery. Even in patients in whom high-grade tumors exist initially, successful cure may be obtained with BCG. Most patients are now given a trial of BCG therapy with follow-up evaluative biopsies before radical surgery is recommended.

When BCG fails in stage B disease, and in patients who present with stage C disease, radical cystectomy is the treatment of choice. Some stage D patients additionally undergo surgery, as stage D1 bladder cancer with nodal metastases may not be diagnosed until the pathology report is received after radical surgery.

Partial cystectomy is an option for a select group of patients. Only about 10% to 15% of patients having invasive bladder cancer are suitable candidates (Catalona, 1991). Those patients with a solitary lesion who do not have evidence of malignancy or dysplasia elsewhere in the bladder meet the criteria for partial cystectomy. Vigilant follow-up remains necessary for this group of patients, because the 70% recurrence rate still applies, as for all transitional cell tumors.

Most patients with stage B, C, or early stage D bladder cancer undergo radical cystectomy. Numerous surgical options are currently available for both male and female patients. Although the standard surgical procedure remains radical cystectomy and ileal conduit urinary diversion, many types of continent urinary diversions are performed throughout the country. The most information available about long-term results and complications concerns the standard ileal conduit surgical procedure. Data about the risks and benefits of continent urinary diversions continue to be collected as the procedures are refined and performed in greater numbers. Lifestyle implications for the patient are significant with either type of procedure, requiring much patient education and counseling. Nursing plays an essential role in the rehabilitation of patients after radical cystectomy.

Radical cystectomy in men includes removal of the bladder, prostate, and seminal vesicles. A total urethrectomy is usually not performed in men, unless the tumor is near the urethra, to preserve the distal urethra. In women, this surgery includes removal of the bladder, the urethra, the uterus, and the anterior vaginal wall. In both men and women, the pelvic lymph nodes are dissected for pathologic evaluation.

This section discusses the three major types of urinary diversions performed along with radical cystectomy for invasive bladder cancer: ileal conduit urinary diversion, continent cutaneous urinary diversion, and orthotopic bladder replacement anastomosed to the urethra.

## ILEAL CONDUIT URINARY DIVERSIONS

Bricker (1950) first described the technique for ileal conduit urinary diversion that is still used today. Some refinements in operative technique have evolved over the years; however, the procedure remains essentially unchanged (Boyd et al., 1987; deKernion et al., 1991). A 12-cm segment of ileum is used to make the conduit, which is closed off at the proximal end. The ureters are implanted into the segment of ileum, which drains through an abdominal stoma (Fig. 9–3). An everted and well-placed stoma is essential to the long-term success of the surgery.

Complications associated with the ileal conduit include early complications such as wound dehiscence and infection, as well as intestinal obstruction or ileus (deKernion et al., 1991). The most significant late complication of the ileal conduit is renal deterioration, which is believed to occur in 18% to 56% of patients (deKernion et al., 1991; Doughty & Lightner, 1992; Skinner et al., 1987). Chronic reflux in patients without other conduit-related complications is believed to be the cause of decreased renal function. Other causes of renal deterioration in patients with an ileal conduit include

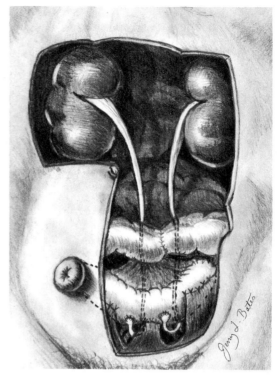

*FIGURE 9–3* Standard ileal conduit urinary diversion.

stomal stenosis, ureteroileal anastomotic strictures, and persistent residual urine within the conduit.

Small, flexible ureteral stents are routinely placed after construction of the ileal conduit and are left in place for 10 to 21 days. The use of stents has reduced the incidence of anastomotic leakage, formerly a frequently occurring early complication.

Other late complications seen in patients after ileal conduit urinary diversion include recurrent or chronic urinary tract infection, and in some patients recurrent bouts of pyelonephritis requiring aggressive antibiotic therapy. Also, stone formation with resultant obstruction and electrolyte disturbances is possible (Doughty & Lightner, 1992; McDougal, 1991).

The use of colon to construct a conduit is necessary in some patients. Usually, these are patients who have undergone radiation therapy and who have significant radiation changes in the ileum and portions of the large bowel. Preoperatively, these patients require a thorough evaluation of their bowel function. An advantage to the use of colon is the decreased incidence of stomal stenosis; however, the incidence of serious complications requiring surgical repair after colon conduit construc-

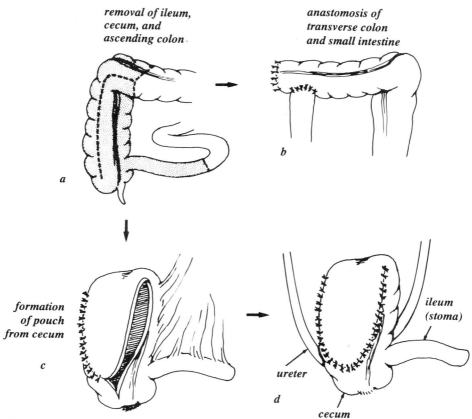

*removal of ileum, cecum, and ascending colon*

*anastomosis of transverse colon and small intestine*

*b*

*a*

*formation of pouch from cecum*

*c*

*ileum (stoma)*

*ureter*

*d*

*cecum*

FIGURE 9–4 The Indiana pouch. (From Cavas, M., & MaKay, S. [1991]. The Indiana pouch: A continent urinary diversion system. *AORN Journal, 54*(3), 494–519. Copyright © AORN Inc., 10170 East Mississippi Avenue, Denver, CO 80231. Reprinted by permission.)

tion is higher than in the ileal conduit (de-Kernion et al., 1991).

## CONTINENT CUTANEOUS URINARY DIVERSIONS

Continent cutaneous urinary diversions have gained popularity in recent years, and several forms of the surgery are performed throughout the country. The obvious primary advantage of these diversions is that the patient does not have to wear an external appliance to collect urine. With the cutaneous diversions, a small, flush abdominal stoma is catheterized regularly to empty urine from the internal pouch.

The most commonly performed continent cutaneous diversions differ mainly in the technique used for construction of the internal pouch and in the segments of ileum or colon used to create the pouch. Ideally, the pouch should be able to hold a high capacity of urine at a low pressure, there should be minimal refluxing of urine, the continence valve should

prevent leakage of urine from the stoma, and the stoma should allow for easy catheterization (Cavas & Makay, 1991; Choudhury, 1989).

Most of the continent urinary diversions performed currently involve the detubularization of the segments of bowel used to create the pouch. This component of the surgery prevents the bowel from contracting (or eliminates peristalsis), an important factor in maintaining continence. Most continent diversions also involve an intricate mechanism for preventing ureteral reflux, usually with an intussuscepted nipple valve or the implantation of ureters into the tenia of the colon segment used. These modifications are further described as each procedure is discussed.

According to Rowland (1988), the Indiana pouch is a modification of the Gilchrist procedure; first described in 1950. The Indiana pouch uses 20 to 24 cm of cecum and ascending colon along with 15 to 18 cm of terminal ileum. The section of colon used is opened and detubularized to then create the pouch (Fig. 9–4).

The ureters are tunneled through the posterior wall of the pouch, allowing the surgeon to use the tenia of the colon for ureteral implantation. This technique of ureteral implantation is designed to minimize reflux (Fig. 9–5). The continence mechanism in the Indiana pouch is created through intricate tapering of the efferent limb, which terminates at the pre-existing ileocecal valve. This tapering makes it difficult for urine to flow freely outward toward the stoma. Finally, a flush stoma is created on the abdominal wall that is used to catheterize the Indiana pouch.

Several drains are placed during the surgery (Fig. 9–6). A "cecostomy" tube is placed into the pouch through a separate stab wound on the abdominal wall. A 20 to 24 Fr Malecot catheter is used for this purpose. The cecostomy tube stays in place for at least 3 weeks after the surgery, and the patient is taught to irrigate it regularly to prevent obstruction with mucus. A Penrose or Jackson-Pratt drain is placed to drain the pelvic cavity, often also staying in place for as long as 3 weeks. Bilateral ureteral stents are placed and brought out either through the stoma or through a separate stab wound, draining urine from the kidneys for as long as 3 weeks. Some surgeons additionally place a small Foley catheter into the pouch through the stoma, although it does not drain and may be removed at any time.

After surgery, patients with an Indiana

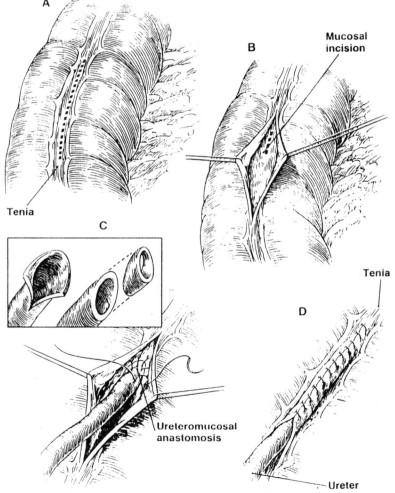

**FIGURE 9–5** Implantation of the ureters: Tunneling through the tenia of the colon. An incision is made along the tenia equal to 3 or 4 diameters of the ureter (A). Tenial flaps are raised. Dash line indicates the mucosal incision (B). The ureter is prepared by spatulation or cutting obliquely as shown in the inset, and a full-thickness ureteromucosal anastomosis is completed with 5-0 synthetic monofilament absorbable suture (C). The tenia is closed over the ureter with a 5-0 nonabsorbable suture (D). (From Rowland, R. G. [1990]. A straightforward surgical approach to urinary diversion. *Contemporary Urology*, 2(1), 13–19, copyright Medical Economics Publishing. Reprinted by permission.)

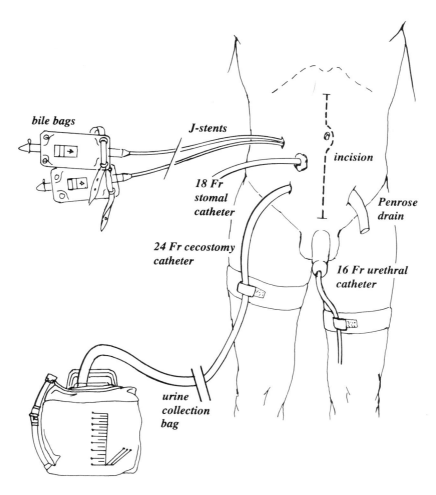

*bile bags*

*J-stents*

*incision*

*18 Fr stomal catheter*

*Penrose drain*

*24 Fr cecostomy catheter*

*16 Fr urethral catheter*

*urine collection bag*

*FIGURE 9–6* Drainage tubes present after Indiana pouch surgery. The J ureteral diversion stents are shown slightly higher than the actual surgical placement for illustration purposes. (From Cavas, M., & MaKay, S. [1991]. The Indiana pouch: A continent urinary diversion system. *AORN Journal, 54*(3), 494–519. Copyright © AORN Inc., 10170 East Mississippi Avenue, Denver, CO 80231. Reprinted by permission.)

pouch go home with the cecostomy tube and possibly the pelvic drain in place. They return to the hospital or clinic 3 weeks later, undergo a radiologic study with contrast material ("pouch-o-gram") to confirm that all anastomoses have healed and to have their tubes removed. They are also taught to catheterize the pouch. Specifics of the catheterization procedure and schedule are found in the section on intervention.

Results with the Indiana pouch have been favorable. It is the simplest of the continent urinary diversions in terms of operative technique and the time required to complete the surgery. Most patients catheterize their pouch four to five times a day for volumes of 400 to 600 mL (Rowland, 1990). Reported complica-

tions include reflux and ureteral obstruction, along with the complications associated with any major abdominal procedure. Long-term results for this procedure are unknown.

Another accepted type of continent cutaneous urinary diversion is the Kock pouch. The Kock urinary pouch was developed as a variation of the Kock continent ileostomy (deKernion et al., 1986). The Kock urinary pouch is constructed of 60 to 80 cm of ileum, all used to create both the pouch and the efferent and afferent limbs (deKernion et al., 1991; Rolstad & Hoyman, 1992). Both limbs are intussuscepted to create a nipple valve. The efferent limb is brought out to the skin as a catheterizable stoma; the afferent limb allows for the nonrefluxing implantation of the ureters into

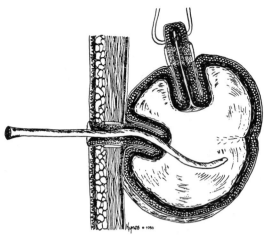

*FIGURE 9–7* The Kock continent reservoir. A No. 20 or 22 Fr coudé catheter is angled over the fascia, then down through the valve into the pouch to accomplish emptying of the pouch. (Courtesy of McNamara & Associates, Fanwood, NJ.)

the pouch (Fig. 9–7). A notable feature of the construction of the nipple valves in the Kock pouch is the use of mesh to secure them and to prevent desussception of the mechanism (deKernion et al., 1991).

Following construction of the Kock continent urinary pouch, a 30 Fr Medina catheter is sutured in place through the efferent limb; it drains urine continuously out the stoma for 3 weeks, requiring temporary use of an external urostomy appliance. A Penrose drain is placed in the pelvic cavity that also remains in place during healing. The patients return to the hospital or clinic after 3 weeks, undergo a radiologic study with contrast material, and have their Medina catheter and Penrose drain removed once the continuity of the pouch is confirmed.

Technically, construction of the cutaneous urinary Kock pouch is a more difficult and lengthy surgical procedure than creation of the Indiana pouch. Results with the Kock pouch have shown loss of continence as the most serious complication and a reoperation rate of 10% to 30% (deKernion et al., 1985).

Other types of continent cutaneous urinary diversions include the Mainz and the "UCLA" pouches. The Mainz pouch uses 10 to 15 cm of cecum and approximately 30 cm of terminal ileum. The colon segment is detubularized. The ureters are implanted into the colon segment of the pouch by tunneling through the tenia, and the continence mechanism is constructed of intussuscepted ileum. The abdominal stoma is usually brought out at the umbilicus. The UCLA pouch is created from the entire right colon along with approximately 14 cm of terminal ileum. The continence mechanism is similar to the Indiana pouch, with intussuscepted ileum implanted into the pre-existing ileocecal valve. Ureteral implantation is different than for other pouches; it involves the tunneling of the distal ureter into the mucosa of the bowel (deKernion et al., 1991). Postoperative care for these pouches is similar to that required for the other types of continent cutaneous urinary diversions.

## ORTHOTOPIC BLADDER REPLACEMENT

A final form of continent urinary diversion is the category of orthotopic bladder replacements. The major characteristic of these diversions is the absence of an external stoma. The pouch is anastomosed directly to the distal urethra, allowing the patient to "void" through an intact urethra. A limited number of patients meet the criteria for this surgery. First, it is rarely performed on women, because the maintenance of continence depends on preserving the bladder neck, which is not recommended in surgery for invasive bladder cancer. Second, the distal urethra in men must be free of malignancy, further reducing the number of suitable candidates for this procedure.

Most of the descriptions of continent orthotopic pouches report a relatively high incidence of nighttime incontinence. This is often outweighed by the benefits to the patient: absence of the need to wear an external appliance or to catheterize at regular intervals, and the ability to voluntarily empty the internal reservoir or pouch. As with the cutaneous continent diversions, long-term results in terms of complications and renal function are unknown.

The original orthotopic urinary pouch was described by Camey and others (Lilian & Camey, 1984). The Camey procedure (Fig. 9–8) used tubularized bowel, but continued peristalsis of the bowel resulted in a high incidence of continuous incontinence. For that reason the detubularized approaches are preferred for orthotopic bladder replacement.

The Kock (or hemi-Kock) pouch has also been used as a bladder replacement in many patients. As with other types of Kock pouches, approximately 45 cm of ileum is used to construct the pouch itself. The same intussuscepted nipple valve mechanism is used to implant the ureters into the pouch, as previously described. Instead of an efferent limb, the pouch is tapered and anastomosed directly to the distal urethra (Fig. 9–9).

A clear plastic Foley catheter (Simplastic) is placed as a stent through the urethral anastomosis, and bilateral ureteral stents are placed through the efferent limb and secured to the Foley. A pelvic drain (Penrose or Jackson-Pratt) is also put in place. The Foley catheter must be vigilantly irrigated in the immediate postoperative period, and the patient must learn to irrigate it four times a day at home. After being discharged with the Foley catheter and pelvic drain in place, the patient should return to the hospital or clinic after 3 weeks for a radiologic study with contrast material and removal of the catheters. "Voiding training" is then initiated.

Several other types of orthotopic bladder replacement surgical procedures are currently performed, including the ileal neobladder, the Mainz pouch, and the ileocolonic pouch (or "Le Bag"). After all of these procedures, which essentially differ only in the segments of bowel used and surgical technique, patients must relearn how to empty their new "bladders." After orthotopic bladder replacement, voiding is performed by straining or Valsalva's maneuver. Initially, a schedule of frequent voiding (every 2 hours during the day, every 3 hours at night) must be maintained to gradually adapt the pouch to greater amounts of urine. Patients are also taught pelvic floor strengthening exercises, found to be of great help in minimizing daytime incontinence when performed without fail. Finally, all patients are taught to catheter-

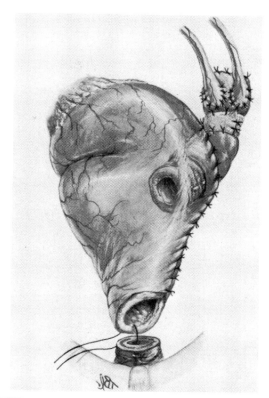

**FIGURE 9–9** The hemi-Kock pouch orthotopic bladder replacement. The opening in the reservoir is sutured to the membranous urethra with interrupted 2-0 chromic. (From Boyd, S. D., Lieskovsky, G., & Skinner, D. G. [1991]. Kock pouch bladder replacement. *Urologic Clinics of North America, 18*[4], 641–648. Reprinted by permission.)

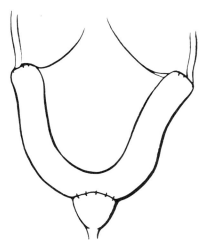

**FIGURE 9–8** The Camey procedure. (From Hinman, F., Jr. (ed.). [1989]. *Atlas of urologic surgery* [p. 567]. Philadelphia: W. B. Saunders. Reprinted by permission.)

ize the pouch in the event that should become necessary. The unlikely patient who is unable to empty the pouch by straining needs to catheterize the pouch intermittently. Self-catheterization is also taught so that the patient can free the urethra of mucus should a mucous plug prevent emptying of the pouch.

Some short-term results after the Kock pouch orthotopic bladder replacement are available. Boyd, Lieskovsky, and Skinner (1991) reported that 94% of their patients with a Kock pouch were continent during the day, whereas 31% reported nighttime continence. The number of those continent throughout the night is increased to 54% when patients who get up once at night to void are added. Long-term complications related to renal function are unknown, although some authors predict that the incidence of renal deterioration will be less than that seen with the ileal conduit because of the intricately created antireflux mechanism in the Kock pouch.

Radical cystectomy provides a cure for bladder cancer in about 50% of patients (Whitmore Jr, 1983). In the other 50%, metastasis has already occurred. Systemic chemotherapy and radiation therapy are options for the management of bladder cancer at this stage. Most chemotherapy regimens for bladder cancer involve cisplatin, methotrexate, doxorubicin, and vinblastine (M-VAC) (Brettschneider & Orihuela, 1990). Approximately 40% of patients experience a positive result from M-VAC, with or without radiation therapy, in terms of prolonging life.

## Approaches to Patient Care

### Assessment

Nursing assessment of the patient with invasive bladder cancer can occur in the office or clinic as hospital admission is arranged, or on admission to the hospital. In the outpatient setting, an assessment of the patients' understanding of their disease and the implications for them after radical surgery is important. Assessment of symptoms is essentially the same as for superficial disease. Assess the patient and family's knowledge about scheduled diagnostic studies (as part of a preoperative metastatic workup) and hospital routines. The nurse may also assess the patient's readiness to learn about the specific type of urinary diversion surgery he or she will have. Often this is a good time to arrange for the patient to speak with another person who has already undergone (and recovered from) the same surgery.

For patients who have been admitted to the hospital, assess their anxiety level and their ability to comprehend all the information they will be asked to learn. Assess their understanding of the need for preoperative bowel preparation, including intravenous therapy, laxatives, and oral antibiotics. This time is also appropriate to assess the support system available to patients as they recover from surgery. Patients without supportive family or friends may need the assistance of a social work professional to assist them after surgery.

Finally, assess the patient's readiness to accept and understand all the procedural and sensory information provided and to prepare for the outcome of surgery.

### Nursing Diagnosis

The nursing diagnoses for the patient with stages B through D bladder cancer may include the following:

1. Fluid volume deficit related to bowel preparation for surgery.

2. Altered pattern of urinary elimination related to
   a. Cystectomy and the creation of a urinary diversion.
   b. Mucous obstruction of the temporary urinary drainage device.
   c. Incontinence caused by the weakness (short term) or impaired effectiveness (long term) of the surgically created continence mechanism.
3. Pain related to the effects of surgery, as well as the placement of multiple surgical drainage devices.
4. Alteration in bowel function related to disruption of bowel integrity through surgery and the presence of decompression tubes.
5. Potential for infection related to disruption of the skin at the surgical site and the placement of surgical drains through stab wounds.
6. Impaired skin integrity related to
   a. Creation of an abdominal stoma.
   b. Leakage of urine from the stoma.
   c. Application of the surgical dressing and the external pouching system.
7. Knowledge deficit related to care of the permanent urinary diversion.
8. Body image disturbance related to
   a. The loss of genitourinary and reproductive structures as a result of radical cystectomy.
   b. The presence of an abdominal stoma.
9. Potential for sexual dysfunction related to postoperative changes affecting self-esteem, body image, and physical ability.

### Plan of Care

Nursing care is directed toward enabling the patient to

1. Adapt to an alternative method of urinary elimination in accordance with the type of urinary diversion created.
2. Remain comfortable as healing progresses after radical cystectomy and urinary diversion.
3. Achieve return of bowel function in a timely fashion after surgery.
4. Prevent infection from occurring in and around the urostomy or continent diversion as well as tracts established for surgical drainage.
5. Prevent skin deterioration around the stoma site.
6. Learn to care for the ileal conduit or continent cutaneous urinary diversion or learn to void with an orthotopic bladder replacement.
7. Integrate the abdominal stoma into the body image in a positive manner.

8. Discuss concerns regarding sexual function and activity following radical cystectomy and urinary diversion.

**Intervention**

An important element in the nursing care of the patient undergoing radical cystectomy and urinary diversion surgery is preoperative education and stoma site marking (when necessary). Often the amount of information a patient may learn in the days preceding major surgery is minimized by anxiety. When possible, an opportunity for the urologic clinical nurse specialist or enterostomal therapy nurse to meet with the patient and family before the hospital admission may be quite beneficial. Information is provided to both the patient and family about postoperative care, recovery time, and what it will be like for the patient, on a daily basis, after the urinary diversion.

Selection of stoma sites is especially important in patients with ileal conduits. Care must be taken so that the permanent stoma is in a location where the patient is able to see and care for it and where it does not interfere with the patient's clothing. The stoma is situated in the abdominal muscles and should lie well away from any skin folds or crevices, the umbilicus, scars, or bony prominences (Smith, 1992). Many surgeons prefer that stoma sites be marked preoperatively on all patients undergoing radical cystectomy (regardless of the type of urinary diversion planned), in the event a standard ileal conduit becomes necessary intraoperatively.

The 48-hour period before surgery is usually spent undergoing a bowel preparation: the patient is allowed only clear liquids, a peripheral intravenous line is started for hydration, and the patient is given a series of laxatives and enemas. Each institution's protocol may differ, but oral and suppository laxatives with tap water or cleansing enemas until clear are often ordered. Monitor the results from the laxatives and enemas to ensure the bowel is clean. Watch the patient for symptoms of fluid volume deficit secondary to excessive loss of fluid from the gastrointestinal tract, including hypotension, dizziness, and nausea. Along with bowel cleansing, antibiotics may be administered (if ordered) for preoperative sterilization of bowel tissue.

Nursing care after any radical cystectomy and urinary diversion must initially be directed toward preventing complications related to major abdominal surgery. The use of pneumatic anti-embolism stockings, early ambulation, and respiratory care, such as incentive spirometry devices for lung expansion and routine turning, coughing and deep breathing, are necessary nursing measures. Careful monitoring of intake and output amounts is also needed to prevent problems with third spacing or excess fluid loss. Monitoring of urinary output amounts every 4 hours initially and then every 8 hours also serves to ensure the patency of urinary drainage catheters.

Postoperative analgesia has evolved in recent years. Many patients with radical cystectomy are now managed with combinations of intermittent or continuous epidural narcotics and patient-controlled analgesia (PCA). These methods are extremely effective in reducing postoperative discomfort and promoting mobility and adequate respiratory function. Nursing interventions with patients using these pain control mechanisms involve the use of a pain assessment tool to determine their response to analgesia, frequent monitoring of vital signs (particularly respiratory rates) in patients receiving epidural medications, and patient instruction in the use of the PCA device. In those situations when newer technologies for pain management are not available, analgesics should be given routinely around the clock for the first 48 hours after surgery.

Gastric decompression tubes are present after radical cystectomy in the form of nasogastric tubes or gastrostomy tubes. Nasogastric tubes are connected to continuous or intermittent suction and should be monitored to ensure they are working. Irrigation and repositioning are sometimes necessary. Gastrostomy tubes are usually placed to straight drainage. In some patients, both types of tubes may be present, with the nasogastric tube being removed during the first few days postoperatively and the gastrostomy tube remaining until just before discharge. The presence of a gastrostomy tube allows for periodic clamping to assess the patient's return of bowel function once oral intake is allowed.

When the method of urinary diversion is an ileal conduit, the stoma should be regularly assessed postoperatively for color and viability. A healthy stoma is beefy red. Bilateral ureteral stents exit from the stoma and drain into the urostomy pouch. It is not unusual for urine to drain both through the stents and around them. Hematuria may be present during the first 48 hours after surgery but should resolve spontaneously.

Among the most important of nursing interventions after radical cystectomy and ileal conduit urinary diversion is teaching the patient how to care for the new urostomy. Instructing the patient on how to care for the pouching system may begin as early as the third postoperative day. A list of tasks to be accomplished by the patient (or caretaker) begins with having the patient just observe the stoma and ends with having the patient independently change the urostomy appliance before discharge (Table 9–4). Other tasks include attaching the appliance to a bedside drainage bag (or container) for nighttime use.

One- and two-piece urostomy pouching systems are available, and patient preference plays a part in determining which system is to be used (Procedure 9–4 and Fig. 9–10). The size, location, and shape of the stoma, individual patient characteristics (e.g., manual dexterity or visual or neurologic deficits), and financial considerations are also involved in the choice of a pouching system. Most pouching systems employ a protective skin barrier and a disposable pouch. Wearing time ranges from 3 to 7 days, depending on the type of pouching system used.

Urostomy stomas tend to decrease in size over time and often end up being flush with the abdominal wall, even when they initially were everted. In cases of flush urostomy stomas, numerous disposable pouches with built-in convexity are available. These convex pouches often readily solve any problems with skin excoriation or leakage of urine the patient may experience.

Patient education also includes a review of the most commonly occurring peristomal skin problems and what to do should they occur. Again, because the amount of information a patient is able to absorb at one time is limited, establishing a relationship with the enterostomal therapy nurse provides the patient with a source of information after hospital discharge as well as a source of help in the event of future problems with urostomy care.

**TABLE 9–4. Tasks for New Urostomy Patients***

1. View stoma.
2. Empty urine from pouch.
3. Change pouch and clean stoma.
4. Prepare new appliance (wafer and pouch†). Measure stoma. Trace pattern onto wafer. Cut out wafer.
5. Change entire appliance, and clean peristomal skin independently.
6. Verbalize appropriate measures to take for skin breakdown and for signs and symptoms of urinary tract infection.

*To be accomplished before discharge.
†For patients using two-piece system.

Altered body image is often a difficult problem for patients with a new urostomy. It may be difficult to adjust to the presence of an abdominal stoma and the need to wear an external collection device. Loss of control and privacy is an additional stressor for the patient, who has no control over urination and who must "share" this normally private bodily function with nursing specialists and staff as well as family or a friend who may be assisting with the care. A consistent, caring attitude by nurses and the patient's gradual independence in his or her own care are beneficial in resolving these issues.

Patients should receive instructions about obtaining their urostomy supplies at home and information about insurance coverage. If possible, the nurse should provide the patient with the names, addresses, and phone numbers of two suppliers of ostomy products. The support of a visiting nurse is helpful for most patients and their families immediately after discharge.

Arranging for an "ostomy visitor" is often an extremely beneficial experience for the patient. Through the United Ostomy Association and the American Cancer Society, most areas have visitation programs in which a fellow urostomate visits the patients, either in the hospital or at home, to talk with them about life with a urostomy. This support mechanism extends beyond recovery from surgery, and many patients eventually become visitors themselves.

When the method of urinary diversion is a continent cutaneous urinary diversion, patient education needs are quite different. Immediately after surgery, multiple drainage tubes are present (see Fig. 9–6). Using the Indiana reservoir as an example, bilateral ureteral stents and a large "cecostomy" tube drain urine from the kidneys and the pouch, respectively. A nasogastric tube or gastrostomy tube, or both, are present. A pelvic drain (Penrose or Jackson-Pratt) is also present. Optional catheters include a urethral and a stomal catheter. Gradually, most of these tubes are removed, and the patient is discharged with the cecostomy tube (or a large-bore catheter that drains the pouch in other cutaneous diversions) and possibly the pelvic drain in place.

Because the pouch is constructed of bowel, mucus is continuously secreted and mixed with the urine. In the immediate postoperative period, it is important to keep the catheters that drain the pouch free of mucous plugs, so regular irrigation is needed. Irrigation of the cecos-

## PROCEDURE 9-4

■

## Application of One-Piece Urinary Pouch*

1. Gather all supplies.
2. Gently remove soiled pouch by pushing down on skin while lifting up on pouch. Discard soiled pouch.
3. Use stoma-measuring guide or established pattern to determine size of stoma.
   a. *Presized pouch.* Check to be sure pouch opening is correct size. Order new supplies if indicated.
   b. *Cut-to-fit pouch.* Trace correctly sized pattern onto back of pouch, and cut stomal opening to match pattern.
   *Note:* Once stomal shrinkage is complete, this step may be omitted. If a cut-to-fit pouch is used, pouch may be cut out before soiled pouch is removed.
4. Remove paper backing from pouch, and lay pouch to one side.
5. Clean stoma and peristomal skin with water; pat dry. *If indicated,* shave or clip peristomal hair.
   *Use wicks against stoma to absorb urine and to keep skin dry for steps 6 and 7.*
6. *Optional:* Apply skin sealant to skin that will be covered by tape. Allow to dry.
7. Remove paper backing from pouch; center pouch opening over stoma and press pouch into place.
8. *Optional:* Apply tape strips to "picture-frame" the pouch–skin junction.

---

*Universal precautions* must be followed when this procedure is performed.
From Hampton, B. G., & Bryant, R. A. (Eds.) (1992). *Ostomies and continent diversions: Nursing management.* St. Louis: Mosby-Year Book. Reprinted by permission.

---

tomy tube with 30 mL of physiologic saline is ordered every 2 hours postoperatively. Later, the patient learns to irrigate this tube at home, at intervals ranging from every 4 hours to four times a day (Cavas & Makay, 1991; Davidson et al., 1990). This maneuver continues to keep the tube patent.

Patients who go home with the pelvic drain in place need to change either the dressing over it daily or a pouch (often a urostomy pouch) over it periodically. The decision about which of these to use is based on the amount of drainage the patient experiences from the pelvic drain.

During the postoperative period, patients should observe and identify their flush abdominal stoma, through which they will catheterize their pouch. Practice catheterization may be helpful. Actual catheterization of the pouch does not begin until healing of the pouch is confirmed by radiographic studies. This may occur 10 to 30 days after surgery, depending on surgeon preference. In many centers, the patients are readmitted to the hospital after having been home for several weeks with the cecostomy tube in place. They are then taught to catheterize the pouch. Procedure 9–5 contains instructions for catheterization of the Indiana pouch.

In addition to the catheterization procedure, reviewing with the patients their schedules for catheterizations is important. By gradually expanding the pouch to hold larger amounts of urine, the continence mechanism is conserved and the pouch adapts well. (Procedure 9–6 contains an example of a catheterization schedule.) Eventually, most Indiana pouches hold between 400 and 600 mL of urine, requiring catheterization four to five times a day.

Finally, patients need information about where to obtain their catheters when they are home and how to care for them. Clean technique applies to catheter care, and either reusable red rubber catheters or disposable plastic catheters may be used.

Patients who have continent cutaneous Kock pouches have slightly different needs than those with Indiana pouches. Patients with a Kock pouch have a large (30 Fr) Medina tube sutured through their abdominal stoma into the pouch during the first few weeks after surgery. An external collection device must be worn during this time. The patient must also learn to irrigate the Medina tube every 4 hours

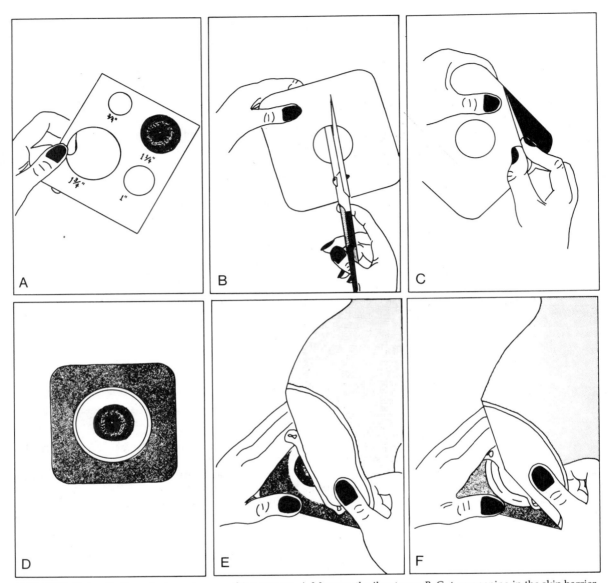

**FIGURE 9–10** Application of a two-piece pouching system. *A*, Measure the ileostomy. *B*, Cut an opening in the skin barrier. *C*, Remove the paper backing. *D*, Center the skin barrier over the stoma. *E*, Snap on the pouch. *F*, Tug on pouch to ensure security. (From Erickson, P. J. [1987]. Ostomies: The art of pouching. *Nursing Clinics of North America, 22*[2], 311–320. Reprinted by permission.)

(Greig, 1986). After radiographic studies confirm healing of the Kock pouch, these patients learn to catheterize with a 20 or 22 Fr red rubber coudé catheter.

Nursing care after an orthotopic bladder replacement also involves maintaining the patency of urinary drainage tubes. These patients have a large Simplastic Foley catheter in place after surgery. Bilateral ureteral stents are present but may not be seen because they are secured to the tip of the Foley. A pelvic drain (Penrose or Jackson-Pratt) is present, as is a nasogastric or gastrostomy tube, or both.

As with other urinary pouches constructed from bowel, mucous secretion may be problematic, so regular irrigation of the Foley catheter is performed every 2 hours postoperatively. The patients are taught to irrigate the catheter every 4 hours to four times a day at home. They are also taught how to use a leg bag and a bedside drainage bag and how to change the external collecting pouch usually applied over the pelvic drain.

Patients with a bladder replacement also return to the hospital or clinic for more instruction once radiographic studies confirm their

## PROCEDURE 9-5

■

## Patient Instructions for Catheterizing the Indiana Pouch

### ■ SUPPLIES

16 or 18 red rubber catheter
A water-soluble lubricant
Saline and a piston syringe

### ■ PROCEDURE

1. Wash your hands!
2. Draw up 30–40 mL of saline in the piston syringe (once a day *only*).
3. Place a small amount of lubricant on the tip of the catheter.
4. Insert the catheter into your stoma, and keep going until urine begins to flow out the catheter. Hold the catheter in place until urine flow stops. Then remove the catheter.
5. Once a day, during your regular catheterization, you should irrigate the pouch with 30–40 mL of saline. Repeat if necessary to clear the pouch of mucus.
6. After catheterization, clean the catheter with mild soap and water. Dry the catheter with a clean paper towel, and store it in an airtight sandwich bag. Use a new bag after each use of the catheter.

### ■ TIPS

You will need to replace the catheters about every 6 months. You may boil the catheters for about 20 minutes in water on the stove once a week if you like.
If your pouch becomes too full, urine will leak out the stoma. You waited too long!
Catheterize more often when your fluid intake is much higher than normal.
Keep a catheter with you at all times.
Occasional flecks of blood in your urine are normal.
If you have leakage from the stoma at night, decrease your fluid intake after 7–8 PM.
You need only a small adhesive bandage over the stoma.

---

pouch is healing. With these patients, the Foley catheter, ureteral stents, and pelvic drain are removed, and the patient is taught how to "void." Most patients instinctively understand they must "push" or "strain" to void, and they have no difficulty doing this. The most disconcerting aspect of this period for the patient is the inevitable urinary incontinence. Instruction in pelvic floor strengthening exercises is needed at this time, and the patient must be reassured that by doing these exercises regularly, the periods of continence will dramatically improve. Instruction in clean urethral catheterization must also be provided, so that the patients can empty the pouch in the event they cannot void or their urethra becomes occluded with mucus.

Patients with orthotopic bladder replacements must also adhere to a strict schedule of pouch emptying for the first few weeks after the tubes are removed. Procedure 9–7 contains a sample voiding schedule, which illustrates that the patient cannot sleep for longer than 3 hours at a time during the first week. Combine the incontinence with the sleep deprivation and this situation makes for an arduous recovery. Continuous reassurance about the eventual outcome is often needed. If possible, arranging for the patient to talk to a previous bladder replacement patient may be beneficial as well.

Male patients who undergo some form of radical cystectomy and urinary diversion are likely to be impotent following the procedure.

## PROCEDURE 9-6
■
### Schedule for Catheterizing the Indiana Pouch

You are now catheterizing your Indiana pouch. For the next few weeks, you must gradually "train" your pouch to hold larger amounts of urine. You should catheterize your pouch according to the following schedule:

| WEEK | DAY | NIGHT |
|---|---|---|
| 1 and 2 | Every 2–3 h | Every 4 h* |
| 3 and 4 | Every 3–4 h | Every 5 h* |
| 5 and 6 | Every 4–5 h | Every 6 h |
| 7 and 8 | Every 4–6 h | Every 7 h |

*Set your alarm clock to wake you up to catheterize your pouch.

Most people get to the point where they catheterize about every 6 hours, or 4 times a day. You will need to catheterize more often if you've had a lot of fluids.

This may be the outcome even when "nerve-sparing" procedures are performed. Surgeons routinely provide the patient and his partner with this information preoperatively, along with options to be considered. The patient often must first deal with the diagnosis of cancer and major surgery and then must recover from the surgery and learn to live with a urinary diversion. Reinforcement of the availability and success of treatment options for sexual dysfunction assists the patient in eventually resolving this problem.

For women undergoing radical cystectomy, a portion of the anterior vaginal wall is re-

## PROCEDURE 9-7
■
### Patient Instructions for "Kock to the Urethra" Voiding Schedule

#### ■ VOIDING SCHEDULE

1st week:  Urinate every 2 hours during the day and every 3 hours at night.
2nd week:  Urinate every 3 hours during the day and every 4 hours at night.
3rd week:  Urinate every 4 hours during the day and every 5 hours at night.
4th week:  Urinate every 5 hours during the day and every 6 hours at night.
5th week:  Urinate every 6 hours during the day and not at all at night.

#### ■ TIPS

Urinating every 6 hours during the day and night is an ideal goal. The above schedule is approximate and represents goals you should try to meet. Some people are not able to hold their urine for 6 hours.

One problem that may occur is nighttime incontinence (or leakage). There are three things you can do to help prevent this if it happens to you:

Drink less fluid in the evening, before going to bed.
Catheterize yourself before going to bed to completely empty your new bladder pouch.
Or, you can set your alarm to wake up during the night to urinate, so the pouch does not become so full that leakage happens.

moved during the surgery. Provide the patient with information about when to resume sexual activity, and the information that, initially, it may be uncomfortable and require additional lubrication. The effects of the hysterectomy on the patient's sexuality must not be overlooked. Often it is the nurse who is in the best position to counsel the patient and her partner.

Caring for patients with a urinary diversion is extremely rewarding. With this group of patients, nursing plays an essential role in postoperative care, education, and rehabilitation. Patients who have an ileal conduit may be restored to near normal daily living, with the addition only of caring for and emptying the external appliance. Patients who undergo continent cutaneous urinary diversion or orthotopic bladder replacement are usually delighted with their results, which have little impact on their lifestyle. Overall, the surgical experience for the patient with invasive bladder cancer may be rewarding for all concerned.

### Patient Outcomes

1. The patient's urinary drainage devices and surgical wound drains remain patent during the postoperative period.
2. The patient states that comfort was maintained during the postoperative period.
3. The patient's normal bowel function returns, with normal oral intake of food and fluids and the regular passage of stool.
4. The patient remains free of infection at the surgical site.
5. The patient learns to change and empty the urostomy appliance, or learns to catheterize the continent urinary diversion, or learns to void with bladder replacement.
6. The patient's skin surface around the stomal site remains intact and free of irritation.
7. The patient verbalizes an acceptance of the abdominal stoma and projects a positive attitude regarding his or her body image.
8. The patient demonstrates a willingness to openly discuss the effects of the surgery on his or her sexuality and sexual function.

## ACKNOWLEDGMENTS

The author thanks S. Bruce Malkowicz, MD, Wendy English, RN, and Carralee Sueppel, CURN, for their assistance in the preparation of this chapter.

## *REFERENCES*

Armstrong, B., & Doll, R. (1975). Bladder cancer mortality in diabetics in relation to saccharin consumption and smoking habits. *British Journal of Prevention, 29,* 73.

Bengtsson, U., Angervall, L., Ekman, H., & Lehmann, L. (1968). Transitional cell tumors of the renal pelvis in analgesic abusers. *Scandinavian Journal of Urology and Nephrology, 2,* 145.

Boyd, S. D., Feinberg, S. M., Skinner, D. G., Lieskovsky, G., Baron, D., & Richardson, J. (1987). Quality of life survey of urinary diversion patients: Comparison of ileal conduits versus continent Kock ileal reservoirs. *Journal of Urology, 138*(6), 1386–1389.

Boyd, S. D., Lieskovsky, G., & Skinner, D. G. (1991). Kock pouch bladder replacement. *Urologic Clinics of North America, 18*(4), 641–648.

Brettschneider, N. R., & Orihuela, E. (1990). Carcinoma of the bladder. *Urologic Nursing, 10*(1), 14–19.

Bricker, E. M. (1950). Bladder substitution after pelvic evisceration. *Surgical Clinics of North America, 30,* 1511.

Brosman, S. A. (1991). Indications for BCG use in carcinoma-in-situ. *Urology, 37*(5), 12–13.

Brosman, S. A., Lamm, D. L., van der Meijden, A. P. M., & DeBruyne, F. M. J. (1991). A practical guide to the use of intravesical BCG for the management of stage Ta, T1, CIS transitional cell cancer. *Urology Times, 19* (Suppl. 1), 31–36.

Catalona, W. J. (1991). Bladder cancer. In J. Y. Gillenwater, J. T. Grayhack, S. S. Howards, & J. W. Duckett (Eds.), *Adult and pediatric urology* (2nd ed., pp. 1135–1177). Chicago: Year Book.

Cavas, M., & Makay, S. (1991). The Indiana pouch: A continent urinary diversion system. *AORN Journal, 54*(3), 494–519.

Choudhury, M. S. (1989). The Indiana pouch: A continent urinary reservoir. *Progressions: Developments in Ostomy and Wound Care, 1,* 12–15.

Cole, P., Monson, R. R., Haning, H., & Friedell, G. H. (1971). Smoking and cancer of the lower urinary tract. *New England Journal of Medicine, 284*:129–134.

Cutler, S. H., & Young, J. L., Jr. (Eds.). (1975). Third national cancer survey: Incidence data. *National Cancer Institute Monographs, 41*:1–454.

Davidson, M. W., Brown, K. A., Freedman, P. A., & Thompson, M. (1990). Continent Indiana reservoir: Nursing management. *Ostomy/Wound Management, 31*(6), 50–57.

deKernion, J. B., Den Besten, L., Kaufman, J. J., & Ehrlich, R. (1985). The Kock pouch as a urinary reservoir: Pitfalls and perspectives. *American Journal of Surgery, 150*(1), 83.

deKernion, J. B., Stenzyl, A., & Mukamel, E. (1991). Urinary diversion and continent reservoir. In J. Y. Gillenwater, J. T. Grayhack, S. S. Howards, & J. W. Duckett (Eds.), *Adult and pediatric urology* (2nd ed., pp. 1185–1209). Chicago: Year Book.

Doughty, D. B., & Lightner, D. J. (1992). Genitourinary surgical procedures. In B. G. Hampton & R. A. Bryant (Eds.), *Ostomies and continent diversions: Nursing management* (pp. 249–263). St. Louis: Mosby-Year Book.

Droller, M. Y. (1986). Transitional cell cancer: Upper tracts and bladder. In P. C. Walsh, R. F. Gittes, A. D. Perlmutter, & T. A. Stamey (Eds.), *Campbell's urology* (5th ed., pp. 1343–1440). Philadelphia: W. B. Saunders.

Greig, B. J. (1986). Interventions of the ET nurse with the continent urinary Koch pouch patient. *Journal of Enterostomal Therapy, 13*(6), 226–231.

Lamm, D. L., Stogdill, V. D., Stogdill, B. J., & Crispin, R. G. (1986). Complications of bacillus Calmette-Guérin immunotherapy in 1,278 patients with bladder cancer. *Journal of Urology, 135*(2), 272–274.

LeBouton, J. (1990). Nursing aspects of bacillus Calmette-Guérin immunotherapy for superficial bladder cancer. *Urologic Nursing, 10*(4), 9–13.

Lilian, O. M., & Camey, M. (1984). 25-year experience with

replacement of the human bladder (Camey procedure). *Journal of Urology, 132,* 886–891.

Malloy, T. R., & Wein A. J. (1987). Laser treatment of bladder carcinoma and genital condylomata. *Urologic Clinics of North America, 14*(1), 121–126.

McDougal, W. (1991). Perioperative care. In J. W. Gillenwater, J. T. Grayhack, S. S. Howards, & J. W. Duckett (Eds.), *Adult and pediatric urology* (2nd ed., pp. 445–474). Chicago: Year Book.

Morales, A., Eidinger, D., & Bruce, A. W. (1976). Intracavitary bacillus Calmette-Guérin in the treatment of superficial bladder tumors. *Journal of Urology, 116,* 180.

Morrison, A. S. (1984). Advances in the etiology of urothelial cancer. *Urologic Clinics of North America, 11,* 557–566.

Rolstad, B. S., & Hoyman, K. (1992). Continent diversions and reservoirs. In B. G. Hamptom & R. A. Bryant (Eds.), *Ostomies and continent diversions: Nursing management* (pp. 129–162). St. Louis: Mosby-Year Book.

Rowland, R. G. (1988). Continent urinary reservoirs. *Surgical Clinics of North America, 68*(5), 891–907.

Rowland, R. G. (1990). A straightforward surgical approach to urinary diversion. *Contemporary Urology, 2*(1), 13–19.

Skinner, D. G., Lieskovsky, G., & Boyd, S. D. (1987). Continuing experience with the continent ileal reservoir (Kock pouch) as an alternative to cutaneous urinary diversion: An update after 250 cases. *Journal of Urology, 137*(6), 1140–1145.

Smith, D. B. (1992). Psychosocial adaptation. In B. G. Hampton & R. A. Bryant (Eds.), *Ostomies and continent diversions: Nursing management* (pp. 1–27). St. Louis: Mosby-Year Book.

Wein, A. J., & Hanno, P. M. (1987). Carcinoma of the genitourinary tract. In P. M. Hanno & A. J. Wein (Eds.), *A clinical manual of urology* (pp. 281–351). Norwalk, CT: Appleton-Century-Crofts.

Whitmore, W. F., Jr. (1983). Management of invasive bladder neoplasms. *Seminars in Urology, 1,* 34–41.

# CHAPTER 10

# Cancer of
# the Male Genitalia

■

*Angela D. Klimaszewski and Karen A. Karlowicz*

Cancer of the Prostate
Cancer of the Testis

Cancer of the Penis
Cancer of the Scrotum

## OVERVIEW

Cancers of the male genitalia are tumors that arise from the prostate, testis, penis, or scrotum. Each of these structures, although located in or near the male pelvis, is primarily affected by a distinct histologic type of cancer.

Ninety-five percent of prostate cancers diagnosed are adenocarcinoma. Forty percent of testis tumors are seminoma, whereas penile and scrotal tumors are predominantly squamous cell carcinoma (National Cancer Institute, 1990).

The medical management for each type of male genital cancer is different and must be individualized. Likewise, nursing care must be focused on the specific needs of the male patient with a tumor arising from a genital structure. This chapter provides information regarding cancer of the prostate, testis, penis, and scrotum. Theories of tumor causation are explored, the course of disease is discussed, and advances in diagnosis and treatment are presented.

## BEHAVIORAL OBJECTIVES

After studying this chapter, the reader should be able to

**1.** Discuss techniques for early detection of prostate cancer.

**2.** Distinguish the most effective treatment alternative for each stage of prostate cancer.

**3.** Describe the basic mechanism of action and side effects of hormonal therapies used to treat prostate cancer.

**4.** Teach testicular self-examination to a young male client.

**5.** Identify at least two nursing interventions for the testicular cancer patient receiving chemotherapy and experiencing nausea and vomiting.

**6.** Analyze the relationship among penile cancer, smegma, and the uncircumcised penis.

## KEY WORDS

**Adjuvant therapy**—a treatment given in addition to the primary modality to enhance its effectiveness.

**Alopecia**—hair loss.

**Alpha-fetoprotein (AFP)**—the dominant serum protein produced by fetal tissue that is found in only trace amounts after 1 year of age.

**Anorexia**—loss of appetite.

**Biopsy**—excision of a tissue sample from a patient for diagnostic study.

**Brachytherapy**—treatment with ionizing radiation in which the radioactive material is applied to the skin surface or placed a short distance from the area requiring therapy.

**Carcinogen**—any substance that causes cancer.

**Carcinoma**—cancer of epithelial cell origin.

**Combination therapy**—the use of more than one method to treat a patient with cancer.

**Grading**—the appearance of tumor cells, specifically concerning their degree of anaplasia.

**Human chorionic gonadotropin (hCG)**—a hormone secreted by the placenta during pregnancy that is not present in significant amounts in normal men.

**Induration**—an abnormal hardening of tissue; often a finding during rectal examination of a diseased prostate.

**Metastasis**—the spread of cancer from one part of the body to another by direct extension or hematogenous and lymphatic pathways.

**Prostate-specific antigen (PSA)**—an antigen produced by the prostate that increases in the presence of benign prostatic hypertrophy and prostatic cancer.

**Prostatic acid phosphatase (PAP)**—an enzyme that increases with the metabolism and catabolism of prostatic cancer cells.

**Sarcoma**—a cancer arising from muscle, bone, fat, or other connective tissue.

**Staging**—a quantification of the extent of a disease that serves as a parameter for determining prognosis and treatment.

**Verrucous**—pertains to the wartlike or papillary growths of squamous cell carcinoma of the penis; this term may also be used to describe lesions of viral origin, often appearing small, round, and raised with a rough, dry surface; the lesions may occur on any body surface.

# CANCER OF THE PROSTATE

## PERSPECTIVE ON DISEASE ENTITY

**Etiology.** Cancer of the prostate is diagnosed in more than 165,000 Americans annually. Although the diagnosis of localized prostate cancer has increased in the last 10 years, it is the second most common cause of cancer among men in the United States, accounting for 18% of all new cases and 11% of cancer deaths each year. It is estimated that 1 in 10 men will develop prostate cancer by age 85. In 1993, it is anticipated that 35,000 deaths will be attributable to the disease (American Cancer Society, 1993; Mettlin, et al., 1993).

The incidence of cancer of the prostate among black Americans is the highest in the world. African blacks have a significantly lower rate, suggesting that genetics are not the only cause. The lowest incidence is among Japanese males, although the risk increases in Japanese migrants to the United States. White Americans have a rate higher than that of Japanese migrants and half the rate of black Americans (Ross et al., 1988).

Age is an important factor in determining the risk of prostate cancer. Rarely found in men younger than 40 years of age, cancer of the prostate is the major cause of cancer deaths in men older than 65 years of age, with a median age at diagnosis of 72 years (Mettlin et al., 1993; National Cancer Institute, 1990). Autopsy studies demonstrate occult disease in 95% of men who are older than 90 years of age at the time of death, suggesting that cancerous changes in the prostate may be part of the aging process (Lind, 1992; Piemme, 1988). In addition to age, males with occupational exposure to cadmium (a metallic element used in welding, electroplating, and the production of alkaline batteries) or a familial history of prostate cancer among first-order blood relatives are also at risk for developing the disease (American Cancer Society, 1993; Piemme, 1988).

The two main factors reported by Ross and associates (1988) to cause prostate cancer are (1) an infectious agent that is sexually transmitted, and (2) stimulation of the prostate with testosterone. The infectious agent hypothesis is supported by the discovery of viruslike particles in prostate tissue and a reported increase in the incidence of cervical cancer in the wives of prostate cancer patients. On the other hand, prostate cancer patients are also known to have higher levels of testosterone than healthy men (Lind & Nakao, 1990; Ross et al., 1988). Ross and associates (1988) reported that blacks have a mean testosterone level that is 15% higher than whites. They found that blacks ingest more dietary fat than whites, and reported that increased dietary fat can increase the level of circulating testosterone. The relationship of dietary fat intake to prostate cancer is supported in several other studies, suggesting a positive correlation between the incidence and mortality of prostate cancer and the per capita consumption of dietary fat (Meikle & Smith, 1990).

A recent study by Giovannucci and coworkers (1993) also suggested a causal relationship between vasectomy and the later development of prostate cancer. Despite the statistically significant findings in this study, which involved 47,855 men, more research is needed to verify that vasectomy poses an increased risk of prostate cancer.

**Pathophysiology.** Adenocarcinomas are typically found in the peripheral and transition zones of the prostate gland. They tend to arise from the epithelial lining of the prostatic acini, small saclike structures terminating into ducts that function as secretory reservoirs for cell matter within the prostate. In the peripheral zone of the prostate, which accounts for almost 70% of gland's tissue volume, the acini and ducts emanate and extend laterally from the distal portion of the prostatic urethra; the epithelial lining within differentiates from the urogenital sinus. Acini and ducts originating from the proximal prostatic urethra constitute the transition zone (Stamey & McNeal, 1992).

Theories abound regarding the nature of premalignant cellular changes that lead to adenocarcinoma. Currently, it is believed that new ductal structures develop and undergo a malignant transformation when the gland begins to hypertrophy. Another hypothesis suggests that there is an increase in the number of cells in preexisting ductoacinar units that exhibit cytologic atypia with abnormal nuclei (Stamey & McNeal, 1992). Most prostate cancers are acinar adenocarcinoma. Ductal adenocarcinoma, mucinous adenocarcinoma, squamous carcinoma, transitional cell carcinoma, neuroendocrine carcinoma, sarcomas, and carcinosarcomas collectively account for about 5% of all other types of prostate cancers (Paulson, 1987; Waisman, 1988).

Prostate tumors are graded based on differentiation and aggressiveness, and there is an established correlation between grade and incidence of metastasis (Paulson, 1987; Waisman, 1988). In general, a well-differentiated cancer cell closely resembles the normal cellular make-up of the prostate gland, whereas a poorly differentiated prostate cancer cell appears disorganized and abnormal, with a tendency for rapid growth. The Gleason scale is the best known and most widely used grading system for prostate cancer. Each area of the prostate containing cancer is graded on a scale of 1 to 5 based on the primary and secondary patterns of tumor cells. The score, which may range from 2 to 10, is obtained from the sum of the two grades assigned to each area. Using the Gleason scale, a score of 2 to 4 represents a well-differentiated tumor; a score of 5 to 7 suggests a moderately differentiated tumor; and a score of 8 to 10 is consistent with a poorly differentiated tumor (Narayan, 1992; Stamey & McNeal, 1992).

Staging is the primary way tumors are classified. In the United States, the most commonly used staging system for prostate cancer is the A-B-C-D system, often referred to as the *Whitmore-Jewett system*, the *American Urological Association's modified Jewett staging system*, or the *American Urological system* (Table 10–1). The most salient feature of this staging method is the division of each stage into substages that define the extent of disease as well as the degree of tumor cell differentiation.

Another method used for the clinical staging of prostate cancer is the tumor, node, and metastasis (TNM) system (American Joint Committee on Cancer, 1992) (Table 10–2). This classification requires that tumor volume, lymph node involvement, and presence or absence of distant metastases each be evaluated for a more

**TABLE 10–1. A-B-C-D System for Staging Cancer of the Prostate in the United States**

| STAGE | DESCRIPTION |
| --- | --- |
| A | Tumor not clinically palpable but detectable in microscopic sections by biopsy or transurethral resection |
| A1 | 1–3 foci of well-differentiated tumor *or* <5% of specimen is tumor and it is well differentiated |
| A2 | >3 foci *or* >5% well differentiated *or* any moderately or poorly differentiated tumor |
| B | Palpable tumor confined to the prostatic capsule |
| B1 | Nodule confined to the prostate and involving less than one lobe |
| B2 | Nodule confined to prostate involving one whole lobe, both lobes, or bilateral nodules |
| C | Local extension of tumor beyond the prostate, with or without invasion of contiguous organs, but with no distant metastases |
| C1 | Lateral extension only |
| C2 | Seminal extension only |
| C3 | Both lateral and seminal vesicle extension |
| D | Cancer has spread to regional lymph nodes or beyond the pelvis to the bone or other organs |
| D0 | Local disease rectally, elevated serum enzymatic acid phosphatase, bone scan normal |
| D1 | Local disease rectally; positive obturator, hypogastric, external, or common iliac lymph nodes; bone scan normal |
| D2 | Nodal disease outside pelvis; bone or soft-tissue metastases |
| D3 | Progression of disease after hormonal therapy for metastasizing tumor |

Adapted from Donahue, R. E., & Miller, G. J. (1991). Adenocarcinoma of the prostate: Biopsy to whole mount. *Urologic Clinics of North America, 18*(3), 450.

comprehensive determination of the extent of a prostate tumor.

Locally, prostate cancer spreads by direct extension to the seminal vesicles, bladder, and peritoneum. Metastasis is accomplished through lymphatic and hematogenous routes to the lymph nodes, bones, lung, liver, and kidneys (Lind, 1992). Patients with metastatic disease often are found to have involvement of the supraclavicular or scalene lymph nodes. This is because lymph is routed from the pelvis to the thoracic duct into the left subclavian and left internal jugular veins (Lind, 1992; Waisman, 1988).

Signs and symptoms occur when the disease has spread from the periphery of the prostate throughout the gland or to adjacent structures. They include urinary frequency, dysuria, slow urine stream, and urgency. Later signs include hematuria and urinary retention. If a patient has advanced disease at diagnosis, bone pain, anemia, neuritic pain, weight loss, and lethargy may be present (Lind & Nakao, 1990; Piemme, 1988).

## Medical-Surgical Management

*Early Detection and Diagnosis.* Prostate cancer screening is accomplished using one or more of three tests: digital rectal examination, transrectal ultrasonography, or measurement of serum biochemical markers. Although it is acknowledged that no single examination has proved to be unequivocally specific for prostate cancer, it is agreed that these techniques for early detection have enabled physicians to begin treatment for prostate tumors in earlier stages of the disease to decrease associated mortality rates. The American Cancer Society (ACS) recommends an annual screening for prostate cancer consisting of digital rectal examination (DRE) for men 40 years of age and older, and DRE and measurement of prostate-specific antigen (PSA) for all men older than 50 years of age. High-risk individuals, including black men and men who have first-degree relatives with prostate cancer, should begin annual screening at age 40. The report of the ACS National Prostate Cancer Detection Project suggests that screening with a combination of DRE and PSA provides the least costly approach to prostate cancer early detection (Littrup et al., 1993) (Procedure 10–1).

DRE of the prostate is the most commonly used technique for the early detection of prostate cancer. It is a simple procedure that requires that the physician palpate the prostate for asymmetry, induration, or nodularity. When the examination is performed annually

### TABLE 10–2. Definition of TNM in Prostate Cancer

**PRIMARY TUMOR (T)**

| | |
|---|---|
| TX | Primary tumor cannot be assessed |
| T0 | No evidence of primary tumor |
| T1 | Clinically inapparent tumor not palpable or visible by imaging |
| T1a | Tumor incidental histologic finding in 5% or less of tissue resected |
| T1b | Tumor incidental histologic finding in more than 5% of tissue resected |
| T1c | Tumor identified by needle biopsy (e.g, because of elevated PSA) |
| T2 | Tumor confined within the prostate* |
| T2a | Tumor involves half of a lobe or less |
| T2b | Tumor involves more than half of a lobe, but not both lobes |
| T2c | Tumor involves both lobes |
| T3 | Tumor extends through the prostatic capsule† |
| T3a | Unilateral extracapsular extension |
| T3b | Bilateral extracapsular extension |
| T3c | Tumor invades the seminal vesicle(s) |
| T4 | Tumor is fixed or invades adjacent structures other than the seminal vesicles |
| T4a | Tumor invades any of: bladder neck, external sphincter, or rectum |
| T4b | Tumor invades levator muscles and/or is fixed to the pelvic wall |

**REGIONAL LYMPH NODES (N)**

| | |
|---|---|
| NX | Regional lymph nodes cannot be assessed |
| N0 | No regional lymph node metastasis |
| N1 | Metastasis in a single lymph node, 2 cm or less in greatest dimension |
| N2 | Metastasis in a single lymph node, more than 2 cm but not more than 5 cm in greatest dimension; or multiple lymph node metastases, none more than 5 cm in greatest dimension |
| N3 | Metastasis in a lymph node more than 5 cm in greatest dimension |

**DISTANT METASTASES‡ (M)**

| | |
|---|---|
| MX | Presence of distant metastasis cannot be assessed |
| M0 | No distant metastasis |
| M1 | Distant metastases |
| M1a | Nonregional lymph node(s) |
| M1b | Bone(s) |
| M1c | Other site(s) |

*Note: Tumor found in one or both lobes by needle biopsy, but not palpable or visible by imaging, is classified as T1c.
†Note: Invasion into the prostatic apex or into (but not beyond) the prostatic capsule is not classified as T3, but as T2.
‡Note: When more than one site of metastasis is present, the most advanced category (pM1c) is used.
PSA, prostate-specific antigen.
From American Joint Committee on Cancer. (1992). *Manual for Staging of Cancer* (4th ed., p. 182). Philadelphia: J. B. Lippincott. Reprinted by permission.

in men older than 40 years of age, the disease is likely to be identified at a more curable stage (Lind & Nakao, 1990; National Cancer Institute, 1990).

Transrectal ultrasonography has been used as a screening technique for prostate cancer for more than a decade. Tumor detection rates using this test have varied. Although it is generally agreed that transrectal ultrasonography may be more sensitive than digital examination in identifying nonpalpable, suspicious areas in the prostate gland, it is less specific in recognizing the type of abnormality (Optenberg & Thompson, 1990). The value of transrectal ultrasonography as a primary screening test for prostate cancer is called into question with reports that abnormal results are confirmed by biopsy in only 5% of patients (Hernandez & Smith, 1990). Its value is compromised further

by the cost of the procedure compared with other screening tests.

The measurement of serum biochemical markers as a method of detecting prostate cancer is an advancement in the quest for a simple, cost-effective way to screen the male population. Prostatic acid phosphatase (PAP) is a normal enzyme that elevates metabolism and catabolism of prostate cancer cells. It is increased in 80% of men with stage D prostate cancer (Lind, 1992). The use of PAP as a diagnostic test has declined 13% between 1984 and 1990, and recent studies raise questions about the use of this less accurate assay in the future (Burnett et al., 1992; Mettlin et al., 1993). PSA is a glycoprotein produced by the epithelial cells of the prostate that elevates in the presence of a prostate tumor or benign prostatic hypertrophy. Increased levels may aid in establishing a diag-

## PROCEDURE 10-1

■

### Prostate Cancer Screening Programs:
### Urologic Nurses Make It Happen

Each year in September, health care providers across the United States observe **Prostate Cancer Awareness Week**. The week-long focus on prostate cancer is designed to increase public awareness about the disease, including the methods and benefits of early detection, current treatment options, and research efforts. Prostate cancer screening clinics, which provide men with educational information along with the opportunity for a digital rectal examination and PSA test, are among the many activities offered to the public—often free of charge.

Urologic nurses, because of their knowledge of urologic diseases, educational resources, expertise in patient education, and organizational skills, have assumed an integral role in developing and coordinating these programs in their communities. Through their efforts, collaboration among health care professionals and institutions is remarkable, and response from the community is overwhelming.

Are you interested in setting up a prostate cancer screening program in your community? If yes, begin by reviewing the articles listed below to learn how other urologic nurses planned successful programs for their communities. You may also want to contact the American Cancer Society and American Foundation for Urologic Diseases for additional information. Then, meet the challenge and make it happen! Approach your institution and physicians with a proposal and guidelines for a local screening program. Once the program is approved . . . the rest is up to you.

1. Aspholm, D. (1991). Primary intervention—a rewarding challenge in nursing. *Urologic Nursing, 11*(4), 21–23.
2. Coyne, C. L. (1991). Early screening programs for prostate cancer. *Innovations in Urology Nursing, 11*(3), 4–5.
3. Lang, B. A. (1991). Implementation of a screening program for carcinoma of the prostate. *Urologic Nursing, 11*(4), 24–27.
4. Moore, S., Kuhrik, M., Kuhrik, N., & Shea, L. (1992). Screening for prostate cancer: PSA, blood test, rectal examination, and ultrasound. *Urologic Nursing, 12*(3), 106–107.
5. Wilkinson, G. B., & Meacham, A. R. (1991). Prostate awareness week: How we did it! *Urologic Nursing, 11*(4), 19–20.

nosis of prostate cancer, or be considered as a marker of disease progression (Lind, 1992). PSA is a more reliable indicator of the presence of prostate cancer with a detection rate of approximately 55%, despite the fact that other nonmalignant types of prostate disease may elevate the blood level. The use of PSA for the diagnosis of prostate cancer has increased nearly 63% in the last 10 years (Mettlin et al., 1993). The normal value for PAP is less than 3 ng/mL. The normal value for PSA is less than 4 ng/mL.*

*Normal values for PAP and PSA may vary and depend on techniques and standards used by the testing laboratory.

To confirm the diagnosis of prostate cancer, the patient is required to submit to a variety of diagnostic studies. The physician's initial work-up includes a complete history and physical examination; laboratory studies (complete blood count, serum alkaline phosphatase, serum acid phosphatase, and PAP and PSA levels); biopsy of the prostate; and cytologic examination of urine and expressed prostatic fluid.

A prostate biopsy is necessary to verify the presence of malignant cells. The procedure is usually done on an outpatient basis (often in conjunction with cystoscopy) using local anesthesia; it may also be performed in a surgical setting as an open biopsy. Tissue samples are most commonly obtained by either fine-needle aspiration or core-needle biopsy. Fine-needle aspiration requires a device consisting of a flexible 23-gauge aspiration needle, needle guide, and aspiration syringe (Narayan, 1992). Often guided by transrectal ultrasonography, the needle is inserted through the perineum and into the prostate (transperineal biopsy) to aspirate tissue for analysis. Core-needle biopsy is performed with a manual Tru-Cut needle or a spring-powered biopsy gun that uses the Tru-Cut needle design. The advantage of the biopsy gun is that it allows for multiple transrectal or transperineal prostate tissue samples to be obtained quickly and with minimal discomfort to the patient (Carter, 1992; Narayan, 1992).

Individual staging of confirmed prostate cancer and evaluation for metastatic disease require that some or all of the following procedures be performed: chest radiography; intravenous excretory urography (intravenous pyelography [IVP]); transrectal ultrasonography; computed tomography (CT) scan; magnetic resonance imaging (MRI); bone, liver, and brain scans (if clinically indicated); and lymphangiography, pelvic lymphadenectomy, or laparoscopic pelvic lymph node dissection.

*Treatment.* Prostate cancer is treated with one or more of the following approaches: surgery, radiation therapy, hormonal manipulation, and chemotherapy. Although controversy exists regarding the most effective treatment for a given stage, localized disease is usually treated with surgery or radiation therapy, whereas advanced and metastatic disease is treated with hormonal manipulation or chemotherapy. The use of prostatectomy for stage B prostate cancer has increased nearly 13% (to 27.5%) since 1984 (Lind, 1992; Mettlin et al., 1993).

Surgical approaches to prostate cancer include suprapubic, retropubic, or perineal prostatectomy. These procedures all are considered to be radical. The anatomic approach to radical retropubic prostatectomy is now the most common procedure for stages $A_2$ and B disease. The procedure is characterized by the precise control of bleeding from the dorsal vein complex that makes possible preservation of the pelvic plexus and the branches that innervate the corpora cavernosa. It requires that the surgeon carefully dissect adjacent structures while excising pelvic lymph nodes, seminal vesicles, and the prostate gland. The protection of neurovascular bundles during the procedure contributes to the preservation of sexual function and urinary continence, heretofore frequent complications of radical prostatectomy (Walsh, 1992).

Perineal prostatectomy has long been used as an alternative surgical approach to the retropubic technique. The combined approach of laparoscopic pelvic lymph node dissection, followed by perineal prostatectomy, is used in some centers. By initially performing the lymph node dissection laparoscopically, patients with positive lymph nodes are identified before a major surgical incision is required, sparing them from a lengthy postoperative recovery. The rates of postoperative complications of sexual dysfunction and rectal injury are higher in perineal prostatectomy; however, some urologists consider this approach to be technically easier with less blood loss.

Radiation therapy is used primarily to treat patients with stages B and C prostate cancer (Mettlin et al., 1993). Those patients with stage A, $B_1$, or $B_2$ disease who refuse surgery or for whom surgery is contraindicated may also benefit from this treatment modality (Greenburg et al., 1990; Mahon et al., 1990). External beam radiotherapy may be used alone or with brachytherapy, using radioactive gold ($^{198}$Au) or radioactive iodine ($^{125}$I) (Lind & Nakao, 1990). In external beam therapy, radiation is delivered to a target area that includes the prostate gland and adjacent lymph nodes. Treatments are usually continued for 5 days each week for 6 to 8 weeks (Mahon et al., 1990). Improved techniques have lessened the rate and severity of complications associated with external beam radiotherapy (Fallon & Williams, 1990). However, it is possible for contiguous tissues and organs to be affected by the exposure. Cellular damage to the skin, bladder, or lower intestinal tract may manifest as irritative voiding symptoms, bladder spasms, hematuria, rectal bleeding, cystitis, proctitis, diarrhea, bowel obstruction, bowel perforation, fistula, genital edema, or dermatitis (Lind & Nakao, 1990; Mahon et al., 1990). Erectile dysfunction has been reported as a persistent problem for some men following external beam radiotherapy.

Another method for irradiating prostate cancer consists of implanting $^{125}$I, $^{198}$Au, or iridium-192 ($^{192}$Ir) seeds directly into the interstitium of the prostate by suprapubic, retropubic, or transperineal incision; lymphadenectomy may or may not be performed at the same time. In some centers, the radioactive seeds are implanted in the gland through multiple surgically placed needles, the position of which is verified by prostate ultrasonography. The needles are removed after the injection is completed, leaving behind a row of radioactive seeds. This technique, referred to as *brachytherapy* or *interstitial therapy,* allows for radiation to be delivered more closely and precisely to the tumor, thereby protecting the surrounding tissues from excess radiation. Sexual function is maintained in 70% to 90% of men who were potent before treatment (Fallon & Williams, 1990; Lind & Nakao, 1990).

Hormonal manipulation is an effective treatment for prostate cancer because nearly 85% of prostatic cancers are androgen dependent (Lind & Nakao, 1990). It has been shown to be the most effective initial therapy for 70% to 80% of patients with advanced disease, and is effective for palliation in stage D prostate cancer. Treatments are designed to cause androgen deprivation in the prostate gland, thereby inhibiting the growth of androgen-dependent prostate tumors. Regardless of the method of hormonal manipulation, the goal of treatment is to block androgen production to decrease circulating androgens, thereby arresting the prostate cancer (Taylor, 1991). Treatment approaches employed to block androgen production include the following:

1. Bilateral orchiectomy
2. Estrogen therapy, such as diethylstilbestrol
3. Antiandrogens, such as flutamide
4. Gonadotropin-releasing hormone analogues, such as leuprolide acetate (Lupron) and goserelin acetate (Zoladex)
5. Adrenalectomy, surgical or chemical (with aminoglutethimide)

Table 10–3 summarizes the options for hormonal therapy.

Chemotherapy may offer palliation for men with hormone-resistant disease. Single and combination regimens are equally effective. Drugs used alone include cyclophosphamide, methotrexate, doxorubicin, 5-fluorouracil, cisplatin, mitomycin C, and decarbazine. Mitomycin C, 5-fluorouracil, and doxorubicin are used in combination chemotherapy regimens (Lind & Nakao, 1990). Estramustine phosphate sodium (Emcyt), a hormonal-chemotherapeutic drug combination, is now available; however, it is believed that the drug's effectiveness is no better than that of diethylstilbestrol (Stamey & McNeal, 1992).

## APPROACHES TO PATIENT CARE

### Assessment

A thorough assessment of the patient with prostate cancer is a key responsibility of the nurse. Begin every assessment with questions specifically related to the history of the suspected disease process. Assess or inquire about the following:

Age: Is the patient older than 50 years of age?
Ethnicity: What are the patient's race and national origin?
Family history: Does the patient have a first-order blood relative who has died of or been diagnosed with prostate cancer?
Diet: Does the patient eat a high-fat diet?
Occupation: Does the patient work in an environment where he is exposed to cadmium?
Symptoms: Has the patient experienced urinary frequency, dysuria, slow stream, urgency, or urinary retention? Has the patient experienced hematuria? Does the patient currently have bone pain, back pain, or neuritic pain? Is the patient pale or lethargic? Has the patient experienced any weight loss? Does the patient experience erectile dysfunction? Does the patient perceive an altered libido?

Physical examination is an important means of assessing the patient's current status. Begin at the head and work down, looking for clues that indicate metastatic disease.

Head: assess the patient's skin color for signs of anemia. Thoroughly examine the head, eyes, ears, nose, and throat, including an assessment of the cranial nerves.
Neck: palpate for firm, fixed, enlarged, or tender supraclavicular and scalene lymph nodes.
Chest: auscultate lungs for decreased breath sounds. Monitor respiratory rate.
Back: palpate the vertebrae for tenderness. If spinal cord compression is suspected, complete a thorough neurologic examination.
Abdomen: palpate for hepatomegaly.
Pelvis: palpate the groin for hard, firm, enlarged, fixed, or tender lymph nodes.
Rectum: prepare the patient for a DRE to identify asymmetry, induration, or nodularity of the prostate.
Legs: inspect the legs for edema.

As part of the nursing assessment, be sure to ascertain that the patient has had blood samples collected for all necessary laboratory studies *before* rectal examination or prostatic biopsy is performed. This ensures an accurate measurement of biochemical markers. Finally, assess the patient's knowledge of prostate cancer. Does he know that the disease occurs in vary-

**TABLE 10–3. Hormonal Manipulation: Therapeutic Options for Advanced Stage D Prostate Cancer**

| TREATMENT | DOSAGE/THERAPEUTIC ACTION | SIDE EFFECTS | ADVANTAGES | DISADVANTAGES |
|---|---|---|---|---|
| Orchiectomy (surgical removal of the testes) | Removes the organ most responsible for testosterone production | Erectile dysfunction<br>Decreased libido<br>Hot flashes<br>Incisional bleeding<br>Infection<br>Pain | Procedure can often be performed using local anesthesia | Surgical procedure<br>Irreversible<br>Psychological impact<br>Grief reaction<br>Depression |
| Estrogens (diethylstilbestrol) | 3 mg/day<br>Feedback inhibition of circulating testosterone accomplished by a reduction in the level of gonadotropins secreted by the pituitary gland | Gynecomastia<br>Edema<br>Myocardial infarction<br>Hypertension<br>Cerebrovascular accident<br>Thrombophlebitis<br>Pulmonary embolus<br>Nausea and vomiting<br>Abdominal cramping<br>Erectile dysfunction<br>Decreased libido | May be orally administered<br>Effects may be reversed if therapy is continued for less than 2 years | Patient compliance with therapy always uncertain |
| Antiandrogens (flutamide) | 250 mg three times daily<br>Acts on specific DNA sites in the nuclei of prostate cells to inhibit the binding of dihydrotestosterone and testosterone to receptor proteins; blocks the 10% of circulating androgens produced by the adrenal glands | Gynecomastia<br>Diarrhea<br>Erectile dysfunction | Administered by oral capsule<br>May increase the effectiveness of other hormonal therapies when used concomitantly | Medical or surgical castration may be required in conjunction with the use of this drug; often not covered by insurance |
| Luteinizing hormone–releasing hormone agonists (leuprolide acetate, goserelin acetate) | Leuprolide acetate 1 mg/day by subcutaneous injection<br>Leuprolide acetate depot suspension: 7.5 mg or 3.75 mg/month by intramuscular injection<br>Goserelin acetate: 3.6 mg/28 days by subcutaneous injection<br>Causes stimulation, then suppression of pituitary gonadotropins that eventually results in the reduction of testosterone to castrate levels | Symptoms of advanced disease (pain) may worsen during the first week or two of therapy; other reported side effects include:<br>Edema<br>Nausea and vomiting<br>Decreased testicular size<br>Hot flashes/sweats<br>Erectile dysfunction<br>Anorexia<br>Lethargy | May be administered as simple monthly injection; effects are reversible | Monthly office visits required for those receiving time-release injections |

Adapted from Taylor, T. K. (1991). Endocrine therapy for advanced stage D prostate cancer. *Urologic Nursing, 11*(3), 22–26. Reprinted by permission.

ing stages? Does he know that a number of laboratory studies and diagnostic procedures must be performed to confirm the diagnosis of prostate cancer? Does he understand that the method of treatment is defined by the extensiveness of the disease? Is he aware of the alternatives for treatment of prostate cancer? Is he aware that loss of sexual function may not be an inevitable result of radical surgery for prostate cancer (Waxman, 1993)?

**Nursing Diagnosis**

Nursing diagnoses for the patient with cancer of the prostate may include the following:

1. Knowledge deficit related to
   a. Causes and course of prostate cancer.
   b. Diagnostic procedures performed to confirm prostate cancer.
   c. Treatment alternatives for prostate cancer, including surgery, radiation therapy, hormonal therapy, and chemotherapy.
2. Fear related to
   a. Effect of treatments on quality of life.
   b. Perceived threat of death.
3. Altered pattern of urinary elimination related to
   a. Prostatic enlargement caused by the presence of a tumor or a transient inflammatory response following biopsy.
   b. Postoperative placement of urinary drainage devices.
   c. Tissue damage to bladder caused by radiation treatments.
4. Alteration in bowel elimination related to
   a. Radical prostatectomy
   b. Radiation therapy
5. Pain related to
   a. Effects of surgery to excise diseased prostate.
   b. Bladder spasms due to the presence of a urethral catheter causing irritation to the bladder mucosa or traction on the catheter balloon.
   c. Metastasis of prostate cancer to bone.
6. Impaired tissue integrity related to
   a. Presence of an abdominal wound (surgical incision).
   b. Effects of external beam radiotherapy or interstitial radiation on the skin, lower urinary tract, or lower intestinal tract.
7. Fluid volume deficit related to blood loss during radical prostatectomy.
8. Altered sexuality patterns related to the cancer, and the effects of surgery, radiation, or hormonal therapy characterized by a decrease in libido, erectile dysfunction, or infertility.
9. Activity intolerance (potential) related to

   a. Effects of radiation or hormonal therapy.
   b. Impaired sensory or motor function caused by disease progression or spinal cord compression.
10. Body image disturbance related to orchiectomy or pharmacologic hormonal manipulation.
11. Noncompliance (potential) with hormonal therapy related to the side effects of medications.

**Plan of Care**

Nursing care is directed toward enabling the patient to

1. Increase his knowledge of the causes of prostate cancer, prognosis for the disease, diagnostic procedures, and treatment goals and alternatives.
2. Participate in decisions related to his treatment regimen.
3. Express a lessening sense of fear regarding the diagnosis of prostate cancer.
4. Maintain a normal pattern of urinary and bowel elimination.
5. Obtain relief from pain.
6. Verbalize concerns regarding sexual functioning and satisfaction, and physical appearance.
7. Avoid complications associated with radical prostatectomy, radiation, or hormonal manipulation.
8. Plan and participate in daily activities that permit a balance between exertion and rest.
9. Comply with the dosage schedule of medications prescribed for hormonal therapy.

**Interventions**

The patient diagnosed with prostate cancer has a critical need for information. Therefore, initial nursing interventions should be directed toward dispeling any misconceptions the patient may have about cancer of the prostate, explaining diagnostic procedures, and clarifying differences about various treatment options, as well as reinforcing treatment goals. Ask the patient what his physician has told him about prostate cancer so that you may support the information given. Written materials from the National Cancer Institute and the ACS are helpful to newly diagnosed patients. These exceptional resources explain the disease, diagnostic procedures, and treatment options in lay terms. Because questions will continually arise during the course of treatment, suggest to the patient that he write his questions in a notebook. This process helps him remember issues that he will want to discuss during meetings with the physician.

Encourage the patient to verbalize his fears about the diagnosis of cancer, planned treatment, masculinity, sexuality, and even death. Identify family and friends the patient may turn to for support, and encourage them to express their feelings and concerns. Remember that clear, concise, and factual information regarding special care needs before and after diagnostic procedures and treatments helps lessen the concerns and fears of everyone. Although the urologic nurse will be the patient's primary resource, keep in mind that a social worker, psychologist, or members of a support group may also offer helpful information and reassurance to the patient and family.

Of all the psychosocial issues confronting the patient with prostate cancer, many people consider the threat to sexual function to be the most important. Nurses must understand that surgical, radiation, and hormonal therapy all have the potential to diminish a man's libido as well as cause erectile dysfunction and infertility. Because most men remain sexually active throughout life, education and counseling about matters concerning sexual activity are important, regardless of the patient's age. Help patients understand the effects of prostate cancer therapies by initiating discussions about their planned treatment and its possible risk to sexual function. Be sure to include their partners in your sessions because they also share in the apprehension a potential alteration in sexual function may produce.

If radical prostatectomy is planned, explain to the patient that recovery of a full erection, or an erection sufficient for penetration, may take from 6 months to 1 year. Reassure the patient that once he resumes sexual activity, there should be no change in orgasmic feelings. He will, however, experience a "dry orgasm," as no semen will ejaculate from the penis (Reilly, 1991). In the event that the patient experiences persistent postoperative problems with erectile dysfunction, offer assurance that counseling and assistance will be available to help him explore techniques, treatments, or devices that may enable him and his partner to experience mutual sexual satisfaction. If orchiectomy is planned, advise patients that they will lose their ability to produce viable sperm. Men who wish to father a child may want to look into sperm banking prior to surgery (see Chapters 12 and 13 for a more detailed discussion about treatments of sexual dysfunction).

***Prostate Biopsy.*** All patients suspected of having prostate cancer will undergo tissue biopsy, usually as an outpatient procedure. A prostate biopsy requires no special preparation by the patient. However, it is important to identify and alert the urologist to those patients who regularly take aspirin, aspirin-containing products, or anticoagulant medication so that these drugs may be temporarily discontinued, or dosages reduced, to prevent excessive bleeding of the biopsy site.

For a transperineal prostate biopsy, the patient will be placed on a table in the lithotomy position. A sedative may be administered before the procedure if the patient appears apprehensive or fidgety. Depending on the technique that is used to obtain tissue samples, the urologist may choose to administer a local anesthetic to numb the biopsy site. Patients should be reminded to lie still throughout the procedure; the slightest movement may cause deflection of the biopsy needle away from the area the physician desires to sample. Explain that it will be necessary for the physician to place a finger in the patient's rectum (or insert an ultrasound probe) to guide the biopsy needle, thus creating a sensation of fullness or pressure. During the procedure, the nurse may be asked to assist the physician by raising the patient's scrotum off the perineum to permit unobstructed access to the biopsy site. The nurse will also assist with the collection and labeling of the tissue samples.

Immediately after the biopsy, fluids are encouraged, and patients are usually asked to remain in the office or clinic until they are able to void. This gives the urologic staff an opportunity to collect a urine specimen and examine it for signs of excessive bleeding. It also permits early intervention for urinary retention if the patient experiences swelling of the biopsy site sufficient to obstruct urine flow from the bladder.

Home care instructions for patients after prostate biopsy should include the following information (Mahon et al., 1990):

1. Urine may be blood tinged for as long as 24 hours after the procedure; a few blood clots may also be noted.
2. Bleeding and bruising may be noticed at the biopsy site.
3. Avoid strenuous activity and, if necessary, rest in a recumbent position for the remainder of the day.
4. Increase oral fluid intake (unless medically contraindicated) for 24 hours after the procedure, or until bleeding subsides; alcoholic beverages should be avoided during this time.
5. Contact the physician if fever and chills de-

velop or if difficulty in urinating or an inability to urinate occurs.

6. Resume aspirin or anticoagulant medication when directed by the physician.
7. Hematospermia may be noticed for as long as 6 months after the procedure.

***Radical Retropubic Prostatectomy.*** Radical retropubic prostatectomy is the surgical procedure most often performed to eradicate localized prostate cancer. Nursing interventions the night before surgery usually include the administration of an enema, as well as the management of intravenous fluids for hydration (Walsh, 1992). Postoperative nursing care of the patient who has undergone this procedure includes interventions to promote comfort, facilitate urinary elimination, support wound healing, maintain fluid and electrolyte balance, and prevent possible complications such as thrombophlebitis and pulmonary embolism.

*Pain management* is a consideration after radical retropubic prostatectomy. During the 48 to 72 hours after surgery, the patient experiences moderate to severe pain from the incision and wound drains, as well as from the intraurethral urinary drainage catheter. In most instances, the patient's pain can be controlled with opioid analgesics administered through an epidural catheter or intravenous line and regulated by a patient-controlled analgesia (PCA) pump. Some centers employ a continuous infusion for the first 24 hours postoperatively. If such devices are unavailable, the nurse should administer intravenous or intramuscular analgesics on a regular schedule around-the-clock for at least 36 hours; the patient may be advanced to oral analgesics as soon as fluid intake is tolerated. Ongoing assessment of the intensity (using a pain scale), type, and location of the patient's pain is important. At regular intervals, the nurse should also determine the efficacy of the medication, presence of side effects, and the need for adjustments in dosage or schedule, as well as the need for supplemental analgesics for breakthrough pain (AHCPR, 1992). Antispasmodics such as oxybutynin chloride (Ditropan) and propantheline bromide (Pro-Banthine) may be administered to relieve painful bladder spasms that result when receptors in the bladder wall are stimulated to cause involuntary bladder contractions. Often, it is the presence of the urethral catheter, causing irritation to the bladder mucosa, which prompts the bladder to repeatedly respond to the false sense of fullness. The application of 10% lidocaine jelly to the urethral meatus may

also provide relief for patients who complain of penile discomfort (Reilly, 1991).

*Urinary elimination* is accomplished by maintenance of a closed urethral catheter drainage system. The urethral catheter acts as a splint for urethral anastomosis following radical prostatectomy. To promote adequate drainage and avoid excessive manipulation, the catheter should be secured to the patient's inner thigh, and excess tubing should be coiled on the bed; the drainage bag should be affixed below bladder level. Careful measurement of urinary output is important. Observe the urinary drainage for color and consistency. Although bleeding is common for the first 24 hours following surgery, excessive or continued bleeding or the presence of clots should be reported to the urologist. In some instances, manual irrigation of the catheter is required to restore patency. Always check with the physician before initiating this procedure, then proceed gently to flush the catheter. Continue the irrigation until the clots have been dislodged, the drainage is free flowing, and the urine is clot free (Reilly, 1991).

*Wound care* is also a consideration. The patient returns from surgery with a midline lower abdominal incision that extends from the umbilicus to the pubis; skin clips are used to keep the surgical wound closed. Small suction-type drains, positioned in the pelvic area, will also be observed projecting outward from the primary incision or through a separate incision. Regularly inspect the surgical site for evidence of wound healing or signs of infection. If a dressing covers the incision, reinforce or change it according to the physician's orders. If drainage is excessive, remember to weigh the dressings before discard to estimate the amount of output. Pelvic drains ooze a serous, blood-tinged fluid until about the 4th or 5th postoperative day (Walsh, 1992). Until this drainage subsides, output should be carefully measured and recorded, and the physician should be notified if the drains stop functioning. Wound irrigations, sitz baths, or heat lamp treatments may be ordered to facilitate wound healing.

*Restoration of fluid volume* must be planned carefully. Excessive bleeding is a common intraoperative problem that requires replacement with intravenous fluids or blood products for at least 48 to 72 hours following surgery, or until the patient can tolerate oral fluids. A fluid intake of 2500 to 3000 mL/day should be maintained unless medically contraindicated. Laboratory studies such as the patient's hemoglobin, hematocrit, and serum electrolyte levels should be monitored and used to calculate the patient's fluid replacement needs. In addition, be alert to signs of dehydration or hypovolemia (increased pulse and respiration, decreased blood pressure, diaphoresis, pallor, delayed capillary refill, dry mucous membranes, and restlessness or confusion), which may be early indications of the development of shock.

*Prevention of complications* is an important consideration after radical retropubic prostatectomy. Thrombophlebitis and pulmonary embolism are among the most common and most serious complications after radical retropubic prostatectomy. Nursing interventions to decrease venous stasis and prevent the occurrence of these problems include (1) assisting the patient to begin ambulation on the first postoperative day; (2) encouraging the patient to perform dorsiflexion exercises 100 times every hour, while awake; (3) encouraging the patient to perform deep-breathing exercises hourly; (4) using elastic stockings or pneumatic compression stockings; and (5) maintaining the patient in a resting position that will permit elevation of the feet and legs above heart level (Kaut, 1992; Walsh, 1992). Additionally, anticoagulant therapy with either warfarin sodium (Coumadin) or heparin may be prescribed prophylactically.

*Discharge and home care planning* is a concern after radical retropubic prostatectomy. Patients who have undergone radical retropubic prostatectomy are usually discharged from the hospital 7 or 8 days after surgery with a Foley catheter connected to a drainage device. Instructions for home care should include the following information:

1. Guidelines for home maintenance of an indwelling catheter, including catheter and meatal cleansing with soap and water twice daily and, if a closed drainage system is not used, daytime use of a leg bag, and connection to and emptying of a nighttime drainage bag.
2. Instructions to maintain an oral fluid intake of 2000 to 3000 mL/day.
3. Review of the signs and symptoms of urinary tract infection.
4. Review of the signs and symptoms of wound complications, such as swelling, tenderness, redness, discolored or foul-smelling drainage, and wound separation.
5. Instructions to notify the physician if the catheter comes out, if the urine becomes bloody, or if the patient is experiencing chills or fever higher than 100°F (38°C).

6. Recommended use of a shower for bathing—allowing the incision to be gently cleansed with warm soapy water and patted dry.
7. Recommended use of high-fiber foods and stool softeners (if necessary) to prevent constipation and straining with bowel movements.
8. Avoidance of strenuous exercise, heavy lifting (more than 25 pounds), or driving an automobile or tractor for 6 weeks after surgery.
9. Instructions to avoid sitting with legs in a dependent position for 3 to 4 weeks after surgery (Walsh, 1992).
10. Avoidance of sexual intercourse for 6 weeks after surgery.
11. Appointment with the urologist for postoperative evaluation and catheter removal 3 weeks after surgery.

*Other potential problems* should be noted. For a period after catheter removal, patients experience irritative voiding symptoms including frequency, urgency, urge incontinence, and dysuria. Some men may also experience stress incontinence. Although these symptoms are bothersome, reassure the patient that they will subside in within a few weeks. Products such as drip collectors, condom catheters, and pads may be recommended to contain the small amount of urine leakage during this transient period.

Bladder neck contracture, total incontinence, and impotence are potential long-term complications after radical retropubic prostatectomy. Fortunately, new surgical techniques have enabled physicians to avoid injury to pelvic floor musculature, preserve neurovascular bundles, and reconstruct the bladder neck to reduce the incidence of these most dreaded complications.

***Radiation Therapy.*** This is an alternative to surgery for prostate cancer. External beam radiotherapy is usually administered on an outpatient basis in an institution's radiation oncology department. Urologic nursing interventions for these patients are therefore limited to monitoring their overall response to the treatment and signs of disease progression. On the other hand, interstitial radiation therapy requires a limited hospital stay and a more active role for the urologic nurse.

Preoperatively, the urologic nurse should provide the patient with information regarding the procedure, type of anesthesia to be used (either spinal or general), postoperative care activities, and radiation precautions established by the institution. Brandt (1991) studied the informational needs of patients receiving brachytherapy and found that 54% requested the following preimplant information: (1) how to manage side affects; (2) activity restrictions while the implant is in place; (3) pain management and comfort measures; (4) the cause of current symptoms; and (5) how the implant might affect current symptoms. The postimplant information most desired included (1) when to call the doctor; (2) possible side effects of radiation implant therapy; (3) how to manage side effects; and (4) what symptoms to expect at home. In addition to the usual routine surgical preparations (such as diet restrictions, discontinuance of aspirin or aspirin-containing products, and NPO after midnight), the patient should also be advised to use a cleansing enema to clear the rectum of stool to enhance the clarity of ultrasound images during the procedure (Greenburg et al., 1990). Admission to the hospital is usually planned for the same day the implantation procedure is scheduled.

Postoperative management of the patient following interstitial implantation of [198]Au, [125]I, or [192]Ir includes the following:

1. Monitoring the perineum for signs of bruising, edema, or drainage twice each day; an ice bag may be applied to the area to reduce swelling and increase comfort.
2. Monitoring and recording intake and output throughout the hospital stay; fluids are encouraged, and diet is advanced as tolerated.
3. Maintaining the patency of the urethral catheter and straight drainage system for as long as 24 hours after procedure; when the catheter is removed, the tube and bag should be inspected and scanned to detect any dislodged seeds that may have drained into the collection system.
4. Monitoring the time, amount, and characteristic of each void after removal of the catheter and until the patient's normal pattern of urination is re-established; urine will be blood tinged for the first 24 hours; the physician should be notified if gross hematuria is present or if the patient is experiencing dysuria.
5. Straining all urine emptied from the catheter drainage bag or voided to collect any dislodged seeds; the number of seeds obtained should be recorded on the intake and output record each shift.
6. Encouraging ambulation in the room once the patient has recovered from the effects of anesthesia; during the first 24 hours after

the procedure, the nurse should be alert to postural changes in blood pressure.
7. Administering intramuscular or oral analgesics as needed for discomfort.
8. Administering intravenous or oral antibiotics, if prescribed.
9. Monitoring bowel movements daily.
10. Monitoring the patient's adaptation to isolation (if required by institutional policy); a referral to an activity therapist may be beneficial in stimulating interest in diversional activities (Greenburg et al., 1990; University of Iowa, 1992).

Safety precautions specific to the implantation of radioactive seeds into the prostate require that the clothing of operating room personnel, linens used during the procedure, and accumulated waste be checked for contamination by stray seeds. Once the patient is transferred to the inpatient unit, linens and waste are checked by an appropriate official (e.g., the radiation safety officer) daily until the patient is discharged. The patient's room should contain a lead receptacle and forceps for recovering dislodged seeds. Lost seeds are to be picked up by forceps, not retrieved with a bare hand; they are deposited into the lead receptacle and disposed of by the radiation safety officer. Urinals or strainers contaminated by lost seeds should be discarded and replaced.

[198]Au seeds have a half-life of 2.7 days and are inert within about 21 days (University of Iowa, 1992). [125]I seeds have a half-life of 60 days and are inactive after 1 year (Greenburg, 1990). Gamma radiation is emitted while the isotopes are active, necessitating that family and visitors limit contact with the patient during hospitalization and for a period after discharge. General guidelines employed to minimize radiation exposure include the following:

1. Family and visitors *older than 45 years* of age should maintain a distance of at least 3 feet between themselves and the patient at all times and visit for periods of only 2 or 3 hours for the first 3 to 6 days; close contact is permitted for a short period for usual greetings or care activities.
2. Family and visitors *younger than 45 years* of age should avoid remaining in the same room with the patient or maintain a distance of 9 feet or further between themselves and the patient for only a few minutes each day.
3. Pregnant or possibly pregnant women, infants, and children *younger than 18 years of age* should avoid any contact with the pa-

tient while the isotope is most active. When radioactivity has sufficiently decreased (6 days for $^{198}$Au, 2 months for $^{125}$I), brief visits are permitted as long as a distance of 9 feet or more away from the patient is maintained (University of Iowa, 1992).

On discharge from the hospital, CT dosimetry may be performed to verify the number of seeds still present in the prostate as well as the amount of radiation being emitted. At this time, the patient is scheduled for follow-up visits with the urologist and radiation oncologist. Other important discharge instructions include the following:

1. If possible, retrieve seeds lost at home by using a pair of tweezers. The recovered seeds should be wrapped in aluminum foil and returned to the institution's radiation oncology department (Greenburg et al., 1990).
2. Notify the physician if experiencing chills or a fever higher than 100°F (38°C), irritative voiding symptoms, difficulty with urination, excessive bleeding or clots in the urine, or rectal bleeding.

*Hormonal Manipulation.* Nursing management of the patient undergoing hormonal manipulation for advanced prostate cancer is first directed toward promoting patient compliance with the prescribed regimen. Instruct the patient about the treatment he will be receiving, including any known side effects that should be anticipated. Men choosing to have an orchiectomy should be advised about body image changes and the loss of sperm production capabilities. If questions arise about the chance for reconstructive surgery, the nurse should acknowledge the patients' feelings and the possible psychological benefit of such a procedure but explain to them that testicular prostheses are no longer available, having just recently been taken off the market (Lind, 1990; Polomano, 1991). Those men choosing to participate in pharmacologic hormonal manipulation should also be advised of the importance of maintaining therapeutic blood levels of the medication to prolong the period of palliation.

Throughout the treatment period, it is important for the urologic nurse to monitor the patient with prostate cancer for signs of disease progression. Results of laboratory tests, radiographic procedures, as well as examination of the patient's physical and psychological status, should be obtained to determine the overall response to hormonal manipulation (Table 10–4).

**TABLE 10–4. Monitoring Patients With Prostate Cancer**

1. Monitor serum tumor markers: prostate-specific antigen (PSA) and prostatic acid phosphatase (PAP), especially noting any upward trend.
2. Monitor bone scan, CT scan, and/or radiographic results, comparing them to previous reports and noting any changes.
3. Monitor for signs and symptoms of anemia ( ↓ Hgb, ↓ Hct, pallor, ↑ fatigue) which can indicate progression of bone metastases.
4. Monitor for signs and symptoms of urinary retention and/or lymphedema, which can indicate local disease progression.
5. Monitor for ↓ appetite, weight loss, nausea, vomiting, ↑ pain, and/or ↓ performance status, which can indicate systemic disease progression.
6. Monitor for signs and symptoms of impending spinal cord compression in patients with bone metastases—numbness, tingling, or weakness of the limbs, especially legs; ↓ bowel or bladder function; ↑ back pain, especially along the spinal cord.
7. Correlate all observations, lab values, and radiologic reports to determine response to treatment.

CT, computed tomography; Hgb, hemoglobin; Hct, hematocrit.
Taylor, T. (1991). Accurate patient monitoring improves quality of life. *Innovations in Urology Nursing, 2*(2), 2. Reprinted by permission.

As the disease progresses, interventions for the relief of symptoms and overall comfort of the patient are a key responsibility of the nurse. If bony metastasis is present, pain and unstable bone may alter the patient's ability to ambulate. A referral to physical therapy and rehabilitation personnel may enable the patient to reach his ambulating potential with a program for strengthening muscles aided by the use of crutches, a walker, or a wheelchair. Radiation therapy may be employed to palliate the prostate cancer patient with bone pain. Pain relief from radiation therapy is gradual; therefore, analgesics and other comfort measures should be used until the radiation treatments begin to take effect.

Spinal cord compression is an oncologic emergency that may occur in the patient with advanced prostate cancer. Frequent neurologic examinations should be performed on those persons with spinal metastasis to detect any changes in sensation, pain, bowel or bladder function, or limb strength, and abnormal findings should be reported to the physician immediately (Held & Peahota, 1993). Palliative surgical instrumentation may be required to stabilize the spine and control pain (Dyck, 1991).

**Patient Outcomes**
1. The patient can verbalize an understanding

of prostate cancer, including its causes, method of diagnosis, and treatment options.

2. The patient can verbalize his treatment goals and willingness to comply with the planned therapeutic regimen.
3. The patient verbalizes an acceptance of the diagnosis of prostate cancer.
4. The patient maintains a normal pattern of urinary elimination without irritative voiding symptoms, hematuria, dysuria, incomplete bladder emptying, or incontinence.
5. The patient expresses relief from pain with the implementation of appropriate comfort measures.
6. The patient exhibits complete healing of the surgical wound.
7. The patient is free of long-term complications associated with radical prostatectomy or radiation therapy.
8. The patient regains sexual function or experiences sexual satisfaction using an alternative method of expression, if necessary.
9. The patient is mobile within the limits of his disease.
10. The patient verbalizes an understanding of the side effects and safety precautions related to radiation therapy.
11. The patient verbalizes an acceptance of body image changes necessitated by orchiectomy or resulting from pharmacologic hormonal manipulation.
12. The patient observes the dosing schedule of hormonal medication he is taking to achieve palliation.
13. The patient verbalizes an awareness of the signs and symptoms of disease progression and the importance of notifying the physician, especially if symptoms of spinal cord compression occur.

## CANCER OF THE TESTIS

### PERSPECTIVE ON DISEASE ENTITY

**Etiology.** Testicular cancer is uncommon for two important reasons: (1) it accounts for less than 1% of all cancers found in males, and (2) unlike other cancers, it is potentially curable in an advanced stage (Henderson et al., 1988; Richie, 1993). The incidence of cancer of the testis peaks between ages 15 and 40 years; it is the most common solid tumor in men ages 20 to 34 years. Occasionally, it is found in children younger than 10 years of age and men older than 60 years (Richie, 1992, 1993).

Worldwide, testicular cancer has the highest incidence in Scandinavian countries (6.4 to 6.7 per 100,000) and the lowest in Africa and Asia. The incidence for young white European and North American males (3.7 per 100,000) has been steadily increasing during the last few decades. Although the incidence of testicular cancer is now comparable between Hispanics and whites, it is unexplainably low in black Americans (0.9 per 100,00), who have one third the rate of whites (Henderson, 1988; Richie, 1992). In Israel, the incidence of testicular tumors in Jewish men is eight times higher than in non-Jewish men. The incidence of testicular tumors also differs among the various ethnic populations in Hawaii (Richie, 1992).

Cancer of the testis is a disease of high socioeconomic groups. For every two high socioeconomic group males diagnosed with testicular cancer, one male will be diagnosed from a low socioeconomic group (Henderson et al., 1988). Data also suggest a higher incidence among professional men (Graham & Gibson, 1972).

Known risk factors for testicular cancer include a family history of testicular cancer, a cryptorchid testis, and exogenous estrogen exposure. The relationship between testicular maldescent and tumor formation is well established. The degree of risk for bilateral testicular cancer due to unilateral or bilateral cryptorchidism is estimated to be 50% (Richie, 1993). An increasing incidence of right-sided cryptorchidism correlates with reports that testicular tumors occur more commonly in the right testis than in the left (Presti & Herr, 1992; Richie, 1992). The increased incidence of cryptorchidism is linked to the maternal exposure to diethylstilbestrol (DES) and oral contraceptives during pregnancy, as well as low birth weight and prematurity (Cosgrove et al., 1977; Depue et al., 1983; Henderson et al., 1988; Rothman & Lovik, 1978). Studies that examined the relationship between estrogens and testicular cancer suggest an increased risk of tumors (2.8% to 5.3%) in the sons of women exposed to DES, estrogen, or estrogen-progestin combinations in the first 2 months of pregnancy. The first full-term male child born to any woman who required treatment for excessive nausea during the first 2 months of pregnancy—when estrogens levels are rapidly increasing—is also at risk for testicular cancer. The high level of unbound estrogen during this critical period of development may be a causal factor in the later growth of a testis tumor (Henderson et al., 1988).

Trauma, inguinal hernia, and vasectomy have been suggested as other possible risk factors for testicular cancer, although studies examining these risks have not supported the hypotheses linking them to a greater incidence of testis tumors (Nienhuis et al., 1992; West, 1992).

**Pathophysiology.** Testis tumors are predominately germ cell cancers; they possess characteristics similar to germ cell tumors also found in the ovaries and extragonadal sites. To understand the origin of these tumors, it is important, first, to realize that during normal embryonal development of the male, germ cells differentiate to become spermatocytes (Presti & Herr, 1992). However, when germ cells undergo an abnormal pattern of differentiation, they become tumor cells. The most accepted theory of the histogenesis of testicular cancers suggests that all types of tumors initially arise from germ cells that differentiate along a single neoplastic path to become either seminoma or nonseminoma (totipotential) tumor cells (Fig. 10–1). Although germ cell tumors tend to be of one cell type, it is not uncommon for a testicular tumor to have multiple cell types. Furthermore, metastatic lesions may have different or more mature cell types than the primary tumor in the testis (Skinner & Lieskovsky, 1988). Testicular tumors arising from the abnormal differentiation of germ cells account for approximately 95% to 97% of all malignancies.

Non–germ cell type tumors represent less than 5% of all testicular malignancies. Leydig cell tumors, Sertoli cell tumors, and gonadoblastomas are the three most common tumors in this category. On rare occasions, tumors develop in the testis secondary to other disease processes such as lymphoma and leukemia. Metastasis from a primary site in the prostate, lung, gastrointestinal tract, melanoma, and kidney may also lead to the development of a testis tumor (Presti & Herr, 1992). See Table 10–5 for a comparative analysis of all types of testis tumors.

Several pathologic and clinical staging systems have been developed to assist practitioners in determining the extent of disease from a testis tumor. Pathologic staging systems are based primarily on surgical findings and histologic examination of retroperitoneal lymph nodes. Clinical staging systems rely on noninvasive diagnostic procedures to provide information about the appearance, predicted aggressiveness, and metastatic tendency of the tumor at the time of diagnosis, during the course of treatment, and at follow-up (Morse & Whitmore, 1986; Richie, 1993). All are variations of a system first proposed in 1951 (Boden & Gibb) that identified three basic stages of disease:

A (I)—tumor confined to testis
B (II)—tumor spread to regional lymph nodes
C (III)—spread beyond retroperitoneal nodes

The TNM classification developed by the American Joint Committee on Cancer (1992) reflects the most recent effort to standardize clinical staging for all types of testis tumors (Table 10–6). The pathologic staging system proposed by Skinner (1969) is still used for classifying nonseminomatous testis tumors (Table 10–7).

Metastasis from testicular tumors occurs primarily through the lymphatics. (The exception to this is choriocarcinoma, which spreads by way of the blood stream.) The spread of disease follows in a stepwise pattern via the primary route of lymphatic drainage from each testis. In the right testis, primary lymphatic drainage is to the interaortal caval lymph nodes, then to the precaval, preaortic, paracaval, right common iliac, and right external iliac lymph nodes. Because it is common for disease to spread

*FIGURE 10–1* Tumorigenic model for germ cell tumors of the testis. (From Presti, J. C., & Herr, H. W. [1992]. Genital tumors. In E. A. Tanagho & J. W. McAninch [Eds.], *Smith's general urology* [13th ed., p. 414]. Norwalk, CT: Appleton & Lange. Reprinted by permission.)

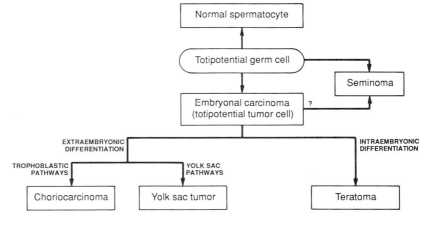

## TABLE 10-5. Types of Testis Tumors

| TUMOR TYPE | DIAGNOSTIC FREQUENCY | COMMENTS |
|---|---|---|
| **Germ Cell Tumors**<br>*Seminomas* | Approximately 27–35% of all testis tumors are of this type | |
| Classic seminoma | 82–85% of seminomas | Slow-growing tumor; most commonly seen in the 4th decade of life |
| Anaplastic seminoma | 5–10% of seminomas | An aggressive tumor with an increased potential for metastasis that tends to present at a higher stage than does classic seminoma |
| Spermatocytic seminoma | 5–10% of seminomas | More than half of the men diagnosed with this tumor are older than 50 years of age; although tumor may be 5 cm or larger at the time of detection, it has a low potential for metastasis and prognosis is favorable with treatment |
| *Nonseminomas* | Approximately 50–65% of all testis tumors are of this type | |
| Embryonal cell carcinoma | 5–10% of nonseminomas | Occurrence in pure form is rare; usually presents as a painless testicular mass that extends beyond the testis in 30% of cases; in adults this type is often a feature in mixed cell tumors |
| Endodermal sinus tumor | 10–20% of nonseminomas | Also called "yolk sac tumor"; it is the most common testis tumor in infants and children up to age 3; often presents as a rapidly enlarging painless scrotal mass—metastasis to retroperitoneal lymph nodes is possible; in adults, rarely seen in pure form but is a component of mixed cell tumors in 30% of cases |
| Teratoma | 10% of nonseminomas | Represents the second most common germ cell tumor in boys younger than 4 years of age; usually larger than other germ cell tumors, ranging 5–10 cm in diameter, but with no tendency for metastasis; pure lesion is rare in adults |
| Choriocarcinoma | <1% of nonseminomas | Very rare but aggressive tumor that first presents as a small (<5 cm) palpable nodule along with signs of distant metastasis or gynecomastia; often spreads by way of the blood stream to lung or central nervous system; median age of onset is early 20s |
| Mixed cell type | 60–80% of nonseminomas | Majority of mixed cell tumors are combination of teratoma and embryonal cell carcinoma, also called *teratocarcinoma*; presentation and metastatic tendency depend on the various cell types composing the tumor |
| **Non–Germ Cell Tumors**<br>Leydig cell tumors | 1–3% of all testis tumors | Most common non–germ cell tumor; 25% occur in children ages 5 to 9 with tumors that are usually benign; 75% are diagnosed in men ages 25 to 35 with a 10% malignancy rate |
| Sertoli cell tumors | <1% of all testis tumors | Very rare tumor that most commonly presents as an undefined mass, 1 to 20 cm in size; one third of tumors occur in children younger than 12 years of age, two thirds in men 20 to 45 years of age; 10% of lesions are malignant |
| Gonadoblastomas | <0.5% of all testis tumors | Usually seen in patients under 30 years of age with some form of gonadal dysgenesis; tumor tends to be bilateral in 50% of cases |

Information and data compiled from Brodsky, 1991; Presti & Herr, 1992; Richie, 1992.

from the right to the left, there may also be involvement of the left common iliac and left external iliac nodes. Lymphatic drainage of the left testis is to the preaortic, left common iliac, and left external iliac lymph nodes. If the tumor extends to the epididymis or spermatic cord, there may be metastasis to the iliac or obturator lymph nodes. Inguinal metastasis is possible if the tumor involves the tunica albuginea or if lymphatic drainage has been altered by previous scrotal surgery (Presti & Herr, 1992; Richie, 1993).

Clinically, involvement of the retroperitoneal lymph nodes may result in back or abdominal pain, nausea, anorexia, or bowel and bladder changes. Distant metastasis is most common to

## TABLE 10–6. Definition of TNM in Testis Cancer

### PRIMARY TUMOR (T)

The extent of primary tumor is classified after radical orchiectomy.

| | |
|---|---|
| pTX | Primary tumor cannot be assessed (if no radical orchiectomy has been performed, TX is used) |
| pT0 | No evidence of primary tumor (e.g., histologic scar in testis) |
| pTis | Intratubular tumor: preinvasive cancer |
| pT1 | Tumor limited to the testis, including the rete testis |
| pT2 | Tumor invades beyond the tunica albuginea or into the epididymis |
| pT3 | Tumor invades spermatic cord |
| pT4 | Tumor invades the scrotum |

### REGIONAL LYMPH NODES (N)

| | |
|---|---|
| NX | Regional lymph nodes cannot be assessed |
| N0 | No regional lymph node metastasis |
| N1 | Metastasis in a single lymph node, 2 cm or less in greatest dimension |
| N2 | Metastasis in a single lymph node, more than 2 cm but not more than 5 cm in greatest dimension; or multiple lymph nodes, none more than 5 cm in greatest dimension |
| N3 | Metastasis in a lymph node more than 5 cm in greatest dimension |

### DISTANT METASTASIS (M)

| | |
|---|---|
| MX | Presence of distant metastasis cannot be assessed |
| M0 | No distant metastasis |
| M1 | Distant metastasis |

From American Joint Committee on Cancer. (1992). *Manual for Staging of Cancer* (4th ed., p. 188). Philadelphia: J. B. Lippincott. Reprinted with permission.

the lung and may manifest as a cough, dyspnea, or hemoptysis. Other less common sites of distant metastasis, often seen in only advanced stages of the disease, include the liver, viscera, brain, and bone.

### Medical-Surgical Management

*Diagnosis.* A visit to the urologist is most often prompted by the discovery of a mass or lump on the testis along with painless enlargement of the hemiscrotum. Some patients may describe a feeling of heaviness in the scrotum, inguinal area, or lower abdomen, whereas others may complain of a backache, abdominal pain, weight loss, generalized weakness, or a neck mass.

When physical examination confirms the presence of a testicular mass, the urologist will request that several laboratory and radiographic tests be performed to distinguish a malignant testis tumor from other benign scrotal masses. Testicular ultrasonography is often the first diagnostic study performed. If the mass is presumed to be cancerous, chest radiographs (posteroanterior and lateral) are performed to identify any pulmonary metastasis, whereas CT scans are used to examine the patient for evidence of metastasis to the retroperitoneal lymph nodes. Liver, brain, and bone scans may also be done if there is a specific clinical indication of metastasis to these areas.

As part of the medical evaluation, blood is drawn to measure tumor markers. Tumor markers are "substances produced and secreted by tumor cells that are found in the serum of patients" (Ostchega & Culnane, 1985). The tumor marker levels for germinal testicular tumors elevate when disease is present and return to normal when the tumor is eradicated. Thus, the physician can use these biochemical measurements to aid in the diagnosis of testicular cancer, to monitor results of treatment, and as evidence of tumor recurrence. The serum tumor markers for testicular cancer are beta-human chorionic gonadotropin (beta-hCG), alpha-fetoprotein (AFP), and lactic acid dehydrogenase (LDH). Placental alkaline phosphatase (PLAP) is currently being studied as another possible marker for seminoma (Richie, 1993).

Beta-hCG is a glycoprotein usually produced by trophoblastic cells in the fetal placenta (Pagana & Pagana, 1990). The serum level of beta-hCG is normally elevated in the pregnant female yet is undetectable at birth. However, ab-

## TABLE 10–7. Pathologic Staging of Nonseminomatous Testis Tumors

Stage A—tumor confined to the scrotum, chest radiograph and excretory urogram negative, no positive nodes on lymph node dissection

Stage B—tumor metastases present below the diaphragm, chest radiograph and mediastinum normal

Stage B₁—gross or microscopic involvement of <6 nodes that are well encapsulated with no evidence of tumor extending through the capsule of the node involving the retroperitoneal fat

Stage B₂—gross or microscopic involvement of >6 nodes or tumor extending through the capsule of the node involving the retroperitoneal fat

Stage B₃—bulky, palpable abdominal mass (>5 cm)

Stage C—metastases above diaphragm or liver involvement

Adapted from Skinner, D. G. (1969). Non-seminomatous testis tumors: A plan of management based on 96 patients to improve survival in all stages by combined therapeutic modalities. *Journal of Urology, 115,* 65–69. © Williams & Wilkins, 1969. Reprinted by permission.

normal elevations of beta-hCG occur in men with seminomatous testis tumors; an increase in beta-hCG levels may also be associated with nonseminomatous tumors, such as embryonal carcinoma, yolk sac carcinoma, and choriocarcinoma. Gynecomastia, a frequent physical finding in males with a testicular tumor, is thought to be caused by an elevated level of beta-hCG.

AFP is also a serum glycoprotein. High levels of AFP may be found in infants for as long as a year after birth but thereafter in only trace amounts. Elevated levels of AFP may be seen with nonseminomatous germ cell tumors but not in patients with seminomas (Presti & Herr, 1992; Richie, 1993).

LDH is a cellular enzyme normally produced in muscles as well as in the liver, kidney, and brain. Levels of total LDH, and more specifically LDH isoenzyme-1, elevate in germinal testicular tumors because of the increased metabolism and catabolism of cancer cells. Although an elevated LDH level is not considered diagnostic for a primary tumor in the testis, it may raise suspicions about the presence of metastatic disease associated with a testicular malignancy (Ostchega & Culnane, 1985; Richie, 1993).

The diagnosis of testicular cancer is verified by inguinal exploration of the testis. In those instances when direct inspection of the testis neither confirms nor excludes the presence of cancerous tissue, biopsy of the mass for frozen-section analysis is performed. If a negative result cannot be verified, a radical orchiectomy is still advised (Presti & Herr, 1992; Skinner & Skinner, 1992). Radical inguinal orchiectomy involves removal of the testis, epididymis, and vas deferens, with ligation of the spermatic cord just inside the internal inguinal ring.

Until recently, insertion of a testicular prosthesis into the affected hemiscrotum was an option for men who had undergone radical orchiectomy. However, urologists are no longer performing the procedure because the prosthesis has been withdrawn from the market and is unavailable.

*Treatment.* A characteristic of low-stage seminoma that differentiates it from other germ cells tumors is that it is radiosensitive (Findlay & Glatstein, 1986; Richie, 1993; Smith, 1988). Patients with stage I or IIA disease are treated with radical orchiectomy, followed by postoperative radiation therapy to the retroperitoneal lymph nodes. Because this type of tumor is so responsive to irradiation, the dosage and number of treatments needed to eradicate disease

are comparatively low; as a result, side effects are minimal (Presti & Herr, 1992; Steinfeld, 1990). Treatment of low-stage seminomas in this manner has resulted in a 5-year survival rate of almost 95%.

Advanced-stage (IIB or higher) seminomas are more chemosensitive. Therefore, primary treatment with chemotherapy following radical orchiectomy is usually recommended. The administration of cisplatinum in combination with other drugs such as vinblastine and bleomycin results in a disease-free survival rate of approximately 85% (Richie, 1993). In this group of patients, radiation therapy is employed only when chemotherapy has failed.

Nonseminomatous germ cell tumors confined to the testis (stages A and $B_1$ disease) are treated with radical orchiectomy followed by retroperitoneal lymph node dissection. A transabdominal or thoracoabdominal approach to retroperitoneal lymphadenectomy along with modified dissection techniques is advocated to protect ejaculatory function and preserve fertility, the loss of which is a frequent complication when other surgical approaches are employed (Skinner & Lieskovsky, 1988). More recently, endoscopic surgical techniques have been adapted by urologists, enabling them to perform laparoscopic lymph node dissection through a much smaller incision and with few complications (Clayman, 1991). A period of surveillance after orchiectomy and lymphadenectomy is mandatory to detect tumor recurrence. At each follow-up visit, the patient should undergo a thorough physical examination, chest radiograph, and measurement of serum tumor markers; these are performed monthly for the first year, every 2 months for the second year, then every 3 to 6 months for as long as 5 years. To assess the retroperitoneum, a CT scan 1 year postoperatively is required (Richie, 1993). Five-year survival rates following treatment for stage A nonseminomatous tumors are reported to be 96%; stage $B_1$ disease has a 5-year survival of 90% (Presti & Herr, 1992).

Patients with a stage $B_2$ or higher nonseminomatous germ cell tumors are treated with radical orchiectomy followed by cisplatinum-based, multidrug chemotherapy. Patients with partial response to this treatment may eventually require retroperitoneal lymph node dissection, whereas disease progression requires several more cycles of chemotherapy and possibly bone marrow transplantation (Richie, 1992). Survival rates for nonseminomatous tumors stage $B_2$ or higher range from 55% to 80% (Presti & Herr, 1992).

## APPROACHES TO PATIENT CARE

### Assessment

A thorough assessment of the patient with testicular cancer is a key responsibility of the nurse. Begin every assessment with question specifically related to the history of the disease process. Assess or inquire about the following:

Age: How old is the patient?

Ethnicity: What is the patient's race and national origin?

Socioeconomics: What is the socioeconomic status of the patient's family? What type of job does the patient hold, and where is he employed?

Birth history: Did the patient's mother have extreme nausea that required treatment during pregnancy? Was the patient's mother exposed to oral contraceptives, drugs for threatened abortion, or hormonal injection for determining if she was pregnant? Is the patient the first full-term male child born by his mother, or was he born prematurely, with a low birth weight? Were both testes descended at birth? If no, was orchidopexy performed, and at what age?

Family history: Is there a family history of testicular cancer or any other urogenital abnormality?

Detection: How was the current problem first discovered? Does the patient currently practice monthly testicular self-examination (TSE)?

Symptoms: Has the patient experienced any pain, heaviness, or other discomfort in the testicle or scrotum? If yes, how long? Has the patient experienced any breast tenderness, backache, nausea, anorexia, abdominal pain, or bowel or bladder changes? Has the patient experienced persistent coughing, dyspnea, or hemoptysis? Has the patient experienced any visual or mental status changes? Has he had any seizures? Has he experienced any recent weight loss?

Physical examination is an important means of assessing the patient's current status. Begin at the head and work down, looking for clues that would be indicative of metastatic disease.

Head: Do a thorough examination of the head, eyes, ears, nose, and throat, including an assessment of the cranial nerves.

Neck: Palpate for any firm, fixed, enlarged, or tender cervical or supraclavicular lymph nodes.

Chest: Auscultate the lungs for decreased breath sounds. Monitor the rate and depth of respirations. Inspect the breasts for gynecomastia, and palpate for any tenderness.

Back: Palpate the vertebrae, flank, and lower back for tenderness.

Abdomen: Palpate for masses and hepatomegaly.

Pelvis: Inspect for inguinal adenopathy, then palpate the groin for firm, fixed, enlarged, or tender lymph nodes. Inspect both sides of the scrotal sac for gross asymmetry or enlargement. Palpate the testicle to isolate the mass. Transilluminate the scrotum to determine if the lump is fluid (hydrocele) or a solid mass.

Legs: Inspect the legs for edema (Jenkins, 1988).

Issues pertaining to the patient's psychosocial needs, as well as concerns about sexual function and body image, should also be explored during the nursing assessment. What is his reaction to the diagnosis of testicular cancer? Is he able to express fears, and to whom? How is his spouse, or companion, reacting to the diagnosis? What will be the impact of the diagnosis and treatment on the couple's relationship and that of their immediate family? Has the patient fathered any children, or are there future plans for children? Does the patient understand that infertility may be a consequence of treatment? Is the patient familiar with sperm banking and other reproductive technologies? How does he envision his appearance after radical orchiectomy, and what affect does he expect this will have on him as an individual—and as a man (Smith & Babaian, 1992). Finally, assess the patient's educational needs concerning testicular cancer. Can he simply describe the procedure and purpose for radical orchiectomy? Does he understand that subsequent treatment is determined by the type of tumor and stage of disease? Does he understand the differences among radiation therapy, chemotherapy, and lymph node dissection? Does he realize that most types of testis tumors have a 5-year survival rate of 85% or higher? Is he able to demonstrate the procedure for TSE, and can he state the importance of performing it monthly?

### Nursing Diagnosis

The nursing diagnoses for the patient with cancer of the testis may include the following:

1. Knowledge deficit related to
   a. Causes and course of testicular cancer.
   b. Diagnostic procedures performed to confirm testicular cancer, including inguinal exploration.

  c. Indications for radical orchiectomy.
  d. Treatment approaches after radical orchiectomy, including retroperitoneal lymph node dissection, radiation therapy, and chemotherapy.
2. Fear related to the effect of treatments on virility, quality of life, and life expectancy.
3. Pain related to
  a. Surgical excision of diseased testis.
  b. Retroperitoneal lymphadenectomy.
  c. Metastasis of testis cancer.
4. Body image disturbance related to
  a. Development of gynecomastia.
  b. Appearance of scrotum after radical orchiectomy.
5. Ineffective airway clearance (potential) related to discomfort associated with a thoracoabdominal or transabdominal incision for retroperitoneal lymph node dissection and the presence of chest drainage system.
6. Altered peripheral tissue perfusion (potential) related to the development of hypovolemic shock caused by injury to a blood vessel during excision of lymph nodes.
7. Altered sexuality patterns (potential) related to
  a. Loss of ejaculatory function.
  b. Infertility.
8. Noncompliance (potential) related to prolonged periods of therapy or medical follow-up.
9. Health-seeking behavior: technique for monthly TSE related to the lack of knowledge of need for regular self-assessment of the contralateral (unaffected) testis, *or* use of the procedure as a screening technique for all men aged 15 to 40 years.

### Plan of Care

Nursing care is directed toward enabling the patient to

1. Demonstrate an understanding of the risk and causes of testicular cancer, prognosis for the disease, diagnostic procedures, and treatment goals and alternatives.
2. Express a lessening sense of fear regarding the diagnosis of testicular cancer and any perceived threat to virility.
3. Obtain relief from pain.
4. Cope with changes in body image.
5. Verbalize concerns regarding sexual functioning and fertility.
6. Comply with protocol for radiation therapy or chemotherapy, as well as rigorous follow-up schedule.
7. Correctly perform the procedure for TSE.

### Interventions

*Radical Orchiectomy.* The interval between discovery of a lump in the testis, medical evaluation, and radical orchiectomy is often no longer than 1 week. Therefore, patient teaching by the urologic nurse must be well organized and concise yet designed to dispel myths and provide reassurance. Begin with one-on-one discussion to answer questions about the diagnosis of testis cancer and the proposed treatment regimen, as well as explain hospital procedures and nursing care related to radical orchiectomy. Written materials and videotape instruction foster an atmosphere of informed consent while helping to reinforce information presented verbally by the health care team. A referral to the National Cancer Institute or American Cancer Society will provide the patient and his family with additional helpful resources, including support groups.

In most health care institutions, radical orchiectomy is performed as same-day surgery with an overnight hospital stay. It is a relatively short and uncomplicated procedure accomplished through an inguinal incision. Postoperatively, the surgical site is approximated with Steri-Strips or staples that remain in place for 7 to 10 days. Serosanguineous drainage may be observed oozing from the surgical site for as long as 24 hours after the procedure; excessive bleeding or wound separation is uncommon and should be reported to the urologist immediately. On inspection, the scrotum is tender and slightly swollen. Ice bags may be applied to the scrotal area for the first 12 hours after surgery, as tolerated (Flannery, 1992). The formation of a hematoma with severe edema suggests bleeding from the spermatic cord stump; therefore, frequent examination of the scrotum is advised to detect this rare, but serious, condition. To manage the pain associated with radical orchiectomy, analgesics are administered by intramuscular injection until oral analgesics can be tolerated. In addition, patients are usually provided with a scrotal support, which should be worn at all times (particularly when ambulating) to alleviate discomfort and prevent edema. Before discharge, patients are given an appointment for a follow-up visit to the urologist. They are also instructed to contact the physician if unusual symptoms occur, such as fever, chills, excessive weakness, and increased scrotal edema.

*Retroperitoneal Lymph Node Dissection.* This procedure is performed either as open or laparoscopic. Depending on the approach used by the surgeon, hospitalization may be required for as long as 7 days (Skinner & Skinner, 1992). Preoperatively, the urologic nurse provides appropriate teaching about the procedure and postoperative care activities. This should include a discussion about the possible effects of the surgery on future fertility. If needed, a consultation with a reproductive specialist may be arranged for the patient (and his spouse, if married) to discuss sperm banking. Postoperative nursing care following retroperitoneal lymph node dissection may include any or all of the following:

Monitoring the patency and output from the urethral catheter, nasogastric tube, or chest tube.

Monitoring the effectiveness of pain management—during the first 24 to 48 hours, this is usually accomplished via an epidural infusion or PCA pump.

Administering prophylactic antibiotics, if ordered.

Monitoring intravenous fluid therapy to ensure adequate hydration.

Observing the surgical site for signs of wound infection.

Being alert to changes in vital signs—hypovolemic shock is a rare, but possible, complication caused by the inadvertent injury to a blood vessel during the dissection and excision of lymph nodes.

Examining the abdomen for return of bowel sounds or for signs of complications such as peritonitis and bleeding.

Ensuring effective airway clearance by assisting the patient to perform coughing and deep-breathing exercises.

Applying and maintaining elastic stockings or pneumatic compression devices to prevent venous stasis.

Assisting the patient with ambulation beginning on the first postoperative night, advancing the frequency and distance of ambulation on subsequent days.

In preparation for discharge, the nurse should ascertain that the patient is familiar with the signs and symptoms of possible postoperative complications such as infection, ileus, and atelectasis and pneumonia. Provide the patient with information about his postoperative visit to the urologist, and emphasize the need for continued medical evaluation.

*Other Treatments.* Radiation therapy and chemotherapy are usually coordinated by the medical oncologist and administered in settings outside the urology inpatient unit, office, or clinic. As is often the case, the urologic nurse will not be directly involved in either of these treatments. Instead, the urologic nurse assumes the role of advocate and liaison for the patient by offering support, providing information, and coordinating long-term follow-up appointments with the urologist.

*TSE* is a simple technique that any adolescent or adult male is capable of performing. However, few men in the 15- to 40-year age group are aware of the facts about testicular cancer, much less the need and procedure for monthly TSE. This is unfortunate because testicular cancer, if detected early, is among the most curable solid tumors (Willson, 1991).

Why is it that men do not regularly perform TSE? Several reasons have been suggested, including the following: (1) lack of or inadequate instruction by health care professionals; (2) skills required to perform TSE are too complicated, thus difficult to learn; (3) TSE is a time-consuming procedure; and, (4) men are uninformed, misinformed, or do not comprehend information about testis cancer (Friman & Finney, 1990; Sheley, 1991). There are also some who believe that the health maintenance needs of men are less important in our society as compared with the attention devoted to women's issues. Consequently, men do not receive enough encouragement to annually visit their physician for a thorough physical examination, nor are they invited to candidly discuss health care needs and concerns. Whatever the reason, there is an unequivocal need for testicular cancer education.

Urologic nurses possess the knowledge, skills, and resources necessary to provide health education about testicular cancer. Each must assume the responsibility to educate their patients and the public about the incidence, risks, and symptoms of the disease. This includes instructing all men 15 to 40 years of age about the correct technique and time for performing TSE. Although TSE is most widely advocated as a screening technique for testis cancer, those men who have been treated for the disease should perform the procedure on the unaffected testis to monitor for tumor recurrence. Procedure 10–2 illustrates the proper technique for TSE.

**Patient Outcomes**

1. The patient verbalizes an understanding of the causes, diagnostic protocol, and treatment options for testis cancer.
2. The patient states that information provided to him about testis cancer has reduced or alleviated his fears about the disease and the effect of treatments.

3. The patient expresses relief from pain.
4. The patient avoids complications associated with surgical removal of a testis or retroperitoneal lymph node dissection.
5. The patient expresses an understanding and demonstrates acceptance of body image changes.
6. The patient seeks advice concerning future fertility.

7. The patient experiences sexual satisfaction despite the effects of surgery, radiation, or chemotherapy.
8. The patient observes the schedules for radiation therapy, chemotherapy, and routine surveillance after treatments.
9. The patient reiterates the procedure for TSE; the patient performs TSE monthly, as instructed.

---

## PROCEDURE 10-2
■
### Testicular Self-Examination (TSE)

TSE is a simple, 2- to 3-minute procedure that should be performed *every month*. All men 15 years of age and older are encouraged to make TSE a life-time practice.

### ■ TSE: WARNING SIGNS

1. A lump on the testis, often small, hard, and painless
2. Enlargement of the testis
3. Pain in the testis
4. Heaviness in the testis or scrotum
5. Pulling, discomfort, or pain in the lower abdomen or groin
6. Breast enlargement or nipple tenderness
7. Any noticeable difference in the way the testis feels from one month to the next

### ■ TSE STEP BY STEP

TSE is best performed during or immediately folllowing a warm shower or bath, when hands are warm and the scrotum is relaxed and descended. To increase finger sensitivity, hands should be well lathered with soap. Throughout the procedure, use gentle pressure to examine each structure within the scrotum.

1. Gently raise the penis upward and note that the left side of the scrotum is lower than the right side. Observe and compare each side of the scrotum for any differences in size or shape *(A)*.

2. Hold the scrotum in the palm of both hands and compare the weight of each side. Both halves of the scrotal sac should have the same degree of heaviness. Continue with the procedure, examining *each side of the scrotum separately*.

3. With the thumb on top and the index and middle fingers underneath, slowly and gently roll the testicle between the fingers. Feel for any lumps or areas that seem hard or enlarged *(B)*.

4. Locate the epididymis. Sperm collect in this comma-shaped organ, which feels soft and slightly tender; notice that it extends downward from the top to behind the testis. Be sure to also examine the space between the front of the testis and back of the epididymis—this is done by pressing the thumb and fingers into the grooved area between the two structures *(C)*.

5. Move the thumb, index, and middle fingers upward from the epididymis to examine the spermatic cord. The spermatic cord is shaped like a tube and usually feels smooth and firm, yet moveable *(D)*.

Immediate evaluation by a physician is recommended if any lumps or other changes are detected by TSE.

## PROCEDURE 10-2 *Continued*
■
## Testicular Self-Examination (TSE)

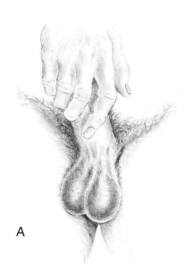

A

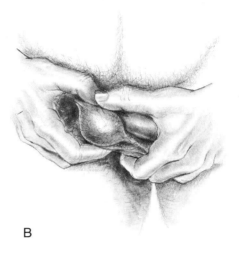

B

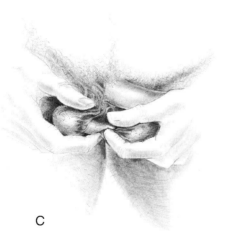

C

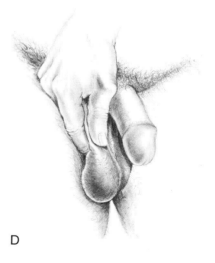

D

(Drawings by Jerry L. Bates)

# CANCER OF THE PENIS

## PERSPECTIVE ON DISEASE ENTITY

**Etiology.** Cancer of the penis is rare in the United States, where less than 1% of all male cancers are penile in origin (Crawford & Dawkins, 1988). The incidence is higher (10% to 20%) in African, South American, and Far Eastern countries (Black, 1986; Crawford & Dawkins, 1988; Livne & Pontes, 1986). Men migrating to regions where the incidence of squamous cell cancer of the penis is high tend to assume the incidence of the region (Persky, 1977).

Penile cancers occur in males aged 20 to 90 years, with a mean age at diagnosis of 58 years (Burgers et al., 1992; Crawford & Dawkins, 1988; Persky, 1977). In the United States, cancer of the penis rarely occurs before the age of 40 years; however, a case has been reported involving a 2-year-old child (Kini, 1944).

Risk factors include late or lack of circumcision and poor hygiene. Studies indicate that cancer of the penis is rare in males circumcised at birth, low in males circumcised before puberty, and high in uncircumcised males (Nichols, 1988). This explains the low incidence of the disease in Israel, where males are circumcised at birth, and the high incidence in Uganda, where circumcision of males is uncommon (Crawford & Dawkins, 1988). In the 1980s, many Americans withheld consent for circumcision despite evidence that circumcision protects men from developing cancer of the penis. Eighty-five percent of newborn males were circumcised in 1970 compared with 59% in 1985. Unfortunately, "the long-term effects of this trend may not be realized for fifty or sixty years" (Black, 1986).

Phimosis or paraphimosis is present in most males with cancer of the penis, suggesting that a carcinogen is produced or contained under the foreskin. Smegma has been associated with carcinogenesis in animal models, but specific carcinogenic components of smegma have not been identified (Flannery, 1992; Persky, 1977; Persky & de Kernion, 1986). Because smegma can be removed by retracting the foreskin and washing the area regularly and thoroughly, it has been theorized that the low incidence of cancer of the penis in some countries may be directly attributed to good hygiene and early circumcision.

Several studies have identified a link between cancer of the penis and cancer of the uterine cervix. One study reported an increased risk of cervical cancer in the wives of men with penile cancer—particularly in China, where both types of cancer are common (Li et al., 1982, 1983; Nichols, 1988).

During the 1950s and 1970s, venereal disease was thought to be a contributing factor to the development of penile cancer. At that time, as many as 25% of patients with cancer of the penis had a history of venereal disease. Studies conducted since then have shown no known association between cancer of the penis and venereal disease. Trauma to the penis has also been dismissed as a possible risk factor (Black, 1986; Livne & Pontes, 1986).

**Pathophysiology.** By far, the most common type of penile cancer is squamous cell carcinoma; it accounts for approximately 95% of all penile malignancies (Burgers et al., 1992). Other types of penile cancers, which collectively represent less than 5% of all cases reported, include (1) sarcomas, particularly Kaposi's sarcoma associated with acquired immunodeficiency syndrome, malignant hemangioendothelioma, schwannoma, leiomyoma, leiomyosarcoma, and rhabdomyosarcoma; (2) mesenchymal tumors, which arise from the stromal or connective tissues; (3) basal cell carcinoma; and (4) melanoma (Livne & Pontes, 1986; Nichols, 1988; Persky & de Kernion, 1986).

Additionally, there are several types of premalignant-type lesions that develop on the penis: These include (1) condylomata acuminata; (2) Buschke-Löwenstein's tumor, also referred to as *giant condyloma acuminata* or *verrucous carcinoma*; (3) Bowen's disease or *carcinoma-in-situ*; and (4) leukoplakia (Wein & Hanno, 1987).

j20Tumors may originate anywhere on the penis: 48% of primary penile cancers develop in the glans; 21% in the prepuce; 9% in both the glans and prepuce; 6% in the coronal sulcus; and less than 2% in the penile shaft (Burgers et al., 1992).

Penile cancers initially appear as one or more papillary or flat lesions. Papillary lesions are wartlike—small, round, and raised. Flat lesions are usually small, superficial ulcerations. In the early stages of the disease, the patient may complain of itching or burning beneath the foreskin. The penis may exhibit only a simple nodule that appears as a pimple or wart, or there may be a small, shallow ulceration on the glans or prepuce; phimosis is often apparent. As the disease progresses and the lesion extends, a foul-smelling, purulent discharge may be evident from underneath the prepuce. If left untreated, tissue erosion of the glans, shaft, and corpora leads to the eventual destruction of the phallus (Burgers et al., 1992; Schellhammer et al., 1992) (Fig. 10–2).

Primary carcinoma of the penis spreads via the lymphatics. The extension of disease to regional lymph nodes correlates with the type of lesion, as well as with the degree to which the shaft of the penis is affected. "Patients with 75% involvement of the shaft and a flat growth pattern have a greater incidence of inguinal lymph node involvement" (Burgers et al., 1992, p. 249). More than half of the patients with penile carcinoma present with some sort of lymphadenopathy—either cancer in the nodes or inflammation due to infection of the lesion. Distant metastasis from penile cancers, although uncommon, occurs very late in the disease and may involve the bone, lung, or liver.

Primary cancers, especially genitourinary cancers, do metastasize to the penis. Sixty percent of all cancers metastatic to the penis originate in the bladder or prostate (Nichols, 1988). Metastasis from primary tumors in the kidney, testis, and lung are seen with less frequency,

followed by tumors originating in the rectosigmoid colon, pancreas, and ureter (Livne & Pontes, 1986; Nichols, 1988; Persky & de Kernion, 1986). Penile metastasis has prognostic significance in that patients usually die within 6 months of the discovery of the lesion (Livne & Pontes, 1986).

The most popular staging system for penile squamous cell carcinoma is a clinical classification first proposed by Jackson in 1966 (Table 10–8). The TNM staging system adopted by the American Joint Committee on Cancer (1992) relies on the histopathology of the penile lesion and the degree of lymph node involvement for prognosis (Table 10–9). Neither method, however, is universally accepted by practitioners because of the difficulties encountered in trying to standardize descriptions of the penile tumors (Burgers et al., 1992; Schellhammer et al., 1992).

**Medical-Surgical Management.** Medical evaluation of a penile lesion requires that the urologist first perform a thorough history and physical examination. Laboratory studies, such as cultures, tissue stains, skin tests, and syphilis

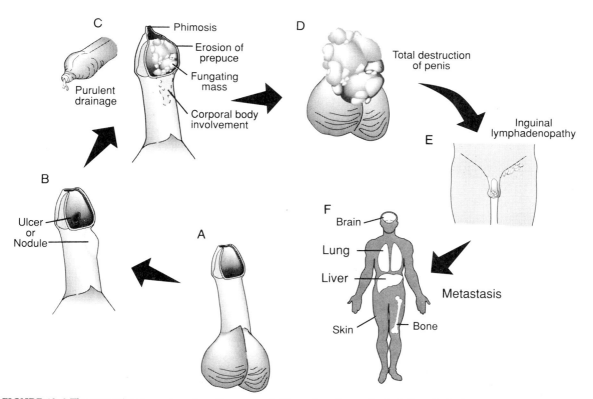

*FIGURE 10–2* The natural progression of penile cancer. *A,* Normal uncircumcised phallus. *B,* Early stage with formation of either an ulcer or a nodule. *C,* Purulent, fungating mass below a phimotic prepuce. *D,* Complete phallic destruction. *E,* Inguinal lymph node metastasis. *F,* Distant metastases; most commonly to lung and liver, followed by bone, brain, and skin. (Copyright © by the Division of Urology, The Ohio State University. Reprinted by permission.)

TABLE 10–8. Jackson Classification for
Squamous Penile Cancer

| STAGE | DESCRIPTION |
|-------|-------------|
| I | Tumor confined to glans or prepuce |
| II | Invasion into shaft or corpora; no nodal or distant metastases |
| III | Tumor confined to penis; operable inguinal nodal metastases |
| IV | Tumor involves adjacent structures; inoperable inguinal nodes and/or distant metastasis(es) |

From Burgers, J. K., Badalament, R. A., & Drago, J. R.
(1992). Penile cancer: Clinical presentation, diagnosis, and
staging. *Urologic Clinics of North America 19*(2), 247. Reprinted by permission.

serology, are performed next to determine if
the lesion may be caused by an infectious
agent. A tissue biopsy is required for histologic
examination and confirmation of a malignant
lesion. Specimens are usually obtained by deep
incision of the periphery of the lesion; however, a dorsal slit or circumcision may be necessary to obtain tissue from underneath the
prepuce (Burgers et al., 1992). Cavernosography, ultrasonography, CT scan, and MRI all
may be employed to identify tumor extension
into the corporal bodies.

Cancer of the penis may be treated with surgery, radiation, or chemotherapy. Treatment
selection is based on extent of disease, lymph
node involvement, and presence of distant metastasis (Crawford & Dawkins, 1988; Johnson &
Lo, 1987; Livne & Pontes, 1986).

Many agree that circumcision is the treatment of choice for noninvasive squamous cell
carcinoma of the penis that is limited to the
foreskin. Unfortunately, this treatment is associated with a tumor recurrence rate that may
be as high as 50% (Schellhammer et al., 1992).
Therefore, external beam radiation is often recommended for patients who have recurrent or
residual disease following circumcision for a
malignant penile lesion (Johnson & Lo, 1987).

A partial penectomy is usually recommended for superficial lesions of 2 to 5 cm in
diameter that are located on the glans or distal
third of the penile shaft (Crawford & Dawkins,
1988; Johnson & Lo, 1987). A 2-cm tumor-free
margin proximal to the lesion is advised to reduce local recurrence of disease (Schellhammer
et al., 1992). Local recurrence in patients treated
with partial penectomy is reported to range
from 1% to 6%. Five-year survival is approximately 70% to 80% as long as there is no inguinal lymph node metastasis (Schellhammer

et al., 1992). In many instances, the remaining
penile length is sufficient for the patient to direct his urinary stream while standing, and
most will be able to have satisfactory sexual
intercourse (Johnson & Lo, 1987).

The use of $CO_2$ and Nd:YAG lasers has been
applied to the treatment of premalignant penile
lesions such as condylomata acuminata, verrucous carcinomas, and carcinoma-in-situ. Depending on the location of the tumor and the
degree of tumor development, the effects of
laser therapy may be comparable to partial penectomy. Patients treated in this manner require close observation and regular follow-up,
because tumor recurrences may require additional laser treatments or an alternative therapy
(Schellhammer et al., 1992).

Total penectomy is performed when cancer
originates on the proximal shaft or at the base
of the penis. It may also be considered if curative surgery would create a penis too short for
standing urination (Johnson & Lo, 1987; Livne
& Pontes, 1986). The procedure includes the
formation of a perineal urethrostomy to facilitate bladder emptying.

Metastatic nodal disease is present in one
third of all patients with penile cancer at the
time of diagnosis (Grabstald, 1980). On the
other hand, as many as 50% of patients have

TABLE 10–9. Definition of TNM in Carcinoma of
the Penis

**PRIMARY TUMOR (T)**

| | |
|-----|-----|
| TX | Primary tumor cannot be assessed |
| T0 | No evidence of primary tumor |
| Tis | Carcinoma-in-situ |
| Ts | Noninvasive verrucous carcinoma |
| T1 | Tumor invades subepithelial connective tissue |
| T2 | Tumor invades the corpus spongiosum or cavernosum |
| T3 | Tumor invades urethra or prostate |
| T4 | Tumor invades other adjacent structures |

**REGIONAL LYMPH NODES (N)**

| | |
|-----|-----|
| NX | Regional lymph nodes cannot be assessed |
| N0 | No regional lymph node metastasis |
| N1 | Metastasis in a single superficial, inguinal lymph node |
| N2 | Metastasis in multiple or bilateral superficial inguinal lymph nodes |
| N3 | Metastasis in deep inguinal or pelvic lymph node(s), unilateral or bilateral |

**DISTANT METASTASIS (M)**

| | |
|-----|-----|
| MX | Presence of distant metastasis cannot be assessed |
| M0 | No distant metastasis |
| M1 | Distant metastasis |

From American Joint Committee on Cancer. (1992).
*Manual for Staging of Cancer* (4th ed., pp. 191–192). Philadelphia: J. B. Lippincott. Reprinted by permission.

palpable lymphadenopathy secondary to a superimposed infection of the cancerous penile lesion. Evaluation of inguinal lymph nodes is difficult because no single radiologic test can adequately differentiate metastatic from infectious lymphadenopathy. Lymphangiography is limited because of the variability of the radiographic appearance of inguinal nodes, whereas CT scanning is not sensitive enough to locate subclinical disease (Johnson & Lo, 1987).

Currently, three techniques less invasive than complete inguinal lymphadenectomy are used to identify nodal metastasis due to cancer of the penis. The first is percutaneous fine-needle aspiration cytology of the sentinel lymph node and several regional lymph nodes. This approach requires that fluoroscopy or CT scanning be used to guide sampling of selected lymph nodes. It is a technically difficult procedure, except when nodes are grossly enlarged and readily identifiable, with an estimated false-negative rate of 20% (Schellhammer et al., 1992). The second technique is excisional biopsy of the sentinel lymph node and two or three surrounding nodes. Although histologic examination of the sentinel lymph node was thought to be a reliable indicator of the presence of metastatic disease, many are now questioning the accuracy of this approach based on evidence that the false-negative rate may be as high as 50% (McDougal et al., 1986). The third technique for evaluating inguinal lymph nodes is superficial inguinal node dissection. This procedure is less complex, has fewer complications, and offers more reliable information than the others previously described.

Confirmed regional lymph node metastasis requires ilioinguinal lymphadenectomy. Controversy exists, however, regarding the timing and extent of prophylactic or adjunctive ilioinguinal lymph node dissection, in part because inguinal lymphadenectomy has a morbidity rate of 30% to 50% and a mortality rate of 1% to 3%. There are also several complications associated with the procedure, including chronic leg edema, flap necrosis, seroma, scrotal edema, wound infection, lymphocele, thrombophlebitis, and postoperative bleeding (Johnson & Lo, 1987). Nonetheless, bilateral ilioinguinal lymphadenectomy is generally recommended if one or more of the following conditions is present:

1. Lymphadenopathy persisting longer than 4 weeks after penectomy and adequate antimicrobial therapy
2. Pathologic confirmation of nodal metastases
3. Development of adenopathy in a patient with a history of penile cancer who has no actual inflammatory or infective process
4. Presentation with extensive lesions at the base of the penis
5. Any lesion involving the corpora cavernosa (Crawford & Dawkins, 1988)

Treatment of penile cancer with radiotherapy has advantages and disadvantages. The major advantage is that the structure and function of the penis are spared. Disadvantages cited include the risk of tumor recurrence or failure of the treatment necessitating salvage penectomy, as well as complications such as tissue necrosis and urethral stricture. A greater concern is that radiotherapy delays assessment of and possible intervention for regional lymph nodes involved with disease (Johnson & Lo, 1987).

Radiation therapy is usually reserved for young patients with noninvasive cancers that have low metastatic potential. It is most effective when circumcision precedes treatment and when limited to tumors smaller than 4 cm in diameter that do not invade the corpora cavernosa (Gerbaulet & Lambin, 1992). Interstitial brachytherapy is considered the best means of achieving local control of penile cancer. Wires containing $^{192}$Ir are introduced into several nonradioactive needles that have been surgically implanted in parallel fashion, perpendicular to the penis, and directly into the lesion (Gerbaulet & Lambin, 1992). Delivery of the radiation dosage is often completed in 5 to 7 days. When interstitial brachytherapy is not possible, external beam radiotherapy may be employed as a primary treatment. However, this technique is more likely to be used as a treatment for postoperative tumor recurrence or palliation of symptoms caused by extension of the tumor (Gerbaulet & Lambin, 1992).

The rarity of cancer of the penis has made it impossible to conduct multicenter trials that can adequately evaluate the role of chemotherapy in the treatment of the disease. Medical literature has sporadic reports of responses from four drugs: bleomycin, methotrexate, cisplatin, and 5-fluorouracil. In clinical trials, each has been shown to be individually effective against squamous cell carcinomas of various primary sites. Studies conducted to determine the efficacy of these drugs against penile squamous cell carcinoma have concluded that these tumors are responsive to chemotherapy. However, combination drug regimens are likely to be more successful than treatment with a single agent (Eisenberger, 1992). The role of chemotherapy in treating cancer of the penis will neither be fully appreciated nor share the success of surgery as an established treatment modality until multicenter, prospective, and randomized trials can prove its usefulness.

## APPROACHES TO PATIENT CARE

### Assessment

A thorough assessment of the patient with cancer of the penis is a key responsibility of the nurse. Begin every assessment with questions specifically related to the history of the disease process. Inquire about the following:

Age: How old is the patient?

Ethnicity: Was the patient born outside the United States?

Family history: Has the patient's wife or partner had problems with cervical dysplasia? Has she ever been treated for cervical cancer?

Circumcision: Has the patient been circumcised? If so, at what age?

Hygiene: How often does the patient bathe? Does routine bathing include thorough cleansing of the penis? Is the foreskin retracted and the glans cleansed?

Symptoms: Does the patient experience any itching or burning anywhere on the penis? If so, for how long? Can the patient retract the foreskin of his penis? Does he experience any pain when he tries to retract the foreskin? Once the foreskin is retracted, can the patient return it to its normal position? Is this a painful process? Is there a foul smell from the penis? Has the patient noticed any irritation, inflammation, or ulcerations of the penis? (If so, for how long?) Is there a discharge from the penis, or from an ulcer on the penis? Any bleeding? Has the patient noticed any swelling in his groin? If so, which side? Is it a painful swelling? How long has the patient experienced discomfort?

Self-examination: Does the patient routinely practice penile self-examination? Can he describe the procedure he uses to inspect the penis? How long has the patient be performing penile self-examination, and when was the current problem first discovered?

Physical examination is a valuable means of collecting data about the patient's present health problem. Complete a thorough physical examination, focusing on signs that are indicative of metastatic disease.

Chest: Auscultate lungs for signs of decreased breath sounds.

Back: Palpate vertebrae for tenderness and pain.

Abdomen: Palpate for abdominal tenderness or masses; palpate for hepatomegaly.

Pelvis: Inspect the penis for wartlike or ulcerative lesions. Retract the foreskin to thoroughly examine the glans, then return it to its normal position; determine the location and size of each lesion, as well as the presence of any superimposed infection—lesions that appear infected should be cultured at this time; palpate the penis and scrotum to ascertain tumor boundaries; inspect and palpate for inguinal lymphadenopathy.

Legs: Inspect the legs for edema.

Additionally, verify the results of laboratory tests such as syphilis serology, HIV testing, skin tests, cultures, and tissue stains. Review the findings of chest and pelvic radiographs, as well as liver and bone scans. Correlate the results of these diagnostic tests with information collected during the history and physical examination to formulate an overall impression of the patient's health status.

As part of the nursing assessment, determine the patient's aptitude to comprehend information pertaining to the diagnosis and treatment of cancer of the penis. Assess his ability to cope with body image changes that are the inevitable result of partial or total surgical amputation of the penis. Also, consider the ability of his wife or partner to cope with the diagnosis and planned treatment. Identify sources of support, including family, friends, support groups, and marriage or sexual counselors to whom each may turn during the treatment and recovery period.

### Nursing Diagnosis

Nursing diagnoses for the patient with cancer of the penis may include the following:

1. Knowledge deficit related to
   a. Causes and course of penile cancer.
   b. Treatment alternatives for penile cancer, including surgery, radiation therapy, and chemotherapy.
2. Fear related to
   a. Diagnosis of penile cancer and the perceived threat of death.
   b. Effect of treatments on ability to empty bladder and engage in sexual intercourse.
3. Altered health maintenance related to a lack of information about the need and procedure for regular cleansing of the penis.
4. Infection, high risk for, related to

a. Inadequate personal hygiene.
b. Tendency of malignant penile lesions to harbor bacteria.
5. Pain related to
a. Effects of circumcision.
b. Effects of partial or total penectomy.
c. Effects of laser destruction of malignant penile lesions.
d. Inguinal lymphadenectomy.
e. Metastatic disease.
6. Altered pattern of urinary elimination related to total penectomy and formation of perineal urethrostomy.
7. Impaired tissue integrity related to
a. Bacterial infection of malignant penile lesion.
b. Surgical excision or laser destruction of malignant lesion.
c. Effects of radiation therapy to penile lesion.
8. Body image disturbance related to disfigurement caused by treatments, including partial or total amputation of the penis and radiation therapy.
9. Altered sexuality patterns related to structural changes in the penis due to partial or total penectomy or radiation therapy.
10. Ineffective individual or family coping related to understanding and acceptance of disease, treatments, and physical alterations resulting from treatments.
11. Health-seeking behavior: technique for penile self-examination, related to the lack of knowledge of need to practice regular screening.
12. Health-seeking behavior: technique for penile hygiene, related to the lack of knowledge of complete personal hygiene.

**Plan of Care**

Nursing care is directed toward enabling the patient to

1. Increase his knowledge of the causes of penile cancer, prognosis for the disease, diagnostic procedures, and treatment goals and alternatives.
2. Express a lessening sense of fear regarding the diagnosis of cancer of the penis.
3. State the importance of and practice good bathing and hygiene techniques.
4. Recognize and report signs and symptoms of infection.
5. Obtain relief from pain.
6. Adapt to changes in normal pattern of urination as a result of the creation of a perineal urethrostomy.
7. Employ measures to promote tissue heal-

ing and minimize infection or other adverse reactions.
8. Verbalize a positive perception of himself and his physical appearance following treatments for cancer of the penis.
9. Verbalize concerns regarding sexual functioning and alternatives for sexual satisfaction.
10. Perform monthly penile self-examination.

**Interventions**

The diagnosis of cancer of the penis is devastating news for any man. It can create an immense sense of loss and have a profound impact on the male patient's perception of his self-image and his anticipated quality of life after treatment. For his partner, the diagnosis of cancer of the penis may evoke feelings of pain and sadness as she realizes that the couple's sexual relationship will be compromised because of the physical difficulty or inability to participate in sexual intercourse. Feelings such as these are common and might be compared with the intense emotions felt by the breast cancer patient and her partner. For the nurse caring for a patient with cancer of the penis, it is important to remember that emotions run high during the diagnosis and treatment period. Therefore, encourage the patient and his partner to express their fears and concerns to health care providers as well as to each other. Provide factual and straightforward information as you explain the disease process, treatments, and care needs following therapy. Emphasize to them that it is important to ask questions if they do not understand what is being taught. Encourage each to seek support from sources such as social workers, marriage or sexual counselors, or support groups to help them accept and adapt to changes in the patient's physical appearance and sexual functioning (Smith & Babaian, 1992).

All patients should be instructed about the importance of good perineal hygiene, regardless of the therapy selected for treating their cancerous penile lesion. Daily cleansing of the glans and shaft of the penis, as well as the entire perineum, is essential to prevent infection and promote tissue healing. Patients are advised to use a mild soap, warm water, and a soft cloth for bathing. When cleansing the penis, the entire surface should be washed; the foreskin, if present, should be retracted to cleanse the glans and remove any residue trapped beneath it (Flannery, 1992). Be sure that the patient understands to return the foreskin to its normal protracted position after cleansing. For those who have undergone par-

## PROCEDURE 10-3

■

## Technique for Penile Self-Examination

1. Perform penile self-examination monthly while bathing or in the shower.
2. Visually examine the entire length of the shaft, looking for any rashes, white patches (leukoplakia), growths, or ulcers.
3. Palpate the penile shaft by using two fingers to slowly move over the entire surface of the shaft, feeling for any lumps or abnormalities.
4. Completely retract the foreskin (if present).
5. Thoroughly examine the glans visually, checking for rashes, white patches, growths, or ulcers.
6. Palpate the glans by slowly moving a fingertip over the entire surface, feeling for lumps or abnormalities.
7. Return the foreskin to its normal protracted position.

---

tial or total penectomy, good perineal hygiene is especially important and should be stressed when providing discharge teaching and home care instructions.

A teaching session about bathing and hygiene should also include instruction on the technique for penile self-examination (Procedure 10–3). This uncomplicated procedure may be performed in less than 5 minutes and enables men to recognize the signs of a cancerous or precancerous lesion (Table 10–10). Because studies indicate that men have a tendency to delay treatment for as long as 1 year after the discovery of a suspicious lesion or growth on the penis, it is also important that they be taught to seek immediate medical advice for any abnormalities detected during penile self-examination.

Instructions concerning antibiotic therapy are important because almost 50% of patients with cancer of the penis also have a superimposed infection of the lesion that requires treatment. Antibiotic therapy may be prescribed for as long as 4 to 6 weeks. Therefore, stress to the patient that antibiotics must be taken until the prescribed amount is finished. In addition to providing information about the drug itself and any possible side effects, make certain that the patient is familiar with the signs and symptoms of an infection.

Postoperative nursing care activities for men who have had partial or total penectomy are essentially the same as for any other urologic surgical procedure, with a few exceptions. The patient who has undergone a partial penectomy returns from surgery with an indwelling urethral catheter connected to a straight-drainage system, one or more surgical drains, and a dressing covering the penis; these are usually removed within 4 or 5 days after surgery. Although the patient should be able to void in the standing position without too much difficulty, it is important that the nurse watch his first few attempts at urination after catheter removal to verify his ability to empty his bladder and direct his stream. Any discomfort or difficulties should be reported to the urologist prior to discharge.

The patient who has had a total penectomy returns from surgery with an indwelling catheter that has been inserted through the newly created perineal urethrostomy. The catheter is connected to a straight-drainage system until it is removed, usually within 4 or 5 days after surgery. A dressing covers the perineum at the site where the penis was amputated; surgical drains may also have been placed. With a physician's order, sitz baths may be used to relieve

**TABLE 10–10. Precancerous Lesions of the Penis**

| TYPE | APPEARANCE |
| --- | --- |
| Leukoplakia | Patches of white plaques |
| Erythroplasia | Distinct, velvety-red plaques |
| Bowen's disease | Ulcerating, crusting plaques |
| Balanitis xerotica obliterans | Thin, scaly epidermis |
| Buschke-Loewenstein tumor | Large, exophytic lesion |
| Bowenoid papulosis | Erythematous papules |

discomfort of the perineal urethrostomy and promote tissue healing. Prior to discharge, the surgical drains and catheter will be removed. Remind the patient that he will now have to urinate while *sitting* on the toilet. Again, it is a good idea for the nurse to observe the patient's first few attempts at urination; he may need to be cued when his urinary stream has stopped because of the initial inability to feel urine escaping from the perineal urethrostomy. Leakage from the perineal urethrostomy may also be a problem for a few weeks following surgery. To contain urine leakage until control of the perineal urethrostomy is attained, the nurse may want to suggest the temporary use of protective undergarments. Remember that the patient requires lots of support to accept his new pattern of urination. Encourage him to allow himself the time to heal and to adapt to his urinary diversion. A referral to a professional counselor may be needed to help him through this difficult period of adjustment.

**Patient Outcomes**

1. The patient can verbalize an understanding of cancer of the penis and its causes and treatment options.
2. The patient states that fear is reduced or alleviated as a result of health teaching or referrals to outside sources of support.
3. The patient demonstrates improved self-care practices such as personal hygiene.
4. The patient verbalizes (1) the importance of completing antibiotic therapy; (2) an understanding of the signs and symptoms of infection; and (3) an awareness of the need to seek health care if infected lesions do not respond to antibiotic therapy or if infection recurs.
5. The patient states relief of pain or discomfort.
6. The patient resumes a normal voiding pattern following partial penectomy, *or* the patient adapts to changes in his pattern of urination necessitated by the creation of a perineal urethrostomy following total penectomy.
7. The patient's surgical wounds exhibit signs of normal healing.
8. The patient demonstrates self-respect, self-confidence, and self-worth in interactions with his partner and others.
9. The patient describes the procedure and performs routine penile self-examination.
10. The patient states that he and his partner are experiencing sexual satisfaction through new or different methods of expression.

# CANCER OF THE SCROTUM

## PERSPECTIVE ON DISEASE ENTITY

**Etiology.** Primary cancer of the scrotum is rare. Historically, it was found to be caused by soot in the clothing of chimney sweeps and thus became the first known environmentally related cancer. The disease is often referred to as *chimney-sweep's cancer* or *Pott's cancer*, named after the Englishman who first described it in 1775 (Livne & Pontes, 1986; Lowe, 1992).

Over the last two centuries, occupational exposure to many carcinogens has been associated with cancer of the scrotum (Table 10–11). Today, however, the primary risk factors for scrotal cancer are not environmental but poor hygienic and chronic inflammatory conditions (Johnson & Lo, 1987; Livne & Pontes, 1986). Psoriasis has been recently linked to the development of scrotal cancer. The chronic irritation and inflammatory changes of the skin caused by the disease, coupled with abrasive treatments for psoriasis, such as the use of compounds containing arsenic or ultraviolet A radiation, significantly increase the risk of scrotal cancer (Love, 1992; Ray & Whitmore, 1977). Studies are also being conducted to determine the relationship between human papillomavirus and scrotal cancer.

Scrotal cancer is a disease that is seen in men older than 35 years of age; however, it primarily manifests in men 50 to 70 years old. In 1976, the incidence of scrotal cancer in the United States was estimated to be approximately 10 cases per year. In the United Kingdom, where the disease is most prevalent, the incidence is 20 times that of the United States. Men in higher economic classes, professional white collar workers, and those dwelling in rural areas are less likely to develop scrotal cancer. Race may also be a factor because the disease is reported to occur more frequently in white than in black men (Lowe, 1992).

**Pathophysiology.** Scrotal cancers are predominantly squamous cell carcinomas, although adenocarcinoma (Paget's disease) and basal cell carcinoma can occur. Isolated cases

**TABLE 10–11. Carcinogens Associated with Cancer of the Scrotum**

| | |
|---|---|
| Coal tar | Grease |
| Pitch | Solvents |
| Mineral oils | Wood oil |
| Petroleum | Paraffin |
| Shale | |

of melanoma, lymphoma, and sarcoma have also been reported in the literature (Johnson & Lo, 1987; Livne & Pontes, 1986).

Although cancer of the scrotum can occur anywhere on the scrotal surface, most lesions are found on the anterolateral aspects of the scrotum. McDonald (1982) noted a predominance for the left side of the scrotum.

Scrotal cancers begin as a solitary lump, nodule, pimple, or sore that may be associated with pruritus. Initially, they are painless, but pain does occur late in the disease. Ulceration with an associated discharge may occur after 6 months, and because scrotal cancers are slow growing, superimposed infections are frequently encountered.

Tumors tend to remain localized and unfixed to the scrotal contents, although direct extension into the scrotal sac and penis may be seen. Invasion into the perineum with extravasation of urine has also been reported (McDonald, 1982).

As many as 50% of all patients who present with palpable inguinal lymphadenopathy have metastatic disease in the nodes. Inguinal metastases tend to occur on the same side as the primary tumor, with spread to the contralateral side, deep inguinal nodes, iliac nodes, and lung occurring in advanced disease.

Staging of scrotal cancer is based on a system first proposed in 1977 by Ray and Whitmore. Modifications to this classification have since been made (Lowe, 1992) (Table 10–12).

The stage of the disease at the time of diagnosis is the most significant factor affecting survival. Most patients are aware of a lesion anywhere from 2 to 12 months before seeking medical advice. During this interim period, they are using conventional home remedies such as over-the-counter ointments to treat the

**TABLE 10–12. Staging System for Scrotal Carcinoma**

| STAGE | DESCRIPTION |
| --- | --- |
| A1 | Localized to scrotal wall |
| A2 | Locally extensive tumor invading adjacent structures (testis, spermatic cord, penis, pubis, perineum) |
| B | Metastatic disease involving inguinal lymph nodes only |
| C | Metastatic disease involving pelvic lymph nodes without evidence of distant spread |
| D | Metastatic disease beyond the pelvic lymph nodes involving distant organs |

From Lowe, F. C. (1992). Squamous cell carcinoma of the scrotum. *Urologic Clinics of North America, 19*(2), 404. Reprinted by permission.

lesion (Lowe, 1992). As with other types of genitourinary cancers, the likelihood of 5-year survival is best when treatment is begun in the earlier stages of the disease. Patients with stage A scrotal cancer have an estimated survival rate of 70%, whereas only 44% of those with stage B disease may survive. The survival rate is very poor for patients presenting with stage C or D scrotal tumors (Lowe, 1992; Ray & Whitmore, 1977).

**Medical-Surgical Management.** Medical evaluation of the patient with a scrotal mass requires that the physician first complete a thorough history and physical examination. Diagnostic studies employed to confirm the diagnosis of scrotal cancer, as well as determine the extent of disease, are performed after the initiation of a broad-spectrum antibiotic and include excisional biopsy of the lesion; sentinel node biopsy and lymphography or CT scanning, if regional nodes are suspicious; and chest radiographs to rule out lung metastasis.

Surgery is the treatment of choice for scrotal cancers. Many agree that a wide local excision of the lesion, with a 2- to 3-cm margin of both skin and subcutaneous tissue, is required for curative treatment. In most instances, this approach enables the urologist to easily approximate scrotal wall tissue for primary closure of the area excised (Johnson & Lo, 1987; Livne & Pontes, 1986; Lowe, 1992). Sometimes a portion of the penile skin may need to be removed if the tumor involves the penile shaft at the penoscrotal junction (Johnson & Lo, 1987). A local recurrence rate of 20% 1 to 10 years after the initial surgery has been reported (Ray & Whitmore, 1977).

The management of regional lymph node metastasis is similar to that of penile cancer. Generally, biopsy of the ipsilateral sentinel lymph node is recommended for any patient with suspected groin disease due to scrotal carcinoma. If the biopsied node shows metastasis, unilateral ilioinguinal lymphadenectomy is performed; a bilateral dissection is done only when inguinal metastasis is validated by biopsy in both groins and there is no pelvic lymph node involvement. Patients with scrotal cancer found to have nodal disease beyond the inguinal region have a poor prognosis and therefore are usually not candidates for lymphadenectomy (Johnson & Lo, 1987; Livne & Pontes, 1986; Lowe, 1992).

Neither radiation therapy nor chemotherapy has been shown to be effective primary treatments for scrotal cancer. Currently, these treatment approaches are reserved for patients requiring palliative therapy because of tumor recurrence after surgical excision, or those not candidates for surgery because of advanced disease. Of the two treatment modalities, chemotherapy may someday be a viable alternative to surgical resection of the scrotum; in part, this is because of the reported response of squamous cell carcinomas to drugs such as bleomycin, cisplatin, methotrexate, cyclophosphamide, vincristine, and 5-fluorouracil. However, as in the case of penile cancer, prospective trials are needed to identify agents and regimens that will increase survival for men with disseminated scrotal cancers.

## APPROACHES TO PATIENT CARE

### Assessment

Nursing assessment of the patient with suspected cancer of the scrotum begins with a thorough medical history specifically related to the disease process. During the interview, solicit answers to these questions:

Occupation: How is the patient employed? Does he work in an environment where he may be exposed to industrial carcinogens?

Lifestyle: Does the patient live in an urban or rural area?

Hygiene: How often does the patient bathe? Does routine bathing include a thorough cleansing of the scrotum?

Dermatologic history: Does the patient have scrotal eczema? psoriasis? chronic superficial fungal infections? cutaneous nevi? sebaceous cysts? How have these conditions been treated?

Symptoms: Does the patient have a "sore" on the scrotum? What does it look like? Is there any drainage from the lesion? Does the lesion ever bleed? Does he experience chronic itching of the scrotum? Is there a foul smell from the scrotum? Is there any pain associated with a red, itchy lesion? What methods has he used to treat the scrotal lesion? Has the patient noticed any swelling in his groin? (If so, which side? For how long?) Is it a painful swelling?

Self-examination: Does the patient routinely perform a monthly self-examination? How was the lesion first discovered? How long has he known about the scrotal lesion?

Complete your initial assessment with a physical examination. With the patient lying on an examination table, inspect and palpate the scrotum. Begin with a visual inspection of the entire scrotum, noting any masses, lesions, rashes, or ulcerations. Next, use light palpation to determine the borders of the lesion or mass. Use deep palpation to detect fixation to internal structures. Drainage from an open lesion should be cultured. Visually inspect the groin, looking for obvious lymphadenopathy. Proceed to light, then deep palpation of lymph nodes in the inguinal area. Note any firm, hard, tender, ulcerated, or fixed lesions. Throughout the physical examination, observe the patient for manifestations of discomfort.

During the nursing assessment, also try to discern the patient's understanding of his illness. Did he anticipate being told that the scrotal lesion was cancerous? What were his expectations regarding treatment alternatives for the lesion? What does he know about scrotal cancer and his chances for survival if treatment is delayed? Does he understand what risk factors may have predisposed him to this disease? What are his fears and concerns regarding the diagnosis and treatment of scrotal cancer?

### Nursing Diagnosis

The nursing diagnoses for the patient with cancer of the scrotum may include the following:

1. Knowledge deficit related to
   a. Causes and course of scrotal cancer.
   b. Diagnostic procedures used to confirm scrotal cancer.
   c. Treatment approach for scrotal cancer.
2. Fear related to
   a. Diagnosis of scrotal cancer and perceived threat of death.
   b. Effects of surgery on quality of life and life expectancy.
3. Pain related to
   a. Irritation or infection of the scrotal lesion.
   b. Surgical excision of malignant scrotal lesion.
   c. Lymphadenopathy due to scrotal cancer.
4. Infection, high risk for, related to
   a. Tendency of scrotal of lesions to harbor bacteria.
   b. Contamination of the surgical wound due to inadequate personal hygiene.
5. Altered health maintenance related to inadequate personal hygiene.

### Plan of Care

Nursing care is directed toward enabling the patient to

1. Increase his knowledge of the cause, prognosis, and treatment approach for scrotal cancer.
2. Relate increased feelings of psychological

comfort after receiving information about scrotal cancer.

3. Experience relief of the pain and discomfort associated with surgery or metastatic disease.
4. Recognize the relationship between good hygiene and the prevention of infection.
5. Recognize and report the signs and symptoms of an infected scrotal lesion.
6. Employ techniques for good personal hygiene with regular bathing.

### Interventions

Nursing interventions specific for the patient diagnosed with cancer of the scrotum are similar to those described for the patient with penile cancer. Patient teaching about the likely cause of scrotal cancer, as well as the disease course, should be among the nurse's first priorities. It is often helpful to provide the patient with pamphlets from the National Cancer Institute and ACS to help reinforce this general information.

Encourage the patient to ask questions so that you may dispel any misconceptions he has about scrotal cancer. This should help to alleviate some of his fears and concerns about the disease prior to treatment.

Preoperatively, the nurse should explain the procedure and postoperative care activities for surgical excision of the scrotal lesion. This is also a good time to reinforce treatment goals outlined by the physician. Postoperatively, the nurse will need to care for the patient's scrotal dressing and any surgical drains that may have been inserted. Also, administer antibiotics as prescribed, and pain medication as needed. To prevent excess scrotal swelling, elevate the scrotum on a small rolled towel while the patient is in bed; when the patient ambulates, he should be encouraged to use a scrotal support. As with any postoperative urologic patient, ascertain that there are no difficulties with urination, monitor intake and output, and be alert for signs of infection.

Before discharge, instruct the patient about the importance of cleanliness, regular bathing, and careful washing of the perineum, including the penis and the scrotum. Teach the patient about care of the surgical wound and the technique for dressing change, if one is to be retained over the surgical site. Explain the importance of antibiotic therapy, and stress that the entire amount of medication must be taken for the length of time prescribed. Identify the signs and symptoms of infection, and instruct the patient to notify the physician at once if any of these occur. In addition, advise the pa-

tient to contact the physician if swelling or pain develops in the groin area. Finally, encourage the patient to keep appointments for follow-up visits with the physician.

### Patient Outcomes

1. The patient verbalizes an understanding of cancer of the scrotum and its causes and treatment.
2. The patient expresses feelings of increased psychological comfort after receiving information about scrotal cancer.
3. The patient indicates relief of postoperative and metastatic pain and discomfort after analgesics are administered or other pain management techniques are implemented.
4. The patient expresses an understanding of the rationale for continued antibiotic therapy, even when symptoms of infection are not apparent.
5. The patient describes the signs and symptoms of infection and is aware of the need to seek health care if any of those signs and symptoms develop.
6. The patient acknowledges the relationship between good hygiene and prevention of infection.
7. The patient demonstrates a willingness to improve personal hygiene practices by complying with the recommendation for regular bathing and perineal cleansing.

## REFERENCES

Agency for Health Care Policy and Research. (1992). *Quick reference guide for clinicians—acute pain management in adults: Operative procedures* (DHHS Publication No. AHCPR 92-0019). Rockville, MD: U.S. Department of Health and Human Services.

American Cancer Society. (1993). *Cancer facts & figures— 1993* (Publication No. 5008-93). Atlanta: Author.

American Joint Committee on Cancer. (1992). *Manual for staging of cancer* (4th ed.). Philadelphia: J. B. Lippincott.

Berthelsen, J. G., Skakkebaek, N. E., Sorensen, B. C., Mogensen, P. (1982). Screening for carcinoma in situ of the contralateral testis in patients with germinal testicular cancer. *British Journal of Medicine, 285,* 1683.

Black, B. (1986). Penile cancer. *Uro-Gram, 14*(4), 5.

Boden, G., Gibb, R. (1951). Radiotherapy and testicular neoplasms. *Lancet, 2,* 1195–1197.

Brandt, B. (1991). Informational needs and selected variables in patients receiving brachytherapy. *Oncology Nursing Forum, 18*(7), 1221–1227.

Burgers, J. K., Badalament, R. A., Drago, J. R. (1992). Penile cancer: Clinical presentation, diagnosis, and staging. *Urologic Clinics of North America, 19*(2), 247–256.

Burnett, A. L., Chan, D. W., Brendler, C. B., & Walsh, P. C. (1992). The value of serum enzymatic acid phosphatase in the staging of localized prostate cancer. *Journal of Urology, 148,* 1832–1834.

Carter, H. B. (1992). Evaluation of the urologic patient. In P. C. Walsh, A. B. Retik, T. A. Stamey, & E. D. Vaughan

(Eds.), *Campbell's Urology* (6th ed., pp. 307–341). Philadelphia: W. B. Saunders.

Clayman, R. V. (1991). Laparoscopy: New yet familiar [Symposium]. *Contemporary Urology, 3*(10), 34–50.

Cosgrove, M. D., Benton, B., Henderson, B. E. (1977). Male genitourinary abnormalities and maternal diethylstilbestrol. *Journal of Urology, 117*, 220–222.

Crawford, E. D., Dawkins, C. A. (1988). Cancer of the penis. In D. G. Skinner & G. Lieskovsky (Eds.), *Diagnosis and management of genitourinary cancer* (pp. 549–563). Philadelphia: W. B. Saunders.

Depue, R. H., Pike, M. C., Henderson, B. E. (1983). Estrogen exposure during gestation and risk of testicular cancer. *Journal of the National Cancer Institute, 71*, 1151–1155.

Dyck, S. (1991). Surgical instrumentation as a palliative treatment for spinal cord compression. *Oncology Nursing Forum, 18*(3), 515–521.

Eisenberger, M. A. (1992). Chemotherapy for carcinomas of the penis and urethra. *Urologic Clinics of North America, 19*(2), 333–338.

Fallon, B., Williams, R. D. (1990). Current options in the management of clinical stage C prostatic carcinoma. *Urologic Clinics of North America, 17*(4), 853.

Findlay, P. A., Glatstein, E. (1986). Principles of radiation therapy. In S. D. Graham, Jr. (Ed.), *Urologic oncology* (pp. 183–203). New York: Raven Press.

Flannery, M. (1992). Reproductive cancers. In J. C. Clark & R. F. McGee (Eds.), *Core Curriculum for oncology nursing* (2nd ed., pp. 451–469), Philadelphia: W. B. Saunders.

Friman, P. C., and Finney, J. W. (1990). Health education for testicular cancer. *Health Education Quarterly, 17*(4), 443–453.

Gerbaulet, A., and Lambin, P. (1992). Radiation therapy of cancer of the penis. *Urologic Clinics of North America, 19*(2), 325–332.

Giovannucci, E., Ascherio, A., Rimm, B., Colditz, G. A., Stampher, M. J., Willett, W. C. (1993). A prospective cohort study of vasectomy and prostate cancer in US men. *JAMA, 269*(7), 873–877.

Grabstald, H. (1980). Controversies concerning lymph node dissection for cancer of the penis. *Urologic Clinics of North America, 7*, 793–799.

Graham, S., Gibson, R. (1972). Social epidemiology of cancer of the testis. *Cancer, 29*, 1324.

Greenburg, S., Petersen, J., Hansen-Peters, I., Baylinson, W. (1990). Interstitially implanted $I^{125}$ for prostate cancer using transrectal ultrasound. *Oncology Nursing Forum, 17*(6), 849–854.

Held, J. L., & Peahota, A. (1993). Nursing care of the patient with spinal cord compression. *Oncology Nursing Forum, 20*(10), 1507–1514.

Henderson B. E., Ross, R. K., Pike, M. C. (1988). Epidemiology of testicular cancer. In D. G. Skinner & G. Lieskovsky (Eds.), *Diagnosis and management of genitourinary cancer* (pp. 46–52). Philadelphia: W. B. Saunders.

Hernandez, A. D., Smith, J. A. (1990). Transrectal ultrasonography for early detection and staging of prostate cancer. *Urologic Clinics of North America, 17*(4), 745.

Jackson, S. M. (1966). The treatment of carcinoma of the penis. *British Journal of Surgery, 53*, 33–35.

Jenkins, J. (1988). Testicular cancer. In S. B. Baird (Ed.), *Decision making in oncology nursing* (pp. 18–19). Toronto: B. C. Decker.

Johnson, D. E., Lo, R. K. (1987). Tumors of the penis, urethra, and scrotum. In J. B. de Kernion & D. F. Paulson (Eds.), *Genitourinary cancer management* (pp. 219–258). Philadelphia: Lea & Febiger.

Kaut, K. J. (1992). Assessment and management of patients with vascular disorders and problems of peripheral circulation. In S. C. Smeltzer & B. G. Bare (Eds.), *Brunner*

*and Suddarth's medical surgical nursing* (7th ed., pp. 737–779). Philadelphia: J. B. Lippincott.

Kini, M. G. (1944). Cancer of the penis in a child, aged 2 years. *Indian Medical Gazette, 79*, 66–68.

Li, J. Y., Li, F. P., Blot, W. J., Miller, R. W., Fraumeni, J. F., Jr. (1982). Correlation between cancers of the uterine cervix and penis in China. *Journal of the National Cancer Institute, 69*, 1063–1065.

Li, J. Y., Li, F. P., Blot, W. J., Miller, R. W., Fraumeni, J. F., Jr. (1983). Correlation between cancers of the uterine cervix and penis. *Journal of the National Cancer Institute, 71*, 427–428.

Lind, J. (1992). Genitourinary cancers. In J. C. Clark & R. F. McGee (Eds.), *Core curriculum for oncology nursing* (2nd ed., pp. 428–450). Philadelphia: W. B. Saunders.

Lind, J., & Nakao, S. L. (1990). Urologic and male genital cancers. In S. L. Groenwald, M. H. Frogge, M. Goodman, & C. Henke Yarbro (Eds.), *Cancer nursing: Principles and practice* (2nd ed., pp. 1026–1073). Boston: Jones and Bartlett.

Littrup, P. J., Goodman, A. C., & Mettlin, C. J. (1993). The benefit and cost of prostate cancer early detection. *CA, 43*(3), 134–149.

Livne, P. M., Pontes, J. E. (1986). Tumors of the penis, scrotum, and spermatic cord. In S. D. Graham, Jr. (Ed.), *Urologic oncology* (pp. 369–382). New York: Raven Press.

Lowe, F. C. (1992). Squamous cell carcinoma of the scrotum. *Urologic Clinics of North America, 19*(2), 397–405.

Mahon, S. M., Casperson, D., Wozniak-Petrofsky, J. (1990). Prostate cancer: Screening through treatment and nursing implications. *Urologic Nursing, 10*(2), 5–11.

McDonald, M. W. (1982). Carcinoma of the scrotum. *Urology, 19*, 268–274.

McDougal, W. S., Kirchner, F. K., Jr., Edwards, R. H., Killion, L. T. (1986). Treatment of carcinoma of the penis: The case of primary lymphadenectomy. *Journal of Urology, 136*, 38.

Meikle, A. W., Smith, J. A. (1990). Epidemiology of prostate cancer. *Urologic Clinics of North America, 17*(4), 709.

Mettlin, C., Jones, G. W., & Murphy, G. P. (1993). Trends in prostate cancer care in the United States, 1974–1990: Observations from the patient care evaluation studies of the American College of Surgeons Commission on Cancer. *CA, 43*(2), 83–91.

Morse, M. J., Whitmore, W. F. (1986). Neoplasms of the testis. In P. C. Walsh, R. F. Gittes, A. D. Perlmutter, T. A. Stamey (Eds.), *Campbell's urology* (5th ed., pp. 1535–1582). Philadelphia: W. B. Saunders.

Müller, K. (1962). *Cancer testis* [Thesis]. Copenhagen, Munksgaard.

Narayan, P. (1992). Neoplasms of the prostate gland. In E. A. Tanagho & J. W. McAninch (Eds.), *Smith's general urology* (13th ed., pp. 378–412). Norwalk, CT: Appleton & Lange.

National Cancer Institute. (1990). *Cancer of the prostate: Research report* (NIH Publication No. 91-528). Bethesda, MD: National Cancer Institute.

Nichols, P. (1988). Pathology of cancer of the penis. In D. G. Skinner & G. Lieskovsky (Eds.), *Diagnosis and management of genitourinary cancer* (pp. 207–214). Philadelphia: W. B. Saunders.

Nienhuis, H., Goldacre, M., Seagroatt, V., Gill, L., Vessey, M. (1992). Incidence of disease after vasectomy: A record linkage retrospective cohort study. *British Medical Journal, 304*(6829), 743–746.

Optenberg, S. A., Thompson, I. M. (1990). Economics of screening for carcinoma of the prostate. *Urologic Clinics of North America, 17*(4), 719.

Ostchega, Y., Culnane, M. (1985). Tumor markers. *Nursing 85, 15*, 48–51.

Pagana, K. D., Pagana, T. J. (1990). *Diagnostic testing and nursing implications.* St. Louis: C. V. Mosby.

Paulson, D. F. (1987). Management of prostatic malignancy. In J. B. de Kernion & D. F. Paulson (Eds.), *Genitourinary cancer management.* Philadelphia: Lea & Febiger.

Persky, L. (1977). Epidemiology of cancer of the penis—recent results. *Cancer Research, 60,* 97–109.

Persky, L., de Kernion, J. (1986). Carcinoma of the penis. *CA, 36*(5), 258–273.

Piemme, J. A. (1988). Prostate cancer. In S. B. Baird (Ed.), *Decision making in oncology nursing* (pp. 16–17). Toronto: B. C. Decker.

Polomano, R. C. (1991). Quality of life issues with metastatic prostate cancer. *Innovations in Urology Nursing, 2*(1), 2–4.

Presti, J. C., Herr, H. W. (1992). Genital tumors. In E. A. Tanagho & J. W. McAninch (Eds.), *Smith's general urology* (13th ed., pp. 413–425). Norwalk, CT: Appleton & Lange.

Ray, B., Whitmore, W., Jr. (1977). Experience with cancer of the scrotum. *Journal of Urology, 117,* 741–745.

Reilly, N. J. (1991). Questions about prostate surgery. *Innovations in Urology Nursing, 2*(1), 10.

Richie, J. P. (1988). Diagnosis and staging of testicular tumors. In D. G. Skinner & G. Lieskovsky (Eds.), *Diagnosis and management of genitourinary cancer* (pp. 498–507). Philadelphia: W. B. Saunders.

Richie, J. P. (1992). Neoplasms of the testis. In P. C. Walsh, A. B. Retik, T. A. Stamey, E. D. Vaughan (Eds.), *Campbell's urology* (6th ed., pp. 1222–1263). Philadelphia: W. B. Saunders.

Richie, J. P. (1993). Detection and treatment of testicular cancer. *CA, 43*(3), 151–175.

Ross, R. N., Paganini-Hill, A., Henderson, B. E. (1988). Epidemiology of prostatic cancer. In D. G. Skinner & G. Lieskovsky (Eds.), *Diagnosis and management of genitourinary cancer* (pp. 40–45). Philadelphia: W. B. Saunders.

Rothman, K. J., Lovik, C. (1978). Oral contraceptives and birth defects. *New England Journal of Medicine, 229,* 522–524.

Schellhammer, P. F., Jordan, G. H., Schlossberg, S. M. (1992). Tumors of the penis. In P. C. Walsh, A. B. Retik, T. A. Stamey, & E. D. Vaughn (Eds.), *Campbell's urology* (6th ed., pp. 1264–1298). Philadelphia: W. B. Saunders.

Sheley, J. F. (1991). Limited impact of testicular self-examination promotion. *Journal of Community Health, 16*(2), 117–124.

Skinner, D. G. (1969). Non-seminomatous testis tumors: A plan of management based on 96 patients to improve survival in all stages by combined therapeutic modalities. *Journal of Urology, 115,* 65–69.

Skinner, D. G., Lieskovsky, G. (1988). Management of early-stage nonseminomatous germ cell tumors of the testis. In D. G. Skinner & G. Lieskovsky (Eds.), *Diagnosis and management of genitourinary cancer* (pp. 516–525). Philadelphia: W. B. Saunders.

Skinner, E. C., Skinner, D. G. (1992). Surgery of testicular neoplasms. In P. C. Walsh, A. B. Retik, T. A. Stamey, & E. D. Vaughn (Eds.), *Campbell's urology* (6th ed., pp. 3090–3113)). Philadelphia: W. B. Saunders.

Smith, D. B., & Babaian, R. J. (1992). The effect of treatment for cancer on male fertility and sexuality. *Cancer Nursing 15*(4), 271–275.

Smith, R. B. (1988). Testicular seminoma. In D. G. Skinner & G. Lieskovsky (Eds.), *Diagnosis and management of genitourinary cancer* (pp. 508–515). Philadelphia: W. B. Saunders.

Stamey, T. A., McNeal, J. E. (1992). Adenocarcinoma of the prostate. In P. C. Walsh, A. B. Retik, T. A. Stamey, & E. D. Vaughan (Eds.), *Campbell's urology* (6th ed., pp. 1159–1199)). Philadelphia: W. B. Saunders.

Steinfeld, A. D. (1990). Testicular germ cell tumors: Review of contemporary evaluation and management. *Radiology, 175,* 603–606.

Taylor, T. K. (1991). Endocrine therapy for advanced stage D prostate cancer. *Urologic Nursing, 11*(3), 22–26.

University of Iowa Hospital and Clinics, Department of Nursing. (1992). *Standard care plan: Transperineal placement of radioactive gold (Au$^{198}$) seeds.* Iowa City: Author.

Waisman, P. (1988). Pathology of neoplasms of the prostate gland. In D. G. Skinner & G. Lieskovsky (Eds.), *Diagnosis and management of genitourinary cancer* (pp. 150–194). Philadelphia: W. B. Saunders.

Walsh, P. C. (1992). Radical retropubic prostatectomy. In P. C. Walsh, A. B. Retik, T. A. Stamey, & E. D. Vaughan (Eds.), *Campbell's urology* (6th ed., pp. 2865–2886). Philadelphia: W. B. Saunders.

Waxman, E. S. (1993). Sexual dysfunction following treatment for prostate cancer: Nursing assessment and interventions. *Oncology Nursing Forum, 20*(10), 1567–1571.

Wein, A. J., Hanno, P.M. (1987). Carcinoma of the genitourinary tract. In P. M. Hanno & A. J. Wein (Eds.), *A clinical manual of urology* (pp. 281–351). Norwalk, CT: Appleton-Century-Crofts.

West, R. R. (1992). Vasectomy and testicular cancer. *British Medical Journal, 304*(6829), 729.

Willson, P. (1991). Testicular, prostate and penile cancers in primary care settings: The importance of early detection. *Nurse Practitioner, 16*(11), 18–26.

# PART IV

# External Genital Disorders and Sexual Dysfunction

# CHAPTER 11

# External Genital Disorders

◼

*Patricia Bates*

**Disorders of the Penis**
> Phimosis and Paraphimosis
> Priapism
> Peyronie's Disease and Chordee

**Disorders of the Scrotum**
> Hydrocele, Inguinal Hernia, Hematocele,
> Spermatocele, and Varicocele

**Genital Skin Conditions**
> Infections, Dermatitis, Benign and
> Malignant Growths, Vascular Lesions,
> Pigmentary Disorders, Diseases Due to
> Animal Parasites, and Other Skin
> Disorders

## OVERVIEW

This chapter describes external genital disorders common to adults. Most afflictions, although a source of worry and aggravation, are not serious and can be treated by relatively simple medical or surgical means. Other conditions, however, are emergencies needing immediate attention. The nurse has to differentiate to give correct advice and care. Conditions discussed include disorders of the penis, disorders of the scrotum, and genital skin conditions. Information on cancer, infection, sexually transmitted disease involving the external genitalia, and genital disorders commonly seen in children can be found in other chapters.

Patients may seek medical attention at urology offices, but nurses often find external genital disorders when caring for patients in other settings. Sexual partners may also ask for a nurse's professional advice. It is important to convey accurate information about these diseases because fear and rumors are common. Physician follow-up for ongoing evaluation of external genital disorders should be strongly encouraged.

Psychological aspects of genital problems can be overwhelming for patients. Often patients, although worried, delay seeking treatment because they are embarrassed and hesitant to talk about their genital conditions. Counseling, teaching, and reassurance are the primary ways nurses help these patients and their families. When surgical procedures are necessary, preoperative and postoperative nursing care follow basic nursing concepts. Specific points of care are discussed throughout the chapter. As with any surgical procedure, nursing observation and documentation are extremely important.

## BEHAVIORAL OBJECTIVES

After studying this chapter, the reader should be able to

1. Describe a method for manually reducing a paraphimotic foreskin.
2. Differentiate the types of benign scrotal masses.
3. Identify the presenting signs and symptoms of testicular torsion.
4. Explain one medical and one surgical technique for treating priapism.
5. Compare and contrast treatments for inflammatory genital skin conditions.

## KEY WORDS

**Cavernous bodies**—anatomic cylinders of erectile tissue that, when filled with blood, become the rigid structures of a penile erection.

**Chordee**—curvature of the penis.

**Condylomata acuminata**—soft, warty nodules of viral origin occurring on the penis and around the anus.

**Hematocele**—a collection of blood in the cavity of the tunica vaginalis.

**Hydrocele**—an accumulation of fluid within the cavity of the tunica vaginalis.

**Inguinal hernia**—abdominal protrusion of the bowel through the inguinal canal.

**Paraphimosis**—retraction of a narrow or inflamed foreskin that cannot be replaced into its normal position.

**Peyronie's disease**—a condition characterized by the development of fibrous thickening or plaques within the fascia around the corpora.

**Phimosis**—tightening of the foreskin so that it cannot be drawn back over the glans.

**Priapism**—persistent abnormal erection of the penis, usually without sexual desire.

**Smegma**—a thick, cheesy substance consisting of secretions of the preputial sebaceous glands and desquamative cellular debris.

**Spermatocele**—cystic dilatation of a duct in the head of the epididymis or in the rete testis.

**Tinea cruris**—a fungal infection involving the skin of the groin, perineum, and perianal areas.

**Varicocele**—dilatation of the veins of the pampiniform plexus of the spermatic cord

---

## DISORDERS OF THE PENIS

### Perspective on Disease Entities

Pathologic changes can distort the appearance of the penis and cause annoying or debilitating symptoms. Common disorders of the penis are phimosis, paraphimosis, priapism, Peyronie's disease, and chordee. Genital warts, rapidly becoming a disease of serious concern, are mentioned under genital skin conditions and more thoroughly discussed in Chapter 7. The disorders have different causes. Treatments may be controversial or may not guar-

antee successful resolution. In some cases, the lack of complete cure or additional problems caused by treatment add to a patient's frustration. Each condition is discussed separately.

### PHIMOSIS AND PARAPHIMOSIS

**Etiology and Pathophysiology.** Phimosis describes a constricted foreskin that cannot be retracted over the glans penis. Although it may be a congenital abnormality of the penis, chronic subpreputial infections with consequent adhesions and fibrotic changes also lead to this disorder (Sonda & Wang, 1988). Urination is seldom impeded, but phimosis may interfere with intercourse. Movement of the foreskin may cause pain or bleeding if adhesions are torn.

Men with phimotic foreskins may find it impossible to clean this area adequately, so that the problem worsens. Smegma, a normal cottage cheese–like secretion of the sebaceous glands of the prepuce, is retained under these conditions and becomes an excellent medium in which organisms grow. Bacterial and monilial infections, as well as condylomata, can develop readily in the warm, moist environment. Posthitis (inflammation of the prepuce) or balanitis (inflammation of the glans) occurs. If phimosis is not corrected, more infection, scarring, and even tumors can result from the chronic irritation. Squamous cell carcinoma of the penis, for instance, occurs more often in uncircumcised men (Gikas, 1976). This association is seen mostly in Latin, African, and South Asian countries. Less than 1% of penile cancer occurs in the United States (Nichols, 1988).

Paraphimosis is a condition in which the foreskin is constricted behind the glans so that it cannot be replaced to its normal position over the glans. The resultant constriction compresses the dorsal veins and lymphatics of the distal penis, causing increasing edema and pain of the glans and foreskin. Mild, preexisting phimosis or unawareness of its potential occurrence predisposes men to develop the condition. Paraphimosis happens when uncircumcised men do not replace the foreskin immediately after intercourse or bathing. Health providers caring for uncircumcised patients who are unable to perform their own perineal care should be particularly aware of this problem. A man's foreskin may be pulled back during a bath or while applying a condom catheter and inadvertently left retracted. Because the presence of a foreskin also makes it difficult to keep a condom in place, circumcision may be recommended if condom drainage is desired.

Paraphimosis is a medical emergency. The longer the situation continues, the harder it is to rectify. If it is allowed to continue, arterial blood is blocked and gangrene of the glans will occur.

**Medical-Surgical Management.** Because inflammation and infection are often associated with phimosis, conservative measures such as antibiotics and warm soaks are ordered initially. The physician may cut the foreskin vertically (dorsal slit) to gain access to the infected area if there is marked infection.

After tissues heal, circumcision may be performed. Surgery in the adult is performed under general or local anesthesia. The foreskin is

incised around the dorsal surface of the corona; hemostasis is achieved by use of hemostats, ligatures, or cautery, and the foreskin around the glans is removed. Because adults have larger vessels, Gomco or Plastibell clamps, which are used for small children, do not provide adequate hemostasis. A petroleum jelly or antibiotic-embedded dressing is usually wrapped loosely around the incision for protection and ease of removal a few days after surgery.

After circumcision, a patient may experience temporary hyperesthesia or have minor cosmetic imperfections. If a hematoma forms, it can be treated with evacuation, ligation of the bleeding vessel if necessary, and application of a compression dressing (Malloy & Wein, 1986). Barbiturates may be ordered to be taken at bedtime postoperatively to prevent rapid eye movement (REM) sleep erections that could break sutures before the incision is healed (Lerner & Khan, 1982). An amyl nitrite ampule may also be prescribed to prevent erections, and placed at the bedside.

Paraphimosis first requires pushing the edematous fluid out of the foreskin and glans, then manually pulling the foreskin back to its normal position. Nurses can perform this maneuver without a physician's order by firmly squeezing the glans for several minutes before attempting to reposition the foreskin back over the glans (Fig. 11–1).

Manual reduction is uncomfortable for the patient. If the procedure described in Figure 11–1 does not remedy the situation, the physician should be called immediately. He or she may inject lidocaine into the dorsal nerve of the penis before performing the maneuver to help alleviate some of the discomfort (Krause, 1985). The physician may also use a method described by Ganti et al. (1985) to compress edema in which a 2-inch elastic bandage is firmly wrapped from the glans to the base of the penis for 5 to 7 minutes. This method is not used if there is ulceration or chronic balanitis because the potential compromise of blood supply would make such conditions worse. A circumcision may be performed after the acute incident of paraphimosis to prevent recurrences.

## Approaches to Patient Care

### Assessment

A patient with symptomatic phimosis or paraphimosis will describe difficulty moving his foreskin. A patient with phimosis may relate

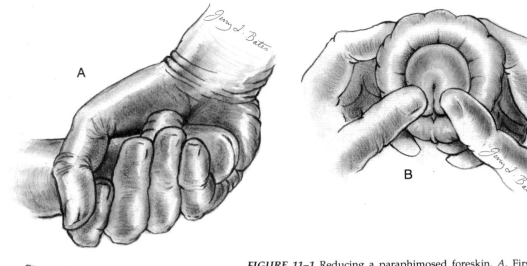

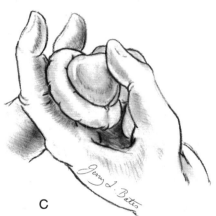

*FIGURE 11–1* Reducing a paraphimosed foreskin. *A,* First, grab the glans and edematous prepuce inside a fistlike grip of the hand, much like a handshake. Squeeze the glans with firm, steady pressure for a few minutes to redistribute edematous fluid from the distal penis back into the area proximal to the constriction. *B,* Using two hands (required for most adults), grasp the foreskin with your middle and index fingers, pulling them toward you. At the same time, push the glans back with your thumbs. Maintain firm, steady pressure for at least 5 minutes. *C,* If the penis is small, the same maneuver can be done by placing the penis between the second and third fingers of one hand and pushing back on the glans with your thumb. If reduction is successful, grasp and squeeze the end of the penis in the same fistlike manner as in *A* to ensure that the prepuce will remain in its normal position.

episodes of tearing the foreskin and bleeding during attempts to retract it. If inflammation or infection is present, he will complain of soreness in the glans and foreskin and may describe a burning or itching sensation. A patient with paraphimosis complains of pain in the glans and along the penile shaft; the degree depends on the amount of edema present.

Patients who are asymptomatic, which is sometimes the case with phimosis, or those who have impaired sensory or perceptual abilities may not be aware that a problem exists. Some men never learn to retract the foreskin when bathing. Others fear discomfort and bleeding.

Observe the glans and foreskin for signs of inflammation, ulceration, edema, adhesions, or purulent discharge. The glans may be discolored in some cases of paraphimosis because of a compromised blood supply. If a discharge is present, culture it. Small, gravel-like stones or polypoid growths around the corona may be signs of chronic infection. Small, pearly-appearing papules surrounding the corona may also be normal benign lesions.

Ask the patient how long the condition has lasted and about his perineal hygiene habits. Also, ask about previous treatment, medical or self-prescribed. If the patient cannot perform his own hygienic care, find out who the caregivers are and include them in any teaching session.

**Nursing Diagnosis**

Nursing diagnoses for the patient with phimosis or paraphimosis may include the following:

1. Pain related to inflammation, infection, or edema of glans or foreskin.
2. Alteration in health maintenance related to lack of knowledge about perineal hygiene and preventive measures.
3. Potential for infection related to chronic ir-

ritation of the glans, inadequate cleansing of the foreskin, or constriction and tearing of the foreskin.

4. Impaired integrity of foreskin tissue related to altered blood supply caused by constriction, tearing, and scarring or surgical incision.

### Plan of Care

Nursing care is directed toward enabling the patient to

1. Express relief of pain.
2. Verbalize comprehension of information presented about treatment regimes and preventive measures.
3. Successfully demonstrate proper genital hygiene.
4. Exhibit no postoperative signs of infection, hematoma, or abnormal healing.

### Interventions

Patients or their caregivers are responsible for compliance with medical treatments because patients are not hospitalized specifically for phimosis or paraphimosis. The success of treatment depends on instruction and patient compliance. Give clear instructions about how to take the prescribed antibiotics or other medications. Explain the drug's actions and potential side effects. Generic names may be ordered when possible to decrease costs, and the regimen should be incorporated into the patient's daily routine to improve compliance.

If a medication is topical, tell the patient to use it sparingly as prescribed. Seeking fast relief of discomfort, he may believe that if a little medication helps, more would be better. Such a practice is wasteful, costly, and ineffective.

Teach about warm soaks to the penis. A 10-minute soak (either in a bath or with a warm, wet towel) two or three times a day is sufficient to promote healing. Caution against using very hot water to avoid tissue damage. Patients follow these instructions easily because of the pain relief warm soaks bring. Monitor treatment effectiveness and document the results on his record.

Explain the necessity of gentle, daily cleansing of the penis with soap and water to prevent recurrence of infection. Demonstrate how to retract the foreskin, exposing surfaces prone to irritation and infection, and how to replace it back to its normal position over the glans. Use written materials, illustrations, or other teaching materials to reemphasize information.

Encourage follow-up visits with the physician. As soon as the glans heals and the patient

is free from infection, circumcision will be recommended to prevent further problems.

A dressing is usually in place after surgery and often removed the following day. If the dressing falls off, do not replace it. Check the dressing or suture line and the head of the penis for circulatory changes, signs of bleeding, drainage, or edema. Instruct the patient to check his temperature at least every 8 hours for the first 48 hours. Tell him to report his response to pain medication and any significant changes to the physician.

Although petroleum or Telfa dressings are usually employed, tell the patient to soak off the dressing if necessary to prevent pulling the suture line. Caution him against applying any medication to the incision unless it is prescribed. Topical medications may be occlusive and trap bacteria. Tell the patient when he should return to the office for a follow-up visit with the physician.

### Patient Outcomes

1. The patient relates feelings of comfort after treatments or surgery
2. The patient states the cause-and-effect relationship between inadequate hygiene or not replacing the foreskin and the development of symptoms of either condition.
3. The patient verbalizes his knowledge of the prescribed medications and treatments and demonstrates compliance with instructions.
4. The patient is able to retract and replace his foreskin without difficulty.
5. The patient exhibits signs of good penile circulation and healing.
6. The patient has no fever or abnormal wound conditions after surgery.

## PRIAPISM

**Etiology and Pathophysiology.** Priapism represents a medical emergency. It consists of a sustained, painful erection that lasts over a period, usually longer than 4 hours. Although priapism can happen after prolonged sexual activity, it is not related to sexual desire. Priapism may interfere with urination if the erection persists for longer than 8 to 12 hours. Etiologic factors identified include sickle cell disease, leukemia, metastatic cancer, and spinal cord trauma or lesion. Localized infectious masses, such as pelvic abscesses, may cause abnormal neural stimulation to erectile tissues, but this is rare (McConnell & Zimmerman, 1983; Yealy & Hogya, 1988). Certain pharmacologic agents such as papaverine, psychotropic drugs, alcohol, and marijuana may also cause priapism (Pantaleo-Gandais et al., 1984). It usually affects men between 20 and 50 years of age.

The actual pathophysiology involves obstruction or venospasm of the small veins draining the corpora cavernosa, usually caused by one of the previously mentioned conditions. Alteration in outflow may also occur at the level of major collecting veins, but circulation to and from the corpus spongiosum or glans penis is not affected. When the venous channels are closed by either obstruction or venospasm, blood trapped in the corpora rapidly loses its oxygen content and sludges cell fragments. These fragments and the high carbon dioxide concentration increase viscosity. As ischemic changes progress, the corporeal bodies lose their muscle contractility, becoming edematous and eventually fibrotic (Pantaleo-Gandais et al., 1984).

There are two types of priapism: ischemic and nonischemic. Other terms used are, respectively, low-flow and high-flow priapism. Various degrees of the disease can occur between these two extremes. The amount of ischemia is related to the number of veins involved, the severity of the pathophysiology, and the duration of the abnormal erection (Lue et al., 1986). Classification and initial treatment are often determined by results of tests performed during evaluation.

The pain experienced by patients is acute in either situation. It is thought to be caused by these ischemic changes and the prolonged stretching of the bulbocavernous and ischiocavernous muscles during an abnormal erection (Lue et al., 1986).

Varying degrees of impotence may result, even after priapism. Impotency rates after appropriate treatment can be as high as 50% (Bertram et al., 1985). The degree of ischemic changes and the degree of intracorporeal pressure before and after treatment seem to be the factors most affecting potency after an episode of priapism (Lue et al., 1986). Early intervention should be encouraged.

Because impotence is a common sequela, patients should understand that the disease process, and not the therapy, causes impotence. Signed statements are often required to ensure legal protection for the caregivers.

**Medical-Surgical Management.** Priapism necessitates rapid and complex treatment. Patients are given sedation and analgesics, meperidine often being used because of its hypotensive effect. At times, spinal or epidural anesthesia is needed. Initial medical treatments may include ice packs to the penis, warm or ice water enemas, local anesthetic infiltration of erectile tissues, or vigorous prostatic massage to relax the neurovascular mechanisms causing the priapism. Intravenous fluids, oxygen, and blood alkalinizers are supportive measures instituted as necessary (Macaluso & Sullivan, 1985). Drugs such as amyl nitrite, propranolol, phentolamine, or heparin are systemically injected to increase venous dilation and outflow of the trapped blood (Bertram et al., 1985). If a definite cause for priapism is found, treatment is directed toward that cause.

If the erection is not reversed, a second stage of care involves needle aspiration and irrigation of the corpora to evacuate sludged blood. After local anesthesia, a needle is inserted into one corpus. Alternate aspiration and irrigation are performed until bright red blood appears, clots are no longer seen, and (it is hoped) the penis becomes flaccid. Saline, norepinephrine, or anticoagulants are used as irrigants (McConnell & Zimmerman, 1983). Some physicians use needle aspiration and irrigation initially to relieve priapism, in the belief that other measures do not often work and can delay surgical treatment (Winter, 1991).

When aspiration and irrigation are not successful, surgical diversion of blood from the corpora is necessary. When priapism is determined to be the ischemic type, the urologist may proceed directly to a shunting procedure, of which Winter's procedure is the simplest. After local anesthesia, a biopsy needle is inserted through the glans into the distal corpora, and a core of tissue is removed. Several fistulas are created to help achieve penile detumescence. The skin opening is sutured closed after the procedure is completed (Winter, 1991). Other operations involve anastomosing the corpora cavernosa to the corpus spongiosum or to the saphenous vein (Macaluso & Sullivan, 1985).

Because there is a semipermeable membrane between the two corpora, both drain when blood is diverted from only one side. Some physicians apply intermittent pressure on the penis, using a pediatric blood pressure cuff, to help maintain adequate shunt flow during these procedures (Bertram et al., 1985).

Shunts should spontaneously thrombose after an acute episode, but surgical correction is occasionally needed (Malloy & Wein, 1986). Hematoma and minor tissue trauma are expected after shunting procedures, but shunts can be problematic. Skin necrosis may occur after Winter's procedure. Permanent fistulas, stricture, and gangrene can follow corpora cavernosa–corpus spongiosum anastomosis (Winter, 1991). Although not as common, pulmonary emboli have been reported after saphenous vein shunts (Macaluso & Sullivan, 1985). Sepsis can happen after any procedure.

## Approaches to Patient Care

### Assessment
A patient's history influences the choice of treatment. The amount of information obtained from a patient seeking help for priapism will assist the physician in determining which treatment(s) to use and may even influence the outcome. Question the patient about his erection. How long has it lasted? What precipitated it? Is this the first time a prolonged erection has occurred? Has he experienced prolonged erections during sexual activity?

What is the medical history? Not only are you looking for diseases recognized as predisposing to priapism, but you are identifying diseases that could contraindicate the use of certain drugs in treatment. For example, a patient with a known cardiovascular condition is not given alpha-adrenergic blockers because cardiac arrhythmias might occur. What medications, prescribed or otherwise, is the patient currently taking?

Observe the penis. How much of an erection do you see? Does the dorsal side feel firm, while the glans appears soft? Do you see ischemic color changes?

Blood is drawn to help detect possible causes of the priapism. A complete blood count, coagulation and sickle cell studies, and a chemical analysis are the most common tests. Others may be ordered if specific diseases are suspected (e.g., renal failure). Ischemic changes are evaluated by performing intracavernosal and arterial blood gas studies for comparison. If severe ischemia occurs, treatment is initially more aggressive. Tissue or fluid samples, such as prostatic fluid for culture, may be taken if an infectious process is suspected.

Computed tomography (CT) scanning may be ordered to help detect spinal cord lesions, tumors, pelvic abscesses, or other causes of priapism. Infusion cavernosography via the pudendal arteries may be used to discover clots or fibrosis within the cavernosal bodies.

Intracavernosal blood flow is evaluated by penile Doppler flow studies, before and after treatment, to determine the effectiveness of therapy and predict the chances of consequent

impotence. An arterial pressure monitor is connected to a scalp vein needle inserted into one corpus, and the pressure is recorded. This needle is often the one used to draw blood for blood gas studies. Normal intracorporeal pressure is less than 40 mm Hg.

### Nursing Diagnosis
Nursing diagnoses for the patient with priapism may include the following:

1. Pain related to ischemia and prolonged stretching of supporting penile musculature.
2. Anxiety related to lack of knowledge regarding the significance and consequence of a prolonged erection.
3. Altered sexuality patterns related to
   a. fear and embarrassment about priapism.
   b. the risk of impotence after treatment for priapism.
4. Potential for impaired skin integrity related to ischemia or edema of penile tissues.

### Plan of Care
Nursing care is directed toward enabling the patient to

1. Relate feelings of comfort.
2. Cope effectively with the acute episode.
3. Exhibit no adverse reactions to medications used in treatment.
4. Exhibit no postoperative signs of vascular impairment or infection.
5. Verbalize awareness of impotence as a probable result of priapism, even when the disease is successfully treated.

### Interventions
Although the patient with priapism is experiencing acute pain, he will also be embarrassed about his erection. He may have delayed seeking medical attention and may be reluctant to talk about details surrounding the incident. Allay embarrassment by explaining that an erection caused by priapism cannot be voluntarily corrected by the patient alone. Assure him that he was right in seeking medical assistance. This assurance and acceptance will help him feel trust and confidence. Provide as much privacy as possible. If the patient is awake (although sedated) during procedures, explain what is being done and why. After the initial crisis, the patient may need more psychosocial support.

Treatment for priapism is usually provided in an emergency or surgery department. Constantly monitor the patient for changes in blood pressure (treatment can cause blood pressure to increase or decrease), cardiac arrhythmias, and possible chest pain. Document intracorporeal pressures, if taken, and urinary output. Other parameters may need to be measured if treatment is directed toward specific diseases causing the priapism, and are ordered by the physician. Maintain oxygen and intravenous hydration, administer sedatives and analgesics as prescribed, and assist with tests and procedures as requested. After any needles are removed from the corporeal bodies, digital compression is necessary for at least 5 minutes to prevent the formation of a hematoma. Ecchymosis and mild edema are common because of the invasive nature of diagnostic and treatment maneuvers.

The penis should be checked for flaccidity and changes in color or temperature after surgery. Any degree of tumescence, duskiness, coldness, drainage, or increased swelling should be reported immediately to the physician. Such observations may indicate that a dressing is too tight, priapism is recurring, or a fistula has formed. Monitor the patient's temperature; an elevation may be a sign of emboli or infection.

Potent broad-spectrum antibiotics such as aminoglycosides, cephalosporins, and fluoroquinolones are continued postoperatively, and the patient is observed for adverse effects. Nephrotoxicity, ototoxicity, and neurotoxicity are the more serious reactions that can occur to aminoglycosides. Hepatotoxicity and colitis can follow administration of cephalosporins. Other medications may be given to prevent erections while the penis heals or to counter specific diseases that originally caused the priapism.

After the initial crisis, the patient may relate more fears about the priapism and its consequences. Impotence can occur despite successful treatment, and this concern may be foremost on his mind. Listen to the patient, and encourage him to express his feelings or to ask questions. The patient's sexual partner, if present, should be encouraged to ask questions also. Impotence is common but may not happen. Assure the patient of the need to recuperate from the acute episode first.

Accepting the loss of sexual function can be difficult. Refer the patient to other appropriate members of the health team or to an impotence support group.

Whether the patient is hospitalized or not depends on the severity of priapism and the extent of treatment. A patient who achieves penile detumescence after aspiration and irrigation may be discharged from the emergency department, whereas a surgical patient will be admitted for inpatient care. Before discharge, explain about any medication to be taken at home and the necessity of follow-up visits with the urologist. Teach the patient to check the dressing and report any fever, increased pain, or unusual symptoms to his physician. Reassure him that the appearance of the penis will improve as tissues heal. Tell him about any restrictions on sexual activities.

**Patient Outcomes**

1. The patient relates feelings of comfort and appears relaxed.
2. The patient verbalizes feelings reflecting a sense of well-being.
3. The patient's penis is flaccid, with signs of good penile circulation.
4. The patient's vital signs are stable.
5. The patient exhibits no signs of infection, skin necrosis, or fistula after surgery.
6. The patient relates feelings about the possible loss of sexual function.

## PEYRONIE'S DISEASE AND CHORDEE

**Etiology and Pathophysiology.** In Peyronie's disease, fibrous thickening or plaques develop in the sheath of the tunica albuginea, mainly on the dorsal surface of the penis. The cause is unknown, but inflammatory changes are implicated. Vasculitis in the connective tissue is thought to spread to surrounding tissue components, which heal by means of fibrosis. Infrequently, the process involves actual ossification (Langemo, 1985). Some studies suggest histocompatible antigens and heredity as factors (Krane, 1992).

Chordee, a curvature of the erect penis, can be seen with Peyronie's disease (although not necessarily) or with hypospadias and other penile anomalies. Occasionally, it is caused by urethral strictures or penile scarring (Devine, 1983). Fibrotic areas or plaques of Peyronie's disease pull on the corpora and angulate the penis toward the affected side. The curvature is usually dorsal or dorsolateral. The shortened muscle fibers of an undeveloped corpus spongiosum in hypospadias, on the other hand, pull the penis in a ventral direction. Lateral curvature is possible with some congenital abnormalities and with penile scarring.

Peyronie's disease and chordee usually do not cause impotence because plaque or fibrotic scarring do not, or only partially, block blood flow through the corpora. However, severe pain and deviation can cause impotence, and concurrent organic causes should also be ruled out (Horton et al., 1987).

**Medical-Surgical Management.** For unknown reasons, spontaneous regression of Peyronie's disease can occur, and patients are often encouraged to wait 6 to 12 months before considering surgery for the disease. Surgery does not guarantee a permanent cure for this disease, and resultant scarring may make further surgery more difficult. The longer the disease continues, however, the more likely it is that inflammatory changes will lessen and fibrotic changes increase (Malloy & Wein, 1986).

Several treatments have been advocated, each carrying successes and risks. Various medications include vitamin E, cortisone, para-aminobenzoic acid, dimethyl sulfoxide, and procarbazine. Radiotherapy and ultrasonography have also been used (Krane, 1992; Langemo, 1985).

When plaques calcify, improvement does not occur. Surgery involves excision of the plaques and, usually, placement of dermal grafts. Dermal grafting corrects penile deviation and relieves pain in most patients (Horton et al., 1987).

There are different local operative approaches. A surgeon can incise around the distal penile shaft (circumcision incision) or along the dorsal midline of the penis. The neurovascular bundle extending along the midline is retracted away, and the plaques are excised. In some instances, the entire tunica albuginea is excised to prevent further occurrences (Devine, 1983). A dermal graft is taken from a donor site, usually the patient's groin area or skin over the iliac crest. Fat, subcutaneous tissue, and epidermis are removed before the graft is sutured in place.

When organic impotence is a concurrent problem, a penile prosthesis may be inserted at the time of grafting (Horton et al., 1987). Some urologists prefer to wait until a second operation (Devine, 1983), but fibrosis often makes further surgery complicated (Malloy & Wein, 1986).

Correction of chordee is accomplished at the same time as that of Peyronie's disease, hypospadias, or strictures. The penis is incised and fibrotic tissue removed (Devine, 1983; Kroovand, 1987). If chordee is associated with a congenital weakness of the fascia surrounding one corpus cavernosum, several vertical excisions of tissue are made on the convex side, which are then closed with suture. The result is a shortening of the convex side and straightening of the penis (Stewart, 1982).

# Approaches to Patient Care

### Assessment

When obtaining a history from a patient with suspected chordee or Peyronie's disease, ask him to describe the lesion or curvature. Most patients seek medical attention when they feel a firm, painless lump in their penis, mistakenly thinking it to be a warning sign of cancer. There may be more than one lesion. If the penis curves, ascertain in which direction.

Ask how long the lesion has been present and if there have been any changes over the duration. Is there discomfort or difficulty with intercourse? How has this problem affected the patient's life?

When palpating the penis, note the number, size, and location of indurated areas. Are they soft or firm? After a physical examination, the urologist may inject saline intracavernously to mimic erection and directly observe any curvature of the penis.

### Nursing Diagnosis

Nursing diagnoses for the patient with Peyronie's disease or chordee may include the following:

1. Anxiety related to
   a. An erroneous fear of cancer.
   b. The causes and treatment of Peyronie's disease.
2. Altered sexuality patterns related to
   a. The curvature of the penis and pain characteristic of Peyronie's disease.
   b. The fear of rejection by the sexual partner.
3. Potential for infection related to surgical correction of chordee associated with Peyronie's disease.

### Plan of Care

Nursing care is directed toward enabling the patient to

1. Verbalize an understanding of the possible causes and treatment of Peyronie's disease.
2. Verbalize knowledge that impotence may be a possible sequela and that alternative means of sexual expression are possible.
3. Exhibit no postoperative signs of neurovascular impairment or infection.

### Interventions

The patient with Peyronie's disease may have many fears and questions. He may fear rejection by his sexual partner or inability to perform sexual intercourse. Penile curvature may cause him to feel less masculine and may make intercourse impossible. The nurse can help by listening to the patient and his sexual partner and encouraging them to express their feelings. If the patient fears that the penile "lumps" are a sign of cancer, reassure him that Peyronie's disease is an inflammatory process and not a malignant one.

Reassure the patient about the possibility of spontaneous resolution if the urologist recommends a waiting period without treatment. Tell him that pain can be relieved for most patients and that medications such as vitamin E and steroids prescribed by the physician may help achieve this purpose. Caution him that all medications must be taken as prescribed; taking more than prescribed does not hasten improvement and may cause untoward side effects. Vitamin E, for instance, is a fat-soluble vitamin that can accumulate in the body and cause thrombophlebitis if taken in megadoses. Fungal infections occur when too much oral steroid is taken, and if steroids are stopped abruptly, adrenal insufficiency can result. Tell the patient to take steroid pills with food or milk to prevent gastric irritability and to watch for unusual signs or symptoms such as nausea, fever, weakness, lethargy, skin infections, or leg pain. Steroids injected into plaque can cause increased local fibrotic changes.

If chordee is present and the pain is not severe, sexual intercourse may still be possible. Increased amounts of lubrication and different positions help. A patient and his partner must be willing to experiment, and other forms of sexual expression can be explored. Books on human sexuality are available that detail approaches for sexual intercourse and alternative activities. Psychological factors greatly influence choices in sexual activity, and referral to a sex therapist or counselor is helpful.

The patient undergoing surgery for Peyronie's disease returns from the operating room with a light pressure dressing, which is kept in place for several days. A drain is often used. Observe the dressing for bleeding or purulent drainage. Monitor vital signs. Because local nerve or vessel damage is possible during surgery, check the penis closely for color and temperature changes. Immediately report signs of duskiness, coldness, or edema to the urologist.

Sedatives or amyl nitrite are ordered postoperatively to prevent erections. Watch for their effectiveness and for inadvertent systemic responses. Amyl nitrite is inhaled to produce less systemic vascular resistance, and even more important, less penile vascular resistance. Orthostatic hypotension, heart palpitations,

and a throbbing headache are the most common adverse reactions. Diazepam is the sedative usually given to patients after penile surgery. It depresses the central nervous system and thus may cause such reactions as drowsiness, lethargy, bradycardia, and hypotension. Warn the patient to avoid activities that require alertness and not to take the drug with alcohol or other sedatives at home.

Before discharge, teach the patient about checking the penis and reporting fever, increased pain, or unusual symptoms to the urologist. Explain the purpose and side effects of any prescribed medication. Tell him about any restrictions on activities, especially sexual activities. Many urologists want patients to avoid having erections for at least 2 weeks after surgery or having intercourse for about 6 to 8 weeks. Tell the patient when follow-up appointments should be made with the urologist. Supplement verbal instructions with written ones and encourage him to reread these when he gets home. Patients who have had surgery on their sexual organs often are too anxious to comprehend all verbal instructions given at discharge.

**Patient Outcomes**

1. There is verbal or behavioral indication that the patient is coping with his current situation and participates in decisions about the treatment regimen.
2. The patient expresses feelings about possible impotence.
3. The patient describes and understands alternative methods for sexual expression.
4. The patient exhibits no signs of postoperative neurovascular impairment or infection.

# DISORDERS OF THE SCROTUM
## Perspective on Disease Entities

Many scrotal disorders are benign conditions, but it is important to differentiate these from tumors or infectious processes. Hydrocele, inguinal hernia, hematocele, spermatocele, and varicocele are common. Testicular torsion is another condition that presents itself as a scrotal mass and is discussed separately in Chapter 19.

### HYDROCELE, INGUINAL HERNIA, HEMATOCELE, SPERMATOCELE, AND VARICOCELE

**Etiology and Pathophysiology.** A hydrocele is a collection of fluid within the scrotum (Fig.

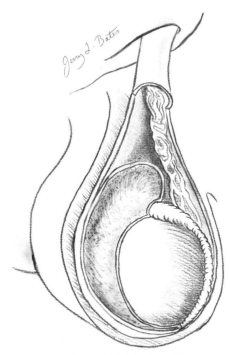

*FIGURE 11–2* Hydrocele.

11–2). The causes of hydroceles that develop in children are different from those that result in hydroceles in adults. Variations of hydroceles present since childhood may be identified on clinical notes and are briefly differentiated in this discussion.

As the embryonic testis descends, it can bring fluid with it. If this fluid is trapped in the scrotum after closure of the processus vaginalis, a hydrocele of the tunica vaginalis occurs. A small opening between the peritoneal cavity and the tunica vaginalis causes a communicating hydrocele. Fluid shifts from one area to the other, depending on changes in body position or intraabdominal pressure. A young man usually comments on his scrotum being small and soft when he gets up in the morning and becoming large and more tense as the day continues. A third type, hydrocele of the cord, represents a collection of fluid enclosed only around the spermatic cord ("Overlooked anatomy," 1984).

It is postulated that hydroceles developing later in life are caused by an imbalance between production and reabsorption of fluid within the layers of the tunica vaginalis (Bodner, 1987). This imbalance may be the reason that aspiration techniques are not very successful. Occasionally, trauma causes hydroceles (Tanagho & McAninch, 1992).

Hydroceles are not dangerous. Treatment is pursued only when a large hydrocele causes constant discomfort, patient embarrassment, or a threat to testicular blood supply by virtue of its size. A hydrocele may camouflage an inguinal hernia, but this is a relatively benign condition. Danger does exist when a hydrocele conceals a testicular tumor.

An inguinal hernia occurs when a loop of bowel slips into the scrotum through the inguinal ring (Fig. 11–3). There are no symptoms, but the mass feels soft and separate from the testicle. The mass can usually be pushed up into the peritoneal cavity. An incarcerated hernia, however, is one that is trapped in the inguinal ring, and its blood supply is threatened by strangulation. This type causes pain and tenderness and is impossible to reduce; surgery is indicated.

A hematocele is a collection of blood in the scrotum, usually the result of trauma from a direct blow to the scrotum or to scrotal surgery. It is not harmful and requires only drainage of the bloody contents.

A spermatocele is a painless, mobile, usually

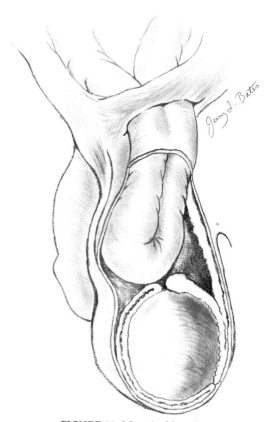

*FIGURE 11–3* Inguinal hernia.

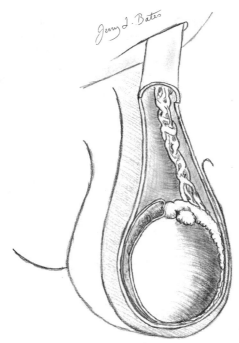

*FIGURE 11–4* Spermatocele.

cystic mass that contains white fluid and dead sperm (Fig. 11–4). Trauma or infection may produce the initial leakage of sperm. The spermatocele usually appears behind the testicle and is separate from it. Surgery is not necessary unless the condition worries the patient.

Large varicose veins can appear on the scrotum. The patient usually has leg varicosities and a family history of varicose veins. They rarely cause problems.

A varicocele is a varicose condition of the veins of the pampiniform plexus and, sometimes, the spermatic vein (Fig. 11–5). Varicoceles are commonly described as feeling like a "bag of worms." They develop slowly and may or may not be symptomatic. Most occur on the left side because the left spermatic vein enters the left renal vein at a 90-degree angle. If back-pressure becomes too high for the valves to compensate, the veins dilate. The right spermatic vein enters the vena cava at a smaller angle, so back-pressure is not as high. If a varicocele appears on the right side, or if the onset is sudden, there may be pathologic causes. A renal tumor and retroperitoneal fibrosis are two such causes ("When your patient," 1985).

Infertility occurs three times more often in men with a varicocele than in the general population. Hypoxia, elevated testicular temperature, reflux of renal or adrenal metabolites, and hormonal imbalances are some of the theories used to explain this phenomenon (La Nasa & Lewis, 1987). If the condition is progressively painful or if infertility is a possibility, varicocelectomy is performed.

**Medical-Surgical Management.** Hydroceles can be treated by aspiration, injection of sclerosing agents after aspiration, or surgery. They often recur after aspiration, so the other two methods are employed more often.

Sclerosing agents obliterate a hydrocele sac after aspiration, but the procedure often needs to be repeated as many as three or four times. Tetracycline is a common sclerosing agent that is injected directly into the hydrocele sac after aspiration of its fluid contents. Sometimes the drug is combined with tetradecyl sulfate, quinine, or urea solutions, which are also sclerosing agents (Bodner, 1987). Infection and fibrosis are complications that have occurred after injection of sclerosing agents (Thomson & Odell, 1979). Mild to moderate pain and fever are usual postprocedural occurrences.

The hydrocele sac can be drained, everted, and sutured during a hydrocelectomy so that it cannot accumulate more fluid, or it can be completely removed. Although hydrocelectomy is considered a minor procedure, hematoma, abscess, or injury to scrotal structures may occur (Bunce, 1983; Kay & Stewart, 1982). A scrotal drain may be left in place for 2 or 3 days post-

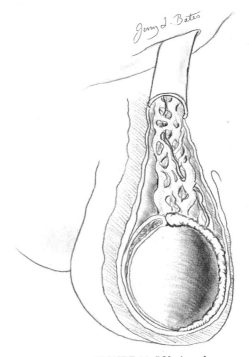

*FIGURE 11–5* Varicocele.

operatively; fluff dressings and a scrotal support are usually ordered by the physician. Oral anti-inflammatory drugs may be used to minimize edema, and analgesics to alleviate pain. Some physicians also require ice bags to be applied to the scrotum for the first 24 hours to keep edema in check.

Hematocelectomy and spermatocelectomy also require a scrotal approach. After blood and blood clots are evacuated during hematocelectomy, the surgeon examines the testicle for injury. A spermatocele is simply dissected from the epididymis, and the site of the resection closed (Bunce, 1983). Postoperative orders are similar to those discussed earlier.

An inguinal incision or an incision above the superior iliac spine is made for varicocelectomy so that the trunks of the spermatic vein can be better identified and ligated (McConnell & Zimmerman, 1983). Stewart (1983) described experimental techniques in which some urologists insert a small balloon through the femoral vein into the internal spermatic vein and either inject sclerosing agents or inflate the balloon to occlude the vein. This technique will not work if there are collateral vessels or if there is concern about malfunction of the balloon or risk of pulmonary embolism. Therefore, surgery is still considered the standard form of therapy. In recent years, urologists have adapted laparoscopic techniques to correct varicoceles.

An inguinal incision is also used to repair an inguinal hernia. If the loop of bowel appears viable, it is replaced into the abdominal cavity after the sac is dissected. Muscle and fascial layers are closed to prevent recurrence.

## Approaches to Patient Care

### Assessment

A patient with a scrotal mass may or may not seek medical attention. This may not be necessary if the mass is benign and not causing significant symptoms, but if concern is voiced, the patient should be encouraged to see a doctor.

If the patient seeks help, question him about the onset and any changes in size over time. Was there any predisposing event? Does a change in position affect how the mass feels? Is he experiencing any discomfort, or is he asymptomatic? Patients with hydroceles or varicoceles, for instance, often describe a vague aching or heavy feeling in the scrotum because of the increasing pressure on scrotal structures, whereas trauma, torsion, or infection causes more acute scrotal pain. Are there any other symptoms? Note which side of the scrotum is affected.

Note any obvious signs of swelling in the scrotum. Check whether a soft or turgid mass is present and, if so, determine its size and whether it is separate from the testicle. Auscultation may reveal bowel sounds if an inguinal hernia is present. Physical examination may be performed with the patient in a supine position or standing and doing a Valsalva maneuver to detect changes in the scrotal contents. A varicocele or an inguinal hernia, for example, may not be as apparent in a supine position.

Hydroceles are initially differentiated from solid masses by transillumination. A light is held against the scrotum to see if it shines through. A cystic mass transilluminates, but a solid mass, such as a tumor or hernia, does not.

Ultrasonography is appropriate when there is a doubt about a scrotal mass after the physical examination. This is a highly accurate way to distinguish solid from cystic masses, and it can help differentiate a possible tumor or other scrotal conditions when the results are correlated with other diagnostic findings. When a varicocele appears on the right side, intravenous pyelography (IVP) or CT may be ordered to help identify the cause.

### Nursing Diagnosis

Nursing diagnoses for the patient with a hydrocele, inguinal hernia, hematocele, spermatocele, or varicocele may include the following:

1. Anxiety related to fear of cancer or potential altered sexuality.
2. Potential for pain related to the collection of fluid or blood within the scrotum.
3. Potential for infection related to inflammation and edema after surgical repair of hydrocele, inguinal hernia, hematocele, spermatocele, or varicocele.

### Plan of Care

Nursing care is directed toward enabling the patient to

1. Relate feelings of comfort.
2. Verbalize awareness that the condition is benign.
3. Show no postoperative signs of infection, bleeding, or other complications.

### Interventions

Patients with scrotal or penile disorders often are concerned about the appearance of their sexual organs, and this is why many asymptomatic men seek medical advice. They may also be worried about cancer because public education emphasizes the fact that painless "lumps" may be a sign of testicular cancer. Listen to the patient and encourage him to express his feelings. To minimize embarrassment and anxiety, provide as much privacy as possible. Explain which diagnostic procedures will be performed and why. Assure him that many scrotal conditions are benign or infectious processes. Just knowing that his condition may not be serious can reduce a patient's psychological discomfort.

When a scrotal condition causes physical discomfort, the physician usually orders a scrotal support. Physicians differ in their choice. A support that holds the scrotum close to the body may be preferred to an elastic suspensory or jockey shorts. Oral analgesics are ordered to minimize discomfort, and elevating the scrotum on an ice pack may provide relief. Teach the patient about the medication's actions or side effects, and give clear instructions about how to take them. Encourage follow-up visits with the urologist when indicated.

Surgery is often the only means to correct the scrotal disorder, and standard postoperative nursing care is needed. Check the dressing for signs of bleeding or other drainage, and change it as needed. If a drain is present, take care not to dislodge it. Monitor the patient's temperature. Report any significant changes to the physician. Make sure that the patient wears the scrotal support at all times to reduce scrotal edema and that he elevates it on a towel or ice pack when sitting or lying down. Document observations and treatment effectiveness. Tell the patient when the physician will need to see him in the office.

**Patient Outcomes**

1. The patient relates feelings of comfort after treatment or surgery.
2. The patient is able to verbalize his knowledge of the prescribed treatments and demonstrate compliance with the instructions.
3. The patient expresses an understanding that his condition is benign and may not need treating.
4. The patient shows no signs of bleeding, fever, or abnormal wound conditions.

## GENITAL SKIN CONDITIONS

### Perspective on Disease Entities

Many skin disorders appear in the genital or anogenital area. Some are localized diseases; others are manifestations of systemic disease or generalized dermatologic conditions. The natural warmth, perspiration, and constant contact of opposing skin surfaces of this area create an environment conducive to invading organisms and skin breakdown. Even bacteria normal to the genital area can be pathogenic when skin integrity is impaired. Tight-fitting clothes, nylon pantyhose, incontinence, vaginal drainage, and vigorous hygienic measures increase the suseptibility to many genital skin conditions.

Dermatologic diagnosis of genital lesions can be confusing. Diseases can be categorized according to cause, presentation, symptoms, and whether they are contagious. Some texts use different terminology for the same condition. To confuse matters further, many skin disorders appear similar, yet require detailed histories and tests to differentiate them. Sometimes the appearance of a lesion changes as the disease progresses.

Genital lesions are rarely life-threatening, but they do cause patients concern because of cosmetic appearance, discomfort, or the fear of their being contagious or cancerous. The earlier a suspicious lesion is examined and treated, the better the chances are for detecting a possible genital skin cancer. The following discussion identifies common genital skin disorders in broad categories according to cause. Venereal diseases are discussed in Chapter 7.

### INFECTIONS, DERMATITIS, BENIGN AND MALIGNANT GROWTHS, VASCULAR LESIONS, PIGMENTARY DISORDERS, DISEASES DUE TO ANIMAL PARASITES, AND OTHER SKIN DISORDERS

**Etiology and Pathophysiology.** Infectious organisms account for many genital skin disorders. They affect epidermal, dermal, or subcutaneous skin layers. Bacteria, usually staphylococci or streptococci, can cause a generalized macular rash, serous vesicles, or crusting lesions. Individual lesions can also appear around hair follicles as superficial pustules pierced by the hair; if a deeper abscess forms, they are called *furuncles.* When these abscesses spread under the skin, they interconnect to form carbuncles. Carbuncles discharge pus to the surface of the skin at more than one site (Collins & Rosen, 1984). Localized inflammation and pain accompany these lesions. Bacterial infections also occur secondary to other infections that break down skin defenses; these are discussed later. Balanitis, produced by several different kinds of organisms, is an example of a genital condition frequently caused by bacteria.

Viruses also cause skin lesions. Herpes simplex, which causes herpes progenitalis (so named because of location), is a virus that produces small vesicular eruptions on the glans, prepuce, or penile shaft. In women, the lesions may appear on the labia majora, labia minora, clitoris, or near the urethral meatus. Burning and itching accompany the lesions. Local hyperalgesia or paresthesia and fever may precede the appearance of genital lesions.

When these lesions burst, a thin crust develops. The skin around the lesions may appear reddened or normal. As lesions multiply and coalesce, irregular erosions result. Lesions usually heal within 6 to 10 days, but recurrences are frequent. Scars rarely form. Secondary bacterial infections compound the problem. Febrile episodes or even intercourse may trigger a recurrence (Callomon & Wilson, 1956).

Molluscum contagiosum is another virus that invades the epithelial cells. Lesions may occur on the thighs as well as on genital skin, although they rarely affect the vulva or vagina (Korting, 1981). The lesions are small, round, smooth nodules that have a natural skin color but a pearly, almost transparent appearance. Fully developed lesions become centrally indented and may appear to have minute dark openings in the center of the depressions. They may be isolated lesions, but molluscum often appears in clusters. On examination a cheesy mass can be expressed containing the infecting virus.

Warts (verrucae) are another virus-caused skin condition. Condylomata acuminata are warts that occur in the genital region. They may first appear as reddish or white elevations and rapidly form into pedunculated masses or cauliflower-like forms. In fact, a variety of presentations are now recognized for the papillomavirus infection, adding to the confusion in making a diagnosis. Genital warts grow around the genital and anal openings, may become quite large, and can be sexually transmitted. Some become an overgrowth of hardened callous tissue. They appear more often than genital herpes lesions and are difficult to eradicate (Coldiron & Jacobson, 1988).

The most serious concern is the association of papillomavirus with cancer. Different subtypes have been discovered, some of which have been linked with genital and cervical cancer (Coldiron & Jacobson, 1988).

Fungi cause superficial lesions on genital skin, usually producing generalized inflammation. Fungi release an enzyme that digests keratin and causes the skin to scale and disintegrate. It is thought that the subsequent vesicle formation and erythema are due to an exotoxin that the fungi release (Sauer, 1985). Other signs and symptoms differ with each organism.

Tinea cruris ("jock itch") is a common genital fungal infection. It is caused by *Trichophyton rubrum* and appears as bilateral red patches with papules and vesicles around well delineated margins. The lesions are first seen on the thighfold and perineal area. Tinea cruris usually does not involve the penis or scrotum (Bickers & Carney, 1987). As the lesions slowly spread, they can extend over the lower abdomen or down the thighs, often accompanied by intense itching. Tinea may appear at the same time on the feet. Skin thickening occurs as the disease becomes chronic (Sauer, 1985).

In contrast, candidiasis (yeast infection) has no sharp border. Skin appears red and oozing with satellite pustules or vesicles around the edges (Sauer, 1985). *Candida albicans* is the offending organism.

Patients who are immunosuppressed, are obese, have diabetes, or have taken long-term antibiotics are more susceptible to yeast infection. If the infection originates in the vagina, a white cottage cheese–like discharge may be noticeable. A white discharge may also be apparent with yeast-caused balanitis (Korting, 1981).

Parasites also cause genital skin lesions and may be contagious. Scabies and pubic lice are more common in populations in which personal hygiene is not a priority. The female mite, *Sarcoptes scabiei*, favors the warm environment of the genitalia, lower abdomen, and back. This microscopic mite burrows under the skin, advancing a few millimeters each day, and forms linear ducts containing eggs, debris, and feces. There is intense itching and excoriation due to scratching. Secondary infection is common (Sauer, 1985).

*Phthirus pubis*, the crab louse, causes pediculosis and can infest the entire body, including the genital area. Lice attach themselves to skin near hair follicles, bite the skin, and lay their eggs on the hair. They also cause intense itching (Nickel & Plumb, 1986).

Psoriasis occasionally involves the genital area, but the lesions are also seen elsewhere on the body. The most common genital site is the preputial glans (Coldiron & Jacobson, 1988). Although the cause and cure are unknown, genetic and environmental factors seem to be involved in the pathophysiology (Nasemann et al., 1983). Psoriasis appears as erythematous, ringlike plaques covered with loosely adhering silvery-white scales on most parts of the body. However, silvery scales are usually absent in genital lesions (Korting, 1981; Nickel & Plumb, 1986). Instead, lesions appear as red, soft plaques. Psoriasis can appear on the vulva, groin, or male genitalia.

Dermatitis literally means inflammation of the skin, although other skin changes occur as the condition progresses. Dermatitis in the genital area suggests contact with a substance that either directly irritates the skin or causes an allergic reaction. Use of over-the-counter medication on the groin, perineum, or scrotum that inadvertently produces a chemical burn is an example of this type of genital dermatitis. Allergic contact dermatitis, on the other hand, requires sensitization and then exposure to the offending substance in order to produce the inflammation and other symptoms. When genital dermatitis is caused by allergy factors, dermatitis may also develop on other body sites.

Poison ivy, nickel, and synthetic rubber or latex products (e.g., condoms and catheters) are a few examples of substances that cause allergic contact dermatitis. Poison ivy and poison oak excrete an oleoresin, the actual allergen, that binds readily to skin surfaces. Men may transfer this allergen from their hands to their penis when urinating and develop severe balanitis (Epstein, 1983). Sometimes the entire penis and scrotum become edematous (Coldiron & Jacobson, 1988).

The chemicals added to synthetic rubber to keep the material from hardening or oxidizing can also cause allergic skin reactions. Nickel in belt buckles or fasteners on jeans can cause dermatitis in the genital area, similar to reactions experienced with nickel content in jewelry when a person is sensitized. Friction, heat, and perspiration cause the nickel to leach out (Rosen, 1988). Other common allergens are douches, feminine hygiene sprays, dusting powders, toilet paper, and home remedies for itching (Sauer, 1985).

Redness, edema, weeping, and skin erosion are the presenting signs of dermatitis. Vesicles or crusting may be present. In chronic stages, papular eruptions and fissures are seen (Korting, 1981). Bacterial infection can superimpose on skin affected by dermatitis and complicate treatment.

Allergies to drugs can cause splotchy, itching skin rashes or dermatitis that may involve the genitalia, but these conditions are usually seen elsewhere on the body as well. The redness in these cases is caused by vasodilatation. Purpura (purplish skin discolorations) represent a more severe reaction. Drug-related dermatitis can occur even after a patient has taken a drug previously without incident. Time for sensitization varies. Penicillin, sulfonamides, antihistamines, neomycin, iodoform, and local anesthetics are common causes (Durgin, 1983).

A fixed drug eruption is a round, red or purple lesion that appears in only one or a few spots on the body, commonly on the penis, and less often on the scrotum or vulva (Callomon & Wilson, 1956; Coldiron & Jacobson, 1988). Sometimes blistering occurs, making the lesion appear similar to one caused by herpes infection. Itching and burning are common complaints. The lesions occur at the same location soon after a person takes the drug, but disappear a few weeks after it is discontinued. The area, however, may remain lightly pigmented. Sulfa, tetracycline, phenolphthalein, and barbiturates are common offenders (Rosen, 1986).

Angiokeratomas are small, benign, vascular lesions that appear on the scrotum, penis, or vulva. There may be one or more that appear red or bluish-red. They may bleed if injured or may thrombose. When these lesions extend to other areas of the body, Fabry-type angiokeratoma should be suspected (Korting, 1981; Nickel & Plumb, 1986).

A urethral caruncle, not to be confused with a carbuncle (a deep-seated infection described earlier), is a red, fleshy, papillary mass that protrudes from the urethral meatus. It occurs only in women. The benign lesions may be very tender or, in some cases, asymptomatic. Women frequently complain of dysuria, frequency, dyspareunia, perineal pressure, and hematuria (Hopkins & Grabstald, 1986).

Epithelial inclusion cysts, or sebaceous cysts, are harmless raised lesions that appear on the scrotum. They are white or yellow and may be soft or firm. Often multiple, they contain accumulations of keratin.

Bartholin's cysts, which result from chronic infection or irritation of Bartholin's glands, may also be seen on perineal examination. They contain clear or suppurative fluid.

Another nonmalignant lesion that appears less frequently in the genital area of both men and women is seborrheic keratosis. This lesion is a warty-looking growth caused by hyperplasia of the epidermis.

Pearl-like papules surrounding the corona of the penis are common in young men. They are classified as angiofibromas and have no clinical significance (Nickel & Plumb, 1986).

Malignant skin lesions are rare in the genital area. If a lesion is irregular, is dark, or has changed in color and consistency, a physician should examine it. Epitheliomas can appear on the penis or vulva and spread to the inguinal lymph nodes late in the disease (Epstein, 1984). Genital melanoma, although uncommon, is seen four times more often in women, mostly on the vulvar surfaces (Korting, 1981).

**Medical-Surgical Management.** A variety of treatments are available for genital skin disorders, depending on their cause, symptoms, and the stage of disease. Not all are successful in curing genital skin conditions, but they do help alleviate symptoms.

Bacterial infections are treated with systemic and sometimes local antibiotics. Warm, dry heat may be prescribed as adjuvant therapy. When lesions such as furuncles or abscesses contain pus, they should be incised and drained to promote healing. A local anesthetic may be used for this minor procedure, but it should not contain epinephrine, because there is some evidence that this agent's vasoconstricting action provokes an infection to spread (Epstein, 1983).

Topical, oral, and intravenous acyclovir is the drug of choice for treating and reducing symptoms of herpes (Berger, 1992). Antibiotic-corticosteroid ointments also help relieve pain and inflammation and prevent secondary infection. Some physicians order wet compresses when the herpes lesions are crusted (Sauer, 1985).

Cantharidin, a blistering agent, is sometimes used on lesions of molluscum contagiosum, but it must be applied only on the lesions themselves and not on the surrounding skin, and must be allowed to dry thoroughly. Repeated applications may be necessary (Epstein, 1983). Cryotherapy and curettage are other popular treatments (Berger, 1992).

Podophyllin and dichloroacetic acid are blistering agents used for condylomata acuminata on external skin. Care must be taken not to apply the medication on surrounding skin or mucous membrane surfaces because of a localized reaction or systemic toxicity. Intraurethral warts may be treated with 5-fluorouracil cream. Warts tend to recur, so repeated applications may be necessary. Condylomata can also be treated by fulguration, liquid nitrogen application, excision, or (more recently) by laser surgery (Malloy & Wein, 1987; Smith, 1987).

Medications are used to treat fungal and yeast infections, as well as parasitic infesta-

tions. Tolnaftate powder and Whitfield's (benzoic and salicylic acids) ointment are over-the-counter fungicides that are often effective for fungal infections in the groin. The physician may prescribe broad-spectrum fungicides such as miconazole, clotrimazole, and haloprogin creams instead. If dermatitis coexists with the fungal infection, a topical corticosteroid may be ordered to reduce acute inflammation before an antifungal drug is prescribed (Epstein, 1983). Griseofulvin or ketoconazole may be given orally for difficult infections, but blood studies (particularly liver) must be closely monitored (Nickel & Plumb, 1986).

Miconazole, clotrimazole, nystatin, and terconazole are other medications used for *Candida* infections. These medications are available in the form of creams and vaginal suppositories. Hydrocortisone cream is often used in conjunction with one of these drugs to treat candidal balanitis (Nasemann et al., 1983).

Gamma benzene hexachloride (lindane) lotions are the most effective treatment for scabies and lice but should be used only once or twice because of their neurotoxic side effects. Crotamiton cream is an alternative agent used in pregnant women and small children. Other pediculicides are available. Patients are instructed to leave the medication on their entire bodies for 8 to 18 hours before bathing and to wash their clothes and bedding. A tapering course of oral prednisone may be prescribed to alleviate itching (Epstein, 1983; Sauer, 1985).

Genital psoriasis is more resistant to treatments generally used for the disease (Nickel & Plumb, 1986). In addition, many of the agents irritate genital skin. Tar compounds, for instance, must be greatly diluted in lotion bases (Coldiron & Jacobson, 1988). Hydrocortisone cream is effective, but fluorinated corticosteroids are avoided because they cause skin thinning and atrophy (Epstein, 1983). Ultraviolet light may be of some value.

Dermatitis, as discussed, has a variety of causes. Often it is the type of lesion, rather than the cause, that directs the type of treatment, but both are important. Sauer (1985) offered the following guidelines for treating dermatitis. When a lesion is irritated and oozing, the physician orders wet soaks such as Burow's (aluminum acetate) or dilute vinegar solutions. Topical lotions or aerosol sprays are better tolerated and do not trap bacteria on irritated skin surfaces. Topical ointments and creams lubricate and penetrate dry, scaly lesions more effectively. Topical medications are generally prescribed at lower concentrations and increased or changed if the lesions are not healing.

Oral antihistamines and tapering doses of systemic steroids are prescribed for allergic contact dermatitis (Rosen, 1988). Patients are instructed to avoid soaps, topical anesthetic creams, and calamine lotions that contain diphenhydramine. Topical anesthetics and diphenhydramine are potential allergens themselves and can cause a dermatitis to worsen. Once sensitized to these substances, a patient may not be able to tolerate them in other forms in the future (e.g., cold medications and systemic anesthetics) (Rosen, 1986). Avoidance of identified irritants or allergens is an obvious way to cure the condition and prevent recurrences.

Treatment is not necessary for vascular or other nonmalignant genital lesions except for cosmetic purposes or when there are repeated bleeding episodes. Electrosurgical desiccation is used to destroy angiokeratomas. Surgical excision and laser are employed with other lesions. Cryosurgery is a common treatment for seborrheic keratoses (Nickel & Plumb, 1986).

## Approaches to Patient Care

### Assessment

Patients' descriptions of their dermatologic condition will help the health care team to make a diagnosis and select treatment. Ask when the lesions first appeared and what they looked like. Have they changed and, if so, how? Was there any predisposing event? Do the lesions appear elsewhere on the body?

Question patients about the medications they are taking. Have they tried any self-treatment and, if so, with which products? Do they use perfumes or powders in the genital area? What type of clothes do they wear (e.g., tight jeans, pantyhose)? Is there a history of other diseases? Do other family members or contacts have similar problems? What specific symptoms are patients experiencing: pain, itching, burning, bleeding, or discharge? Ask them about other factors they may believe are important to know about the condition.

During a physical examination, observe the patient's general appearance and cleanliness. Note the characteristics of the lesions. Where do they appear in the genital area? Are they hard or soft, flat or elevated? Is there any redness, edema, dryness, oozing, pus, or discharge? What is the color? Do they have well-delineated borders or are they diffuse?

It is necessary to examine the skin elsewhere on the body as well to see if lesions are present. Sometimes patients are too embarrassed to mention this fact or are unaware that other lesions exist (e.g., on the back). Check their temperature. More often than not, it will be normal, but fever may indicate an infectious process.

Cultures or tissue scrapings are often taken, especially if bacterial, viral, or yeast infection or parasitic infestation is suspected. Biopsies are done on warts or unusual-looking lesions that may be malignant. Occasionally, skin biopsies are performed for purposes of differential diagnosis. When condylomata are suspected, but lesions are difficult to see, a 5% acetic acid solution soak may be placed on the genital skin for 5 minutes to make the lesions more visible. Condylomata are supposed to turn white, but the change is not always dramatic enough to make a clear diagnosis.

Looking at lesions through a magnifying glass may help make observation easier. Urethroscopy or direct vaginal examinations are performed when lesions are intraurethral or intravaginal. The physician may order blood tests to rule out systemic or venereal diseases.

### Nursing Diagnosis

The nursing diagnoses for the patient with a genital skin condition may include the following:

1. Impaired skin integrity related to the presence of genital lesions associated with infection or inflammation.
2. Anxiety related to fear of cancer or contagion.
3. Sexual dysfunction related to the effects of an actual or perceived limitation imposed by a dermatologic condition of the external genitalia.
4. Knowledge deficit related to an unfamiliarity with health and hygiene practices that prevent genital skin conditions.

### Plan of Care

Nursing care is directed toward enabling the patient to

1. Exhibit an improvement in the condition of the genital skin area with the healing of lesions.
2. Verbalize an awareness that the genital skin condition is benign and not contagious, as appropriate.
3. Cope effectively with the acute episode of a dermatologic condition of the external genitalia.

4. Share feelings about the effects of skin condition on self-perception and sexual function.
5. Exhibit no signs of adverse reactions to treatments.
6. Verbalize comprehension of information regarding health and hygiene practice to prevent recurrence of a genital skin condition.

**Interventions**

Patients with genital lesions are often anxious and physically uncomfortable. Initial interventions must be directed toward alleviating their distress. Assure them that most genital skin conditions are benign processes that appear more serious during acute episodes. Most can be cured or controlled given time and appropriate medical attention. If skin conditions are not contagious, inform patients so that they will not worry. If they are contagious, recommend that family members or sexual contacts, as appropriate, be examined and treated also. The use of condoms should be advised during acute episodes of herpes infections or when condylomata are present. All bedding and clothes must be washed when parasitic infestations are identified.

Systemic and topical medications are ordered for most genital skin diseases. These include antibiotics, antifungals, antivirals, antihistamines, and sedatives taken internally, as well as external-use antibiotics, antifungals, blistering agents, and pediculicides. Because most patients with genital skin lesions are treated as outpatients, give clear, detailed instructions about how to take the prescriptions. Explain each drug's action and potential side effects. To decrease cost, order generic names when possible, and fit the regimen into the patient's daily routine to improve compliance.

Topical medications should be used sparingly as prescribed. Creams and lotions should be rubbed in thoroughly. Ointments or powders, on the other hand, have a protective value and should be lightly applied to the skin. Patients may need a protective dressing to prevent soiling of clothes.

Topical medications are usually costly. Emphasize the need to follow directions exactly. Tell patients that if medications are not used often enough, they may be ineffective in curing or controlling the disease. The use of increased amounts, however, does not increase their effectiveness. In fact, topical medications can create problems. For example, cortisone cream, if used for an extensive period, can thin the skin and make it more susceptible to irritation and infection. The systemic toxicity of some drugs

such as podophyllin, gamma benzene hexachloride, and antifungal medications has already been mentioned, and possible sensitization and consequent allergic reaction has been discussed.

Physical measures also promote comfort. Warm, dry heat or warm soaks are prescribed when there is infection. Heat increases circulation to the affected area and enhances healing. Caution patients against very hot temperatures so as to avoid tissue damage to skin that is already injured. When itching or burning is a symptom (e.g., in dermatitis), cold compresses or tepid baths provide comfort. Cold temperature causes vasoconstriction and decreases localized inflammatory responses. Instruct patients to use soft material such as gauze fluffs or soft toweling and to keep the compresses wet. Warm or cold compresses applied for about 15 minutes several times a day should help relieve symptoms.

Explain the necessity of gentle contact in treating genital skin conditions and preventing extension of the lesions. Patients should avoid rubbing or scratching. Mild soap should be used for bathing. Suggest the daily use of an antibacterial soap if a patient is prone to carbuncles or furuncles. The genital area should be blotted dry after bathing and be thoroughly dry before applying topical medications. A hand-held blow dryer can be used to facilitate drying, but teach patients safety precautions to prevent burns. When blistering agents such as podophyllin or cantharidin are ordered, care must be taken to prevent damage to the surrounding skin. These medications should be applied to the lesions only for the prescribed time. Petroleum jelly can be applied to the skin around the lesions for protection before applying the medication.

Advise patients to eliminate predisposing factors that increase perspiration, humidity, and irritation from clothing. In noninflammatory conditions such as tinea cruris, witch hazel and cornstarch help reduce moisture in the perineal area. Nonperfumed talcs can also be applied. Cotton underwear absorbs perspiration better than does synthetic material. Soft, loose-fitting clothes may be more comfortable and reduce skin friction.

Tell patients to avoid factors that seem to aggravate symptoms. These may include stressful encounters, alcohol, caffeinated beverages, or spices, depending on the disease process. Direct contact with known irritants or allergens should be avoided.

Patients with genital skin conditions may feel

embarrassed, dirty, disgusted, and ashamed. The nurse's attitude will affect how they cope with the condition. Do not show revulsion or hesitate to touch patients. Listen to them and allow them to express feelings and ask questions. When a condition is chronic, such as psoriasis, patients will need constant encouragement to continue treatments.

Use written or other teaching materials to reemphasize information and instructions, and to serve as a reference for patients. Monitor treatment effectiveness and document objective signs regarding the appearance of the skin condition as well as patients' emotional response.

Instruct patients to notify the physician of any unusual reactions, either systemic or localized. Encourage follow-up visits with the physician and explain the necessity of additional tests that he or she may suggest (e.g., proctoscopy when perianal condylomata are present). A gynecologic examination, including a Pap smear, helps detect other lesions, especially because an increased risk of cervical cancer is a recognized potential sequela. Any genital skin condition that does not heal or improve within several weeks needs further investigation by a urologist or dermatologist.

**Patient Outcomes**

1. The patient relates feelings of comfort after treatments.
2. The patient exhibits no signs of adverse reaction to the treatments.
3. The patient shows signs of skin improvement by the healing of genital lesions.
4. The patient verbalizes knowledge of the prescribed medications and treatments and demonstrates compliance with instructions for home care of a genital skin condition.
5. The patient expresses reduced feelings of anxiety about the genital skin disorder.
6. The patient expresses feelings about the genital skin condition and how it has affected sexual function and activity.
7. The patient is able to state the cause-and-effect relationship between predisposing factors and the skin condition, when appropriate, and indicate preventive action.

## REFERENCES

Allen, T. D. (1984). Testicular torsion: To avert a tragedy, don't wait for a diagnosis. *Consultant, 24*(3), 301–305.

Berger, R. E. (1992). Sexually transmitted diseases. In P. C. Walsh, A. B. Retik, T. A. Stamey, & E. D. Vaughan (Eds.), *Campbell's urology* (6th ed., pp. 823–846). Philadelphia: W. B. Saunders.

Bertram, R. A., Webster, G. D., & Carson, C. C. III. (1985). Priapism: Etiology, treatment, and results in series of 35 presentations. *Urology, 26*(3), 229–232.

Bickers, D. R., & Carney, P. S. (1987). Dermatologic diseases of the genitalia. In E. D. Kursh & M. I. Resnick (Eds.), *Urology* (pp. 85–99). Oradell, NJ: Medical Economics Books.

Bodner, D. R. (1987). Hydrocele in adults. In M. I. Resnick & E. Kursh (Eds.), *Current therapy in genitourinary surgery* (pp. 306–307). Philadelphia: B. C. Decker.

Bunce, P. L. (1983). Scrotal and intrascrotal surgery. In J. F. Glenn (Ed.), *Urologic surgery* (3rd ed., pp. 1099–1108). Philadelphia: J. B. Lippincott.

Callomon, F. T., & Wilson, J. F. (1956). *The nonvenereal diseases of the genitals.* Springfield, IL: Charles C Thomas.

Coldiron, B. M., & Jacobson, C. (1988). Common penile lesions. *Urology Clinics of North America, 15*(4), 671–685.

Collins, W. E., & Rosen, T. (1984). Pyoderma: Differentiating the infectious processes. *Consultant, 24*(9), 181–192.

Devine, P. C. (1991). Peyronie's disease. In J. F.Glenn (Ed.), *Urologic surgery* (4th ed., pp. 864–875). Philadelphia: J. B. Lippincott.

Durgin, J. M. (1983). Common dermatologic-drug reactions. *Journal of Practical Nursing, 33*(8), 21–25.

Edelsberg, J. S., & Surh, Y. S. (1988). The acute scrotum. *Emergency Medicine Clinics of North America, 6*(3), 521–546.

Epstein, E. (1983). *Common skin disorders* (2nd ed.). Oradell, NJ: Medical Economics Books.

Epstein, E. (1984). *Regional dermatology: A system of diagnosis.* New York: Grune & Stratton.

Finnerty, D. P. (1983). Orchiopexy and herniorrhaphy. In J. F. Glenn (Ed.), *Urologic surgery* (3rd ed., pp. 1061–1066). Philadelphia: J. B. Lippincott.

Ganti, S. W., Sayegh, N., & Addonizio, J. C. (1985). Simple method for reduction of paraphimosis. *Urology, 25*(1), 77.

Gikas, P. W. (1976). Uropathology. In J. Lapides (Ed.), *Fundamentals of urology* (pp. 110–165). Philadelphia: W. B. Saunders.

Harrison, R. M. III. (1983). Testicular torsion. In J. F. Glenn (Ed.), *Urologic surgery* (3rd ed., pp. 1067–1076). Philadelphia: J. B. Lippincott.

Hopkins, S. C., & Grabstald, H. (1986). Benign and malignant tumors of the male and female urethra. In P. C. Walsh, R. F. Gittes, A. D. Perlmutter, & T. A. Stamey (Eds.), *Campbell's urology* (5th ed., pp. 1441–1443). Philadelphia: W. B. Saunders.

Horton, C. E., Sadove, R. C., & Devine, C. J. (1987). Peyronie's disease. *Annals of Plastic Surgery, 18*(2), 122–127.

Kay, R., & Stewart, B. H. (1982). Hydrocelectomy. In B. H. Stewart (Ed.), *Operative urology: Lower urinary tract, pelvic structures and male reproductive system* (pp. 356–357). Baltimore: Williams & Wilkins.

Korting, G. W. (1981). *Practical dermatology of the genital region.* Philadelphia: W. B. Saunders.

Krane, R. J. (1992). Diagnosis and therapy of erectile dysfunction. In P. C. Walsh, T. A. Stamey, A. B. Retik, & E. D. Vaughan (Eds.), *Campbell's urology* (6th ed., pp. 3033–3072). Philadelphia: W. B. Saunders.

Krauss, D. J. (1985). Reduction of paraphimosis (letter to editor). *Urology, 26*(3), 337.

Kroovand, R. L. (1987). Hypospadias and chordee. In M. I. Resnick & E. Kursh (Eds.), *Current therapy in genitourinary surgery* (pp. 270–278). Philadelphia: B. C. Decker.

La Nasa, J. A., Jr., & Lewis, R.W. (1987). Varicocele and its surgical management. *Urology Clinics of North America, 14*(1), 127–135.

Langemo, D. V. (1985). Peyronie's disease. *AUAA Journal, 5*(3), 4–6.

Lerner, J., & Khan, Z. (1982). *Mosby's manual of urologic nursing.* St. Louis: C. V. Mosby.

Lue, T. F., Hellstrom, W. J. G., McAninch, J. W., & Tanagho, E. A. (1986). Priapism: A refined approach to diagnosis and treatment. *Journal of Urology, 136*(1), 104–106.

Macaluso, J. N., & Sullivan, J. W. (1985). Priapism: Review of 34 cases. *Urology, 26*(3), 233–236.

Malloy, T. R., & Wein, A. J. (1986). Surgery of the penis. In P. C. Walsh, R. F. Gittes, A.D. Perlmutter, & T. A. Stamey (Eds.), *Campbell's urology* (5th ed., pp. 2888–2914). Philadelphia: W. B. Saunders.

Malloy, T. R., & Wein, A. J. (1987). Laser treatment of bladder carcinoma and genital condylomata. *Urologic Clinics of North America, 14*(1), 121–126.

McConnell, E. A., & Zimmerman, M. F. (1983). *Care of patients with urologic problems* (pp. 174–175). Philadelphia: J. B. Lippincott.

Nasemann, T., Sauerbrey, W., & Burgdorf, W. H. C. (1983). *Fundamentals of dermatology*. New York: Springer-Verlag.

Nichols, P. (1988). Pathology of cancer of penis. In D. G. Skinner & G. Lieskovsky (Eds.), *Diagnosis and management of genitourinary cancer* (pp. 207–214). Philadelphia: W. B. Saunders.

Nickel, W. R., & Plumb, R. T. (1986). Cutaneous diseases of external genitalia. In P. C. Walsh, R. F. Gittes, A. D. Perlmutter, & T. A. Stamey (Eds.), *Campbell's urology* (5th ed., pp. 956–982). Philadelphia: W. B. Saunders.

Overlooked anatomy. (1984, April 15). *Emergency Medicine, 16*(7), 152–184.

Pantaleo-Gandais, M., Chalbaud, R., Chacon, O., & Plaza, N. (1984). Priapism: Evaluation and treatment. *Urology, 24*(4), 345–346.

Rosen, T. (1986). The alarming dermatoses. *Emergency Medicine, 18*(15), 22–60.

Rosen, T. (1988). Allergic contact dermatitis. *Emergency Medicine Reports, 9*(1), 1–7.

Sauer, G. C. (1985). *Manual of skin dermatology* (5th ed.). Philadelphia: J. B. Lippincott.

Smith, J. A., Jr. (1987). Condylomata acuminata. In M. I. Resnick & E. Kursh (Eds.), *Current therapy in genitourinary surgery* (pp. 129–131). Philadelphia: B. C. Decker.

Sonda, L. P., & Wang, S. (1988). Evaluation of male external genital diseases in the emergency room setting. *Emergency Medicine Clinics of North America, 6*(3), 473–486.

Stewart, B. H. (1982). Correction of lateral chordee. In B. H. Stewart (Ed.), *Operative urology: lower urinary tract, pelvic structures and male reproductive system* (pp. 374–375). Baltimore: Williams & Wilkins.

Stewart, B. H. (1983). Infertility and vas reconstruction. In J. F. Glenn (Ed.), *Urologic surgery* (3rd ed., pp. 1077–1097). Philadelphia: J. B. Lippincott.

Tanagho, E. A., & McAninch, J. W. (Eds.). (1992). *Smith's general urology* (13th ed.). Norwall, CT: Appleton & Lange.

Thomson, H., & Odell, M. (1979). Sclerosant treatment for hydrocoele and epididymal cysts. *British Medical Journal, 2*, 704.

When your patient has a scrotal problem. (1985, January 15). *Patient Care, 19*(1), 50–71.

Winter, C. C. (1991). Priapism. In J. F. Glenn (Ed.), *Urologic surgery* (4th ed., pp. 845–853). Philadelphia, J. B. Lippincott.

Yealy, D. M., & Hogya, P. T. (1988). Priapism. *Emergency Medicine Clinics of North America, 6*(3), 509–520.

# CHAPTER 12

# Erectile Dysfunction

■

*Cindy E. Meredith*

## OVERVIEW

Impotence, the inability to achieve or maintain a usable erection, has been a stigmatized subject for centuries. After years of relative neglect, this topic is just beginning to receive widespread attention from health care professionals (Gee, 1975).

Nurses play a unique role in working with men who are experiencing sexual dysfunction such as impotence. They are often the primary educators in hospitals and community settings and the caregivers after medical interventions such as surgery and pharmacologic treatment. There is a great need for nurses to be aware of cues patients may give that indicate a sexual concern, such as noncompliance with prescribed medications, anger or withdrawal from their partner, sexual acting out, multiple partners who do not satisfy their sexual needs, and blaming others for problems. Letting men know that they are not alone and that there are solutions for their problem is a major step in getting them to seek treatment. In addition, recognizing that the major cause of impotency is *physical* rather than emotional brings considerable relief to a couple.

Nurses should also be aware of the emotional impact of a physical problem—it can become a Catch-22 of disappointment and denial. Impotence is a complex problem to diagnose and treat. Treatment may take months and sometimes years to complete, and there are no guarantees. Emotional counseling is often needed for patients experiencing the evaluation process and may also be indicated following treatment.

This chapter discusses the care of impotent men from a urologic nursing perspective. Because the focus is urologic, treatment interventions are directed toward those men with physiologic rather than psychological impotence.

## BEHAVIORAL OBJECTIVES

After studying this chapter, the reader should be able to

1. Identify physiologic factors involved in the sexual dysfunction known as impotence.

2. Distinguish frequently prescribed diagnostic tests used to assess impotence.

3. Differentiate between approved and experimental forms of treatment.

4. Formulate appropriate nursing diagnosis and treatment plans for the patient experiencing impotence.

## KEY WORDS

**Ejaculation**—the muscular propulsion of semen (containing sperm) down the urethra, often accompanied by an orgasmic sensation.

**Erection**—a firmness of the penis resulting from the corpora cavernosa's filling with blood. It is generally caused by the interaction of emotions, hormones, nerves, and blood flow.

**Impotence**—the inability to achieve or maintain a usable penile erection. It is not infertility or the inability to ejaculate.

**Orgasm**—a pleasurable sensation generally associated with rhythmic contractions of the perineal muscles and the base of the penis. It may also be a psychological means of achieving pleasure, as in the absence of tactile sensations or loss of ejaculation.

**Sexual intercourse**—the physical union of the genitalia, often ending in an orgasm for one or both partners.

## PERSPECTIVE ON ERECTILE DYSFUNCTION

The diagnosis and treatment of impotence have changed radically in the past 5 to 10 years. In the 1970s it was believed that 80% to 90% of all impotence was psychologically induced. Because of technologic advances, physical causes of impotence are now being identified in more than 50% of the documented cases.

As other areas of medical science have advanced in treatment modalities, physical impotence has been the secondary result. The causes are increasing at an alarming rate for all levels of the age continuum.

In the older male population, quality of life has allowed men to stay active in their 70s, 80s, and even 90s. Along with these positive changes has come an increasing desire to stay sexually active, regardless of the physiologic changes associated with aging (e.g., arteriosclerosis and an increased need for medications). The middle-aged group is being affected by the advances medical science has made in such areas as organ transplants, chemotherapy, and radical surgical techniques. Young men are increasingly experiencing the problem owing in part to traumatic injuries and problems with substance abuse.

The problem of impotence now affects 1 in 8 men in the United States. Each year the number of cases increases. It is imperative that health care professionals remain informed about the problem of physical impotence and its impact on people's lives.

## Etiology

The factors involved in producing a penile erection sufficient for sexual intercourse are complex and involve both the mind and the body. The mind may be willing and ready for intercourse, but if the body is incapable of producing an erection owing to a physiologic problem, then all the wishing in the world will not produce a satisfactory response. The converse situation may exist when the body is physically capable of functioning but the mind is occupied with stress or depression. It is important to examine both the psychological and physical components of sexual functioning to provide optimal patient care.

## PSYCHOLOGICAL CAUSES OF IMPOTENCE

Stress, fear of failure, performance anxiety, anger, depression, loss of self-esteem, and breakdown in communication are some of the many emotional factors that may interfere with achieving an erection. Unfortunately, a Catch-22 situation often results, because one episode of failure often leads to a second or third, until the behavior becomes self-defeating. To avoid failure, the man may withdraw emotionally from the partner, thus creating additional stressors in his life. When a man fails to achieve an erection, he perceives himself as a failure not only in his own eyes but in those of the partner as well. A man cannot fake an erection—it is either present and usable, or it is not. When lack of erection occurs, both partners are painfully aware of the failure.

Women in all age categories expect and often even demand sexual satisfaction. A tremendous burden is placed on a man to engage in sex more frequently and with greater skill. If he is unable to satisfy the partner, additional anxiety is experienced, and impotence is often the result. The harder he tries, the more likely he is to fail. According to Brooks and Brooks (1985, p. 59), "Throughout history the single most consistent factor contributing to impotence has been the level of cultural demand for male sexual performance. At no time has this demand been greater than it is today."

Negative psychological factors may interfere with any man's ability to function. He may be in excellent physical condition, but unless his mind is also experiencing good health, then psychological impotence often occurs. High levels of stress may actually cause a physiologic response by increasing catecholamines and blocking sympathetic response.

Much of the psychological component of male sexual functioning may be summed up in the following statement:

In our society, as in almost every other society that has ever existed, manhood is a conditional attribute. The possession of a penis is necessary but not sufficient; you still had to prove, and keep on proving, that you were worthy (Zilbergeld, 1978, p. 15).

Zilbergeld (1978) discussed what he labels the fantasy model of sex. Included in the discussion is a presentation of 10 male myths. It is helpful to become aware of these myths when approaching the topic of loss of sexual functioning. Unless one understands some of the underlying thinking of many men, and some women as well, it is difficult to know how to assess the problem, much less develop a plan of care or interventions. The first myth discusses the age-old concept of "big boys don't cry." Many men have great difficulty expressing their feelings, both verbally and sexually. The result is a lack of knowing how to express concerns related to sexual function or dysfunction. Women rarely experience difficulty in communicating the need for a hug or a kiss or wanting to be left alone—the old "not tonight" routine.

The second myth addresses the issue of performance. Books are filled with techniques and national averages related to topics such as frequency of intercourse, achieving high levels of pleasure, and finding the "G spot." Unfortunately, most authors do not point out that sexual expression and even degrees of pleasure are very individualized. Time, the aging process, medical conditions, environmental factors, emotional issues, and stressors all play a part in the ability to function and enjoy the sexual experience. Most women indicate that the elements of foreplay—not the erectness of the penis—provide them with the greatest amount of pleasure. "Sex can be whatever you and your partner want it to be at the moment, whatever best expresses and satisfies the two of you" (Zilbergeld, 1978, p. 38).

Many men are still operating under the misconception of the third myth, which relates to the man taking charge of and orchestrating sexual performance. Today women are beginning to change many of the old traditions concerning dating and taking the initiative to begin sexual activity. However, many men still feel they should be in charge and be able to provide all that is needed for sexual pleasure. This situation creates tremendous tension for both partners and further accentuates any sexual dysfunction that may exist.

The fourth myth, a popular one for most people, especially since the advent of James Bond, is the notion that a man is always ready, willing, and able to engage in sexual activity. Television is constantly promoting the image of this type of man and begins to convince us that this is fact rather than Madison Avenue hype. It is perfectly normal for a man to be interested or concerned with issues other than sexual intercourse. We need to start being more realistic about our expectations. The magazines are full of articles discussing "burn out" and eliminating the myth of "Super Mom, Super Woman." When are we going to allow men the freedom to eliminate the myth of "Super Jock?"

The fifth myth was perpetuated in the warning given every young girl as she reached puberty; that is, "all physical contact must lead to sex." It is the old adage of "don't sit on a guy's lap or turn him on unless you're ready to deal with the consequences." Although it is true that young men in their adolescent years are easily aroused by contact with the opposite sex, these factors change over time. Unfortunately, the concept is so ingrained in us that when intercourse is not possible, many men will withdraw all physical contact from their partner and avoid any form of intimacy. At a time when human touching between two people should bring a sense of caring and warmth, it is withheld to avoid more "pain."

A popular myth is the one that simply states "sex equals intercourse." This is an instance in which it is so important to understand definitions. What do we mean by sex, and what does intercourse convey? Sex, defined most broadly, is how we view ourselves as male or female, that is, gender identification. We choose to express it in a variety of ways, such as by our clothes, manners, and associations. Intercourse, on the other hand, is the physical union of the genitalia, often ending in an orgasm for one or both partners.

The seventh myth follows the previous one in that it promotes the idea that an erection is necessary for sexual activity. Although sexual intercourse generally is performed with an erect penis, other techniques such as oral stimulation, sexual devices, and manual stimulation can achieve the same goal: an orgasm or a pleasurable sensation. Again, an undue amount of pressure may be placed on a man if the only form of sexual pleasure the couple has experienced is through intercourse.

The eighth myth is related to intensity. It indicates that as the pleasurable feelings one experiences through foreplay accelerate, the ultimate pleasure is achieved through intercourse. Stories abound on the subject of overwhelming passion and the ultimate release that takes place as a result of ejaculation and orgasm. There are also high school stories handed down from each generation about "blue balls" or "lover's nuts" as a consequence of not completing the act after becoming excited. What about patients with a spinal cord injury or diabetic neuropathy or those who have had prostate surgery? Does this mean they can never experience sexual pleasure? If this myth is believed, then there is no joy of sex for them.

Sex should be natural and spontaneous—this is another myth that may be somewhat controversial. Many people may argue that spontaneous sexual activity is the most fun. However, we need to learn about sexual functioning and how to experience the greatest pleasure before it can be truly enjoyed. The first sexual encounter may no doubt be memorable but not necessarily pleasurable. Patients experiencing disabilities related to factors such as immobility, cardiac limitations, and ostomies often must make sexual activities a planned event to fully enjoy the experience.

The final myth states that the preceding myths no longer influence people; this is the most unfortunate one of all. Without a doubt, many of the other myths not only still exist but also influence much of our thinking about sexual activity. Hopefully, through education and discussion, positive changes can be brought about for today's sexually active couples.

## PHYSIOLOGIC CAUSES OF IMPOTENCE

### Vascular Causes

The diameter of the vessels inside the corpora cavernosa has been stated to be the size of a pencil lead. It is no wonder that trauma or arteriosclerotic changes may prevent an adequate flow of blood into the penis. An occlusion of the blood supply to the penis at either the proximal or the distal end may cause erectile dysfunction (Baum, 1987b).

Arteriosclerosis of pelvic blood vessels interferes with blood flowing into the corpora cavernosa. It is a gradual process, generally associated with increased age. However, today's stressful lifestyles and poor dietary habits are contributing to an increase in the incidence of vascular problems at an earlier age. Any time a patient demonstrates evidence of arteriosclerotic changes, regardless of age, a thorough pelvic and penile circulatory examination should be performed.

Hypertension has often been viewed as a primary factor in physiologic impotence (Shrom, 1979). The question generally arises as to whether the problem is actually a result of decreased blood flow or the effects of the antihypertensive medication. When evaluating a patient with hypertension, careful consideration should be given to the timing of the onset of erectile dysfunction. Did the problem occur gradually or in direct connection with the implementation of a medication? A change in medication may bring about the desired results. It should be carefully emphasized to the patient that he should not experiment or change medications without supervision from his physician.

Cerebrovascular disease as well as cerebrovascular accidents have been implicated as a cause of impotence, most likely related to a decrease in cerebral cortical output (Fletcher & Martin, 1982). Aortic aneurysm, although located in a completely different area of the body, is another vascular problem that may affect penile erections. Less common vascular diseases that may result in impotency are Leriche's syndrome, sickle cell anemia, leukemia, and Hodgkin's disease.

In addition, it should be kept in mind that *anything* that interferes with blood flow into or out of the penis results in erectile dysfunction. According to Zorgniotti (1989, p. 468), "Insufficient blood flow to the corpus cavernosum or insufficiency in outflow restriction is the ultimate cause of all erectile failure, regardless of which etiology is assigned to the impotence." Most often in the past, problems were identified with inadequate amounts of blood flowing into the penis. Today, not only the filling process but also the need for adequate internal pressure to maintain the erection is being evaluated.

It is easy to understand the role of obstructed blood flow in not achieving an adequate erection, as in arteriosclerosis. Without the dilatation and increased flow of blood under pressure into the corpora cavernosa, an adequate erection does not occur. A discovery in the early 1980s demonstrated a phenomenon known as the *pelvic steal syndrome* that indicates a problem in maintaining an erection. According to Goldstein, Siroky, Nath, McMillan, Menzoian, and Krane (1982) and Goldwasser, Carson, Braun, and McCann (1985), the pelvic steal syndrome occurs when exercise, such as coital movement in the "missionary position," requires blood to be shunted into the lower extremities, diverting it from the pelvic arteries. The result is loss of erection. This particular problem may now be diagnosed using a simulation exercise technique before testing penile blood flow.

A similar but somewhat different problem is the venous or cavernous leak. Lack of venous compression creates this problem. The blood flowing into the arteries may be sufficient to achieve an erection, but there is not enough pressure exerted on the veins to compress them and prevent the blood from leaving the area. The venous or cavernous leak is now the most widely recognized problem, although the exact cause is unknown (Zorgniotti, 1989). A few cases have been attributed to congenital anomalies of the cavernous veins, fibrosis of the sinusoids due to aging, Peyronie's disease, traumatic lesion of the artery, or inadequate production of cavernous neurotransmitters such as norepinephrine and vasoactive intestinal polypeptide (Blanco et al., 1990; Krauss, 1983; Wespes & Schulman, 1987).

In the category of vascular causes of impotence, the effects of nicotine and caffeine on the blood supply to the penis should be considered. It is widely accepted that nicotine and caffeine act as vasoconstrictors. However, until recently, no strong conclusions have been made to link these factors independently to impotence. In a study by Condra, Morales, Owen, Surridge, and Fenemore (1986), the percentage of heavy smokers among the impotent population was more than twice the level that could be predicted from available population data. Further testing demonstrated a statistically significant difference on a measure of penile vascular functioning between smokers and nonsmokers. Smokers had lower penile blood flow than nonsmokers. Another interesting finding was that a large number of impotent men who were nonsmokers at the time of their impotency evaluation workup had long-standing histories of heavy smoking (more than two packs per day). The primary effects of nicotine and caffeine are on the small vessels and certainly should be considered as possible contributing factors in an impotency evaluation (Shabsigh et al., 1991).

## Neurologic Causes

Both the sympathetic and parasympathetic nervous systems are involved in achieving a usable erection along with various neurotransmitter substances (e.g., nitric oxide, guanylate cyclase cyclic system).

The loss of nerve innervation, injury such as trauma or surgery, and intervention with various medications interfere with normal physiologic functioning.

Conditions most closely associated with nerve impairment are indicated in Table 12–1.

**TABLE 12–1. Neurologic Causes of Impotence**

Multiple sclerosis
Parkinson's disease
Peripheral neuropathies
Sympathectomy
Trauma to spinal cord
Tumors or transection of the spinal cord
Spina bifida
Electroshock therapy
Temporal lobe lesions
Tabes dorsalis
Cerebral palsy
Amyotrophic lateral sclerosis
Myasthenia gravis

## Genitourinary Causes

Under the topic of genitourinary causes of impotence is included a variety of conditions affecting only males. The most transient of the group is prostatitis, because the resultant impotence is often resolved following antibiotic therapy. Unfortunately, prostatitis that recurs over a period of years generally leads to permanent problems with erection. Although it must be noted that fear of failure is a factor in repeated cases of loss of erection, such as those associated with prostatitis, it should not be eliminated from the list of *physiologic* causes of impotency.

Peyronie's disease is a common cause in the list of genitourinary disorders. A simple definition of Peyronie's disease indicates a decrease in blood flow into one or both corporal bodies causing a bent or crooked penis. The cause is uncertain, ranging from traumatic injury to the penis to sclerotic changes in the area around the corporal bodies (Vorstman & Lockhart, 1987). Men as young as 17 years of age have experienced the condition; however, it can occur at any age. The condition may have existed for years before a man seeks help. Generally, help is sought only after the erection becomes impossible to use because of pain or a curvature so severe that penetration cannot take place.

Prolonged priapism that must be medically or surgically reversed can also lead to permanent impotence. The factor in this instance is generally the tissue damage resulting from blood clotting in the vascular spaces that leads to fibrosis or necrosis.

Conditions such as phimosis, testicular torsion, varicocele, and hydrocele also appear in the literature but lack substantial numbers to warrant further discussion (Mims, 1980; Shrom, 1979).

## Endocrine Causes

The primary endocrine cause of impotence is diabetes mellitus, followed by pituitary disorders (resulting in a low testosterone or high prolactin level), primary gonadal failure, thyroid and adrenal abnormalities, ingestion of female hormones, and obesity (Braunstein, 1983; Cooper, 1984).

It is estimated that as many as 60% of diabetic men will eventually become impotent (Cooper, 1984; Newman & Marcus, 1985). There is controversy as to whether the primary cause is the vascular changes resulting from diabetes or whether neuropathy is the mediating factor (Bovington, 1983; Lehman & Jacobs, 1983; Lin & Bradley, 1985; Mims & Swenson, 1980). Other effects of diabetes on sexual functioning may include retrograde ejaculation and a lack of tactile sensation in feeling a climax or orgasm. These factors should be kept in mind when discussing treatment options with a diabetic man who has become impotent. Often there may be unrealistic expectations as to the extent of functional restoration that is possible following the onset of physical impotence related to diabetes.

Abnormalities of the hypothalamus-pituitary-gonad axis are the second most prevalent endocrine factors related to male impotence. Within this category are pituitary tumors, hypopituitarism-hypogonadism (i.e., hypoandrogenism), and hyperprolactinemia (Baum, 1987a; Braunstein, 1983; McConnell & Zimmerman, 1983). The primary element within this category is the lowering of testosterone levels by an increase in prolactin production. When prolactin levels are elevated, a decrease in testosterone production results (normal plasma testosterone level is 350–800 ng/mL). Hyperprolactinemia may result from pituitary tumors, trauma, surgery, drugs, hypothyroidism, renal disease, hemodialysis, or idiopathic causes (Baum, 1987a; Maatman & Montague, 1986).

Primary hypogonadism is rarely a cause of impotence. Klinefelter's syndrome is one of the few recognized congenital causes of hypogonadism. Secondary hypogonadism may be the result of mumps, orchitis, radiation, cytotoxic chemotherapy, vascular disease, or surgical intervention (Braunstein, 1983; McKendry et al., 1983).

Cushing's syndrome and Addison's disease are two additional endocrine disorders that often result in impotence, possibly owing to reduced plasma testosterone levels (McKendry et al., 1983). Hyperthyroidism is another condition that results in 40% to 56% of the men becoming impotent; an increase in the plasma-free estradiol–plasma-free testosterone ratio is believed to be the contributing factor (Braunstein, 1983; McKendry et al., 1983).

In men with gross obesity (body weight exceeding the ideal by 160% or more), there is a significant decrease in plasma testosterone and an increase in estradiol levels (Kley et al., 1980; McKendry et al., 1983). These negative changes may generally be reversed and testosterone levels returned to normal after weight loss.

## Cardiorespiratory Causes

For a usable erection to occur, there must be adequate blood flow to the pelvic region and the penis in particular. Problems with an erection may be the result of inadequate blood flow into the penis or insufficient vascular pressure within the penis that permits the blood to stay trapped in the corporeal bodies until sexual activity is completed. This means that any factor that restricts penile blood flow or promotes venous leak will result in physical impotence.

Although arteriosclerosis is a well-established factor in reducing blood flow, there are numerous other culprits in this scheme, including myocardial infarction, angina, coronary insufficiency, and congestive heart failure. Many of the disease processes are further complicated by medications that may also cause impotence (see section on medications and substance abuse).

The chronic obstructive type of emphysema has also been implicated in impotence; however, it remains a question as to whether activity intolerance and shortness of breath or the disease process itself is the primary agent. Many of the patients with emphysema are not only limited in their activity but also may face psychological and medication factors. In a study conducted by Fletcher and Martin (1982), it was found that sexual dysfunction worsened as lung disease progressed and that in the absence of other commonly known causes, chronic obstructive pulmonary disease may indeed be associated with impotence.

## Anatomic Causes

Anatomic factors that may contribute to impotence are congenital anomalies of the penis such as epispadias, hypospadias, chordee, microphallus, or a short penis associated with bladder exstrophy. With the advances in pediatric urologic surgery to correct these conditions, many men may be spared the trauma of impotence later.

## Medications and Substance Abuse

The pathophysiology of medications and substance abuse as it relates to impotence is highly controversial. What may cause a lack of erection in one man may have no impact on another. There are five basic levels at which medications may affect the sexual cascade (Tables 12–2 and 12–3): (1) libido, (2) the erection itself, (3) ejaculation, (4) orgasm, and (5) detumescence.

Any patient who suspects that a medication is the cause of his sexual dysfunction must be instructed to consult with his physician. Discontinuing any medication without advice from a physician may result in negative consequences for the patient's overall health.

Table 12–4 lists a variety of medications that have been known to cause impotency. The list is far from being exhaustive and, unfortunately, continues to grow as new medications are developed.

## Surgical Interventions

There are few surgeries that are recognized as being a direct cause of erectile dysfunction. However, questions have been raised concerning certain surgical procedures that may indirectly result in a decreased blood flow to or nerve innervation of the penis.

The surgical procedures that most often result in impotency are abdominoperineal resection, cystectomy, radical prostatectomy (generally excluding the Walsh technique) (Walsh et al., 1983), pelvic lymphadenectomy, renal transplantation (Nghiem et al., 1983), sympathectomy, and transection of the spinal cord. All result in decreased penile blood flow or nerve innervation.

Other types of surgery have been implicated indirectly and need further investigation because of questionable findings. These procedures are transurethral resection of the prostate (Shrom, 1979), laminectomy, orchiectomy, herniorrhaphy, vasectomy, and heart bypass surgery (Nghiem, et al., 1983). It is indeed unfortunate that many lifesaving techniques have resulted in a loss of ability to function sexually in some men. The exact mechanisms creating the loss are not always known, but patients

TABLE 12–2. Effects of Medication on the Sexual Cascade

| SEXUAL CASCADE | DRUGS BY CLASS | EFFECTS ON SEXUAL FUNCTION |
|---|---|---|
| 1. Libido | Antihistamines | Sedation; anticholinergic |
| | Antidepressants | Sedation, mood alteration |
| | Antipsychotics (phenothiazines) | Alteration in perception, sedation; also cause increase in prolactin production |
| | Anxiolytics | Sedation, mood alteration |
| | Narcotic analgesics | Sedation, mood alteration |
| | Drugs of habituation | Change in object of desire |
| 2. Erection | Antihistamines | Sedation; anticholinergic |
| | Antihypertensives | Alteration in blood flow |
| | Anticholinergics | Block parasympathetic nerve transmission |
| | Antidepressants | Block sympathetic and parasympathetic nerve transmission |
| | Antipsychotics | Block neurotransmitters in brain |
| | Anxiolytics | Alteration in neurotransmitters, decreased muscle tone |
| | Narcotic analgesics | Block neurotransmitters, decreased muscle tone |
| | Drugs of habituation | Decrease physical condition |
| 3. Ejaculation | Antihypertensives | |
| | Antidepressants | |
| | Anxiolytics | Inhibit urethral contraction |
| | Narcotic analgesics | |
| | Drugs of habituation | |
| 4. Orgasm | Antihistamines | |
| | Antidepressants | |
| | Antipsychotics | |
| | Anxiolytics | Mood alteration via sedation |
| | Narcotic analgesics | |
| | Drugs of habituation | |
| 5. Detumescence | Antihypertensives | Alteration in blood flow |
| | Anxiolytics | Alteration in blood flow |
| | Narcotic analgesics | Alteration in neurotransmitters |
| | Drugs of habituation | |

TABLE 12–3. Medications That Decrease Male Libido

| CLASSIFICATION | EXAMPLES | USAGE |
|---|---|---|
| Hormones | Estrogens | Prostatic cancer |
| Steroids | Androgens | Muscle building |
| | Anabolic steroids | Deficiency replacement |
| Sedatives and hypnotics | Chloral hydrate, flurazepam (Dalmane), triazolam (Halcion), temazepam (Restoril), secobarbital (Seconal), pentobarbital (Nembutal), diazepam (Valium), alprazolam (Xanax), oxazepam (Serax), chlorazepate (Tranxene), chlordiazepoxide (Librium), meprobamate (Equanil, Miltown) | Anxiety, insomnia, muscle relaxant |
| Antidepressants | Amitriptyline (Elavil), lithium | Depression |
| Beta-blockers | Propranolol (Inderal), atenolol (Tenormin), labetalol (Normodyne), metoprolol (Lopressor) | Angina, arrhythmias, hypertension, migraine |
| Antihypertensives | Methyldopate (Aldomet), reserpine | Hypertension |
| Antilipemics | Gemfibrozil (Lopid), clofibrate (Atromide–S) | Hyperlipoproteinemia |

### TABLE 12–4. Medications That May Cause Impotence

| TYPE | AGENT* | TYPE | AGENT* |
|---|---|---|---|
| Antihypertensives and diuretics | Chlorothiazide (Diuril) | Antineoplastics | Busulfan (MyLeran) |
| | Hydrochlorothiazide (Esidrix) | | Cyclophosphamide (Cytoxan) |
| | Chlorthalidone (Hygroton) | Antiparkinsonians | Biperiden (Akineton) |
| | Triamterene, hydrochlorothiazide | | Bromocriptine (Parlodel) |
| | Dyazide, (Maxzide) | | Procyclidine (Kemadrin) |
| | Spironolactone (Aldactone) | | Trihexyphenidyl (Artane) |
| | Hydralazine (Apresoline†) | | Benztropine (Cogentin) |
| | Minoxidil (Loniten†) | | Levodopa (Larodopa, Sinemet) |
| | Methyldopate (Aldomet) | Antihistamines | Dimenhydrinate (Dramamine) |
| | Clonidine (Catapres) | | Diphenhydramine (Benadryl) |
| | Reserpine (Serpasil) | | Hydroxyzine (Vistaril) |
| | Guanethidine (Ismelin) | | Meclizine (Antivert, Bonine) |
| | Pargyline (Eutonyl) | | Promethazine (Phenergan) |
| | Phenoxybenzamine (Dibenzyline) | Muscle relaxants | Cyclobenzaprine (Flexeril) |
| | Phentolamine (Regitine) | | Orphenadrine (Norflex) |
| | Prazosin (Minipress†) | Commonly abused drugs | Alcohol |
| | Propranolol (Inderal) | | Amphetamines |
| | Metoprolol (Lopressor) | | Barbiturates |
| | Labetalol (Normodyne) | | Cocaine |
| | Guanfacine (Tenex) | | Marijuana |
| | Enalapril (Vasotec) | | Methadone |
| | Guanabenz (Wytensin) | | Narcotics (heroin, morphine) |
| | Atenolol (Tenormin) | | Nicotine |
| Anxiolytics | Chlordiazepoxide (Librium) | | Opiates |
| | Oxazepam (Serax) | | |
| | Diazepam (Valium) | Miscellaneous | Cimetidine (Tagamet) |
| | Clorazepate (Tranxene) | | Clofibrate (Atromide–S) |
| | Meprobamate (Miltown, Equanil) | | Ranitidine (Zantac) |
| | Lorazepam (Ativan) | | Disopyramide (Norpace) |
| | Buspirone (BuSpar) | | Digoxin (Lanoxin) |
| Antidepressants | Nortriptyline (Pamelor) | | Indomethacin (Indocin) |
| | Amitriptyline (Elavil) | | Aminocaproic acid (Amicar) |
| | Desipramine (Norpramin) | | Various estrogens |
| | Doxepin (Sinequan) | | Furazolidine (Furoxone) |
| | Fluoxetine (Prozac) | | Verapamil (Calan) |
| | Imipramine (Tofranil) | | |
| | Isocarboxazid (Marplan) | | |
| | Phenelzine (Nardil) | | |
| | Tranylcypromine (Parnate) | | |
| Major tranquilizers | Fluphenazine (Prolixin) | | |
| | Trifluoperazine (Stelazine) | | |
| | Prochlorperazine (Compazine) | | |
| | Mesoridazine (Serentil) | | |
| | Promazine (Sparine) | | |
| | Chlorpromazine (Thorazine) | | |
| | Thioridazine (Mellaril) | | |
| | Haloperidol (Haldol) | | |
| | Fentanyl (Innovar) | | |
| | Thiothixene (Navane) | | |
| | Chlorprothixene (Taractan) | | |

*Generic name is shown with example of trade name following in parentheses.
†Least likely to cause potency problems.

need to be alerted to the possible outcome of impotence.

Age and general physical condition must also be considered as contributing factors along with the surgical intervention. A surgical episode that may have no negative effects on a younger man may result in impotence in an older man.

## Other Causes

Some causes of impotence may result in a temporary loss of erectile dysfunction, whereas others seem to have a permanent effect. Among more unusual causes is long-distance bicycling or riding a stationary bicycle (Solomon & Cappa, 1987; Weiss, 1985). Although the condition appears to be temporary, the resultant paresthesias and loss of erection are nonetheless frightening to the men who have had the experience. It is postulated that the impotence may have resulted from bilateral compression of the pudendal nerves or constriction of the blood supply to the penis. Some preventive suggestions offered by the authors were to lower the angle of the seat horn or to change positions frequently to relieve the pressure to the pudendal nerve and promote adequate blood flow.

Traumatic injury to the pelvic region or penis owing to auto or motorcycle accidents or even blows that are delivered during contact sports, such as football and basketball, may result in compression of the nerve or internal arteries (Kerstein et al., 1982; St. Louis et al., 1983). The most radical result of traumatic injury, whether surgical or accidental, is complete loss of the penis. In those cases in which the loss is self-inflicted owing to psychological factors, surgical repair generally is not performed.

## Pathophysiology of Impotence

To fully appreciate the problems associated with impotence, it is necessary to understand the basic physiology involved in a normal erection. As discussed in the section on etiology, erections result from a complex set of interactive components, yet the components need to be examined separately to diagnose and treat the problem accurately.

### PSYCHOLOGICAL COMPONENTS OF ERECTION

The brain is ultimately the sexiest organ in the body, for it is in the brain that the thoughts and desires for sexual activity begin. The libido—the sexual drive or desire for pleasure and satisfaction—is orchestrated by the limbic system in the brain.

The limbic system, the location of the libido in the brain, is responsible for a variety of automatic and somatic responses. Sensory sexual stimuli such as sight, hearing, touch, smell, and taste all are integrated in the brain and not only arouse pleasurable sensations but also stimulate an erection. Many men are "turned on" sexually by the smell, touch, or sound of a lover. The exact mechanism of this phenomenon is unknown.

Certain medications have been known to suppress the limbic system and libido and thus lower the desire to engage in sexual activities.

The hypothalamus is another important center in the brain that directly affects sexual functioning. By the release of luteinizing hormone, influence is exerted on the testicles to produce testosterone, which is a requirement for normal sexual functioning. Testosterone influences a man's desire for sexual activities. Lowered testosterone levels significantly decrease a man's willingness and ability to engage in sexual activities. He becomes much less aggressive in his behavior as it relates to sexual intercourse.

It must be kept in mind that a man may be capable of achieving a physical erection, but if he is psychologically distressed, or the libido is repressed, then a conscious erection may not occur. There is sufficient evidence to demonstrate that the mind and body work together as a unit.

### VASCULOGENIC COMPONENT OF ERECTION

To recognize how circulation affects an erection, it is important to understand the anatomy of the penis.

The blood supply to the penis originates from the hypogastric and internal pudendal arteries. The glans penis receives its main blood supply from the dorsal arteries. The fasciae and skin also receive most of their blood supply from the dorsal artery in addition to some from the external pudendal arteries. The paired cavernous arteries supply the corpora cavernosa, and the urethral arteries affect the corpus spongiosa (Fig. 12–1) (Klein, 1988; Newman & Northup, 1981).

The main areas that engorge with blood during an erection are the corpora cavernosa and, to a lesser extent, the corpora spongiosa (Fig. 12–2). The corpora cavernosa is a pair of spongy chambers that fill with blood during an erection. The function of the corpora cavernosa is purely erectile. Normally, the arterioles supplying these chambers are constricted, allowing little blood to flow in and keeping the penis in a flaccid state. When excitement or direct stimulation occurs, the arterioles dilate, the cavernous bodies fill with blood, the veins are constricted, trapping the blood in, and an erection occurs. An erect penis holds about eight times as much blood as does a flaccid one (Berger & Berger, 1987). In a full erection, the average pressure in the corpora cavernosa is approximately 90 to 100 mm Hg, and in the glans penis it is 40 to 50 mm Hg.

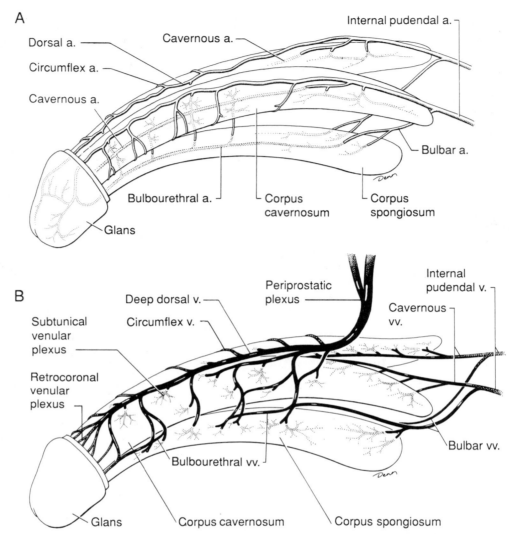

**FIGURE 12–1** Circulatory system of the penis. *A,* Arterial supply. *B,* Venous drainage. (From Lue, T. F. [1992]. Physiology of erection and pathophysiology of impotence. In Walsh, P. C., Retik, A. B., Stamey, T. A., & Vaughan, E. D., Jr. [Eds.], *Campbell's urology* [p. 710]. Philadelphia: W. B. Saunders. Reprinted by permission.)

There is some controversy as to the exact physiology of the circulatory system involved in achieving and maintaining an erection. According to Lue and Tanagho (1987), during erection, the sinusoids and arterioles relax, allowing more blood to flow into the corpora, distending the sinusoidal spaces and compressing the subtunical venous plexus against the tunica albuginea. An erection, therefore, is created when there is an increase in arterial blood flow, a relaxation of the sinuses, and an increase in venous resistance. Muscular contraction at the base of the penis further enhances the erection. Detumescence occurs when the arteries constrict, allowing the veins to empty the

penis. Lue and Tanagho (1987) use the following mathematical formula to denote the hemodynamic factors involved in an erection:

$$T = C / (A - B)$$

where A is arterial flow, B is venous flow, C is the total capacity of sinusoidal spaces, and T is the time required to achieve an erection.

## NEURONAL ELEMENTS

In the male, nerves receive signals from the senses and send messages to the brain, initiating the arousal process that results in an erection. The senses have a powerful influence over

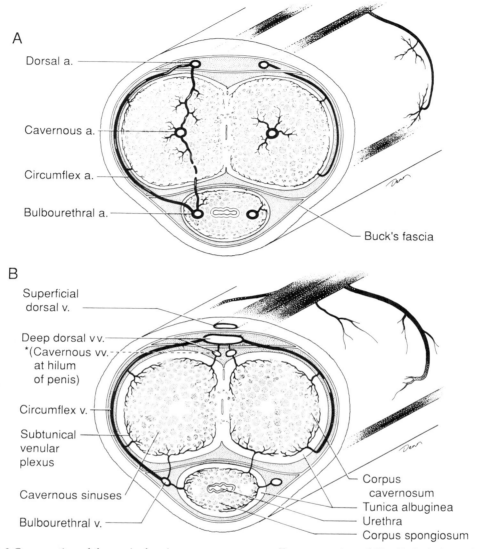

A

Dorsal a.

Cavernous a.

Circumflex a.

Bulbourethral a.

Buck's fascia

B

Superficial
dorsal v.

Deep dorsal vv.
*(Cavernous vv.
  at hilum
  of penis)

Circumflex v.

Subtunical
venular
plexus

Cavernous sinuses

Bulbourethral v.

Corpus
cavernosum

Tunica albuginea

Urethra

Corpus spongiosum

*FIGURE 12–2* Cross section of the penis showing corpora cavernosa. Transverse view of Fig. 12–1. *A,* Arterial supply. *B,* Venous drainage. (From Lue, T. F. [1992]. Physiology of erection and pathophysiology of impotence. In Walsh, P. C., Retik, A. B., Stamey, T. A., & Vaughan, Jr. [Eds.], *Campbell's urology* [p. 711]. Philadelphia: W. B. Saunders. Reprinted by permission.)

bodily responses—both males and females are often stimulated into an aroused state by the sight or touch of a lover. Smell, taste, and the sound of intimate communication may also initiate the process. In the male, the parasympathetic nervous system begins sending the signal to the penile arteries to expand, and the corpora cavernosa begin to fill with blood. If the nervous system is intact, and the penile circulation is normal, an erection occurs.

While awake, a man's senses and thought processes contribute to his ability to have an erection. Erections also occur during rapid-eye-

movement (REM) or dream sleep. The process begins at birth and should continue until the end of life. Because these involuntary erections occur during sleep, it is possible to differentiate nerve impairment from psychological impotence using monitoring devices. It is also possible to elicit a reflexogenic erection, as in the patient with a spinal cord injury.

The actual process of achieving an erection is innervated by the dorsal, perineal, and ilioinguinal nerves at the levels of S2, S3, and S4. The pudendal nerve provides the somatosensory aspect to the penis. There is an abundance of neural receptors located in the glans, pre-puce, and mucosa as well as the connective tissue of the skin and urethra.

Researchers are currently investigating the existence of multiple neurotransmitters in the corpus cavernosum, including prostaglandins, vasoactive intestinal polypeptide, acetylcho-line, nitric oxide, and other adrenergic sub-stances. Their exact action is not clearly under-stood at this time.

## HORMONAL BALANCES

There are three basic male hormones that in-fluence potency. The primary hormone is tes-tosterone. In males, the normal testosterone level ranges from 350 to 800 ng/dL. Functional levels vary for each individual. Testosterone generally remains at a normal level until ap-proximately 70 years of age, when it begins to decline gradually (Baum, 1987a). Testosterone is known to exert a strong influence on sexual desire or drive; it is not totally understood how testosterone affects an erection.

Two hormones produced in the pituitary gland also exert an influence on potency: Lu-teinizing hormone (normally in a range of 5–18 mIU/mL) stimulates testicular produc-tion of testosterone, and prolactin (normally <15 ng/mL), in large amounts, blocks the ef-fectiveness of testosterone and decreases sexual desire.

Studies are currently under way to investi-gate the influence of the hypothalamus-pitui-tary-gonad axis on sexual functioning. The physician may often evaluate the prolactin level or thyroid gland function to determine the cause of a low testosterone level. Any time hyperprolactinemia is found, a complete pitui-tary evaluation should be performed.

## Medical-Surgical Management

Most men experiencing impotence are look-ing for magic pills or potions. For this reason, it is important that health care professionals are knowledgeable about not only the effects of the treatment but also any possible complications or side effects. Unfortunately, there is no ideal treatment option.

### PHARMACOLOGIC THERAPY
#### Hormone Therapy

When a testosterone deficiency is present, ef-forts are first made to determine the cause of the deficiency, then treatment is begun. If the cause is a pituitary tumor or thyroid abnormal-ity, correction of these disorders often results in the restoration of normal testosterone levels. In the event that age or idiopathic causes are factors, hormone replacement therapy is the treatment of choice.

Testosterone is available as either an oral agent or an intramuscular (IM) injection. Do-sages range from 200 to 400 mg IM every 2 to 4 weeks, depending on the response. The first indication of a positive response is generally an acknowledgment on the part of the man that the intensity of the desire for sexual activity has increased and an overall sense of well-being is pervasive. It may take several weeks until a therapeutic level of testosterone is achieved.

It must be kept in mind that administering testosterone to a man with normal levels will act to suppress natural production and possibly make the problem of impotence more complex. Therefore, testosterone therapy should not be provided arbitrarily for erectile failure but should be used only for those men who are actually lacking in their own natural produc-tion of testosterone. Further, testosterone is contraindicated in men with cancer of the pros-tate or breast. A final drawback may be that desire may increase but the inability to func-tion may remain. Human chorionic gonadotro-pin, which stimulates the testicular secretion of testosterone, is another treatment option. In some instances it has been found to be more effective than treatment with androgens (Buvat et al., 1987).

If the problem is associated with an abnor-mality in the pituitary gland, such as a tumor, then surgery on the pituitary gland is indi-cated. Bromocriptine (Parlodel), a second form of treatment for high prolactin levels, is consid-ered experimental because the medication is not yet approved by the Food and Drug Ad-ministration. The dosage is 2.5 to 5 mg given three times a day at mealtime (Spark, 1983).

### Intracorporeal Injection Therapy

Papaverine or prostaglandin $E_1$ ($PGE_1$; al-prostadil) injections and, as yet untested, vaso-active intestinal polypeptide are nonsurgical treatment alternatives as well as diagnostic in-dicators (Kursh et al., 1988; Lakin, 1988; Nel-lans et al., 1987; Nelson, 1988. Papaverine is discussed first, because the greatest body of knowledge exists on this medication. The drug was first introduced in Europe in the early

1980s and was brought to the United States shortly thereafter. It was discovered that an injection directly into the penis would cause an erection. Papaverine, often used in conjunction with phentolamine (Regitine), acts locally on penile tissue by relaxing the arterioles (causing dilatation) and cavernous muscles and by increasing the compliance of the sinusoidal system. The result is a lowering of peripheral resistance, thereby allowing an initial inflow of blood to the cavernous bodies and then a trapping action that maintains the erection. The erection may last from 30 minutes to 4 hours. The usual injection dosage ranges from 30 to 90 mg of papaverine with or without 0.5 to 1 mg of phentolamine using a 26- or 27-gauge needle. The medication is injected at the base of the corpora cavernosa, alternating sites for subsequent injections. Some physicians advocate the use of a tourniquet at the base of the penis prior to injection to prevent systemic absorption of the drug (Zorgniotti & Lefleur, 1985). A reduction to 25 mg of papaverine mixed with 0.83 mg of phentolamine is generally indicated in neurogenic patients (Sidi et al., 1986). The most serious side effects of papaverine injection therapy are priapism and fibrosis of the corpora cavernosa (Larsen et al., 1987). Priapism (an erection lasting longer than 6–8 hours) generally responds to aspiration and irrigation with saline or intracavernous irrigation with combinations that may include epinephrine, dopamine, levodopa, phenylephrine, or metanephrine. The most severe form of priapism must be reversed surgically or the result will be edema, thrombosis, and, finally, tissue death. Other complications of papaverine injection may be transient paresthesia and hematoma at the injection site (Lue & Zorgniotti, 1987). Because of the potential complications involved, this form of therapy requires a well-controlled, well-monitored program and long-term follow-up (Lakin, 1988). Most of the intracorporeal injection therapy is currently initiated in an office or clinic setting, and after satisfactory results are achieved, the injection method is taught to patients for home use (Lue & Zorgniotti, 1987). Patients generally are limited to a maximum of three injections per week. Those patients with nearly normal arterial and sinusoidal systems have the best results. According to Lue and Tanagho (1987),

In theory this treatment will be effective in patients with psychogenic, neurogenic or hormonal impotence, and in those with a slight degree of vascular disease. In practice, of course, hormonal deficiency should be treated with hormones and psychogenic impotence with psychological consultation (p. 834).

Patients participating in any form of new treatment should be screened carefully and may be required to sign special consent forms acknowledging possible risks and complications. Careful patient selection is important. Lue and Tanagho (1987) have concluded that

This therapy is *not* recommended in antisocial, aggressive or suicidal patients, patients with sickle cell disease or trait, or a severe coagulation defect and users of aspirin or Persantine [dipyridamole], extremely nervous and anxious patients, or those who have dizziness, facial flushing or a decrease in blood pressure after an initial test dose (p. 834).

Even though $PGE_1$ is a newer form of intracavernous injection therapy (introduced in the mid-1980s), it requires guidelines similar to those for papaverine. The drug is available as Prostin VR, 500 µg/mL. The usual dosage ranges from 0.5 to 20 µg/mL diluted in saline and injected into the corpora. Trials with dosages as high as 100 µg/mL have shown good results and few side effects (Lee et al., 1989). It is believed the side effects will be minimal with prostaglandin, because it is a naturally occurring substance in the body. There have been no serious complications, such as priapism and fibrosis, among those patients using $PGE_1$, but the results of this treatment option should be followed. A newer combination of papaverine, phentolamine, and prostaglandin has resulted in good responses with lower dosages. The combination helps overcome the sympathetic responses. Papaverine and $PGE_1$ are also used as diagnostic indicators, often in conjunction with cavernosometry and cavernosography (Bookstein et al., 1987; Goldstein, 1987; Wespes & Schulman, 1987), to distinguish vascular from neurogenic impotence. When impotence is attributed to a severe vasculogenic problem, papaverine is generally incapable of creating an erection (Williams et al., 1988).

## Yohimbine

Yohimbine (Yocon, Yohimex) is derived from the bark of the West African *Corynanthe yohimbe* tree. According to the 1986 meeting of the International Society for Impotence Research held in Prague, Czechoslovakia, there is controversy within the medical community as to whether the medication is an aphrodisiac and mild vasodilator or simply a placebo. It is most often prescribed for those patients who are considered borderline cases, when it cannot be determined whether the origin is physical or psychological (Morales et al., 1987). For some men it has provided the measure of confidence needed to resume sexual activity. The basic ingredients of the drug may be found in most health food stores or mail order catalogs, under a variety of names. The danger in purchasing the medication from these sources is that often the exact ingredients and dosage are not listed on the label. If a patient is interested in trying this form of treatment, it is suggested that he obtain a physician's prescription and have it filled by a reputable pharmacist.

The basic action of the drug is to block presynaptic alpha$_2$-adrenergic receptors and decrease the outflow of blood from the corporeal bodies (Baum, 1987b). The usual dosage is 5 mg three times a day. As with any medication, patients should be instructed to inform their physician if any side effects occur. The most serious side effect to watch for is orthostatic hypotension owing to vasodilation.

## OTHER NONSURGICAL SOLUTIONS

### Home Remedies

There are a wide variety of techniques and remedies men have devised to achieve an erection. Unfortunately, many of them are either unsuccessful or may produce serious damage to the penile tissue. Among the various solutions men have tried are vacuum cleaners or a variety of objects such as swizzle sticks, pens, pencils, or eyedroppers inserted into the urethra (Berger & Berger, 1987), all of which may be unsuccessful and cause injury.

Among the less invasive remedies are high-powered vitamins (e.g., "Big Ox"), vitamin E and zinc, ginseng, oysters (high in zinc), or the age-old "Spanish fly," which can actually be dangerous or even fatal if ingested in large amounts (Brooks & Brooks, 1985).

Some men have spent hundreds of dollars on pills, potions, and books that claim to be a miracle cure. Health care professionals need to take an active role in educating the public about fraudulent and dangerous practices that are being advertised to men through the mail and in catalogs.

### Sexual Devices and Techniques

Sexual devices and techniques represent another noninvasive option for impotent men. The biggest impediment to this form of treatment may be the value system of the man or his partner or the inaccessibility of the products. Although visual imagery is available to any man, it may not be as effective as when it is combined with actual instruction, sensate focusing, or videotapes. Many of these techniques are enhanced when combined with sexual therapy and counseling. Sexual pleasure may also be experienced through the use of oral-genital stimulation or the penile-vaginal stuffing technique. Again, without some form of instruction, these methods may actually become additional forms of frustration.

The availability of penile rings, dildos, vibrators, and other devices may be limited in certain geographic areas, and some patients may not be aware of legitimate catalog sources. There are many people in this country who are trying to sell inferior products and services to these men through the mail. Nurses as health care professionals need to be alert to fraudulent products and educate the lay public to investigate all claims carefully before investing any money in a product, book, or pill that claims to restore normal sexual functioning.

### Suction Devices

There are a variety of devices, such as that shown in Figure 12–3, on the market that attempt to create an erection through the use of suction. A well-lubricated cylinder with a penile ring or tourniquet at the base is placed over the penis. Suction is applied to create a vacuum in the cylinder. Once an erection is achieved, the penile ring or compression device is slipped down onto the base of the penis, trapping blood in the corporeal bodies. The cylinder is gently removed, and the man is ready to engage in sexual activity. Caution should be exercised to remove the ring within 30 to 40 minutes to avoid tissue damage. Other side effects may be ecchymosis, priapism, and coldness of the penile skin. The device is most successful in men who have adequate penile blood flow. It is also considered a viable option for men who are poor surgical candidates. With a physician's prescription, the cost is generally covered by major insurance companies (Nadig, 1986; Turner et al., 1991).

Another device places a ring around the base of the penis and scrotum and then blood is pumped manually into the penis by exerting pressure in the perineal area. As with any device, patients should be advised to consult their physician before the initial use.

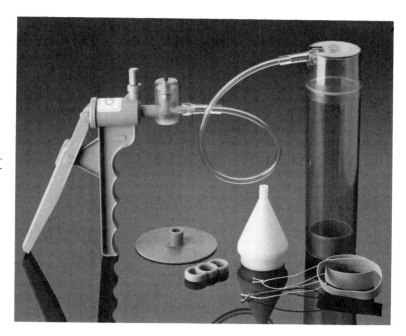

*FIGURE 12–3* VED vacuum device. (Courtesy of Mission Pharmacal Company, San Antonio, TX.)

## SURGICAL INTERVENTIONS

### Revascularization and Other Surgical Techniques

There are a variety of surgical techniques to achieve revascularization (Goldstein, 1987; McDougal & Killion, 1988; Wespes & Schulman, 1987; Schramek, et al., 1992). The primary goal is to re-establish circulation to the corporeal bodies. This may be accomplished through anastomosis of the inferior epigastric artery to the corporeal body or to the deep dorsal vein of the penis. Other methods may be employed to accomplish arterialization of patent distal penile arteries (Baum, 1987b; Bennett et al., 1986).

When proximal occlusion is present, the approach may be transluminal balloon angioplasty, endarterectomy, or bypass graft. An important factor to consider in any attempt to revascularize is the age of the patient. The older the patient, the greater the potential for arteriosclerosis. Attempting revascularization is temporary at best. Although the immediate results may be increased blood flow to a particular area, health factors, lifestyle, and medications may quickly reverse the process. The highest success rate for this type of surgery has been in the younger age group. New techniques involving laser and microsurgery are showing great promise but have yet to be tested over time.

Venous incompetence, or "venous leak," is most often treated by ligating the dorsal vein (Reiss, 1987) or combinations of veins (Williams et al., 1988). The success of vein ligation is questionable, and the long-term results are proving to be disappointing. The primary cause of failure is related to the body's natural tendency to form collateral circulation around blocked veins and arteries. Thus, the leak reforms as the collateral vessels develop.

The Nesbit operation is another surgical technique designed to overcome the impotence problem created by Peyronie's disease (Lemberger et al., 1984). The procedure basically requires excision of the plaque and sometimes placement of a dermal or synthetic graft. Success of the procedure often depends on the severity of the disease process.

### Penile Prosthesis

Penile prosthesis represents another surgical approach to the treatment of impotence. Generally, this treatment option is limited to those patients who are experiencing physiologic rather than psychological impotence. The primary rationale is that treatments for psychological impotence generally do not quality for insurance reimbursement, and a secondary consideration is the desire to try psychological counseling first if the problem is psychological in nature.

A penile implant is an efficient method of restoring erectile function. It should be empha-

## TABLE 12–5. Comparison of Penile Prostheses

| TYPE | ADVANTAGES | DISADVANTAGES |
|---|---|---|
| **Semirigid** | | |
| Small-Carrion | Simple surgery<br>Minimal complications<br>Low cost | Positionally always erect<br>Harder to conceal in daily activities |
| Hinged Finney | Simple surgery<br>Minimal complications<br>Can be concealed in daily activities<br>Firm penis hangs in downward position<br>Low cost | When in downward position, remains firm |
| **Malleable** | | |
| Jonas-Silver<br>Mentor<br>AMS 600<br>DuraPhase | Simple surgery<br>Minimal complication<br>Simplicity of design that closely approximates normal function<br>Malleability enables normal positioning in downward state<br>Low cost | When in downward position, remains firm |
| **Inflatable** | | |
| Scott-Bradley (AMS-700)<br>Mentor<br>GFS<br>UniFlate 1000 | Mimics the natural process of erection<br>Control over erections<br>More natural appearance | Mechanical failure (replacement may be necessary)<br>More expensive<br>Most involved surgical procedure |
| **Self-Contained** | | |
| Hydroflex<br>OmniPhase<br>FlexFlate | Same as inflatable<br>Less complicated surgery<br>Fewer mechanical parts | No increase in girth<br>Long-term complications unknown<br>Most expensive |

sized, however, that patients need to be carefully evaluated before being allowed to consider a penile implant as a treatment option. Unrealistic expectations can often lead to disappointment after surgery if a patient is not informed of all the advantages and disadvantages (Montague, 1989). No surgery can make a man 21 years old again, restore a bad relationship, or reverse retrograde ejaculation or neuropathy. A man must be aware of the limitations as well as the benefits of implant surgery. Another important issue to consider is the man's partner, if present. Satisfaction rates among recipients of penile implants tend to be highest when the partner has been involved in the decision-making process (Beutler et al., 1984). Penile implant surgery has been available in various forms for many years (Bretan, 1989; Gee, 1975); however, it was not until the early 1970s that technology made this a truly desirable option. For purposes of discussion, the implants are divided into three basic categories: (1) the noninflatables (rigid or semirigid), (2) the inflatable, and (3) the self-con-

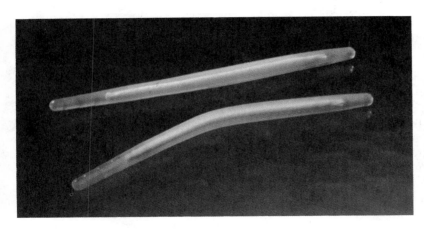

*FIGURE 12–4* Malleable ESKA-Jonas penile prosthesis. (Courtesy of Bard Urological, Bard, Inc., Spring Hill, NJ.)

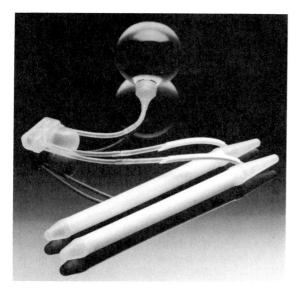

*FIGURE 12–5* AMS Inflatable 700CX three-piece penile prosthesis. (Courtesy of American Medical Systems, Inc., Minnetonka, MN.)

tained. Table 12–5 shows a comparison of the advantages and disadvantages among the types of prostheses, and Figures 12–4 to 12–7 illustrate the various products available. They all provide a usable erection after being implanted in the corpora cavernosa.

The surgical technique for implanting the devices may now be performed under local anesthesia in an outpatient setting on preselected patients (Scott, 1987). Special precautions are generally taken for diabetic and cardiac patients to prevent intraoperative and postoperative complications. All patients are placed on prophylactic antibiotics before surgery and 24 to 72 hours after surgery. All the penile implants are inserted into the spongy tissue of the penis (corpora cavernosa) that fills with blood under normal conditions. Because the penis of an impotent man does not adequately fill with blood, the space normally occupied by blood can be used for the implant instead.

The semirigid rods are made of silicone and may have a flexible metal core that allows the wearer to bend his penis down and fit it comfortably and inconspicuously into his clothing. Semirigid rods involve a simpler and less expensive surgical procedure than does the inflatable prosthesis (Nielsen & Bruskewitz, 1989).

The inflatable prosthesis is composed of two hollow silicone cylinders that are placed into the penis, a pump and valve that are placed into the scrotum, and a reservoir of liquid that is placed in the lower abdomen. A man can

discreetly fill the cylinders by gently squeezing the pump. A newer version of the inflatable prosthesis combines the pump and reservoir into one system that then activates the cylinders. Although inflatable prostheses are more complex, they more closely resemble a natural erection (Furlow et al. 1988, Merrill, 1989).

The self-contained prostheses are of two types: self-contained inflatable and self-contained mechanical. The former contains a fluid reservoir and pump within its cylinders, and the latter contains plastic segments, a spring, and a cable within its cylinders (Mulcahy, 1989; Stanisic & Dean, 1989).

## Alternative or Experimental Treatment Options

Technology in the area of impotence treatment options has accelerated greatly in the past 5 years. Tremendous mental and financial resources are being devoted to the area.

Several major drug companies are developing medications aimed at increasing libido. In

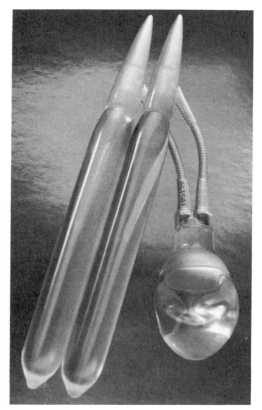

*FIGURE 12–6* GFS two-piece inflatable penile prosthesis. (Courtesy of Mentor Urology, Santa Barbara, CA.)

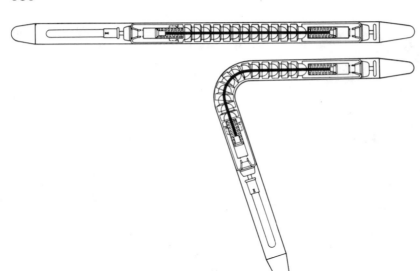

*FIGURE 12–7* OmniPhase self-contained penile prosthesis. (Courtesy of Dacomed Corporation, Minneapolis, MN.)

Germany, work is continuing on the development of an implantable device that will dispense papaverine or other substances directly into the corpora to produce an erection when the pump is activated.

Work is progressing in the development of an electronic genital stimulator. The primary beneficiaries will be patients with multiple sclerosis or spinal cord injuries. The device is expected to permit direct stimulation of the nerves by activation of a rectal probe to produce an erection.

# APPROACHES TO PATIENT CARE

Because the most widely used treatment options currently are implant surgery and intra-

corporeal injection therapy, these areas are the focus of this section.

## Penile Implant

### Assessment

In obtaining a medical-sexual history from the patient, care should be taken to ensure privacy and confidentiality before beginning the process. If the man is not a good historian, it may be helpful to ask his partner, if the patient permits, to verify surgical dates or major illnesses.

The information in Table 12–6 may be helpful in guiding the assessment and establishing the causes of the impotency, thereby providing evidence as to the appropriate treatment option for this person. The primary areas to be con-

**TABLE 12–6. Initial Medical and Sexual History**

| HISTORY | FINDINGS |
| --- | --- |
| Medical | Cardiac problems, diabetes mellitus, endocrine disorder, epilepsy, neurologic diseases (e.g., Parkinson's, multiple sclerosis), neuropathy, back problems (injury or surgery) |
| Surgical or medical treatment | Any surgery that interferes with blood flow or nerves to the groin area; radiation treatment |
| Genitourinary | Congenital anomalies, varicocele, hydrocele, Peyronie's disease, prostatitis, benign prostatic hypertrophy, neurogenic bladder, sexually transmitted disease, kidney disease or dialysis |
| Medication | Prescription and over-the-counter |
| Substance abuse | History and current use, type of substance, e.g., alcohol or recreational drugs |
| Lifestyle | Tobacco use, caffeine intake, exercise/weight patterns, change in job, stress factors, mental health care history, performance anxiety, depression |
| Sexual | Loss of erection with partner of at least 3–6 months; number and type of sexual partners; loss of nocturnal erections; methods used to achieve or sustain erections; level of sex drive |

cerned with in the history and physical examination focus on the medical-surgical history, genitourinary patterns, medications, evidence of substance abuse, general lifestyle patterns, and a sexual history. The examiner is compiling data that will indicate vasculogenic, neurologic, endocrine, and psychological factors. A thorough assessment must involve examination of both physical and emotional factors. To treat one without the other often results in dissatisfied patients and may contribute to the termination of a relationship of a patient with his partner.

The physical examination of the patient involves inspection and palpation of the genital organs for evidence of congenital anomalies, hormonal imbalance, or surgical interventions. The pulses and reflexes of all extremities are also examined for evidence of diminished or absent pulses or loss of nerve innervation.

New technology has greatly enhanced the diagnostic capability of the urologist in diagnosing erectile dysfunction. Basic testing begins with a blood profile, often including an SMA-18, testosterone, prolactin, triiodothyronine-thyroxine, fasting blood glucose or glycosolated hemoglobin, prostate-specific antigen, and prostatic acid phosphatase levels and others according to the patient history. Doppler studies such as the duplex-pulsed Doppler analysis with high-resolution ultrasonography may be used to rule out fibrosis plaque or calcification. The introduction of dynamic corpora cavernosography, cavernosometry combined with intracorporeal injections, and pudendal arteriography has advanced the diagnosis of venous leaks and filling deficiencies to a level of greater precision and permits a clear picture of the feasibility of microsurgery. Penile brachial pressure index or waveform analysis and penile plethysmography have also emerged as diagnostic indicators of circulatory function.

In the evaluation of nerve conduction, the biothesiometer, a simple electronic vibratory device that attempts to elicit the level of tactile sensation felt by a patient, is usable in any office setting. A more sophisticated level of assessment uses sleep tumescence monitoring. The most basic level of technology is a snap-gauge device placed at the base of the penis by the patient before sleep that is then observed the following morning to count the number of threads that may be broken. The next level of technology involves an electronic monitoring device placed at the tip and the base of the penis to measure changes occurring during REM sleep. The device is worn at home by the

patient and brought back to the physician's office for computer analysis of the results. Sleep laboratory studies are at present the highest level of technology in evaluating changes in nerve conduction that affect penile tumescence. Patients are required to spend 2 or 3 nights in a sleep laboratory center where they are monitored for not only tumescence or rigidity changes but also the presence or absence of REM sleep episodes. They may also be monitored for sleep apnea, electrocardiographic and electroencephalographic changes, and sleep patterns. Cost and availability of the studies generally determine the level of diagnostic testing performed before the implementation of a treatment plan.

Psychological evaluation is often a component in the diagnostic process. The evaluation may consist of an informal interview conducted by the urologist or require a complete psychological profile under the direction of a therapist or mental health care professional. Individual or couple counseling may be desirable before any medical intervention is implemented to achieve the highest possible level of satisfaction.

**Nursing Diagnosis**

The nursing diagnoses for the patient scheduled for implant surgery may include the following:

1. Altered health maintenance related to insufficient knowledge of surgical implantation of a penile prosthesis.
2. Altered comfort related to edema and ecchymosis of the penis and scrotum following implant surgery.
3. Self-concept disturbance related to perceived change in body image caused by penile implant surgery.

**Plan of Care**

Nursing care is directed toward enabling the patient to

1. Understand the preoperative and postoperative events involved in penile implant surgery.
2. Cooperate with nursing care plans to facilitate the healing process.
3. Implement measures to provide comfort to the perineal and penile areas.
4. Support a positive self-image regarding male identity and the return of erectile functioning.

**Interventions**

Penile implant patients should be allowed to view, touch, and ask questions about the various types of implants before making a final decision. Their decision may be guided by a health care professional who evaluates the lifestyle, physical and emotional limitations, and availability of their sexual partner. Participation in an educational self-help program designed for impotent men and their partners is often therapeutic. These programs are available in most states.

Urologists, sexual treatment centers, and some of the companies that sell implant devices have postoperative instruction materials and videotapes demonstrating the use of prostheses after surgery. Copies of these instructions may be obtained by contacting the implant companies or various sexual treatment centers. Patients should be informed about these instructions and review them with their physician to develop an individualized postoperative regimen (e.g., inflating and deflating schedule for the inflatable implants).

Medical identification cards are available with some of the implants. Patients should be instructed to carry these cards in their wallet at all times. In case of a medical emergency, this card could help medical personnel administer safe medical treatment to patients (e.g., by avoiding misinterpretation of x-ray study results owing to radiopaque fluid in inflatables or mistaking semirigid implants for priapism).

Preoperative and postoperative teaching for implant patients should include comfort measures and emotional support. They need to know that pain medication will be available after surgery. Encourage them to use medication before their pain becomes severe. They should be encouraged to keep their pain under control, which will allow them to relax, rest better, ambulate more freely, and promote faster healing. Instruct patients to support their penises on their abdomen using snug briefs or a supporter during ambulation. While they are lying down, the scrotal area should be elevated using ice bags for the first 48 hours postoperatively. Administration of analgesics or anti-inflammatory agents also alleviates discomfort. Individual postoperative instructions should be given to each patient by his physician in regard to resuming normal activities, hygiene habits, and resumption of sexual activities. Sexual intercourse is generally allowed 4 to 8 weeks postoperatively, depending on the patient's general health as well as the condition of the operative site. When intercourse is resumed, the patient should be instructed in the use of a water-soluble lubricant and possible positions that facilitate penetration with the

least amount of discomfort for both partners. If the female partner is menopausal and has not had vaginal penetration for a period exceeding 1 year, she may need to see her gynecologist for estrogen therapy or vaginal dilatation.

Penile implant patients need to be supported emotionally by their partners and members of the health care team. This is not a surgery for which they receive cards, flowers, or visits from friends because of the secrecy surrounding the problem. The nursing staff plays a key role in providing verbal encouragement concerning their decision regarding implant surgery. Patients should be provided with privacy and the opportunity to discuss their feelings and possible concerns surrounding their surgery. If possible, arrange for other patients who have had positive surgical experiences to talk with the patients before and after surgery. When patients demonstrate signs of maladjustment or unrealistic expectations, have a referral list ready to provide them with names of mental health care professionals who specialize in this area. The possible complications after implant surgery may be either physical or emotional.

*Emotional Complications.* Emotional complications may include the following:

1. Partner rejection: This may be related to the partner's not having been included in the decision-making process. Also, an infantile dependency relationship may disappear after potency is restored, and a partner's emotional reference points may be destroyed. In some instances the wife or partner never enjoyed sexual intercourse to begin with and does not welcome the thought of renewed sexuality. There have been cases in which implants were obtained for the benefit of girlfriends and not wives.
2. Depression due to unrealistic expectations of the implant or loss of the implant.

*Physical Complications.* The physical complications after penile implant surgery may include the following:

1. Pain postoperatively, which may last several months.
2. Genital edema and bruising, making it difficult for the patient to sit or wear normal clothing or to urinate normally.
3. Removal of implant due to infection, surgical complications, extrusion of implant, and mechanical failures. (Many of these patients may receive another implant later but must be prepared to deal with extreme depression [Meredith et al., 1987]).

### Patient Outcomes

1. The patient verbalizes a basic understanding of his preoperative and postoperative course.
2. The patient states relief of or decrease in pain.
3. The patient verbalizes reasonable satisfaction with the appearance and anticipated function of his penile implant.

## Intracorporeal Injection Therapy

### Assessment

Patients with neurologic disorders, mild circulatory problems, or lack of self-confidence appear to have the best response to injection therapy. Assessment for a patient who is a candidate for penile intracorporeal injections is basically the same as for penile implant surgery (refer to Table 12–6). Additional tests may also include an electrocardiogram, prothrombin and partial prothrombin times, and liver enzyme measurements to avoid potential cardiac or liver complications. Although the diagnostic screening is generally less extensive than for implant surgery (e.g., sleep studies may not be included), a careful psychological evaluation is extremely important. Any time a self-administered drug is used, the potential for abuse exists. Patients with a history of substance abuse or mental illness must be evaluated before instruction in home injection therapy is provided and may require continued monitoring before obtaining a refill of the prescription. Health care professionals need to be alert to the potential harm that may be self-inflicted (priapism) or other directed (rape). Patients who exhibit symptoms of anxiety, fear of needles, or low self-confidence may require several teaching sessions, assistance from a therapist or partner, or, in severe cases, exclusion from the program.

The patient is tested first with a low dosage of the medication to assess the effectiveness in achieving an erection and to determine the appropriate dosage. The goal is to achieve an erection that is sufficient for penetration and intercourse yet will subside within a reasonable period. An erection lasting less than 30 minutes is generally considered inadequate, whereas an erection lasting longer than 2½ hours is approaching the uncomfortable stage.

### Nursing Diagnosis

The nursing diagnoses for the patient receiving intracorporeal injection therapy may include the following:

1. Altered health maintenance related to insufficient knowledge of administration of intracorporeal medication to achieve an erection.
2. Self-concept disturbance related to dependency on injection therapy to achieve an erection.
3. Self-harm, high risk related to complications of intracorporeal injection therapy, such as priapism, fibrosis, and bruising.

### Plan of Care

Nursing care is directed toward enabling the patient to

1. Achieve a usable erection following self-injection therapy teaching.
2. Verbalize satisfaction with sexual performance.
3. Avoid obtaining an erection lasting longer than 2½ to 4 hours, without evidence of fibrosis or bruising.

### Interventions

Because the use of papaverine combination therapy or $PGE_1$ for intracorporeal injection therapy is considered experimental, it is highly advised that a detailed consent form be signed before any trial of the therapy. Consult the institution's legal affairs or risk management personnel for their recommendations.

After the patient's dosage requirements have been successfully determined and the appropriate level of medication has been prescribed for him, teaching may begin. Instructions should be presented in a clear manner, with written and visual illustrations used. It is also highly recommended that the patient demonstrate the complete procedure (using sterile saline) before any medication or supplies are dispensed. Patient teaching guidelines have been developed at various sexual treatment centers and may be available to assist in the presentation.

The number of intracorporeal injections currently is limited to a maximum of three per week to reduce the incidence of fibrosis. Patients should be assessed at regular intervals for evidence of fibrosis or indications of liver dysfunction. Having patients maintain a log of their injections will provide evidence as to the success of therapy, any complications, and validation of the current dosage. It should be noted that $PGE_1$ is light- and heat-sensitive and requires special handling, both in the clinic and by the patient. Patients should be instructed to keep their medicine bottle in the refrigerator, wrapped in foil or placed in a compartment with a door covering. Use of an insulated container facilitates traveling with the medication.

## PROCEDURE 12-1

■

## Reversal of Prolonged Erection

### ■ PURPOSE

To cause detumescence of an erection lasting longer than 1–2 hours under supervision, or 4 hours without supervision, or reduction of any erection that may compromise penile tissue.

### ■ EQUIPMENT

**Phenylephrine Method (Neo-Synephrine)**

1. Needles: (2) 19-gauge butterfly; (2) 27 gauge
2. Syringes: (2) 10 mL; (2) 20 mL with Luer tips; (1) tuberculin
3. Three-way stopcock
4. (2) Sterile kidney basins
5. (1) Straight catheter set with No. 14 Robinson Foley catheter
6. Medications
   a. Phenylephrine 10 mg mixed in 500 mL of physiologic saline
   b. Lidocaine 1% injection (without epinephrine)
7. Optional: IV connector tubing

**Metaraminol Method (Aramine)**

1. Needles: (2) 27 gauge
2. Syringes: (2) tuberculin
3. Medications
   a. Metaraminol 1 mg injection
   b. Lidocaine 1% injection (without epinephrine)

### ■ RESPONSIBLE PERSON

Physician assisted by trained personnel.

### ■ PROCEDURE

1. Assemble equipment.
2. Explain basics of procedure to patient; allay anxiety and gain cooperation.
3. Place patient in supine position with blood pressure cuff on arm; blood pressure must be monitored every 15 minutes during injection of medication.
4. Inject 1–2 mL of lidocaine 1% injection into base of penis and allow for penetration; assess patient comfort.

5. *Phenylephrine method*
   a. Aspirate 20 to 40 mL of blood from corporeal bodies.
   b. Replace same amount with phenylephrine irrigating solution, if detumescence has not occurred. (A tourniquet may be placed at the base of the penis before injection to minimize systemic absorption.)
   c. Irrigate corpora gently until detumescence has occurred.
   d. Monitor patient's vital signs every 15 minutes until stable.

5. *Metaraminol method*
   a. Inject metaraminol 1 mg injection into corporeal body, using 27-gauge needle.
   b. Monitor patient's vital signs every 15 minutes until stable.

## PROCEDURE 12-2

■

### Self-Injection Procedure

### ■ SUPPLIES

Alcohol swab or cotton ball
Medicine bottle
mL Syringe

### ■ PROCEDURE

1. After washing your hands, clean the rubber top of the bottle with alcohol.
2. Fill syringe with air by pulling the plunger back to the 1-cc mark.
3. Carefully take the cover off the needle.
4. Push the needle through the rubber top of the bottle and push the air in the syringe into the bottle.

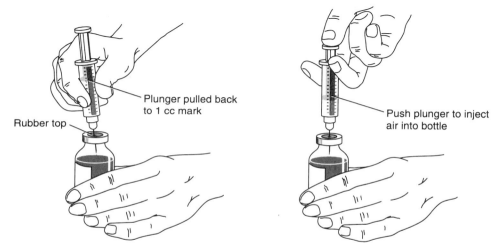

5. Turn the bottle upside down, keeping the needle inside the bottle.
6. Keep the tip of the needle in the medicine and pull the plunger back to the amount of medicine ordered by your doctor.

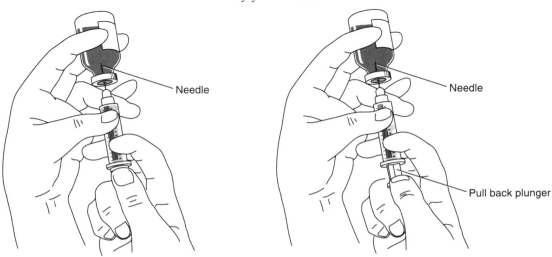

*Procedure continued on following page*

## Self-Injection Procedure

7. Push any air bubbles out of the syringe back into the bottle. Remember to pull the plunger back to the right amount of medicine.

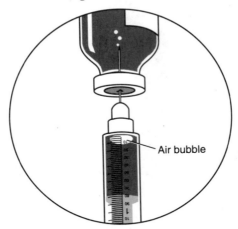

Air bubble

8. Take the needle out of the bottle and loosely put the cover back on the needle. (If you are using the shot at a later time, replace the cover tightly.)
9. Placing two fingers under the penis and your thumb on top, hold the penis against the side of your leg to provide support. Be sure not to twist or turn the penis. This will help you put the shot in the right place.
10. Clean the injection site off with alcohol.
11. Pick up the syringe and remove the cover. Inject the medicine directly into the side of the penis near the base (closer to the body).

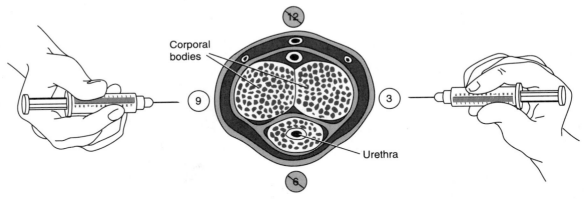

Corporal bodies

Urethra

   Picture a clock when injecting. Inject only at the 3 or 9 o'clock position. Use either hand to inject, and try to change sides with each injection.
12. Remove the needle; press the alcohol swab firmly over the site for 2–4 min.
13. Throw the syringe away carefully. Do not re-use the syringe and never put a dirty needle into your medicine bottle.
14. If you are using prostaglandin $E_1$ (PGE$_1$), return it to the proper storage area as soon as possible. Remember, it must be protected from heat and light.
15. Record the results of the medicine and report them to your doctor/nurse. If the results were not satisfactory you may need a change in your medicine dose or more practice in giving the shot.

An additional preventive measure for patients traveling out of their state or country is to provide them with written guidelines for the reversal of priapism (Procedure 12–1). In the event that such a problem might occur, they are directed to find the nearest emergency department and give the staff a copy of the reversal procedure (physician and clinic phone numbers should be included).

Initially, when a patient begins injection therapy, he may have concerns about the naturalness of the erections or the impact the resumption of sexual activities will have on his partner. Both of these concerns are valid and should be dealt with in a sensitive manner. Evidence is beginning to indicate that following injection of the medication, the erection response mimics the natural process, to the extent that any external distraction or emotional upset will diminish or eliminate the erection. An intervention that may be beneficial to both partners is a session with a therapist to discuss love-making techniques and encourage communication about sexual expressions as well as the relationship in general. Without communication between partners and realistic expectations as to sexual functioning, the treatment will not succeed. Medical science can now guarantee almost every man the ability to achieve a physical erection, but emotional satisfaction may be more difficult to achieve. Once successful intercourse has been resumed, self-confidence generally returns, leading to greater satisfaction.

Patients should be instructed carefully about selecting the proper injection sites and technique. Written instructions, including illustrations, will facilitate patient compliance (Procedure 12–2). Aseptic technique, using small-gauge (27–30) needles and site rotation, will reduce the risk of fibrosis. Instructing the patient to apply firm pressure over the injection site for 3 to 5 minutes will prevent bruising. Although bruising is not dangerous, it is not aesthetically pleasing.

There are various techniques for reversing priapism, beginning with conservative approaches such as localized cold packs, prostatic massage, masturbation, sedatives, analgesics, antispasmodics, or anticoagulants. Rapid treatment may include corporal aspiration and irrigation and the administration of epinephrine or metaraminol (Aramine) (see Procedure 12–1). The final approach involves surgical ligation or shunting and is generally reserved for extreme cases. If the patient's dosage requirements have been determined appropriately,

priapism should not occur, and reversal should not be necessary.

**Patient Outcomes**

1. The patient demonstrates proper injection technique using sterile saline.
2. The patient's log verifies the success of the injection therapy.
3. The patient states that emotionally satisfactory intercourse has been achieved.
4. There is no evidence of priapism, fibrosis, or bruising.

## REFERENCES

Anabolic steroid abuse. (October, 1987). *FDA Drug Bulletin, 17*(3), 26–30.

Baum, N. (1987a). Treatment of impotence: I. Nonsurgical methods. *Postgraduate Medicine, 81*(7), 133–136.

Baum, N. (1987b). Treatment of impotence: II. Surgical methods. *Postgraduate Medicine, 81*(7), 137–140.

Bennett, A. H., Rivard, D. J., Raymond, P. B., & Moran, M. (1986). Reconstructive surgery for vasculogenic impotence. *Journal of Urology, 136*, 599–601.

Berger, R. E., & Berger, D. (1987). *BioPotency: A guide to sexual success.* Emmaus, PA: Rodale Press.

Beutler, L. E., Scott, F. B., Karacan, I., Baer, P. E., Roger, R. R., & Morris J. (1984). Women's satisfaction with partner's penile implant. *Urology, 24*(6), 552–558.

Blanco, R., Saenz de Tejada, I., Goldstein, I., Krane, R. J., Wotiz, H. H., & Cohen, R. A. (1990). Dysfunctional penile cholinergic nerves in diabetic impotent men. *Journal of Neurology, 144*, 278–280.

Bookstein, J. J., Valji, K., Parsons, L., & Kessler, W. (1987). Penile pharmacocavernosography and cavernosometry in the evaluation of impotence. *Journal of Urology, 137*(4), 772–776.

Bovington, M. M. (1983). Neurologic complications in diabetes mellitus. *Nursing Clinics of North America, 18*(4), 735–746.

Bretan, P. N. (1989). History of the prosthetic treatment of impotence. *Urologic Clinics of North America, 16*(1), 1–5.

Brooks, M. B., & Brooks, S. W. (1985). *The lifelong lover.* New York: Doubleday.

Buvat, J., Lemaire, A., & Buvat-Herbaut, M. (1987). Human chorionic gonadotropin treatment of nonorganic erectile failure and lack of sexual desire: A double-blind study. *Urology, 30*(3), 216–219.

Condra, M., Morales, A. J. A., Owen, J. A., Surridge, D. H., & Fenemore, J. (1986). Prevalence and significance of tobacco smoking in impotence. *Urology, 27*(6), 495–498.

Cooper, A. J. (1984). Advances in the diagnosis and management of endocrine impotence. *The Practitioner, 228*, 865–870.

Fletcher, E. C., & Martin, R. J. (1982). Sexual dysfunction and erectile impotence in chronic obstructive pulmonary disease. *Chest, 81*(4), 413–421.

Furlow, W. L., Goldwasser, B., & Gundian, J. C. (1988). Implantation of model AMS 700 penile prosthesis: Long-term results. *Journal of Urology, 139*(4), 741–742.

Gee, W. F. (1975). A history of surgical treatment of impotence. *Urology, 5*, 401–405.

Goldstein, I. (1987). Vasculogenic impotence: Its diagnosis and treatment. *Problems in Urology, 1*(3), 547–562.

Goldstein, I., Siroky, M. B., Nath, R. L., McMillan, T. N.,

Menzoian, J. O., & Krane, R. J. (1982). Vasculogenic impotence: Role of the pelvic steal test. *Journal of Urology, 128,* 300–306.

Goldwasser, B., Carson, C. C., III, Braun, S. D., & McCann, R. L. (1985). Impotence due to the pelvic steal syndrome: Treatment by iliac transluminal angioplasty. *Journal of Urology, 133,* 860–861.

Kerstein, M. D., Gould, S. A., French-Sherry, E., & Pirman, C. (1982). Perineal trauma and vasculogenic impotence. *Journal of Urology, 127,* 57.

Klein, E. A. (1988). The anatomy and physiology of normal male sexual function. In D. K. Montague (Ed.), *Disorders of male sexual function* (pp. 2–19). Chicago: Year Book Medical Publishers.

Kley, H. K., Edelman, P., & Kruskemper, H. L. (1980). Relationship of plasma sex hormones to different parameters of obesity in male subjects. *Metabolism, 29,* 1041–1045.

Krauss, D. J. (1983). The physiologic basis of male sexual dysfunction. *Hospital Practice,* February, 193–222.

Kursh, E. D., Bodner, D. R., Resnick, M. I., Althof, S. E., Turner, L., Risen, C., & Levine, S. B. (1988). Injection therapy for impotence. *Urologic Clinics of North America, 15,* 625–629.

Larsen, E. H., Gasser, T. C., & Bruskewitz, R. C. (1987). Fibrosis of corpus cavernosum after intracavernous injection of phentolamine-papaverine. *Journal of Urology, 137,* 292–294.

Lakin, M. M. (1988). Therapeutic pharmacologic erections. In D. K. Montague (Ed.), *Disorders of male sexual function* (pp. 223–229). Chicago: Year Book Medical Publishers.

Lee, L. M., Stevenson, R. W., & Szasz, G. (1989). Prostaglandin E₁ versus phentolamine/papaverine for the treatment of erectile impotence: A double-blind comparison. *Journal of Urology, 14*(3), 549–550.

Lehman, T. P., & Jacobs, J. A. (1983). Etiology of diabetic impotence. *Journal of Urology, 129,* 291–293.

Lemberger, R. J., Bishop, M. C., & Bates, C. P. (1984). Nesbit's operation for Peyronie's disease. *British Journal of Urology, 56*(5), 467–478.

Lin, J. T., & Bradley, W. E. (1985). Penile neuropathy in insulin-dependent diabetes mellitus. *Journal of Urology, 133,* 213–215.

Lue, T. F., & Tanagho, E. A. (1987). Physiology of erection and pharmacological management of impotence. *Journal of Urology, 137,* 829–836.

Lue, T. F., & Zorgniotti, A. W. (1987). Patient guide: Treatment for impotence. *Medical Aspects of Human Sexuality, 21*(3), 29–30.

Maatman, T. J., & Montague, D. K. (1986). Routine endocrine screening in impotence. *Urology, 27*(6), 499–502.

McConnell, E. A., & Zimmerman, M. F. (1983). *Care of patients with urologic problems.* Philadelphia: J. B. Lippincott.

McDougal, W. S., & Killion, L. T. (1988). Corporeal arterial and venous insufficiency. In D. K. Montague (Ed.), *Disorders of male sexual function* (pp. 210–222). Chicago: Year Book Medical Publishers.

McKendry, J. B. R., Collins, W. E., Silverman, M., Krul, L. E., Collins, J. P., & Irvine, A. H. (1983). Erectile impotence: A clinical challenge. *Canadian Medical Association Journal, 128,* 653–662.

Meredith, C. E., Zaleski, S. M., & Fitzgerald, J. T. (1987). *ROMP coordinator's manual* (pp. 25–27). Detroit: Grace Hospital.

Merrill, D. C. (1989). Mentor inflatable penile prostheses. *Urologic Clinics of North America, 16*(1), 51–66.

Mims, F. H., & Swenson, M. (1980). *Sexuality: A nursing perspective.* New York: McGraw-Hill.

Montague, D. K. (1987). *Disorders of the male sexual function.* Chicago: Year Book Medical Publishers.

Montague, D. K. (1989). Penile prosthesis: An overview. *Urologic Clinics of North America, 16*(1), 7–11.

Morales, A., Condra, M., Owen, J. A., Surridge, D. H., Fenemore, J., & Harris, C. (1987). Is yohimbine effective in the treatment of organic impotence? Results of a controlled trial. *Journal of Urology, 137*(6), 1168–1172.

Mulcahy, J. J. (1989). The OmniPhase and DuraPhase penile prostheses. *Urologic Clinics of North America, 16*(1), 25–31.

Nadig, P. W. (1991). Vacuum devices for erectile dysfunction. *Problems in Urology, 5*(4), 559–565.

Nadig, P. W., Ware, J. C., & Blumoff, R. (1986). Noninvasive device to produce and maintain an erection-like state. *Urology, 27*(2), 126–131.

Nellans, R. E., Ellis, L. R., & Kramer-Levien, D. (1987). New treatment for impotence: Pharmacologic erection. *Medical Aspects of Human Sexuality, 21*(3), 20–28.

Nelson, R. P. (1988). Nonoperative management of impotence. *Journal of Urology, 139,* 2–5.

Newman, H. F., & Marcus, H. (1985). Erectile dysfunction in diabetes and hypertension. *Urology, 26*(2), 135–137.

Newman, H. F., & Northup, J. D. (1981). Mechanism of human penile erection: An overview. *Urology, 17*(5), 399–408.

Nghiem, D. D., Corry, R. J., Picon-Mendez, G., & Lee, H. M. (1983). Factors influencing male sexual impotence after renal transplantation. *Urology, 21*(1), 49–52.

Nielsen, K. T., & Bruskewitz, R. C. (1989). Semirigid and malleable rod penile prostheses. *Urologic Clinics of North America, 16*(1), 13–23.

Reiss, H. (1987). Role of spongiosography in study of penile veins. *Urology, 29*(2), 146–149.

Schramek, P., Engelmann, U., & Kaufmann, F. (1992). Microsurgical arteriovenous revascularization in the treatment of vasculogenic impotence. *Journal of Urology, 147,* 1028–1031.

Scott, F. B. (1987). Outpatient implantation of penile prosthesis under local anesthesia. *Urologic Clinics of North America, 14*(1), 177–185.

Shabsigh, R., Fishman, I. J., Schum, C., & Dunn, J. K. (1991). Cigarette smoking and other vascular risk factors in vasculogenic impotence. *Urology, 38*(3), 227–231.

Shrom, S. (1979). Clinical conference: Evaluation and treatment of impotence. *Medical Aspects of Human Sexuality,* 89–104.

Sidi, A. A., Cameron, J. S., Duffy, L. M., & Lange, P. H. (1986). Intravenous drug-induced erections in the management of male erectile dysfunction: Experience with 100 patients. *Journal of Urology, 135,* 704–706.

Solomon, S., & Cappa, K. G. (1987). Impotence and bicycling: A seldom-reported connection. *Postgraduate Medicine, 81*(1), 99–102.

Spark, R. F. (1983). Neuroendocrinology and impotence. *Annals of Internal Medicine, 98*(1), 103–145.

Stanisic, T. H., & Dean, J. C. (1989). The Flexi-Flate and Flexi-Flate II penile prostheses. *Urologic Clinics of North America, 16*(1), 39–49.

St. Louis, E. L., Jewett, M. A., Gray, R. R., & Grosman, H. (1983). Basketball-related impotence (Letter). *New England Journal of Medicine, 308*(10), 595–596.

Turner, L. A., Althof, S. E., Levine, S. B., Bodner, D. R., Kursh, E. D., & Resnick, M. I. (1991). External vacuum devices in the treatment of erectile dysfunction: A one-year study of sexual and psychosocial impact. *Journal of Sex Marital and Therapy, 17*(2), 81–93.

Vorstman, B., & Lockhart, J. (1987). Peyronie's disease. *Problems in Urology, 1,* 507–517.

Walsh, P. C., Lepor, H., & Eggleston, S. C. (1983). Radical prostatectomy with preservation of sexual function: Anatomical and pathological considerations. *Prostate, 4,* 473–485.

Weiss, B. D. (1985). Nontraumatic injuries in amateur long distance bicyclists. *American Journal of Sports Medicine, 13*(3), 187–192.

Wespes, E., & Schulman, C. C. (1987). Cavernous leakage. *Problems in Urology, 1*(3), 487–494.

Wespes, E., & Schulman, C. C. (1988). Systemic complication of intracavernous papaverine injection in patients with venous leakage. *Urology, 31*(2), 114–115.

Williams, G., Mulcahy, M. J., Hartnell, G., & Kiely, E. (1988). Diagnosis and treatment of venous leakage: A curable cause of impotence. *British Journal of Urology, 61,* 151–155.

Zilbergeld, B. (1978). *Male sexuality: A guide to sexual fulfillment.* Boston: Little, Brown.

Zorgniotti, A. W. (1989). Vascular insufficiency: A significant factor in impotence. *New York State Journal of Medicine, 89*(11), 614–617.

Zorgniotti, A. W., & Lefleur, R. S. (1985). Auto-injection of the corpus cavernosum with a vasoactive drug combination for vasculogenic impotence. *Journal of Urology, 133,* 39–41.

# CHAPTER 13

# Male Infertility

■

*Cindy E. Meredith*

## OVERVIEW

This chapter examines the factors that contribute to problems of male infertility. Before approaching a discussion of reproductive issues, it is imperative that a distinction be made between the terms *infertility* and *impotence*. Impotence is defined as the inability to achieve or maintain an erection satisfactory for sexual intercourse. Infertility is generally defined as the inability to induce pregnancy after 1 year of regular, unprotected intercourse. While impotence may cause the problem of infertility, the fact that a man is impotent does not necessarily mean that he is infertile. On the other hand, men who are infertile are rarely impotent.

This chapter will aid the nurse in identifying the physiologic factors necessary for a functional male reproductive system and in recognizing how deviations caused by disease, medical interventions, congenital factors, chemical substances, or injuries may result in infertility. Since the primary focus of nursing is directed toward enabling patients to achieve optimal health potentials, a discussion of diagnostic testing and treatment options is presented. A portion of the chapter also focuses attention on the emotional care that must be combined with the physical interventions.

## BEHAVIORAL OBJECTIVES

After studying this chapter, the reader should be able to

1. Distinguish among the unique physiologic factors related to male infertility.

2. Interact with patients in a manner that reflects an understanding of the physical and emotional components of male infertility.

**3.** Correlate diagnostic testing for male infertility with the appropriate treatment modality.

**4.** Provide educational counseling or resources to couples for whom male infertility is a primary factor.

## KEY WORDS

**Agglutination**—the clumping of sperm and other particles in the semen, which may indicate the presence of antisperm antibodies.

**Azoospermia**—the absence of live sperm in the semen.

**Cryptorchidism**—a congenital failure of descent of one or both testicles.

**Density**—the ratio of sperm to the volume of semen.

**Hamster test**—a test that measures the penetration ability of the sperm on a hamster ovum. A predictor of the ability of the sperm to penetrate a human ovum.

**Infertility**—the inability to cause conception after 1 year of regular, unprotected sexual intercourse.

**Morphology**—the normal structure. In the case of the sperm there should be an oval head, a normal midpiece, and a single tail.

**Motility**—the ability to move in a forward direction. Necessary for the sperm to reach and penetrate the ovum.

**Varicocele**—the abnormal dilation of the veins of the spermatic cord.

**Vasoepididymostomy**—anastomosis of the vas deferens to the epididymis.

**Vasovasostomy**—anastomosis of the vas deferens generally after surgical separation has taken place (vasectomy).

## PERSPECTIVE ON MALE INFERTILITY

Infertility is generally acknowledged to be present if conception has not occurred after 1 year of regular, unprotected sexual intercourse. The problem of infertility has become increasingly widespread in the United States over the past two decades. Because many of today's couples wait until their late 20s and 30s to start a family, the problem is frequently unknown until the female uterine clock has begun ticking, and the situation becomes a desperate race against time. It is estimated that 15% of all marriages encounter a problem of infertility; one third of the cases are related to the male partner, one third are related to the female, and one third are a combination of both (Baum, 1987; Suarez et al., 1987).

Modern technology has increasingly allowed both the gynecologist–infertility specialist and the urologist to make more accurate diagnoses and prescribe treatment modalities that were only dreamt of a generation ago. In vitro fertilization and surgical reconstruction of severed fallopian tubes or the vas deferens have

brought new hope to previously hopeless infertile couples.

## Etiology

The physical causes of male infertility can be divided into three general categories: endocrine (or pretesticular), testicular, and posttesticular. Each of these areas should be examined in the process of determining the etiology.

### PRETESTICULAR (ENDOCRINE) FACTORS

Endocrine causes of infertility are fairly rare and account for approximately 3% (McClure, 1987a; McNally, 1987) to 25% (Baskin, 1989) of the cases of infertility. The endocrine factors related to infertility involve the hypothalamic-pituitary-testicular axis, particularly luteinizing hormone (LH), follicle-stimulating hormone (FSH), and testosterone, and are extremely complex (Fig. 13–1). Within this category are those with pituitary or adrenal tumors, thyroid disease, and diabetes mellitus (Table 13–1). If a

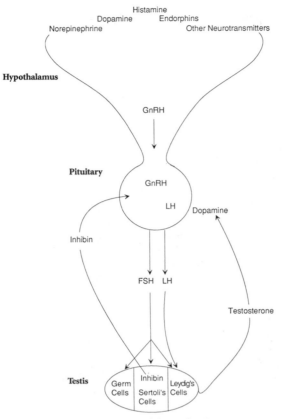

*FIGURE 13–1* Anatomy of the endocrine system.

man's overall health status is good, these endocrine causes can generally be treated with medication or surgery, or both, to correct the problem.

## TESTICULAR FACTORS

Two of the three most common causes of infertility come under the category of testicular factors. It is currently believed that the number one cause of male infertility is varicocele (40–50%), followed by idiopathic causes (40%), and testicular failure (10%). The remaining causes are related to other factors, which will be discussed later in this chapter.

**Varicocele.** A varicocele is defined as a varicosity or swelling of the veins that drain the testes. Varicoceles are the result of retrograde venous flow related anatomically to blood flow from the renal vein. The vast majority (60%) occur on the left side, whereas 39% are bilateral, and only 1% appear on the right side (Lipshultz, 1987). There are numerous theories related to how a varicocele actually causes lowered sperm levels; the causes are classified

under the categories of thermoregulatory, hormonal, and hemodynamic (Nagler & Kaufman, 1987).

**Congenital Anomalies.** An example of a congenital anomaly is Klinefelter's syndrome, a chromosomal disorder (XXY) exhibiting defective development of the seminiferous tubules and elevated gonadotropins. Another condition is cryptorchidism, or undescended testicles, which can occur unilaterally or bilaterally. Cryptorchidism may produce atrophy or hypertrophy of the undescended testis (Wing et al., 1986). Within the area of congenital anomalies is a nondescript category labeled maturational arrest. A portion of the reproductive system fails to develop owing to unknown etiology, which in turn leads to infertility. This maturational arrest may occur at any point in utero and be caused by prenatal exposure to diethylstilbestrol (DES) (McClure, 1987a), or it may occur just prior to puberty.

**Infections and Inflammatory Processes.** Disease or inflammatory processes may lead to testicular damage, resulting in sperm degeneration. Bacteria, especially large concentrations of gram-negative bacteria, may directly affect semen quality by inducing phagocytosis or may produce epididymal obstruction or injury to the seminiferous epithelium (McConnell, 1987; Megory et al., 1987; Suarez et al., 1987). The most identifiable infection is orchitis—generally induced by the mumps virus, but rarely by leprosy, syphilis, gonorrhea, tuberculosis, or fungal organisms. Any fever or illness can impair spermatogenesis. The effects on the sperm may not be noticed until 3 months or more after the event. This is due to the fact that spermatogenesis takes approximately 74 days for completion.

The role of antisperm antibodies in male in-

---

**TABLE 13–1. Endocrine Causes of Male Infertility**

1. Hypogonadotropism—resulting in ↓ testosterone, LH, and FSH
   a. Pituitary tumors, cysts, or injury
   b. Genetic defects
2. Estrogen excess
   a. Adrenal or pituitary tumors
   b. Cirrhosis of the liver
3. Androgen excess
4. Hyperprolactinemia
5. Hyperthyroidism
6. Hypothyroidism
7. Glucocorticoid excess
   a. Cushing's syndrome
   b. Treatment for ulcerative colitis, rheumatoid arthritis, bronchitis, or asthma
8. Diabetes mellitus

fertility remains a complex and controversial issue. Because of this controversy, the role of antisperm antibodies will not be discussed in this section. According to Hellstrom and colleagues (1987), immunologic infertility is an important area of research; however, they do not consider the condition to be an absolute one, but rather a relative impediment to fertilization.

**Medications, Radiation, Substance Abuse, and Environmental Hazards.** There is a wide variety of chemical substances that may influence sperm quality, quantity, or delivery process (i.e., interference with erection or ejaculation; see Chapter 12). The most well-known chemical substances associated with infertility are anabolic steroids, cimetidine, sulfasalazine, spironolactone, antineoplastic agents (dose related), and recreational drugs (Conrad & Ross, 1985; McClure, 1987a). For an extended listing of medications refer to Table 13–2. Exposure to hazards such as Agent Orange, pesticides, and radiation remains controversial and is still under investigation (Gerber et al., 1988; Hecht, 1987). Radiation damage tends to be dose related. Permanent sterility is thought to occur following a single-dose exposure of 10 to 20 Gy. On the other hand, complete recovery often occurs within 9 to 18 months after less than 1 Gy of exposure.

## POSTTESTICULAR FACTORS

**Congenital Factors.** There is a variety of congenital anomalies that often lead to infertility. In some congenital disorders the vas deferens, seminal vesicles, and some of the epididymis may be absent. One example is cystic fibrosis, in which the vas deferens or epididymis is absent (McClure, 1987a). Wolffian duct malformation has also been identified in some subfertile males (Pryor & Hendry, 1991).

**Infection.** The condition known as epididymitis is an example of posttesticular infection that may cause infertility. Epididymitis is generally associated with *Chlamydia trachomatis* or other sexually transmitted diseases. Asymptomatic infection, fever, or both may also result in decreased sperm motility (McConnell, 1987).

**Surgical Procedures.** Surgical interventions such as bladder neck reconstruction, anterior and posterior resections, retroperitoneal lymph node dissection, or prostatic surgery performed in cases of advanced cancer generally cause retrograde ejaculation or absent emission. For this reason it is important that men faced with this surgery, who are contemplating having children, are counseled preoperatively concerning the possibility of utilizing a sperm bank. Bilateral lumbar sympathectomy will also result in retrograde ejaculation owing to the fact that peristalsis of the distal epididymis and vas deferens at the time of ejaculation is mediated by the sympathetic nerves (Howards, 1987b). Iatrogenic injury during inguinal herniorrhaphy (e.g., ligation of the vas deferens) has on occasion been a factor in preventing sperm transport. Ligation of the vas deferens, whether voluntary or iatrogenic, results in infertility. In the case of couples today, a vasectomy may have

---

**TABLE 13–2. Some Medications Affecting Fertility***

| | |
|---|---|
| **Antihypertensive** | **Toxins** |
| Aldomet (methyldopa) | Agent Orange |
| Dibenzyline (phenoxybenzamine hydrochloride) | Lead poisoning |
| Ismelin (guanethidine monosulfate) | Pesticides |
| Mellaril (thioridazine) | |
| Reserpine | **Other** |
| | Anabolic steroids |
| **Chemotherapy—Dose-dependent** | Aspirin (excessive) |
| Bleomycin | Azaline (sulfasalazine) |
| Cytoxan (cyclophosphamide) | Azulfidine (sulfasalazine) |
| Leukeran (chlorambucil) | Colchicine |
| Methotrexate | DES—maternal use |
| Mitomycin | Dilantin (phenytoin) |
| Myleran (busulfan) | Furadantin (nitrofurantoin) |
| Neosar (cyclophosphamide) | Monoamine oxidase (MAO) inhibitors |
| Nitrogen mustard | Tagamet (cimetidine) |
| Procarbazine | Testosterone (excessive) |
| | Thiotepa |
| **Substance Abuse** | |
| Alcohol | |
| Caffeine (excessive) | |
| Marijuana | |
| Nicotine | |

*Product trade name is followed by generic name in parentheses.

been performed as a method of birth control in a first marriage, whereas a second marriage may bring about a desire for more offspring. Any condition that causes a disruption of the internal sphincter, altered function of the bladder neck, or dyssynergia between the internal and the external sphincters may result in retrograde ejaculation.

**Miscellaneous Causes.** Under the category of miscellaneous are a wide variety of conditions that may result in infertility: sickle cell anemia, chronic liver disease, renal disease, prostatitis, obesity, cachexia, myotonic dystrophy, seizure disorders, paraplegia, traumatic testicular injury, spinal cord injury, retrograde ejaculation, premature ejaculation, abnormality of prostatic or seminal vesicular secretions, impotence, extreme stress, increased testicular heat, sexual techniques, frequency of intercourse, and idiopathic oligospermia. The exact mechanisms are not clearly understood, underscoring the need for a complete history and physical examination with specific diagnostic tests that are indicators of sperm morphology and delivery of the ejaculate.

**Emotional Factors.** A condition such as infertility is emotionally charged and, in itself, may produce stress and emotional disturbances that can lower hormonal levels (Spencer, 1987). Stress can also interfere with a man's ability to obtain or maintain an erection and may further aggravate conditions such as premature ejaculation. When a man is forced to "perform" at set times of the month or in a prescribed manner, he may experience a lack of desire or pleasure. Increased frustration over the failure of the woman to become pregnant can result in anger, fear, anxiety, despair, and depression in her partner, with a resultant decrease in his libido. There is a direct correlation between mind and body where sexual functioning is concerned.

## Pathophysiology

The physiology involved in the male reproductive system is complex and could fill several chapters. In an attempt to make the material understandable and applicable, the discussion is kept to a minimum, and more material is devoted to the diagnosis and treatment of male infertility.

A basic understanding of the mechanisms involved in facilitating conception will help clarify the mechanisms of infertility. The fundamental factors leading to conception are endocrine function involving the hypothalamic-pituitary-gonadal axis sufficient to promote spermatogenesis, at least one testicle that produces spermatozoa, an ability to mature the sperm in the epididymis, a ductal system to transport the sperm from the testes to the outside of the body, secretory glands for seminal fluid, and an intact nervous system that produces an erection and ejaculation (Bernstein, 1986). The semen itself must demonstrate at least 50% to 60% motile sperm cells, with a concentration of at least $20 \times 10^6$ cells per mL in 1.5 to 5 mL of volume (Table 13–3). In normal semen, 60% to 80% of the sperm should demonstrate a normal configuration of oval head, midpiece, and tail of high quality. A small amount of fructose should be present in the semen as well as a demonstrated ability to coagulate (McClure, 1987a).

The primary factors specifically related to semen are sperm concentration (or density), motility, and morphology. Other factors are the presence of fructose and coagulation factors (antibody and deoxyribonucleic acid [DNA] issues will not be discussed because of the controversial and conflicting reports in the literature).

A "normal" male has approximately $425 \times 10^6$ mature spermatozoa available for ejaculation (Howards, 1987a). It is the general opinion that the sperm concentration must be at a minimum of $20 \times 10^6$ cells per mL, and normal sperm volume should range from 1.5 to 5.0 mL. A volume of less than 1.5 mL may indicate poor collection technique, retrograde ejaculation, obstruction of the ejaculatory ducts, congenital absence of the seminal vesicles, Leydig's cells, or pituitary deficiency. A large volume (>6 mL) may indicate prolonged sexual abstinence or accessory gland overactivity. Too little semen decreases the odds of the sperm's reaching the ovum; too much semen can dilute the sperm count and reduce the chances of impregnation.

**TABLE 13–3. Normal Standards of Semen Analysis**

| |
|---|
| Volume: 1.5–5 mL |
| Density: >20 million cells/mL |
| Motility: >60% grade 2 or higher (scale 1–4) |
| Morphology: >60% normal |
| pH: 7.2–7.8 |
| Color: grayish white |
| Odor: oxidation produces strong odor |
| Fructose: positive |
| Agglutination: may indicate antisperm antibodies |
| White blood cells: if present, suspect infection |

Assessment of forward progressive motility should demonstrate between 50% and 60% motile cells and a sperm quality greater than 2 (on a scale of 0 [no movement] to 4 [excellent forward progression]). The factors affecting motility are heat, cold, drugs, certain bacteria, and possibly the presence of antisperm antibodies. Men with sperm motility problems may also be experiencing abnormal epididymal dysfunction or varicocele. Adequate sperm motility not only is required for sperm transport into the vagina but also aids in penetration of the ovum. According to McClure (1987a), "motility is the single most important measure of semen quality," and it may compensate for a low sperm count. The motility factors are rated in two ways: the first is the total percentage of motile sperm, the second is how fast and straight the sperm swim. Modern technology, including video cameras and computers, has greatly enhanced the accuracy and objectivity with which these factors are evaluated.

Morphology of the sperm is based on stained seminal smears and is usually scored as a percentage of normal cells. Infertility is generally associated with a normal sperm configuration score of 60% or lower. To be classified as normal, a sperm cell must have an oval head, a normal midpiece, and a tail. These structures potentiate penetration of the ovum. Sperm cells that have tapered heads, microheads, or amorphous spermatozoa may be indicative of poor testicular function. When morphology factors and a test known as the zona free hamster ova penetration assay or sperm penetration assay (SPA) are combined, the predictability of infertility versus fertility has a much higher degree of accuracy (Kruger et al., 1987).

If there is an abnormality in the semen viscosity, it may indicate a disorder of the accessory glands (i.e., prostate) and may affect the accuracy of assessment of both the sperm motility and the sperm density. Occasional clumps of agglutinated sperm are not that unusual, but increased clumping may indicate inflammatory or immunologic processes.

Coagulation is another factor that is sometimes evaluated. Normal semen should first coagulate, then liquefy over the next 5 to 20 minutes. A delay in this process may also indicate a disorder of the accessory glands.

Fructose, which is androgen dependent and produced in the seminal vesicles, should be present in the semen. Its absence from the semen may indicate obstruction of the ejaculatory ducts or congenital absence of the seminal vesicles or vas deferens. Fructose levels should be assessed in men with azoospermia and those with an ejaculation volume of less than 1 mL.

Small semen volume, failure of the semen to coagulate, or absence of fructose from the semen may indicate either a congenital absence of the seminal vesicles and vas deferens or an obstruction of the ejaculatory duct (McClure, 1987a).

## Medical-Surgical Management

Technologic advances have raised the hopes of and opportunities for infertile couples. With the advent of in vitro fertilization and laser repair, a whole new generation of children have been brought into this world.

### CONSERVATIVE LIFESTYLE CHANGES

On the conservative side of treatment are the issues we refer to as lifestyle changes. These may include decreasing excessive nicotine or caffeine consumption. Although the exact mechanisms are not understood, consumption of these substances can interfere with normal rest patterns and erectile functioning (see Chapter 12). Men should also avoid using large quantities of alcohol and marijuana, as these substances are potential gonadotoxins (Suarez, et al., 1987). Further recommendations may be made concerning exposure to excessive heat as a result of wearing tight underwear or jeans or the use of a hot tub or sauna. It is known that increased temperatures of the scrotal contents interfere with the sperm storage function of the epididymis and may cause infertility. Identification of stress factors and the implemention of relaxation and stress-management techniques may also prove very helpful during the evaluation process. Education as to the optimal time for fertilization, as evidenced by the female's basal body temperature record, may further enhance the chances of pregnancy. Sexual practices and positions may also need to be reviewed. For instance, the couple may be engaging in intercourse too frequently, resulting in a reduced sperm count. Prolonged abstinence may have also occurred, leading to decreased sperm motility. The couple should avoid the use of vaginal lubricants and jellies, most of which are spermicidal or contribute to decreased sperm motility. Female positioning, with her supine and a pillow under the hips after intercourse, may maximize semen contact with the cervical os.

## MEDICATIONS

When infertility is the result of an infectious process, the primary organism should be isolated, and a microbe-specific drug administered. Careful culturing of all secretions and urine will validate the presence of a bacterial factor. Medication such as nitrofurantoin (Furadantin) should be avoided because of the negative side effects on the sperm. The most frequently recommended antibiotic for the treatment of sexually transmitted diseases and urinary tract infections in men is tetracycline.

If the etiology is endocrine, then treatment may take the form of thyroid supplements as in the case of hypothyroidism. Treatment of hypothalamic-pituitary disorders depends on the cause of the abnormality. If a pituitary tumor is present, it is generally removed. Prolactin-secreting tumors are usually treated with bromocriptine (Parlodel), which suppresses prolactin secretion at the pituitary level. The side effects, however, may outweigh the benefits of this therapy. Men with non–prolactin-secreting tumors may be treated with a combination of human menopausal gonadotropins, such as menotropins (Pergonal) and human chorionic gonadotropin (hCG) (McNally, 1987; Sokol, 1987). Men with hypogonadotropic hypogonadism are deficient in LH and FSH secretion; the secretion of these hormones can be restored with administration of hCG. Therapy may consist of hCG 2000 to 4000 IU intramuscularly (IM) two or three times per week for 3 to 12 months before sperm may appear in the ejaculate. If therapy is unsuccessful after this period of time, an additional dosage of FSH 38 to 75 IU IM three times a week may be required. The gonadotropin-releasing hormone (GnRH) may also be utilized to stimulate spermatogenesis. It is usually administered as low-dose, long-term therapy given by repeated subcutaneous injections. Androgen therapy (administration of testosterone 200 to 250 mg IM every 2 weeks) has been tried in some men to achieve what is known as rebound therapy. The testosterone, when administered, actually suppresses LH and spermatogenesis; however, when it is withdrawn, the sperm concentration in some men may rebound to a level higher than that before initiation of the therapy. However, questions regarding the efficacy of androgen therapy have caused practitioners to dis-

courage this form of treatment in favor of other recommended options.

In cases of retrograde ejaculation that may be due to such factors as peripheral neuropathy, antihypertensive medicines, and spinal cord injury, administration of epinephrine, pseudoephedrine hydrochloride (Sudafed), phenylpropanolamine (Ornade), or imipramine hydrochloride (Tofranil) to promote forward ejaculation has proved effective in some men.

Trials of drugs known as antiestrogens are also being conducted in cases of male infertility. The two most commonly known drugs are clomiphene (Clomid) and tamoxifen (Nolvadex). These medications act as competitive inhibitors of estrogen action by occupying estrogen receptors. Clomid is generally administered in doses of 25 to 100 mg orally every day for approximately 6 months; tamoxifen is given 10 mg orally twice a day for 6 months. The results of this form of therapy have been mixed, with no firm conclusions being drawn as to the true level of effectiveness of these drugs (Salisz & Goldman, 1990; Check et al., Sokol, 1987; Urry & Middleton, 1986). Clomid is not approved by the U.S. Food and Drug Administration (FDA) for use in the treatment of male infertility, so it may be wise to obtain written consent prior to administration. Also inform patients that their insurance may not cover the cost of the medication. Another drug category under investigation is prostaglandin E (PGE) or $E_2$ synthetase inhibitors (e.g., indomethacin). A few studies have demonstrated increased serum levels of LH and FSH, as well as increased sperm concentration and motility after administration of indomethacin 75 mg orally daily.

Other medications such as amino acids (arginine), vitamin-like compounds (carnitine), vitamins A, E, and C, zinc, thyroxine, nucleotides (cyclic adenosine monophosphate), proteolytic enzymes (kallikrein), methylxanthines, caffeine in moderation, and relaxin all have been attempted. Success rates are questionable in the absence of a specific deficiency state.

## IN VITRO SPERM MANIPULATION AND SPERM BANKING

Perhaps one of the most promising methods of treatment for male infertility has been sperm manipulation or artificial insemination. When the sperm is present but lacks density or has diminished motility, manipulation of the sperm in a controlled manner has greatly facilitated pregnancy.

What are now known as assisted reproductive treatments include in vitro fertilization and embryo transfer (IVFET), gamete intrafallopian transfer (GIFT), intrauterine insemination (IUI), and ZIFT (zygote intrafallopian transfer). IVFET is a technique that involves hyperstimulation of the female ovum to obtain multiple, mature, fertilizable oocytes. The oocytes are obtained by laparoscopy or ultrasound-directed follicular aspiration at the height of ovulation and are incubated in vitro with spermatozoa that have been specially processed. Sperm processing separates out the functional, motile sperm from immotile sperm, seminal plasma, and what is known as cellular debris. The sperm is, in fact, concentrated, high quality, viable sperm. The concentration of motile sperm in the oligospermic male may be as high as 1 million cells per mL. The oocyte and the sperm are then incubated in a volume of less than 2 mL of specialized media that may also have been treated with human follicular fluid (hFF). In addition, the cumulus may be mechanically dissected from the corona-oocyte complex to further aid in sperm penetration (Batzofin et al., 1987; Lipshultz, 1987). It may also be facilitated with a technique called zona drilling. Several openings are made into the ova to allow easier sperm penetration. After approximately 24 to 72 hours, the fertilized embryos (usually up to four) are placed transcervically into the uterus via a catheter, to await natural development. If sufficient sperm have been obtained, excess sperm or embryos may be banked (cryopreserved) for future use. Success rates range from 8% to 20% per completed cycle. The GIFT procedure again involves hyperstimulation of the female ovum; however, instead of the ova being removed from the body, they are mixed with the processed sperm in a specialized catheter and immediately transferred into the fallopian tubes. The success rates for GIFT range from 25% to 40% per completed cycle. ZIFT, a newer technique, involves controlling the uterine environment with medications such as leuprolide acetate (Lupron), Pergonal, progesterone, estradiol, and hCG. The egg is then placed in the presence of either single or mixed donor sperm that have been processed. The oocyte and sperm are then incubated for 35 to 38 hours. Reimplantation is accomplished directly into the fallopian tubes during a laparoscopic procedure. Success rates are approximately 40% to 50%, with the cost averaging $5500. The technique of IUI, on the other hand, requires less manipulation of the ovum and basically involves deposition of a large number of processed spermatozoa in the fundus of the uterus at the optimal point in the menstrual cycle. The success rate ranges from 8% to 10% per treatment cycle. There are other variations in the process of assisted reproduction (e.g., micromanipulation and microinjection of sperm, alloplastic spermatocele, and direct intraepididymal aspiration of sperm); these remain somewhat experimental. One important consideration before involvement in this treatment option is the cost factor. These forms of treatment are not covered by insurance plans and may run $6000 or more, with no guarantee of success. Another option that may be suggested to the couple with severe male factor infertility is artificial insemination by a donor (AID). Counseling and careful screening of individual responses would certainly be recommended prior to any form of in vitro fertilization.

There are various methods used to process sperm to accomplish optimal fertilization goals. The methods utilized most frequently are (1) direct swim-up separation, (2) two-step washing with swim-up separation, and (3) Percoll discontinuous gradient separation techniques (Batzofin et al., 1987). The direct swim-up technique allows the first portion of the ejaculate with highly motile sperm to be collected. Unfortunately, this technique may also collect ejaculate debris, and there are significantly fewer sperm collected compared with the two-step washing and Percoll techniques. The two-step washing procedure, which is most frequently used, provides the highest sperm recovery rate but still contains some nonviable sperm and debris. The Percoll gradient separation technique is most often utilized when there is normal sperm density but very low motility or with increased concentrations of white blood cells or immature sperm. Ideally, sperm processing is an attempt to select and concentrate the best specimen of highly motile, morphologically normal sperm with as little debris and white blood cells as possible to provide for maximum penetration capability. The sperm penetration assay (SPA) will be discussed in the diagnostic section of this chapter.

Another form of sperm manipulation involves the retrieval of retrograde ejaculate. In some cases, discontinuing the causative drugs or treating with sympathetic-acting agents may be the solution (see the section on medication). Two nonsurgical alternative methods for sperm recovery involve retrieval of semen from the bladder. Prior to extraction, the urine should first be alkalized by taking 1 teaspoon of sodium bicarbonate four times a day for 2 days prior to ejaculation. After ejaculation, the bladder is emptied by having the patient urinate or by catheterization. The contents are centrifuged for 10 minutes and 1 to 2 mL of sediment is aspirated. Various methods may be used for disposition of the sperm with the ova. In addition, a technique involving electro-ejaculation has been available to spinal cord patients since 1948. Transrectal electrical stimulation of the seminal vesicles stimulates ejaculation; unfortunately, some of the possible side effects may be rectal injury or induction of autonomic dysreflexia.

Sperm banking, or the storage of processed sperm, has opened the doors for thousands of infertile couples. In the past few years, however, sperm banks themselves have come under close scrutiny as more centers for infertility are established. At present, the only regulatory agency for such centers is the American Association of Tissue Banks (AATB), with headquarters in McLean, Virginia. It is strongly recommended that any inquiries as to the practices within any given center be made to the AATB.

## SURGICAL INTERVENTIONS

**Varicocele Balloon Occlusion or Repair.** Medical science is always looking for inventive ways of treating "old problems," and infertility treatment modalities are no different in this respect. Just as cardiologists are experimenting with balloon occlusion-dilation to achieve homeostasis in cardiac conditions, so urologists are exploring the use of this technique in the treatment of varicoceles. The advent of percutaneous venographic occlusion of the internal spermatic vein with a detachable balloon allows the physician not only to diagnose the presence of a varicocele but also to provide treatment. There is definitely a cost savings and decreased risk to the patient related to anesthesia. However, during the early stages of development of this technique there were isolated reports of balloons migrating to the lungs. As the level of expertise increases, such occurrences should become a thing of the past.

Surgical repair of a varicocele—varicocelectomy—consists of high ligation of the internal spermatic vein in the retroperitoneal area, low ligation of the branches of the internal spermatic vein in the inguinal area, or a scrotal approach (the most difficult and least popular). Ligation of the spermatic vein may be accom-

plished as an open or laparoscopic procedure. It is generally performed on an outpatient basis. The success rates vary from 30% to 55%. The results are basically unknown for the first 3 to 6 months because of the length of time needed for spermatogenesis to occur.

Another method of intervention in the treatment of a varicocele, although rather controversial, involves sclerosing of the spermatic veins with a solution such as sodium morrhuate. Extreme care must be taken in the administration of the sclerosing agent to avoid damage to the surrounding structures.

**Vasovasostomy.** The incidence of vasovasostomy has greatly increased in the past 20 years owing in part to the increasing number of men who underwent vasectomy surgery, subsequently remarried, and desired offspring. The procedure involves microsurgery (with or without lasers) to perform the anastomosis. In one group under investigation by Howards (1987b), if spermatozoa were present in fluid from the distal vas deferens at the time of surgery, more than 90% of the men had spermatozoa in their postoperative ejaculate. In the wives of these men, the pregnancy success rate was 40% to 70%. One factor that influences the success rate is the length of time between the initial vasectomy and the reanastomosis. The longer the time interval, the lower the success rate.

The surgery is generally performed on an outpatient basis, and the patient can return to work 1 or 2 days postoperatively. He is advised to wear a scrotal support and to avoid heavy lifting and ejaculation for 2 weeks. Semen analysis is generally performed at 3-month and 6-month intervals to assess sperm count and sperm motility. If spermatozoa do not appear intraoperatively or 6 months postoperatively, a second surgery (vasoepididymostomy) may be advised (Belker, 1987).

**Vasoepididymostomy.** In cases in which epididymal obstruction has occurred as the result of vasovasostomy, congenital defects, cystic abnormalities, or postinflammatory obstructive lesions, microsurgical anastomosis between the vas and an epididymal tubule may prove successful. The anastomosis is made as low as possible in the epididymis because of the fact that sperm maturation and motility increase as sperm move down the epididymis. The creation of a spermatocele can then facilitate the aspiration of sperm percutaneously.

If a vasectomy was performed less than 10 years previously, it is generally recommended that a vasovasostomy be performed. If, however, more than 10 years have elapsed since the vasectomy and the vasectomy was performed high in the scrotum, the patient may be advised to have a vasoepididymostomy to increase the chances of success (McClure, 1987b). A good diagnostic evaluation should precede any surgical consideration.

**Testicular Transplantation.** Because of tissue rejection difficulties and the lack of willing donors, the option of a testicular transplantation is extremely rare. It bears mentioning, however, owing to the fact that at least one successful case was presented in the literature that involved a set of identical twins. Another reason for inclusion of testicular transplantation as a possible treatment is the significant strides that have been made in antirejection medication as it relates to organ donation. We are seeing increasing numbers of transplantation operations being performed, including heart, lung, liver, and kidney transplantation, and it is not beyond the realm of medical science to consider the possibility of future research into the area of testicular transplantation as a means of infertility treatment.

# APPROACHES TO PATIENT CARE

One of the most important aspects in the care of a man experiencing infertility is a careful, thorough diagnostic evaluation. Without proper diagnosis, treatment options either may take a long time to achieve any measure of success or may be totally ineffective and leave the patient with additional emotional difficulties to overcome.

## Assessment

An infertility evaluation should begin with a specifically designed history and physical examination. This is followed by a series of diagnostic tests that further examine the possible cause for infertility.

The history should elicit information related to the following:

*Sexual Practices.* Previous successful impregnations, frequency of intercourse (including positioning and timing), sexual habits (e.g., masturbation), problems with premature ejaculation or erectile dysfunction, use of lubricants or birth control methods, understanding of ovulation cycle.

*Lifestyle.* Weight training; long-distance bicycling; hot tubs or saunas; exposure to high heat; tight jeans; use of caffeine, nicotine, alcohol, marijuana, steroids. Desire for children (does it fit "economic plan?").

*Occupation.* High stress; long periods of sitting; exposure to radiation; exposure to pesticides or Agent Orange.

*Medical-Surgical History.* Inquire about previous infertility evaluations, prostatic disease, genitourinary tract infections, sexually transmitted diseases, human immunodeficiency virus (HIV) testing, diabetes, thyroid or pituitary disorders; conditions such as the onset of puberty, mumps, cryptorchidism, testicular trauma or torsion, varicocele, hydrocele, infectious mononucleosis, hepatitis, liver disease, respiratory illness, cancer, hernias, back injuries, tuberculosis, cystic fibrosis, renal disease, sickle cell disease; treatments such as medications (including maternal use of DES), radiographs, chemotherapy, operations.

The physical examination should begin with an observation of secondary sex characteristics (i.e., muscle mass, upper and lower body proportions, hair patterns and amount, presence of gynecomastia). Examination of the penis should look for evidence of Peyronie's disease or hypospadias, which interferes with deposition of sperm into the vagina. Testicular size, shape, and consistency should be evaluated; on average, a normal testis measures $4 \times 3$ cm and has a volume greater than 15 to 20 mL (an orchidometer may be used for measurement). Careful examination of the testicles should be performed to determine the presence of a varicocele. This can be ascertained by having the man stand while the entire contents of the scrotum are palpated. To further assess for a varicocele, epididymal induration, cystic changes, or swelling or nodules on the vas deferens, ask the man to perform a Valsalva maneuver, and repeat the palpation. The increase in intra-abdominal pressure will accentuate any enlarged veins along the cord if a varicocele is present. If a varicocele is suspected, a more extensive examination may be performed using Doppler scrotal thermography or venography to facilitate visualization.

If an infection is suspected, prostatic massage and culture of the prostate secretions may be indicated along with the routine urinalysis. A postejaculation urinalysis may also be performed to assess for retrograde ejaculation.

The following are descriptions of the most commonly performed diagnostic tests used in the assessment of male infertility.

*Endocrine Evaluation.* Endocrine evaluation may include measurement of the following: FSH, LH, testosterone (total and free), prolactin, estradiol, and adrenocorticotropic hormone (ACTH). Measurement should be made of GnRH and fasting blood sugar (FBS), as well as 24-hour urine testing for free cortisol. A low testosterone level is a good indicator of hypogonadism of either hypothalamic, pituitary, or congenital origin. Abnormalities in FSH, LH, and prolactin indicate pituitary dysfunction. ACTH and GnRH should be evaluated in terms of thyroid functioning. An FBS may be indicated in an uncontrolled diabetic patient, which may lead to further evaluation of neuropathy or erectile dysfunction. Depending on the findings, more extensive testing may be required; however, since endocrine factors are rarely the cause of infertility, more time should be spent assessing other areas.

*Semen Analysis.* Procedural semen analysis provides information on the quality and quantity of the sperm (see Table 13–3). Accuracy in the collection of semen is extremely important in order to obtain accurate results. Specimens that are collected over 2 or 3 weeks may vary as much as 200% in their results (Suarez et al., 1987). Semen samples should be analyzed by a laboratory that specializes in screening large numbers of samples and has established its own reference values (Wing et al., 1986). The use of sophisticated computers, lasers, and video cameras has greatly enhanced the ability to assess density simultaneously with motility factors.

Careful written instructions should be given to the patient prior to collection of the semen specimen. It is generally recommended that the man refrain from any form of ejaculation for 3 days prior to sample collection, because frequent ejaculations may reduce sperm concentration and semen volume and increase the chances of obtaining sperm with abnormal morphology. Ideally, three separate specimens should be collected in sterile containers over a period of 4 to 6 days and taken to the laboratory for analysis within 1 hour of collection. Masturbation is the preferred method of obtaining the ejaculate, as coitus interruptus may result in some loss of the specimen in the vagina and the first portion of the ejaculate has the highest concentration of sperm and contains the most motile sperm. Patients should also be instructed to refrain from using a condom or lubricant, as these may render the sperm immotile. The specimen collected should be kept as close to body temperature as possible. If it is not collected in a laboratory or office setting, the semen specimen should be transported to the testing area within 1 hour,

with a warm environment being maintained around it.

*Sperm Penetration Assay.* After a semen analysis has been completed and if the results are within normal limits, the next test is often the SPA, also known as the zona-free hamster ova penetration assay. It is one of the most reliable indicators of the spermatozoa's ability to penetrate and fertilize a human ovum (short of actually using a human ovum) (Lipshultz, 1987). In this test the spermatozoa are placed with hamster ova to calculate the percentage of spermatozoa that can penetrate the ova. When fewer than 10% of the spermatozoa penetrate the ova, sperm dysfunction and male infertility are considered to exist, and further investigation into sperm morphology is required. A positive SPA result implies good semen, while poor results imply a cervical factor, the presence of antisperm antibodies, or postfertilization factors. A postcoital test may be necessary if cervical factors are suspected. In this case cervical mucus is removed 2 to 12 hours after intercourse and evaluated.

The SPA is able to detect sperm function not assessed by semen analysis; however, the test does not measure motility and transport factors that may be present in the female genital tract. The SPA is generally used, prior to attempting any in vitro–in vivo fertilization, as a predictor of possible success. In light of the cost involved in performing in vitro–in vivo fertilization, it is highly recommended that the SPA be performed first.

*Antisperm Antibodies.* Although testing in this area remains controversial, it is generally conceded that antibody factors should be considered in couples when repeated postcoital tests are abnormal or when infertility persists after the man has had a vasovasostomy that results in normal sperm counts and motility. Immunologic factors are believed to play a part in 10% to 30% of the unexplained cases of infertility. A history of testicular trauma (surgical or otherwise), torsion or maldescent, persistent pyospermia, or repeated genital infections may be cause for conducting antibody testing (Hellstrom et al., 1987). Some of the more frequently recommended antibody tests are found in Table 13–4.

*Testicular Biopsy.* Testicular biopsy is generally restricted to men who have normal hormone levels and fructose in the semen and demonstrate azoospermia or severe oligospermia based on at least two semen analyses. Retrograde ejaculation should also be ruled out by postejaculatory urinalysis prior to biopsy.

**TABLE 13–4. Antisperm Antibody Tests**

Simple serum sample
Enzyme-linked immunosorbent assay (ELISA)
Immunobead rosette test (IBT)
Indirect immunofluorescence
Mixed agglutination reaction (MAR)
Radiolabeled antiglobulin assay
Sperm agglutination test (Franklin-Dukes, Kibrick)
Sperm immobilization test (Isojima)

Great care must be taken in the biopsy technique, tissue handling, and processing of the testicular biopsy. Any invasion into the testicles runs the risk of disturbing spermatogenesis and causing possible antibody formation. The sample size is generally 2 mm or less and should be placed immediately into a fixative solution, such as Bouin's, Zenker's, and Conroy's, with a minimum of handling. Testicular biopsy can give a tissue diagnosis of normal spermatogenesis, maturational arrest, hypospermatogenesis, or germinal aplasia (McClure, 1987b).

*Radiologic Studies.* Radiologic procedures are utilized after all other noninvasive diagnostic modalities have been exhausted or as a method of pinpointing obstruction prior to an invasive procedure.

A vasogram may be performed to determine whether the ejaculatory ducts or abdominal end of the vasa are patent. This procedure is generally reserved for patients who have normal testicular biopsies but severe impairment of sperm density on semen analysis. Care must be taken during the procedure to prevent the possibility of sclerosing the vas or rupturing the epididymal tubule when injecting the contrast medium. A technique using dilute methylene blue irrigation solution and observing the color of the urine via a Foley catheter may prevent such damage.

Spermatic venography, although somewhat controversial and requiring specialized skills and equipment, is performed to identify subclinical varicoceles in men who remain infertile after surgical ligation of the internal spermatic vein. In some cases the physician may embolize the spermatic vein during the course of spermatic venography (Pochaczevsky et al., 1988).

Other radiologic procedures that may be performed in the quest for answers are Doppler sonography (to identify subclinical varicoceles), ultrasound (to detect intrascrotal abnormalities by visualizing both testicles and surrounding structures), scrotal thermography (to support the diagnosis of suspected varicocele),

and magnetic resonance imaging (for pelvic evaluation, including seminal vesicles and prostate; or to detect hemorrhage, congenital abnormalities, tumors, infective processes, and abscesses). A pertinent consideration before proceeding with any of these diagnostic studies should be the cost factor. Accurate diagnosis still does not guarantee treatment success and a final outcome of fertility. Another issue involved here is the emotional capacity of the couple to deal with uncertainties. At what point should the physician suggest alternative methods of having children? How can you, as the nurse, support and guide such decision-making for the couple?

**Nursing Diagnosis**

The nursing diagnosis for the man experiencing infertility may include

1. Powerlessness, related to the inability to control the infertility evaluation process.

**Plan of Care**

Nursing care is directed toward enabling the patient to

1. Verbalize feelings associated with powerlessness, for example, loss of control, anger, depression, frustration, hopelessness, and helplessness.
2. Interact in the decision-making process of the diagnostic and treatment plan.
3. Examine alternative treatment options.

**Intervention**

Infertility evokes a high level of emotional response from both partners and provides ample opportunity for nursing intervention. Some of the more common feelings experienced by the patient are those similar to any grief response, such as anger, fear, anxiety, depression, despair, and frustration (Davis, 1987). Similarly, issues related to the self, body image, and locus of control are brought to bear on the situation. For these patients, a diagnosis of knowledge deficit related to infertility is only scratching the surface of the areas for intervention.

These patients not only need encouragement to verbalize their feelings about the situation but also need to develop interactive communication skills with each other. A tremendous amount of laying blame and frustration is evident when the issue of infertility is first brought to light. The man may ask himself: Is it her fault, my fault, or both? How does this make me feel as a person? Each partner may wonder: Will I still be loved if it's my fault? With encouragement a couple may be able to resolve these issues alone; for other couples the assistance of a marriage-family therapist or a support group may be necessary. Both partners need a "safe environment" in which to think and share their feelings. Too often, well-meaning friends and relatives add additional pressures by constantly referring to their childless state or endlessly asking how the infertility evaluation process is proceeding. This may also create a situation of social isolation that places additional stress on the couple.

The diagnostic testing itself can cause emotional trauma by seemingly taking control away from the patient (Carpenito, 1992). Many adults function under the auspices of what is known as an internal locus of control. We control our immediate environment and what is happening to us. In the situation of infertility, however, feelings of lack of control over the desired outcome may be strong. Often, the patient must submit to diagnostic testing, prescribed treatments, and rigid sexual routines in order to satisfy the medical regimen for infertility. The couple may also sense a lack of control about how to go about organizing and making decisions about their future.

An important role of the nurse is to utilize all available methods of providing information concerning the diagnostic testing and treatment options, thereby allowing the couple to gain knowledge and make reasonable decisions. It may also be extremely helpful if the nurse and physician are aware of when it may be necessary to intervene and give the couple permission to withdraw from further testing and look at other alternatives. Both partners may be so emotionally involved in the situation as to fear rejection if they suggest calling a halt to further medical intervention. The couple may also feel a sense of obligation to the physician to succeed, since he or she is trying so hard to help them. Information should also be shared with the couple as to their alternatives, such as artificial insemination, adoption, and becoming foster parents.

Infertility has the potential to affect every aspect of the man's life. Every effort should be made to alleviate the sense of powerlessness that accompanies infertility.

### Patient Outcome

The patient verbalizes a sense of control and a lack of frustration over the infertility evaluation and treatment process.

## REFERENCES

Baskin, H. J. (1989). Endocrinologic evaluation of impotence. *Southern Medical Journal, 82*(4), 446–449.

Batzofin, J. H., Marrs, R. P., Serafini, P. C., & Lipshultz, L. I. (1987). Assisted reproductive treatments for male factor infertility. *Problems in Urology, 1*(3), 430–442.

Baum, N. (1987). Introduction: Male Infertility. *Postgraduate Medicine, 81*(2), 191.

Belker, A. M. (1987). Vasectomy reversal. *Urologic Clinics of North America, 14*(1), 155–165.

Bernstein, G. S. (1986). Male factor in infertility. In D. R. Mishell & V. Davajan (Eds.), *Infertility, contraception & reproductive endocrinology* (2nd ed., p. 423). Oradell, NJ Medical Economics Books.

Carpenito, L. J. (1992). *Nursing diagnosis: Application to clinical practice.* (3rd ed., pp. 591–594). Philadelphia: Lippincott.

Check, J. H., Chase, J. S., Nowroozi, K., Wa, C. H. & Adelson, H. G. (1989). Empirical therapy of the male with clomiphene in couples with unexplained infertility. *International Journal of Infertility 34*(2), 120–122.

Conrad, M. J., & Ross, L. S. (1985). Evaluation and treatment of the infertile male. *Primary Care, 12*(4), 687–701.

Davis, D. C. (1987). A conceptual framework for infertility. *Journal of Obstetric, Gynecologic, and Neonatal Nursing,* January/February, 30–35.

Gerber, W. L., de la Pena, V. E., & Mobley, W. C. (1988). Infertility, chemical exposure, and farming in Iowa: Absence of an association. *Urology, 31*(1), 46–50.

Hecht, N. B. (1987). Detecting the effects of toxic agents on spermatogenesis using DNA probes. *Environmental Health Perspectives, 74,* 31–40.

Hellstrom, W. J. G., Overstreet, J. W., & Lewis, E. L. (1987). The clinical significance of antibodies in the treatment of male infertility. *Problems in Urology, 1*(3), 418–429.

Howards, S. S. (1987a). Epididymal sperm maturation. In *The male factor in infertility: Pathophysiology, evaluation and treatment.* The American Fertility Society, 20th Annual Postgraduate Course, Sept. 26–27, 1987, 21–42.

Howards, S. S. (1987b). Microsurgery for male infertility. In *The male factor in infertility: Pathophysiology, evaluation and treatment.* The American Fertility Society, 20th Annual Postgraduate Course, Sept. 26–27, 1987, 269–283.

Kruger, T. F., Acosta, A. A., Simmons, K. F., Swanson, R. J., Matta, J. F., Veeck, L. L., Morshedi, M., & Brugo, S. B. (1987). New method of evaluating sperm morphology with predictive value for human in vitro fertilization. *Urology, 30*(3), 248–251.

Lipshultz, L. I. (1987). In vitro fertilization as therapy for male factor infertility. In *The male factor in infertility: Pathophysiology, evaluation and treatment.* The American Fertility Society, 20th Annual Postgraduate Course, Sept. 26–27, 1987, 229–240.

McClure, R. D. (1987a). Evaluation of the infertile male. *Problems in Urology, 1*(3), 443–459.

McClure, R. D. (1987b). Vasoepididymostomy. In *The male factor in infertility: Pathophysiology, evaluation and treatment.* The American Fertility Society, 20th Annual Postgraduate Course, Sept. 26–27, 1987, 287–301.

McConnell, J. D. (1987). The role of infection in male infertility. *Problems in Urology, 1*(3), 467–475.

McNally, M. R. (1987). Male infertility: Endocrine causes. *Postgraduate Medicine, 81*(2), 207–213.

Megory, E., Zuckerman, H., Shoham (Schwartz), Z., & Lunenfeld, B. (1987). Infections and male infertility. *Obstetrical and Gynecological Survey, 42*(5), 283–290.

Nagler, H. M., & Kaufman, D. G. (1987). Pathophysiology of a varicocele. *Problems in Urology, 1*(3), 411–417.

Pochaczevsky, R., Lee, W. J., & Mallett, E. (1988). Management of male infertility: Role of contact thermography, spermatic venography and embolization. *American Journal of Roentgenology, 147,* 97–102.

Pryor, J. P., & Hendry, W. F. (1991). Ejaculatory duct obstruction in subfertile males: Analysis of 87 patients. *Fertility and Sterility, 56*(4), 725–730.

Salisz, J. A., & Goldman, K. A. (1990). Testicular calcifications and neoplasia in patients treated for subfertility. *Urology, 36*(6), 557–560.

Sokol, R. Z. (1987). Pharmacological treatment of infertility. *Problems in Urology, 1*(3), 461–466.

Spencer, L. (1987). Male infertility: Psychological correlates. *Postgraduate Medicine, 81*(2), 223–228.

Suarez, G., Swartz, R., & Baum, N. (1987). Male infertility: Patient evaluation. *Postgraduate Medicine, 81*(2), 193–198.

Urry, R. L., & Middleton, R. G. (1986). Modern concepts in the diagnosis and treatment of male infertility. *Urologic Clinics of North America, 13*(3), 455–463.

Wing, R. L., Sloan, C. S., & Hammond, M. E. G. (1986). Male infertility. *Emergency Medicine,* Jan. 30, 105–112.

# PART V

# Voiding Disorders

# CHAPTER 14

# Adult Voiding Dysfunction

■

*Karen A. Karlowicz and Cindy E. Meredith*

## OVERVIEW

Dysfunctional voiding problems in adults manifest clinically as either urinary incontinence or urinary retention. *Urinary incontinence* is defined as ``the involuntary loss of urine so severe as to have social and/or hygienic consequences'' (NIH Consensus Development Conference Statement, 1988, p. 1). *Urinary retention* is defined as the inability to completely empty the bladder during attempts at micturition. Both conditions are considered symptoms of other more complex problems, such as anatomic or mechanical defects of the lower urinary tract, neurologic diseases or injuries, gynecologic conditions, as well as transient or functional disorders.

Various types of urinary incontinence constitute the majority of adult voiding disorders. Statistics suggest that about 10 million Americans are affected by this problem (Agency for Health Care Policy Research (AHCPR), 1992). Interest in adult voiding disorders, particularly urinary incontinence, has grown over the past 15 years. This is evidenced by the increasing number of professional books, journal articles, and conferences (such as the American Urological Association Allied's National Multispecialty Nursing Conference on Urinary Continence) devoted solely to the subject. In addition, the 1988 National Institutes of Health Consensus Development Conference on Urinary Incontinence in Adults, followed by the release of the Agency for Health Care Policy and Research Clinical Practice Guideline on Urinary Incontinence in Adults in 1992, has helped to heighten the awareness of the health care community about issues associated with the diagnosis, treatment, and management of adult voiding disorders.

Similarly, public attention and acceptance of the prevalence of bladder control problems has improved. Television and print ads for incontinence products appear regularly, as do articles in publications such as *Time* (Toufexis, 1986) and *The Washington Post* (Rovner, 1992). Even "Dear Abby" (1990) columns occasionally feature letters from readers who suffer with urinary incontinence. It seems that the message is finally getting out—treatments for dysfunctional voiding problems such as urinary incontinence can improve or cure the symptoms of most patients!

This chapter is designed to provide the reader with a general overview of adult voiding dysfunction. It begins with a discussion of the causes of voiding dysfunction in adults, differentiating neurogenic from nonneurogenic diseases and disorders. Methods of diagnosis and treatment alternatives are described, as are the complications of untreated or poorly managed voiding problems. Finally, the unique role and options that nurses have in the assessment and long-term management of patients with voiding dysfunction are highlighted.

## BEHAVIORAL OBJECTIVES

After studying this chapter, the reader should be able to

1. Predict the type of vesicourethral dysfunction that may occur with neurogenic and nonneurogenic diseases and disorders.
2. Explain the diagnostic value of various urodynamic measurements in the assessment of adult voiding dysfunction.
3. Describe treatment options for adult voiding dysfunction, including indications for the use of

pharmacologic, surgical, and behavioral therapies, as well as supportive measures and devices.
4. Develop a protocol for the nursing assessment of individuals with problems of urinary elimination.
5. Implement appropriate nursing management techniques for individuals with urinary incontinence or urinary retention.

## KEY WORDS

**Detrusor**—smooth muscle of the bladder.
**Detrusor areflexia**—acontractility of the bladder due to an abnormality of nervous control.
**Detrusor hyperreflexia**—overactivity of the bladder due to a disturbance of the nervous control mechanisms that is characterized by involuntary contractions.
**Detrusor-sphincter dyssynergia**—detrusor contraction concurrent with the

involuntary contraction of the urethral or periurethral striated muscle; a sign of a neurologic voiding disorder.
**Dyssynergia**—muscular incoordination.
**Micturition**—the act of urination.
**Urodynamics**—a series of diagnostic tests that use measurements of pressure, flow, and electrical response to evaluate physiologic functioning of the lower urinary tract.

## PERSPECTIVE ON DISEASE ENTITY

### Etiology

There are an assortment of neurogenic and nonneurogenic conditions that are known to affect the physiologic functioning of the lower

urinary tract. The most common of these are summarized in Table 14–1. Neurologic conditions are listed beginning with intracranial disorders and progress to include conditions affecting the spinal cord and peripheral nerves. Keep in mind, however, that this listing is not inclusive. Given that micturition is considered a nerve-mediated event, any disease or disor-

## TABLE 14–1. Causes of Adult Voiding Dysfunction

| CONDITION | DESCRIPTION | EFFECT ON LOWER URINARY TRACT | COMMENTS |
|---|---|---|---|
| **Neurogenic Disorders** | | | |
| Cerebrovascular accident | A hemorrhagic or ischemic event in the brain that causes damage to one of the areas or neurologic pathways responsible for regulating urinary function. | During the first 2 weeks poststroke, most patients will exhibit complete urinary retention due to detrusor areflexia. As poststroke recovery continues, sensory urgency with urinary incontinence due to detrusor hyperreflexia (w/normal, underactive, overactive, or dyssynergic striated sphincter activity) becomes the most common voiding problem. | Post-CVA voiding dysfunction may also be an exacerbation of a preexisting problem with urinary elimination, a complication of pharmaco-therapy, or the result of other stroke-related deficits. Indwelling catheter drainage required for at least the first 2 weeks post-CVA. |
| Cerebellar ataxia | A gait disturbance associated with pathologic degenerative diseases or disorders of the cerebellum. Patients exhibit wide-based, staggering, lurching, or uncoordinated gait. | Usually urinary incontinence due to detrusor hyperreflexia. Striated sphincter activity is synergistic, unless disease extends to the spinal cord to cause dyssynergia and high volume residual urine. | None |
| Cerebral trauma | Injury to the brain caused by a direct impact to the head. The extent of injury relates to the degree of acceleration-deceleration and rotation of brain tissue at the time of insult. | Similar to the effects post-CVA. There is an initial period of detrusor areflexia that requires indwelling catheter drainage preceding the development of urinary incontinence due to detrusor hyperreflexia. | Irritative voiding symptoms, usually associated with UTI, often complicate voiding dysfunction in the brain-injured patient. |
| Dementia | A generalized slowing and widespread deterioration of all acquired cognitive functions, particularly memory, which results from an interference with cellular metabolism and progressive atrophy of brain tissue. | Urinary incontinence may be precipitated by detrusor hyperreflexia, by a function of an inappropriately timed micturition reflex, or result because the individual has lost any awareness of his/her ability to voluntarily control bladder function. | Causes of dementia include diseases of the CNS (Alzheimer's disease, Pick's disease); metabolic disorders (chronic hypoglycemia); vascular disorders; hypoxia or anoxia; environmental toxins; drugs; or infections (meningitis, AIDS). |
| Parkinson's disease | A degenerative disorder of the basal ganglia associated with a deficiency of dopamine, a neurotransmitter. Progression of the disease leads to difficulties with behavior, and fine motor movements characterized by bradykinesia, tremors, and skeletal rigidity. | Patients usually exhibit symptoms of frequency, urgency, nocturia, and urge incontinence associated with detrusor hyperreflexia and poor voluntary sphincter control. | Voiding difficulties are often complicated by anatomic obstruction (i.e., BPH) or effects of various treatments for the Parkinson's. |
| Shy-Drager syndrome | A rare, progressively degenerative disorder affecting both the autonomic and central nervous systems, caused by the loss of neurons and the development of neurologic lesions in the midbrain, caudate nuclei, & intermediolateral column of the thoracic and sacral spinal cord. Symptoms of the disease include severe, orthostatic hypotension, cerebellar dysfunction, and impotence, along with voiding dysfunction. | Initially, patients experience frequency, urgency and nocturia; with disease progression there is urge incontinence due to detrusor hyperreflexia and sphincter incompetence during bladder filling; eventually urinary retention develops because of a poorly sustained or absent detrusor contraction. | CISC and anticholinergics or antispasmodics are usually ineffective in patients w/advanced disease; thus, an indwelling catheter remains the only viable treatment option. |

*Table continued on following page*

**379**

TABLE 14–1. Causes of Adult Voiding Dysfunction *Continued*

| CONDITION | DESCRIPTION | EFFECT ON LOWER URINARY TRACT | COMMENTS |
|---|---|---|---|
| Spinal cord injury | Any insult to the spinal column that results in partial or complete anatomic transection of the cord. Causes of injury include "high-velocity missile fracture or dislocation of the spinal column secondary to motor vehicle or diving accidents, vascular injuries, infection, disc prolapse, or sudden or severe hyperextension" (Wein, 1992). | *Suprasacral injuries.* After recovery from spinal shock, the detrusor becomes hyperreflexic with poorly sustained bladder contractions; striated sphincter dyssynergia results in patients w/complete lesions, while those with partial lesions will exhibit varying degrees of striated sphincter dysfunction. *Sacral injuries.* With recovery from spinal shock, there is persistent detrusor areflexia with failure of the sphincter to relax during attempts to void by Credé or abdominal straining. | Spinal shock is a period of suppressed autonomic and somatic activity at and below the level of all cord injuries. During this time, the bladder is areflexic, but sphincter tone is present. Still, continuous bladder drainage with an indwelling catheter is needed until recovery begins. |
| Pelvic plexus injuries | Any denervation, defunctionalization, or tethering of the pelvic plexus—an anatomic network of nerves that lies deep in the pelvis, and is formed by branches of the pelvic and hypogastric nerves and a variety of ganglia. Most injuries are iatrogenic, occurring after abdominal-perineal resection, radical hysterectomy, as well as adjuvant treatment such as chemotherapy or radiation therapy. | Compete urinary retention associated with an impaired or absent bladder contraction, and fixed striated sphincter, which creates an anatomic obstruction. | Symptoms are sometimes transient and diminish within 3 to 6 months of the event. During this recovery period, patients are maintained on CISC and reevaluated regularly for recovery of lower tract function. |
| Multiple sclerosis | A chronic, progressive, degenerative disease affecting the white matter of the brain and spinal cord, and caused by the destruction of the myelin sheath along conduction pathways of the central nervous system. The area of demyelination is referred to as a lesion or plaque. | In the initial phase of the disease, patients complain of either irritative or obstructive voiding symptoms, or a combination of both. With disease progression, a predominance of cervical plaques will cause incontinence due to detrusor hyperreflexia with altered bladder sensation, decreased capacity, poorly sustained contraction, and lower postvoid residual. A predominance of lower cord plaques (though less frequent) causes urinary retention due to detrusor areflexia with increased capacity and postvoid, and poor sensation to bladder filling. True striated sphincter dyssynergia is present in only about half of patients with hyperreflexia. | Sexual dysfunction, constipation, and/or bowel incontinence are also associated with lower urinary tract dysfunction. |
| Diabetes | Middle-aged, elderly, or poorly controlled diabetics are most likely to develop a diabetic peripheral neuropathy—a condition resulting from a disturbance in peripheral nerve metabolism, which causes segmental demyelinization and poor nerve conduction. | Characterized by altered sensations to bladder filling, increased bladder capacity, and poor bladder contractility w/increasing residual urine; effects to lower urinary tract similar as for other types of peripheral neuropathy. | Voiding dysfunction is often complicated by chronic urinary tract infection. |

## TABLE 14–1. Causes of Adult Voiding Dysfunction *Continued*

| CONDITION | DESCRIPTION | EFFECT ON LOWER URINARY TRACT | COMMENTS |
|---|---|---|---|
| **Nonneurogenic Disorders** | | | |
| Postprostatectomy incontinence | Urinary leakage that occurs following surgical resection of the prostate. | Incontinence after transurethral prostatectomy is usually due to direct structural damage to the sphincteric mechanisms; leakage after radical prostatectomy is often the result of injury to the nerves innervating the bladder or urethral sphincters. The amount of urine leakage may range from a dribble to total incontinence. | Preexisting voiding difficulties caused by conditions such as diabetes, chronic alcoholism, or CVA may increase the likelihood or aggravate symptoms of postprostatectomy incontinence. |
| Female urethral incompetence | Also termed stress incontinence, this condition occurs because of a weakness that develops in the smooth muscle of the urethral sphincter. Factors contributing to urethral incompetence may include childbearing (# vaginal deliveries), decreased estrogen production w/menopause, iatrogenic interference w/sphincter mechanism during bladder neck surgery, congenital weakness of sphincter, and obesity. | With coughing, sneezing, laughing, or physical effort, there is an increase in intra-abdominal pressure, which is transmitted to the proximal urethra. The involuntary loss of urine, usually in small amounts, is despite the absence of a detrusor contraction or bladder overdistention, and frequently is attributed to hypermobility or significant displacement of the urethra and bladder, as well as a reverse pressure differential between the urethra and bladder with exertion. | Conditions such as anterior vaginal wall prolapse or cystocele may aggravate symptoms of stress incontinence. Symptoms of frequency and urgency often coexist with symptoms of stress urinary leakage. |
| Idiopathic urinary retention | Clinical presentation is either long-standing or recurrent acute episodes of urinary retention. Psychological problems such as hysteria, psychosis, family/marital conflict, family death, occupational problems, reproductive difficulties, or impotence, are often the underlying cause of the complete inability to void. | The total inability to void exists for 24 to 48 hours before the patient seeks health care. Catheter drainage of the distended bladder usually produces a large volume of clear, yellow urine. If a program of CISC is not implemented, repeated overdistention of the bladder will cause diminished tone and sensations to filling. | Psychiatric or behavioral therapies are often combined with medical treatment to restore normal voiding. |
| Frequency/urgency syndrome | Dysfunctional voiding characterized by urinary frequency and urgency, and sometimes accompanied by urge incontinence, suprapubic pain/pressure, dysuria, hesitancy, weak stream, or postvoid urgency. In most patients, there will be no physical evidence of a urologic or neurologic condition, but the onset of symptoms can often be linked to a psychosocial crisis. | Detrusor instability or detrusor areflexia with or without striated sphincter spasm are responsible for symptoms experienced by the patient. In either instance, complications of inconsistent and incomplete bladder emptying will result if treatment is not instituted in a timely manner. | Pharmacologic and psychological therapies are usually combined with other medical-surgical treatments to eventually restore normal voiding. |

UTI, urinary tract infection; CNS, central nervous system; CVA, cerebrovascular accident; BPH, benign prostatic hyperplasia; CISC, clean intermittent self-catheterization.
Sources: Hickey (1992), Wein (1992), and Krane & Siroky (1991).

der that affects or interrupts nerve pathways may potentially produce some type of neurogenic voiding dysfunction. The list of nonneurogenic causes for voiding dysfunction includes the most common functional disorders in men and women, as well as postprostatectomy incontinence. Outlet obstruction, a common cause of nonneurogenic voiding dysfunction in adults, has been omitted from this listing because the topic is extensively discussed in Chapter 4.

## Pathophysiology

In order to understand the impact of ineffective voiding on the urinary tract, it is essential that one first appreciate the highly coordinated and complicated process known as micturition. The normal micturition cycle can be simply separated into two phases: urine storage and bladder emptying. Both phases are controlled and coordinated through innervation by the sympathetic, parasympathetic, and central nervous systems. The following is an oversimplified summary of the events that constitute the micturition cycle.

During urine storage (or the filling phase), there is a slow rise in intravesical pressure owing to the increasing volume of urine in the bladder. As pressure increases, stretch receptors in the bladder wall convey afferent impulses via the pelvic nerve to the spinal cord. This action stimulates the sympathetic efferent supply, located in spinal cord segments T11 to L2, to convey impulses back to the bladder and urethra via the hypogastric nerve. The result is stimulation of the smooth muscle of the bladder neck and proximal urethra (or a tightening of the internal sphincter) to maintain continence and the inhibition of vesical contraction to allow for more complete bladder filling. Additionally, efferent impulses through the pudendal nerve stimulate increased activity of the striated sphincter.

When intravesical pressure reaches a critical point and the bladder is sufficiently distended, nerve impulses are transmitted from the spinal cord to the brain. Although many areas of the brain may be involved in the voiding process, it is the brain stem that is considered to be the actual organization center for micturition.

Bladder emptying (or voiding) occurs by parasympathetic facilitation and sympathetic inhibition. Initiation of voiding is achieved when the efferent pelvic nerve, which originates in spinal cord segments S2 to S4, stimu-

lates the bladder to contract and permits the bladder neck and urethra to funnel open. This action coincides with relaxation of the internal and external urethral sphincters, and perineal muscles, through inhibition of the pudendal nerve, which originates in the sacral spinal cord.

There are other factors that also contribute to normal micturition. Urine storage requires appropriate sensations to bladder filling, a bladder outlet that remains closed at rest and with increased intra-abdominal pressure, and the absence of involuntary detrusor contractions. Bladder emptying requires a coordinated and strong, sustained detrusor contraction; simultaneous lowering of resistance of the smooth and striated sphincters; as well as the absence of anatomic obstruction. Conditions that singularly or in combination interfere or alter these requirements jeopardize normal voiding (Van Arsdalen & Wein, 1991; Wein, 1992).

### CLASSIFICATION OF VOIDING DISORDERS

When a disease or disorder compromises the normal micturition cycle, it manifests as urinary incontinence, urinary retention, or both. Despite the descriptiveness and familiarity of these terms, urologic practitioners have for years sought a more precise means for characterizing difficulties in urinary elimination. Classification schemes proposed by Bradley (1986), Gibbons (1976), and Bors and Comarr (1971) used a variety of neuroanatomic terms to describe voiding dysfunction. The system first proposed by McClennan (1939), then refined and popularized by Lapides (1967), combined urodynamic findings with neuroanatomic terms to explain voiding dysfunction, whereas the classification scheme developed by Krane and Siroky (1979) is based entirely on objective urodynamic findings. The current trend, however, is to describe voiding dysfunction using a functional approach. For example, the Wein functional classification system (1981) simply classifies voiding dysfunction as either the failure to store (urinary incontinence) or the failure to empty (urinary retention), whereas the classification system proposed by the International Continence Society uses the terms *overactive, normoactive,* or *underactive* to explain voiding dysfunction (Tables 14–2 and 14–3).

Admittedly, there are strengths and weaknesses inherent to each classification scheme. For this reason, urologic health care professionals may find it helpful to employ more than

## TABLE 14–2. Major Classification Schemes for Voiding Dysfunction

| BRADLEY | BORS/COMARR | GIBBONS | LAPIDES | KRANE & SIROKY | WEIN |
|---|---|---|---|---|---|
| | ← Neurologic | | | Functional → | |
| Loop 1:<br>Frontal lobe–brain stem<br>Loop 2:<br>Brain stem–detrusor nucleus (sacral cord) | Upper motor neuron lesion<br>Complete vs. incomplete<br>Balanced vs. imbalanced | Suprasacral lesion | Uninhibited neurogenic bladder<br>Reflex neurogenic bladder | Detrusor hyperreflexia (or normoreflexia)<br>Coordinated sphincters<br>Striated sphincter dyssynergia<br>Smooth sphincter dyssynergia | Failure to store<br>Bladder<br>Outlet |
| Loop 3:<br>Detrusor–pudendal nucleus (sacral cord) | Lower motor neuron lesion<br>Complete vs. incomplete<br>Balanced vs. imbalanced | Sacral lesion<br>Motor<br>Sensory | Autonomous neurogenic bladder<br>Motor paralytic bladder<br>Sensory neurogenic bladder | Detrusor areflexia<br>Coordinated sphincters<br>Nonrelaxing striated sphincter<br>Nonrelaxing smooth sphincter | Failure to empty<br>Bladder<br>Outlet |
| Loop 4A:<br>Frontal lobe–pudendal nucleus<br>Loop 4B:<br>Pudendal–pudendal | Mixed lesion | Mixed lesion | | Denervated striated sphincter | |
| S = Helps practitioners to understand and apply neuro-urophysiology concepts to diagnostic techniques | S = Useful to predict detrusor function in spinal cord injured patients w/complete lesions, after spinal shock only | S = Simplification of Bors/Comarr system | S = Classic neuro-urologic classification system; uses objective measurements of bladder function combined w/functional description of neurologic lesions | S = Neuro-urologically derived; urodynamically based; functionally oriented; classifies both detrusor and sphincter dysfunction | S = Provides framework of treatment of neurogenic and nonneurogenic disorders |
| W = Difficult to predict urinary tract dysfunction solely by anatomic location of lesion in relation to reflex pathway | W = Unable to predict urinary tract dysfunction due to other types of neurologic lesions; cannot be used to classify non-neurogenic voiding dysfunction | W = Same as Bors/Comarr | W = Sphincter function not considered | W = Difficult to apply to non-neurogenic voiding dysfunction | W = Does not require diagnosis in order to classify voiding dysfunction; does not provide framework to derive diagnosis |

S = strengths; W = weaknesses.
Adapted from Krane, R. J., & Siroky, M. B. (1984). Classification of voiding dysfunction: Value of classification systems. In D. M. Barrett & A. J. Wein (Eds.). Controversies in *neuro-urology* (p. 234). New York: Churchill Livingstone.

one method. To determine which classification schemes will best suit your clinical needs, consider (1) the underlying concepts guiding the development of each scheme, (2) the patient population to which the nomenclature will be applied, (3) your diagnostic capabilities, and (4) information to be communicated (Gray, 1992a; Staskin, 1991).

## COMPLICATIONS OF VOIDING DYSFUNCTION

If voiding dysfunction goes undetected or untreated, there may be untoward effects to the entire urinary system. Chronic infection is a common problem associated with ineffective, low-pressure bladder emptying and persistent residual urine. Infections that go unresolved predispose the patient to the development of urinary calculi, recurrent pyelonephritis, and, ultimately, urinary sepsis. Bladder trabeculation, detrusor hypertrophy and decreased compliance, vesicoureteral reflux, hydronephrosis, and eventual deterioration of the upper urinary tract with altered renal function are problems associated with high-pressure urine storage and bladder emptying; these result from long-standing anatomic (e.g., benign prostatic hy-

**TABLE 14–3. International Continence Society
Classification**

Overactive bladder
  Uninhibited bladder contractions
    Detrusor hyperreflexia secondary to suprasacral
      neurologic lesion
    Coexistent urologic conditions
      Detrusor instability (nonneurogenic)
      Outlet overactivity (obstruction)
  Decreased (low) bladder compliance
    Bladder fibrosis (infection, indwelling catheter)
    Neurogenic
Normoactive bladder
Underactive bladder
  Absent or impaired detrusor contractility
    Neurogenic
      Sacral or infrasacral lesion
      Spinal shock
    Pharmacologic
      Anticholinergic therapy
      Smooth muscle relaxants (direct, $Ca^{2+}$ channel)
    Musculogenic
      Overdistention
      Fibrosis
Mixed detrusor dysfunction
  Detrusor hyperreflexia with impaired contractility
    Poor sustained detrusor contraction (neurogenic)
      Loss of facilitation
      Inhibition by pelvic floor reflex
    Decreased detrusor contractility (myogenic)
  Noncontractile bladder with low compliance

From Krane, R. J., & Siroky, M. B. (1991). *Clinical neuro-
urology* (2nd ed.). Boston: Little, Brown.

perplasia) or physiologic (e.g., smooth or
striated sphincter dyssynergia) obstruction of
the urinary outlet. Finally, perineal skin irritation and breakdown may result from incessant
urine leakage and the lack of regular, adequate
hygiene measures. (See Chapters 4 and 5 for
further information and discussion.)

## Medical-Surgical Management

### DIAGNOSIS OF VOIDING DISORDERS

Medical evaluation of the patient with complaints of voiding dysfunction often begins
with routine laboratory studies, including urinalysis, urine culture and sensitivity, and selected blood chemistries (serum creatinine,
blood urea nitrogen, prostate-specific antigen,
and prostatic acid phosphatase). During an initial assessment, residual urine volume may
also be measured. This is a traditional yet valuable means of assessment that may be performed when obtaining a urine sample for cul-

ture or in conjunction with other diagnostic
studies.

To assess the anatomic integrity of the urinary tract, the patient is required to undergo
one or more imaging procedures, including an
excretory urography, cystogram, voiding cystourethrogram (VCUG), and bladder ultrasonography. When voiding dysfunction has been
a long-standing problem and imaging studies
suggest upper tract deterioration, a dimercaptosuccinic acid (DMSA) or diethylenetriamine
acid (DPTA) radionuclide scan also is performed to assess renal function. Cystourethroscopy is an important component of the medical
evaluation and is performed to identify pathologic changes in the lower urinary tract that
may be the cause or result of voiding dysfunction.

To distinguish stress incontinence from other
conditions, the physician may perform what is
traditionally referred to as a *stress test* (also
called the Marshall–Marchetti or Bonney test).
This test is usually performed with the patient
in an upright position and the bladder moderately distended. Using two fingers or two
clamps, the physician lifts the bladder neck upward toward the symphysis pubis, then asks
the patient to cough or strain. The absence of
urinary leakage with this maneuver suggests
that continence could be achieved with added
support to the bladder neck (Tanagho, 1992).

When a vesicovaginal fistula is suspected as
the cause of urinary incontinence, but not con-
clusively demonstrated by other diagnostic
techniques, the physician may perform a *methylene blue test*. The test involves placing a tampon into the vagina, then instilling a solution
containing methylene blue into the bladder.
The patient is asked to hold the solution and
encouraged to assume an upright position;
walking is recommended, if possible. After a
short period, the tampon is removed and examined. Blue staining of the middle or proximal third of the tampon confirms the presence
of a vesicovaginal fistula, whereas staining of
the distal portion of the tampon suggests urethral leakage. To perform this assessment on
an outpatient basis, the patient may be prescribed a drug such as phenazopyridine (Pyridium), which is known to discolor the urine.
Tampons are worn for several days, with
stained inserts saved and returned to the office
or clinic for analysis.

### URODYNAMIC TESTING

*Urodynamics* is the broad term that refers to
a series of diagnostic techniques used to evalu-

ate the process of micturition in a patient with complaints of voiding dysfunction. The use of urodynamic procedures to measure lower urinary tract function is analogous to pulmonary function tests that measure lung function in that the procedures incorporate measures of flow, volume, and pressure, in addition to electrical response.

The need for urodynamic testing is based, in part, on findings from the history, physical examination, imaging studies, and cystourethroscopy. The extent of testing required depends on the complexity of the patient's problem, the urologist's preference for various procedures, and the availability of urodynamic testing equipment. In some instances, the knowledge, skill, and experience of the urodynamicist may be important when determining whether the patient is studied using simple office or bedside procedures or is referred to a large medical center where more sophisticated testing techniques are used. In some settings, urodynamic testing may require a physician's order, although the procedures are most frequently performed by a professional nurse or trained urologic technician.

**Urinary Flow Rate.** The urinary flow rate is an assessment of the joint action of the bladder and outlet. It is a measure of the volume of urine expelled from the bladder via the urethra over a given period; it is calculated and expressed as milliliters per second. This test allows the practitioner to gather information about one's micturition abilities with a minimum of discomfort, thus making the urinary flow rate the easiest, most informative, most cost-effective, and the only noninvasive urodynamic procedure. As a general rule, the measurement of residual urine is not a routine component of urinary flow rate testing.

The urinary flow rate is used to assess patients with symptoms of outflow obstruction (benign prostatic hyperplasia or urethral stricture); before and after any surgical procedure designed to improve urine flow or that may compromise lower urinary tract function; before and during pharmacotherapy for lower urinary tract dysfunction; and as a screening procedure for those with dysfunctional voiding prior to initiating other invasive urodynamic tests (Rollema, 1991).

In most settings, the urinary flow rate is measured using an electronic device with a container placed on it, which then is positioned beneath a free-standing commode. However, there are some nonelectronic devices commercially available that permit measurement of urinary flow with color-indicator strips or chambers.

Preparation for the procedure requires that the patient delay voiding until the bladder is comfortably full so that a valid and reliable study may be obtained. Asking the patient to increase his or her fluid intake prior to uroflometry sometimes helps ensure an adequate voided volume. For the urinary flow rate study to be considered valid and reliable, a voided volume larger than 150 mL should be obtained (Wein, 1992). Many practitioners also recommend the measurement of two flow events for a comparative assessment of a patient's voiding capabilities, with the first urinary flow rate performed before any lower urinary tract instrumentation. Subjectively, the patient must feel as though these voiding attempts are similar to those in other settings at other times.

The urinary flow rate is analyzed according to the following parameters: maximum (or peak) flow rate, total voided volume, time to maximum flow, total flow time, and average flow rate (Fig. 14–1). A normal maximum flow rate is considered to be 20 to 25 mL/s for men and 25 to 30 mL/s for women (Tanagho, 1992). The usual average flow rate ranges from 15 to 25 mL/s and is calculated by dividing the total volume voided by the total flow time. Variations from these normal parameters are common and are dependent on the voided volume, voiding time, and age of the patient (Wein, 1992).

In addition to the numeric measurements involving volume and time, the urinary flow rate is analyzed for its graphic pattern. The normal urinary flow rate is graphically depicted as a bell-shaped curve. Outlet obstruction is typically characterized by a weak and prolonged

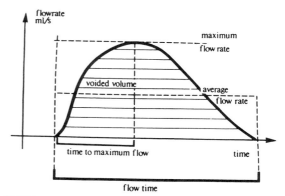

*FIGURE 14–1* Graphic depiction of urinary flow rate. (From Wein, A. J., English, W. E., & Whitmore, K. E. [1988]. Office urodynamics. *Urologic Clinics of North America, 15,* 609. Reprinted by permission.)

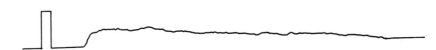

*FIGURE 14–2* Flow trace in outflow tract obstruction. (From Abrams, P. H. [1983]. *Urodynamics.* [p. 37]. New York: Springer-Verlag. Reprinted by permission.)

urinary flow rate pattern that may span several minutes (Fig. 14–2). Detrusor weakness assisted by abdominal straining produces an intermittent flow pattern, characterized by repeated starts and stops during the attempt at voiding (Fig. 14–3). Detrusor-sphincter dyssynergia is displayed as a continuous but irregular urinary flow pattern with rapid fluctuations in the maximum flow rate (Fig. 14–4). An explosive urine stream, in which the maximum flow rate may approach 40 to 50 mL/s, and the voiding time is comparatively short for the amount voided, is typically associated with stress urinary incontinence in women (Gray, 1990) (Fig. 14–5).

**Cystometrogram.** The cystometrogram (CMG) is a measure of bladder capacity and pressure during the filling and storage phases of micturition. This procedure requires that an intraurethral or suprapubic catheter be inserted and the bladder filled. The size of the catheter used depends on the sophistication of measurement techniques, as well as the type of recording equipment being used. For example, a simple bedside CMG may require that a single 14 Fr catheter be used. This approach requires that bladder filling and the simultaneous measurement of bladder pressure be accomplished through the same lumen. On the other hand, combined filling and voiding cystometry requires the use of either a multilumen catheter, a microtransducer-tipped catheter, or dual catheters (i.e., 14 Fr plus a 5 Fr inserted together). This approach enables the urodynamicist to fill the bladder through one lumen while measuring pressure separately through another.

The debate continues as to whether the best filling medium for cystometry is gas (carbon dioxide) or liquid. Many practitioners find gas filling is useful for quick screening studies and bedside cystometry. Disadvantages to this approach are that patients may perceive sensations of fullness more quickly and subsequent voiding measurements cannot be performed. On the other hand, there are those practitioners who consider the use of liquid (sterile water, saline solution, or water-soluble radiographic contrast solution) to be absolutely critical; it is more physiologic and more versatile in that pressure-flow studies are easily performed after bladder filling has been completed.

Bladder filling during cystometry may be continuous or in increments. The International Continence Society (ICS) defines the following filling rates:

Up to 10 mL/min is slow-fill cystometry.
Ten to 100 mL/min is medium-fill cystometry.
Over 100 mL/min is rapid-fill cystometry (Abrams, et al., 1991).

An infusion rate of approximately 20 mL/min is desirable for most adult cystometric studies. When trying to provoke uninhibited bladder contractions, or when challenging bladder compliance, a rapid-fill cystometry may be employed.

Cystometry may be performed in either the supine or upright position, with comparative studies performed in some patients in both positions. The upright position is thought to be better, however, if trying to evaluate bladder instability or to demonstrate stress incontinence. In addition, progression to pressure-flow studies is more easily accomplished when bladder filling is performed in an upright position, because the patient will often be situated standing near or sitting on the commode.

Patient cooperation and communication are extremely important during cystometry. Not only are they asked to assume a variety of awkward positions with numerous devices and tubes attached to them, but they must avoid any excessive movement (such as coughing, sneezing, straining, and moving their extremities) unless directed by the urodynamicist. (It is not uncommon for patients to be asked to cough, or bounce on their heels, during cystometry to provoke an incontinent episode or demonstrate an uninhibited bladder contraction.) During the procedure, patients are also asked to indicate their (1) first sensation of bladder filling, (2) first sensation of a comfort-

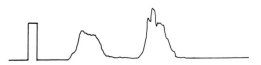

*FIGURE 14–3* Irregular urinary flow due to straining. (From Abrams, P. H. [1983]. *Urodynamics* [p. 38]. New York: Springer-Verlag. Reprinted by permission.)

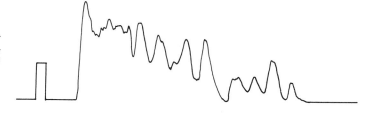

**FIGURE 14–4** Irregular urinary flow due to detrusor-sphincter dyssynergia. (From Abrams, P. H. [1983]. *Urodynamics* [p. 38]. New York: Springer-Verlag. Reprinted by permission.)

able or moderate degree of bladder fullness, and (3) definite fullness with an absolute need to void. In most adults, the first sensation of bladder filling occurs after a volume of 90 to 150 mL has been infused, and fullness occurs at a volume of 300 to 600 mL (Gray, 1991). For patients unable to communicate this information, close observation for behavioral changes that may be indicators of bladder fullness is required.

The following features are analyzed from the CMG: bladder capacity; volume at which the first, second, and third sensations of filling occurred; overall compliance of the detrusor (changes in pressure to corresponding changes in volume); presence or absence of involuntary contractions; and leakage of fluid with provocative maneuvers. Many physicians consider the inability to generate a voluntary detrusor contraction at the conclusion of bladder filling to be an abnormal finding of cystometry. This, though, is simply not true. In fact, the most that can be made of this observation is that either fear of leakage, embarrassment, intimidation of the testing environment, or supine positioning prevented the patient from voluntarily contracting his or her bladder. Often, placing the patient in a more natural voiding position (i.e., on the commode) is enough to demonstrate a voluntary bladder contraction. Figure 14–6 illustrates the various filling patterns for adult cystometry.

**Urethral Profilometry.** The urethral pressure profile (UPP) is a graphic representation of in-

traurethral pressure measurements either at rest, during coughing or straining, or during the process of voiding (Abrams et al., 1991). This urodynamic test is used to assess functional urethral length, as well as the general competency of the urethra and sphincter. In

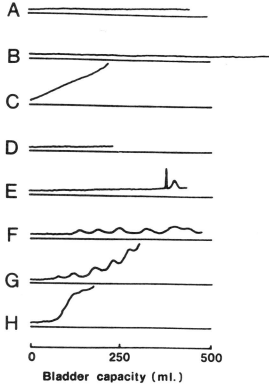

**FIGURE 14–6** Various representative adult cystometrograms. *A,* Normal filling curve in a patient with a bladder capacity of 450 mL, normal compliance, and no involuntary bladder contractions. *B,* Large-capacity bladder with increased compliance at medium fill rate. *C,* Decreased compliance. *D,* Small-capacity bladder secondary to hypersensitivity without decreased compliance or involuntary bladder contraction. *E,* Bladder contraction provoked by cough. *F,* Low-amplitude detrusor contractions. *G,* Decreased compliance and involuntary bladder contractions. *H,* High-amplitude early involuntary bladder contraction. (From Wein, A. J., English, W. E., & Whitmore, K. E. [1988]. Office urodynamics. *Urologic Clinics of North America, 15,* 609. Reprinted by permission.)

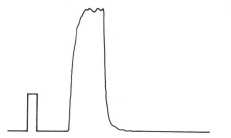

**FIGURE 14–5** Explosive urinary stream. (From Abrams, P. H. [1983]. *Urodynamics* [p. 37]. New York: Springer-Verlag. Reprinted by permission.)

most instances, the UPP is performed as a static procedure, meaning that a pressure-sensing device (usually a microtransducer catheter) is slowly withdrawn through the urethra while pressure measurements are made at regular intervals until the device reaches the meatus. This is often performed with the bladder empty and the patient at rest and thus is referred to as a *resting UPP*. A stress UPP is performed using the same technique, but with the addition of stress measures such as a cough or Valsalva maneuver (Abrams et al., 1991).

Urethral pressure may also be measured simultaneously with intravesical pressure during provocative cystometry, as well as during pressure-flow studies. When measuring urethral pressure in this manner, the pressure sensing device is usually stationary in the urethra. Fluoroscopic monitoring adds another diagnostic dimension to the measurement of UPP and has proved quite useful in the assessment of stress incontinence.

Analysis of the UPP requires an understanding of the following definitions established by the ICS:

1. Maximum urethral pressure—maximum pressure of the measured profile, regardless of where in the measurement that peak occurred.
2. Maximum urethral closure pressure—maximum difference between urethral and intravesical pressure.
3. Functional profile length—length of the urethra from the point where urethral pressure exceeds intravesical pressure to the meatus; when performing a stress UPP, *functional profile length* refers to the length over which the urethral pressure exceeds intravesical pressure on stress (Abrams et al., 1991).

Figure 14–7 depicts a static urethral pressure profile in a female.

Another measurement technique, similar to the UPP, used to differentiate intrinsic sphincter incompetence from pelvic descent is called the *Valsalva leak point pressure* (LPP) (Gray, 1993). To perform this test, the patient's bladder should be filled to a moderate capacity (150 to 250 mL). Bladder and urethral pressure measurements are recorded as the patient is instructed to increase abdominal pressure by tightening abdominal muscles and bearing down. The LPP is the amount of pressure generated by Valsalva that results in urinary leakage. When slow Valsalva fails to produce urine leakage, then the patient may be asked to cough. The amount of pressure generated by a cough that produces urine leakage is considered the LPP. A diagnosis of stress incontinence related to intrinsic sphincter incompetence should be suspected when the Valsalva LPP is 70 cm $H_2O$ or less (Gray, 1993).

**Electromyography.** The recording of electrical activity generated by the striated muscles of the pelvic floor is called *electromyography* (EMG). Also referred to as *sphincter EMG*, it is used as an adjunct to other urodynamic measurements to evaluate the coordination of the external urethral sphincter and pelvic floor musculature with detrusor activity during bladder filling and emptying.

To establish an EMG recording, two needle or wire electrodes are inserted into the periurethral muscles or anal sphincter: One needle is placed at approximately the 10 o'clock position, and the other at approximately the 2 o'clock position. Another approach is to apply two patch surface electrodes (neonatal electrocardiogram leads or cup electroencephalogram leads) to the anal sphincter. When using surface electrodes, it is imperative that the skin is cleaned and dried thoroughly before application of the electrodes; otherwise, the EMG recording may be weak or plagued by artifact. A reference or ground electrode is also needed and is usually taped to the patient's inner thigh or groin.

The EMG chart display and accompanying audio signal from most urodynamic recording devices represent the action potentials from groups of motor units. This type of measurement enables the urodynamicist to make only general conclusions about the coordination, or lack thereof, of striated muscle activity.

An EMG recording is analyzed for the extent to which the groups of motor units are coordinated with bladder filling and emptying. A normal EMG response is subtle at rest, yet steadily increases to a feverish pitch as the bladder reaches capacity; this represents the tightening of the external sphincter to maintain continence. With the initiation of a voluntary detrusor contraction, EMG activity is completely silenced; this represents relaxation of the external sphincter to facilitate bladder emptying (Fig. 14–8). Additionally, the EMG chart display can confirm a positive bulbocavernosus reflex (depicted as an acceleration in EMG activity) when elicited by either gently squeezing the clitoris in females or the glans in males, or placing light traction against a Foley catheter balloon during filling (Gray, 1991).

The absence of increasing EMG activity with bladder filling may be indicative of pelvic floor

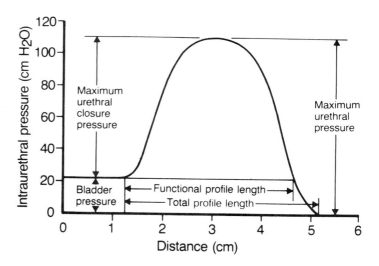

*FIGURE 14–7* Diagram of female urethral pressure profile. (From International Continence Society Committee on Standardisation of Terminology. [1976]. First report on the standardisation of terminology of lower urinary tract function. *British Journal of Urology, 48,* 39–42.)

denervation, whereas an increase in EMG activity concurrent with voiding suggests detrusor-sphincter dyssynergia. These findings must be correlated with the patient's history and physical examination and should be interpreted with caution because patient-induced artifacts can often produce similar results.

**Combined Studies.** Combined studies offer the clinician the opportunity to evaluate the entire micturition cycle. During bladder filling, all or some of the following parameters may be simultaneously measured: intra-abdominal pressure (usually via a rectal probe), intravesical pressure (via a transurethral or suprapubic catheter), subtracted detrusor pressure (intra-abdominal minus intravesical pressure), ure-

thral pressure, and sphincter EMG. To evaluate the effectiveness of bladder emptying, the urinary flow rate is an added component to the pressure-flow study.

In instances of complicated voiding dysfunction, the synchronous recording of urodynamic parameters with cystourethrography, also called *video urodynamics,* has proved beneficial. These procedures must be performed in a radiologic suite and involve the use of a television camera, an image intensifier, and a mixer unit that allows the urodynamic recording and fluoroscopic image to be synchronously recorded to videotape for more careful analysis. Recent advances in technology also permit the creation of a computerized record

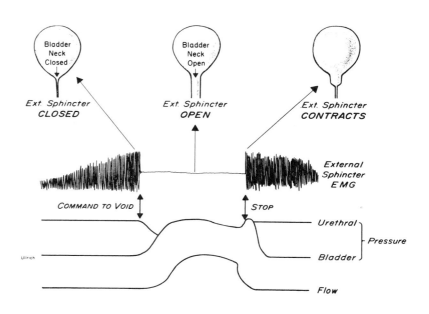

*FIGURE 14–8* Schematic of micturition reflex. (From Blaivas, J. G. [1985]. Pathophysiology of lower urinary tract dysfunction. *Urologic Clinics of North America, 12,* 215. Reprinted by permission.)

in which the urodynamic measurements and fluoroscopic images may be stored and analyzed. This type of study is most helpful when urodynamic findings differ from the clinical impression given by the patient's history and physical examination, when medications and surgery produce unsuccessful therapeutic results, or when the patient presents with complex neurologic symptoms.

## TREATMENT OF VOIDING DISORDERS

This section highlights pharmacologic and surgical treatments for adult voiding dysfunction. The choice of a particular treatment for an adult with voiding dysfunction depends on (1) the patient's symptoms, (2) results of diagnostic testing, (3) analysis of alternative therapies, (4) reversibility and side effects of treatments, (5) ability of patient to comply with the recommended therapy, (6) cost of therapy, (7) access to treatment, and (8) patient and family preference (Wein, 1992). In many instances, it is not uncommon for the physician to decide to use a combination of therapeutic modalities (including behavioral therapies or assistive devices) for maximum benefit.

**Pharmacotherapy.** A variety of pharmacologic agents are available to treat voiding disorders. Although not every patient is a candidate for pharmacotherapy, many benefit from the therapeutic effects pharmacologic agents exert on the lower urinary tract. In addition to those most commonly prescribed medications highlighted in Table 14–4, studies are under way to determine the role and efficacy of calcium agonists, potassium channel openers, and prostaglandin inhibitors in the treatment of voiding dysfunction.

**Surgical Interventions.** Another alternative in the treatment of adult voiding disorders is surgical intervention. As a general rule, surgery is reserved for those patients whose voiding dysfunction does not improve after conservative therapy by means such as medications or behavioral training. The most commonly performed surgical procedures for adult voiding dysfunction are listed and defined below. A more in-depth discussion of each procedure is not within the scope of this chapter, and the reader is referred to a urologic surgery text for further explanation.

I. Surgery for uncomplicated female stress incontinence (urethral hypermobility)
   A. Anterior colporrhaphy (anterior repair)—a transvaginal procedure in which horizontal sutures are placed from the distal suburethral area to the bladder neck, so as to tighten the pubocervical fascia and elevate the urethra. This is the most commonly performed gynecologic procedure (Leach & Raz, 1991).
   B. Marshall-Marchetti-Krantz (MMK) cystourethropexy—a transabdominal vesicourethral suspension in which sutures are placed through the anterior vaginal wall, and anterior and lateral portions of the bladder base are secured to the periosteum of the symphysis pubis and rectus abdominis muscles to lift and support the urethra and bladder neck.
   C. Burch colposuspension—a modified MMK in which sutures placed through the anterior vaginal wall are fixed to the ligament of Cooper to provide support to the urethra and bladder neck (Lam & Hadley, 1991; Leach & Raz, 1991).
   D. Stamey endoscopic vesical neck suspension—a procedure first described in 1973 that involves two small suprapubic incisions on each side of the symphysis pubis, a T incision through the anterior vaginal wall, and the use of a long suspension needle for the placement of sutures to elevate and support each side of the bladder neck (Lam & Hadley, 1991; Stamey, 1992).
   E. Modified Pereyra needle bladder neck suspension—the transvaginal placement of suspension sutures through a U-shaped vaginal incision, with needle transfer and fixation of each suture through a small suprapubic incision to the rectus fascia (Leach & Raz, 1991).

II. Surgery for intrinsic sphincter deficiency (male or female)
   A. Vaginal wall/pubovaginal sling procedure—a procedure whereby a fascial (or synthetic) sling is positioned underneath the urethrovesical junction, then secured to retropubic or abdominal structures. This technique may be combined with needle suspension and is sometimes used when other surgical procedures have failed.
   B. Insertion of artificial urinary sphincter—involves the insertion of a prosthetic device consisting of a cuff, a pump, and a reservoir. In adult females, the cuff of the artificial sphincter is placed around the bladder neck. In adult males, it may be placed either

## TABLE 14–4. Medications to Treat Voiding Disorders

| DRUG CLASS | ACTION | ADVERSE EFFECTS | NURSING CONSIDERATIONS |
|---|---|---|---|
| **Drugs That Inhibit Contractility and Promote Urine Storage** | | | |
| Anticholinergics (propantheline bromide, hyoscyamine, methantheline bromide, dicyclomine hydrochloride, tincture of belladonna, atropine sulfate, glycopyrrolate) | Reduces spasm or smooth muscle contraction by blocking or inhibiting the effects of acetylcholine at the muscarinic receptor | Dizziness, drowsiness, blurred vision, dry mouth; ↑ HR; contraindicated in many disease states—check before administration | Give 30–60 min before meals and at bedtime; monitor vital signs and urine output; use gum or sugarless candies to relieve dry mouth |
| Antispasmodics/direct smooth muscle relaxants (oxybutynin chloride, flavoxate hydrochloride, belladonna & opium [B & O] suppositories) | Inhibits muscarinic action of acetylcholine on smooth muscle; direct antispasmodic effect on detrusor smooth muscle | Same as for anticholinergics | Same as for anticholinergics |
| Beta-adrenergics (terbutaline) | Increases bladder capacity through beta-stimulatory effect on bladder body | Palpitations, insomnia, hypertension | Monitor pulse and blood pressure |
| Tricyclic antidepressants (imipramine, doxepin) | Anesthetic-like action at nerve terminals; produces strong inhibitory effect on bladder smooth muscle | Weakness, fatigue, sedation, postural hypotension, rash, parkinsonian effect, fine tremors, abdominal distress, nausea and vomiting, headache, lethargy, irritability | Elderly require close observation; inform patient of possible side effects |
| **Drugs That Increase Bladder Outlet Resistance** | | | |
| Alpha-adrenergics (ephedrine sulfate, imipramine, phenylpropanolamine hydrochloride, pseudoephedrine) | Exaggerate alpha response in the bladder neck and urethra to increase bladder outlet resistance | Tachycardia, precordial pain, cardiac arrhythmias, vertigo, headache | Used to treat stress urinary incontinence, postprostatectomy incontinence; monitor vital signs |
| Beta-adrenergic blockers (propranolol) | Blocks beta-adrenergic receptors in the urethra, thereby increasing urethral pressure | Bradycardia, lightheadedness | Used when alpha-adrenergics are contraindicated |
| Estrogens | Increases periurethral blood flow; strengthens periurethral tissues | Headache, edema, hypertension, nausea, weight changes, breast tenderness | Assess for vaginal bleeding, GU, or abdominal pain; monitor blood pressure and weight |
| **Drugs That Stimulate Detrusor Contractility and Promote Bladder Emptying** | | | |
| Cholinergics (bethanecol chloride, neostigmine methylsulfate, myotonachol, carbachol) | Stimulates muscarinic cholinergic receptors in the bladder to increase bladder tone and sensations to bladder filling | Increased GI motility; vasodilation; decreased HR | Used for postoperative and nonobstructive urinary retention; do not give bethanecol IM or IV; give oral bethanecol on empty stomach; monitor vital signs; contraindicated in many disease states—check before administering |
| **Drugs That Decrease Bladder Outlet Resistance** | | | |
| Alpha-adrenergic blockers (phenoxybenzamine hydrochloride, phentolamine, reserpine, prazosin, terazosin, doxasozin) | Blocks alpha-adrenergic receptors of the bladder neck, posterior urethra, and external sphincter | Postural hypotension | Have patient change positions slowly; give with food or milk; avoid use with alcohol; avoid cold products containing sympathomimetics |
| External sphincter/striated muscle relaxants (baclofen, diazepam, dantrolene sodium) | Relaxes the external sphincter by inhibiting polysynaptic reflexes of striated muscles | Weakness; sedation | Often used in patients with multiple sclerosis or high-cord lesions; implement safety precautions |

HR, heart rate; GU, genitourinary; GI, gastrointestinal; IV, intravenous; IM, intramuscular.

around the bladder neck or the bulbar urethra (Mitchell et al., 1992). (See Chapter 22 for additional information about the artificial urinary sphincter.)

C. Contigen injections—the use of injectable collagen is gaining popularity as a treatment for urinary incontinence, especially since contigen was approved in September 1993 by the Food and Drug Administration for widespread use in the United States. Contigen is glutaraldehyde cross-linked bovine collagen, a biocompatible product that is used to add bulk to the bladder neck area to increase resistance to urine loss in women with stress incontinence type III (intrinsic sphincter incompetence) (Stricker & Haylen, 1993). It is administered by periurethral or transurethral injection using a fine-gauge spinal needle. The implant is often performed as an outpatient procedure under local or regional anesthesia. Stricker and Haylen (1993) reported an overall success rate of 82% with the use of injectable contigen to treat type III stress incontinence. In their study, 21 of 50 patients experienced no incontinent episodes following the implant, and 20 of 50 patients noted a marked reduction in the number of incontinent episodes. Although contigen appears to be a safe alternative for the treatment of stress incontinence, there are no data on the long-term effectiveness of this therapy.

III. Other surgical approaches

A. Augmentation cystoplasty—this type of reconstructive surgery is reserved for the individual whose bladder is structurally and functionally contracted. The primary goals of surgery are to increase bladder capacity and to reestablish low-pressure urine storage. Bowel segments are used to replace a portion of the diseased bladder. The decision as to whether a segment of the small or large intestine is used depends on the overall health of the patient's bowel, the desired shape of the cystoplasty, the condition of other lower urinary tract structures, and the planned method for bladder emptying (Mitchell et al., 1992).

B. Urinary diversion—this surgical approach is reserved for patients with severe neurogenic bladder disease. Indications for this form of treatment include (1) long-standing, unresolved upper tract obstruction associated with bladder instability; (2) detrusor hypertrophy; and (3) vesicorenal reflux with renal deterioration associated with a bladder capacity of less than 150 mL (Jonas & Truss, 1991). Cutaneous ureterostomy, ileal conduit, Kock pouch, orthotopic hemi-Kock pouch, Mainz pouch, and the Indiana pouch are but a few of the types of urinary diversions that may be performed. (See Chapter 9 for additional information about urinary diversions.)

C. Transurethral resection/incision of the bladder neck—a surgical technique, performed most frequently in males, requiring that the bladder neck be incised from the bladder base to the verumontanum at either the 5 o'clock or 7 o'clock position. Indications for the procedure are bladder neck obstruction or smooth sphincter dyssynergia confirmed by video-urodynamic testing (Wein, 1992). (See Chapter 4 for information about other therapies for outlet obstruction.)

D. Sphincterotomy—surgical destruction of the external urethral sphincter with an incision at the 12 o'clock position. This procedure results in total urinary incontinence and therefore is reserved for male patients with documented detrusor-striated sphincter dyssynergia in whom other management techniques have been unsuccessful or are inappropriate (Wein, 1992).

E. Procedures to interrupt innervation to the bladder—techniques in this category include the subarachnoid block, sacral rhizotomy, and dorsal rhizotomy. In each instance, selective nerve section is performed to diminish or eliminate involuntary detrusor contractions, thereby increasing bladder capacity in patients with detrusor hyperreflexia associated with profound neurologic deficits (Wein, 1992).

# APPROACHES TO PATIENT CARE

## The Patient Undergoing Urodynamic Testing

### Assessment

The patient about to undergo urodynamic testing must first be assessed for any signs or symptoms that indicate the presence of a urinary tract infection (UTI). Does the patient have a fever? Does the patient's urine have a pungent odor? Has there been a previous positive urine culture? If the answer is yes to any of these questions, the urodynamic testing should be postponed until verification of a negative urine culture. As a general rule, urodynamic testing should never be done when a UTI is suspected; irritation of the urinary tract from infection will adversely alter test results and repeated instrumentation could lead to sepsis.

The patient's physical condition must also be assessed as multiple position changes are usually required during the course of urodynamic testing. Can the patient transfer from a bed to a commode with ease? Is the patient able to walk alone, or is assistance needed? Does the patient have the strength to undergo testing at the time it is scheduled? Although urodynamic testing is often performed in patients with impaired mobility, such as those with spinal cord injury, cerebrovascular accident, and debilitating neurologic disease, a more complete evaluation can be obtained if the patient feels physically able to cooperate with the testing. Also, keep in mind that urodynamic testing is not a priority when the patient's condition is critical but is best performed during the rehabilitative phase of an illness or injury.

Because communication and cooperation are integral to successful urodynamic testing, a patient who is disoriented, confused, or unable to respond appropriately may not be a candidate for the procedures. Therefore, it is helpful to assess the patient's overall mental status and then schedule testing for a time when the patient will be able to tolerate instrumentation and comply with instructions.

Finally, medications currently prescribed for the patient should be reviewed for any that may directly alter bladder function. Special note should be made of cholinergic and anticholinergic agents, musculotropic relaxants, polysynaptic inhibitors, beta-adrenergic stimulants, and tricyclic antidepressants. These groups of drugs are frequently prescribed for other medical problems, yet may produce an effect on the urinary tract that could interfere with urodynamic test results and prevent evaluation of true lower urinary tract function.

### Nursing Diagnosis

Nursing diagnosis for the patient undergoing urodynamic testing may include the following:

1. Noncompliance related to a lack of knowledge about urodynamic testing techniques.
2. High risk for infection related to diagnostic instrumentation of the urinary tract.
3. High risk for alteration in pattern of urinary elimination related to diagnostic instrumentation of the urinary tract.

### Plan of Care

Nursing care is directed toward enabling the patient to

1. Cooperate with urodynamic testing to obtain accurate test results.
2. Verbalize an understanding of the purpose for urodynamic testing as well as procedure techniques.
3. Tolerate testing without serious discomfort or complications.
4. Implement measures to reduce urethral irritation and prevent UTI.

### Interventions

An explanation of each urodynamic procedure is extremely important. If you will not be performing these tests but are referring the patient to another center, it is wise to call the urodynamic facility to inquire about any special testing techniques used so that these may be explained to the patient. When explaining urodynamic testing, it is also important to emphasize that these studies are neither passed nor failed; rather, they are used to collect information about a person's voiding pattern.

Prior to testing, the patient should be dressed in a hospital gown only. The limited clothing is necessary due to the amount of equipment attached to the patient during the urodynamic procedures.

Although premedicating patients with sedatives or analgesics is common prior to many procedures, it should never be done prior to urodynamic testing unless ordered for a specific reason. These drugs can affect bladder function, but more importantly, they alter a patient's perception and threaten his or her safety during the procedures.

After urodynamic testing, the patient experiences some perineal discomfort, generally as a result of repeated instrumentation. Because of this irritation, the patient may also be reluctant to void. An increased fluid intake for 24 to 36 hours after urodynamic testing is helpful to (1) increase urine output and stimulate voiding and (2) dilute urine and flush out bacteria.

Because UTI can occur after urodynamic testing, the patient should be instructed to report suggestive signs and symptoms. For those who

### TABLE 14–5. Nursing History

Characteristics of incontinence
   Onset and duration
   Frequency
   Timing (day, night, or both)
   Precipitating circumstances (cough, sneeze, laugh,
      exercise, positional changes, hand washing, other)
   Associated urgency
   Amount of leakage
   Type of loss (spurt or stream, or continuous
      dribbling)
   Use of pads/protective briefs (number of pads or
      clothing changes per day)
Toileting patterns
   Diurnal frequency
   Nocturnal frequency
Associated genitourinary symptoms
   Awareness of bladder fullness
   Ability to delay voiding
   Sensation of incomplete bladder emptying
   Dribbling after urination
   Obstructive symptoms (hesitancy, slow or interrupted
      stream, straining)
   Symptoms of urinary tract infection (dysuria,
      hematuria)
Past genitourinary history
   Childbirth
   Surgery (pelvic or lower urinary tract)
   Recurrent urinary tract infections
   Previous incontinence treatment and results (drugs,
      pelvic floor exercises, surgery, dilatations)
Relevant medical history
   Acute illness
   Depression
   Diabetes mellitus
   Neurologic disease (e.g., cerebrovascular accident,
      Parkinson's disease, dementia)
   Cardiovascular disease (e.g., hypertension, congestive
      heart disease)
   Renal disease
   Bowel disorders (constipation, impaction, fecal
      incontinence)
   Psychological disorders (depression, mental illness)
   Cancer
Medications (including nonprescription drugs)
Patient's/caregiver's perceptions of incontinence
   Perception of cause and severity
   Interference with daily activities
   Expectations for cure
Environmental factors
   Accessible bathrooms
   Distance to bathrooms
   Use of toileting aids

From Wyman, J. F. (1988). Nursing assessment of incontinent, geriatric outpatients. *Nursing Clinics of North America*, 23(1), 178–179. Reprinted by permission.

are prone to developing a UTI, prophylactic antibiotics may be ordered and administered to safeguard against infection.

### Patient Outcomes

1. The patient complies with instructions in preparation for and during the course of urodynamic testing.

2. The patient's anxiety is reduced enough to permit completion of testing with reliable test results.
3. The patient denies irritative voiding symptoms following the testing.
4. The patient increases fluid intake in the 24 to 36 hours following the completion of testing with a relative urinary output.
5. The patient resumes his or her normal voiding pattern without dysuria.

## Specific Nursing Strategies to Manage Adult Voiding Dysfunction

### Assessment

Assessment of lower urinary tract status by the nurse is a necessary and important first step when he or she is caring for adult patients with a known or suspected voiding disorder. A thorough assessment includes a urologic health history (Table 14–5), physical examination (Table 14–6), determination of postvoid residual volume, review of findings from perti-

### TABLE 14–6. Physical Examination

Cognitive and affective status
   Mental status
   Mood
   Motivation
Mobility status
   Manual dexterity (ability to disrobe for toileting)
   Gait and balance (walking speed, use of assistive
      devices)
Neurologic examination
   Focal signs
   Signs of Parkinson's disease
Abdominal examination
   Scars
   Distended bladder
   Suprapubic tenderness
   Mass
Genital examination
   Skin condition
   Signs of infection
   Bulbocavernous reflex
   Women—atrophic vaginitis, pelvic relaxation, or
      other abnormality
Rectal examination
   Sphincteric tone
   Fecal impaction
   Masses
   Men—prostatic size
Stress test (with full bladder)
   Supine and standing
Other
   Signs of congestive heart failure

From Wyman, J. F. (1988). Nursing assessment of incontinent geriatric outpatients. *Nursing Clinics of North America*, 23(1), 181. Reprinted by permission.

nent laboratory tests (urinalysis, urine culture and sensitivity, blood urea nitrogen, and creatinine), analysis of urodynamic study results, analysis of the voiding diary, and perineal pad test.

A voiding diary is a written record of the time, frequency, voided volume, and other factors associated with urinary elimination (AHCPR, 1992). Also called a *bladder record,* it enables the patient and the patient's caregiver to provide the nurse with objective information about urinary elimination patterns over a 24-hour period. In an institutional setting, such as a hospital or long-term care facility, the record should be maintained for at least 3 days consecutively. For office or clinic patients, a diary maintained for 7 to 14 days is desirable and most useful. When carefully analyzed, data obtained from the voiding diary can help to guide the selection of the most appropriate nursing management technique for voiding dysfunction. (The reader is referred to the 1992 AHCPR *Clinical Practice Guideline—Urinary Incontinence in Adults*—for examples of voiding diaries [records] that may be used in institutional and office settings.)

For patients who complain of urinary incontinence, a perineal pad test is an objective method for determining the severity of urine leakage. One way to perform the test is to fill the patient's bladder via a sterile catheter, then ask the patient to wear a preweighed pad while performing a variety of provocative maneuvers. The pad is weighed afterward to determine the amount of fluid lost during the exercises (Wyman, 1988).

On completion of this assessment, the nurse should be able to correlate the patient's symptoms with the type of voiding dysfunction he or she is most likely experiencing (Table 14–7). In addition, the nurse should be able to answer these questions: (1) What is the patient's current pattern of urinary elimination? (2) How do the symptoms and current pattern of urinary elimination differ from what the patient considers to be a normal routine or pattern for urinary elimination? (3) What key factors or influences appear to be related to the changes in urine storage or bladder emptying? (4) If an intervention can be identified to help manage the voiding disorder, what degree of success would the patient expect from the therapy?

**Nursing Diagnosis**

Nursing diagnoses for the adult with dysfunctional voiding may include the following:

1. Alteration in pattern of urinary elimination related to
   a. Anatomic obstruction of the outlet
   b. Neurogenic disorder or injury
   c. Drug therapy
   d. Stress and anxiety
2. Functional incontinence related to
   a. Progressive dementia
   b. Drug therapy
   c. Impaired mobility
   d. Environmental barriers to toileting
3. Stress incontinence related to
   a. Estrogen deficiency
   b. Loss of muscle tone with aging
   c. Obesity
   d. Pregnancy
   e. Effects of pelvic surgery (prostatic, hysterectomy)
4. Total incontinence related to
   a. Presence of urinary fistula
   b. Radical pelvic surgery
   c. Decreased attention to bladder cues
5. Overflow incontinence related to bladder overdistention due to obstruction or acontractility
6. Urge incontinence related to
   a. Presence of urinary tract infection
   b. Irritation following instrumentation
   c. Neurogenic disease or injury
   d. Diminished bladder capacity associated with self-induced deconditioning
7. Urinary retention related to
   a. Anatomic obstruction (prostatic enlargement, bladder neck obstruction)
   b. General or spinal anesthesia
   c. Drug therapy
   d. Spinal cord injury
   e. Childbirth
   f. Depression, confusion
   g. Increased bladder capacity associated with self-induced deconditioning
8. Knowledge deficit related to causes of voiding dysfunction and options for treatment and management
9. Sexuality patterns, altered, related to
   a. Feelings of embarrassment associated with urinary incontinence
   b. Long-term use of an indwelling urethral catheter
10. High risk for social isolation related to urinary incontinence
11. High risk for impaired skin integrity related to
    a. Improper hygiene following incontinent episodes
    b. Use of external urinary catheters
    c. Maceration related to repeated contact with urine
12. High risk for infection related to

TABLE 14–7. Relationship of Symptoms to Voiding Dysfunction*

| PRESENTING SYMPTOMS | MOST LIKELY VOIDING DYSFUNCTION | COMMON ASSOCIATED OR CAUSATIVE FACTORS | FACTORS LIKELY TO EXACERBATE SYMPTOMS |
|---|---|---|---|
| Urinary frequency; urgency, urge incontinence; nocturia | Detrusor instability | Neurologic disorders: brain (CVA, closed head injury, tumor), spinal cord (injury, spinovascular disease); irritative bladder disorder; bladder outlet obstruction; stress urinary incontinence; idiopathic factors | Immobility, impaired dexterity; visual deficit; poorly designed environment; anxiety; urinary tract infection |
| Stress incontinence (subjective report of leakage with physical exertion) | Genuine stress incontinence | Pelvic descent: multiple vaginal deliveries, estrogen deficiency; urethral sphincter incompetence: radical prostatectomy, transurethral prostatectomy, trauma denervation | Chronic cough; obesity |
| Poor force of stream; hesitancy; dribbling incontinence; urinary frequency, nocturia | Deficient detrusor function or bladder outlet obstruction | Deficient detrusor function: sacral spinal cord disorders, peripheral polyneuropathies, pelvic trauma, herpes zoster, chronic anemia; obstruction: prostatic enlargement (prostatic hyperplasia, cancer, inflammation), bladder neck hypertrophy, contracture or dyssynergia, detrusor-striated sphincter, dyssynergia, urethral stricture or distortion | Fecal impaction; acute, debilitating illness, immobility |
| Continuous incontinence (absent warning or sensations of urgency) | Extraurethral leakage: vesicovaginal, urethrovaginal; urethrocutaneous fistula; urethral ectopia; epispadias, bladder exstrophy | Urinary ectopia, fistula; severe urethal sphincter incompetence; sphincteric incompetence: urethral trauma, iatrogenic trauma (multiple anti-incontinence procedures, etc.), denervation | Fecal impaction; acute, debilitating illness; immobility |
| Unpredictable incontinence; no apparent reason | Functional incontinence | Alzheimer's disease | Disorientation, unfamiliar surroundings; immobility, deficient dexterity, vision; caregiver unaware of patient needs; depression, poor motivation; institutionalization or other crisis |

*The relationships presented here are broad generalizations only.
CVA, cerebrovascular accident.
From Jeter, K., Faller, N., & Norton, C. (Eds). (1990). *Nursing for continence.* Philadelphia: W. B. Saunders. Reprinted by permission.

a. Incomplete bladder emptying and urine stasis
b. Urinary tract instrumentation for diagnostic testing
c. Long-term use of an indwelling urethral/suprapubic catheter
13. High risk for noncompliance with nursing management strategies for urinary incontinence and urinary retention related to embarrassment, fear, and frustration

**Plan of Care**
Nursing care is directed toward enabling the patient to

1. Resume a normal pattern of urinary elimination.
2. Eliminate or reduce incontinence episodes.
3. Facilitate effective bladder emptying.
4. Verbalize an understanding of the cause for voiding dysfunction and rationale for selected therapy.
5. Express concerns regarding the impact of his or her voiding disorder on sexual functioning.
6. Resolve feelings regarding the need for social isolation because of a voiding disorder.
7. Prevent skin breakdown.

8. Reduce the incidence of urinary tract infection.
9. Comply with recommended nursing management techniques for urinary incontinence and urinary retention.

### Interventions

This section highlights those interventions for adult voiding disorders that are coordinated and managed by the urologic nurse. Included are discussions about self-assisting measures, behavioral therapy, pelvic muscle reeducation (including Kegel exercises, vaginal cones, biofeedback, and electrical stimulation), external collection devices, absorbent products, skin care, and catheter drainage.

## Self-Assisting Measures

Self-assisting measures are the simplest, and perhaps the oldest, interventions for voiding dysfunction associated with a failure to empty. Included in this category are the techniques of Credé or Valsalva voiding and trigger voiding.

The purpose of the Credé method is to aid in the passage of urine out of the bladder. The patient or caregiver applies a gentle massage to the bladder in a downward direction toward the pubic bone during and after urination. The patient may also be instructed to rock back and forth while sitting on the toilet. A third method is to have the patient bear down as in passing stool (the Valsalva maneuver); however, this is not recommended for cardiac or elderly patients in poor health. The Credé method may be used in conjunction with clean intermittent self-catheterization to facilitate complete bladder emptying. Patients with neurogenic bladders, particularly those with multiple sclerosis or paralysis, are especially encouraged to practice the technique.

Trigger voiding relies on a variety of techniques to achieve voiding on cue. Mothers have often used the simple trigger technique of turning on a water faucet while trying to toilet train a young child. Similar kinds of trigger mechanisms may also be used on adult patients experiencing difficulty in starting the process of urination. Among the techniques utilized are stroking the inner thighs or abdomen, gently pulling the pubic hair, suprapubic tapping, oil of wintergreen in the bedpan, dilating the anus or vagina along with the Valsalva maneuver, using an alarm clock or timer, running water in a slow stream from the faucet, as well as dipping the hands in warm water. Individual assessment must be made as to which trigger mechanism is most likely to succeed. A combination of techniques may be necessary to initiate and achieve bladder emptying.

## Behavioral Therapy

Behavioral techniques are low-risk interventions that are based on the premise that voiding is a learned behavior (AHCPR, 1992). Based on the principles of operant learning, this management approach presumes that adults with urinary incontinence can relearn those behaviors necessary for urinary storage and bladder emptying to regain continence and to establish control over urinary elimination (Wyman & Fantl, 1991). As with any behavioral training program, behavioral techniques for the management of urinary incontinence rely on (1) identification of a target behavior (i.e., continence), (2) development of a meaningful stimulus (i.e., prompted or scheduled voiding), and (3) reinforcement or reward for appropriate behavior (i.e., praise for dry interval or decrease in incontinent episodes) (Wyman & Fantl, 1991).

Studies have shown that behavioral interventions are successful in improving or curing symptoms of urinary incontinence in 50% to 80% of adults treated by either bladder training, habit training, timed voiding, prompted voiding, or contingency management (McCormick et al., 1988). Success, however, depends on the establishment of a therapeutic relationship and caregiver commitment, as well as appropriate training and education (Table 14–8).

## Pelvic Muscle Reeducation

**Kegel or Pelvic Floor Exercises.** The Kegel or pelvic floor exercise method of controlling involuntary loss of urine was first developed in the early 1940s to help women regain urinary control following childbirth. Now, 50 years later, it is a proven, noninvasive management technique recommended for women with stress incontinence and for some men following prostate surgery. Performance of the technique on a regular basis for 4 to 6 weeks is designed to improve urethral resistance through strengthening of the periurethral muscles of the pelvic floor, primarily the pubococcygeus muscle (AHCPR, 1992; Newman & Smith, 1992).

The most difficult aspect of performing pelvic floor exercise is identification of the pelvic muscle. One method is to instruct the patient to stop the flow of urine while urinating on the toilet. Another approach is to insert a gloved

TABLE 14–8. Behavioral Interventions and Nursing Interventions for Urinary Incontinence

| BEHAVIORAL INTERVENTION | TYPE OF INCONTINENCE USUALLY AFFECTED | NURSING INTERVENTIONS |
|---|---|---|
| **Bladder Training** | | |
| Begin by establishing the patient's voiding behavior by observing wetness and dryness pattern for several days. This training regimen starts with a preestablished interval of time (usually 1–2 hours). The patient is prompted to go to the bathroom. During the interval of time between toileting the patient may ask to use the bathroom or may use the bathroom independent of staff. As the patient becomes drier, the interval is progressively lengthened. If there is no improvement on the 2-hour interval, the interval of time may be decreased to 1 hour. | Urge; neurogenic bladder | Assess the patient's ability to use toilet or toilet substitute. Assess the patient's voiding pattern. Utilize proper communication skills. Provide positive reinforcement for any desired behavior (e.g., a dry pad, urinating in the toilet, asking for help or assistance to go to the bathroom). Keep toilet schedule consistent. Inform patients when you will be back to take them to the bathroom again. Encourage self-care management. Assess environment for accessibility of bathrooms or toilet substitute. |
| **Habit Training** | | |
| This training regimen starts with preestablished assigned times for toileting (usually, every 3 hours). Patients are encouraged to use the bathroom or ask for assistance. During the 3-hour interval, if they feel the urge to go, use the bathroom, and urinate, the toileting schedule is adjusted. The next time the patients are scheduled to be prompted to the bathroom would be 3 hours from the time they last voided on their own. If the patients do not use the bathroom during a 3-hour interval, the staff prompts them to use the bathroom. | Urge; functional | Focus on the patient's ability to request the bathroom or use it independently. Strongly reinforce this behavior. |
| **Timed Voiding** | | |
| A fixed voiding schedule is established that remains unchanged during training. For instance, if a voiding interval of 3 hours is set, then the patient is toileted every 3 hours regardless of pattern of wetness or dryness. | Urge incontinence; overflow incontinence (especially if infrequent voiding is contributing to overflow leakage) | Commitment to the established "routine or regular" toileting times is critical. Encourage patient to monitor the clock in order to promote awareness of schedule. |
| **Prompted Voiding** | | |
| A behavioral method designed to teach the incontinent person to perceive wetness or dryness, and to request toileting assistance. The person is checked on a regular basis by the caregiver and prompted to void. However, assistance is provided only if the person requests to void. | Urge, functional incontinence | Praise for maintaining continence, and for asking and attempting to void is critical. Prompt response by caregiver when request for toileting is initiated is essential. |
| **Contingency Management** | | |
| This method involves a systematic reinforcement of appropriate toileting through the use of verbal praise and punishment of unsuccessful toileting with verbal disapproval | Functional, stress, urge | Consistency is essential in this treatment so that positive reinforcement is used to reinforce desired behaviors. |

Adapted from McCormick, K. A., Scheve, A. A. S., & Leahy, E. (1988). Nursing management of urinary incontinence in geriatric inpatients. *Nursing Clinics of North America, 3*(1), 253–254.

finger into the female patient's vagina and instruct her to tighten as if holding back urine. For male patients, the nurse can insert a gloved finger into the patient's rectum and ask him to tighten his anus (Newman & Smith, 1992). The goal is to draw in or tighten the pelvic floor muscles without using the abdominal, buttock, or inner thigh muscles (AHCPR, 1992) (Procedure 14–1).

Once the correct group of muscles for tightening has been identified, patients are instructed to tighten and hold the contraction for as long as 10 seconds; an equal period of relaxation should then follow. This constitutes one exercise sequence. For pelvic floor exercises to be effective, this sequence should be performed about 30 to 80 times per day (AHCPR, 1992). One exercise program recommends that the patient perform 15 exercises 3 times/day for a total of 45 exercises each day, with 15 sequences performed lying down, 15 sequences performed sitting, and 15 sequences performed standing. Improvement-cure rates for patients practicing Kegel exercises range from 54% to 77% (AHCPR, 1992; Newman & Smith, 1992).

**Vaginal Cones.** The use of vaginal cones for pelvic muscle reeducation is considered an assistive technique for pelvic exercise. A vaginal cone is a weighted device that is inserted into the vagina and held for as long as 15 minutes twice per day. To retain the weighted cone for that period of time, a sustained contraction is required. The weight of the cone is assumed to provide heightened proprioceptive feedback for the desired pelvic contraction (AHCPR, 1992). Vaginal cones are marketed in sets of five, each with a different weight, ranging from 20 to 70 g (Newman & Smith, 1992). Patients usually begin training with the lightest cone and advance to the heavier cones as they become proficient with contraction of the pubococcygeal muscle.

**Biofeedback.** The purpose of biofeedback is to provide the patient with positive rewards for accomplishing a certain task. For patients who wish to achieve control over the involuntary loss of urine, it is a method that uses auditory or visual displays from various electronic instruments to reinforce teaching about physiologic responses to bladder control. The most frequently used measures for biofeedback training are either pelvic or abdominal EMG recording and measurement of detrusor pressure.

To initiate biofeedback training, baseline measurements are done to establish bladder ca-

pacity, the interval between voids, and the number of incontinent episodes. As the patient achieves greater ability to contract the pelvic floor muscles and to hold urine for longer periods of time, the rewards become more satisfying. A positive reward may be the visible cues of more response from the electronic instruments, or evidence of increasing time between voiding or decreased episodes of urine loss in the patient's daily bladder record. For biofeedback to be successful, the patient must be goal oriented and value self-care. Moreover, this technique appears to be most effective when combined with other behavioral therapies.

**Electrical Stimulation.** Electrical stimulation is a technique whereby low-voltage current is administered to the nerve fibers of pelvic muscles and structures (Gray, 1992b). The excitation of the neuromuscular units can either interrupt or quicken electrical signals to strengthen or alter neuromuscular function of the bladder and urethra. For example, when detrusor afferent fibers are stimulated, bladder sensation is altered to facilitate urine storage. Likewise, when detrusor efferent fibers are stimulated, bladder contractility is enhanced. Additionally, electrical stimulation has been shown to influence the sacral micturition reflex and thus to inhibit detrusor overactivity (AHCPR, 1992). In a recent case report, stimulation of the smooth muscle of the bladder neck was employed as a means to stimulate detrusor contractility, since stimulation of either the bladder neck or detrusor produces the same efferent impulses (Moore et al., 1993).

The electric current may be delivered via needle electrodes, intra-anal and/or intravaginal plug electrodes, as well as transcutaneous, percutaneous, or implanted electrodes (Newman & Smith, 1992). There is disparity, however, regarding (1) the optimal location for placement of electrodes; (2) frequency, duration, and amplitude of voltage; (3) type of stimulation (i.e., phasic, intermittent, or continuous) (AHCPR, 1992).

The use of electric stimulation for the treatment of adult voiding dysfunction is limited primarily to patients with stress and urge incontinence and those with interstitial cystitis (Gray, 1992b). Research is ongoing to understand the physiologic effects of electric stimulation as well as the role this therapeutic modality will have in the future treatment of voiding dysfunction.

## PROCEDURE 14-1
■
## Patient Teaching Instruction: Pelvic Muscle (Kegel) Exercises

### ■ How to Find the Pelvic (PC) Muscle

To find the muscle, imagine you are at a party and the rich food you have just consumed causes you to have gas. The muscle that you use to hold back gas is the one you want to exercise. Some people find this muscle by voluntarily stopping the stream of urine. Another way to find the muscle is by pulling your rectum, vagina, and urethra up inside. Try to think about the area around the vagina.

### ■ Exercising the Muscle

Begin by emptying your bladder. Then try to relax completely. Tighten this muscle and hold for a count of 10, or 10 seconds, then relax the muscle completely for a count of 10, or 10 seconds. You should feel a sensation of lifting of the area around your vagina or of pulling around your rectum.

### ■ When to Exercise

Do 10 exercises in the morning, 10 in the afternoon, and 15 at night. Or else you can exercise for 10 minutes three times a day. Set your kitchen timer for 10 minutes three times a day. Initially, you may not be able to hold this contraction for the complete count of 10. However you will slowly build to 10-second contractions over time. The muscle may start to tire after six or eight exercises. If this happens, stop and go back to exercising later.

### ■ Where to Practice These Exercises

These exercises can be practiced anywhere and anytime. Most people seem to prefer exercising lying on their bed or sitting in a chair. Women can try doing these exercises during intercourse. Tighten pelvic muscles to grip your partner's penis and then relax. Your partner should be able to feel an increase in pressure.

### ■ Common Mistakes

Never use your stomach, legs, or buttocks muscles. To find out if you are also contracting your stomach muscle, place your hand on your abdomen while you squeeze your pelvic muscle. If you feel your abdomen move, then you are also using these muscles. In time, you will learn to practice effortlessly. Eventually, work these exercises in as part of your lifestyle; tighten the muscle when you walk, before you sneeze, on the way to the bathroom, and when you stand up.

### ■ When Will I Notice a Change?

After 4 to 6 weeks of consistent daily exercise, you will notice less urinary accidents; after 3 months you will see an even bigger difference.

### ■ Can These Exercises Harm Me?

No! These exercises cannot harm you in any way. Most patients find them relaxing and easy. If you get back pain or stomach pain after your exercise, then you are probably trying too hard and using stomach and/or back muscles. Go back and find the PC muscle, and remember this exercise should feel easy. If you experience headaches, then you are also tensing your chest muscles and probably holding your breath.

---

## External Devices

The term *external collection device* generally refers to use of the condom catheter for management of male urinary incontinence. External (condom) catheters are a disposable-type product that come in a variety of sizes and are made from either latex rubber, polyvinyl, or silicone (AHCPR, 1992). A sizing template should be used to aid in the selection of the condom catheter that will best fit the patient. Careful cleansing, thorough drying, and inspection of the penis are required before applying the device. To apply a condom catheter, the penis should be stretched as the condom is unrolled completely along the penile shaft. Care should be taken to keep the foreskin in place in uncircumcised men; failure to do so can result in phimosis. Depending on the design of the condom catheter, it is held in place with an adhesive strap or self-adhesive lining, or attached to a pouching system in instances when the penis is retracted (Jeter, 1990). All condom catheters should be removed and the skin inspected every 24 to 72 hours.

A penile clamp is another type of external device that is applied directly on the shaft of the penis to stop the urinary flow. It is cost effective but must be used only with men who are aware of tactile sensations and will remember to remove it every 2 hours to empty the bladder. Paraplegic and quadriplegic patients will find it extremely useful when swimming, because it stays in place even when wet.

External collecting devices for women are generally considered to be ineffective and uncomfortable for those who are ambulatory. However, for nonambulatory, institutionalized, incontinent women this method of containment may be useful. Because a truly reliable and satisfactory device has not been developed for the female, research continues in this area.

## Absorbent Products

Several manufacturers are producing disposable, absorbent products for the management of incontinence. They range from small male drip collectors and perineal shields or inserts to large diaper-like products and bed pads. The absorbency rates for these items differ depending on the size and fiber content of the product. The variation in absorbency is matched by the variation in the overall quality, cost, and effectiveness of each product.

When considering the use of an absorbent product, these factors should be considered:

functional ability of the patient, type and severity of incontinence, gender, availability of caregivers, failure with previous treatment programs, patient preference, and comorbidity (AHCPR, 1992).

The male drip collectors are small pockets of absorbent padding with a waterproof backing that are designed to be held on the penis by close-fitting underwear. They are intended for the management of mild postvoid dribbling and transient postoperative leakage. The next level of management available for males and females is absorbent pads or liners that are worn inside continence pants or held in place with adhesive strips inside tight-fitting underwear. A second type of liner or undergarment is held in place by its own straps, which fit around the hips.

Absorbent adult briefs (adult diapers) are an alternative for those with total incontinence who cannot be managed by other methods. These garments are usually sized small, medium, large, and extra large and should fit securely. Furthermore, they should be absorbent enough to contain a full voiding of at least 300 mL (many products can hold well over this volume), or constant dribbling over several hours. Gathers around the legs are also important, as they prevent leakage when the brief is compressed, that is, when positioning or transferring the patient (Jeter, 1990). The use of absorbent briefs does not encourage self-help techniques and often has a negative emotional and social impact on the patient. Moreover, the long-term use of these products can be a financial strain for the patient and family.

Reusable undergarments offer the patient a sense of dignity in that they are wearing underpants as well as saving costs over the purely disposable kind. The pants are made of washable material, often with a waterproof crotch panel. They are designed to hold reusable or disposable liners or pads in place by snaps, loops, pockets, or self-adhesive strips. A benefit of most reusable undergarments is that they do not totally encompass the patient in a plastic liner, which can hold in moisture and lead to skin breakdown. The pants also promote independence and are socially more acceptable than adult briefs. Like all continence products, they are easily obtained through local medical supply companies, drug stores, department stores, and mail order catalogs.

Underpads, drawsheets, and chair liners are designed for patients who have very limited mobility. Often made of an absorbent material with a waterproof backing, they may be disposable or reusable. An added benefit of some of the new products on the market is their ability to pull moisture away from the surface layer, often within a few short minutes of an incontinent episode; this protects the patient's skin from prolonged contact with a wet surface. Again, the length of time the problem exists and the financial ability of the patient will determine which product is most applicable. Disposable underpads and chair liners tend to be expensive if not used carefully in combination with other products or toileting techniques. "Homemade" pads, such as flannel-backed tablecloths, shower curtain liners covered with a flannel sheet, or newspaper, may be an alternative for those with limited financial resources. Reusable drawsheets may provide a secondary purpose of not only protecting the linen or furniture but also serving as a lift sheet when turning or moving an immobile patient. Care should be taken when using any of the underpads so as to not interfere with any pressure-relieving devices (e.g., flotation pad) that may be used on a bed or in a wheelchair.

## Skin Care

An important adjunct to the care of the adult with voiding dysfunction is meticulous skin care. This involves regular cleansing, moisturizing, and protecting (Faller & Jeter, 1992). In addition, careful daily inspection of vulnerable, high-risk areas is essential, especially for incontinent persons.

Cleansing the perineum with soap and water is not sufficient to remove irritants deposited on the skin from urine and feces. The use of specially formulated incontinence cleaners, in either spray or spout containers, is an essential first step in maintaining skin integrity. This should be followed by the application of a water-soluble moisturizing cream, which prevents the skin from drying and cracking. Finally, a water-insoluble barrier cream or ointment should be applied to promote healing of damaged skin as well as to protect it from the harsh effects of repeated excrement contamination (Faller & Jeter, 1992). One word of caution though—petrolatum-based moisturizers and barrier creams or ointments should be used sparingly because they have been found to interfere with the absorbency of some disposable incontinence products (Grove et al., 1994). Because of the variety of skin care products that are available, the urologic nurse is advised to use several different formulations

on a trial basis, then select the combination of products that, in your estimation, perform best.

## Catheter Drainage

**Indwelling Catheters.** Indwelling catheters are used for the continuous drainage of urine from the bladder. They may be employed temporarily following a surgical procedure, used to monitor fluid balance in an acutely ill person, be required for long-term management of urinary retention that cannot be otherwise treated or for which an alternative therapy is not feasible, or used to manage incontinence in the terminally ill or severely impaired patient (AHCPR, 1992). Regardless of use, all indwelling catheters should be maintained as a sterile, closed-drainage system and should be inserted using strict aseptic technique by qualified personnel.

Indwelling catheters can lead to many negative side effects; among them are inflammation of the urethra, strictures, urinary tract infections, renal and bladder calculi, and hydronephrosis, and in males, epididymitis and penoscrotal complications. To minimize the complications associated with indwelling urinary catheters, the nurse should keep in mind the following guidelines (Wong, 1983):

1. Aseptic technique must be utilized in catheter insertion.
2. The appropriate type and size of catheter should be determined before insertion. Lubricant must be used for all male catheterizations and in females who experience decreased lubrication.
3. A closed drainage system should be employed. If irrigations are ordered, all efforts must be made to prevent contamination of the system.
4. The drainage bag must stay below the level of the bladder at all times.
5. An indwelling catheter should be removed as soon as is possible.
6. Urine samples should be taken from the aspiration port utilizing aseptic technique. Avoid clamping catheters for this or any other purpose.
7. A catheter should be changed only when it becomes obstructed or contaminated; catheters should not be changed on a routine basis.
8. Routine catheter care consists of daily cleansing of the meatus with mild soap and water.
9. The drainage bag should be emptied every

8 hours, or less if volume is excessive. The outlet valve should be cleaned each time and care taken to prevent contact contamination by the measuring container.

10. Each catheterized patient in an inpatient setting should have a separate, labeled measuring container.

11. Adequate hydration must be maintained in all catheterized patients; 2 to 3 L/day of water is recommended, except in the presence of cardiac insufficiency or renal failure.

12. The catheter must be securely anchored to the leg or lower abdomen using tape or a catheter strap.

13. Assessment of the catheterized patient should be done on a routine basis and should include intake and output levels, patency of the system, color, odor, evidence of sediment, presence or absence of patient discomfort, fever, or hematuria.

14. Catheter removal should be done by aspirating fluid from the inflation port with a syringe. As varied amounts of fluid are used to inflate catheter balloons, be sure to check the insertion record to determine the amount of fluid used before aspiration. Also, there is no evidence to suggest that a schedule of catheter clamping prior to catheter removal will aid in the reestablishment of a normal voiding pattern.

Bacteriuria will be present within 24 to 72 hours after insertion of an indwelling catheter. In the acute care setting, 66% to 86% of nosocomial urinary tract infections may be attributed to urethral catheterization (Wong, 1983). Patients most at risk for infection are pregnant women, the elderly, diabetics, and those who are immunosuppressed. Routine cultures are indicated only when symptoms of an upper urinary tract or systemic infection are present. Routine catheter changes, once done to impede bacterial growth, are also not necessary unless the closed drainage system has been broken. While continuous bladder irrigations are common after transurethral surgery, routine bladder irrigations are contraindicated, except when specifically ordered by the physician when clots or other residue have blocked catheter drainage.

Nursing measures such as the application of antimicrobial agents at the urethral meatus have proved ineffective in reducing the risk of catheter-related infections and may, in fact, promote infections by acting as an irritant to meatal tissue. In addition, repeated washing of the meatus with soap and water also increases the risk of infection, due in part to the manipulation of the catheter and the introduction of exogenous bacteria into the bladder. Instillation of antiseptic solutions, such as hydrogen peroxide and chlorhexidine, into the urinary drainage bag has also proved to be ineffective in reducing catheter-induced urinary tract infections. Thus, routine perineal care during the daily bath is generally sufficient to minimize infection from the indwelling catheter (Burke et al., 1981, 1983).

For patients requiring catheter drainage at home, a low-dose prophylactic antibiotic may be prescribed to control bacterial growth, and vitamin C or mandelamine may be used to help acidify urine. Cranberry juice is often recommended as a supplemental fluid in addition to water. Although cranberry juice does aid in kidney filtration, 1 g of vitamin C lowers the pH the same as 1 gal of cranberry juice. Either method is contraindicated in patients with a history of renal calculi or sensitivity to sulfa drugs.

Patients with indwelling catheters may require an occasional catheter change; the usual practice is to change indwelling catheters every 30 days; however, there is no research that has established the optimal frequency for catheter changes (AHCPR, 1992). Catheter irrigation may also be occasionally necessary to prevent occlusion of the catheter from crystals that tend to form on the tip. However, if the tube is patent and draining well, there is really no reason to change or irrigate it. The only exception to this rule is when a sterile urine specimen must be obtained for culture and sensitivity testing and the catheter and tubing are littered with debris. In this instance, an indwelling catheter that has been maintained for 30 days or longer should be removed, a new drainage system inserted, and a specimen collected from urine draining through the clear, sterile system. This procedure will permit a more accurate analysis of bacteria present in the urinary tract without the risk of contamination. In addition, patients should be instructed on the procedure for transferring the catheter from a drain bag to a urinary leg bag (Procedure 14–2).

**Suprapubic Catheters.** A suprapubic catheter may be used as an alternative to long-term urethral catheterization in men when there is urethral injury, prostatic obstruction, or strictures; it is also used after gynecologic surgery and for long-term catheterization (AHCPR, 1992). Insertion of the catheter may be done intraoperatively, during cystoscopy, or at the

## PROCEDURE 14-2

■

## Patient Instructions: How to Care for the Catheter Drainage Bags

An overnight drainage bag is a larger bag with a long tubing, which should be used during the night. Hang the bag over the side of the bed below the level of your catheter so that the urine will flow easily.

A leg bag is a smaller collection bag for use at home or when you go out of your house. The smaller bag is easily hidden beneath your clothing. Take care of the leg bag as you would the larger drainage bag.

To disconnect or change your drainage bag follow these steps:

1. Pinch the catheter tubing above the drainage bag connection between your fingers to stop the flow of urine.
2. Using a twisting motion, disconnect the tubing and bag from the catheter.
3. Take an alcohol pad and clean the end of the new tubing and the connection site of the catheter and insert the new tubing into the catheter.
4. Using an alcohol pad, clean the end of the tubing that was removed.
5. Replace the protective cap and clean the drainage bag.

Drainage bags can be cleaned and deodorized by filling the bag with a solution of 2 parts vinegar and 3 parts water and letting it soak for 20 minutes. The drainage bag can be dried by hanging it with the emptying spout pointing downward. Do not hang the bag over the heat of an oven or radiator.

When dry, recap the bag until ready to use.

Replace the bag if it starts to wear out or deteriorate.

If you get repeated bladder infections, spasms, and pain, you may be told by your nurse not to ever disconnect the catheter from the bag. If you get repeat infections, spasms, and other problems, you should use only the overnight drainage bag.

Remember, a catheter may leak on occasion. This is normal and is caused by bladder spasms. There is no reason to be alarmed unless the catheter leaks all the time if there is no urine in the drainage bag.

Notify your nurse or doctor for any of the following:

The urine has a strong odor or becomes cloudy.

You experience chills, fever above 99.4°F, lower back pain, and/or leakage around the catheter.

Swelling at the catheter insertion site, especially in males.

The catheter is not draining any urine.

Copyright 1991: Golden Horizons, Inc., St. Davids, PA.

---

bedside. The catheter is inserted into the bladder using a trocar or cannula device that is inserted directly above the pubic bone. The catheter is held in place either internally by the design of the catheter or externally by a disk or sutures. Initially, the insertion site needs to be cleaned and redressed every day; after healing has occurred, the permanent suprapubic opening should be cleaned and observed about every other day. Catheters should be changed only by qualified personnel and if they become obstructed or show evidence of obstruction. Irrigations may be ordered to maintain patency

and should be performed using clean technique.

The suprapubic catheter must be connected to either a drain bag or a urinary leg bag. Use of the leg bag is beneficial to patients who are ambulatory or wish to sit in a wheelchair without having a cumbersome drain bag present for everyone to see. One advantage of the suprapubic catheter is that it does not interfere with sexual activity, as does an indwelling catheter. Potential problems associated with the use of a suprapubic catheter that urologic nurses should be alert to include uncontrolled urine leakage, skin erosion, hematoma formation, and problems with catheter reinsertion (AHCPR, 1992).

**Intermittent Self-Catheterization.** Generally referred to as clean intermittent self-catheterization (CISC), the technique was reinstituted in the early 1970s as an alternative to indwelling catheterization. The procedure may be used on a long- or short-term basis depending on the bladder's ability to return to normal function. Paraplegic or quadriplegic patients are seldom able to discontinue the process, but some patients with transient neurologic deficits or following gynecologic surgery may use the program for only a few weeks or months.

The theory behind the effectiveness of CISC is the physiologic capacity of the bladder to hold approximately 300 mL. When the amount goes over 300 mL, two problems can occur: (1) the blood flow to the bladder is decreased, lowering the defense mechanisms of the bladder wall; (2) bacteria present in the urine will multiply at a rate of 100 times per hour (Lapides et al., 1972). The longer contaminating urine is allowed to stay in the bladder, the higher the bacterial count. Consequently, the natural defense mechanism of the bladder wall is decreased as the fluid volume increases, contributing to bladder infections. For this reason, patients should be taught the importance of regular and complete bladder emptying to prevent recurrent urinary tract infection.

The goals of CISC are the prevention of urinary tract infection and the preservation of normal renal function, as well as the elimination of urinary incontinence and the need for permanent catheters, diapers, or external devices (Rosen & Ravalli, 1990). It is important that patients understand the necessity of learning the procedure and that without their compliance, the desired results will not occur. Self-care and the willingness to overcome fears (i.e., pain, failure, body image changes) must be within the value system of the person for a self-catheterization program to succeed.

Both male and female patients should be instructed in the location of basic anatomic structures and be allowed to visualize them in a comfortable environment. Do not assume patients know or understand how the urinary tract functions or have ever really viewed, much less handled, their genital organs (particularly elderly females). In addition, older men may have a poor understanding of the location or function of the prostate gland.

To perform CISC, clear catheters of varying sizes are available. A size 14 Fr, 6-inch catheter is recommended for most women; however, for those who are bedridden, chair-bound, or obese, a longer length 14 Fr catheter connected to a urinary leg bag may greatly enhance their ability to perform the procedure. For male patients, urologic nurses usually recommend the use of a size 14 Fr, coudé-tipped catheter. Because plastic catheters for CISC are a disposable product that may not be covered by all insurance plans, it is not uncommon for urologic nurses to instead recommend the use of the basic red rubber catheter for this procedure. The only other supplies necessary to perform the procedure are water-soluble lubricant and a storage container for the catheter (i.e., plastic sandwich bag, make-up case, or toothbrush holder). In emergency situations, water may be substituted for lubricant.

Gloves should be worn by all health care professionals assisting patients with the procedure and by those patients who are immunosuppressed, have genital lesions, or are in long-term care facilities.

When instructing the female patient, a mirror should be used initially to aid in the location of the urinary meatal opening. After initial location is made, it is *strongly recommended* that the palpation method be used in locating the urinary meatus rather than relying on a mirror. This technique involves spreading the labia with the second and fourth fingers, while the middle finger is used locate the meatus (Rosen & Ravalli, 1990). Exceptions may need to be made for patients experiencing paresthesia in the perineal area. The female patient is then instructed to insert the catheter in an upward direction, toward the umbilicus. In situations in which a vaginal prolapse is evident, it may be necessary to perform the procedure in a recumbent position or to use a pessary for proper placement of the internal organs. Once the catheter has been inserted into the meatus (approximately 2 to 3 inches), urine will begin to flow. At this point, the Credé procedure may be employed to facilitate complete bladder emptying.

The male patient is instructed to hold the penis on the sides, perpendicular to the body, to facilitate passage of the catheter. The catheter may meet with resistance at the level of the prostate, at which time it may be helpful to institute deep-breathing relaxation exercises. Once urine starts to flow, the male patient should advance the catheter 1 inch farther to adequately drain the bladder (Rosen & Ravalli, 1990).

After the catheter has been inserted, it is held in place until all urine has been allowed to drain out of the bladder. To remove the catheter, advise patients to slowly withdraw it from the bladder in short increments, and in a rotating fashion, to ensure complete bladder emptying. Once the catheter has been withdrawn from the bladder, patients should be instructed to wash it with soap and water, rinse it in clear water, dry the outside area of the catheter, and then place it in a convenient storage container (Rosen & Ravalli, 1990).

A routine catheterization schedule encourages compliance on the part of the patient. Initially, catheterization should be done four times per day—before each meal and at bedtime—to establish a voiding pattern. Adjustments in this schedule may need to be made according to output. For instance, if the amount of urine drained is consistently more than 300 mL, the patient will need to catheterize more often or decrease fluid intake. The catheterization schedule should be individualized to achieve the highest level of compliance. Patients are taught to monitor their own intake and output to determine progress and to establish a routine. Whenever possible, patients should also be encouraged to urinate independent of the catheter.

When instructing patients on CISC, emphasis should be placed on performing the procedure according to scheduled need rather than convenience. Too often women, in particular, avoid performing CISC in a public bathroom if they view it as an unclean facility. In this situation, it is more important that the patient perform the catheterization rather than worry about the cleanliness of the facility. As an alternative, the patient should be encouraged to catheterize standing up with one foot on the toilet seat to maintain balance using as clean a technique as is possible. ·

A single catheter may be reused for 2 to 4 weeks. Although simple cleansing with soap and water should be sufficient catheter care, patients may also want to soak their catheters in a white vinegar and water solution overnight once per week to clean out exudate or odors. However, they must be cautioned to thoroughly rinse the catheters with clear water before use. To prevent stiffness and cracking, patients should be advised not to store their catheters in sunlight, near an oven, or near a radiator (Rosen & Ravalli, 1990).

### Patient Outcomes

1. The patient states an understanding of the cause for his or her voiding dysfunction.
2. The patient participates in decision making regarding the most appropriate therapeutic intervention for the voiding disorder.
3. The patient verbalizes expectations for suc-

cess of the selected treatment method(s) for his or her voiding dysfunction.
4. The patient resumes a normal pattern of urinary elimination following pharmacologic, surgical, or nursing intervention for a voiding disorder.
5. The patient verbalizes that episodes of urinary incontinence have been reduced or eliminated following pharmacologic, surgical, or nursing intervention.
6. The patient achieves complete bladder emptying with each void or when performing clean intermittent self-catheterization.
7. The patient and his or her partner confront concerns regarding the impact of voiding dysfunction on their sexual relationship and functioning.
8. The patient's attitude and response to bladder management methods enables him or her to resume usual social activities.
9. The patient exhibits no signs of perineal skin breakdown associated with urinary incontinence.
10. The patient remains free of urinary tract infection or implements measures to reduce the incidence of symptomatic urinary tract infection.
11. The patient demonstrates compliance and success with recommended nursing management techniques for urinary incontinence and urinary retention.

## SUMMARY

Nursing care of the adult with voiding dysfunction is an area of urologic nursing practice that continues to expand. In recent years, significant progress has been made toward professional and public education about the options and benefits of nursing interventions for voiding disorders. In addition, there are increasing opportunities for research, collaborative clinical practice, and direct nursing service to patients, families, and health care facilities. The urologic nurse, as a trained and experienced caregiver in matters associated with adult voiding dysfunction, is a needed and valuable member of the health care team, not only in our current system of health care delivery, but in the reformed health care delivery system of the future.

## *REFERENCES*

Abrams, P., Blaivis, J. G., Stanton, S. L., & Andersen, J. T. (1991). Appendix: Standardization of terminology of lower urinary tract function. In R. J. Krane & M. B. Siroky (Eds.), *Clinical neuro-urology* (2nd ed., pp. 651–669). Boston: Little, Brown.

Agency for Health Care Policy and Research. (1992). *Clinical practice guideline: Urinary incontinence in adults* (AHCPR 92-0038). Rockville, MD: Department of Health and Human Services.

Bors, E., & Comarr, A. E. (1971). *Neurological urology.* Baltimore: University Park Press.

Bradley, W. E. (1986). Physiology of the urinary bladder. In P. C. Walsh, R. F. Gittes, A. D. Perlmutter, & T. A. Stamey (Eds.), *Campbell's urology* (5th ed., pp. 129–185). Philadelphia: W. B. Saunders.

Burke, J. P., Garibaldi, R. A., Britt, M., Jacobson, J. A., Conti, M., & Ailling, D. W. (1981). Prevention of catheter-associated urinary tract infections: Efficacy of daily meatal care regimens. *American Journal of Medicine, 70*(2), 227–232.

Burke, J. P., Jacobson, J. A., Garibaldi, R. A., Conti, M., and Alling, D. W. (1983). Evaluation of daily meatal care with poly-antibiotic ointment in prevention of urinary catheter–associated bacteriuria. *Journal of Urology, 129,* 331–334.

Dear Abby. (1990). Incontinence problem that can be solved. Copyright: Universal Press Syndicate.

Faller, N., & Jeter, K. F. (1992). The ABC's of product selection. *Urologic Nursing, 12*(1), 52–54.

Gibbons, N. O. K. (1976). Nomenclature of neurogenic bladder. *Urology, 8,* 423.

Gray, M. (1990). Assessment and investigation of urinary incontinence. In K. Jeter, N. Faller, & C. Norton (Eds.), *Nursing for continence* (pp. 25–63). Philadelphia: W. B. Saunders.

Gray, M. (1991). Assessment of patients with urinary incontinence. In D. B. Doughty (Ed.), *Urinary and fecal incontinence: Nursing management* (pp. 47–94). St. Louis: Mosby-Year Book.

Gray, M. (1992a). *Genitourinary disorders.* St. Louis: Mosby-Year Book.

Gray, M. (1992b). Electrostimulation in the management of voiding dysfunction. *Urologic Nursing, 12*(2), 73–74.

Gray, M., & King, C. J. (1993). Urodynamic evaluation of the intrinsically incompetent sphincter. *Urologic Nursing, 13*(2), 67–69.

Grove, G. L., Lutz, J. B., Burton, S. A., & Tucker, J. A. (1994). Assessment of diaper clogging potential of petrolatum based skin barriers. Poster presentation at the 2nd National Multi-Specialty Nursing Conference on Urinary Continence, Phoenix, AZ.

Hickey, J. V. (1992). *The clinical practice of neurological and neurosurgical nursing* (3rd ed.). Philadelphia: J. B. Lippincott.

Jeter, K. (1990). The use of incontinence products. In K. Jeter, N. Faller, & C. Norton (Eds.), *Nursing for continence* (pp. 209–222). Philadelphia: W. B. Saunders.

Jonas, U., & Truss, M. (1991). Continent urinary reservoir in neurogenic bladder disease. In R. J. Krane & M. B. Siroky (Eds.), *Clinical neuro-urology* (2nd ed., pp. 575–592). Boston: Little, Brown.

Krane, R. J., Siroky, M. B. (1979). Classification of neuro-urologic disorders. In R. J. Krane & M. B. Siroky (Eds.), *Clinical neuro-urology* (pp. 143–158). Boston: Little, Brown.

Krane, R. J., & Siroky, M. B. (Eds.). (1991). *Clinical neuro-urology* (2nd ed.). Boston: Little, Brown.

Lam, T. C., & Hadley, H. R. (1991). Surgical procedures for uncomplicated ("routine") female stress incontinence. *Urologic Clinics of North America, 18*(2), 327–337.

Lapides, J. (1967). Cystometry. *Journal of the American Medical Association, 201,* 618.

Lapides, J., Diokno, A. C., Silber, S. J., & Lowe, B. S. (1972).

Clean, intermittent self-catheterization in the treatment of urinary tract disease. *Journal of Urology, 107*(3), 458–461.

Leach, G. E., & Raz, S. (1991). Surgery for stress incontinence. In R. J. Krane & M. B. Siroky (Eds.), *Clinical neuro-urology* (2nd ed., pp. 627–641). Boston: Little, Brown.

McClellan, F. C. (1939). *The neurogenic bladder* (pp. 57–70, 116–185). Springfield, IL: Charles C. Thomas.

McCormick, K. A., Scheve, A. A. S., & Leahy, E. (1988). Nursing management of urinary incontinence in geriatric inpatients. *Nursing Clinics of North America, 23*(1), 231–264.

Mitchell, M. E., Rink, R. C., & Adams, M. C. (1992). Augmentation cystoplasty and reconstruction. In P. C. Walsh, A. B. Retik, T. A. Stamey, & E. D. Vaughan, Jr. (Eds.), *Campbell's urology* (6th ed., pp. 2630–2653). Philadelphia: W. B. Saunders.

Moore, K. N., Griffiths, D. J., Metcalfe, J. B., & McCracken, P. N. (1993). Electrostimulation of the bladder neck in acontractile bladder: Two case reports. *Urologic Nursing, 13*(4), 113–115.

National Institutes of Health Consensus Development Conference Statement. (1988). *Urinary incontinence in adults* (Vol. 7, no. 5). Bethesda, MD: Office of Medical Applications of Research.

Newman, D. K., & Smith, D. A. (1992). Pelvic muscle reeducation as a nursing treatment for incontinence. *Urologic Nursing, 12*(1), 9–15.

Rollema, H. J. (1991). Uroflowmetry. In R. J. Krane & M. B. Siroky (Eds.), *Clinical neuro-urology* (2nd ed., pp. 201–244). Boston: Little, Brown.

Rosen N., & Ravalli, R. (1990). Intermittent self-catheterization. *Clinics in Geriatric Medicine, 6*(1), 101.

Rovner, S. (1992, March 24). Bladder training can stop incontinence. *Washington Post Health,* p. 11.

Stamey, T. (1992). Urinary incontinence in the female. In P. C. Walsh, A. B. Retik, T. A. Stamey, & E. D. Vaughan, Jr. (Eds.), *Campbell's urology* (6th ed., pp. 2829–2850). Philadelphia: W. B. Saunders.

Staskin, D. R. (1991). Classification of voiding dysfunction. In R. J. Krane & M. B. Siroky (Eds.), *Clinical neuro-urology* (2nd ed., pp. 411–424). Boston: Little, Brown.

Stricker, P., & Haylen, B. (18 January, 1993). Injectable collagen for type 3 female stress incontinence: The first 50 Australian patients. *Medical Journal of Australia, 158,* 89–91.

Tanagho, E. A. (1992). Urodynamic studies. In E. A. Tanagho & J. W. McAninch (Eds.), *Smith's general urology* (13th ed., pp. 473–494). Norwalk, CT: Appleton & Lange.

Toufexis, A. (December 1986). The last of the closet issues. *Time,* p. 69.

Van Arsdalen, K. & Wein, A. J. (1991). Physiology of micturition and continence. In R. J. Krane & M. B. Siroky (Eds.), *Clinical neuro-urology* (2nd ed., pp. 25–82). Boston: Little, Brown.

Wein, A. J. (1981). Classification of neurogenic voiding dysfunction. *Journal of Urology, 125,* 605.

Wein, A. J. (1992). Neuromuscular dysfunction of the lower urinary tract. In P. C. Walsh, A. B. Retik, T. A. Stamey, & E. D. Vaughan, Jr. (Eds.), *Campbell's urology* (6th ed., pp. 573–642). Philadelphia: W. B. Saunders.

Wong, E. S. (1983). Guideline for prevention of catheter-associated urinary tract infections. *American Journal of Infection Control, 11*(1), 28–33.

Wyman, J. (1988). Nursing assessment of the incontinent geriatric outpatient population. *Nursing Clinics of North America, 23*(1), 169–187.

Wyman, J. F., & Fantl, J. A. (1991). Bladder training in ambulatory care management of urinary incontinence. *Urologic Nursing, 11*(3), pp. 11–17.

# Trauma

# Genitourinary Trauma

■

*Nancy J. Reilly*

## OVERVIEW

Like all bodily systems, the genitourinary tract is subject to injury from external sources. Any number of incidents, both accidental and intentional, can disrupt the integrity of the urinary system and the male reproductive organs. At risk are the essential functions of the kidney and the ability of the human body to eliminate waste by way of the urinary tract. Reproductive and sexual functioning in men is also at risk. Overall, genitourinary trauma accounts for only 2% to 3% of all total admissions on a major trauma service (Charles & Hanno, 1987).

The assessment and evaluation of genitourinary injuries must take their appropriate place after assessment and stabilization of trauma to other, more vital systems. Blaisdell (1982) described the priorities in assessing the multiple trauma patient by systems. Assessment of the respiratory system with establishment of an adequate airway is the first priority. Second is the evaluation of the cardiovascular system, followed by the central nervous system. Fourth is the abdominal contents, including the genitourinary organs.

Trauma from external sources is usually categorized as either blunt or penetrating (or a combination of both). The usual causes of blunt trauma include falls from heights, motor vehicle accidents (or sudden deceleration injuries), and sporting injuries. Trauma sustained during blunt-type incidents is less obvious than penetrating trauma. Initial evaluation involves assessing a myriad of signs and symptoms and the use of radiographic studies and minor invasive techniques, such as peritoneal lavage. Any incidence of significant internal bleeding necessitates surgical intervention.

In most cases involving penetrating trauma, usually gunshot and stab wounds, the patient is moved expeditiously to surgery after initial resuscitation and stabilization. Diagnosis of injuries often takes place by direct observation and through radiographic techniques employed in the operating room.

This chapter first discusses the principles of triage and the initial assessment of the trauma victim. These topics are followed by discussions of upper urinary tract trauma, which includes injuries to the kidneys and ureters, and lower urinary tract traumatic injuries to the bladder and urethra. Finally, trauma to the external genitalia in men is

**411**

described. Each section covers the etiology, pathophysiology, medical and surgical management, and nursing care appropriate for each type of injury and the patient's recovery from it.

## BEHAVIORAL OBJECTIVES

After studying this chapter, the reader should be able to

1. List the types of injuries that are likely to result in renal trauma.
2. Differentiate between intraperitoneal and extraperitoneal bladder rupture.
3. Identify the cause of most ureteral injuries.
4. Discuss the reliability of the degree of hematuria as an indicator of the severity of trauma to the genitourinary tract.
5. Define posterior versus anterior urethral rupture and the clinical implications of each type.

## KEY WORDS

**Anterior urethral injury**—injury to the bulbous or penile male urethra, below the urogenital diaphragm.

**Avulsion injury**—a forcible tearing away of a part or structure.

**Blunt trauma**—the transfer of energy to the victim by application of external forces, without penetration of the body.

**Contusion**—a bruise; an injury to a part without disruption of it.

**Extraperitoneal bladder rupture**—a rupture on the anterior lateral wall of the bladder; urine extravasates into the perivesical tissue and the pelvic cavity.

**High-velocity gunshot wound**—the result of a bullet's being fired from a rifle or gun with great power and speed; the bullet tumbles over and over, creating a large cavity and extensive tissue damage. Some semiautomatic weapons fire at high velocity.

**Intraperitoneal bladder rupture**—a rupture of the dome of the bladder; urine extravasates into the peritoneal cavity.

**Low-velocity gunshot wound**—the result of a bullet's being fired from a handgun, but at lower power and speed than a high-velocity weapon; the bullet usually cores out a hole through tissue.

**Penetrating trauma**—the transfer of energy from a projectile, which breaks the skin and passes into or through the victim.

**Penile fracture**—rupture of the tunica albuginea; may or may not involve the corporal bodies, the urethra, or Buck's fascia.

**Peritoneal lavage**—the introduction of saline into the peritoneal cavity through a dialysis catheter; used to evaluate for the presence of intra-abdominal bleeding.

**Posterior urethral injury**—an injury to the prostatic or membranous male urethra, above and including the urogenital diaphragm.

**Sudden deceleration**—a mechanism of injury in blunt trauma; the body is moving at a rate of speed and suddenly stops, as in a fall or motor vehicle accident.

**Trauma**—an acute transfer of energy from an external source to the victim.

## TRIAGE AND INITIAL ASSESSMENT

Victims of genitourinary trauma are often the victims of trauma to other systems. It is difficult, if not impossible, to separate the treatment of genitourinary injuries from the treatment of hypovolemic shock, organ hypoperfusion, and the cardiogenic and cerebral complications of multiple trauma. Such a discussion is certainly beyond the scope of this chapter. The reader is referred to textbooks on

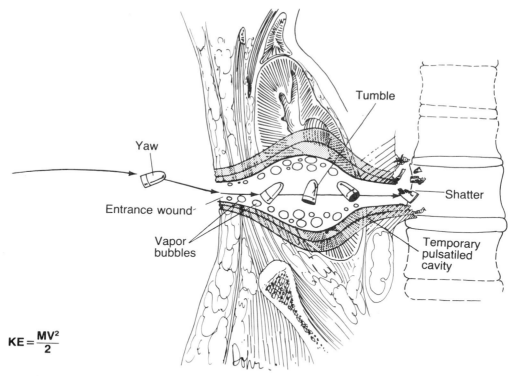

Yaw

Entrance wound

Vapor bubbles

Tumble

Shatter

Temporary pulsatiled cavity

$$KE = \frac{MV^2}{2}$$

*FIGURE 15–1* Effects of a high-velocity gunshot wound. (From McAninch JW. In *Urogenital Trauma*, Trauma Management Series, Volume II, Blaisdell FW and Trunkey DD [eds.], New York, Thieme Medical Publishers, Inc. Reprinted by permission.)

trauma and critical care nursing for more extensive information. This chapter provides knowledge of specific genitourinary injuries, and should be approached with the understanding that injuries to other organ systems may or may not exist and that the initial resuscitation and stabilization of victims must occur before an intervention for genitourinary trauma.

## UPPER URINARY TRACT TRAUMA

### Renal Trauma

#### PERSPECTIVE ON DISEASE ENTITY

**Etiology.** Most authors agree that blunt trauma is the cause of 80% to 90% of renal injuries (Carroll & McAninch, 1989; Hanno & Wein, 1984; McAninch, 1987). Fortunately, most renal injuries from blunt trauma are classified as minor and are often managed without surgery. Blunt renal trauma results from automobile accidents, falls, contact sports, assaults,

and personal violence (McAninch, 1987) (Fig. 15–1).

Penetrating renal trauma from stab or gunshot wounds accounts for 10% to 20% of all renal injuries. This statistic is likely to increase in large urban areas (Peters & Sagalowsky, 1986). Victims of gunshot wounds rarely sustain injury only to a kidney. McAninch (1987) reported an 8% incidence of associated intraabdominal injuries from gunshot wounds affecting a kidney. Stab wounds can similarly damage other organs, although less often. Together, blunt and penetrating renal trauma account for nearly half of all genitourinary trauma (Charles & Hanno, 1987).

**Pathophysiology.** The location and position of the kidneys in the retroperitoneum normally provide great protection from injury. Both kidneys are surrounded by fat within Gerota's fascia. They are fixed in place only by the attachments of the renal artery and vein to the aorta and the attachment of the ureter to the kidney. The lower rib cage provides additional protection, as does the outer renal capsule, which is tough and fibrous and resists rupture.

None of this protective anatomy will save

the kidney from penetrating trauma. The force and velocity of a gunshot wound may cause significant trauma as the bullet makes its way through or near the kidney (Fig. 15–1). A knife or other sharp instrument may cause similar damage, although its pathway is better defined.

All the kidney's protective anatomy is employed in cases of blunt trauma, as is evidenced by the fact that 80% of blunt renal injuries are classified as minor (Hanno & Wein, 1987; McAninch, 1987). Blunt trauma to the kidney occurs when the force of impact causes the kidney to move upward and forward, thrusting it against the ribs. This event can result in injuries as minor as a contusion or, if the force is great enough, a major vascular injury as the renal artery is torn away from the pedicle (vascular pedicle injury). Major renal parenchymal damage is additionally possible from blunt trauma.

The kidney is also at risk for injury when fractures to nearby bones occur. Rib fractures or a fracture of the transverse process of one of the upper lumbar vertebrae may damage the kidney with bone fragments (Hanno & Wein, 1984).

**Medical-Surgical Management.** Decisions about the appropriate management of a renal injury are often made after staging of the injury, if time permits. In the event of severe injury, staging takes place in the operating room when the victim's condition requires immediate surgical intervention. In cases in which the victim may be stabilized in the trauma bay or emergency department, a sequence of examinations and diagnostic studies is performed to evaluate and stage renal trauma.

Urinalysis to evaluate for the presence of hematuria is essential. Most patients with renal injury will have hematuria, either gross or microscopic; however, the degree of hematuria present *does not* correlate with the severity of renal trauma (Carroll & McAninch, 1989; Hanno & Wein, 1984; Nicholaisen & McAninch, 1985). Although hematuria alone is the best indicator of renal injury, 10% to 40% of patients with significant renal injury from blunt trauma do not have hematuria (Hanno & Wein, 1984). Conversely, many patients with minor renal injuries have gross hematuria.

Intravenous urography (IVU) provides valuable information when evaluating victims of blunt trauma. Contrast material (2 mL/kg) may be administered during the initial phase of evaluation of the injury, with serial abdominal films being taken in the trauma bay. A nor-

mal IVU in the presence of hematuria suggests a minor injury that can be treated nonsurgically. Poor visualization of a kidney or extravasation of contrast material requires further evaluation.

In the clinically stable patient, computed tomography (CT) scanning is preferred by some clinicians for definitive initial evaluation of renal injury. At the same time, potential injuries to other organs or vessels are diagnosed. The results of the CT scan may ultimately stage the renal injury and determine the appropriate method of management. Arteriography is occasionally used when the kidney is not visualized on IVU and vascular damage is suspected, or when CT scan is unavailable (McAninch, 1987). Magnetic resonance image (MRI) scanning may also be useful.

Blunt renal trauma is classified or staged into one of the four following groups, according to McAninch (1987) (Fig. 15–2):

*Contusions*—bruises or subcapsular hematomas; the renal capsule and collecting system are intact.

*Minor lacerations*—superficial cortical disruptions that do not involve the deep renal medulla or the collecting system.

*Major lacerations*—parenchymal disruptions extending through the cortex and into the deep medulla; the collecting system may be involved.

*Vascular injuries*—occlusions or tears of the renal artery or vein.

Contusions are usually managed conservatively. In patients with a normal IVU study and microscopic hematuria, hospitalization is not always necessary. When contusion with gross hematuria or a minor laceration is present, hospitalization with bed rest, monitoring of vital signs, serial physical examinations, and serial urine sample testing are recommended (Hanno & Wein, 1984). Such minor injuries generally resolve without specific treatment over time. The renal capsule and Gerota's fascia both provide a mechanism of tamponade to control bleeding.

Major lacerations are the subject of some controversy regarding decisions about management. Some urologists advocate a conservative approach to all but the most severe and life-threatening renal injuries. Others routinely surgically explore and repair major lacerations. The results of either approach seem to be generally favorable, although surgeons who rou-

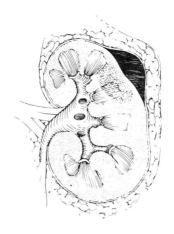

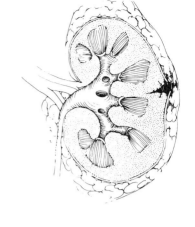

**RENAL CONTUSIONS**

**MINOR LACERATIONS**

*FIGURE 15–2* Classification of renal injuries. (From Mee, S. L., & McAninch, J. W. [1989]. Indications for radiographic assessment in suspected renal trauma. *Urologic Clinics of North America, 16,* 189. Reprinted by permission.)

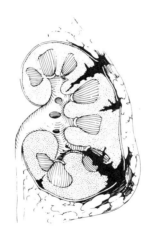

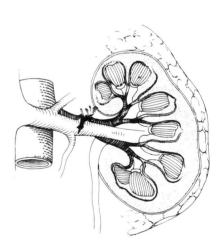

**MAJOR LACERATIONS**

**VASCULAR INJURIES**

tinely explore and repair major lacerations report a lower incidence of late complications, including nephrectomy.

Vascular injuries to the kidney include a tear of the renal artery, vein, or both, and total avulsion of the renal artery and vein. Any renal vascular injury involves serious hemorrhage and is life threatening. The victim often is in shock and requires aggressive resuscitation. If time permits, IVU is performed in the trauma bay. More often, it is carried out when the patient is on the operating table. Knowledge of the presence and function of the contralateral kidney is needed by the surgeon before reconstruction of the injured kidney begins.

Penetrating renal injuries are almost always surgically explored (Hanno & Wein, 1984; McAninch, 1987; Peterson, 1987). A small percentage of patients with penetrating wounds affecting the kidney have injuries that are classified as minor. These patients are usually victims of posterior or flank stab wounds and can be managed without surgery. Treatment is identical to that described for minor blunt renal trauma.

Surgery to evaluate penetrating trauma is performed through a midline abdominal incision. This approach facilitates repair to other abdominal organs. The pathway of the stab or gunshot wound is explored with débridement of devitalized tissue. After the retroperitoneum is entered, renal parenchymal defects are closed with peritoneal grafts or omental grafts, and the renal capsule is replaced if possible. The renal vessels are repaired and reconstructed using grafts from the saphenous vein or hypogastric artery. When renal parenchymal damage is too great to repair, partial or total nephrectomy may be necessary.

## APPROACHES TO PATIENT CARE

### Assessment

The professional nurse is a member of the trauma team. The team works together when a trauma victim is brought to a hospital or trauma center for treatment. Efforts to stabilize the patient must take first priority. Portions of the nursing assessment may have to be postponed until the patient is stable or even until after surgery. Much information necessary for a nursing assessment is obtained during resuscitation and stabilization, and should be documented and passed on to subsequent nurses caring for the patient.

Determination of the mechanism of *blunt injury* is vital in assessing the renal trauma victim. Find out exactly what happened to the patient to guide assessment. Table 15–1 outlines nursing assessment data that should be obtained for all trauma victims. To obtain more specific assessment data for the suspected blunt renal trauma victim, ask if the patient sustained a sports injury or was the victim of an assault or personal violence. If so, were any blows delivered to the kidney area, or did the patient fall onto either flank?

Victims of *penetrating trauma* are usually moved to the operating room immediately following stabilization. Information about the mechanism of injury is obtained through observation and paramedic or police reports. Count the number of entrance and exit wounds, and document them. Wounds in the posterior flank areas certainly lead to suspicion of renal damage. Plain abdominal films performed in the trauma bay or emergency department will localize any bullets or foreign objects remaining in the abdomen or retroperitoneum.

Physical assessment of blunt trauma victims should include looking at both flanks for the presence of pulsating or expanding masses, indicating retroperitoneal hematoma. Assess also for tenderness in the flank area. If the patient has lower rib fractures or a vertebral fracture in the lumbar spine, the status of the kidneys needs to be evaluated.

**TABLE 15–1. Nursing Assessment Data for Trauma Victims**

For victims of a motor vehicle accident:
____ Position of the victim (passenger or driver)
____ Use of seat belts (lap, shoulder, or both)
____ Speed of vehicle at impact
____ Entrapment and details of extrication
____ Condition of other victims
____ Pedestrian: type of vehicle; was the victim thrown or run over?

For victims of a gunshot wound(s):
____ Type of gun and caliber of bullet
____ Number of shots fired
____ Distance from the victim that the gun was fired
____ Number and location of entrance and exit wounds

For victims of a knife wound(s):
____ Type and length of the knife
____ Victim's distance from the assailant
____ Assailant's height and sex
____ Number and location of entrance and exit wounds

For victims of a fall:
____ Distance of the fall
____ Position of victim on landing
____ Type of surface on which the victim landed
____ Striking anything during descent
____ Reason for fall: deliberate or accidental

Sources of information:
____ Patient (if possible)
____ Family or witnesses
____ Police or police report
____ Paramedics or flight team

Adapted from Wagner, M. M. (1990). The patient with abdominal injuries. *Nursing Clinics of North America, 25*(1), 45–55. Reprinted by permission.

Urinalysis is necessary as part of the evaluation for renal injury. Urine is obtained either by catheterization or by having the patient void when possible. A "dipstick" check of the urine is not considered adequate; the urine must be examined under a microscope. The absence of gross or microscopic hematuria does not rule out renal injury.

Assessment of the patient's fear and anxiety is essential if the patient is conscious during evaluation of the injury. Altered levels of consciousness may also result in confusion, lethargy, or agitation.

### Nursing Diagnosis

The nursing diagnoses for the patient with renal trauma may include the following:

1. Fluid volume deficit: actual, related to blood loss from disrupted vessels.
2. Alteration in tissue perfusion: renal, related to disrupted blood flow to the kidney.
3. Alteration in patterns of urinary elimination related to hematuria.

4. Alteration in comfort: pain related to bruising or laceration of the kidney.
5. Fear related to uncertain outcome of physical trauma.

### Plan of Care

Nursing care is directed toward enabling the patient to

1. Achieve hemostasis through interventions designed to control or stop bleeding.
2. Be restored to maximum possible renal functioning.
3. Eventually achieve normal urine production without hematuria.
4. Remain comfortable throughout treatment.
5. Comply with restriction on activity.
6. Have his or her fears allayed through increased knowledge of the injuries and expected recovery.

### Intervention

Nursing interventions during the initial evaluation of injury are directed toward resuscitation. Monitor vital signs, administer intravenous fluids and blood products, obtain laboratory samples of blood or urine, and monitor the patient for signs of shock.

In the less severely injured patient, time permits more extensive nursing interventions. Explain procedures and diagnostic tests to the patient. Plain films and an IVU may be done in the emergency area. Prepare the patient for other diagnostic studies, such as CT scan, MRI, renal scan, or ultrasonography. Keep the family informed of the patient's status.

Once renal trauma is diagnosed, nursing interventions depend on whether or not surgery is necessary. When conservative treatment is recommended, monitor vital signs, administer intravenous fluids and analgesic medications, and monitor urine output. The evaluation of urine output should include the amount and color or consistency. The amount of urine output per hour is a good indication of renal function. "Serial urines" may be ordered to monitor successive voidings for clearing of hematuria. In some areas this practice is called "racking urines." A sample of each voiding, usually approximately 30 mL, is separated and placed in a transparent glass container, usually a test tube or blood vial. It is then labeled with the date and time and placed on a rack next to the sample from the previous void. If a rack is unavailable, the samples may be taped to the wall in the patient's bathroom. This method allows for "at a glance" evaluation of lessening hematuria by all involved in caring for the patient. The patient also may see his or her progress rather clearly.

Bed rest is usually ordered for patients who are hospitalized for blunt renal trauma. If a fall, motor vehicle accident, or assault was the cause of injury, the patient is likely to have muscular aches and pains, bruises, and contusions that are uncomfortable. Maintaining bed rest may be difficult in conjunction with other injuries. Explain the necessity of rest to the patient, and elicit his or her cooperation and that of the family.

Monitor the patient for symptoms of infection. Urinary tract infection is possible, as are localized infectious processes from urine extravasation, such as peritonitis or perinephric abscess formation. Laboratory values should be watched, particularly the levels of hemoglobin and hematocrit (for bleeding), blood urea nitrogen and creatinine (for renal function), and white blood cell count (for infection).

When surgery is necessary, the nurse may be caring for a postoperative patient who has undergone surgical repair or partial or total nephrectomy. Monitor the incision for drainage of pus, blood, or serous fluid. Continued bleeding is a potential complication, as is perinephric abscess formation. Administer analgesic medications to relieve pain. Maintain a closed urinary drainage system, and monitor the degree of hematuria. Watch the patient's vital signs and laboratory values. Hypertension is a possible complication of any renal surgery, but is usually a late complication of renal injury.

The patient and family need to be educated about postoperative care and long-term complications. Teach them about care of the incision and the importance of a good fluid intake. Describe the symptoms of late complications, including chronic renal insufficiency, hypertension, and calculus formation. In patients who have had a nephrectomy, educate them on good fluid intake and, if the physician concurs, wearing a Medic Alert bracelet. Encourage patients to comply with long term follow-up to help avoid any complications.

### Patient Outcomes

1. The patient is restored to hemodynamic stability or is transferred to surgery.
2. The patient's vital signs are stable.
3. The patient is relieved of pain.
4. The patient complies with activity restrictions.
5. The patient's hematuria slowly resolves.
6. The patient verbalizes an understanding of the purpose of diagnostic studies.
7. The patient describes symptoms of late com-

plications, including hypertension and calculus formation.
8. The patient verbalizes the importance of maintaining adequate fluid intake (at least eight 8-ounce glasses per day).

## Ureteral Trauma

### PERSPECTIVE ON DISEASE ENTITY

**Etiology.** Penetrating trauma and accidental injury during surgery are the most frequently seen causes of trauma to the ureter (Corriere, 1987b). Blunt trauma rarely results in ureteral injury; however, severe sudden deceleration accidents may cause an avulsion of the upper third of the ureter (Hill, 1988). Overall, ureteral trauma accounts for only 4% of all genitourinary trauma.

Gunshot wounds constitute 95% of ureteral injuries from penetrating trauma (Blaisdell, 1982; Corriere, 1987b; Peters & Sagalowsky, 1986). Stab wounds rarely affect the ureter, primarily because of its location deep within the retroperitoneum.

Accidental injury to the ureter occurs in fewer than 1% of all pelvic surgeries. Approximately 50% of these ureteral injuries occur during gynecologic surgery, and 30% during urologic surgery (Corriere, 1987b). Among the operations most commonly involving accidental injury to the ureter are abdominal hysterectomy, vesical suspension procedures, cesarean sections, and ureterolithotomy (Peters & Sagalowsky, 1986).

**Pathophysiology.** The ureter is protected anteriorly by the abdominal wall, colon, and pelvic organs, and posteriorly by the vertebral column and the large muscles of the back (Hanno & Wein, 1984). Each ureter lies completely within the retroperitoneum. Its only firm connections are at the ureteropelvic and ureterovesical junctions (Guerriero, 1988).

Penetrating trauma and surgical injury represent the usual threats to this well-protected structure. The effects of gunshot or stab wounds on the ureter range from contusions to complete transections. Accidental surgical injuries to the ureter may cause a similar range of trauma, from a small puncture wound to a complete transection. Most iatrogenic ureteral injuries occur in the lower half of the ureter. Most ureteral injuries from penetrating trauma are discovered during surgical exploration following injury; hence, there are no specific symptoms or signs to watch for. When surgical injury to the ureter is not recognized intraoperatively, certain signs and symptoms become part of the pathophysiologic process. The leakage of urine into the periureteral tissues causes flank pain and fever. If such leakage is left undetected, fistulas are likely to develop.

**Medical-Surgical Management.** IVU is routinely performed when penetrating trauma suggests possible injury to the genitourinary tract and the victim's condition is hemodynamically stable. Ninety percent of ureteral injuries are diagnosed by IVU (Charles & Hanno, 1987; Guerriero, 1988). Hematuria may or may not be present. If present, the amount of hematuria is not a good indicator of the severity of the injury. CT scanning is an accurate method of evaluating trauma to the ureter; however, when penetrating trauma is present, either IVU is quickly followed by exploratory surgery or IVU is performed on the operating table.

If the patient's condition permits, the surgeon may place a ureteral stent preoperatively, which simplifies intraoperative location of the ureter. This task is accomplished through either antegrade or retrograde methods. In some instances, a percutaneous nephrostomy may also be performed. Both of these interventions divert urine away from the injured area.

In many cases of penetrating trauma, surgery must be performed expeditiously. The surgeon frees up and inspects the entire ureter. Indigo carmine, given intravenously, is often useful in locating areas of urinary extravasation intraoperatively. An injection of 5 mL of indigo carmine causes a bluish discoloration of periureteral tissue within 7 to 10 minutes. Several different types of surgical procedures are used to repair ureteral trauma; the type performed depends on the location of the injury in the ureter.

The simplest surgical repair of the ureter involves repair of a partial laceration when the affected area remains viable. The laceration is closed and the ureter is stented. Indwelling or double-J stents are usually used.

Trauma to the upper third of the ureter is repaired by various pyeloplasty techniques (Hanno & Wein, 1984). Injury to the middle third of the ureter is repaired by end-to-end anastomosis, or ureteroureterostomy. Ureteroneocystostomy, which reimplants the ureter into the bladder, is often used to repair trauma to the lower third of the ureter (Fig. 15–3).

Alternative types of repair are necessary when an area of the ureter is devitalized and must be débrided. The bladder may be brought closer to the lower ureter through a technique

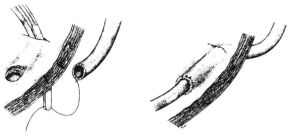

FIGURE 15–3 Ureteroneocystostomy, or reimplantation of the ureter into the bladder wall; for trauma to the lower third of the ureter. (From Corriere, J. N. [1987b]. Ureteral injuries. In J. Y. Gillenwater, J. T. Grayhack, S. S. Howards, & J. W. Duckett [Eds.], *Adult and pediatric urology* [p. 439]. Chicago: Year Book Medical Publishers. Reprinted by permission.)

called a bladder flap (Fig. 15–4). If a large section of the ureter is nonviable, a transureteroureterostomy may be performed. This procedure involves crossing the viable section of the traumatized ureter over to the healthy contralateral ureter and anastomosing them together so that they both drain into the bladder through the lower third of the noninjured ureter. Other surgeons replace larger sections of nonviable ureter with ileum. When damage to the ureter is severe and multiple trauma exists, nephrectomy may be necessary.

Ureteral stenting is used postoperatively with all types of ureteral repair, diverting urine flow away from areas of anastomoses. Indwelling ureteral stents are later removed cystoscopically. Percutaneous nephrostomy is also an option for diverting urine away from an injured ureter. It may be used in conjunction with ureteral stents when the upper half of the ureter is damaged. Nephrostomy additionally provides for renal drainage when ureteral damage is severe and later repair is planned.

Repair of ureteral injury that occurs acciden-

tally during pelvic or abdominal surgery is accomplished by the same types of surgery. Diagnosis of this type of ureteral injury usually involves more extensive studies, including retrograde pyelography and CT scanning. Percutaneous nephrostomy and ureteral stenting are used preoperatively not only to allow for diversion of urine but also to provide time for resolution of the effects of urine extravasation into the periureteral tissues and, if necessary, healing of fistulas.

## APPROACHES TO PATIENT CARE

### Assessment

As in all cases of traumatic injury, nursing assessment must include obtaining as much information as is possible about the incident or accident that caused the patient's injuries. When the patient is unable to provide any information, family members, witnesses or paramedic reports may provide valuable assessment data (see Table 15–1).

Ureteral injury should be suspected when gunshot entrance or exit wounds are present in the lower abdominal or flank area. Assessment of both the anterior and posterior trunk is important. Entrance and exit wounds should be counted and documented. Anterior stab wounds rarely affect the ureter; however, posterior stab wounds may. The flank should be inspected for an expanding hematoma in the retroperitoneum. Any urine output should be assessed for the presence of gross or microhematuria. Because most penetrating injuries involve other organ systems, symptoms are usually not specific to the ureteral injury in and of itself.

If ureteral trauma is not diagnosed at the

FIGURE 15–4 Bladder flap procedure for reimplantation of the ureter into the bladder. (From Corriere, J. N. [1987b]. Ureteral injuries. In J. Y. Gillenwater, J. T. Grayhack, S. S. Howards, & J. W. Duckett [Eds.], *Adult and pediatric urology* [p. 440]. Chicago: Year Book Medical Publishers. Reprinted by permission.)

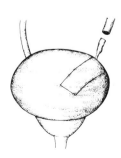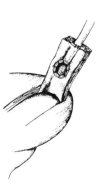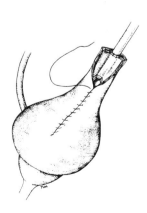

time of injury, later symptoms will develop. Assess the patient for flank or abdominal pain, abdominal tenderness, and signs of peritonitis, paralytic ileus, and fever. Assess the patient for urine leakage from wounds, the surgical incision, or surgically placed drains. Spiking fevers and unstable vital signs occur if sepsis develops.

Fistulas may develop when undetected ureteral injury exists but are more likely to develop when injuries to other organs occurred at the same time as ureteral injury. Vaginal, cutaneous, and enteric fistulas are all possible (Corriere, 1987b). Assess the female patient for leakage of urine from the vagina.

**Nursing Diagnosis**

The nursing diagnosis for the patient with ureteral trauma may include the following:

1. Fluid volume deficit: actual, related to blood loss from interrupted blood vessels.
2. Alteration in comfort: pain related to intra-abdominal or retroperitoneal extravasation of urine.
3. Alteration in patterns of urinary elimination
   a. related to ureteral interruption.
   b. related to placement of urinary drainage tubes.
4. Fear related to uncertain outcome of physical trauma.

**Plan of Care**

Nursing care is directed toward enabling the patient to

1. Achieve hemodynamic stability through interventions that replace fluids and control bleeding.
2. Assist (when possible) in evaluation of injuries by describing and localizing areas of pain.
3. Be restored to normal urinary elimination by way of an intact urinary tract.
4. Understand diagnostic and surgical interventions and be reassured by information provided about his or her prognosis.

**Intervention**

During the initial evaluation of injury phase, nursing interventions are directed toward participating in a team approach to stabilize and resuscitate the victim. Assessing the victim, obtaining historical data, and performing nursing interventions often take place simultaneously. Vital signs must be monitored very closely, intravenous fluids and blood products are given as ordered, and blood and urine samples are sent for laboratory evaluation. When possible, information and reassurance should be provided to allay patient fears and anxieties.

When the patient is being evaluated for suspected ureteral injury in a non–emergency situation, nursing interventions include monitoring vital signs with a watchful eye toward patterns of temperature elevation. Interventions directed toward relieving pain, other than the administration of analgesia, will comfort the patient when analgesics are withheld so that symptoms are not masked (i.e., positioning, relaxation techniques, and distractions). Output of both urinary and gastrointestinal fluids is measured; vomiting may occur if an ileus is forming. Intake of fluids must also be monitored. During the evaluation period, the nurse provides information to the patient and family about diagnostic studies. This may be a particularly anxious time for the patient, especially when he or she has recently undergone surgery. A ureteral injury usually involves additional surgical intervention. Postoperative nursing care of the patient who has undergone repair of a ureteral injury includes the following:

1. Maintaining patency of ureteral and Foley catheters and nephrostomy tubes, if present.
2. Closely monitoring intake and output at least every 8 hours.
3. Monitoring vital signs at least every 4 hours.
4. Administering medication to relieve pain and monitor the patient's response.
5. Administering antibiotics to prevent the development of a urinary tract infection.
6. Teaching the patient and family to care for indwelling nephrostomy tubes, stents, or Foley catheters.

**Patient Outcomes**

1. The patient is resuscitated to a state of hemodynamic stability or is transferred to the operating room.
2. The patient remains afebrile.
3. The patient is relieved of pain.
4. The patient's urine remains sterile.
5. The patient verbalizes an understanding of the purpose of diagnostic studies.
6. The patient expresses an understanding of the need for good fluid intake.
7. The patient verbalizes side effects of antibiotic therapy.
8. The patient and family learn to care for indwelling urinary catheters that may remain in place at discharge.

# LOWER URINARY TRACT TRAUMA

## Bladder Trauma

### PERSPECTIVE ON DISEASE ENTITY

**Etiology.** When empty, the bladder is a well-protected structure. It lies deep within the bony pelvis, which provides protection from injury. It is as the bladder fills that it becomes more vulnerable to injury. The type of injury a bladder sustains often depends on the amount of urine contained within it at the time of injury (Peters & Sagalowsky, 1986).

Blunt trauma is the cause of most bladder injuries, with motor vehicle accidents being the most common source of the blunt force. Other sources include pedestrian–motor vehicle accidents, falls, and blows to the abdomen. Seat belts are often implicated when motor vehicle accidents result in bladder trauma. The lap portion of the seat belt, while restraining the wearer, becomes a source of force to the lower abdomen when sudden deceleration occurs, especially when a shoulder harness is not worn.

Pelvic fracture is present in more than 70% of blunt trauma resulting in bladder damage (Wiegel, 1982). However, only 5% to 10% of patients with a pelvic fracture will have a severe bladder injury (Hanno & Wein, 1984). Bone fragments from the fracture of the pelvis may bruise or lacerate the bladder. The most significant traumatic bladder injuries are ruptures that occur when the force of the blunt insult causes a section of the full bladder's wall to erupt.

Penetrating trauma accounts for only a small percentage of bladder injuries. Gunshot wounds are the usual cause (Corriere, 1987a; Peters & Sagalowsky, 1986). Stab wounds and iatrogenic injuries are additional sources of penetrating trauma to the bladder.

**Pathophysiology.** The urinary bladder is firmly attached to the urogenital diaphragm at its base. In men, this fixation is more pronounced with the attachments of the prostate to the pubic bone (Wiegel, 1982). The dome of the bladder is its most mobile area, becoming more so as it fills with urine and rises up out of the pelvis. The muscular bladder wall stretches and becomes thinner with distention.

When blunt trauma to the lower abdomen is sustained, a variety of bladder injuries may result, depending on the force of the blow and the amount of urine in the bladder (Table 15–2). Contusion occurs when the bladder wall sustains an incomplete tear, often the result of nearby bone fractures or fragments from a pelvic fracture. "Teardrop bladder" is also a result of pelvic fracture but does not represent an actual injury to the bladder itself. Teardrop bladder refers to the bilateral compression of the bladder by pelvic hematoma, so that the bladder assumes a "teardrop" configuration seen on cystogram.

Intraperitoneal bladder rupture may be caused when the victim sustains a blow to the lower abdomen while the bladder is full. The bladder ruptures at its weakest point: the dome (Fig. 15–5). Urine extravasates into the peritoneal cavity and continues to flow into the peritoneum if unrecognized. The patient may develop what appears to be ascites. If the urine is infected, peritonitis quickly ensues.

Extraperitoneal bladder rupture is far more common than intraperitoneal rupture and is a serious consequence of pelvic fracture. The bladder ruptures near its base, usually on the anterior lateral wall (Corriere, 1987a) (see Fig. 15–5). Urine extravasates into the perivesical tissue but does not extend beyond the urogenital diaphragm or into the peritoneal cavity (Peters & Sagalowsky, 1986).

Penetrating trauma from gunshot or stab wounds may strike the bladder. Again, the full bladder is more at risk. High-velocity gunshot injuries with significant blast effect may cause major damage to nearby structures and require a team approach to surgical repair (Wiegel, 1982).

**Medical-Surgical Management.** Bladder trauma is suspected whenever there is a history of lower abdominal trauma, blunt or penetrating. Specific symptoms are usually not present, although the patient may experience suprapubic pain and is unable to void (Corriere, 1987a). Unlike other genitourinary injuries, hematuria is almost always present with bladder trauma. Because the patient may be unable to void, the first urine obtained may be in the course of performing diagnostic studies. Patients with

**TABLE 15–2. Classification of Bladder Trauma**

| TYPE | CAUSE |
|---|---|
| Contusion | Incomplete tear of bladder wall |
| Teardrop bladder | Compression from pelvic hematoma |
| Intraperitoneal rupture | Rupture at bladder's dome into peritoneal cavity |
| Extraperitoneal rupture | Rupture near base of bladder into perivesical space |

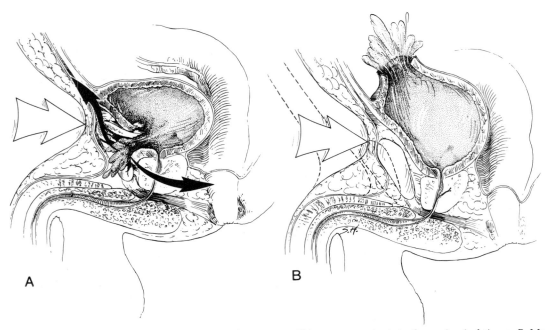

**FIGURE 15–5** *A*, Mechanism of extraperitoneal bladder rupture. Urine extravasates into the perivesical tissue. *B*, Mechanism of intraperitoneal bladder rupture. Urine extravasates into the peritoneal cavity. (From Peters, P. C., & Sagalowsky, A. I. [1986]. Genitourinary trauma. In P. C. Walsh, R. E. Gittes, A. D. Perlmutter, & T. A. Stamey [Eds.], *Campbell's urology* [Vol. 1, 5th ed., p. 1212]. Philadelphia: W. B. Saunders. Reprinted by permission.)

pelvic fracture often have symptomatology specific to that injury.

IVU may be performed when multiple blunt trauma exists but usually is not sufficient to diagnose bladder injury. Cystography is necessary for diagnosis. In the absence of urethral injury, cystography is performed through a Foley catheter. Contrast material is infused through the catheter, and several films are taken as the bladder is filled. A cystogram is not deemed normal until the bladder is completely filled and no extravasation is seen. Films are also taken after the bladder is emptied of contrast material; small posterior bladder ruptures may be seen only on these films. If a bladder injury is present, extravasation of contrast material is readily seen radiographically.

When urethral injury is suspected, a retrograde urethrogram must be performed prior to cystography. If urethral continuity has been disrupted, cystography is performed via suprapubic cystotomy.

Treatment of bladder injuries, once they are confirmed, depends on their severity. Small tears or ruptures as well as partial lacerations may often heal without surgery. All bladder injuries require diversion of urine away from the injury. For contusions, partial lacerations,

and some small ruptures, this is achieved through Foley catheterization. If the physician prefers, or if the injury is near the base of the bladder, suprapubic cystotomy may be performed. Seven to 10 days of catheter drainage and bed rest may be all that are necessary for the bladder to heal.

Small tears in the bladder wall may be repaired surgically when the patient must undergo surgery for other injuries. In these instances, diagnosis of injury may take place by direct observation of the bladder by the surgeon. An incision in the bladder is necessary to observe the bladder base and bladder neck area.

Most urologists agree that intraperitoneal ruptures must be surgically repaired. When blunt trauma is the cause of the injury, there is a significantly sized rupture at the bladder's dome. Devitalized tissue is débrided and the bladder wall closed. Urine and blood, which have accumulated in the peritoneal cavity, are evacuated. Penrose drains may be placed on either side. A suprapubic tube is placed during surgery and left in place for 7 to 10 days. A cystogram is usually performed prior to removal of the suprapubic catheter to confirm that healing is complete.

Large extraperitoneal ruptures are repaired

surgically in a manner similar to that described for intraperitoneal ruptures. An incision is made into the superior aspect of the bladder wall to allow for visualization and repair of the base of the bladder. Some urologists prefer to treat small extraperitoneal ruptures by catheter drainage alone, when the following conditions are met: (1) the patient has no associated injuries that require surgical exploration, (2) the diagnosis has been made within 12 hours of injury, and (3) there is no evidence of urinary tract infection (Hanno, 1987). Catheter drainage continues for ten days. A cystogram confirms healing before the catheter is removed.

Occasionally a pelvic fracture patient is found to have both intraperitoneal and extraperitoneal bladder ruptures. When this occurs, surgery is performed to repair all ruptures in the bladder wall.

Late complications of surgical repair of bladder ruptures include formation of a vesicocutaneous fistula at the site of the suprapubic catheter, stricture formation near the urethra, and voiding dysfunction.

## APPROACHES TO PATIENT CARE

### Assessment

Injury to the urinary bladder should be suspected in any patient who has sustained blunt trauma to the lower abdomen or pelvic area and is more likely when a pelvic fracture has occurred. Penetrating trauma to the lower abdomen should also lead to suspicion of bladder trauma.

As with any form of trauma, obtain as much information as is possible about the mechanism of injury (see Table 15–1). Assess the patient for suprapubic pain and determine if the patient has been able to void. If not, does he or she feel the need to void? Try to determine when the patient last voided before the injury. Gross hematuria is almost always present and is obvious when catheterization is achieved. If the patient has a large intraperitoneal or extraperitoneal rupture, it may be difficult to obtain any urine for laboratory studies.

Continued, prolonged drainage of frank blood into the pelvis or through any successfully placed urinary catheters indicates a significant hemorrhagic event. The patient should be assessed for deteriorating vital signs and other evidence of ensuing shock. Assess the patient for symptoms of peritonitis: auscultate for bowel sounds (which may be absent), and palpate for abdominal pain, tenderness, or rigidity.

Patients with intraperitoneal ruptures that have allowed the accumulation of large amounts of urine in the peritoneal cavity develop uroascites. The abdomen is markedly distended, but nontender. If enough fluid has accumulated so that there is pressure on the diaphragm, respiratory effort may be compromised.

### Nursing Diagnosis

The nursing diagnoses for the patient with trauma to the bladder may include the following:

1. Alteration in pattern of urinary elimination secondary to traumatic injury to the bladder.
2. Alteration in comfort: pain related to traumatic physical injury.
3. Alteration in tissue perfusion related to disrupted blood vessels and possible pelvic hematoma.
4. Fear and anxiety related to unknown outcomes of injury.
5. Potential for infection related to
   a. traumatic injury of bladder tissue
   b. disruption of the integrity of the urinary system.

### Plan of Care

Nursing care is directed toward enabling the patient to

1. Be returned to a state of hemodynamic stability.
2. Be relieved of pain through analgesic medication.
3. Verbalize an understanding of his or her injury and the interventions used to repair it.
4. Maintain a patent and closed urinary drainage system.
5. Eventually resume normal voiding patterns.
6. State the dosage schedule and side effects of antibiotic therapy.
7. Verbalize knowledge of the care of indwelling urinary catheters.
8. State the signs and symptoms of urinary tract infection.

### Intervention

Nursing interventions after initial stabilization are directed toward assisting in the establishment of a method of urinary drainage. This plan may mean assisting with placement of a Foley catheter or suprapubic cystotomy, or it may mean preparing the patient for surgery.

When an intraperitoneal or extraperitoneal rupture of the bladder has been diagnosed, the patient should be monitored for symptoms of sepsis or peritonitis. Monitor vital signs for deterioration of blood pressure, elevated pulse rate, and fever. Absent bowel sounds and nausea and vomiting, accompanied by abdominal pain and rigidity, are indicative of peritonitis.

Administer antibiotic drugs, and monitor the patient for side effects. Give intravenous fluids and blood products. Watch laboratory values for a decreasing hemoglobin level or deteriorating renal function.

After surgery to repair a bladder rupture, relief of pain and maintenance of urinary drainage catheters are priorities. Administer pain medication and evaluate pain relief. Monitor urine output and assess for degree of hematuria. Urine and blood should not be allowed to distend the repaired bladder, which would jeopardize the sutured incision. Make sure catheters do not become occluded. Manual irrigation of urinary catheters should not be attempted without permission of the urologist.

Patients may need to learn to care for indwelling urinary catheters. This involves learning to change from leg bag to bedside drainage containers, learning measures to inhibit bacterial growth, and learning the signs and symptoms of urinary tract infection.

Bladder tissue heals rapidly and well. After the removal of catheters, most patients resume normal voiding within a few weeks but may experience frequency and nocturia for a short while.

**Patient Outcomes**

1. The patient is restored to hemodynamic stability.
2. The patient is relieved of pain.
3. The patient demonstrates the ability to care for an indwelling urinary drainage system.
4. The patient verbalizes measures to remain free of urinary tract infection.
5. The patient states the signs and symptoms of urinary tract infection.
6. The patient eventually resumes normal voiding patterns.

## Urethral Trauma

### PERSPECTIVE ON DISEASE ENTITY

**Etiology.** Trauma to the male urethra may be the result of numerous accidental events. Blunt trauma to the lower abdominal or pelvic area is usually involved. Penetrating trauma in the form of projectile missiles of various types can also injure the anterior male urethra, although this type of injury is rare (Corriere, 1987a; McAninch, 1985). Urethral trauma may also be the result of accidental perforation during

endoscopic procedures or selfmanipulation. Female urethral injuries are extremely rare (Corriere, 1987a; Hanno & Wein, 1984; Wiegel, 1982).

Any discussion of trauma to the male urethra must begin with a definition of the two major classifications: posterior and anterior urethral injuries.

Posterior urethral injuries are defined as involving the prostatic or membranous urethra; or the area of the urethra that is superior to the urogenital diaphragm (Fig. 15–6). Bleeding and extravasation of urine from a posterior urethral injury occur into the *pelvis.*

Anterior urethral injuries involve the bulbar or penile urethra, or the area of the urethra that is *inferior* to the urogenital diaphragm. Bleeding and extravasation take place within the *perineum* when the anterior urethra is injured (Hanno & Wein, 1984).

Posterior urethral injuries almost always occur in conjunction with a pelvic fracture (Corriere, 1987a; Devine & Devine, 1982; McAninch, 1985). This type of injury is often the result of a motor vehicle accident, a fall from a height, or industrial or sporting injuries.

Anterior urethral injuries are commonly found in patients with a history of blunt trauma to the perineum. Typical causes include falling astride an object (straddle-type injury) or sustaining a blow to the perineum. Less

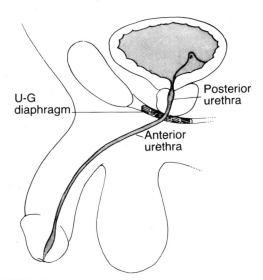

*FIGURE 15–6* Anatomy of the anterior and posterior male urethra in relation to the urogenital diaphragm. (From McAninch, J. W. [1985]. Urogenital trauma. In R. W. Blaisdell & D. D. Trunkey [Eds.], *Trauma management series* [Vol. 2]. New York: Thieme Medical Publishers. Reprinted by permission.)

**TABLE 15–3. Etiology of Urethral Injuries**

**Posterior Urethral Injuries**
Fracture of the pelvis
  Motor vehicle accidents
  Fall, crush
  Sporting accidents
Penetrating injuries
  External violence
    Gunshot
    Stab
  Urethral instrumentation
    Resectoscope
    Sounds
    Filiforms, followers
Lateral pelvic blow

**Anterior Urethral Injuries**
Straddle injury
  Fall
  Fence, ladder
  Kick
  Bicycle
Penetrating injury
  Gunshot
  Machine injury
  Knife wound
Urethral instrumentation
  Catheter
  Cystoscope
  Sounds
  Filiforms, followers
  Self-instrumentation
Penile surgery
  Prosthesis placement,
    erosion
  Circumcision
Sexual intercourse
  Urethral laceration
  Fracture of the penis

common causes of anterior urethral injuries include damage from urethral instrumentation, such as inflation of a Foley catheter balloon in the bulbous urethra and from the insertion of foreign bodies into the urethra for erotic stimulation (Corriere, 1987a; Hanno & Wein, 1984; Peters & Sagalowsky, 1986). Table 15–3 lists the many possible causes of urethral trauma.

**Pathophysiology.** Posterior urethral injuries usually occur as a result of the shearing force of pelvic fracture. The prostate and its ligaments are pulled in one direction while the membranous urethra is pulled in the other. The result is a partial or complete urethral disruption. The collection of blood and urine at the site of a complete posterior urethral disruption causes the bladder and prostate to be superiorly displaced (Fig. 15–7). When the puboprostatic ligaments remain uninjured, the degree of displacement is minimal, despite a complete urethral rupture. Partial disruptions usually do

not cause prostatic displacement (McAninch, 1985).

Patients with posterior urethral injuries usually exhibit a classic triad of symptoms along with a history suggestive of such an injury. Blood at the urinary meatus, an inability to void, and a distended bladder are together indicative of a posterior urethral injury. Evidence of a pelvic fracture is usually present. If the prostate and bladder have become superiorly displaced, rectal examination by the physician will note the absence of the prostate, with only a "boggy mass" being felt. No external evidence of bleeding—other than at the urinary meatus—will be present as blood will collect as a pelvic hematoma above the urogenital diaphragm (Hanno, 1987; McAninch, 1985; Peters & Sagalowsky, 1986).

Anterior urethral injuries often result from the external force of a straddle-type injury or any type of blunt trauma to the perineum. The urethra is penetrated and crushed, most often deep in the perineum where the urethra is relatively fixed in position (McAninch, 1985). As

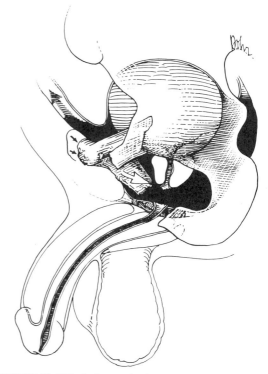

*FIGURE 15–7* Posterior urethral rupture with superior displacement of the bladder and prostate. (From McAninch, J. W. [1985]. Urogenital trauma. In R. W. Blaisdell & D. D. Trunkey [Eds.], *Trauma management series* [Vol. 2]. New York: Thieme Medical Publishers. Reprinted by permission.)

with posterior injuries, the urethra may be partially or completely disrupted. When this type of injury occurs in the bulbous urethra, blood and urine collect along fascial planes and hematoma is evident. If Buck's fascia is intact, blood and urine collect along the penile sheath. If Buck's fascia is disrupted, bleeding and extravasation collect along Colles' fascia involving the scrotum and, eventually, the abdominal wall. A butterfly-shaped hematoma (Fig. 15–8) is characteristic of bleeding along Colles' fascia.

Penetrating injuries of the anterior urethra may involve either the bulbous or the pendulous urethra. The urethra may be penetrated from within during endoscopic urethral manipulation, by a Foley catheter balloon inflated in the urethra, or by sharp objects inserted into the urethra. Penetrating missiles, such as gunshot or stab wounds, may penetrate the urethra from outside the penis.

Depending on the severity of the urethral injury, the patient may or may not be able to void. If the patient is able, urine will extravasate through the injured area. Perineal hematoma or contusion and penile hematoma and edema are frequently evident. Bleeding from the urethral meatus is also frequently present. The penis and perineal area will be tender. When the pendulous urethra is involved, a fluid-filled mass is palpable along the penis. Infection is a possibility, especially when self-inflicted injuries are not reported for several days.

**Medical-Surgical Management.** In both anterior and posterior urethral injuries, blood at the urinary meatus should alert the trauma team to the possibility of urethral injury. Despite the need for monitoring of urinary output in the multiple trauma patient, urethral catheterization should not be attempted until urethral continuity is confirmed. When radiologic equipment is available in the trauma bay or emergency department, a retrograde urethrogram can be quickly and easily performed. Stable patients should be taken to the radiographic suite if necessary. Unstable patients may require a method of supravesical urinary diversion. Any attempt to catheterize an injured urethra may convert a partial disruption into a complete one or may infect a previously sterile hematoma (Corriere, 1987a).

A retrograde urethrogram is performed by injecting 15 to 25 mL of contrast material into the urethra, usually through a Foley catheter that has been inserted 2 to 3 cm into the urethral meatus. Fluoroscopic monitoring during the injection of contrast material shows extravasation (if present). If no extravasation is found, the catheter can be advanced into the bladder. Diagnosis of the type and severity of urethral injury present is based primarily on the results of the retrograde urethrogram.

When a posterior urethral injury is found on x-ray studies, rectal examination may reveal an absence of the prostate if superior displacement has occurred.

Surgical repair is approached in one of two ways when posterior urethral injury exists: immediate repair and delayed repair with suprapubic cystotomy. Some urologists prefer to repair the posterior urethra immediately, particularly when other injuries necessitate surgery. After placement of a suprapubic catheter, the urethra is realigned using interlocking

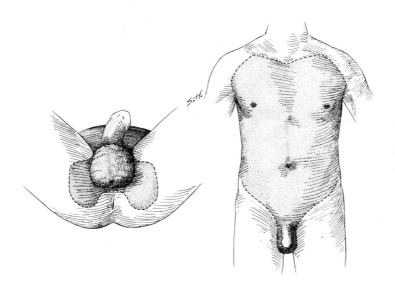

*FIGURE 15–8* Areas of potential urine extravasation extending along Colles' fascial attachments in anterior urethral injury. (From Peters, P. C., & Sagalowsky, A. I. [1986]. Genitourinary trauma. In P. C. Walsh, R. E. Gittes, A. D. Perlmutter, & T. A. Stamey [Eds.], *Campbell's urology* [Vol. 1, 5th ed., p. 1212]. Philadelphia: W. B. Saunders. Reprinted by permission.)

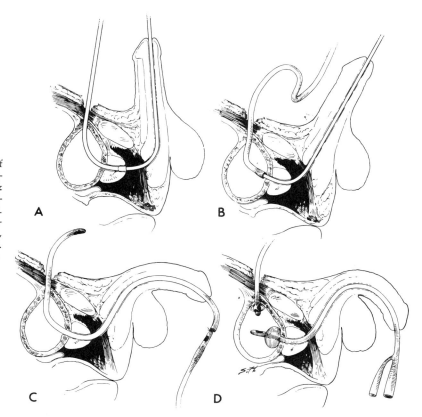

*FIGURE 15–9* Sequential method of urethral realignment with interlocking sounds. (From Peters, P. C., & Sagalowsky, A. I. [1986]. Genitourinary trauma. In P. C. Walsh, R. E. Gittes, A. D. Perlmutter, & T. A. Stamey [Eds.], *Campbell's urology* [Vol. 1, 5th ed., p. 1224]. Philadelphia: W. B. Saunders. Reprinted by permission.)

sounds or catheters (Fig. 15–9). In this manner, the continuity of the urethra is re-established. Traction is used to reapproximate the edges of the ruptured urethra. Some clinicians place traction on the urethral catheter; others place perineal traction sutures through the bladder neck (Corriere, 1987a; Hanno & Wein, 1984; Peters & Sagalowsky, 1986).

Delayed surgical repair is more often the procedure favored for almost all patients with posterior urethral injuries. Evidence now exists that this method carries a lower risk of the long-term complications of impotence, incontinence, and urethral strictures (Corriere, 1987a).

Delayed surgical repair involves placing a suprapubic cystotomy tube at the time of the injury, then doing nothing more for 3 to 9 months. Among the advantages to this approach is the natural resolution of hematoma, with the prostate and bladder gradually resuming their natural anatomic positions. Also, the posterior urethra heals during the 3- to 9-month interim period; however, a stricture will almost certainly develop. The delayed repair actually involves surgical intervention for the resulting stricture. Several methods are used for this purpose, including urethral reconstruc-

tion with a transpubic urethroplasty, or several variations on the classic Johanson two-stage urethroplasty (Fig. 15–10).

After the delayed repair is completed, urethral catheterization with an indwelling Silastic Foley catheter is maintained for up to 1 month. Long-term complications include recurrent urethral stricture, impotence (in approximately 10%), and incontinence.

Anterior urethral injuries are treated in much the same manner as posterior injuries. When complete disruption is present, a suprapubic cystotomy is put in place, and the injured area is allowed to heal for 4 to 6 months. With healing, the urethra becomes scarred and stricture formation occurs. The stricture is later repaired with urethroplasty.

What follows is a description of the general procedure for a two-stage urethroplasty. This surgical procedure is the same as that used for urethral stricture, and, in fact, the same scenario prompts its use after healing of a urethral injury. Urethroplasty is used for strictures of either the anterior or posterior urethra; however, its description here highlights repair of the anterior urethra.

Following the 4- to 6-month interim period

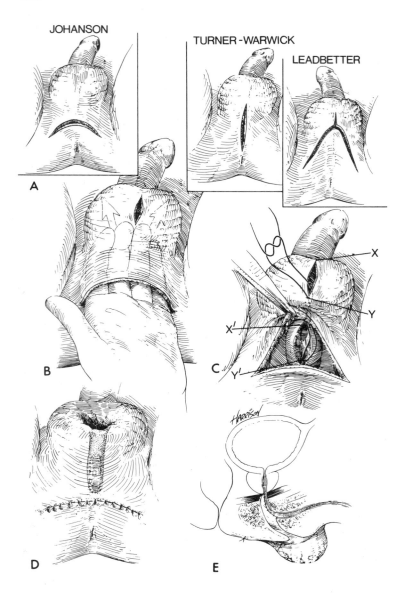

**JOHANSON**

**TURNER-WARWICK**

**LEADBETTER**

A

B

C

D

E

*FIGURE 15–10* Johanson urethroplasty, first stage for posterior urethral repair. *A*, Skin incision (*inset* shows alternative incisions). *B*, Mobilization of scrotal flap. *C*, Edge of scrotal skin approximated to urethral mucosa ($X^1$ to X; $Y^1$ to Y). *D*, Finished inlay. *E*, Cross-sectional view. (From Peters, P. C., & Bright, T. C. [1976]. Management of trauma to the urinary tract. *Advances in Surgery, 10,* 232. Reprinted by permission.)

postinjury, the patient is evaluated by a combined cystogram–retrograde urethrogram to confirm an intact bladder and to delineate the urethral defect. Some physicians order urodynamic testing, particularly a cystometrogram to evaluate bladder function preoperatively (Corriere, 1987a).

At surgery, the urethra is incised vertically at the area of the stricture. The edges of the skin incision are then sutured to the edges of the incised urethra after removal of excess scar tissue. The wound is then left open. This first-stage technique essentially marsupializes the strictured urethra (Corriere, 1987a) (Fig. 15–11). The tissue gradually heals and softens, making it more pliable. Another three-month

period is allowed for the first stage to heal. The second stage involves closure of the wound, the urethra, then the periurethral tissue, and finally, the skin (Fig. 15–12). A Silastic Foley catheter is placed as a stent and left in place for 2 to 4 weeks. The catheter is removed after a voiding cystourethrogram confirms urethral continuity.

Other surgical interventions for strictures resulting from urethral injury include (1) one-stage urethroplasty using urethral intussusception, (2) one-stage repair using end-to-end prostatourethral anastomosis, (3) transpubic urethroplasty, (4) patch-graft urethroplasty, and (5) endoscopic re-establishment of urethral continuity.

Long-term complications of surgery to repair the injured urethra by immediate repair include a high incidence of urethral strictures, impotence, and incontinence. The incidence rates of these complications are lower with delayed repair; however, stricture formation is a certainty, and impotence and incontinence remain a possibility. Impotence may take more than a year to resolve after injury. Additionally, patients must learn to live with an indwelling suprapubic catheter for many months, as well as with the potential complications of long-term catheterization.

## APPROACHES TO PATIENT CARE

### Assessment

Any available information about the mechanism behind the patient's injury as well as his overall status should be obtained first (see Table 15–1). Patients with severe posterior urethral injury may experience significant blood loss because of pelvic hematoma and may present in shock. Orthopedic injuries often accompany posterior urethral trauma and are more evident in the trauma bay.

Nursing assessment of the unstable patient includes participation as a member of the trauma team in efforts to hemodynamically stabilize the patient. The external genitalia should

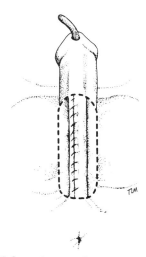

FIGURE 15–12 Second stage of a two-stage urethroplasty for anterior urethral stricture. (From Corriere, J. N. [1987a]. Trauma to the lower third of the urinary tract. In J. Y. Gillenwater, J. T. Grayhack, S. S. Howards, & J. W. Duckett [Eds.], *Adult and pediatric urology* [p. 457]. Chicago: Year Book Medical Publishers. Reprinted by permission.)

be inspected for any obvious injury and for the presence of blood at the urethral meatus. If the patient is conscious, determine if he has voided or feels as though his bladder is full but is unable to void. A rectal examination by the physician, which reveals an absent or displaced prostate, should alert the team to posterior urethral injury. At this point, a retrograde urethrogram should confirm the diagnosis, and a suprapubic catheter is placed to facilitate urine drainage. Further urologic assessment is usually deferred while hemodynamic stability is restored and the pelvic fracture is treated, along with other injuries.

Patients with incomplete disruptions of the posterior urethra may exhibit similar symptoms but may have actually voided. Some urine traverses the urethra, and gross hematuria is present. Some urine extravasates into the pelvis. In some cases of pelvic fracture, the posterior urethra is compressed by pelvic hematoma, making it difficult or impossible to void. Retrograde urethrogram confirms an intact urethra, and a Foley catheter may then be placed to allow urine drainage.

Anterior urethral injuries are often more evident to inspection. The penis may be ecchymotic and edematous, as may the scrotum. Assessment of the perineal area and lower abdominal wall may reveal hematoma and edema along Colles' fascial attachments. The area, particularly the penis, is quite painful. When urethral perforation has been caused by

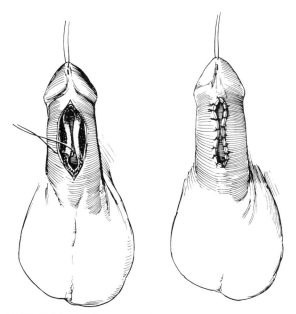

FIGURE 15–11 Johanson urethroplasty, first stage for anterior urethral stricture. (From Hinman, F., Jr. [1989]. *Atlas of urologic surgery* [p. 177]. Philadelphia: W. B. Saunders. Reprinted by permission.)

the placement of a foreign body into the urethra, it is important to determine how much time has passed since the incident. Local infection may already be present, causing marked inflammation and discomfort. Hematuria is often present along with bacteriuria and numerous white blood cells, making the urine appear cloudy. Vital signs should be monitored for temperature evaluation and, in the acute postinjury phase, signs of blood loss.

**Nursing Diagnosis**

The nursing diagnoses for the patient with urethral trauma may include the following:

1. Fluid volume deficit: actual, related to blood loss and hematoma formation.
2. Alteration in pattern of urinary elimination related to urethral disruption.
3. Alteration in comfort: pain related to traumatic injury.
4. Anxiety and fear related to uncertain outcome and loss of control.

**Plan of Care**

Nursing care is directed toward enabling the patient to

1. Be restored to hemodynamic stability.
2. Receive treatment for accompanying orthopedic injuries or lower abdominal injuries.
3. Adapt to suprapubic urinary drainage, if necessary.
4. Eventually resume normal voiding patterns.
5. Obtain relief of pain through analgesic medication.
6. Become knowledgeable about the injury he sustained and the rationale for treatment.
7. Participate in decision making about his care.
8. Verbalize an understanding of his prognosis and the likelihood of recurrent urethral strictures.

**Intervention**

During the initial evaluation of injury phase, nursing interventions are directed toward stabilizing the patient in cooperation with the trauma team. Monitor vital signs continuously, and administer intravenous fluids and blood products as needed. Monitor the patient's state of consciousness, and perform neurologic checks frequently. Respiratory status must also be monitored when multiple trauma exists.

After stabilization has been achieved, nursing interventions specific to urethral trauma are appropriate. Look at the urinary meatus. Is blood present? If so, an important nursing intervention is to avoid inserting a Foley catheter.

Once diagnosed, nursing interventions for the urethral trauma patient include maintaining the patency of urinary catheters and protecting closed drainage systems. Monitor intake and output at least every 8 hours. Assess for signs of urinary tract infection. Promote patient comfort by administering analgesic medication and suppositories for bladder spasms, if present. Administer and monitor intravenous fluids, encourage oral fluid intake, or both.

In the stable patient with urethral injury, fear and anxiety are likely to be understandably high. Discomfort is great, as may be the patient's embarrassment over an injury to the genitalia. Fear of loss of penile function is certainly real. Provide the patient with as much privacy as is possible, and keep him informed at all times.

Patients who will undergo delayed repair must be taught to care for their suprapubic catheter. This includes daily dressing changes, changing from leg bag to bedside drainage at night, the mechanics of emptying both systems, hygienic and antiseptic measures to inhibit bacteria growth, and learning the signs and symptoms of urinary tract infection. Some patients may take prophylactic antibiotics and should learn the dosage and side effects of these drugs. Likewise, some patients may require antispasmodic medication. Learning to irrigate retention catheters may be necessary for some patients whose catheters frequently become occluded. All patients should know what to do in the event of an occluded catheter.

Patients who have undergone the first stage of a two-stage urethroplasty procedure must also learn to care for their penile or scrotal wound. This usually involves dressing changes and efforts to promote healing and prevent bacterial growth. A variety of dressings may be used; however, eventually the area is left open to air. Any dressing that may become incorporated into the wound should not be used.

Following a second-stage urethroplasty (or immediate repair), an indwelling urethral catheter is usually present, and the patient must learn to care for it. The suprapubic sinus (after the suprapubic catheter is removed) heals and seals off over a period of several days, often depending on how long it was in place. Nursing interventions to protect lower abdominal skin from maceration (such as moisture barrier ointments, dressing changes, or, in dire cases, pouching) are needed until the sinus seals itself off.

**Patient Outcomes**

1. The patient is restored to hemodynamic stability.

2. The patient is relieved of pain.

3. The patient's urine remains sterile.

4. The patient verbalizes an understanding of the type of injury he sustained and the treatment being provided.

5. The patient and family learn to care for the indwelling suprapubic catheter, if present.

6. The patient verbalizes measures to remain free of urinary tract infection.

7. The patient and family demonstrate the ability to perform dressing changes when necessary.

8. The patient's fears and anxieties are decreased by an increased knowledge of his prognosis and his potential for later complications.

# MALE GENITAL INJURIES

## PERSPECTIVE ON DISEASE ENTITY

**Etiology.** Any number of blunt or penetrating injuries can traumatize the male genitalia. Although the penis and scrotum are normally well protected by their anatomic location, they are highly mobile external organs subject to injury from external forces. Such injuries can be devastating by virtue of the great vascularity of these organs, with the potential for severe blood loss, and by virtue of the implications of permanent loss of function.

Throughout this section, the following categories of external genital trauma will be used: (1) nonpenetrating (blunt, contusions, fractures), (2) penetrating, (3) avulsions, (4) burns, and (5) radiation injuries. The overall incidence of any of these categories of injuries is relatively low. Although all genitourinary trauma accounts for only 2% to 3% of admissions to a large trauma center, male genital trauma accounts for approximately one fifth of that 2% to 3% (Atkins, 1988; Charles & Hanno, 1987).

**Pathophysiology.** Nonpenetrating genital injuries result from the application of a sudden force to the scrotum or the penis. Often this force is crushing in nature. Underlying structures are ruptured or fractured. Superficial skin may or may not be intact. Examples of nonpenetrating injuries from blunt trauma include bruises, contusions, penile fractures, and crush injuries. Straddle-type injuries also fall into this category (see the section on urethral trauma).

*Penile fracture* refers to a rupture of the tunica albuginea, which surrounds and covers the corpora cavernosa. A loud snap is felt and heard at the time of injury, with rapid onset of pain

and edema. Penile fracture often occurs during rigorous intercourse, from an abnormal bending of the erect organ during sleep (rolling over onto the penis), or from a direct blow to the erect penis. If Buck's fascia is disrupted, hematoma will expand beyond the penile shaft along Colles' fascial attachments (see Fig. 15–8) (Atkins, 1988; Jordan & Gilbert, 1985).

Another type of nonpenetrating penile injury occurs when the distal end of the penis is strangulated by an object placed around it. Among the offending objects that may cause significant necrosis and damage are erroneously applied condom catheters, a piece of string or thread, or metal rings or bands placed for erotic purposes (Fig. 15–13).

Scrotal trauma due to crushing or straddle-type injuries can cause varying degrees of injury. Contusions of the scrotum are often conservatively managed. More severe trauma may cause rupture of the testicles and tubules with significant hematoma formation as well as complete posterior urethral disruption.

Penetrating injuries usually involve gunshot or knife wounds. This category of genital trauma also includes those unfortunate cases of attempts at self-emasculation or penile (and scrotal) amputation. Bullets and knives may traverse and damage the scrotal contents and the penis. Amputation attempts may be partially or totally successful.

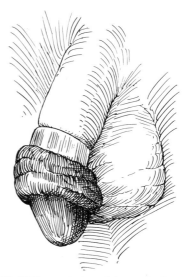

*FIGURE 15–13* Strangulation of the penis due to constricting band. (From Peters, P. C., & Sagalowsky, A. I. [1986]. Genitourinary trauma. In P. C. Walsh, R. E. Gittes, A. D. Perlmutter, & T. A. Stamey [Eds.], *Campbell's urology* [Vol. 1, 5th ed., p. 1237]. Philadelphia: W. B. Saunders. Reprinted by permission.)

Avulsion injuries, or "power take-off" injuries, occur when the patient's clothing and genital skin become trapped in some kind of rotating machinery. This can occur with automobile, farming, or industrial machinery. Avulsion injuries usually tear the skin away from the penis and scrotum, usually just superficial to Buck's fascia in the penis and just beneath the dartos fascia of the scrotum (Atkins, 1988). More severe avulsion injuries may include total or partial amputation of the penis, testicles, or both. The condition of the amputated organs usually prevents replantation.

Burns of the external genitalia can occur in the same manner as any burn. The urethra may or may not be involved. Chemical burns usually involve only the skin. Electrical burns cause damage along the route of the electrical current. An entrance and exit site can often be identified in the electrical burns, with significant damage and necrosis in between. When necrosis is extensive, partial or total amputation may be necessary.

Radiation injuries to the genitalia are unusual when radiation exposure has taken place in a therapeutic setting. The genital area is routinely shielded when radiation is delivered to any area of the body. It is rare to encounter a disorder that requires direct delivery of radiation therapy to the genitalia. Malignant lesions on the skin of the penis may be treated with radiation if partial penectomy is refused. Chronic lymphedema of the genitalia is the most common result, occasionally requiring excision of edematous tissue (Jordan & Gilbert, 1985).

**Medical-Surgical Management.** When penile and scrotal injury have occurred, hemorrhage must be immediately controlled by direct compression, pressure dressings, or occlusion of arteries at pressure points in the groin. During transport, moist saline dressings are applied (Atkins, 1988). Once the patient is in the trauma bay or emergency department, the extent of injury is evaluated. A retrograde urethrogram is done to rule out urethral injury. If the urethra is uninjured, a Foley catheter is placed. Scrotal injury is often evaluated by sonogram. Plain films identify foreign objects or soft tissue masses. Blood studies are important, especially when massive bleeding has occurred, or when several days have passed since the injury and infection is likely.

Penile fracture may be managed conservatively or surgically. Conservative treatment includes catheterization, compression dressings, ice packs, antibiotics, and thrombolytic ther-

apy, ranging from aspirin to streptokinase. Jordan and Gilbert (1985) advocate a surgical approach, stating that the incidence of chordee is lower. Surgical intervention evacuates the hematoma and repairs the disrupted tunica albuginea. Surgery is usually performed when urethral rupture occurs along with penile fracture. An end-to-end urethral reanastomosis is performed with a Foley catheter placed as a stent for 10 to 14 days.

Bruises and contusions of the penis are managed conservatively with rest, cold packs, analgesia, and scrotal elevation. Minor scrotal contusions are treated similarly. When fracture of the testicle is suspected, scrotal exploration is usually performed to evacuate hematoma, débride damage to the tubules, and repair the testes.

Strangulation of the penis can result in ischemia, necrosis, and gangrene. The object causing strangulation must be removed immediately. When edema distal to the object is severe and the object is metal (or made of another inflexible substance), general anesthesia and metal-cutting tools must be used. Treatment of the distal penis depends on the amount of necrosis. Most cases are treated only conservatively. Débridement of necrotic tissue is occasionally necessary.

Penetrating injuries to the penis are treated in a manner similar to penetrating trauma elsewhere in the body. The same is true for penetrating scrotal injuries. A retrograde urethrogram is performed, and the appropriate methods of urinary catheterization instituted, after which the wound is surgically cleaned and débrided, hemostasis is achieved, damage is repaired, and, finally, the wound is closed. Antibiotics are often used postoperatively for prophylaxis, and urinary catheterization is maintained until healing occurs (Atkins, 1988; Hanno & Wein, 1984). When the urethra is involved and repair is performed, subsequent urethral stricture is almost a certainty, and later urethroplasty techniques will be needed.

Management of the amputated penis is best accomplished through microneurovascular replantation surgery. When this technology is not available, the amputated section of the penis may still be attached through surgical reanastomosis of the major blood vessels, corporal bodies, and urethra. Long-term results with this method are favorable, with survival of the corporal bodies and the spongy erectile tissue of the glans (Jordan & Gilbert, 1989).

Microneurovascular replantation was first performed successfully in 1976. Currently used

surgical techniques involve débridement, urethral reanastomosis, then reapproximation of
the erectile tissue, the tunica albuginea, and the
corpora cavernosa. Arteries, veins, and nerves
are then reanastomosed. Finally, the dartos fascia and the skin are closed. The urethra is
stented with a Silastic Foley catheter, and a
suprapubic cystotomy catheter is placed. The
patient must be kept warm and well hydrated;
bed rest is necessary for about 1 week. Doppler
ultrasonography is used to monitor blood flow
(Jordan & Gilbert, 1989).

Avulsion injuries to the external genitalia require immediate surgical intervention. During
transport to the trauma center, moist saline
dressings can be applied to the area. Pain relief
is immediately necessary, and antibiotics are
started expeditiously. Tetanus and gas gangrene antitoxin should be given (Hanno &
Wein, 1984). When penile and scrotal skin is
torn away, but the organs remain relatively intact, surgical repair consists of replacing the
skin. Scrotal tissue regenerates itself; if sufficient skin remains to cover the testicles, it
should be used. Eighty percent or more of the
scrotal skin must be absent to require alternate
methods of closing the scrotum. When this is
the case, the testes are salvaged by surgically
implanting them into subcutaneous thigh
pouches created in both thighs (Fig. 15–14).
This protects the testes and envelops them in
an environment with a temperature similar to
that of the scrotum, allowing spermatogenesis
to continue. Four to 6 weeks are allowed to
pass so that scrotal regeneration can take place.
Reconstruction of the scrotum with replacement of the testes is then performed.

Skin torn away from the penis is replaced
with split-thickness skin grafts. Skin distal to
the avulsion, but below the corona, must also
be excised and replaced with the grafts. If this
is not done, distal lymphedema of the penis
will ensue.

Burns to the external genitalia are treated in
the same manner as burns to any bodily area.
Antibiotic creams and a continuing process of
débridement and skin grafts are used. Urinary
catheterization is necessary to quantify fluid resuscitation and is achieved either through
Foley catheterization or suprapubic cystotomy
(if the urethra is damaged). Urethral injury is
repaired later.

## APPROACHES TO PATIENT CARE

### Assessment

Obtain as much information as is possible

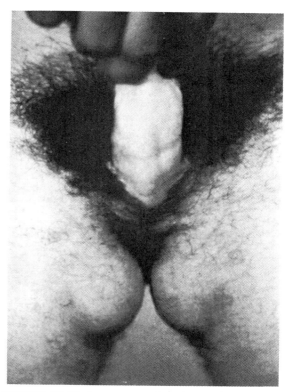

FIGURE 15–14 Appearance of patient with testes im-
planted into subcutaneous thigh pouches. (From Peters, P.
C., & Sagalowsky, A. I. [1986]. Genitourinary trauma. In P.
C. Walsh, R. E. Gittes, A. D. Perlmutter, & T. A. Stamey
[Eds.], *Campbell's urology* [Vol. 1, 5th ed., p. 1242]. Philadel-
phia: W. B. Saunders. Reprinted by permission.)

about the mechanism of injury (see Table 15–
1). Although it may be obvious that some genital injuries have just occurred, others may
have occurred several days before the patient
seeks medical attention. Embarrassment may
make it difficult for the patient to describe exactly what happened; however, accurate information is essential, and the patient should be
encouraged to tell his story.

When serious genital injury has occurred, assessment of the severity of bleeding or hemorrhage is the first priority. Inspection of the genitalia should include noting the presence of
edema and ecchymosis. Look for hematoma
and edema along fascial planes. Determine if
the patient has been able to void. If not, are
there signs and symptoms of bladder distention? If a significant amount of time has passed
since the injury occurred, are there symptoms
of systemic or localized infection? Are any foreign bodies or constricting devices obvious?
When the injury involves penetrating objects or

foreign bodies, the likelihood of contamination is increased (Atkins, 1988).

Fear and anxiety are likely to be major factors in the patient's initial reaction to his injury. The implications of penile and scrotal injuries are profound and may be just as frightening as pain and blood loss. Assessment of the patient's anxiety level is necessary in planning care for patients with genital injuries.

Assessment of patients with penetrating or avulsion injuries also includes inspecting the condition of totally or partially amputated parts, assisting in the determination of amounts of viable skin remaining, assisting with initial attempts at débridement, and achieving hemostasis. Assessing the likelihood of urethral injury is necessary before urinary catheterization is performed.

Burn victims often have burns affecting other bodily areas as well as the genitalia. Initial assessment of fluid status takes priority and is followed by burn treatment. Burn victims are usually stabilized, then transferred (if necessary) to a medical center that specializes in burn treatment.

**Nursing Diagnosis**

The nursing diagnosis for the male patient with genital injuries may include the following:

1. Fluid volume deficit: potential, related to blood loss and hematoma formation.
2. Alteration in comfort: pain related to traumatic injury.
3. Anxiety and fear related to traumatic injury and potential loss of genital function.

**Plan of Care**

Nursing care is directed toward enabling the patient to

1. Achieve hemostasis through control of blood loss and replacement of fluids.
2. Have the option of replantation surgery through proper handling of partially or totally amputated parts.
3. Obtain relief of pain through analgesic medication.
4. Reduce anxiety regarding the extent of his injury, the purpose of diagnostic tests, and the prognosis for recovery of organ function.
5. Participate in decision making about his care (when appropriate).

**Intervention**

When the patient's injury has just occurred and involves significant blood loss, initial nursing interventions must be directed toward achievement of hemostasis. Application of direct pressure and moist saline compression

dressings may be needed. Amputated parts should be kept wrapped in a moist, sterile gauze inside a plastic bag or basin, which should then be placed in an ice bath (Atkins, 1988). Ice should never be allowed to come directly in contact with the amputated part.

Other nursing interventions immediately following severe genital injury may include administering analgesic and antianxiety medications, assisting in the removal of foreign bodies, administering intravenous fluids and blood products, giving tetanus and gas gangrene antitoxins, monitoring vital signs, and preparing the patient for surgery.

For patients with minor nonpenetrating or less severe penetrating genital injuries, nursing interventions are often directed toward pain relief and conservative treatment measures. The patient with a penile fracture or scrotal injury may simply require cold packs, scrotal elevation, and lots of reassurance, or may be prepared for surgery to evacuate the hematoma and evaluate and repair tissue damage. Postoperatively, these patients require continued scrotal elevation, antibiotic therapy, care of their incision and any drains placed during surgery, along with routine postoperative care. Quantify urine output during the postoperative period—initially, the patient will have a Foley or suprapubic cystostomy catheter but may be allowed to void before discharge.

Postoperative nursing care of patients after penile microneurovascular replantation surgery includes frequent inspection of the replanted part, evaluating for color, temperature, and any evidence of infection or necrosis. Also required are maintenance of urethral or suprapubic catheters, administration of antibiotics, local incisional care, penile-scrotal elevation, and administration of analgesics. When the patient has attempted self-emasculation, a psychological or substance abuse problem is likely to be present. Interventions that prevent the patient from handling or disrupting the replanted part may be necessary. Psychological experts should be consulted to assist with the planning of nursing care, and the patient's privacy should be respected and guarded.

When caring for patients being treated for genital injuries, it is important to approach the patient in a professional manner. Any feelings of embarrassment on the part of the nurse are quickly detected by the patient and may undermine the plan of care. These patients need to understand the extent of their injuries and the reasons for treatments or surgeries; they need to have their questions answered and be treated with respect and dignity, regardless of the cause of their injury.

**Patient Outcomes**

1. The patient is restored to hemostasis.
2. The patient's totally or partially amputated genital parts are handled to allow for replantation surgery if possible.
3. The patient is relieved of pain.
4. The patient is free of infection.
5. The patient expresses a lessening sense of fear and anxiety after receiving information and reassurance.

## *REFERENCES*

American College of Surgeons, Committee on Trauma. (1990). *Resources for optimal care of the injured patient.* Chicago: Author.

Atkins, J. (1988). External genital trauma. In E. Howell, L. Widea, & M. G. Hill (Eds.), *Comprehensive trauma nursing: Theory and practice.* Glenview, IL: Scott, Foresman.

Blaisdell, F. W. (1982). General assessment, resuscitation and exploration of penetrating and blunt abdominal trauma. In F. W. Blaisdell & D. D. Trunkey (Eds.), *Trauma management: Abdominal trauma* (Vol. 1, pp 1–7). New York: Thieme-Stratton.

Carroll, P. R., & McAninch, J. W. (1989). Staging of renal trauma. *Urologic Clinics of North America, 16*(2), 193–201.

Charles, R. S., & Hanno, P. M. (1987). Upper urinary tract trauma. In P. M. Hanno & A. J. Wein (Eds.), *A clinical manual of urology* (pp. 189–206). Norwalk: Appleton-Century-Crofts.

Corriere, J. N. (1987a). Trauma to the lower urinary tract. In J. Y. Gillenwater, J. T. Grayhack, S. S. Howards, & J. W. Duckett (Eds.), *Adult and pediatric urology* (pp. 444–464). Chicago: Year Book Medical Publishers.

Corriere, J. N. (1987b). Ureteral injuries. In J. Y. Gillenwater, J. T. Grayhack, S. S. Howards, & J. W. Duckett (Eds.), *Adult and pediatric urology* (pp. 436–443). Chicago: Year Book Medical Publishers.

Devine, P. C., & Devine, C. J., Jr. (1982). Posterior urethral injuries associated with pelvic fractures. *Urology, 20,* 467–470.

Guerriero, W. G. (1988). Etiology, classification, and management of renal trauma. *Surgical Clinics of North America, 68*(5), 1071–1084.

Hanno, P. M. (1987). Lower urinary tract trauma. In P. M. Hanno & A. J. Wein (Eds.), *A clinical manual of urology* (pp. 207–221). Norwalk: Appleton-Century-Crofts.

Hanno, P. M., & Wein, A. J. (1984). Urologic trauma. *Emergency Medicine Clinics of North America, 2*(4), 823–841.

Hill, M. G. (1988). Intra-abdominal trauma. In E. Howell, L. Widea, & M. G. Hill (Eds.), *Comprehensive trauma nursing: Theory and practice* (pp. 618–678). Glenview: Scott, Foresman.

Jordan G. H., & Gilbert D. A. (1985). Male genital trauma. In *AUA update series* (Vol. 4, No. 20). Houston: American Urological Association.

Jordan, G. H., & Gilbert D. A. (1989). Management of amputation injuries of the male genitalia. *Urologic Clinics of North America, 16*(2), 359–367.

Kozimor, A., Hahn, J., Ambrose, S., & Hill, M. G. (1988). Shock. In E. Howell, L. Widea, & M. G. Hill (Eds.), *Comprehensive trauma nursing: Theory and practice* (pp. 251–293). Glenview: Scott, Foresman.

McAninch, J. W. (1985). Assessment and diagnosis of urinary and genital injuries. In F. W. Blaisdell & D. D. Trunkey (Eds.), *Trauma management: Urogenital trauma* (Vol. 2, pp. 1–26). New York: Thieme.

McAninch, J. W. (1987). Renal injuries. In J. Y. Gillenwater, J. T. Grayhack, S. S. Howards, & J. W. Duckett (Eds.), *Adult and pediatric urology* (pp. 421–435). Chicago: Year Book Medical Publishers.

Nicholaisen, G. S., & McAninch, J. W. (1985). Evaluation and management of traumatic renal injuries. In *AUA update series* (Vol. 4, No. 37). Houston: American Urological Association.

Peters, P. C., & Sagalowsky, A. I. (1986). Genitourinary trauma. In P. C. Walsh, R. E. Gittes, A. D. Perlmutter, & T. A. Stamey (Eds.), *Campbell's urology* (5th ed.). Philadelphia: W. B. Saunders.

Peterson, N. E. (1987). Renal trauma. *Urology grand rounds* (No. 16). Kansas City: Marion Laboratories.

Ross, S. E., Morgan, T., & Schwab, C. W. (1988). The emergent phase. In E. Howell, L. Widea, & M. G. Hill (Eds.), *Comprehensive trauma nursing: Theory and practice* (pp. 367–377). Glenview: Scott, Foresman.

Wagner, M. M. (1990). The patient with abdominal injuries. *Nursing Clinics of North America, 25*(1), 45–55.

Wiegel, J. W. (1982). Bladder and urethral trauma. In *AUA update series* (Vol. 1, No. 38). Houston: American Urological Association.

# PART VII

# The Pediatric Urology Patient

# CHAPTER 16

# Health Assessment of the Pediatric Urology Patient

■

*Christine Hoyler-Grant*

## OVERVIEW

The past 30 years have witnessed the emergence of a distinct specialty in pediatric health care: pediatric urology. Advancements in surgical modalities and equipment, coupled with a proliferation of research highlighting the etiology and progression of congenital urologic disorders, have enhanced the favorable outcome produced by surgical intervention. Sophisticated diagnostic imaging allows for early detection of abnormalities, and a dramatic reduction in anesthesia risk among preterm and newborn infants encourages timely reconstructive procedures, often with minimal manipulation. Staged procedures can begin earlier. It is now common for the pediatric urologist to discuss surgical options with prospective parents when the unborn child's obstructive uropathology has been detected by fetal sonography.

Coinciding with the medical achievements afforded to children with urinary tract disorders have been several trends within the health care delivery system. First, nursing has made major strides toward increased professionalism, responsibility, and in-depth educational preparation. Primary nursing promotes continuity of care but demands accountability. Specialization is not only common but necessary owing to fast-paced technologic growth, the complexity of health care needs, and the integration of age-specific psychosocial and developmental concepts in the nursing process.

A second influence has been the humanization of pediatric health care settings toward children and families. Enlightened hospitals encourage parents to direct and participate in all aspects of their child's care; sibling visitation helps to maintain family contact, and child life departments monitor the adjustment of young patients to their hospital environment and their physical condition. Parents naturally remain reluctant to hospitalize their child, but much of their fear dissipates shortly after admission. Pediatric surgery is no longer the ``last resort'' but often is the preferred treatment.

The present era of cost containment is a response to escalating health care costs, propelled by high-tech medical treatment that has improved the prognosis and longevity of patients with chronic or life-threatening diseases. Pediatric nursing in an ambulatory setting (e.g., school or rehabilitation center, home health agency, or outpatient facility) redirects the approach from curative care to health maintenance. It is no longer enough to plan for the hospital discharge; a quality lifestyle must be ensured. Parents of children with long-term disorders, and eventually the children themselves, must acquire skills to be informed health care consumers.

It is likely that pediatric nurses will care for children diagnosed with urologic abnormalities. Whatever the health care setting, nurses must be well acquainted with urologic anatomy, physiology, and pathophysiology, including signs and symptoms that raise suspicion of a urologic anomaly. After the diagnosis of the child's disorder has been established, the nurse needs to have a knowledge of medical and nursing interventions, a methodology to evaluate the child's urologic status, and a foundation of health education principles.

This chapter provides an outline of pediatric urology. The chapter begins with the definition of pediatric urology and its scope of practice, then outlines the health assessment of a child to identify a urologic disorder. Clinical radiologic and diagnostic testing are presented, followed by health maintenance recommendations that refer specifically to the urologic system. A compendium of reference tables that are useful for the health evaluation of a pediatric urologic patient concludes the chapter.

## BEHAVIORAL OBJECTIVES

After studying this chapter, the reader should be able to

1. Comprehend the scope of pediatric urology.
2. Correlate the child's history, symptoms, and physical signs as manifestations of urologic abnormalities.
3. Acquire the ability to perform a pediatric physical examination to assess urologic disease, including the collection of urine samples and anthropometric measurements.
4. Identify various diagnostic procedures and their applications in urologic evaluation.

## KEY WORDS

**Health assessment**—a process used to determine the child's level of physical, developmental, emotional, and social well-being.

**Physiologic parameters**—measurements that present the normal range of structural and physical function.

## PERSPECTIVES ON PEDIATRIC UROLOGY

### Definition

The practice of pediatric urology, in its broadest sense, is considered to be the specialized assessment, diagnosis, and management of children with disorders that affect the structure and function of the genitourinary tract. Pediatric urology is commonly differentiated from pediatric nephrology by its surgical orientation, as opposed to the medical management of disease states, and, indeed, all pediatric urologists are surgeons. However, there is a frequent overlap in practice between the two specialties. Urologic anomalies that compromise kidney function often require the cooperative collaboration of pediatric urologists and nephrologists for optimum health management.

## Scope of the Specialty

Disease entities that are considered a part of pediatric urology run the gamut from minor anomalies, such as inguinal hernia, hydrocele, and urethral meatal stenosis, to complex disorders, including exstrophy, prune belly syndrome, and the massive obstructive uropathy produced by posterior urethral valves. Urologic ramifications that are concomitant to neurologic disease, such as myelomeningocele and neuromuscular dysfunction, or that are sequelae to pelvic tumors, such as rhabdosarcoma and sacral teratoma, constantly influence the child's delicate balance of health equilibrium and mandate the methodical surveillance of the urinary tract. The highest proportion of referrals to pediatric urologists continues to be for treatment of urinary tract infection and childhood enuresis, those age-old problems that remain elusive to the sophistication of current therapy (Abdel-Haleim, 1986; Kroovand & Perlmutter, 1978; Glicklich, 1951; Rabinowitz, 1982; Tudor et al., 1962). In pediatric health care currently, the most heated controversy rages over the need for routine newborn circumcisions (American Academy of Pediatrics, 1989; American Academy of Pediatrics & American College of Obstetricians and Gynecologists, 1983; Anderson & Smey, 1985; Roberts, 1986; Wallerstein, 1985; Wiswell & Roscelli, 1986; Wiswell et al., 1987).

## Demographic Features

### SEX

Urologic anomalies occur in both males and females, but certain disorders have a distinct sex predisposition. For example, urinary tract infections have a far higher prevalence in females (Barratt, 1974; Belman & Kaplan, 1981; Kunin, 1987; Whaley & Wong, 1992) along with vesicoureteral reflux (Belman & Kaplan, 1981; Berry & Chandler, 1986; Carter, 1984). Structural defects of the genitourinary organs found almost exclusively in males include hypospa-

dias, epispadias, cryptorchidism, inguinal hernia, hydrocele, varicocele, and posterior urethral web or valve. An epidemiologic report by Bois, Feingold, Benmaiz, and Briard (1975) indicates a male ratio of 4:1 for lower urinary tract malformations (bladder exstrophy, megacystic-megaureter, and urethral atresia, stenosis, obstruction, or valves). Ureteropelvic junction obstruction has a 67% prevalence in males compared with females (Kelalis, 1985; Snyder et al., 1980). The incidence of inguinal hernia among males is ninefold the rate among females (Waechter et al., 1985).

### AGE

Pediatric urology encompasses the urologic considerations of children from birth through adolescence. Most children in the care of a pediatric urologist are younger than 7 years of age because (1) pediatric urologic disorders are usually congenital and therefore tend to manifest early in life (Berry & Chantler, 1986); (2) urinary tract infections are common in girls until they reach school age, then decrease dramatically either until puberty or the commencement of sexual activity; (3) the current trend is toward early initiation of reconstructive or corrective surgery (Anderson & Smey, 1985; Walker 1985); and (4) premature infants weighing less than 1200 g have a significantly increased incidence of inguinal hernias, which usually require surgical closure when the infant becomes a good surgical candidate (Harper et al., 1975; Peevy et al., 1986; Walsh, 1962).

## Childhood Morbidity

Although the prevalence of urinary tract disorders has not been determined, urologic morbidity among children is significant. The second most common infection of childhood (and the most frequent urologic disorder) is urinary tract infection (Belman, 1985; Waechter, et al., 1985; Whaley & Wong, 1992). Enuresis affects an estimated 15% to 20% of early school-aged children, gradually reducing in frequency until adolescence; approximately 1% to 3% of the adult population is plagued by enuresis (Meadow, 1970; Perlmutter, 1985; Oppel et al., 1968; Thorne, 1944; Waechter et al., 1985). Abdominal masses that require surgery are likely to have a genitourinary cause. In fact, more than two thirds of abdominal masses detected in neonates are either hydronephrosis or renal cystic dysplasia (Kaplan & Brock, 1985; Parrott

& Woodard, 1976; Wedge et al., 1971). In children between 1 month and 1 year of age, abdominal tumors account for a proportion of detected abdominal masses equal to hydronephrosis (40% each), but after 1 year of age, most masses are neoplasms, often Wilms' tumors (Kasper et al., 1976; Schultz et al., 1963; Slim et al., 1969).

Abnormalities of the external male genitalia can be readily identified and are therefore easily monitored. Studies from the United Kingdom (Matlai & Beral, 1985) documented an increased incidence of hypospadias between 1964 and 1983 and a 10-fold increase in hospital admissions to correct cryptorchidism (Chilvers et al., 1984).

The mention of birth defects may bring to mind such images as children with disabling diseases, Down's syndrome, heart defects, or epilepsy. These conditions are certainly important and receive a large measure of concern and financial support from the public as a result of media exposure and established fundraising sources. It is startling that the incidence of genitourinary anomalies outnumbers the *combined* total incidence of clubfoot, cleft lip, congenital hip dislocation, and all gastrointestinal malformations (Burger & Burger, 1974).

## Etiology of Congenital Urologic Abnormalities

Congenital anomalies of the genitourinary tract develop as single gene disorders, by multifactorial action, from additive effects of genetic plus intrauterine influences, or by unknown or nongenetic etiology.

Single gene disorders may result from autosomal dominant, autosomal recessive, or sex-linked inheritance, following classic mendelian patterns of inheritance. These aberrations result from a mutation of an isolated gene locus. Apparently, many gene loci regulate kidney development, more than any organ except the brain (Berry & Chantler, 1986). Kidney changes in the dysmorphic child are therefore common. Under the influence of a genetic mutation arises a syndrome, "a recurrent pattern of multiple malformations that are pathogenetically related" (Rosenbaum, 1985, p. 38). Table 16–1 provides an overview of multisystemic syndromes with genitourinary components.

Multifactorial transmission expresses the interaction between polygenetic inheritance and the intrauterine environment. Characteristics of multifactorial disorders include (1) familial inheritance, including direct-line relatives (not as prominent as single-gene transmission but greater than random effect); (2) regional and ethnic phenomena of anomalies; and (3) involvement of an isolated organ or body system (Rosenbaum, 1985).

Urologic entities that are suspected of having a multifactorial mode of transmission are presented in Table 16–2. The risk factor for occurrence among siblings is also provided.

Prenatal influences have been discovered to inadvertently affect genitourinary development. Teratogenic sources, diethylstilbestrol, and progestin increase the risk of hypospadias or testicular dysplasia (Rosenbaum, 1985). Excessive intake of alcohol during pregnancy may precipitate fetal alcohol syndrome, characterized by multiple organic anomalies, plus microphallus and hypospadias.

## Organic Malformations With Associated Genitourinary Anomalies

Some organic malformations have a greater than expected incidence of associated genitourinary defects (Bashour & Balfe, 1977; Bourne & Benirschke, 1960; Catterall et al., 1971; Curran & Curran, 1972; Engle, 1981; Hilson, 1957; King, 1969; Newman et al., 1969; Potter, 1946; Varsano et al., 1984; Vitko et al., 1972). This relationship is considered an "association," which differs from a syndrome in the reduced number of multiple anomalies and the lack of pathogenetic causation (Rosenbaum, 1985). Organic defects include congenital heart disease, low-set ears, and skeletal anomalies. Knowledge of associated multisystem anomalies is imperative because of the often covert nature of uropathology.

Numerous researchers have also noted abnormalities of the inner urologic system in association with external structural defects, such as hypospadias and cryptorchidism (Bauer et al., 1979; Campbell & Harrison, 1970; Donohue et al., 1973; Dwoskin, 1983; Farrington & Kerr, 1969; Noble & Wacksman, 1980; Shima et al., 1979). The data presented in Table 16–3 summarize the association between organic anomalies and genitourinary defects.

**TABLE 16–1. Multisystemic Anomalies With Genitourinary Pathologic Changes**

| SYNDROME | CARDIO-VASCULAR | GASTRO-INTESTINAL | NEURO-LOGIC | MUSCULO-SKELETAL | INTEGU-MENT | FACIAL | GENITAL | URINARY |
|---|---|---|---|---|---|---|---|---|
| Prune belly | | Occasional | | Abdominal muscles absent | | | Undescended testicles | Hydronephrosis |
| Curran's | | | | Acral anomalies | | | | Renal agenesis Duplication |
| Turner's Winter's | | | Middle ear abnormalities | | | | Vaginal atresia | Renal anomalies |
| Goyer's | | | Hearing loss | | Ichthyosis | | | Renal disease |
| Neonatal ascites | | Portohepatic obstruction Bowel perforation | | | | | | |
| Turner's female (XO) | | | | Wide chest Cubitus valgus | | Webbed neck | | Renal anomalies (70%) |
| Turner's male (Noonan's) | | | | Wide chest Cubitus valgus | | Webbed neck | Small testicles | Renal anomalies (50%) |
| Caudal regression | | Imperforate anus | | Inversion feet Lumbosacral-spine anomalies | | | Uterine and vaginal agenesis | Renal agenesis |
| Vater | Ventricular septal defect | Imperforate anus Tracheo-esophageal fistula | | Vertebral defects Radial dysplasia Polydactyly Syndactyly | | | | Renal agenesis |
| "G" | | Neuromuscular defect of esophagus | | | | Abnormal fascies Low-set ears | Hypospadias | |
| Smith-Lemil-Opitz | | | Retardation | Syndactyly | | Short upturned nose Microcephaly Epicanthal folds | Hypospadias Cryptorchidism | |
| Donohue's "leprechaunism" | | | | | Hirsutism | Elfin face Prominent eyes Thick lips Low-set ears | Enlarged penis or clitoris | |
| Trisomy 13 | Ventricular and atrial septal defects | Omphalocele | Deafness Retardation | Polydactyly | | Low-set ears | Cryptorchidism | Duplication Hydronephrosis |
| Trisomy 18 | Ventricular septal defect Patent ductus arteriosus | Neonatal hepatitis Tracheoesophageal fistula Malrotation | Retardation Hydrocephalus | | | Low-set ears Choanal atresia Cleft palate | Prominent clitoris Cryptorchidism | Horseshoe kidney Duplication Hydronephrosis |
| Trisomy 21 | Increased cardiac anomalies | Duodenal obstruction | Retardation | Muscle hypotonia | | High arched palate | Small penis Cryptorchidism | Renal dysplasia |

Adapted from Kelalis, P. P., King, L. R., & Belman, A. B. (1985). *Clinical pediatric urology* (2nd ed., pp. 6–7). Philadelphia: W. B. Saunders. Reprinted by permission.

TABLE 16–2. Urogenital Disorders With Multifactorial Transmission

| DISORDER | OCCURRENCE IN GENERAL POPULATION (%) | MALE/FEMALE RATIO | SIBLING OCCURRENCE (%) |
|---|---|---|---|
| Hypospadias | 0.3 | — | 9–14 |
| Renal agenesis | 0.1 | 3:1 | 3–5 |
| Ureteral duplication | 1 | 1:2 | 12 |
| Ureteral pelvic junction obstruction | Unknown | 2:1 | 4 |
| Vesicoureteral reflux | 0.5–1 | 1:7 | 10–60 |
| Cryptorchidism | 1–4 (neonates) | — | 9 |

# STRUCTURE AND FUNCTION OF THE DEVELOPING KIDNEY

## Developmental Physiology of the Kidney

In the fifth week of embryologic growth, the metanephros (precursor of the mature kidney) becomes distinguished from the metanephric blastema. During this phase, which continues for the next 15 weeks, the ureteral bud inverts within the metanephric tissue to create the hollow renal pelvis. Further budding forms major calices, branching progressively to create the minor calices. By the fifth fetal month, collecting tubules and the renal pyramid have appeared as the end structures of the caliceal architecture. Collecting tubules are estimated to number 3 million (Behrman & Kliegman, 1990; McCrory, 1972).

The collecting system and the excretory structures are intimately related, as it is the collecting system that stimulates renal vesicle tissue, present in the metanephric blastema, to develop into Bowman's capsule, the glomerulus, and the nephron unit. Nephron formation follows a centrifugal pattern, with inner cortical structures larger and more mature than those found in the peripheral cortex. Nephrogenesis begins in the seventh embryologic week and continues until 32 to 36 weeks; beyond the 36th week, only nephron maturation occurs. Morphologic changes occur throughout the next 3 years (Fetterman et al., 1965). Each kidney comprises about 1 million nephrons (McCrory, 1972). Kidney size is proportionately greater in the infant and child compared with the adult (Engel, 1988).

## Neonatal Considerations

Clamping of the umbilical cord heralds the functional beginning of the newborn's urologic

TABLE 16–3. Congenital Anomalies and Associated Genitourinary Defects

| ANOMALY | ASSOCIATED GENITOURINARY DEFECT | INCIDENCE OF ASSOCIATION (%) |
|---|---|---|
| **Genitourinary System** | | |
| Cryptorchidism | Upper tract defects, contralateral inguinal hernia | 2–3 |
| Hypospadias | Inguinal hernia, ureteral reflux, upper tract defects | 3–25 |
| **Non–Genitourinary System** | | |
| Congenital heart defects | Hydronephrosis, ureteral duplication Renal agenesis or dysplasia | 7–28 |
| Neonatal spontaneous pneumothorax or pneumomediastinum | Renal anomalies | 19 |
| Scoliosis or kyphosis | Upper tract defects | 33 |
| Femoral avascular necrosis | Upper tract defects | 4 |
| Polydactyly, oligodactyly | Renal agenesis, ureteral duplication | Unknown |
| Imperforate anus | Reflux | 17–38 |
| Supernumerary nipples | Ureteropelvic junction obstruction, bilateral polycystic kidneys, double collecting system | Male: 20–40 Female: 5–10 |
| Facial anomalies, oligohydramnios, hypoplastic lungs (Potter's syndrome) | Renal agenesis or posterior ureteral valves | Male: 31 Female: 10 |
| Low-set ears, malformed ears | Hydronephrosis, renal agenesis, duplication, hypospadias | Unknown |
| Single umbilical artery | Renal defects | Variable |

system. Although urine production starts by the third month after conception, it serves the purpose only of maintaining adequate amniotic fluid levels. Blood cleansing, like oxygenation, is accomplished by placental action. Nephrologic function proceeds at an accelerated rate for the first 2 years of life, then slows to mirror somatic growth rates (Hensle, 1985).

Physiologically, the neonatal renal system undergoes a number of significant metabolic and hematologic changes in its transformation to functional responsiveness after birth. Urine production is quickly established; 90% of neonates void within the first day of life, and 99% do so by 48 hours after delivery (Walker, 1985). The glomerular filtration rate at birth is significantly lower than that in adults (mean rate of 38, compared with 117–130 respectively), owing to increased intrarenal vascular resistance, with subsequent reduction in total renal circulation. This lower rate is coupled with a diminished surface area within the juxtamedullary glomerulus and decreased capillary permeability. These effects are almost completely negated by 12 months of age (Gonzales, 1985).

The excretory units are correspondingly underdeveloped, causing disruptions in proximal tubular reabsorption of amino acids and bicarbonate. Neonates, therefore, are in a normal physiologic state of mild acidosis, with a plasma pH of 7.11 to 7.36 and a base excess of −11 to −2 mmol/L (Waechter et al., 1985). When challenged by illness or other bodily stress, the neonate's ability to excrete excessive hydrogen ions is inadequate, potentiating the acidosis. Likewise, the solute threshold is low, and sodium and water overloads equilibrate slowly (Gonzales, 1985). The newborn's metabolic status is fragile, and conditions that upset this balance require careful attention to fluid and electrolyte management.

The mechanisms that concentrate urine are not well established in the newborn; in fact, concentration ability is compromised for several months owing to limitations in urea excretion. During the first year of life, the specific gravity ranges from 1.001 to 1.015, maintaining the upper limit even in states of dehydration. By the child's 12th month, however, elongation of the loop of Henle allows for normal concentration ability (Engel, 1988; Whaley & Wong, 1992).

Obstructive uropathology affects concentration by pathologically affecting the collecting ducts, yet sparing the glomerular structures, causing fluid build-up. Dehydration of an ill newborn can ensue quickly, because urinary diuresis is not compensated or mediated by a reduction in glomerular filtration. Fluid replacement therapy is geared to limiting the renal solute load rather than replacing with large fluid volumes. Nutritionally, breast milk is especially well suited for the infant born with uropathology because of reduced protein, mineral, and electrolyte levels in the milk (Gonzales, 1985).

## PRESENTATION OF THE CHILD WITH UROLOGIC ANOMALIES

Detection of urologic anomalies among the pediatric population requires the thoughtful, concise interplay of detailed historical data and an expert examination. The urinary tract is a uniquely "hidden" body system; its contents are relatively inaccessible by traditional examination techniques. The physical evaluation, therefore, must focus on indicators of urinary function—voiding pattern and stream, signs of appropriate fluid balance, blood pressure levels, and others. In many instances, a carefully pursued history may be more revealing than the physical examination, making it the cornerstone of the health assessment process.

The examiner must remain cognizant that the intertwining of the urinary tract and the genital system is fraught with psychosexual undertones that may adversely influence the history-giving process. A professional attitude, coupled with a nonjudgmental questioning style and careful choices of words, is imperative to collecting a complete and accurate history.

The following sections focus on the urologic-oriented health assessment, a condensed version of the traditional comprehensive physical evaluation. For supplemental reference materials, the reader is directed to standard pediatric nursing textbooks listed in the Additional Readings section at the end of this chapter.

### Urologic Health History

1. *Chief complaint*—an inquiry to ascertain the reason for the child's visit. The information may be presented in the form of symptoms (e.g., "frequent urination") or as a diagnosis (e.g., "I think she has a urinary tract infection"). Note who the historian is and whether this person is the child's primary caretaker; also note the historian's demeanor, communication flow, and consis-

tency in presenting "the child's story." If the child is able to verbalize, he or she should be asked the reason for the health visit. Not only is this interaction useful for assessing the child's receptive and expressive cognition, it exposes any misconceptions or fears held by the child concerning this visit. Steps may then be taken to allay anxiety and clarify the child's understanding of his or her symptoms. Additional information about the chief complaint includes the duration, intensity, and frequency of symptoms, plus associated complaints. Keep in mind that the stated complaint may be a pretense for the underlying concern. For example, a parent may cite enuresis as a problem, when in actuality the real apprehension relates to normalcy of the child's genitalia. Determine the site of the child's primary health care.

2. *Child and family profile*—this section of the health history gathers information about the family unit and the child's lifestyle. The parents' marital and employment status are noted, plus who provides the primary caretaking responsibilities for the child. Does the child attend a day care setting? If the child is of school age, what grade is the child in and how is he or she doing? List other siblings and their ages, plus any other household members. Finally, inquire about the family's financial status and housing arrangement.

3. *History of present illness*—the nurse should initially elicit this information by asking when the child was last well or when the symptom or problem first started. The parent should then be directed to advance through the progression of additional signs and symptoms, constitutional responses, involvement of other systems, treatment recommended by primary care providers, and the child's response to actual treatment given. Symptoms that may be indicators of urologic disease include
   a. Infants and toddlers (0–3 years)—poor growth or weight gain, persistent or intermittent fevers, convulsions, fussiness, poor sleeping pattern, chronic anemia, persistent diaper rash, infrequent voiding (fewer than five times a day), dysuria, diarrhea, vomiting, fatigue, paradoxical voiding (infant voids, yet is always wet in between voidings [ectopic ureter or epispadias]), foul-smelling urine, stranguria, pallor, vaginal discharge, abdominal distention, scrotal edema, groin enlargement or lumps, umbilical discharge,

frequency with small-quantity voiding, for males—thin, forceful urine stream.
   b. Childhood period (3–12 years)—dysuria, frequent stomachaches, intermittent fevers, convulsions, chronic infections (e.g., upper respiratory, otitis media, tonsillitis), frequent voiding (more than 10 times a day) or infrequent voiding (less than three times a day), or holding urine for prolonged time, extreme thirst, poor weight gain, foul-smelling urine, persistent perineal rash, flank pain (especially after large fluid intake), hypertension, hematuria, proteinuria, periorbital edema, stranguria, difficulty in toilet training, relapse after successful toilet training, abdominal distention or masses, easily fatigued, constipation, encopresis.
   c. Adolescent period (12–18 years)—scrotal enlargement or venous engorgement, lumps or pain in the groin, dysmenorrhea, easily fatigued, hematuria, dysuria, proteinuria, foul-smelling urine, weight loss, poor appetite, excessive thirst, chronic fevers, abdominal or flank pain, hypertension. During the physical examination, confidentially question the adolescent about sexual activity and birth control measures.

At this point in the urologic examination, the child needs to be assessed for dysfunctional voiding patterns. Pursuing an accurate voiding assessment from parents requires that the examiner ask explicit questions, as parents are often unaware of what constitutes "normal" micturition and age-appropriate bladder control. The Voiding Profile Questionnaire (Table 16–4), to be completed while the parent waits for the child's visit, may be an efficient tool to glean details of the voiding process and possibly to suggest clues on the cause of voiding malfunctions. For example, it would not be surprising to discover that the child who lists "iced tea" as a preferred drink also experiences frequency or nocturnal enuresis. Likewise, frequent voiding may be less significant after determining that the child maintains a high fluid intake throughout the day (estimate the daily output to be approximately ⅓ to ½ of daily intake).

4. *Child's past health history*—the focus of this section is to identify coinciding conditions that may alert the nurse to urologic problems.
   a. Prenatal history—maternal history of polyhydramnios or oligohydramnios,

## TABLE 16–4. Voiding Profile

1. Do you feel your child has difficulty with bladder control? _____

2. Does your child feel there is a problem with bladder control? _____

3. Has there been a change in bladder control since the last visit? _____

4. List the times when your child urinates on an average day (for example, immediately when awakening, after lunch, etc.) _____

5. Does your child wet the bed? Yes _____ No _____. If yes, Nightly? _____Times a week? _____
   Times a month? _____

6. Does your child wet during the day? Yes _____ No _____. If yes, Constantly? _____ Times a day? _____
   Times a week? _____

7. What has been your child's longest dry period (for example, 1 month, 6 months, never)? _____

8. Have you tried to treat the wetting problem? Yes _____ No _____. How? _____

9. Does your child dribble urine? Yes _____ No _____. Before urinating? _____ After urinating? _____

10. Has your child ever had a urinary tract infection (UTI)? Yes _____ No _____. How many? _____
    Most recent? _____

11. Has your child ever experienced a fever that the doctor couldn't explain? _____

12. Does your child complain of any of these symptoms during urinating:
    _____ Burning?
    _____ Strains to start or maintain stream?
    _____ Urgency (can't hold urine when feels urge)?
    _____ Needs to urinate shortly after completed urinating (within 5 minutes)?
    _____ Frequency (more often than every hour)?

13. Does your child have frequent stomachaches? _____

14. Does your child have lower abdominal pressure when urinating? _____

15. Does your child's urine ever look "red" or cloudy or have a bad odor? _____

16. Is your child frequently constipated? _____ Other bowel problems? _____

17. How much fluid does your child drink on an average day (include all liquids, such as milk, water, soup, etc.)? _____

18. How often does your child drink Kool-Aid, carbonated beverages, tea, or coffee (for example, daily, on occasion)? _____

19. If your child is a girl, does she usually take a bath or shower? _____
    Use bubble bath? _____

sonogram evaluation, maternal diabetes, hypertension, use of nephrotoxic drugs (gentamicin, heavy metals), toxemia, alcohol ingestion, in utero cocaine exposure.

b. Neonatal history—birth weight, gestational age, asphyxia, presence of a single umbilical artery, abdominal mass, abnormal screening test results, sickle cell dis-

ease, chromosome anomaly, spina bifida, malformations (cardiac, esophageal, or rectal), circumcision (if male), bronchopulmonary dysplasia, nephrocalcinosis of prematurity.

c. Childhood history—congenital anomalies (see Table 16–1), bleeding disorders, previous illnesses, history of streptococcal throat infection and treatment, previous hospitalization or surgery. Note the child's response to the experience, regularly administered medication, allergies.

    d. Developmental history—note the child's progress in the areas of gross motor, fine motor, adaptive, language-speech, and social skills, by either report or direct observation. Several screening tools are available that may be used in the office setting (see chapter Appendices). Note older child's school progress and peer and family relationships.

5. *Family medical history*—a history of renal disease or uropathology among parents, siblings, or immediate relatives; family history of type I insulin-dependent diabetes mellitus, hypertension, chronic urinary tract infection, renal calculi; one or both parents who experienced enuresis, and age at resolution.

6. *Review of systems*—the review of systems is a wrap-up of the elicited history and an opportunity for the nurse to ensure a complete documentation of symptoms. In head-to-toe fashion, an inquiry is made regarding the functioning of body systems. Emphasize the symptoms that may disclose organ involvement in response to urologic malfunction.

## Physical Examination

    The urologic physical examination uses the classic techniques of observation, inspection, palpation, percussion, and auscultation—generally accomplished in a head-to-toe systematic style. Special consideration of age and developmental level of the child may alter this regimen. Table 16–5 summarizes various approaches to physical examination, recognizing that cooperation of the child and the parent during physical examination is essential. Allowing the child to become familiar with medical equipment used for the examination and including the parents in the process of physical examination may make the physical examination less upsetting and more efficient (Fig. 16–1). Needless to say, assessment of parts of the body that are painful or anxiety-laden should be performed last.

    Similar to the health history, this description of the urologic physical examination focuses on signs that possibly indicate a urologic abnormality. For information on conducting a complete pediatric physical examination, the reader is directed to sources listed in the Additional Readings section at the end of this chapter.

1. *General appearance*
   a. Activity level—does child look sick, listless?
   b. Nutritional status.
   c. Degree of comfort—is the child in pain?
   d. Race—blacks historically have a low incidence of uropathology; the presence of sickle cell disease may be associated with urologic complications (priapism, hematuria); glucose-6-phosphate dehydrogenase deficiency may be found.

2. *Vital signs and other parameters* (see Appendix 16A–1 for normal values of urine output)
   a. Temperature—if subnormal or elevated, may indicate infection. Check for sepsis if child is very ill.
   b. Pulse—rapid, irregular pulse may indicate fluid overload.
   c. Respirations—rapid or deep breathing may be a sign of respiratory compensation for acidosis; deep breathing may indicate diabetes mellitus.
   d. Blood pressure—elevated blood pressure may be caused by renal disease or fluid retention. Be sure to use proper-sized cuff.
   e. Weight and height—plot on growth curve (Appendix 16A–2). Poor growth may occur from chronic urinary tract infection, obstructive uropathology, or renal disease. Sudden weight gain indicates possible fluid retention. Sudden weight loss indicates possible diabetes mellitus.
   f. Head circumference (measure in children up to 2 years of age)—microcephaly may be associated with obstructive uropathy; hydrocephaly in conjunction with meningomyelocele may be associated with bladder incompetence.

3. *Skin*
   a. Pale—suggests anemia; may have renal etiology (lack of erythropoietin).
   b. Sallow, dry, pruritic—may result from uremia.
   c. Poor turgor, "doughiness"—poor nutritional status, malabsorption, possible renal disease.

4. *Face*
   a. Potter's facies—facial configuration of neonate with widened eyes; broad, flat nose; large, low-set ears; and prominent inner canthal folds. Occurs in conjunction with renal agenesis, posterior urethral valves.

5. *Eyes*

TABLE 16–5. Strategies for Gaining Cooperation During Physical Assessment

| AGE AND TYPE | STRATEGY |
|---|---|
| **Newborn–Infant—Age 0–6 Months** | |
| Developmental influences | Not upset with strangers, easily quieted |
| Parental involvement | Parents present during examination for teaching, to help restrain movement (especially of head) |
| Child preparation | Undress to diaper, if room is warm |
| Position of infant | May be prone or supine, or held by parent |
| Sequence of data collection | 1. Auscultate heart, lungs, and abdomen, record apical pulse and respiratory rate (make note if infant is crying) |
| | 2. Palpate and/or percuss heart, lungs, and abdomen |
| | 3. Primitive reflexes obtained when examining body parts |
| | 4. Generalized reflexes elicited |
| | 5. Head examination performed last |
| | 6. Axillary temperature tolerated well; rectal temperature disliked; may stimulate stool |
| Distractions | Bottle of water; toy or rattle; coo or play with baby, mobile, or mirror above examination table |
| **Older Infant—Age 6–12 Months** | |
| Developmental influences | Anxiety with strangers, negative reaction to touch by strangers |
| Parental involvement | Same as Newborn–Infant |
| Child preparation | Same as Newborn–Infant |
| Position of infant | Held by parent; nurse can sit directly opposite parent so larger infant lies in laps of both |
| Sequence of data collection | Same as Newborn–Infant |
| Distractions | Same as Newborn–Infant, plus finger food for older infant |
| **Toddler—Age 1–3 Years** | |
| Developmental influences | Separation from parent is upsetting until 2½–3 years |
| Parental involvement | Nurse explains procedure to the parent first; may use parent to demonstrate assessment; parent to remove clothing, expose one part at a time, while holding child; reassure parent that upset behavior is expected |
| Child preparation | Sit or kneel by child; explain examination in simple terms, use doll or stuffed toy to demonstrate; make positive requests; give child choices, as able |
| Position of child | Held by parent or between parent and nurse; older toddler may choose examination table |
| Sequence of data collection | 1. Inspect body parts while playing with child |
| | 2. Percuss and palpate head and trunk |
| | 3. Auscultation |
| | 4. Apical pulse respirations, blood pressure |
| | 5. Examination of oral cavity, ears |
| Distractions | Allow toddler to touch instruments; whisper to toddler during examination; tell child the otologic examination is to look for "chirpy bird," bird is then in mouth and look there; use small car to "drive" over child, palpate at same time with spare hand |
| **Preschool Child—Age 3–6 Years** | |
| Developmental influences | Slight anxiety with strangers, autonomy—allow child to remove clothes; fears of body attack, fantasies surrounding physical examination |
| Parental involvement | Parent present, help child remove clothing, may need to restrain movement |
| Child preparation | Have child at eye level with nurse; use more detailed explanations; allow child to touch equipment, use it on self; offer choices |
| Position of child | Usually enjoys sitting on the examination table (the "throne") with parent close by; supine for abdominal and genital examinations |
| Sequence of data collection | Head to toe, may delay ears and throat until last; oral temperature obtained in most cases |
| Distractions | Make game of examination, but make sure child knows that some comments made are fantasy, not real; blood pressure cuff "gives arm a hug"; have a child "blow out" otoscope light; let child listen to heartbeat; have child place hand over nurse's hand, if abdominal examination is ticklish |

*Table continued on following page*

**TABLE 16–5. Strategies for Gaining Cooperation During Physical Assessment** *Continued*

| AGE AND TYPE | STRATEGY |
|---|---|
| **School-Aged Child—Age 6–12 Years** | |
| Developmental concerns | May be embarrassed about undressing in front of opposite sex parent; can undress self; enjoys learning about body; reality-based, used to strangers |
| Parental involvement | Child usually desires a parent to be present; may prefer to answer own questions |
| Child preparation | Use more detailed explanations, understands cause and effect relationships; can negotiate during difficult aspects of examination; explain findings of examination |
| Position of child | Sitting on table, standing for neurologic signs |
| Sequence of data collection | Head to toe, genitalia last |
| Distractions | Most not necessary; use hand over nurse's hand during abdominal examination if ticklish |
| **Adolescent—Age 13–18 Years** | |
| Developmental concerns | Privacy during all components of examination, expose one body part at a time; very concerned about "normalcy of body"; worried about degree of secondary sexual characteristics |
| Parental involvement | Adolescents prefer to present historical data by themselves, parent not to be present during examination |
| Child preparation | Detailed explanation of examination and instruments used; reassure adolescent of body function, normalcy of sexual development; explain reasons for examination of genitals; if male has erection during examination, explain this is a physiologic response, then continue with examination |
| Position of child | Same as for school-age child |
| Sequence of data collection | Head to toe, genitalia last |

Adapted from Marlow, D., & Redding, B. (1988). *Textbook of pediatric nursing* (6th ed., pp. 85–88). Philadelphia: W. B. Saunders. Reprinted with permission.

a. Periorbital edema—possible fluid retention from urinary tract infection or renal failure.

6. *Ears*
   a. Low-set ears (Fig. 16–2)—to measure ear position, draw an imaginary line from the outer canthus to the most prominent aspect of the occiput. No part of the ear pinna will touch this line if the ears are low set. Clue to multisystem syndrome with urologic component (see Table 16–3).

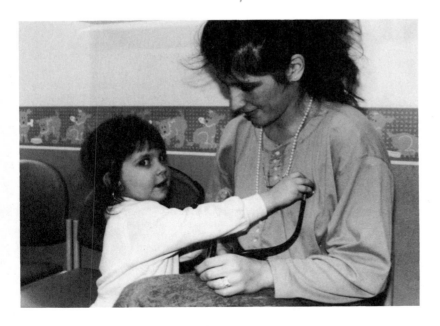

*FIGURE 16–1* Allow the child an opportunity to become familiar with medical equipment.

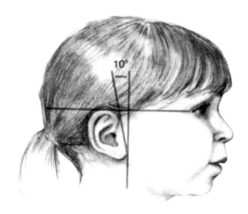
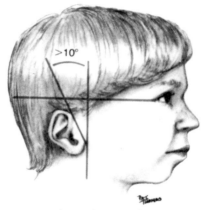

Normal alignment

Low set ears and
deviation in alignment

FIGURE 16–2 Determination of low-set ears. (From Jarvis, C. [1992]. *Physical examination and health assessment* [p. 379]. Philadelphia: W. B. Saunders. Reprinted by permission.)

b. Malformed ears—clue to multisystem syndrome with urologic component (see Table 16–3).
7. *Mouth*
   a. Pale mucosa—anemia.
   b. High-arched palate—possible multisystem syndrome with urologic component.
   c. Circumoral cyanosis—a congenital heart defect may be accompanied by renal anomalies.
8. *Neck*
   a. Webbed neck—Turner's syndrome; Noonan's syndrome; associated with gonad and renal malformations.
9. *Chest*
   a. Laterally placed nipples—Noonan's or Turner's syndrome; associated with gonad and renal malformations.
   b. Supernumerary nipples (accessory nipples)—pigmented nipples located along mammarian line. Associated with increased incidence of uropathology (Varsano et al., 1984).
10. *Cardiovascular system*
   a. Murmur, arrhythmia, thrill—heart defects may be associated with renal pathology.
   b. Venous engorgement, gallop rhythm, thrusting precordium, peripheral cyanosis—cardiac insufficiency secondary to fluid retention and renal failure.
   c. Absent femoral pulses—congenital heart defects may coincide with renal anomalies.
11. *Abdomen*

   a. Technique
      (1) Renal ballottment technique—examiner places own hand that is opposite of side being assessed along the infant's flank area and lifts up, using the opposing hand to palpate the upper quadrant.
      (2) Most effective if performed before feeding, while infant is relaxed. A pacifier is helpful.
   b. Abdominal mass—often has a renal origin, especially in young infants. Suspect hydronephrosis, multicystic kidney; may also be a neuroblastoma or Wilms' tumor, possibly constipation.
   c. Tenderness over costovertebral angle—possible pyelonephritis.
   d. Absent abdominal musculature—prune belly syndrome.
   e. Umbilical drainage—may signal patent urachus.
   f. Hepatic enlargement or hepatosplenomegaly—resulting from circulatory overload and systemic arterial hypertension, due to renal failure.
12. *Pelvis*
   a. Pelvic mass or tenseness—percuss fluid level to outline bladder. Bladder distention may be caused by voluntary retention from dysuria or by urethral obstruction.
   b. Lower abdominal mass, noted with empty bladder—may be an enlarged ovary, obstructed vagina, sarcoma of lower urinary structures, undescended testicle.

c. Inguinal area—bulging may occur as a result of a hernia or communicating hydrocele.

d. Enlarged inguinal lymph nodes—may indicate a urinary tract infection; distinguish from inguinal or femoral hernia.

e. Exposed bladder mucosa—exstrophy.

13. *Male genitalia*

a. Phallus—observe urethral location, hooded prepuce, meatal dimple for hypospadias. Note the shape and size of the penis for microphallus, torsion (penile twisting), or chordee (curvature). Note meatal diameter for possible stenosis by separating the meatus with the thumbs and forefingers. Obese males often have a pubic "fat pad" that buries the penis (Fig. 16–3); this condition is generally outgrown at adolescence (Klauber & Sant, 1985).

b. Prepuce—phimosis is a normal physiologic condition up to 3 years of age. Do not force retraction of the foreskin during examination.

c. Preputial adhesions or remnants—sequelae of improperly performed circumcision. May cause penile curvature during erection.

d. Scrotal sac—note the presence of rugae.
   (1) Underdeveloped, nonpendulous hemiscrotum indicates undescended testis (Fig. 16–4).
   (2) Scrotal edema—sac loses rugae, appears shiny (Fig. 16–5). Differentiate hydrocele from hernia with penlight, as the first will transilluminate. Discolored scrotum—may appear from trauma or infection.
   (3) Scrotal venous engorgement—varicocele.

e. Testes—cremasteric reflex may cause testicle to retract from the scrotal position. To extinguish this reflex, use a gentle "milking action" of the thumb and forefinger to coax the testis into place. Use the opposing hand to block the external inguinal ring during testicular palpation (Fig. 16–6). Place the boy in a squatting or cross-legged position in a warm tub.
   (1) Nonpalpable testis—cryptorchidism. Palpate for testis in the inguinal canal or pubic area.
   (2) Tenderness, pain—may indicate testicular torsion or infection.

A

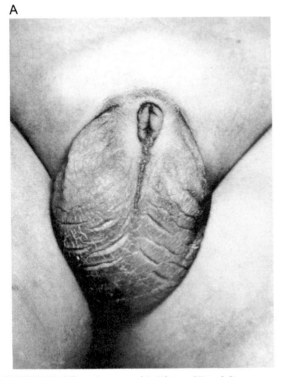

B

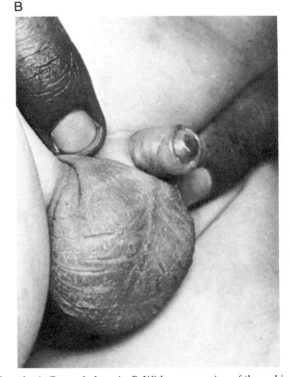

*FIGURE 16–3* Pressing on pubic "fat pad" to delineate penile length. *A,* Concealed penis. *B,* With compression of the pubic fat pad and retraction of the foreskin, a normal penis is visualized. (Adapted from Eckstein, H. B., Hohenfellner, R., & Williams, D. I. [1977]. *Surgical pediatric urology.* Philadelphia: W. B. Saunders. Reprinted by permission.)

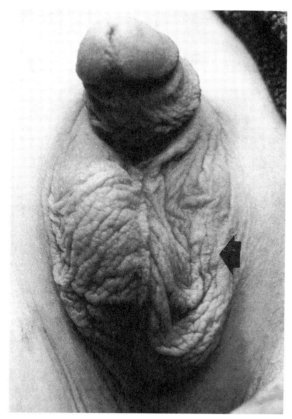

FIGURE 16–4 Empty hemiscrotum *(arrowhead)*. (Photograph courtesy of Carralee Sueppel.)

(3) Testicular mass—any nonpainful enlargement or lumps may suggest cysts or tumors.

14. *Female genitalia*
   a. Labia—fusion of labia minora that may occlude vagina, and in severe cases, the urethral meatus.
   b. Clitoris—note hypertrophy or anterior displacement of urethra.
   c. Urethral meatus—best evaluated by separating labia majora with the thumb and forefinger, using a lateral, downward motion. Note meatal size, location, cleft into clitoris or mons pubis (Fig. 16–7).
   d. Vagina—may be congenitally absent, bifid, or shrouded by imperforate hymen. The hymen may bulge from fluid accumulating behind it. Fusion of urethra–hymenal tissue may direct urinary stream into vagina, causing dribbling, introital irritation, or vaginal discharge.
15. *Rectum*—competence of the anal sphincter can be assessed using a cotton-tipped applicator; swab around rectum to elicit rectal "wink." Lack of rectal tone may be associated with anorectal malformations and possible neurogenic bladder. Rectal fissures and prominences may occur with chronic constipation, becoming an etiologic factor of chronic urinary tract infection or a sign of persistent urethritis or dysuria (due to chronic withholding of urine and stool).
16. *Spine*—spina bifida or meningocele may predispose the child to neurogenic bladder or urologic anomalies.
   a. Tuft of hair over sacrum or sacral dimple may signal spina bifida occulta.
   b. Flattened gluteal region or buttock asymmetry may denote sacral agenesis, with associated uropathology and vesical dysfunction.
17. *Nervous system*
   a. Sluggish or altered neurologic reflexes in lower extremities may occur in conjunction with neurogenic bladder.
   b. Listlessness, poor perceptual skills, and decreased memory may occur with uremia, which depresses central nervous system function.
18. *Developmental assessment*—as with all health encounters, the examiner should ascertain the child's developmental level and emotional well-being while performing the urologic history and physical examination.
   a. This information may be collected formally, using established screening tools, and informally, by noting behavioral cues or during conversation with the child.

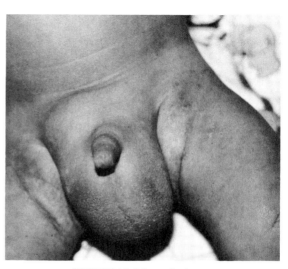

FIGURE 16–5 Scrotal edema.

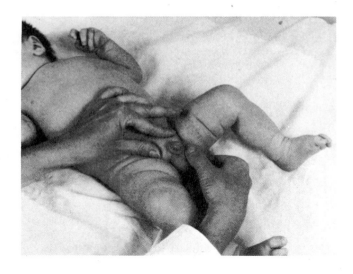

FIGURE 16–6 Use of the hand to block the inguinal ring during palpation of the testicle. (From Jarvis, C. [1992]. *Physical examination and health assessment* [p. 816]. Philadelphia: W. B. Saunders. Reprinted by permission.)

b. Developmental screening tests, to be useful in the office or clinic setting, need to be quick, reliable, and sensitive. Time constraints usually limit the comprehensiveness of testing; abnormal screening results require in-depth testing.
c. Commonly used screening tools:
    (1) Denver II Screening Test—observation test (Appendix 16A–3).
    (2) Revised Denver Prescreening Developmental Questionnaire—parental report (Appendix 16A–4).
    (3) Kansas Infant Development Screen (KIDS)—observation test and parental report.
    (4) Infant Monitoring Questionnaire—parental report (Bricker, 1987).

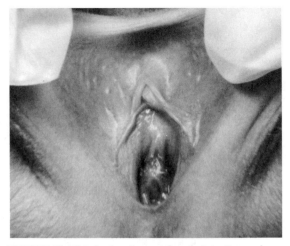

FIGURE 16–7 Method to inspect female introitus and urethral meatus. Gentle labial retraction in a lateroposterior direction affords a clear view of the introitus.

19. *Adolescent sexual development*—refer to Table 16–6 for Tanner's staging of adolescent development.

## EVALUATION OF THE CHILD WITH A UROLOGIC ANOMALY

Once the determination has been made that a child possibly has a urologic dysfunction, more involved testing becomes necessary. This testing includes hematologic, urinary, urodynamic, and radiologic studies. A significant feature of the urinary tract is that pathologic changes are often silent, exhibiting few external signs or physically evident symptoms. Bacteriuria may exist without the classic urinary tract infection complex of frequency, dysuria, and pyuria—this condition is known as *asymptomatic bacteriuria.* Long-term hydronephrosis or extreme urethral obstruction may not be reported by a child who believes that abdominal or pelvic pressure is normal and that "everybody feels this way." Therefore, it is essential that further diagnostic studies be carried out when there is a suspicion of a urologic anomaly and that routine urologic monitoring become a component of every child's routine health maintenance. Various appendices in this textbook detail commonly performed biochemical, urine, and radiologic tests. Chapter 22 concentrates on pediatric voiding disorders, discussing the role of urodynamics in evaluating this phenomenon. Consequently, only the most common clinical studies that are fruitful when evaluating the urinary tract in children are listed here; the reader is directed to appropriate

TABLE 16–6. Tanner's Staging of Adolescent Development

| STAGE | PUBIC HAIR | GENITAL DEVELOPMENT | BREAST DEVELOPMENT | AXILLARY AND FACIAL HAIR |
|---|---|---|---|---|
| **Stage 1**<br>Preadolescent | No pubic hair | Testes, scrotum and penis—no change | Elevation of papilla only | N/A |
| **Stage 2**<br>Male—10–13½ yr<br>Female—8–14 yr | Sparse growth—long, slightly pigmented, downy hair found at base of penis or along labia | Enlargement of testes and scrotum—scrotal tissue reddened and textured. Penis unchanged | Breast bud as a small mound, areola enlarges in diameter | N/A |
| **Stage 3**<br>Male—11–14½ yr<br>Female—9–15 yr | Considerably darker, coarser and more curled hair, found at pubic junction | Penile lengthening. Further growth of testes and scrotum | Enlargement and elevation of breasts and areola, contours not distinct | Facial hair appears on upper lip, axillary hair develops |
| **Stage 4**<br>Male—13–16½ yr<br>Female—9½–15½ yr | Adult-like in type, area smaller, Not found on thighs | Penile growth in breadth, glandular development. Further enlargement of testes and scrotum, scrotal skin darkens | Projection of areola and papilla to form secondary mound on breast | Facial hair on cheeks and midline lower lip |
| **Stage 5—Mature**<br>Male—14–18 yr<br>Female—11–17½ yr | Adult in quantity and distribution | Adult in size and shape, slight decrease in penile size after adolescence | Areola recedes to general contour of breast, projection of papilla only | Facial hair on sides and lower border of chin |

From Tanner, J. M. (1962). *Growth in adolescence* (2nd ed.). Oxford: Blackwell Scientific Publications. Reprinted with permission.

texts for a complete description of tests, findings, methodology, and significance.

### Urine Studies

1. Urinalysis—determine the presence of hemoglobin, protein, glucose, ketones, nitrates, urobilinogen. Measure the pH and specific gravity. Note odor, color.
2. Microscopic Study—examine centrifuged urine for bacteria, red blood cells, white blood cells, casts, epithelial cells, yeast, crystals.
3. Urine culture—to identify bacteria, perform colony count and determine antibiotic sensitivity.

### Hematologic Values

1. Complete blood count—white blood cell count with differential, hemoglobin, hematocrit, sedimentation rate, platelets.
2. Clotting Studies—prothrombin and partial thromboplastin times, sickle cell test.
3. Chemistry—sodium, potassium, chloride, calcium, blood urea nitrogen, creatinine,

phosphate, bilirubin, total protein, albumin.
4. Serology—antistreptolysin O titer, antinuclear antibodies, $C_3$, alpha-fetoprotein.
5. Blood gases—pH, base excess, $PCO_2$, $PO_2$.

### Radiologic Studies

1. Renal and ureteral evaluation—excretory urography, renal scan, renogram, ultrasonography, computed tomography scan, magnetic resonance imaging, retrograde or antegrade pyelogram or ureterogram, kidney-ureter-bladder film.
2. Bladder and urethra—voiding cystourethrogram, retrograde urethrogram.

### Urodynamics

1. Bladder capacity, flow study, cystometry, bladder pressure, urethral pressure profile.

## Recommendations for Routine Urologic Screening

The value of routine screening for early detection of urologic malfunction is widely ac-

## TABLE 16–7. Schedule for Routine Urologic Screening

| PARAMETER | Pre-natal | Birth | 2 mo | 4 mo | 6 mo | 9 mo | 1 yr | 18 mo | 2 yr | 3 yr | 4 yr | 5–6 yr | 7–12 yr | 13–18 yr |
|---|---|---|---|---|---|---|---|---|---|---|---|---|---|---|
| | | | | | | | | | | | AGE | | | |
| Growth measurement (use growth curve) | | X | X | X | X | X | X | X | X | X | X | X | X | X |
| Blood pressure | | X | | | | | | | X | X | X | X | X | X |
| Urinalysis | | | | | | | X | | X | X | X | X | X | X |
| Urine culture (female) | | | | | | | | | X | X | | X | | |
| Hemoglobin and hematocrit | | | | | | | X | | X | X | | | X | |
| Ultrasound | X | | | | | | | | | | | | | |
| Hernia (male) | | X | | | | | | | | | | | X | X |
| Sex staging | | | | | | | | | | | | | X | X |
| Testicular self-examination | | | | | | | | | | | | | | X |

knowledged (American Academy of Pediatrics, 1989; Belman & Kaplan, 1981; Chow et al., 1984; Kuhn et al., 1988; Kunin, 1987; Retik, 1984; Waechter et al., 1985; Whaley & Wong, 1992). Caregivers in primary care settings are encouraged to adopt a standardized screening schedule (Table 16–7), as most recommended tests are easily performed, require a minimum of equipment and professional time, and are sensitive indicators of uropathology.

More important, early detection of correctable urologic anomalies expedites surgical intervention while the kidney is still salvageable. The kidney at birth is underdeveloped, but it continues to mature throughout the first year of life. Consequently, surgical manipulation within that time not only preserves existing renal function but also promotes parenchymal rejuvenation (Kelalis, 1985).

Studies have reported a significant incidence of obstructive uropathology detected prenatally by sonography (Habif et al., 1982; Kuhn et al., 1988; Sabbagha & Shkolnik, 1980). Routine use of maternal ultrasonography has therefore been recommended as a diagnostic tool as well as a means to gauge the severity of renal compromise. Based on these findings, the mother may be advised on treatment options, such as preterm delivery, pregnancy termination, or surgical intervention early in the neonatal period.

Routine urine culture collection is indicated for preschool-age girls, whose high incidence of infection is also positively correlated with correctable structural abnormalities. Benefits of mass screening programs to detect bacteriuria among school-age girls are questionable, however, because this age group is not a population at risk for initial urinary tract infection.

Uroradiologic screening for siblings of children with congenital urologic anomalies is rapidly gaining acceptance among pediatric health practitioners. Familial studies have demonstrated risks for structural defects as high as 20% to 30% (Dwoskin, 1976; Dwoskin, et al, 1986; Jerkins & Noe, 1982). Affected siblings, especially males, rarely experience suggestive symptoms (even bacteriuria); consequently, renal disease may be more advanced for this group. Recommended testing includes urinalysis, urine culture, voiding cystourethrogram, and ultrasonography.

## REFERENCES

Abdel-Halim, R. E. (1986). Pediatric urology 1,000 years ago. Progress in Pediatric Surgery, 20, 256–264.

American Academy of Pediatrics. (1989). Guidelines for health supervision visits (2nd ed.). Elk Grove, IL: Author.

American Academy of Pediatrics. (1989). Professional Communication.

American Academy of Pediatrics, & American College of Obstetricians and Gynecologists. (1983). In A. W. Brans & R. C. Defalo (Eds.), Guidelines for perinatal care (p. 87). Evanston, IL: American Academy of Pediatrics.

Anderson, G. F., & Smey, P. (1985). Current concepts in the management of common urologic problems in infants and children. Pediatric Clinics of North America 32(5), 1133.

Barratt, T. M. (1974). Urinary tract infections. In D. I. Williams (Ed.), *Urology in childhood*. New York: Springer-Verlag.

Bashour B. N. & Balfe, J. W. (1977). Urinary tract anomalies in neonates with spontaneous pneumothorax and/or pneumomediastinum. *Pediatrics, 59*(Suppl 6, Pt. 2), 1048.

Bauer, S. B., Bull, M. J., & Retik, A. B. (1979). Hypospadias: A familial study. *Journal of Urology, 121,* 474.

Behrman, R. E., & Kliegman, R. (Eds.). (1990). *Nelson essentials of pediatrics*. Philadelphia: W. B. Saunders.

Belman, A. B. (1985). Genitourinary infections—non-specific infections. In P. P. Kelalis, L. R. King, & A. B. Belman (Eds.), *Clinical pediatric urology* (2nd ed., p. 235). Philadelphia: W. B. Saunders.

Belman, A. B., & Kaplan, G. W. (1981). *Genitourinary problems in pediatrics*. Philadelphia: W. B. Saunders.

Berry, A. C., & Chantler, C. (1986). Urogenital malformations and disease. *British Medical Bulletin, 42*(2), 181.

Bois, E., Feingold, J., Benmaiz, H., & Briard, M. L. (1975). Congenital urinary tract malformations: Epidemiologic and genetic aspects. *Clinical Genetics 8,* 37.

Bourne, G. L., & Benirschke, K. (1960). Absent umbilical artery: A review of 113 cases. *Archives of Disease in Childhood, 35,* 534.

Bricker, D. (1987). *Infant monitoring questionnaires for at-risk infants 4 to 26 months.* Unpublished project report, Center On Human Development, University of Oregon, Portland.

Burger, R. H., & Burger, S. E. (1974). Genetic determinants of urologic disease. *Urologic Clinics of North America, 1*(3), 419–440.

Campbell, M. F., & Harrison, J. H. (Eds.). (1970). *Urology* (Vol. 2, 3rd ed.). Philadelphia: W. B. Saunders.

Carter, C. O. (1984). The genetics of urinary tract malformations. *Journal de Genetique Humaine (Geneva) 32*(1), 23.

Catterall, A., Roberts, G. C., & Wynn-Davies, R. (1971). Association of Perthes' disease with congenital anomalies of genitourinary tract and inguinal region. *Lancet, 1,* 996.

Chilvers, C., Pike, M. C., Forman, D., Fogelman, K., & Wadsworth, J. E. J. (1984). Apparent doubling of frequency of undescended testes in England and Wales in 1962–1981. *Lancet, 2,* 330.

Chow, M. P., Durand, B. A., Feldman, M. N., & Mills, M. A. (1984). *Handbook of pediatric primary care* (2nd ed.). New York: John Wiley & Sons.

Curran, A. S., & Curran, J. P. (1972). Associated sacral and renal malformations—a new syndrome? *Pediatrics, 48,* 716.

Donohue, R. E., Utley, W. L. F., & Maling, T. M. (1973). Excretory urography in asymptomatic boys with cryptorchidism. *Journal of Urology, 109,* 912.

Dwoskin, J. Y. (1976). Sibling uropathology. *Journal of Urology, 115,* 726.

Dwoskin, J. Y. (1983). [Incidence of associated genitourinary anomalies in males with hypospadias]. Unpublished raw data.

Dwoskin, J. Y., Noe, H. N., Gonzales, E. T., Firlit, C. F., Chaviano, A. H., & Lebowitz, M. D. (1986). Sibling uropathology. *Dialogues in Pediatric Urology, 9* (6).

Engel, J. (1988). *Pocket guide to pediatric assessment.* St. Louis: C. V. Mosby.

Engle, M. A. (1981). Associated urologic anomalies in infants and children with congenital heart disease. In El-Shafie, M. & C. H. Klippel (Eds.) *Associated congenital anomalies.* Baltimore: Williams & Wilkins.

Farrington, G. H., & Kerr, I. H. (1969). Abnormalities of the upper urinary tract in cryptorchidism. *British Journal of Urology 41,* 77.

Fetterman, G. H., Shuplock, N. A., & Phillip, F. J. (1965). The growth and maturation of human glomeruli and

proximal convolutions from term to adulthood—studies by microdissection. *Pediatrics, 34,* 601.

Glicklich, L. B. (1951). An historical account of enuresis. *Pediatrics, 8,* 859.

Gonzales, E. T., Jr. (1985). Genitourinary disorders in the neonate. In R. H. Whitaker & J. R. Woodward (Eds.), *Pediatric urology.* London: Butterworths.

Habif, D. V., Jr., Berdon, W. E., & Yeh, M. N. (1982). Infantile polycystic kidney disease: In utero sonographic diagnosis. *Radiology, 142,* 475.

Harper, G., Garcia, A., & Sea, C. (1975). Inguinal hernias: A common problem of premature infants weighing 1000 grams or less at birth. *Pediatrics, 56,* 112.

Hensle, T. W. (1985). Metabolic care of the neonate and infant with urologic abnormalities. In P. P. Kelalis, L. R. King, & A. B. Belman (Eds.), *Clinical pediatric urology* (2nd ed., pp. 991–1002). Philadelphia: W. B. Saunders.

Hilson, D. (1957). Malformation of ears as a sign of malformation of the genitourinary tract. *British Medical Journal, 2,* 785.

Holmes, G. E., & Hassanien, R. (1982). The KIDS chart: A simple, reliable infant development screening tool. *American Journal of Diseases of Children, 136,* 997.

Jerkins, G. R., & Noe, H. N. (1982). Familial vesicoureteral reflux: A prospective study. *Journal of Urology, 128,* 774.

Kaplan, G. W., & Brock, W. A. (1985). Abdominal masses. In P. P. Kelalis, L. R. King, & A. B. Belman (Eds.) *Clinical pediatric urology* (2nd ed., pp. 57–75). Philadelphia: W. B. Saunders.

Kasper, T. E., Osborne, R. W., Jr., & Smerdjran, H. S. (1976). Urologic abdominal masses in infants and children. *Journal of Urology, 116,* 629.

Kelalis, P. P. (1985). Ureteropelvic junction. In P. P. Kelalis, L. R. King, & A. B. Belman (Eds.). *Clinical pediatric urology* (2nd ed., p. 450). Philadelphia: W. B. Saunders.

King, L. R. (1969). Other congenital anomalies. In O. Swenson (Ed.), *Pediatric surgery* (Vol. 2, 2nd ed.). New York: Appleton-Century-Crofts.

Klauber, G. T., & Sant, G. R. (1985). Disorders of the male genitalia. In P. P. Kelalis, L. R. King, & A. B. Belman (Eds.), *Clinical pediatric urology* (2nd ed.). Philadelphia: W. B. Saunders.

Kroovand, R. L., & Perlmutter, A. D. (1978). Short-stay surgery in pediatric urology. *Journal of Urology, 120,* 483.

Kunin, C. (1977). Urinary tract infections. In M. Green & R. J. Haggerty (Eds.), *Ambulatory pediatrics II* (pp. 165–174). Philadelphia: W. B. Saunders.

Kunin, C. (1987). *Detection, prevention and management of urinary tract infections* (4th ed.). Philadelphia: Lea & Febiger.

Matlai, P., & Beral, V. (1985). Trends in congenital malformations of external genitalia. *Lancet, 1,* 108.

McCrory, W. W. (1972). *Developmental nephrology.* Cambridge: Harvard University Press.

Meadow, R. C. (1970). Childhood enuresis. *British Medical Journal, 4,* 787.

Newman H., Molthan, M. E., & Osborn, W. F. (1969). Urinary tract anomalies in children with congenital heart disease. *American Journal of Roentgenology, 106,* 52.

Noble, M. J., & Wacksman, J. (1980). Screening excretory urography in patients with cryptorchidism or hypospadias: A survey and review of the literature. *Journal of Urology, 124,* 98.

Oppel, W. C., Harper, P. A., & Rider, R. W. (1968). The age at attaining bladder control. *Pediatrics, 42,* 614.

Parrott, T. S., & Woodard, J. R. (1976). Urologic surgery in neonates. *Journal of Urology, 116,* 506.

Perlmutter, A. D. (1985). Enuresis. In P. P. Kelalis, L. R. King, & A. B. Belman (Eds.), *Clinical pediatric urology* (2nd ed., p. 311). Philadelphia: W. B. Saunders.

Potter, E. L. (1946). Facial characteristics of infants with bilateral renal agenesis. *American Journal of Obstetrics and Gynecology, 15,* 885.

Rabinowitz, R. (1982). Update on outpatient pediatric urology. *Dialogues in Pediatric Urology, 5*(8), 5.

Retik, A. (1984). Urinary tract disorders in children: New approaches. *Hospital Practice, 8,* 121.

Roberts, J. A. (1986). Does circumcision prevent urinary tract infections? *Journal of Urology, 135,* 991.

Rosenbaum, K. N. (1985). Genetics and dysmorphology. In P. P. Kelalis, L. R. King, & A. B. Belman (Eds.), *Clinical pediatric urology* (2nd Ed.). Philadelphia: W. B. Saunders.

Sabbagha, R. E., & Shkolnik, A. (1980). Ultrasound diagnosis of fetal abnormalities. *Seminars in Perinatology, 4,* 213.

Schultz, L. R., Calvert, T. O., & Lemon, H. M. (1963). Solid abdominal tumors in childhood. *Nebraska Medical Journal, 48,* 547.

Shima, H., Ikoma, F., Terakawa, T., Satoh, Y., Nagata, H., Shimada, K., & Nagano, S. (1979). Developmental anomalies associated with hypospadias. *Journal of Urology, 122,* 619.

Slim, M. S., Dabbous, I., Frayha, F., & Issa, P. (1969). Malignant abdominal neoplasms in childhood. *American Journal of Surgery, 118,* 75.

Snyder, H. M., Lebowitz, R. C., Colodny, A. H., Bauer, S. B., & Retik, A. B. (1980). Ureteropelvic junction obstruction in children. *Urologic Clinics of North America, 7*(2), 273.

Steinhart, J. M., Kuhn, J. P., Eisenburg, B., Vaughan, R. L., Maggioli, A. J., & Cozza, T. F. (1988). Ultrasound screening for healthy infants for urinary tract abnormalities. *Pediatrics, 82*(4), 609–614.

Tanner, J. M. (1962). *Growth in adolescence* (2nd ed.). Oxford: Blackwell Scientific Publications.

Thorne, F. (1944). The incidence of nocturnal enuresis after age five. *American Journal of Psychiatry, 100,* 686.

Tudor, J. M., Carter, O. W., McClellen, R. E., & Nesbitt, T. E. (1962). An analysis of 2,403 consecutive pediatric urological consultations. *Journal of Urology, 87,* 68.

Varsano, I. B., Jaber, L., Garty, B. Z., Mukamel, M. M., & Grünebaum, M. (1984). Urinary tract abnormalities in children with supernumerary nipples: Experience and reason. *Pediatrics, 73,* 103.

Vitko, R. J., Cass, A. S., & Winter, R. B. (1972). Anomalies of the genitourinary tract associated with congenital scoliosis and congenital kyphosis. *Journal of Urology, 108,* 655.

Waechter, E. H., Phillips, J., & Holaday, B. (1985). *Nursing care of children.* Philadelphia: J. B. Lippincott.

Walker, R. D. III. (1985). Presentation of urogenital disorders in children. In P. P. Kelalis, L. R. King, & A. B. Belman (Eds.). *Clinical pediatric urology* (Vol. 1, 2nd ed., 1). Philadelphia: W. B. Saunders.

Wallerstein, E. (1985). Circumcision: The uniquely American medical enigma. *Urologic Clinics of North America, 12,* 123.

Walsh, S. Z. (1962). The incidence of external hernias in premature infants. *Acta Paediatrica, 51,* 161.

Wedge, J. J., Grosfeld, J. L., & Smith, J. P. (1971). Abdominal masses in the newborn: 63 cases. *Journal of Urology, 106,* 770.

Whaley, L. F., & Wong, D. L. (1992). *Essentials of pediatric practice* (4th ed.). St. Louis: C. V. Mosby.

Wiswell, T. E., Engenauer, R. W., Cornise, J. D., & Hankins, C. T. (1987). Declining frequency of circumcision: Implications for changes in the absolute incidence and male to female sex ratio of urinary tract infections in early infancy. *Pediatrics, 79*(3), 338.

Wiswell, T. E., & Roscelli, J. D. (1986). Corroborative evidence for the decreased incidence of urinary tract infections in circumcised male infants. *Pediatrics, 78* (1), 96.

### APPENDIX 16A–1. Average 24-Hour Urine Output in Infants and Children

| AGE | URINE OUTPUT (mL) |
| --- | --- |
| Birth–48 h | 15–60 |
| 3–10 d | 100–300 |
| 10 d–2 mo | 250–450 |
| 2 mo–1 yr | 500–600 |
| 1–3 yr | 500–600 |
| 5–8 yr | 650–1000 |
| 8–14 yr | 800–1400 |

Adapted from Campbell, M. F., & Harrison, J. H. (1970). *Urology* (Vol. 2, 3rd ed.). Philadelphia: W. B. Saunders. Reprinted by permission.

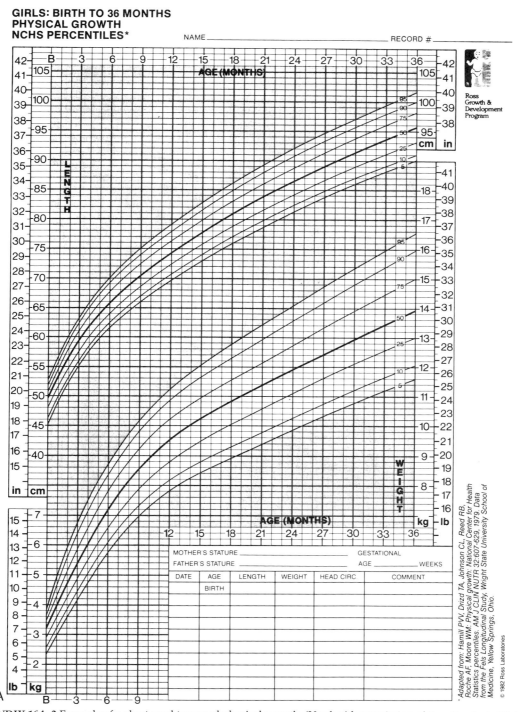

*APPENDIX 16A–2* Example of a chart used to record physical growth. (Used with permission of Ross Products Division, Abbott Laboratories, Columbus, OH 43216. From NCHS Growth Charts © 1982 Ross Products Division, Abbott Laboratories.)

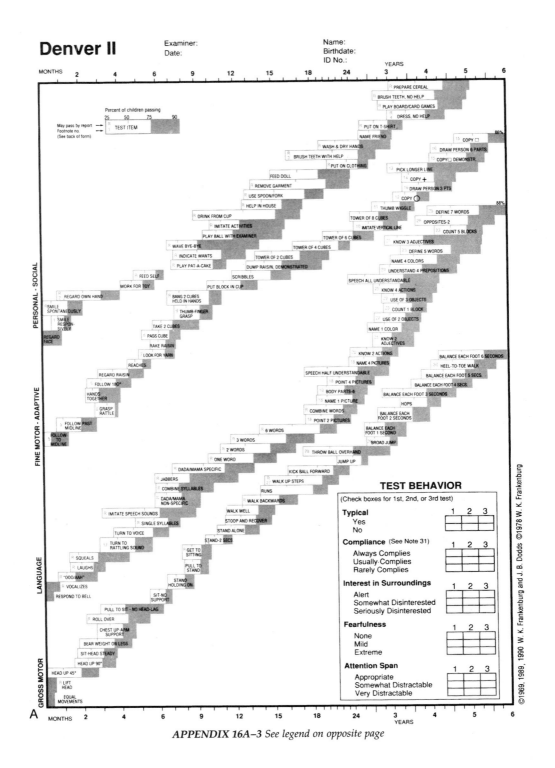

*APPENDIX 16A–3 See legend on opposite page*

# DIRECTIONS FOR ADMINISTRATION

1. Try to get child to smile by smiling, talking or waving. Do not touch him/her.
2. Child must stare at hand several seconds.
3. Parent may help guide toothbrush and put toothpaste on brush.
4. Child does not have to be able to tie shoes or button/zip in the back.
5. Move yarn slowly in an arc from one side to the other, about 8" above child's face.
6. Pass if child grasps rattle when it is touched to the backs or tips of fingers.
7. Pass if child tries to see where yarn went. Yarn should be dropped quickly from sight from tester's hand without arm movement.
8. Child must transfer cube from hand to hand without help of body, mouth, or table.
9. Pass if child picks up raisin with any part of thumb and finger.
10. Line can vary only 30 degrees or less from tester's line. |/
11. Make a fist with thumb pointing upward and wiggle only the thumb. Pass if child imitates and does not move any fingers other than the thumb.

12. Pass any enclosed form. Fail continuous round motions.

13. Which line is longer? (Not bigger.) Turn paper upside down and repeat. ' (pass 3 of 3 or 5 of 6)

14. Pass any lines crossing near midpoint.

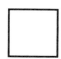

15. Have child copy first. If failed, demonstrate.

When giving items 12, 14, and 15, do not name the forms. Do not demonstrate 12 and 14.

16. When scoring, each pair (2 arms, 2 legs, etc.) counts as one part.
17. Place one cube in cup and shake gently near child's ear, but out of sight. Repeat for other ear.
18. Point to picture and have child name it. (No credit is given for sounds only.)
    If less than 4 pictures are named correctly, have child point to picture as each is named by tester.

 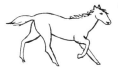   

19. Using doll, tell child: Show me the nose, eyes, ears, mouth, hands, feet, tummy, hair. Pass 6 of 8.
20. Using pictures, ask child: Which one flies?... says meow?... talks?... barks?... gallops? Pass 2 of 5, 4 of 5.
21. Ask child: What do you do when you are cold?... tired?... hungry? Pass 2 of 3, 3 of 3.
22. Ask child: What do you do with a cup? What is a chair used for? What is a pencil used for? Action words must be included in answers.
23. Pass if child correctly places <u>and</u> says how many blocks are on paper. (1, 5).
24. Tell child: Put block **on** table; **under** table; **in front of** me, **behind** me. Pass 4 of 4. (Do not help child by pointing, moving head or eyes.)
25. Ask child: What is a ball?... lake?... desk?... house?... banana?... curtain?... fence?... ceiling? Pass if defined in terms of use, shape, what it is made of, or general category (such as banana is fruit, not just yellow). Pass 5 of 8, 7 of 8.
26. Ask child: If a horse is big, a mouse is __? If fire is hot, ice is __? If the sun shines during the day, the moon shines during the __? Pass 2 of 3.
27. Child may use wall or rail only, not person. May not crawl.
28. Child must throw ball overhand 3 feet to within arm's reach of tester.
29. Child must perform standing broad jump over width of test sheet (8 1/2 inches).
30. Tell child to walk forward, ⟨⟩⟨⟩⟨⟩⟨⟩→ heel within 1 inch of toe. Tester may demonstrate. Child must walk 4 consecutive steps.
31. In the second year, half of normal children are non-compliant.

**OBSERVATIONS:**

B

*APPENDIX 16A–3* Denver II Screening Test. *A*, Front. *B*, Back. (© 1989, Wm. K. Frankenburg, MD. Reprinted by permission.)

# REVISED DENVER PRESCREENING DEVELOPMENTAL QUESTIONNAIRE

**0-9 MONTHS (R-PDQ)**

Child's Name _____

Person Completing R-PDQ: _____

Relation to Child: _____

CONTINUE ANSWERING UNTIL 3 "NOs" ARE CIRCLED

| | | For Office Use |
|---|---|---|

**1. Equal Movements**
When your baby is lying on his/her back, can (s)he move each of his/her arms as easily as the other and each of the legs as easily as the other? Answer **No** if your child makes jerky or uncoordinated movements with one or both of his/her arms or legs.
Yes    No    (0) FMA

**2. Stomach Lifts Head**
When your baby is on his/her stomach on a flat surface, can (s)he lift his/her head off the surface?
Yes    No    (0-3) GM

**3. Regards Face**
When your baby is lying on his/her back, can (s)he look at you and watch your face?
Yes    No    (1) PS

**4. Follows To Midline**
When your child is on his/her back, can (s)he follow your movement by turning his/her head from one side to facing directly forward?
Yes    No    (1-1) FMA

**5. Responds To Bell**
Does your child respond with eye movements, change in breathing or other change in activity to a bell or rattle sounded outside his/her line of vision?
Yes    No    (1-2) L

**6. Vocalizes Not Crying**
Does your child make sounds other than crying, such as gurgling, cooing, or babbling?
Yes    No    (1-3) L

**7. Smiles Responsively**
When you smile and talk to your baby, does (s)he smile back at you?
Yes    No    (1-3) PS

A

**8. Follows Past Midline**
When your child is on his/her back, does (s)he follow your movement by turning his/her head from one side *almost all the way to the other side*?
Yes    No    (2-2) FMA

**9. Stomach, Head Up 45°**
When your baby is on his/her stomach on a flat surface, can (s)he lift his/her head 45°?
Yes    No    (2-2) GM

**10. Stomach, Head Up 90°**
When your baby is on his/her stomach on a flat surface, can (s)he lift his/her head 90°?
Yes    No    (3) GM

**11. Laughs**
Does your baby laugh out loud without being tickled or touched?
Yes    No    (3-1) L

**12. Hands Together**
Does your baby play with his/her hands by touching them together?
Yes    No    (3-3) FMA

**13. Follows 180°**
When your child is on his/her back, does (s)he follow your movement from one side *all the way* to the other side?
Yes    No    (4) FMA

**14. Grasps Rattle**
*It is important that you follow instructions carefully. Do not* place the pencil in the palm of your child's hand. When you touch the pencil to the back or tips of your baby's fingers, does your baby grasp the pencil for a few seconds?
Yes    No    (4) FMA

TRY THIS          NOT THIS

(Please turn page)

**0-9 MONTHS (R-PDQ)**

CONTINUE ANSWERING UNTIL 3 "NOs" ARE CIRCLED

|  | | For Office Use |
|---|---|---|

**15. Sits, Head Steady**
When sitting, can your child hold his/her head upright and steady? Answer **No** if his/her head falls to either side or upon his/her chest.

Yes　　No　　(4)　GM

**16. Stomach Chest Up–Arm Support**
When your baby is on his/her stomach on a flat surface, can (s)he lift his/her chest using his/her arms for support?

Yes　　No　　(4-1)　GM

**17. Squeals**
Does your baby make happy high-pitched squealing sounds which are not crying?

Yes　　No　　(4-2)　L

**18. Rolls Over**
Has your baby rolled over at least 2 times, from stomach to back, or back to stomach?

Yes　　No　　(4-3)　GM

**19. Regards Raisin**
Can your child focus his /her eyes on small objects the size of a pea, a raisin, or a penny?

Yes　　No　　(5)　FMA

**20. Reaches For Object**
Can your child pick up a toy if it is placed within his/her reach?

Yes　　No　　(5)　FMA

**21. Smiles Spontaneously**
Does your child smile at crib toys, pictures, or pets when (s)he is playing by himself/herself?

Yes　　No　　(5)　PS

**22. Pull To Sit, No Headlag**
With your baby on his/her back, gently pull him/her up to a sitting position by his/her wrists. Does your baby hold his/her neck stiffly like the baby in the picture below left? Answer **No** if his/her head falls back like the baby in the picture below right.

Yes　　No　　(6-1)　GM

Yes　　　　　No

**B**

---

**Side # 2**

|  | | For Office Use |
|---|---|---|

**23. Sits, Looks For Yarn**
*Please follow directions carefully.* Get your baby's attention with a scarf, handkerchief, or a tissue and then drop it *out of sight.* Did your baby try to find it? For example, did (s)he look for it under the table or continue to watch where it disappeared?

Yes　　No　　(7-2)　FMA

**24. Passes Cube Hand To Hand**
Can your baby pass something, such as a small block or a small cookie, from one hand to the other? Long objects like a spoon or rattle do not count.

Yes　　No　　(7-2)　FMA

**25. Sits, Takes 2 Cubes**
Can your baby pick up 2 things, such as toys or cookies, and hold one in each hand at the same time?

Yes　　No　　(7-2)　FMA

**26. Bears Some Weight On Legs**
When you hold your baby under his/her arms, can (s)he bear some weight on his/her legs? Answer **Yes** only if (s)he tries to stand on his/her feet and supports some of his/her own weight.

Yes　　No　　(7-3)　GM

**27. Rakes Raisin, Attains**
Can your baby pick up small objects, such as raisins or pieces of food with his/her hand using a raking or grabbing motion?

Yes　　No　　(7-3)　FMA

**28. Sits Without Support**
Without being propped by pillows, a chair, or wall, can your child sit by himself/herself for 60 seconds?

Yes　　No　　(7-3)　GM

**29. Feed Self Crackers**
Can your baby feed himself herself a cracker or cookie? Answer **No** if (s)he has never been given one.

Yes　　No　　(8)　PS

**30. Turns To Voice**
When your child is playing and you come up *quietly* behind him her, does (s)he sometimes turn his/her head as though (s)he heard you? *Loud sounds do not count.*

Yes　　No　　(8-1)　L

©Wm. K. Frankenburg, M.D. 1975, 1986

*APPENDIX 16A–4* Revised Denver Prescreening Developmental Questionnaire. *A*, Page 1. *B*, Page 2. (© 1975, 1986, Wm. K. Frankenburg, MD. Reprinted by permission.)

**463**

# CHAPTER 17

# Growing Up With a Urologic Disorder: Developmental Considerations

■

*Christine Hoyler-Grant*

## OVERVIEW

Child growth and development are processes most distinctly characterized by their orderliness. The progressive sequences of growth, barring any untoward influences, follow the path of cephalocaudal and proximodistal directions. Similarly, development expands from rudimentary to complex skills and from general to specific functions (Nelms & Mullens, 1982). The innate impulse of children is to learn, to explore, and to interact with their surroundings, attempting to gain mastery over their bodies and the environment.

As a manifestation of this orderliness and consistency, a framework of developmental theory has evolved that accommodates the interconnections of component factors and mediating influences. Variables such as uterine environment, family life, social class, and cultural dictates, mediated by inborn genetic and temperament factors, are entwined in a fashion unique to each individual.

To ensure the child's achievement of maximal potential, development needs to be evaluated, rated, and supervised reliably, using standardized tools and employing appropriate interventions. The stepping-stone nature of child development (i.e., that each developmental phase forms a basis for the next step) mandates that any deviations or disruptions in this process be detected and corrected as early as possible, thereby capitalizing on ``critical periods'' of learning as the child is developing.

The impetus of nursing care in the pediatric setting is to build initially on developmental theory, to blend in observational skills and physiologic background, and then to use these concepts to shape the nursing process. Combining an in-depth background of growth and development principles with accessibility to families during the child's formative years, the pediatric nurse can acquire a data base of physical characteristics and environmental influences that forms the foundation of the child's nursing care plan. The pediatric nurse is, thereby, well suited to intervene therapeutically throughout the developmental spectrum, assuming a position of role model, counselor, educator, and child-family advocate.

This chapter expands on the theme of developmental theory to explore the effects of urologic dysfunction on childhood personality development and on familial interrelationships. A brief overview of three widely accepted theories of child development provides a background to explain how urinary tract malfunctions affect the child's emerging personality, with further repercussions on family dynamics. Throughout the chapter, nursing strategies are presented that promote the child's emotional development and augment parental skills and coping abilities.

## BEHAVIORAL OBJECTIVES

After studying this chapter, the reader should be able to

1. Apply the principles of child development during health encounters with the child who has a urologic disorder.
2. Evaluate the effects of urologic dysfunction on the child's psychosocial, sexual, and cognitive development.
3. Analyze the ramifications of a child's urologic disorder on family dynamics.
4. Initiate techniques that foster appropriate coping skills for the child and family.

## KEY WORDS

**Behavior modification**—a training technique founded on the principle of behavioral "shaping." The desired behavior is sequenced in an orderly fashion by the component parts, and as each component behavior is successfully carried out, the person is rewarded (positive reinforcement). A negative reinforcement may be applied to each unsuccessful attempt.

**Concept formation**—the integration of perceived observations, influences, and events within a related framework.

**Coping skill**—activities, attitudes, and behaviors that foster positive adjustment to the trials of living.

**Development**—the progressive changes in skill and behavior in response to genetic and environmental influences.

**Developmental milestone**—a criterion used to evaluate developmental growth, generally a representation of mastered motor tasks or socialization skills

**Family dynamics**—behaviors, roles, and functions of family members as they affect each other and the family unit.

**Growth**—physical changes in size, weight, or structure of an organ or organism during the formation process (a quantitative measure).

**Intellectual-cognitive theory of development**—the orderly progression of problem-solving abilities, following a fixed sequence and representing the increased refinement from simple to complex thinking.

**Maturation**—the ability of an organ, system, or organism to function at its fullest potential, realizing the final level of specialization (a qualitative measure).

**Psychosexual Theory of Personality Formation**—a theory that rests on the power of innate drives, particularly those that promote pleasure, to influence maturation and personality expression.

**Psychosocial Theory of Development**—a theoretical framework of critical periods that involves conflicts; resolution of each conflict is the propelling force that leads to the next critical period.

# EFFECTS OF UROLOGIC DYSFUNCTION ON THE CHILD AND FAMILY

There are multitudinous aspects of a chronic illness or physical disability that impact a child's well-being, such as disease entity, severity of illness or disability, symptom complex, presence of sensory impairment, medical regimen, and prognosis. Additional influences that interface with the physiologic process include family acceptance and caregiving style, cultural supports, and community milieu. Superseding these features is the child's developmental stage, which creates a locus of vulnerability.

Manifestations of the chronic health concerns that emerge during critical periods of growth and development may compromise or delay the attainment of developmental milestones. The child's role within the family structure, among the circle of peers, and throughout the educational process is often disrupted, and assimilation into the mainstream of society may be jeopardized.

Consequences of urologic dysfunction mimic the risks of other chronic disabilities to thwart normal childhood development. However, the uniqueness of the urinary tract plays a special role in modifying the child's developmental outcome; this uniqueness results from an interconnection of the urinary tract in its dual role in excretion and sexual expression. No other body system arouses the depth and range of psychosexual responses, anxieties, myths, and misconceptions.

The nurse who cares for children with urologic disabilities must have a sensitivity to the developmental expression of the disorder as a background to accurately observe for deviations and employ beneficial implementations. Use of behavioral evaluation tools, such as the Behavioral Profile Questionnaire (Table 17–1) by Nelms and Mullen (1982), readily alert the nurse to potentially problematic behaviors that warrant further investigation.

## Features of Urologic Dysfunction That Affect Developmental Growth

### FREQUENT, LONG-TERM HOSPITALIZATION AND SURGICAL INTERVENTION

Numerous studies of the effects of hospitalization on infants, children, and adolescents highlight the potential for emotional trauma (Burling & Collipp, 1969; Douglas, 1975; Vernon et al., 1966). Separation from home, family, peers, familiar surroundings, and school is a major concern, as are pain and bodily mutilation. Children fear loss of control over their body and the environment, as well as a lack of consistency and predictability regarding daily events. Untoward outcomes include regression, withdrawal, nightmares, interrupted development of trust, apathy, temper tantrums, manipulative behavior, and dependence on ritualistic behavior.

### UNCOMFORTABLE HEALTH CARE PROCEDURES

Beginning with the newborn circumcision (usually performed without the numbing effects of a nerve block), and progressing through the performance of urethral catheterizations, meatal dilatations, and diagnostic tests (such as excretory urography, voiding cystourethrograms, urodynamic procedures, suprapubic aspiration, and blood testing), painful procedures are inherent in pediatric urology. The most disruptive time for invasive procedures of the urinary tract (i.e., urethral catheterization or manipulation) is preadolescence or early adolescence, when these procedures are interpreted as sexual assaults on the highly charged genital zone. The second most disruptive time is the toddler years, when psychosexual identity is emerging. Untoward outcomes include extreme fear of the health care provider, which can generalize to fear of strangers (such as people who wear white), extreme anger and hostility, belligerence and anger directed back to parents, shame of the genitalia, and sexual dysfunction.

### IMMOBILITY AND ACTIVITY RESTRICTION

The pediatric urology nurse will, in all probability, encounter children whose urologic dysfunction is a sequel to neurologic deficits. Incapacity to be mobile is a major concern. In a similar manner, some urologically impaired children have assorted tubes, catheters, or leg drainage devices that affect locomotion. Recuperation from urologic surgery (especially penile reconstruction) may require mobility confinement. Untoward outcomes include withdrawal from new situations, altered motor activity, decreased peer interaction, increased frustration, excessive restlessness, disturbed

**TABLE 17–1. Behavioral Profile Questionnaire**

(To be filled out by the Caretaker before the Interview)

Name of Child _____

Birth Date _____ Birthplace _____

1. List all family members living in the house _____

2. Are there other immediate family members *not* living in the house? _____

   Address _____

   Telephone _____

   Is this address an apartment or a house? _____

   Number of Rooms _____

3. Please answer the following questions by checking the appropriate response:

| | YES | NO |
|---|---|---|
| Do you have any difficulty with your child's eating habits or diet? | | |
| Do you have any difficulty with your child's bathroom routine? | | |
| If [your child is] still in diapers, are either bowel or bladder functions of concern to you at this time? | | |
| Is your child toilet-trained? | | |
| Does your child have any sleep problems? | | |
| Do you have any difficulty with your child getting along with his/her sisters or brothers? | | |
| Does your child have any behaviors or habits that bother you? | | |
| Do you have any problems with your living arrangements? | | |
| Are there any other problems or difficulties in your family? | | |

4. Where do you usually go for medical care? _____

5. In the space below, please describe how your child spends his/her day? _____

6. Grade in school _____ Does your child have any problems with either his/her progress in school or his/her playtime activities with his/her schoolmates? _____

   Favorite subject in school? _____

7. What is your child's favorite playtime activity? _____

8. Does your child use a pacifier or have any other "favorite object?" _____

   If so, what is the object? _____

From Nelms, B. C., & Mullins, R. G. (1982). *Growth and development: A primary care approach.* Englewood Cliffs, NJ: Prentice-Hall. Reprinted by permission.

sleep patterns, sluggish bowel patterns, and regression of bowel control.

Another example of how urologic disorders may affect physical activity occurs when the child's urinary tract is vulnerable to possible injury. A youngster who possesses only one of a paired organ is barred from engaging in or-ganized contact sports. For example, if a boy's testicle is damaged because of torsion, nondescent, atrophy, or trauma, or if a child has only one functional kidney, he or she cannot participate in football, basketball, soccer, hockey, wrestling, high jumping, and certain gymnastic activities. Even if both kidneys are present but one has been severely damaged, or if the kidneys are malpositioned (in the case of pelvic or horseshoe kidneys), contact sports may be contraindicated. Activity restrictions are especially traumatic for athletic, highly competitive boys. Untoward outcomes include feelings of deprivation, excessive bargaining behavior and lack of respect for parents or authority figures, overcompensation, or displaced aggression.

## ALTERATIONS IN BODY INTEGRITY AND SELF-ESTEEM

In some instances, urologic dysfunction is manifested by an inability to regulate or control excretory functions. Lagging behind siblings or peers who master this skill without effort, these children believe their bodies have "let them down" and feel inadequate when comparing themselves with others.

Encopresis also may be present in conjunction with chronic urinary tract infection, associated bowel-bladder complexes, or neurologic deficits, adding the further burdens of cleanliness and odor control. During the course of evaluating and treating urologic disorders, attention is focused on body parts or functions that embarrass children. Parental embarrassment of the child's anomaly may be expressed through criticism and lack of acceptance, with devastating effects on the child's development of self-worth and ego formation. This reaction is especially prominent among fathers of boys with a phallic anomaly or sexual ambiguity. Urologic defects that are present during adolescence may create confusion about normal sexual functioning and ignite fears about the adolescent's ability to achieve satisfactory sexual responses. Children suffering from low self-esteem or who lack a sense of body competency may be reluctant to form close friendships, shun opportunities that require independent behavior or group participation, or express feelings of shame and worthlessness. Needing to affirm a masculine identity, some boys develop gender overcompensation techniques and acting-out behaviors.

Children with urologic anomalies, similar to those with other chronic disabilities, may experience bouts of depression and feelings of hopelessness or dejection over their lack of power and control of their bodies. Childhood depression is frequently underdiagnosed, because children lack the expressive skills to communicate their feelings or because adults fail to recognize that aggressive or problem behaviors may be propelled by depression. The Childhood Depression Assessment Tool (Table 17–2), developed by Brady, Nelms, Albright, Murphy, and Rhyne (1984), is a questionnaire that can be easily administered, even to young children. A high score indicates the need for professional intervention.

## SCHOOL CONCERNS

The school environment is often threatening to the child with urologic problems. Having to cope with bathroom stalls that have no doors, using common shower facilities in gym classes, and adapting to inflexible bathroom restrictions are challenges that may appear insurmountable for these children. School phobias, distractions from academic material, timidness, or overaggressive behaviors may result. Close adherence to a daily schedule for personal needs while in school is a frequent recommendation for children with voiding dysfunctions, yet children are developmentally incapable of this task. The child's conflict between developmental unreadiness and the desire for social acceptance becomes manifest as anxiety, inflexible or "ritualistic" behaviors, or feelings of failure at possessing control over oneself and one's surroundings.

## Nursing Interventions to Promote Developmental Growth

Armed with an ensemble of developmental assessment tests, behavioral recognition tools, and observational acumen, the pediatric urology nurse follows through the nursing process by generating nursing diagnoses that reflect potential or actual disruptions from the normal developmental continuum. The formulation of a nursing diagnosis then provides a springboard for the most integral component of the nursing process, the recommendations of effective therapeutic interventions. These interventional strategies are most effective if they become incorporated throughout the total scope of the child's experience—at home, in the hospital, at the clinic or physician's office, in school, and among peers.

Evaluating the outcome of these implementations may be measured by the use of standardized assessment techniques. The experienced pediatric nurse is aware that the most profitable tactic often is the simplest—letting the parent tell you what works and what does not.

## TABLE 17–2. Childhood Depression Assessment Tool Revised

| | SCORING | |
|---|---|---|
| | 0 Point | 1 Point |
| *Withdrawal* | | |
| 1. Do you like to be with other kids? | Yes | No |
| *Self-Concept* | | |
| *2. Do you feel alone even when people are with you? | *No | Yes |
| 3. All kids have problems. Do you have the same problems other kids have? | Yes | No |
| 4. Do you wish you were someone else *most* of the time? | No | Yes |
| 5. Are you glad you are you? | Yes | No |
| *Immobility* | | |
| 6. Are you tired most of the time? | No | Yes |
| 7. Do you like to sit around and not do anything? | No | Yes |
| *Hypochondria* | | |
| 8. Do you get sick a lot (more than other kids)? | No | Yes |
| *Sleep* | | |
| *9. Do you have a hard time getting to sleep at night? | *No | Yes |
| 10. Do you have a hard time sleeping at night? | No | Yes |
| 11. Do you like to take naps during the day? | No | Yes |
| *Eating* | | |
| 12. Do you like to eat? | Yes | No |
| 13. Are you hungry a lot? | Yes | No |
| *Crying/Sadness* | | |
| 14. Do you cry a lot (more than other kids)? | No | Yes |
| 15. Do you often feel like crying? | No | Yes |
| 16. Do you have lots of days when nothing seems like fun? | No | Yes |
| 17. Do you feel sad a lot? | No | Yes |
| 18. Do you have fun a lot of the time? | Yes | No |
| *School Work* | | |
| 19. Do you do as well as most of your friends in school? | Yes | No |
| 20. Do you think school has gotten harder for you lately? | No | Yes |
| *21. Is it hard for you to keep your mind on your school work? | *No | Yes |
| *Other's Concept* | | |
| 22. Do you think other kids like you? | Yes | No |
| 23. Do you think your teacher likes you? | Yes | No |
| 24. Do you feel that someone loves you? | Yes | No |
| *Irritability* | | |
| 25. Do you feel grouchy/crabby/grumpy a lot? | No | Yes |
| *Aggression* | | |
| 26. Do you get mad a lot? | No | Yes |
| 27. Do you get in trouble a lot? | No | Yes |
| 28. Do you have lots of fights with kids other than your brothers and sisters? | No | Yes |
| *29. Do you often hit or kick when you're feeling mad? | *No | Yes |
| 30. Do you feel nervous a lot? | No | Yes |

| | TOTAL SCORES | |
|---|---|---|
| | Range | Mean |
| Normal | 5.20–5.77 | 5.48 |
| Depressed children | 10.06–12.94 | 11.50 |
| Children with behavioral and social problems | 8.62–11.17 | 9.90 |

Forced answer: Ask child if it is more "Yes" or "No."
*Item not included in scoring tool.
Based on research reported in Brady, M. A., Nelms, B. C., Albright, A. J., Murphy, C. M., & Rhyne, M. (1984). Childhood depression: Development of a screening tool. *Pediatric Nursing, 10*(3), 222–225, 227.
Copyright © 1984 by Margaret A. Brady, Barbara Crew Nelms, Angela V. Albright, Carol M. Murphy, and Maureen C. Rhyne, Nursing, Graduate Division, California State University, Long Beach. Reprinted by permission.

The following section describes a variety of nursing interventions, grouped in age-appropriate categories, to foster the development of body awareness and ego integration, cognitive development, and interaction with the environment (family, peers, school, and community). Recommendations for developmental assessment tools plus preprocedural preparation and postprocedural pain management are also included for each age group.

*Text continued on page 482*

---

### Early Infancy: 0–6 Months

#### DEVELOPMENTAL TASKS

1. To maintain body regulatory systems.
2. To recognize and bond with primary caretaker, leading to a trusting relationship.
3. To develop rudimentary skills for communication of body state.

| Developmental Focus | Nursing Intervention |
|---|---|
| *Body Awareness and Ego Integration* | Encourage bonding. |
| |   1. Allow care by parent, open visitation. |
| |   2. Make "greeting card" for parent of newborn using footprints, fingerprints. |
| |   3. Provide tape recordings of parents' voices during hospitalization. |
| |   4. Demonstrate holding technique if infant has tubes, intravenous lines, and dressings. |
| |   5. Remind parent of "normalcy" of infant, even when child has disabilities. Point out developmental accomplishments at each health encounter. |
| | Primary nursing recommended. |
| | Restrain hands only if essential; leave infant's thumb exposed. |
| | Position infant on abdomen whenever possible while in hospital. |
| | Allow parent's presence during procedures, x-ray examinations, and other occasions. |
| *Cognitive Development* | Encourage parent to provide sensory, kinesthetic, and tactile stimulation, e.g., infant massage, use of mobiles, crib toys, musical toys, materials of varying textures, swing. |
| | Use tub for bathing when possible. |
| *Environmental Interaction* | Follow "cluster care" concept. |
| | Establish or mimic home routine while infant is hospitalized. |
| | Maintain comfort-warmth needs during hospital or clinic procedures, e.g., pain management during circumcision or after surgery, swaddling to calm a distraught infant. |
| | Change position—out of hospital room into buggy, infant seat to expand immediate field of vision. |
| *Developmental Assessment*—perform at 1–2-mo intervals | For this age, use Revised Denver Prescreening Developmental Questionnaire (PDQ-R), Denver II Screening Test, Kansas Infant Development Screen (KIDS) Chart, Developmental Profile II, Home Observation for Measurement of Environment (HOME), or other standardized screening tools. Document findings in medical record; make recommendations to parent. |
| | Use Behavioral Profile Questionnaire (see Table 17–1) or adaptation. |
| | Language development—Use Clinical Linguistic and Auditory Milestone Scale (CLAMS) |
| *Preprocedural Teaching* | Focus on parental teaching; use diagrams and simple explanations, repeated often. Parents' anxiety level is high and will remain so until procedure is completed, in spite of nursing and physician reassurance. |
| | Direct parent to another parent whose infant experienced a similar procedure. |
| *Postprocedural Management of Discomfort* | Stroking, touching, rocking. |
| | Sucking thumb or pacifier. |
| | Medication. |
| | Swaddling to provide a feeling of security. |

## Late Infancy: 7–12 Months

### DEVELOPMENTAL TASKS

1. To develop a sense of self as a person separate from the caretaker.
2. To recognize the concept of object permanence.
3. To develop a primitive comprehension of a cause-effect relationship.
4. To acquire skills to meet basic physical needs.

| Developmental Focus | Nursing Intervention |
|---|---|
| *Body Awareness and Ego Integration* | See Early Infancy section. |
| | Explain importance of limit setting, daily schedules, need for infant to have some "alone" time. |
| | Especially important to include parent in caregiving, because anxiety with strangers emerges at this stage. Parent is used for comforting purposes, while nurse performs procedure. |
| | Ascertain infant's temperament and which comforting style is most effective, and incorporate this information when planning care, timing of procedures. |
| *Cognitive Development* | See Early Infancy section. |
| | Provide age-appropriate play materials and experiences to demonstrate the principle of object permanence and to develop sensorimotor learning. |
| *Environmental Interaction* | See Early Infancy section. |
| | Staff of institution should wear colored uniforms. |
| | Allow for exploration of environment—playroom, stroller, playpen, jumping seat. |
| *Developmental Assessment* | Use Home Screening Questionnaire. |
| *Preprocedural Teaching* | See Early Infancy section. |
| *Postprocedural Management of Discomfort* | See Early Infancy section. |

## Toddler: 1–2½ Years

### DEVELOPMENTAL TASKS

1. To develop a sense of autonomy through the use of locomotion skills and comprehension abilities.
2. To expand communication skills through the development of verbalization.
3. To acquire the ability for rudimentary cognitive thinking—symbolization of familiar items and events in the environment.
4. To begin the socialization process through
    a. Control of elimination.
    b. Participation with daily routines.

| Developmental Focus | Nursing Intervention |
|---|---|
| *Body Awareness and Ego Integration* | See Late Infancy section. |
| | Encourage child's participation in health care and during treatments. |
| | Use terminology that is accurate and consistent, yet simple and concise, to describe and identify body parts and functions, procedures, and treatments. |
| | Offer choices that are realistic rather than "Do you want to . . ." questions. Negativism on the part of toddler is common. |
| | Provide security items, such as blanket and doll, during procedures, hospitalization. |
| | Provide parents with toilet-training counseling—assess readiness, relaxed attitude toward this skill. |
| | Accentuate the positive aspects of development by using encouraging statements to child such as "You can" or "Let's try," even when child has a disability or physical dysfunction. |
| | Use of stickers or paper toys that have glue backing encourages drinking postoperatively. |
| | Fill small cups (e.g., medicine cups) with colored liquids, or use "crazy straws" to encourage drinking. |
| *Cognitive Development* | Read books to child; use tape recordings of favorite stories or songs that child wants repeated often. |
| | Constant reassurance and repetition teach cause and effect, predictability of events. |
| | Short attention span—emphasize here and now. |

Has lack of understanding about time passage. Use concrete, familiar events to measure time (e.g., schedule intermittent catheterizations before meals, tell child mother will return to hospital when playroom closes, at suppertime).

*Environmental Interaction*

Allow items from home, e.g., favorite blanket, photos of siblings and pets.

Permit phone calls, audio and video tape recordings from home while child is in hospital.

Provide space and opportunities in hospital or clinics for parallel play with peers.

Modify play if child is not ambulatory or if extremities are immobilized (as with an IV line).
1. Use kicking games—kick balloon or spongelike ball that is suspended from the top of a climber crib or while child is in wheelchair.
2. Punch ball, or use mylar balloon as punching toy.
3. Velcro dartboard.
4. Busyboard.
5. Take bed into playroom.
6. Toe painting, footprints; draw faces on toes.
7. Blowing games—feathers, bubbles, or pinwheels. Especially good to encourage deep breathing postoperatively.

*Developmental Assessment*—perform at 3-mo intervals

See Early Infancy section.

*Preprocedural Preparation*

Use simple explanations—tell child what will be done, then perform procedure immediately.

Tell child if procedure will hurt, then perform it quickly.

Allow child to play with equipment; probably will not understand explanations.

Warn parent that child may be angry or withdrawn after procedure.

Use parent for comforting, not for pain-inducing aspects of procedure, when possible.

*Postprocedural Management of Discomfort*

Soothing, holding.
Praise.
Medication.
Postprocedural play—distraction.

---

## Preschool: 2½–5 Years

### DEVELOPMENTAL TASKS
1. To further expand and refine verbalization.
2. To acquire gender self-identity.
3. To gain mastery of daily habits.
4. To interact with peers, from parallel to participatory play.
5. To identify and define family and societal roles.
6. To develop comprehension of the concepts of discipline and responsibility—a sense of purpose and orderliness of behavior.

**Developmental Focus**

**Nursing Intervention**

*Body Awareness and Ego Integration*

Ritualistic thinking and behavior are common and give child a sense of control over events. Child may fear something "bad" will happen if rituals are not maintained.
1. Identify and respect child's rituals.
2. Communicate the rituals to other staff members.

Gender identity is emerging; child able to recognize body parts. Parental attitude is instrumental.
1. Important for parents to accept child, especially if child has sexual ambiguity.
2. Be sure the parents understand the child's problem and long-range treatment plans.
3. If surgery will be performed on genitalia, state that surgery will allow body part to be "finished," that it was not made completely. Do not say "fixed," or emphasize that there is something "wrong" with the genitalia.

4. During a procedure such as penile dressing change or catheter removal, *never* tell the child that penis will be cut off if he moves.
5. Use of anatomically correct doll for play helps child recreate life situations and role play.

Toilet training is usually accomplished during this stage.
1. Develop routine times.
2. Use child-sized potty so child's feet are flat on the floor.
3. Limit time that child sits on potty. Use a timer or small hourglass.
4. Techniques of behavior modification: reward behaviors as the child progresses toward the desired behavior. For example, if the child is reluctant to use potty, reward for sitting on potty. Use extra reward when child urinates or defecates. Eventually, reward only when child eliminates on potty or toilet.
5. Keep chart of "successes"; do not emphasize "failures."
6. For older preschool child, use of designer underwear may encourage the process.
7. Wake-ups for voiding about 1 1/2 hours after bedtime may help. However, discourage frequent nightly wake-ups unless recommended by physician.
8. Remind parents that relapses are common, that bladder control is a complex process that requires maturation of the lower nervous system.
9. The adage "tincture of thyme" is appropriate—bladder control may take time.
10. Discourage parent from comparing child with siblings or other children, because urologic dysfunction may delay control.

Child believes that illness, hospitalization, or surgery is a punishment for being naughty or for evil thoughts.
1. Emphasize that child is good, that things happen that cannot be helped.
2. Parent should *never* threaten child with visit to the physician, hospital, or clinic if child is bad or state that "I'll tell the doctor/nurse if you . . ."
3. Emphasize positive aspects of hospitalization with child—hospital or clinic play area, card or small gifts that child has received.

Children in this stage often have "pretend" friends—incorporate them in play or teaching.

Allow child the opportunity to express feelings—to be angry, cry.

Encourage participation with procedure or treatment.

Books with specific health theme or about stressful life situations may be useful; teach child coping strategies.

*Cognitive Development*

Thinking is egocentric—child enjoys discussing self, has little tolerance for others. Hospital environment, with other ill or disabled children, helps direct child's thinking away from self.

Child has understanding of numbers—use chart to count down the number of procedures to be performed (Fig. 17–1) or to keep track of fluid intake amounts; use calendar to record days or charts to record amounts (Figs. 17–2 and 17–3).

Has reasoning ability—explain the "why" of procedures and treatments.

Learning at concrete conceptual stage, not global. Use same words or phrases to describe or explain environmental phenomena.

Can follow simple directions; short-term delay of gratification may be understood, as long as parent or health care provider is consistent and reasonable.

*Environmental Interaction*

See Toddler section.

Peers becoming more important.
1. Make-believe and pretending about health problem, health care encounters, or procedures with peers help coping.
2. Manipulative toys or games with health and hospital theme are useful.
3. Integrate child into mainstream of community, and encourage normalcy.

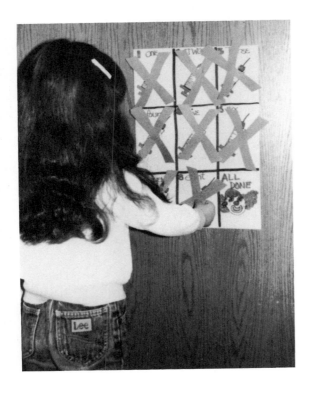

FIGURE 17–1 Using a "countdown" chart to keep track of the number of remaining injections. This child was admitted for parenteral therapy for a complex urinary tract infection.

4. Child may want to tell friends about the urologic problem; friends' parents should be aware, if appropriate.

Encourage sibling visitation policy in the hospital.

For child who needs to drink extra liquids, keep a sport-type water bottle in refrigerator, marked with child's name. Child can obtain liquids by self.

Encourage child to wear own sleepwear or regular clothes while in hospital.

Modify play activities if child is not ambulatory, has restricted use of extremities (see Toddler section).

1. Board games, video games.

*Developmental Assessment*—perform every 3–6 mo

Use PDQ-R, Denver II, McCarthy Scales of Children's Abilities (MCSA), Minnesota Child Development Inventory (MCDI), Pre-School Development Inventory (PDI).

Use Behavioral Profile Questionnaire (see Table 17–1), or assess language development with Denver Articulation Screening Examination (DASE).

*Preprocedural Preparation*

May discuss procedure with child 1–4 days beforehand.

Demonstrate with body figures or doll. Internal parts hard to appreciate; show where incision will be and the location of any external paraphernalia (Fig. 17–4).

Encourage child to touch and play with tubes, catheters, drainage bags, and other equipment beforehand.

Emphasize sensory perception—what child will feel like afterward. If there will be discomfort, honestly explain so, but do not emphasize.

Emphasize that only a specific part of body will be operated on.

Tell child honestly if shots will be necessary and how many, if possible.

Children especially like role playing, use of hospital or operating room doll house, puppets, operating room outfits.

Preoperative teaching program effective, because child has memory and better reasoning power. Books, videotapes, movies, pictures of other children after surgery are helpful.

Teach imagery and relaxation techniques to reduce anxiety.

## Fluid Intake Record — Young Child

My doctor says "drink liquids!"
Be they water, juice, or pop—
Please make sure my cup is full,
So my supply will never stop.
I'll keep track of what I drink,
A quick look at this chart will tell—
I want to do as much as I can
To help myself get well!

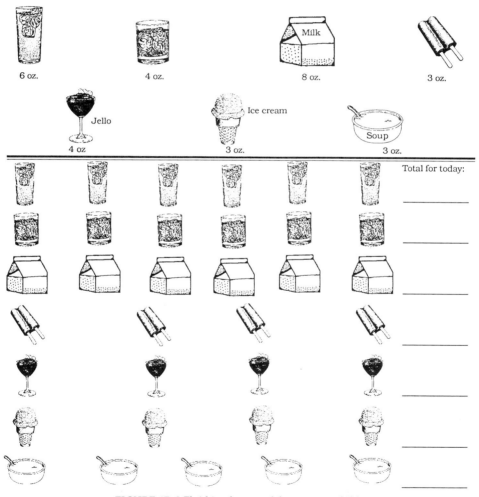

*FIGURE 17–2* Fluid intake record for a young child.

## Fluid Intake Record — Older Child / Teen

Be sure to drink your liquids,
Have your water, juice or pop—
Whatever suits your fancy,
Just make sure supplies don't stop.

Then keep track of what you drink,
This chart will help you tell—
It's up to you to work with us
To help yourself get well.

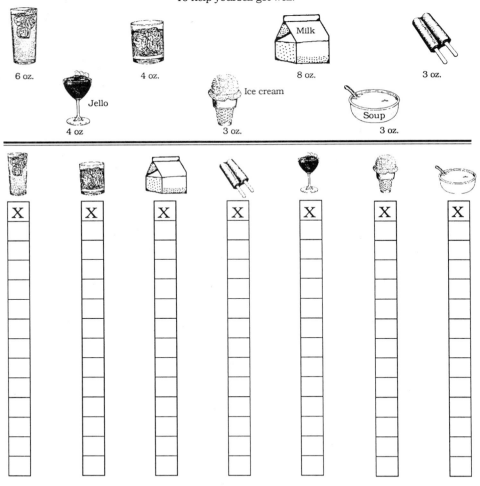

FIGURE 17–3 Fluid intake record for an older child or adolescent.

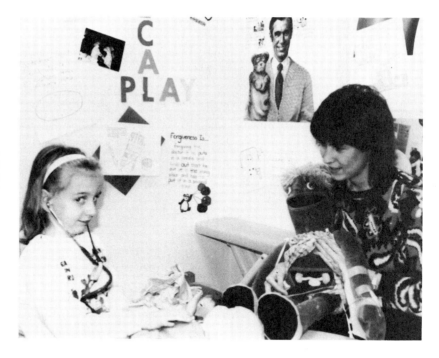

*FIGURE 17–4* Medical play, including a doll with anatomically correct urologic parts, helps the school-aged child understand surgery.

*Postprocedural Management of Discomfort*

Distraction techniques.
Play, especially medical play.
Parental presence.
Partial assistance by child during procedure.
Praise.
Structured verbalization.
Medication.

## School Age: 5–12 Years

### DEVELOPMENTAL TASKS

1. To increase the depth and breadth of understanding cause-effect relationships and logical thinking.
2. To develop a sense of industry and satisfaction through achievement.
3. To recognize right versus wrong.
4. To form more involved and sustained peer relationships, while still remaining aligned with parents.
5. To broaden the child's conceptualization of the world.
6. To gain mastery of gross and fine motor skills.

**Developmental Focus**

*Body Awareness and Ego Integrity*

**Nursing Intervention**

Child is at an industrious stage in development. Recruit child's help with tasks while in hospital or at clinic. Encourage parents to do same at home.

Hero worshiping is prevalent—use signs, games, clothes, posters that feature heroes (e.g., cartoon or television characters, rock singers) as role models to convey health message. For example, urine drainage bag could be painted in camouflage colors to be an army "power pack."

Offer reward certificates—Best Patient of the Day, Super Helper, VIP—Very Important Patient, for skill in accomplishing treatments or procedures.

Use peers in contests, because children in this age group enjoy and thrive on competition (e.g., contest for taking fluids).

Less dependency on parents, often derive sense of accomplishment when a procedure is managed by self, without parent present. Parental support and guidance are still important, however.

If activity restrictions are necessary because of urologic dysfunction (e.g., avoidance of contact sports), direct child into alternative activities, such as swimming, jogging, and tennis.
1. Make these restrictions seem desirable, not punitive.
2. Parents often may participate with child.

Provide group experiences as much as possible to help child learn cooperation and collaboration and to develop tolerance of others and a realistic sense of self and one's capabilities.

Encourage parents to accentuate child's capabilities, not disabilities.
1. Point out talents, skills, and features that are unique about child.
2. Provide parents with appropriate expectations, using positive attitude.

*Cognitive Development*

Child has increased sophistication of concrete concepts—can understand explanations of internal body parts and their function, if pictures, models, and so forth are used to illustrate.

Increased memory skills—can use previous experiences in hospital, in clinic, or from real life more effectively.

Better reasoning power—can accept more detailed explanations about the need for surgical intervention and medical procedures.

Moralistic thinking, also has more sophisticated understanding of cause and effect, of cause of illness and health problem; strives to follow rules.
1. Provide child with reasons why neglecting health care can affect health; may use concepts of germ theory in teaching.
2. Offer rules or guidelines, based on reasons that seem appropriate to child.

Better concept of time—can use specific time span for measuring procedures, e.g., every 4 h.
1. Set up calendar or schedule for hospital, home, or school use.
2. Child can accept responsibility to maintain schedule within limitations.
3. For timing of medications or procedures such as intermittent catheterization, use a wipe-off board with daily or weekly schedule on it. Give child a star when task has been performed. Post the board in a conspicuous spot.
4. Have child wear an alarm watch to remind of times for catheterization, if on timed voids or other routines.

*Environmental Interaction*

School environment extremely important—ensure that child is able to continue with studies, whether in hospital or at home.

Communication with school nurse or teacher is important.
1. Explanation of child's problem, care needs, and limitations helps school personnel maintain consistency in child's life.
2. School may be a continuation of medical regimen; provide instruction to school personnel.
3. Provide guidance to help child devise an explanation of urologic condition for peers.
4. Prevent child from getting unnecessary privileges or restrictions.
5. Help school to devise alternative athletic programs for child, if necessary.

Encourage child to join extracurricular clubs and groups, (e.g., Boy or Girl Scouts, 4-H); especially if they help child achieve mastery over body or environment.
1. Child needs to develop independent skills, which are accomplished as child gains confidence in ability to care for self.

Likes to be with others of similar age, but because of modesty may prefer a private room. Desires privacy during health care encounters.

*Developmental Assessment—*
perform yearly

Developmental Profile III, MCSA, HOME, Goodenough-Harris Drawing Test.
1. Developmental screening tests are often administered in school or under guidance of child psychologist.
2. Refer parents to community agency when child's development seems delayed.

Use Behavioral Profile Questionnaire (see Table 17–1) for adaptation.

Use the Childhood Depression Assessment Scale (see Table 17–2) when child seems to be adjusting poorly to physical problems, social sphere.

*Preprocedural Preparation*

Many similarities to Preschool Age section.
Use more details about internal structures and body systems.
Proper names of organs, procedure.
Mention physical sensations experienced with procedure.
Explain reason for procedure and consequence if not performed.
In general, child has less anxiety during this stage of development.
Discuss with parents that child may exhibit signs of regression.
Accept expression of child's feelings, fears.
Less likely to accept dolls or animals for procedural preparation. Would rather use models, pictures, or discuss with another child who has undergone the procedure.
Allow choices whenever possible; encourage child to participate in procedures.

*Postprocedural Pain Management*

Distraction.
Medication.
Imagery and relaxation techniques.
Preparation and rehearsal.
Tell others; write story or draw picture of experience, feelings.

## Adolescence: 12–18 Years

### DEVELOPMENTAL TASKS

1. To refine conceptual skills and use abstract thought patterns.
2. To create self-identity.
3. To break from parental dependency, forming intense peer interrelationships.
4. To develop a moral code and a personal philosophy of life.
5. To prepare for self-sufficiency.

| Developmental Focus | Nursing Intervention |
|---|---|

*Body Awareness and Ego Integration*

Extremely concerned about physical appearance; fearful of body mutilation.

1. Provide detailed explanation of surgery; stress how surgery will affect physical appearance, that *only* discussed body parts will be operated on.
2. Introduce adolescent to another patient with similar condition, same surgery.
3. Encourage adolescent to use art, drama, drawing, music, poetry to express fears.
4. Recognize that "apparent" disconcern about condition may be a mask for inability to express worries.
5. Because adolescent is reticent to confide in adults, nurse may need to introduce a sensitive subject.

Adolescents are often self-conscious about normal body changes and embarrassed about physical changes due to illness or dysfunction, especially those surrounding elimination or sexual function.

1. Work with adolescent, parents, and schools (if appropriate) to devise methods to maintain privacy during procedures or ways to "cover up" the urologic defect or dysfunction.
2. Encourage parents to respect adolescent's need for confidentiality by not discussing the urologic problem with other friends or relatives.
3. Provide privacy at all times; expose as little of body as is necessary.
4. During physical examinations, mention how the adolescent's body is changing and what is normal about these developments.
5. Provide anticipatory guidance about changes that will be experienced in the future.

Peer identification—need to conform.

1. Adolescent to be scheduled to clinic when other adolescents are to be seen.
2. Use of adolescent unit in hospital or room with patient close to age, if possible.
3. Encourage street clothes when in hospital.
4. Contact a youth member of local support group to interact with adolescent.
5. Discuss with adolescent the possibility of becoming a resource person in the future for other adolescents with similar urologic condition.
6. Ensure that adolescent has opportunity to be alone or alone with peers.

Encourage participation in adolescent discussion groups.

Recognize the adolescent's self-worth by speaking to him or her as an adult. Nurse should maintain the position of "adult" by not using slang or becoming "chummy."

Assist adolescent in acquiring self-care. Offer options; avoid rigid rules.

Adolescent may balk at performing procedures (especially intermittent catheterizations) that are different and emphasize that his or her body is not normal. By not performing the technique, the adolescent is then "redefining" his or her body as normal.

1. Explain consequences of not performing procedure in nonjudgmental way.
2. Shift responsibility for performance of the procedure from parent to adolescent.
3. Encourage use of self-monitoring techniques, use of rewards.
4. Have adolescent devise self-contract with you, to be reviewed at regular intervals.
5. Refer to family counseling if family tension is extreme, on-going, or detrimental to adolescent's health.

Adolescents seek role models separate from parents.

1. The nurse is in a unique position to be a positive role model because of intimate contact with adolescent, especially in hospital.
2. Adolescent should receive hospital care from same-sex nurse when possible.

Sexual identity, sexual functioning heightens.

1. Provide opportunity for speaking with adolescent alone, maintain confidentiality; e.g., stop writing in chart at this point of clinic visit, and just talk with adolescent.
2. Discuss honestly if urologic defect will have any bearing on sexual functioning; reassure if not.

3. Provide counseling for birth control and prevention of sexually transmitted diseases if sexually active.
4. Health care teaching with consideration of the urinary tract, e.g., strategies to reduce incidence of UTI when sexually active, testicular self-examination.
5. Have literature available about menstruation, testicular self-examination, sexually transmitted disease, and other topics.

Allegiance with cultural idols, fads, countercultural behaviors, attitudes, clothing, lifestyles.
1. Work with parents and adolescent to identify which fads and lifestyles may be classified as harmless and which may be detrimental to the adolescent's physical health and emotional development.
2. Encourage tolerance of adolescent's benign acting-out behavior by emphasizing the temporary nature of these incidences.

| | |
|---|---|
| *Cognitive Development* | Adolescent can think in rational terms, understand abstract concepts, and perform complex processes. |

1. Include adolescent in the decision-making process relating to health care or treatment plan. Health care team should speak *with*, not *to*, adolescent.
2. Psychosocial influences and needs often override the adolescent's rational thinking and judgment, causing irrational or risky choices to be made.
3. Health care teaching and expectations should appeal to the adolescent's sense of rational thought, even when adolescent chooses to ignore advice.

Ability to hypothesize and experiment, use deductive reasoning, and project into the future.
1. Use future orientation with health care teaching, more involved cause-effect relationships.

Stage time when adolescent begins to make vocational choices.
1. Nurse serves as a role model as a commonly encountered health professional.
2. Counsel adolescent if the urologic dysfunction has any effect on vocational opportunities (e.g., participating in military service may be prohibitive with kidney disease).

| | |
|---|---|
| *Environmental Interaction* | Maintain contact with school to plan, implement, and evaluate adolescent's health care regimen. |

Peer support critical.
1. Continue educational needs while adolescent is hospitalized or at home to minimize educational and peer group interactional difficulties when returning to school.
2. Encourage extracurricular activities, community group participation.
3. Visitation by peers while adolescent is hospitalized is encouraged.

Assist adolescent in creating meaningful leisure time, e.g., volunteer in hospital, child care setting.

| | |
|---|---|
| *Developmental Assessment—* perform yearly | See School-Age section. |

Especially important to differentiate moodiness from actual depression.
Assess for signs of drug use, which delay developmental growth.

| | |
|---|---|
| *Preprocedural Preparation* | Adolescents like one-on-one teaching, particularly when procedure is of a sensitive nature. |

Health teaching and preparation should be provided by health professionals rather than parents (especially for older adolescents).

When using group teaching for genitourinary procedures, the younger adolescent may prefer group members to be the same sex.

Explain if the procedure will affect physical appearance or have any social ramifications.

Provide details about what will be happening to the body, because adolescents especially need to feel in control of their bodies.

Use of adolescent from local support group can help.

Emphasize that modesty will be maintained, even when adolescent is under anesthesia.

Dispel thoughts that the adolescent will reveal "secrets" or expose self while recovering from anesthesia.

Use of filmed modeling to demonstrate procedural and coping methods.
Systematic desensitization.

| | |
|---|---|
| *Postprocedural Management of Discomfort* | Preparation and reassurance. |

Verbalization.
Distraction.
Medication.
Relaxation and imagery.
Parental presence—adolescents often reject parents, but are deeply hurt if parents seem to reject them or appear inattentive.
Visitation by peers.

| Parental-Family Concern | Intervention |
|---|---|
| Guilt and anger over birth of child with physical defect. Accusations between parents over which one was responsible for defect. | Validate parents' feelings of loss; allow them an opportunity to mourn for unrealized expectation of "perfect child."<br>1. Explain that many urologic problems are a result of multiple gene transmission; causative parent often cannot be pinpointed.<br>2. Use realistic but positive approach when discussing child.<br>3. Encourage parents to maximize child's potential.<br>4. Direct parents to support group, or network parents within patient population. |
| Ability of child to make positive adaptation to social environment—in school, among peers, eventual intimate relationship. | Use realistic but positive approach<br>1. Support groups, parental network within patient population.<br>2. Use of community groups, resources.<br>3. Provide parent-oriented literature, such as "These Special Children" by Jeter (1982). |
| Radiation exposure from multiple uroradiologic studies. | The nurse should encourage parents to be informed consumers—teach them to:<br>1. Question urologist about indication for all diagnostic x-ray studies.<br>2. Discuss radiation concerns with radiologist.<br>3. Understand risk-benefit ratio for all radiologic studies performed on their child. |
| Side effects from long-term medication therapy. | The nurse should encourage parents to be educated consumers—teach them to<br>1. Discuss with urologist or nurse the medication's indications, side effects, and administration details.<br>2. Be sure that the urologist is aware of all medications prescribed by other physicians for their child.<br>3. Use pharmacist as a resource when buying over-the-counter drugs. |
| Concerns about future children—what is the risk of a repeated congenital anomaly? | The nurse should provide parents with information on relative risk of repeated urologic anomaly, based on medical research and clinical experience.<br>1. Refer for genetic counseling. |
| Financial burden—costs of health care visits, surgery and hospitalization, special supplies, medication, other therapeutic interventions, counseling and others. | Direct parents to fully explore their insurance provisions.<br>1. Use community resources (March of Dimes, Crippled Children's Guild).<br>2. Refer to social worker.<br>3. Provide parents with names of local durable supply vendors or names of manufacturers for direct purchasing. |
| Anxiety about child's sexual functioning and acquisition of healthy sexual identity. | Use of parent support groups.<br>1. Refer to psychoendocrinologist, social worker, or sex therapist. |
| Guilt over not recognizing the child's problem in its early stages—especially prominent among parents of children with reflux or hydronephrosis. | Explain etiology of urologic defect.<br>1. Emphasize that urologic dysfunction is often insidious, difficult to diagnosis, mimics other conditions.<br>2. Explain how earlier symptoms may have been masked by child's age or immaturity.<br>3. Emphasize how parents can help child now. |
| Chronic exhaustion from being the child's primary advocate, especially if condition is complex or especially debilitating. | The nurse can intervene as coordinator with schools, rehabilitation team, physical education program, or daycare program.<br>1. Parental stresses and signs of "burn-out" may be assessed by tool such as Chronicity Impact and Coping Instrument, Parent Questionnaire (Hymovich, 1983). |
| Sibling rivalry — resentment of parental attention to symptomatic child, absence from home if frequent hospitalizations are required. | Help parents to be sensitive to needs of siblings.<br>1. Encouraged sibling visitation during child's hospitalization.<br>2. Use of Ronald McDonald House, if available.<br>3. Incorporate siblings in child's care plan. |

## Family Concerns for the Child With a Urologic Dysfunction

Providing supportive care for the child with a chronic urinary tract disorder requires the nurse to focus beyond the symptomatic child's responses to disease and become aware of the family dynamics. It is important to view the child within the context of a family unit and the social environment that shapes the family. Facilitating the child's achievement of optimal growth and development is a primary nursing goal; a secondary aim is to guide parents in their mission to create an environment that nurtures their child's positive adaptation to chronic illness. Offering nursing interventions that are individually tailored to incorporate the family's needs, lifestyles, and capabilities may be accomplished only by a preliminary assessment of the parents' childrearing style, their own personal strengths, and their understanding of the child's disease. An on-going dialogue with the parents must follow to ascertain their degree of acceptance and adjustment to the child's condition. Parents must be effective managers of their child's health care and monitor the impact of the medical regimen on their child's emerging personality development. These demands require parents to possess self-esteem and a knowledge base of the disease, treatment modalities, alternative options and corresponding ramifications, home management techniques, and avenues of support, such as the extended family, friends, and community resources.

The challenges of rearing a child with a long-term health impairment may be overwhelming, as the parents may be consumed with fears of inadequacy and doubts about the child's future. Parents often feel alone and vulnerable, recognizing that decisions made today are often irreversible and may have untoward consequences. Unsure of their judgment and inexperienced in the medical realm, parents turn to the nurse for advice and support. By conveying empathy and sensitivity to the parents' concerns, the nurse is able to anticipate and identify difficulties that, if overlooked, may surface as behaviors that cause parents to undermine their child's physical or emotional response to the medical regimen.

Nurses collaborate with parents of chronically ill children by assuming a role of counselor, observing family interrelationships, assessing the child's behavior, guiding parents to recognize risks that threaten to compromise optimal child and family adjustment, detecting the warning signs of stress build-up, and suggesting strategies to encourage the development of successful coping mechanisms.

Some of the common concerns identified by parents of children with chronic urologic disorders plus possible nursing interventions are listed in the following section.

Along with their families, children and adolescents with chronic urinary tract impairments may be subject to tumultuous stressors that threaten to compromise or adversely shape the child's development and undermine the parent's role in childrearing. The pediatric urology nurse lends expertise in the areas of child and family assessment, formulation of nursing diagnoses, contribution of nursing interventions, and evaluation of these actions, maintaining as a goal the overall support for the family as a unit. The needs of the symptomatic child are intertwined within the composite matrix of the family, and actions that encourage the integrity of the family structure ultimately ensure the positive response of the child.

## REFERENCES

Brady, M. A., Nelms, B. C., Albright, A. J., Murphy, C. M., & Rhyne, M. (1984). Childhood depression: Development of a screening tool. *Pediatric Nursing, 10*(3), 222.

Burling, K. A., & Collipp, A. J. (1969). Emotional responses of hospitalized chidren. *Clinical Pediatrics, 8,* 641.

Douglas, J. (1975). Early hospital admission and later disturbances of behaviour and learning. *Developmental Medicine and Child Neurology, 17,* 456–480.

Hymovich, D. (1983). The chronicity impact and coping instrument: parent questionnaire. *Nursing Research, 32*(5), 275–281.

Jeter, K. (1982). *These special children.* Palo Alto: Bull Publishing.

Nelms, B. C. & Mullens, R. C. (1982). *Growth and development: A primary health care approach.* Englewood Cliffs, NJ: Prentice-Hall.

Vernon, D., Shulman, J., & Foley, J. (1966). Changes in children's behavior after hospitalization. *American Journal of Disease of Childhood, 111,* 581.

# CHAPTER 18

# Urinary Tract Infections in Children

■

*Doris Yukiko Kimura*

## OVERVIEW

Urinary tract infection (UTI) in the pediatric population plays a key role in the practice of urology. With an incidence ranking second only to respiratory infection and a recurrence rate approaching 80% (among girls) (Kunin, 1970), management and prevention of childhood UTI are the cornerstones of pediatric urology. Even more significant is the correlation between UTI and uropathology—between 20% to 50% of the children who develop UTI have underlying structural abnormalities, detected only by radiologic evaluation of the urinary tract (Monahan & Resnick, 1978; Spencer & Schaeffer, 1986). Although detection and correction of these abnormalities are important, to focus our thinking about UTI on this narrow surgical view limits the urologist to the operating room arena and does a disservice to most children presenting with UTI who do not have such abnormalities.

The presence of obstructive anatomic abnormalities such as ureteropelvic or ureterovesical junction obstruction, vesicoureteral reflux, posterior urethral valves, ureterocele, and prune belly syndrome is found most often in childhood and characterizes pediatric from adult UTIs. Functional abnormalities, such as detrusor muscle instability and infrequent voiding, may complicate or promote UTI in childhood. Another difference between pediatric and adult UTI lies in the varied (generalized) clinical presentation of children (especially infants). Fever, malaise, and lethargy may be the only symptoms manifested.

A diagnosis of UTI in the pediatric population is usually defined as ``demonstrated growth of more than $10^5$ colonies per milliliter of a single organism from a clean voided urine specimen or virtually any number of bacteria cultured from a specimen obtained by urethral catheterization or a suprapubic aspiration'' (Spencer & Schaeffer, 1986, p. 661). In western society, prevalence of UTI is influenced by diagnostic methods and varies by age and sex. Winberg (1986) found at least a 5% risk of females getting a symptomatic UTI before the age of 11 years compared with 1% of males. The incidence of asymptomatic bacteriuria in school-aged females is approximately 1% (Eichenwald, 1986). McCracken (1984) estimated that 26% of neonates and, in infants and children, 32% of males and 40% of females will experience recurrent UTIs. The most detrimental result of pediatric UTI is renal scarring caused by prolonged chronic infection, as well as vesicoureteral reflux and hydronephrosis. Eventually, hypertension and renal failure may develop.

The diagnosis of UTI accounts for most of the referrals made to pediatric urologists. Pediatric and urologic nurses must be knowledgeable about the etiology, diagnostic and nursing procedures, treatment modalities, and follow-up protocols to assist in the management of this problem in children of all ages.

## BEHAVIORAL OBJECTIVES

After studying this chapter, the reader should be able to

1. Discuss several characteristics of urinary tract infection in the pediatric population that distinguish it from urinary tract infection in adults.

2. Describe common pediatric urologic problems that may first manifest as a urinary tract infection.

3. Assess the pediatric patient for urinary tract infection, taking into consideration the patient's developmental stage.

4. Recognize commonly accepted treatment protocols for the pediatric patient with urinary tract infection.

5. Communicate with peers and community practitioners the importance of a thorough urologic evaluation for the child with a urinary tract infection.

## KEY WORDS

**Bacteremia**—the presence of bacteria in the blood.

**Constipation**—difficult defecation; infrequent defecation with the passage of unduly hard and dry fecal material; sluggish action of the intestine.

**Dyssynergia, detrusor-sphincter**—a failure in muscular coordination of the detrusor and urinary sphincter.

**Nosocomial infection**—hospital-acquired infection.

**Overactive detrusor**—detrustor that contracts involuntarily at times other than when voiding is mediated by the central nervous system (also termed unstable detrusor or detrusor hyperreflexia, if caused by a disturbance in the nervous system control mechanisms).

**Ureteropelvic junction**—the junction between the ureter and the renal pelvis of the kidney.

# PERSPECTIVE ON DISEASE ENTITY

## Etiology

### PREVALENCE AND INCIDENCE

Urinary tract infection (UTI) is an invasion of bacteria within the organs of the urinary tract, normally a sterile system, that causes local inflammation, distress, involuntary muscle spasm, and in some instances, the systemic effects of an infectious process. Because the classic symptoms of dysuria, frequency, urgency, enuresis, and malodorous urine may be the result of other causes, UTI is reliably diagnosed only with a urine culture collected with great care to avoid contamination from the periurethral zone. Applying the traditional definition of bacteriuria, the presence of more than $10^5$ bacterial colonies per milliliter, as the diagnostic standard of UTI among children is now being questioned, because this measure was derived from studies of adult women and may be irrelevant in the pediatric population (McCracken, 1987). The prevalence of UTIs in the pediatric population is dependent on age, sex, and method of diagnosis.

Although it appears that, among neonates (birth to 30 days of age), boys are more often diagnosed with symptomatic UTI than are girls, this trend seems to reverse by the age of 2 years (Spencer & Schaeffer, 1986). This finding was confirmed in a study by Ginsberg and McCracken (1982) that evaluated 100 infants aged 5 days to 8 months who were hospitalized for UTI. Seventy-five percent of those infants with UTIs were males who were younger than 3 months of age. Preschool- and school-aged girls constitute the largest population at risk, with 3.3% of girls developing symptomatic UTI before the age of 11 years compared with 1.1% of boys in the same age group (Durbin & Peter, 1984). It is estimated that 5% to 6% of girls between first grade and graduation from high school will have at least one episode of bacteriuria (Eichenwald, 1986).

The likelihood of an initial onset of UTI decreases rapidly in males between the ages of 30 days and 1 year. Decline in the female population, although steady, is less pronounced until the age of 11 years. The difference in susceptibility between boys and girls of similar ages is often attributed to the shorter female urethra; however, there may be other influencing factors that explain this phenomenon. The suggested causes include a variable rate of immune system maturation or the resolution with age of other predisposing conditions that differ between the two sexes (Winberg, 1986).

The controversy surrounding UTI and the contributory influence of the foreskin in uncircumcised male neonates has been debated. The 1975 American Academy of Pediatrics (AAP) Ad Hoc Task Force on Circumcision failed to document any medical indications for routine newborn circumcision and therefore discouraged the practice. However, studies by Wiswell and associates (1985, 1987) indicated a 10-fold increase in neonatal UTI in uncircumcised versus circumcised males, along with an increased risk of other problems such as phimosis, paraphimosis, cancer of the penis, and balanoposthitis. Consequently, the AAP modified its position to state that circumcision may have potential medical benefit (see Chap. 19 for a more in-depth discussion regarding circumcision).

### POPULATIONS AT RISK AND ASSOCIATED UROLOGIC PROBLEMS

One characteristic that distinguishes pediatric from adult UTI is its association in the pediatric population with obstructive abnormalities that are anatomic or functional in nature. These abnormalities predispose a child to develop UTI; infection that accompanies renal backflow of urine hastens the development of kidney lesions.

Anatomic abnormalities predisposing to UTI include posterior urethral valves, ureteropelvic (UPJ) or ureterovesical junction (UVJ) obstruction, ureterocele, prune belly syndrome, and vesicoureteral reflux. These abnormalities are found in 3% to 21% of the children with UTI (Spencer & Schaeffer, 1986). To avoid renal deterioration, it is of utmost importance to adequately treat these conditions using appropriate medical and surgical therapies. (Management of these abnormalities is discussed in Chaps. 19 and 20.)

Functional abnormalities predisposing children to UTI include various types of dysfunctional voiding. Residual urine as a consequence of neurogenic bladder or detrusor-sphincter dyssynergia provides a perfect medium for bacterial growth. High intravesical pressures resulting from bladder distention may cause vesical ischemia and a breakdown in the defense mechanisms of the bladder, leading to the development of UTIs. UTI, in turn, exacerbates the pre-existing dysfunction.

"Van Gool and associates stated that the inflammatory reaction associated with urinary tract infection may reflexly elicit detrusor and sphincter hyperactivity, perpetuating the voiding dysfunction" (Spencer & Schaeffer, 1986, p. 663). Prevention of UTI, therefore, is an important component in the treatment of dysfunctional voiding. However, one may also argue that the treatment of dysfunctional voiding is an important component in the prevention of UTI.

Constipation and encopresis are common findings in children with UTI. The exact mechanism for this association is unclear but may be related to ascending bacteria from fecal soiling, outlet obstruction caused by pressure from a large fecal mass, or internal seeding of enteric pathogens from a retained fecal mass. Stools may be withheld as a learned response to the dysuria that a child experiences from poor hygiene or chronic UTI. Several studies (Lindberg et al., 1975; Neumann et al., 1973). have reported that successful control of constipation has resulted in a decrease in the incidence of recurrent UTI.

Even though vesicoureteral reflux is found in as many as 30% to 60% of children with UTIs (Spencer & Schaeffer, 1986), the two conditions may occur independently of each other (Wein & Schoenberg, 1972; Winberg, 1986). Upper urinary tract bacteriuria is found in only 25% to 35% of patients with vesicoureteral reflux (Salvatierra & Tanagho, 1977; Spencer & Schaeffer, 1986). As many as 50% of children who either present with renal scars or acquire renal scars during follow-up do not have vesicoureteral reflux (Spencer & Schaeffer, 1986). Urine refluxing into the renal parenchyma (gross vesicoureteral reflux) associated with intrarenal reflux results in renal scarring, and the process is potentiated by infection. Because a significant proportion of children with UTI are found to have reflux, it has been suggested by Bellinger (1985) that each child who presents with a single UTI should have a voiding cystourethrogram (VCUG) study. If reflux is diagnosed, the child needs to be monitored closely for UTI recurrence.

In summary, UTIs may be caused by preexisting structural or functional abnormalities; likewise, they may also initiate or aggravate these conditions. The pathogenesis of pediatric UTI appears to be related to several factors, including periurethral bacterial colonization, characteristics of the invading bacteria, incomplete emptying of the bladder such as that found in voiding dysfunctions, increased intravesical pressure, and the presence of vesicoureteral or intrarenal reflux. Early detection, treatment, and further prevention of these conditions are necessary to preserve renal function and promote general health.

## COMMONLY IDENTIFIED BACTERIA

Most UTIs are caused by gram-negative anaerobic rods, most commonly *Escherichia coli*. This bacterial organism accounts for more than 90% of acute UTIs in preschool- and school-aged children (Durbin & Peter, 1984). Fewer than 10 of more than 150 identified serogroups of *E. coli* cause approximately two thirds of all UTIs (Winberg, 1986). Also predominately found in fecal flora, these serogroups support the theory of infection through the ascent of fecal flora by the periurethral route. Causative bacterial agents for the remainder of infections are *Proteus*, *Klebsiella*, *Enterobacter*, or *Pseudomonas aeruginosa*. *Proteus* and *Pseudomonas* are involved in most nosocomial infections acquired by instrumentation or catheterization.

In addition to these organisms, gram-positive aerobic cocci have also been identified as pathogenic. The most prominent cocci, group D streptococci (enterococci) and *Staphylococcus saprophyticus*, are commonly found to be the cause of infections in adolescent (especially sexually active) girls.

## ASYMPTOMATIC BACTERIURIA

Asymptomatic bacteriuria may also be described as screening, covert, latent, or symptomless bacteriuria (Winberg, 1986). Often, it is detected by screening of so-called "healthy populations" or in routine monitoring of populations at risk for recurrent infections. Attention must be paid to the sample collection method to distinguish asymptomatic bacilluria from a contaminated urine sample.

Episodes of asymptomatic bacteriuria associated with heavy pyuria have been described as "not uncommon phenomena" (Gonzales, 1985; Winberg, 1986). Although most of these episodes clear spontaneously, asymptomatic bacilluria may be a clinical marker for a child at risk for developing a UTI. Studies by Saxenn and colleagues (1974) and Lindberg and associates (1975) disclosed a correlation of asymptomatic bacilluria with reflux, renal scars, or previous UTI. Children with this finding require further urologic monitoring.

# RECURRENT URINARY TRACT INFECTION

The high rate of UTI recurrence, even after appropriate and complete treatment for the initial infection, causes a great deal of frustration for patients, parents, and clinicians. In a study by Kunin (1970), 80% of school-aged girls with UTI were found to become reinfected within 1 year, many as quickly as 3 months. Most of these reinfections were caused by a new microorganism or a different serologic type of *E. coli.* Similar findings have been demonstrated by Fair and colleagues (1972) and Belman (1978). McCracken (1984) estimated that recurrent bacteriuria should be anticipated in 26% of neonates and in 40% of female infants and children. Approximately one half of recurrent infections are asymptomatic and are diagnosed only during routine urine monitoring.

Multiple infections may alter the inner lining of the bladder, leaving patches that are pale, rough, speckled, and easily reinfected (cystitis follicularis). Long-term prophylaxis with antibiotics (at least 12 months) is necessary to prevent further recurrence and restore the normal bladder mucosa.

Although the rate of recurrence is directly related to the number of previously documented infections, it appears that as the infection-free period lengthens, the rate of recurrence decreases (Kunin, 1986).

Bacteria that enter the bladder are subject to the washout effect of the voiding mechanism, meaning that, in normal circumstances, bacteria are eliminated from the bladder by frequent and complete voiding. Any condition that is conducive to urine retention increases the child's susceptibility to bacterial colonization. This situation places the child with reflux, urethral obstruction, or hydronephrosis at increased risk for UTI. It is now recognized that renal scarring may occur with the reflux of sterile urine; infection potentiates this effect and may induce pyelonephritis. Long-term follow-up with urine cultures and pharmacologic therapy is needed to reduce the morbidity of chronic UTI in these patients.

Another group that appears to be prone to recurrent cystitis is those children with voiding dysfunction. Urodynamic studies may often identify a nonfixed, functional obstruction produced by a voluntary dyssynergic contraction of the internal urinary sphincter while a detrusor contraction is occurring. In the literature, this phenomenon is described as the nonneurogenic neurogenic bladder (also known as the Hinman syndrome) (Hinman, 1986).

As the child tries to gain continence, sphincter activity increases during these contractions, producing increased intravesical pressure. This increased pressure is believed to decrease the defense mechanisms of the bladder by possibly decreasing blood circulation to the vesical wall. Infections resulting from such a situation contribute to a vicious cycle, increasing the bladder's afferent sensitivity and therefore increasing its hyperactivity. Often, children with this problem have displayed normal voiding habits in infancy but present with complaints of dysuria, frequency, urgency, urge incontinence, and appearance of, or worsening of, nocturnal wetting. Another common characteristic is atypical posturing involving leg crossing, squatting, curtsying, and facial grimaces, all employed by the children to suppress the urge to urinate, as well as to keep from wetting their pants.

Although neurologic disease must be ruled out when these symptoms are present, recognition of this pattern and attempts to break the cycle are essential to the provision of quality care and to protect against reinfection in the child with dysfunctional voiding.

## Pathophysiology

It is believed that most cases of UTI are a result of bacterial ascent from the periurethral area. One exception is in the neonate, when a hematogenous (blood-borne) route is considered because of documented evidence of bacteremia preceding bacteriuria (Kunin, 1986). It is thought that the neonate's inability to localize infection causes the kidney to become secondarily seeded with bacteria from a systemic infection. This process may be attributed to the fact that, at any given time, the kidney may receive as much as one fourth of the total cardiac output. Therefore, investigation for UTI should be pursued whenever a neonate presents with fever of unknown origin or failure to thrive.

Development of UTI is dependent on bacterial virulence and host susceptibility. Factors that may influence the development of a UTI include the following:

Age
Sex
Presence of structural abnormalities
Increased receptivity for bacterial attachment
   to human uroepithelial cells
Obstruction of the urine flow resulting in resid-

ual urine, vesicoureteral reflux, or hydrone-phrosis

Defect in the host-defense mechanisms that permits bacteria to adhere to uroepithelial cell receptors, thereby affecting the clearance of bacteria from the bladder and kidneys (Feld et al., 1989; Lomberg et al., 1986).

The five basic stages of development of clinical infection are (1) microorganism–body surface contact with local colonization; (2) organism multiplication resulting in local tissue damage; (3) release of toxins that act locally or systemically against the host; (4) toxic tissue invasion; and (5) dissemination of the organism throughout the body. Virulence factors may affect the ability of the bacteria to invade the host and establish an infection. Because *E. coli* is the most common type of bacteria found in UTI, virulence studies have focused most attention on this organism.

*E. coli* has surface structures called *pili* or *fimbriae*, which are composed of repeating protein subunits. These fimbriae attach to specific polysaccharide receptors on the uroepithelial cells that line the urinary tract. The most commonly found fimbriae on *E. coli* are identified as type 1 fimbriae and are associated with receptors that are mannose-containing glycoproteins. Another fimbria called *P fimbria* is associated with the receptors that are related to the child's P blood group antigens and possess the gal-gal disaccharide. The P fimbriated *E. coli* have been isolated from children with pyelonephritis, and they appear in a higher density in the uroepithelial, periurethral, vaginal, and buccal cells of infection-prone women as compared with noninfection-prone women. This conclusion suggests that density and accessibility at these polysaccharide receptors on the uroepithelial cells may determine susceptibility to infection in children and that susceptible children (especially those with structural abnormalities) possibly possess a higher density of these receptor cells.

Another susceptibility factor may involve a deficient immune response to recurrent infections. It is thought that some children may not maintain a post-UTI increase in urinary immunoglobulin levels, especially secretory IgA. Because these immunoglobulins are the primary defense mechanism of the urinary tract, preventing bacterial adherence, it is possible that this lack of sustained increase contributes to reinfection.

Exploration of the complex concepts of the fimbriae and their relationship with receptors is in the infancy stage, as is our understanding of bacteria-host interaction. Further research is necessary to fully explain the pathogenesis of UTI.

# Medical-Surgical Management

The goals of management of pediatric UTI are renal preservation, symptomatic relief, and elimination of bacteriuria. To achieve these goals, the combination of urologic evaluation, chemotherapy, and vigilant follow-up may need to be used.

Unlike in the adult population, a distinction between upper and lower UTI is not easily made in the pediatric population. Laboratory tests that help determine localization in adults have proved to be either unreliable or impractical (Eichenwald, 1986). Therefore, formulation of the initial management plan must rely primarily on the clinical findings.

## CLINICAL PRESENTATION BY AGE

**Neonate and Infant.** UTI is definitely an indication for urologic evaluation in the newborn. Neonates and infants usually present with nonspecific symptoms that may be confused with respiratory or gastrointestinal infection. Lethargy, irritability, feeding problems, vomiting, diarrhea, fever of unknown origin, unexplained weight loss, failure to thrive, and overall tenderness to touch are the most common signs and symptoms.

Central nervous system symptoms in the neonate with UTI may manifest as generalized convulsions with loss of consciousness, hypotonicity or irritability, respiratory difficulty, and absent or difficult-to-elicit primitive reflexes (Winberg, 1986). An elevated blood urea nitrogen level, oliguria, and temporary increase in renal size may be observed. Bacteremia may be found in these infants, possibly leading to sepsis or meningitis. Neonates do not compartmentalize infection well, leading to a tissue-invasive process in these patients (Burns et al., 1987). Consequently, infants younger than 3 months of age who become febrile require a full sepsis workup, including spinal tap, blood and urine cultures, and parenteral antibiotics. Until culture reports are available, the neonate with a complicated UTI is at great risk of developing gram-negative shock, a physiologic response to bacterial endotoxins that leads to vascular shutdown. Immediate medical intervention and antibiotic therapy may avert this complication.

Of male infants who are diagnosed with UTI, approximately one third have vesicoureteral reflux and one fourth experience reinfection. In contrast, as many as 50% of female infants identified with UTI may have some type of structural abnormalities (Ginsberg & Mc-Cracken, 1982; Gonzales, 1985).

The use of a voiding diary has assisted in establishing an accurate diagnosis of UTI in the infant population. The parents are asked to record the frequency of diapering, the approximate length of time of the dry interval, the voiding stream (especially in male infants), evidence of abdominal tenderness or distention and unexplained fever. Suspicion for UTI is raised if one or more of the following conditions is present: (1) the diaper is dry for an abnormally long period (beyond two feeding times), (2) the presence of urinary frequency with damp rather than wet diapers, (3) an abnormal urinary stream, (4) the presence of recurrent or persistent abdominal distress, and (5) the presence of unexplained fever (Randolph et al., 1975; Spencer & Schaeffer, 1986).

In summary, UTI in the neonate or infant is difficult to assess because of the nonspecific clinical presentation. Care must be taken to rule out other sources of infection while not overlooking the possibility of a UTI in a presenting infant.

**Preschool- and School-Aged Child.** As the child grows older, signs and symptoms of symptomatic UTI become more specific and generally present as a localized illness. The classic manifestations are dysuria, frequency, urgency, incontinence, and foul-smelling urine. Dysuria may also occur with other conditions such as vaginitis or urethritis possibly caused by chemical irritants (e.g., bubble bath), diaper rash, pinworms, or masturbation. Abdominal or flank pain may also be present and is generally indicative of upper UTI. However, there are times when the only evidence of UTI may be a persistent fever of unknown origin.

**Adolescent.** In contrast with the school-aged child, the adolescent may be able to provide the practitioner with a more accurate clinical picture. Signs and symptoms of UTI in this age group are similar to those of the school-aged child; however, differential diagnosis involving dysuria syndromes must be investigated, especially in sexually active young women.

The physical examination should include a gross examination of the perineum and the rectum. Positive findings of flank mass, suprapu-

bic distention, vulvovaginitis, perineal rash, fecal mass, or subtle neurologic deficits may be found in a child with suspected UTI. If possible, actual observation of voiding may give the practitioner helpful information. An abnormal voiding stream may be indicative of obstruction or dysfunctional voiding.

## METHODS OF MEDICAL MANAGEMENT

Formulation of an appropriate management and treatment plan for pediatric UTI depends on clear documentation of infection. The initial task, therefore, is to obtain a urine specimen that will provide the urologist with the most accurate clinical picture.

The four standard methods of obtaining a urine sample or culture are (1) the external bag collection method, (2) the clean-catch method, (3) sterile catheterization, and (4) suprapubic aspiration. The suprapubic aspiration must be performed only by a physician and therefore is described here. The other methods are nursing procedures and are discussed in the section on approaches to patient care. Suprapubic aspiration is recommended only for neonates or infants younger than 1 year of age. The aspiration is done with the infant lying supine and when the bladder is full. The area above the symphysis pubis is prepared antiseptically, and a long needle (e.g., a spinal needle) is inserted into the palpable bladder. Urine is then withdrawn into a syringe attached to the needle. The needle is removed and a small adhesive bandage is placed over the site. (Slight hematuria may occur in a subsequent voiding.) No other specific follow-up is needed. Suprapubic aspiration is a reliable method of obtaining a sterile specimen in a population in which clinical symptoms tend to be nonspecific and accurate diagnosis is critical. However, it does have some disadvantages. Timing the procedure so that the medical staff is available and the infant has a full bladder simultaneously may be difficult. The hazard of puncturing the bowel rather than the bladder is also a concern.

Even when an optimal urine specimen is obtained from the patient, an accurate diagnosis is not guaranteed. Timely transport and proper specimen handling from the clinical site to the laboratory are necessary to ensure the accuracy of laboratory results. If the proper guidelines are not followed, multiplication of bacteria and deterioration of some cellular elements may distort the urine culture results.

When UTI is clearly documented in a child,

the pediatric urologist may then begin a workup to rule out the presence of any anatomic or functional abnormalities. Opinions vary in regard to when such a workup should begin. It has been documented that male children who present with UTI have a high incidence of structural abnormalities. It has also been demonstrated that even after appropriate therapy for structural defects, 80% of female children have recurrent infection. With the potential for renal scar formation in the presence of abnormalities such as vesicoureteral reflux, it is recommended that all children with a clearly documented UTI have a thorough urologic evaluation (Kunin, 1986).

**Diagnostic Studies.** The traditional imaging studies are the VCUG and the excretory urography (IVP). The VCUG examines the lower urinary tract and may reveal vesicoureteral reflux or obstructive lesions, such as posterior urethral valves, ureterocele, trabeculation, and diverticula. This test should be performed after treatment for acute UTI is completed and only after the follow-up culture report is negative. An IVP images the upper urinary tracts, revealing obstructive lesions (UPJ or UVJ obstruction) or the presence of renal scarring. Because of the level of radiation exposure associated with the VCUG and the IVP, debates have arisen as to the necessity for both examinations to be performed routinely.

Ultrasonography has been suggested as a substitute for the IVP because of its noninvasive approach, diagnostic sensitivity (comparable to the IVP for most renal abnormalities), and lack of radiation exposure. A primary drawback to the procedure is that the value and quality of the examination often depend on the pediatric expertise of the sonographer performing the test and the radiologist interpreting the data. Despite these limitations, ultrasonography is a valuable technique that may be used to determine postvoid residual urine in the dysfunctional voider without the invasiveness of catheterization.

Radionuclide tests (dimethylsuccine acid [DMSA] renal scan and diethylenetriamine pentaacetic acid [DTPA] renogram) are best used to assess the degree of function (impact of renal damage) when parenchymal loss and cortical scarring are suspected. A furosemide (Lasix) renal washout study (DTPA with Lasix) is an excellent procedure for assessing renal and ureteral drainage.

Urodynamic studies should be performed if dysfunctional voiding is to be investigated. These studies may document dyssynergia, which may contribute to the presence of infection.

In summary, baseline tests to rule out anatomic and functional abnormalities should be performed after the clear documentation of the first UTI, regardless of the patient's gender. The standard tests requested are the VCUG and the IVP; however ultrasonography may be the test of choice as a substitute for the IVP. If there is any question or concern on review of the ultrasound image, an IVP is then obtained. Radionuclide tests are best used to ascertain the degree of renal function, whereas urodynamic studies best clarify the picture of a suspected voiding dysfunction.

Cystoscopy as a diagnostic tool for evaluation of UTI in the absence of obstruction or other complicating features is generally not recommended (Belman, 1985; Mulholland, 1986; Spencer & Schaffer, 1986).

## CLINICAL CLASSIFICATION

Burns and colleagues (1987) suggest designating UTI as either complicated or uncomplicated to guide medical management. They define complicated UTI as (1) all neonates, (2) most patients with clinical evidence of pyelonephritis, and (3) all patients with an identified mechanical or functional obstruction. Most patients classified according to this criteria are found to need hospitalization for parenteral antibiotic therapy, and they require an evaluation for the presence of significant structural abnormalities.

Appropriate therapy should evidence a quick response, usually producing sterile urine within 48 to 72 hours. The critically ill child who does not respond appropriately has been further compromised by the choice of an incorrect antibacterial agent, an incorrect diagnosis, or an undetected structural abnormality.

The medical-surgical management of children with functional or anatomic abnormalities is addressed in Chapters 19 and 20. Basically, adequate drainage of infected urine is the management goal of children with anatomic or functional abnormalities.

Uncomplicated infections are those that occur in a child with a normal urinary tract. In most instances, uncomplicated UTI may be managed on an outpatient basis, with evaluation for potential abnormalities scheduled at a later date. Follow-up urine culture studies should be performed to ensure resolution of the infection.

## CHEMOTHERAPY

**Acute Urinary Tract Infection.** The choice of antimicrobial agent for the treatment of UTI depends not only on the organism and its sensitivities but also the agent's safety, availability, side effects, cost, and the patient's ability for tolerance. There are several different agents that have similar absorption, urine concentration, and effectiveness against gram-negative bacteria. These agents may be used for acute, uncomplicated infections and include amoxicillin, triple sulfas or sulfisoxazole, trimethoprim-sulfamethoxazole (TMP-SMX), cephalosporins, and nitrofurantoin. Drugs of choice vary from physician to physician. Although short-course (one-day) treatment has proved effective in the adult population, it is not recommended for the pediatric population, excluding the adolescent, because of poor localization of infection in children (Durbin & Peter, 1984; McCracken, 1987). The recommended length of standard treatment continues to be 5 to 14 days.

For complicated infections, hospitalization and parenteral therapy are required. Ampicillin, gentamicin or another aminoglycoside, or a third-generation cephalosporin is usually initiated and continued until repeat urine and blood cultures are sterile, and the child improves to the point of being able to take oral medication.

**Recurrent Infection.** In recurrent infection, the choice of antibiotic therapy should be guided by urine culture results, because the offending organism may differ from that in the initial infection (Kunin, 1986). Breakthrough infections while the child is taking a prophylactic drug may indicate noncompliance or antimicrobial resistance.

**Prophylaxis.** Recommendations for chemoprophylaxis are generally for children younger than 6 or 7 years of age with vesicoureteral reflux or children with frequent recurrent UTIs (more than two episodes in 6 months). In reflux, prophylaxis usually continues until the child is reflux free for 1 year (Spencer & Schaeffer, 1986). The period recommended for prophylaxis to prevent continued recurrence is 3 to 6 months or longer should infections continue. For the greatest effect, once-daily prophylactic medication should be taken at bedtime. Although given in low dosages, long-term antibiotics, such as TMP-SMX and nitrofurantoin, have some disadvantages. TMP-SMX, which is not approved for prophylactic use by the Food and Drug Administration, may cause anemia and precipitate Stevens-Johnson syndrome. Nitrofurantoin may produce some serious toxic reactions, such as allergic reactions and pulmonary fibrosis. Although these problems are occasionally seen in clinical practice, they are rare. Nonetheless, the child's caregiver needs to be warned regarding these facts (Winberg, 1986).

Acidification of urine is another method of prophylaxis for UTI (see the section on approaches to patient care).

## LONG-TERM MANAGEMENT

Recommended follow-up for pediatric UTI includes the following:

1. Routine urine cultures at
   a. Two days *into* the initial treatment (usually 7- to 10-day course) to assess the appropriateness of the treatment plan.
   b. Two days *after* treatment (after the course of treatment is finished) to assess the elimination of bacteriuria.
   c. Regular intervals (every 2–3 months) for as long as 1 year.
2. PRN return to the urologist if culture reports are negative.
3. If follow-up culture reports are positive, further workup may be instituted.

## CLEAN INTERMITTENT CATHETERIZATION AND URINARY TRACT INFECTION

Clean intermittent catheterization (CIC), or an intermittent catheterization program, is a method of ensuring complete bladder emptying when this cannot be achieved by the patient because of neurologic involvement such as traumatic spinal cord injury or myelodysplasia. This method has been practiced since the early 1970s and has decreased the need for surgical interventions, such as ileal diversion, to protect kidney function. CIC consists of the insertion of a catheter into the bladder intermittently throughout the day (usually waking hours) to ensure complete emptying of the bladder.

Although the introduction of bacteria into the bladder occurs, sterile technique is not required because the patient is emptying the medium (urine) in which the bacteria grow. This complete emptying occurs on a regular, timed basis before the bacteria have a chance to multiply to infectious proportions. However, it is common for a nonsymptomatic patient on CIC to grow bacteria when urine is cultured. In these instances, urologic management depends on much more than the urinalysis and culture and sensitivity tests.

First and foremost, diagnosis and treatment are based on the presence or absence of symptoms, including fever, chills, urine with an odor, and cloudy urine. Because of a lack of (or decreased) sensation, patients with spinal cord lesions may not present with dysuria or flank pain. If a patient on a CIC regimen presents with any of the symptoms or signs of a UTI, testing for and treatment of bacteriuria are indicated. Second, if a patient on a CIC regimen has a history of reflux, symptomatic bacteriuria is treated and prophylaxis is employed to protect the upper urinary tracts from infection and renal damage.

The patient on a CIC regimen with asymptomatic bacteriuria may be treated conservatively without antibiotics. Methods used to clear the urine include increasing fluid intake, increasing the number of catheterizations per day (which decreases the time that the urine sits in the bladder), decreasing urine pH (providing a caustic environment), and making the procedure itself more antiseptic (Kimura et al., 1986).

Although bacteriuria is expected in these patients, symptomatic UTI is not. Therefore, routine monitoring with a urine culture every 6 months is recommended for these patients. Also, yearly diagnostic examinations should be done to monitor changes in kidney function and structure. Those patients on a CIC program with a history of UTI may require closer scrutiny, as dictated by their condition.

## APPROACHES TO PATIENT CARE

Variability in sign and symptom presentation is one of the characteristics that distinguishes UTI in the pediatric population from UTI in the adult. In general, the areas discussed in the following paragraphs should be addressed in a nursing interview to assess the pediatric patient presenting with UTI.

*Age of Onset.* Because of the nonspecific presentation in the neonate and infant age group, it is important to rule out UTI versus other sources of infection. An infant may present with lethargy, irritability, feeding problems, vomiting, diarrhea, fever of unknown origin, unexplained weight loss, failure to thrive, and overall tenderness to touch. Generalized convulsions with loss of consciousness, hypotonicity or irritability, respiratory difficulty, and absent or depressed primitive reflexes such as sucking are typical central nervous system symptoms in the neonate with UTI.

As the child grows older and is better able to communicate, the signs and symptoms of UTI become more specific and localized. The most common complaints are dysuria (painful urination), frequency, urgency, enuresis, and foul-smelling urine. The presence of abdominal or flank pain may indicate upper UTI.

In contrast with the school-aged child, the adolescent is able to provide specific, detailed information that aids in establishing a diagnosis. Although signs and symptoms of UTI in adolescents are similar to those in the school-aged child, the differential diagnosis involving a dysuria syndrome should be investigated, especially in sexually active females.

*Number of Infections.* Because the recurrence rate of UTI is directly related to previous infections, documentation of the number of infections is necessary.

*Date of Last Infections and Treatment Plan Employed at That Time.* An increased length of time between infections is directly related to a decreased risk of recurrent infections. Therefore, assessment of this time interval may provide valuable information to perhaps predict which children may have an increased risk of reinfection. Having information about previous treatment regimens may aid the practitioner in the selection of treatment for subsequent episodes, especially if allergic reaction or untoward side effects were experienced. Care must be taken in antibiotic selection when children have been treated multiple times. Antibiotic-resistant strains of bacteria may appear in those children who have been on chronic suppression or multiple antibiotics.

*Presenting Signs and Symptoms.* Presenting signs and symptoms of UTI vary according to age. In the neonate, it is important to rule out other sources of infection. In the older, school-aged child, it is necessary to assess the use of irritation-producing products, such as bubble bath and perfumed soaps. In the adolescent, an evaluation of the sexual activity of the patient is necessary to rule out any sexually transmitted diseases that may cause similar symptoms.

The presence or absence of fever usually determines the acuity of the infection and plays a major role in the immediacy of the treatment plan implementation. Admission to the hospital may be necessary to treat the critically ill child.

*Associated Incontinence: Daytime Versus Nocturnal.* Infection irritates the detrusor itself, causing frequent and involuntary detrusor contractions. This reaction gives the patient a sense of urgency and may be the cause of incontinence. An unusual or sudden onset of incontinence during both the day and night may be indicative of a UTI. Diurnal incontinence past the normal age of toilet training may also be associated with some types of renal anomalies. Infection and anomalies produce both daytime and nighttime wetting versus nighttime wetting alone. Therefore, nocturnal enuresis only is infrequently an indicator of a UTI.

*Age of Toilet Training and Toileting Habits.* It is important to ascertain toileting habits, such as frequency and proper wiping after toileting. Children who void infrequently are more prone to infection because of their irregular habits for bladder emptying. Fecal contamination of the urinary tract may contribute to risk, especially in girls, if improper wiping technique is used. Age and length of time to achieve continence may give some insight to the practitioner who suspects that a cause of recurrent infections may be dysfunctional voiding. An interrupted or stressful toilet-training period may contribute to the development of dysfunctional voiding.

*Associated Constipation and Encopresis.* There is clear evidence that constipation and encopresis are associated with UTI. Because of anatomic arrangement, a constipated colon and rectum may press on the bladder, causing crowding, decreased capacity, and obstruction at the bladder neck. The resulting urinary stasis contributes to the risk of developing UTI. Fecal soiling caused by encopresis is thought to provide the organisms associated with UTI in those children who are dealing with that condition.

*Current Medications and Prophylaxis.* An accurate assessment of the current medication regimen helps the practitioner choose an appropriate drug for treatment of a UTI. Potential drug interactions need to be determined before treatment is started. An assessment of the patient's and family's knowledge about current medications may indicate the need for additional teaching and may provide some insight into their learning abilities and style.

*Previous Radiographic and Laboratory Studies and Date.* Depending on the length of elapsed time, repeated or additional diagnostic workup may be indicated. The quality of previous studies may also necessitate that the studies be repeated. Parents often cannot remember the exact test name but can give a description of the procedure. Basic knowledge about the various tests and what value they have to the diagnostic process perhaps helps identify previous studies performed when information and history are unavailable or sketchy. These previous studies also serve as baselines for the identification of increasing disease or decreasing kidney function. If an infant is being evaluated for UTI, be sure to find out if the mother had ultrasonography testing during pregnancy; these records may be valuable in identifying structural abnormalities that are predisposing the infant to UTIs.

*Previously Identified Renal Abnormalities.* Because of the association between UTI and renal anomalies, previous identification of such anomalies may have some bearing on the current situation. A history of prior surgical corrections or procedures helps determine further diagnostic planning or affects the medical-surgical management of the patient.

*Allergies, Including Medications and Iodine.* It is important to determine allergies to certain medications, especially those often routinely used for treatment or diagnostic purposes. To omit this area of inquiry places the patient at risk for problems with potentially severe consequences.

*Family History of Urinary Tract Infections and Abnormalities.* Some renal abnormalities are genetically linked and may contribute to the risk of developing UTI (see Chaps. 19 and 20 for discussion on renal anomalies).

The nursing interview not only obtains the information necessary for a thorough workup of a UTI but also allows the nurse to assess the patient and family for their learning abilities and style; current knowledge base; the potential for compliance problems with the recommended treatment plan; and the potential need for community resource intervention (e.g., public health nurse, school nurse, and community physician). These factors influence the success of UTI treatment in the pediatric population.

## Obtaining the Proper Urine Specimen

Obtaining an adequate specimen is the key to accurate diagnosis in suspected UTI. Improper transport of the specimen, inadequate specimens, or improper collection methods cause most of the errors in laboratory results. There are four standard methods by which urine is collected (see earlier discussion). Of these methods, the external urinary bag, clean-catch, and sterile catheterization collections may be performed by the nurse.

***Bag Collection Method.*** It is generally believed that a urine specimen obtained from a collection bag is adequate only for screening measures to determine the presence or absence of bacteria (Kunin, 1985). Contamination is the main reason this sampling method is inadequate. With incontinent infants, urine for culture and sensitivity should be obtained by suprapubic aspiration or sterile bladder catheterization. Although invasive, these two methods eliminate the potential for contamination by inadequate perineal cleansing and fecal or vaginal flora. If the collection bag method is employed, the following points should be remembered: (1) meticulous cleansing is essential (to be done every 3 hours if the patient has not voided), (2) the collection bag needs to be removed 15 to 20 minutes after voiding; and (3) if the culture is not done immediately, the specimen should be refrigerated for preservation. Using the collection bag method has an increased risk for giving a false-positive result.

***Clean-Catch Collection Method.*** The clean-catch method is the most popular method for obtaining a urine sample in the toilet-trained child. Accuracy in the results appears to increase with age of the children (Aronson et al., 1973). Midstream collection is the ideal method after proper cleansing of the perineal and periurethral areas has been achieved.

***Sterile Catheterization Method.*** Catheterization is recommended in children who are either too young or unable to produce a reliable clean-catch specimen. Disadvantages identified with this procedure include the possible introduction of bacteria into the bladder, urethral trauma, and possible specimen contamination (although the risk is much lower than with the bag or clean-catch method). Streamlined urethral catheterization kits, which use an 18 Fr feeding tube attached to a covered test tube, may be used safely in infants or young girls. The decreased likelihood of contamination and bowel puncture, as well as the ease of performance by nursing personnel, makes bladder catheterization the preferred sampling method for many practitioners.

**Nursing Diagnosis**

The nursing diagnoses for the child and parent of a child with a UTI may include the following:

***Nursing Diagnoses Involving the Patient***

1. Pain: discomfort related to inflammation of the bladder mucosa and dysuria caused by infection.

2. Fear related to pain and dysuria.
3. Urge incontinence related to bladder irritability caused by bacterial infection.
4. Alteration in health maintenance related to acute or recurrent infection.
5. Alteration in sexuality patterns due to incontinence, foul-smelling urine, or dysuria in the adolescent population, especially those who are chronically disabled.
6. Potential impairment of skin integrity due to incontinence.
7. Potential disturbance in the sleep pattern due to irritative voiding symptoms or nocturnal enuresis.
8. Impaired social interaction due to incontinence and foul-smelling urine.
9. Urinary retention related to a lack of coordination between the sphincter and the detrusor in the patient with dysfunctional voiding.

***Nursing Diagnoses Involving the Parent or Caregiver***

1. Anxiety related to a threat to or change in the child's health status.
2. Potential altered parenting related to the effects or lack of knowledge of the child's urinary tract dysfunction.
3. Knowledge deficit related to
   a. The signs and symptoms of UTI.
   b. The possible causes or functional or structural abnormalities associated with UTI.
   c. The diagnostic procedures and therapeutic approaches to UTI.
   d. The methods of prevention of UTI.

**Plan of Care**

Nursing care is directed toward enabling the child or parent to

1. Reduce acute bladder discomfort.
2. Reduce anxiety associated with discomfort and with diagnostic procedures.
3. Regain control of voiding function and facilitate complete bladder emptying.
4. Express concerns for self-esteem, sexuality, social interaction, and the child's health related to the presenting signs and symptoms.
5. Explore therapeutic options for dealing with concerns regarding self-esteem, sexuality, social interaction, and change in the child's health status.
6. Maintain skin integrity.
7. Obtain restful sleep without interruption.
8. Verbalize an understanding between structural and functional abnormalities and UTI.

9. Maintain compliance with the treatment regimen.
10. Identify signs and symptoms of impending UTI.
11. Institute methods for prevention of recurrent UTI.

### Intervention

As with any prescribed medical treatment, success may depend on the compliance of the patient or parent with the routine. Patient and parent education is the foundation on which compliance is built. A regimen or procedure that is explained and its necessity understood is easier to adhere to than one that is not.

Teaching strategies should be tailored to the child and family's developmental stage, education, coping ability, support network, and learning style. For non–English-speaking families, appropriate interpretive services should be secured to ensure their understanding of the information presented and their informed decision making regarding the treatment plan. The nurse should also be familiar with cultural customs and religious beliefs that may interfere with family's compliance or influence the health team's approach to the family.

Ideally, both verbal and written instructions as well as literature should be provided to facilitate learning. In some instances, play therapy may also be indicated to help the child learn a procedure such as CIC. When teaching a patient or family about UTIs, the areas discussed in the following paragraphs should be incorporated into the teaching care plan.

*Recognition.* Depending on the age of the child, appropriate signs and symptoms of UTI should be reviewed with the family and child.

*Treatment.* To ensure proper treatment and the eradication of bacteria, compliance with the medication schedule should be emphasized. Often, maintenance of a therapeutic drug level must be sustained over time to ensure urine sterility. Patient teaching should stress adherence to the recommended treatment schedule despite the fact that signs and symptoms may disappear sooner. Review of the specific side effects of the prescribed medication allows the patient and family to recognize drug intolerance and contact the physician to alter the treatment plan.

*Control of Pain.* Adjunctive therapy may often need to be employed to provide the patient with relief from the acute pain of infection. Pain medication, massage, meditation and visualization, and warm compresses all are methods that may provide relief.

*Increased Fluid Intake.* Increased fluid intake enhances the flushing mechanism of the bladder. It also reduces the concentration of bacteria. Encourage the child to double the usual daily fluid intake.

*Prevention.* There are several factors that may reduce the risk of recurrent UTIs. In teaching the patient and family about these factors, family economics, dynamics, and lifestyle must be taken into account. Emphasis on items that the family considers a priority helps ensure compliance with treatment and prevention plans.

The first factor is good hygiene and skin care. Although the saying, "cleanliness is next to godliness," may not be true, cleanliness does help prevent infection. The moist environment of the perineal area is an excellent breeding place for bacteria. The most common organism found to cause UTIs is *E. coli*, a normal bowel inhabitant. Thorough cleansing and proper wiping after voiding decrease the likelihood of infection. If possible, showering should be encouraged. A squirt bottle rinses the perineal area well.

Urinary incontinence contributes to skin breakdown, and open skin lesions are a prime site for bacterial growth. The use of skin cleansers that rinse away urine residue and of protective skin barriers by patients who are at risk, such as infants, toddlers, and children with spinal cord lesions, helps deter skin irritation.

The second factor to emphasize in the prevention of recurrent UTIs is regular, complete emptying of the bladder. Because it has been established that urinary retention is related to UTIs, it is essential that the bladder is completely and regularly emptied. This maneuver flushes out organisms before they have a chance to multiply and invade the bladder wall. Patients who normally void only one or two times per day are encouraged to void more often. Youngsters with the tendency to void hurriedly are encouraged to spend more time toileting to ensure proper emptying. Using a timer or a picture book or repeating a nursery rhyme may help the toddler or preschool-aged child prolong toileting time. Blowing on a pinwheel encourages the use of the Valsalva maneuver during voiding.

Tight clothing or diapers may contribute to the harboring of bacteria and its ascent up the urinary tract. Recommended clothing includes loose-fitting garments and diapers that wick the urine away from the skin.

Chemical irritants, such as bubble bath and perfumed soaps, that may cause itching and burning in the perineal area should be avoided, if possible, by children who are prone to UTI. To avoid irritation from chlorinated pools, girls should remove their wet bathing suits after swimming and rinse the introitus.

There have been patients in whom foreign body lodgement in the urinary tract has caused irritation and infection. If this possibility is suspected, immediate care should be sought.

The prevention of constipation decreases the risk of recurrent UTIs. Elimination of constipating foods, such as apples and apple sauce, rice, bananas, Jello and tea, may be enough to change stool consistency and increase defecation efforts. Milk and milk products may also cause constipation, but elimination of these foods from the diet of children must be carefully monitored, and calcium supplements must be provided. Increasing dietary fiber content also changes stool consistency as do some medications, such as psyllium hydrophine mucilloid (Metamucil). Encourage an increased intake of fruit juices, fresh fruits, and vegetables. Problems with chronic constipation and encopresis may require a complete workup, bowel cleansing, and institution of a short-term bowel elimination program to facilitate complete emptying of the rectum and resolution of the constipation.

Because bacterial growth is retarded in acidic environments, it is also helpful to keep the urine pH between 5 and 6. Although urine acidification may not eliminate bacteriuria, bacterial multiplication is decreased, and the natural defense mechanisms of the bladder mucosa are increased. Simple methods to acidify the urine include either the use of ascorbic acid or manipulation of the diet. Diet changes include (1) increasing the fluid intake; (2) reducing the intake of carbonated beverages and citrus products, such as oranges, grapefruit, and tomatoes; and (3) limiting the intake of vegetables and peanuts (Kimura et al., 1986).

Regular urine screening is the final factor that helps prevent recurrent UTIs. Bacilluria may be monitored regularly with home urine tests or formal testing at the local physician's office.

*Psychosocial Aspects of UTIs.* Treatment and evaluation of UTI involve examinations and procedures that are painful or fearful and are performed on areas of the body laden with psychosexual overtones. Children fear for body integrity and social acceptance, whereas parents worry about long-term sexual ramifications. Use of play therapy techniques may help children master their fears and develop their

skills for procedures such as CIC. The nurse, therefore, has a key role in providing education, clarifying misconceptions, counseling the family, and recommending coping techniques to ensure that diagnosis and treatment of a UTI are positive experiences.

*Incorporating Extended Resources.* Nursing intervention among the pediatric population is not isolated to the patient and parents. Implementation of a treatment plan needs to include the extended family (older siblings, grandparents, babysitters, daycare, or school personnel) to ensure compliance and success.

Community resource personnel and professional peers, such as public health nurses, school nurses, teachers and counselors, pediatricians, and family medicine practitioners, all need to be educated regarding the importance of preventing and treating UTIs. Proper education of community professionals only enhances advocacy for the child and family.

If the need is identified, a public health referral to provide a community-based support person or contact with the school nurse to provide advocacy in the school setting for regularly scheduled toileting, privacy, or medication may be necessary. Every effort should be made by the urologic specialists to ensure continued involvement of the primary care provider. Often, follow-up urine culture studies are performed at local facilities; therefore, management and treatment plans need to be communicated clearly to these professionals.

**Patient Outcomes**

1. The patient and parent verbalize feelings about pain and discomfort associated with disease process and with the invasive diagnostic procedures.
2. The patient and parent ask appropriate questions regarding treatment options both for UTI and potential anatomic abnormalities.
3. The patient and parent verbalize concerns about self-esteem, sexuality, and social interactions in light of the presenting signs and symptoms and follow through with the appropriate therapeutic option.
4. The patient and parent state the medication effects and action, including potential side effects.
5. The patient and parent follow the proposed treatment protocol or plan.
6. Dysuria and incontinence are eliminated with the resolution of UTI.
7. The patient's skin remains intact and without local infection.

8. The patient and parent identify the signs and symptoms of UTI.
9. The patient and parent identify ways to prevent reinfection.
10. The repeat culture reports remain negative.
11. The child voids completely and at regular intervals.
12. The parent reports that the child's sleep is not interrupted owing to enuresis or discomfort.

## REFERENCES

Aronson, A. S., Gustafson, B., & Svenningsen, N. W. (1973). Combined suprapubic aspiration and clean voided urine examination in infants and children. *Acta Paediatrica Scandinavica, 62*, 396–400.

Bellinger, M. F. (1985). The management of vesicouretral reflux. *Urologic Clinics of North America, 12*, 23–29.

Belman, A. B. (1978). Clinical significance of cystitis ceptica in girls: Results of a prospective study. *Journal of Urology, 119*, 661.

Burns, M. W., Burns, J. L., & Krieger, J. N. (1987). Pediatric urinary tract infections: Diagnosis, classification, and significance. *Pediatric Clinics of North America, 34*, 1111–1120.

Durbin, W. A., & Peter, G. (1984). Management of urinary tract infections in infants and children. *Pediatric Infectious Disease Journal, 3*, 564–573.

Eichenwald, H. F. (1986). Some aspects of the diagnosis and management of urinary tract infection in children and adolescents. *Pediatric Infectious Disease Journal, 5*, 760–765.

Fair, W. R., Govan, D. E., Friedland, G. W., et al. (1972). Urinary tract infections in children. *Western Journal of Medicine, 121*, 366.

Feld, L. G., Greenfield, S. P., & Ogra, P. L. (1989). Urinary tract infections in infants and children. *Pediatrics in Review, 11* (3), 71–77.

Ginsburg, C. M., & McCracken, G. H. (1982). Urinary tract infections in the young infant. *Pediatrics, 69*, 409–412.

Gonzales, E. T. (1985). Urologic considerations in the newborn. *Urologic Clinics of North America, 12*, 43–51.

Hinman, F. (1986). Nonneurogenic neurogenic bladder (The Hinman syndrome)—15 years later. *Journal of Urology, 136*, 769–775.

Kimura, D. K., Mayo, M., & Shurtleff, D. (1986). Urinary tract management. In D. B. Shurtleff (Ed.), *Myelodysplasias and extrophies: Significance, prevention, and treatment.* Orlando: Grune & Stratton.

Kunin, C. M. (1970). The natural history of recurrent bacteriuria in school girls. *New England Journal of Medicine, 252*, 443–448.

Kunin, C. M. (1985). Urinary tract infection in infancy [Editorial]. *Journal of Pediatrics, 86*, 483–484.

Kunin, C. M. (1986). *Detection, prevention, and management of urinary tract infections* (4th Ed.) Philadelphia: Lea & Febiger.

Lindberg, U., Bjure, J., & Haugstvedt, S., & Jodal, U. (1975). Asymptomatic bacteriuria in school girls: III. Relationship between residual urine volume and recurrence. *Acta Paediatrica Scandinavica, 64*, 437.

Lomberg, H., Eden, C. S., Kaplan, S. L., Uehling, D. T., Roberts, J. A., & Schaeffer, A. J. (1986). Bacterial virulence factors in UTI. *Dialogues in Pediatric Urology, 9*, 1–8.

McCracken, G. H. (1984). Recurrent urinary tract infections in children. *Pediatric Infectious Disease Journal, 3* (Suppl.), S28–S30.

McCracken, G. H. (1987). Diagnosis and management of acute urinary tract infections in infants and children. *Pediatric Infectious Disease Journal, 6*, 107–112.

Monahan, M., & Resnick, J. S. (1978). Urinary tract infections in girls: Age of onset and urinary tract abnormalities. *Pediatrics, 62*(2), 237–239.

Mulholland, S. G. (1986). Controversies in management of urinary tract infection. *Supplement to Urology, 27* 3–8.

Neuman N., P. Z., DeDomenier, I. F., & Smellie, J. M. (1973). Constipation and urinary tract infection. *Pediatrics, 52*, 241.

Randolph, M. F., Morris, K. E., & Gould, E. B. (1975). The first urinary tract infection in the female infant. *Journal of Pediatrics, 86*, 342–348.

Salvatierra O., Jr., & Tanagho, E. A. (1977). Reflux as a cover of end-stage renal disease: Report of 32 cases. *Journal of Urology, 117*, 441–443.

Saxenn, S. R., Collis, A., & Laurance, B. M. (1974). Bacteriuria in preschool children. *Lancet, 2*, 517–518.

Spencer, J. R., & Schaeffer, A. J. (1986). Pediatric urinary tract infections. *Urologic Clinics of North America, 13*, 661–672.

Wein, A. J., & Schoenberg, H. W. (1972). A review of 402 girls with recurrent urinary tract infection. *Journal of Urology, 107*, 329–331.

Winberg, J. (1986). Urinary tract infections in children. In P. C. Walsh, R. F. Gittes, A. D. Perlmutter, & T. A. Stamey (Eds.), *Campbell's Urology* (5th ed., pp. 831–863.) Philadelphia: W. B. Saunders.

Wiswell, T. E., Smith, F. R., & Bass, J. W. (1985). Decreased incidence of urinary tract infections in circumcised male infants. *Pediatrics, 75*, 901–903.

Wiswell, T. E., Enzenauer, T. W., Holton, M. E., Cornish, J. D., & Hankins, C. T. (1987). Declining frequency of circumcision: Implications for changes in the absolute incidence and male to female sex ratio of urinary tract infections in early infancy. *Pediatrics, 79*, 338–342.

# CHAPTER 19

# Disorders of the External Genitalia in Children

∎

*Elayne C. Sugar and Christine Hoyler-Grant*\*

Circumcision
Hernia and Hydrocele
Cryptorchidism

Torsion of the Testicle
Hypospadias
Urethral Obstructive Disorders

## OVERVIEW

Disorders of the external genitalia in children are of major concern because of their effect on the urinary tract, sexual performance, fertility, and self-image. Notwithstanding the physiologic importance of the external genitalia serving as the end organ of the urinary tract, the appearance of the organs shapes the formative image of the child's sexual adequacy. Genital alterations in the child's early years may exert a negative psychological influence with lifelong consequences.

Concerns about anomalies of the external genitalia may cause excessive guilt and anxiety in the parents and precipitate negative psychological and emotional overtones in the child. Therefore, early medical and nursing interventions for these anomalies may facilitate the efforts of parents to provide a positive psychological environment for the child. The disorders discussed in this chapter include cryptorchidism, hydrocele and hernia, torsion of the testicle, hypospadias, urethral obstructive disorders, and the controversy surrounding circumcision.

## BEHAVIORAL OBJECTIVES

After studying this chapter, the reader should be able to

1. Discuss the conflicting points of view surrounding the efficacy of circumcision.

2. Develop teaching guidelines for the uncircumcised male.

---

\*The section entitled "Circumcision" was written by Christine Hoyler-Grant.

3. Describe the etiology and pathophysiology of hernias, hydroceles, cryptorchidism, torsion of the testicle, hypospadias and chordee, and urethral obstructive disorders.

4. Assess the child for indications of disorders of the external genitalia.

5. Create a nursing care plan that reflects the physical and psychosocial needs of pediatric patients with disorders specific to the external genitalia.

6. Provide appropriate nursing interventions specific to the care for children with disorders of the external genitalia.

## KEY WORDS

**Anorchia**—the congenital absence of the testis that may occur unilaterally or bilaterally.

**Anterior urethral valves**—a rare congenital urethral anomaly often associated with mucosal tissue on the ventral aspect of the urethra that may or may not produce some obstruction and may or may not be associated with a urethral diverticulum.

**Cremasteric muscle**—a muscle that arises from the internal oblique muscle, parallels the spermatic cord through the inguinal canal, and inserts on the testicle.

**Dartos fascia**—tunica dartos; a layer of smooth muscle fiber situated in the superficial fascia of the scrotum where the deeper fibers form the septum of the scrotum.

**Ductus (vas) deferens**—the excretory duct of the testicle arising from the tail of the epididymis and terminating obliquely into the seminal vesicle, which forms the ejaculatory duct.

**Fistula**—an abnormal passage that communicates between two internal organs or leads from an internal organ to the surface of the body.

**Monorchism**—having one testis in the scrotum.

**Orchidopexy**—the surgical fixation of an undescended testis into the scrotum.

**Peduncle**—a stemlike supporting structure or tubular connection.

**Processus vaginalis**—a diverticulum of the peritoneal membrane extending into the inguinal canal, accompanying the round ligament in the female or the testis in its descent into the scrotum in the male.

**Torsion**—an abnormal twisting.

**Urethral diverticulum**—a pouch or sac created by herniation of the mucous membrane of the urethra.

**Verumontanum**—seminal colliculus; a portion of the urethral crest on which the opening of the prostatic utricle and the orifices of the ejaculatory ducts are located.

## CIRCUMCISION

### Perspective on Disease Entity

Neonatal circumcision, the most common surgical procedure worldwide, has evolved during the past two decades into the most controversial issue in pediatric health care. Debate focusing on the cost, safety, benefits, risks, and pain associated with the procedure is found in professional journals, lay publications, weekly news magazines, and even in the headlines of the evening news and consumer programs.

Throughout history, newborn circumcision has been ritualized within certain religious or cultural sects; however, in this century, the procedure has been embraced without question by the health community at large and most parents in the United States. In this country, more than 1 million circumcisions are performed annually, representing about 76.4% of all male births (Davenport & Rombert, 1984). In the past decade, thoughtful reconsideration and research have been pursued to shed light on the myths that may have swayed parents' informed decision making on the issue of circumcision. The nurse is in a position to clarify misconceptions and lend counsel as parents ponder how to serve their son's best interests.

**Etiology and Pathophysiology.** The foreskin first appears during the eighth fetal week as a ridge of tissue originating at the glanular corona. It grows into a cloak covering the glans, with the epithelial layers of the glans and prepuce becoming adherent. As birth approaches, clefts form to begin the separation of the glans and the preputial tissue; however, this process is far from complete in the neonate. Fewer than 10% of newborns have retractile foreskins, increasing to 25% by the age of 6 months, 50% by 1 year, and 80% by 2 years (Gardner, 1983).

Separating epithelial tissue between the glans and prepuce dissolves into white clumps called *smegma*. In a natural self-cleansing process, the smegma floats to the preputial opening and is washed away during micturition. Smegma persists into adulthood as a mixture of sebaceous secretions and epithelial discharge.

The purpose of the foreskin is unclear, but it seems to be related to protection of the glans. Meatitis, or glanular ulceration, is nonexistent among noncircumcised infants but affects an estimated 8% to 31% of circumcised infants (Boyce, 1983).

There are two pathologic conditions associated with the foreskin: phimosis and paraphimosis. Until complete separation from the glans has occurred, retraction of the foreskin must be performed cautiously to avoid splitting the orifice. Traumatic retraction creates fibrosis leading to phimosis, which obstructs proper hygiene of the glans. In patients with severe phimosis, the prepuce may balloon during voiding, followed by delayed dribbling. The long-standing irritation to the glans may predispose the child to a leukoplakial precancerous lesion, balanitis xerotica obliterans (Bainbridge et al., 1971).

A more common complication from phimosis is paraphimosis. A stenotic prepuce that has been forcibly retracted for cleansing may slip under the coronal ridge and constrict the glans. Edema and pain quickly ensue. Relief is obtained by compression of the glans through the loop of foreskin. Circumcision is advised to eradicate recurrence of the problem.

**Medical-Surgical Management.** Neonatal circumcision is generally done within the first 24 to 48 hours of life but may safely be performed up through the first month. Beyond that age, the procedure requires general anesthesia, because the skin edges must be approximated with sutures. After placement of the infant on a restraining board, the exposed penis is cleansed and prepared. Bilateral hemostats are placed on the foreskin, and adhesions are lysed. Another hemostat is clamped on the dorsal prepuce, and a dorsal slit is made. The Gomco clamp is applied for 5 minutes to crush the foreskin attachment, and the tissue is then excised. The exposed edges are covered by gauze lubricated with petrolatum or antimicrobial ointment. Some practitioners advocate a "compromise" procedure that is completed after the dorsal slit is made.

Anesthesia has heretofore been denied the infant undergoing circumcision, based on the assumption that the newborn's unmyelinated nerve pathways make pain interpretation impossible. Numerous studies have refuted this supposition. Kirya and Werthman (1978) were early proponents of the dorsal penile nerve block to achieve total local anesthesia (Holve et al., 1983; Rawlings et al., 1980; Stang et al., 1988). Further research by Stang and associates (1988) demonstrated that the dorsal nerve block itself is a relatively pain-free procedure that does not compound the risks inherent in circumcision. Topical lidocaine cream may also be applied before the procedure to induce anesthesia, although with limited effect (Mudge & Younger, 1989).

Aside from ritualistic significance and general appearance, there are some clear indications and advantages to circumcision, along with risks and contraindications associated with the procedure. The discussion that follows is a summary of the issues involved in the debate.

*Pro*

As recently as the mid 1980s, the pediatric community refuted the claims of any medical benefit to circumcision. Two studies, by Ginsburg and McCracken (1982) and Wiswell and colleagues (1987), identified a risk of urinary tract infection (UTI) among uncircumcised infants that is 10 to 20 times higher than the norm. This risk has increased as the population of circumcised males has decreased. Long-term sequelae associated with UTI remain unknown; however, the potential for infection was disturbing enough for the American Academy of Pediatrics (Schiff) to reverse its stance against the procedure in 1989.

Circumcision is the recommended treatment for phimosis and balanitis, paraphimosis, as well as balanoposthitis, a gangrenous lesion of the glans and prepuce.

Squamous cell carcinoma of the penis, which accounts for 1% of all male malignancies, is almost nonexistent in circumcised men. The prevalence of penile cancer in uncircumcised males is 1:600 (Persky & deKernion, 1986).

The necessity of special penile hygienic measures is eliminated by circumcision. Although infants are susceptible to meatal irritation without the protective foreskin, this problem is transient. In contrast, lack of diligence in penile cleansing, because of negligence or poor sanitary conditions, has been implicated in chronic penile inflammation and the possibility of therapeutic circumcision later in life. The estimated risk of an uncircumcised male requiring postneonatal circumcision is 2% to 10% (Kaplan, 1977).

In fact, Ephgrave and Chang (1983) reported an increasing incidence of circumcision among older boys after the number of neonatal procedures had decreased. Given the harshness of delayed circumcision, this phenomenon warrants further exploration.

Psychosexual concerns continue to be raised as an argument for circumcision. In many cultures, the male phallus epitomizes masculinity. Fearing that their son may experience chastisement and feelings of inadequacy if his genitalia appear "different," many parents opt for circumcision.

### Con
Circumcision is contraindicated in the unstable or ill infant. It is generally delayed until the premature infant is ready for hospital discharge.

Circumcision should be avoided among males with hypospadias or a family history of coagulation disorders. Unfortunately, prolonged oozing after the procedure may be the initial indication that the infant has a bleeding dyscrasia.

The rate of complications after circumcision ranges from 1% to 55% (Kaplan, 1983). Both numbers are probably inaccurate and reflect the bias of the reporter. Most untoward consequences are minor, relating to minimal postoperative bleeding or mild infection. Serious complications occur with an incidence rate of 0.2% to 0.6%. The mortality risk is 1 or 2:1 million (Boyce, 1983). Possible complications of circumcision include preputial skin bridging, wound separation, inadequate removal or regrowth of the foreskin, and excision of excessive shaft tissue (concealed penis). More significant consequences, such as urethral fistula and partial penile amputation for necrosis of the glans, are rare (Gearhart & Callan, 1986).

Urethral meatitis may be avoided by retention of the foreskin. Continuous or prolonged irritation may progress to meatal stenosis, requiring medical attention.

Many uncircumcised men claim sexual sensation is enhanced by preputial protection of the glans. Without any reported studies, this idea is purely conjecture.

## Approaches to Patient Care

### Assessment
Before the infant is circumcised, the genitalia must be closely scrutinized for signs of penile anomaly. Observe for chordee, hooded prepuce, or meatal dislocation. Note possible signs of bleeding disorders, including ecchymosis in inappropriate sites or poor clotting after phenylketonuria or bilirubin testing. Inquire about a family history of blood dyscrasia. Palpate the pubic area for bladder distention, and assess voiding.

### Nursing Diagnosis
The nursing diagnosis for the child who undergoes circumcision may include the following:

1. Alteration in comfort related to the procedure and lack of anesthesia.
2. High risk for impaired skin integrity related to infection or bleeding of circumcision site.
3. Knowledge deficit related to postprocedural home instructions.

The nursing diagnosis for the child with intact foreskin may include the following:

1. Health-seeking behavior related to a lack of knowledge about penile care for the uncircumcised male.

### Plan of Care
Nursing care is directed toward enabling the child or the parent to

1. Experience a circumcision with minimal discomfort.
2. Heal after circumcision without complication.
3. Administer proper care after the circumcision.
4. Practice proper penile hygienic measures when the foreskin is retained.

### Intervention
Ideally, the parents should be counseled about the full ramifications of circumcision before the child is born, because the shortened maternity stay and immediacy of the procedure require a decision shortly after delivery. Many parents schedule prebirth conferences with their child's health care provider to discuss such issues. The nurse may enhance this process by providing literature and advice within a multitude of practice settings, such as prenatal clinics, outpatient areas, medical offices, medical or hospital waiting rooms, and the community health sector.

*The Circumcised Male.* There is no doubt that circumcision is painful and the penis remains tender for a variable time after the procedure is completed. Elicited pain among infants appears to disappear within 24 hours, whereas significant discomfort warranting analgesia may continue through the second postoperative day for older children (Tree-Trakarn et al., 1987).

Unanesthetized circumcision has deleterious effects on the infant's fragile cardiovascular, neurologic, and thermoregulatory systems. Attempts to relieve or reduce procedural pain by nursing interventions, including music, intra-uterine sound recordings, and pacifiers, have not been successful (Marchette et al., 1991). Topical lidocaine cream applied 2 hours before circumcision may reduce the discomfort but alone does not alleviate it (Mudge & Younger, 1989). Because dorsal penile nerve block effectively eliminates the pain of circumcision and poses no additional risk or discomfort, nurses should advocate this procedure as an adjunct therapy (Stang et al., 1988).

The nurse should observe the penis for signs of infection, bleeding, urinary retention, necrosis, or insufficient healing. A minimal amount of oozing is normal, but any prolonged oozing or bright-red blood should be reported. Handling of the infant should be minimalized throughout the day of the procedure.

At the time of discharge, the parents receive petrolatum-coated gauze to take home for their infant. They are instructed to wrap gauze around the circumcision for 3 or 4 days and sponge bathe the infant until healing is complete. The older child should maintain restricted activities for 2 or 3 days and avoid tub baths for 5 days. At that time, soaking in the tub dissolves the sutures. Be sure to alert the parents that the penis will appear edematous and possibly ecchymotic for several days postoperatively.

*The Uncircumcised Male.* The choice to leave the foreskin intact mandates a lifetime commitment to attentive penile hygiene. Emphasize to parents that the infant's prepuce is not retractile at birth and may continue to adhere to the glans until the boy is 3 or 4 years old. *Gentle* retraction (until resistance is felt) allows the meatus to be cleansed with soap and water; the foreskin should be returned into position. Infant smegma is expelled naturally and requires no special attention.

When retraction of the foreskin is complete, cleansing of the glans should become part of a boy's hygiene routine. This takes on added significance at puberty as adult smegma is produced. Daily retraction of the foreskin and smegma removal are necessary to prevent problems.

**Patient Outcomes**

1. The infant or child experiences minimal discomfort, based on a verbal report or physiologic responses that indicate comfort.

2. The circumcision heals without complication.

3. Parents verbalizes an understanding of home care for the child who has been circumcised or who has an intact foreskin.

# HERNIA AND HYDROCELE

## Perspective on Disease Entity

**Etiology.** In normal fetal development, the testicle migrates during the seventh month from its retroperitoneal location by the kidney to rest at the inguinal ring directly posterolateral to the processus vaginalis. The processus vaginalis bores its way into the scrotal sac followed by the testis, resting at the scrotal base between the seventh and ninth fetal month. Having completed its role in testicular descent, the processus vaginalis obliterates from its attachment to the peritoneum and blankets the anterior testis and epididymis. It now is known as the *tunica vaginalis.*

Failure of the processus vaginalis to completely sever communication with the peritoneal contents creates a congenital inguinal hernia or hydrocele. The degree of patency in the processus vaginalis distinguishes the hernia from the hydrocele. Resolution of the peritoneal sac initiates in the distal inguinal canal, progressing proximally; the proximal position of obliteration determines the extent of herniation. A patent processus vaginalis that allows passage of abdominal contents, such as the bowel, bladder, and omentum, creates an inguinal hernia. If only peritoneal fluid is allowed to pass into the tunica vaginalis, a hydrocele is present.

A patent processus vaginalis is a normal finding at birth and may be palpated in 50% of boys at 1 year of age (Scorer & Farrington, 1971). Inguinal hernias are a common occurrence among males, with an incidence of 1% to 4%. Only 10% to 20% of hernias in boys are bilateral; the remaining 80% to 90% of hernias are unilateral; of these, nearly two thirds are found on the right side (Klauber & Sant, 1985). Although inguinal hernias are present since birth, some boys fail to show physical findings of the defect until they engage in activities that increase intra-abdominal pressure, such as sports and weight lifting. Hernias are a usual component of the undescended testis.

Premature infants have an increased risk of inguinal hernias, particularly those infants born before testicular descent and processus vaginalis contraction have occurred. Treatment of the preterm infant often increases intra-abdominal pressure; the resultant force exerts further insult to the proximal inguinal canal. The incidence of inguinal hernia is directly proportionate to degree of prematurity; for very-low-birth-weight infants (< 750 g), the rate increases to 40% (Peevy et al., 1986).

Hydroceles are categorized as communicating or noncommunicating, based on whether the patent processus vaginalis allows peritoneal fluid to flow into the scrotum. Contracture at the distal segment of the processus vaginalis creates a noncommunicating hydrocele of the spermatic cord. The communicating hydrocele, also known as a *complete hydrocele*, generally is benign and resolves within the first 12 months of life.

**Pathophysiology.** Although hydroceles and hernias often are self-limiting among the pediatric population, there is a potential for incarceration of the bowel, appendix, or cecum. If a bowel loop becomes plugged in the processus vaginalis, the resultant bowel obstruction may progress to strangulation and gangrene of the intestinal segment. Testicular infarction may occur in conjunction with the incarceration episode.

**Medical-Surgical Management.** The presence of a patent processus vaginalis or a hydrocele may be prognostic of herniation. If spon-

taneous resolution does not occur by the time the infant is 12 months of age, if the hernia or hydrocele is large or increasing in size, or if the infant is in discomfort, surgical repair is indicated at an earlier age to correct this defect. A hydrocelectomy is accomplished through an inguinal skin-crease incision whereby the processus vaginalis is ligated. The distal end of the processus should be opened if necessary, allowing for resorption of scrotal fluid. The repair of an unobstructed inguinal hernia is also performed by a transverse inguinal fold incision, with identification and high ligation of the sac. In some instances, the surgeon chooses to explore the contralateral inguinal canal for an undetected hernia.

Treatment of the child with an incarcerated hernia requires prompt attention. Gastric decompression and administration of intravenous fluids, along with sedation and positioning in the Trendelenburg position, allow the bowel segment to be manually reduced. If the hernia cannot be reduced, emergency surgery is mandatory. Gangrenous bowel should be resected.

## Approaches to Patient Care

### Assessment

The child with a hernia or a hydrocele usually presents with a history of pubic bossing, scrotal swelling, fussiness, and sometimes intestinal irritability, especially when bowel segments slip through the processus vaginalis. Scrotal edema caused by a hydrocele generally decreases as the infant is recumbent, only to rebound when the child assumes an upright position. The older child may complain of persistent groin discomfort, increasing to pain during exercise or bouts of coughing. Partially trapped bowel loops may cause anorexia, abdominal distention, and constipation.

Inspection of the groin and genitalia may reveal an inguinal lump or scrotal edema, either one sided or bilateral (Fig. 19–1). Observe for discoloration or inflammation. Palpation of the scrotal contents, on rare occasions, may elicit "squishy" sounds of bowel contents when a hernia is present; bowel sounds may also be heard by auscultation. The ipsilateral testis may also be undescended. A hydrocele feels tense and full from fluid, without a discernible bump or thickening.

Two assessment techniques are useful to aid the nurse in differentiating a hernia from a hydrocele. Gentle upward pressure on the inguinal or scrotal enlargement reduces a hernia

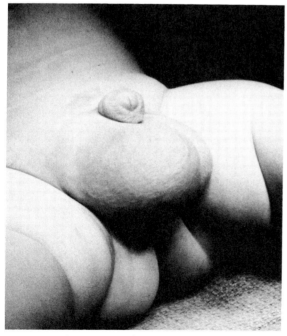

*FIGURE 19–1* Infant with a hydrocele.

but is ineffective for a hydrocele. Transillumination of an engorged scrotum discloses a fluid-filled sac when a hydrocele is present.

The traditional assessment technique to detect a hernia—palpation of the external inguinal ring by insertion of a finger through the scrotum—is unreliable for infants and young children. Because of the intermittent nature of hernias in young children, the examiner may need to rely on the historical report of the parents.

### Nursing Diagnosis

Nursing diagnoses for the child with an inguinal hernia or hydrocele and the parents may include the following:

1. Knowledge deficit related to the etiology and treatment of hernia and hydrocele.
2. Pain related to scrotal swelling or displacement of bowel segments.
3. Potential for constipation related to intestinal irritability.
4. Potential for impaired tissue integrity of the bowel related to bowel incarceration.

### Plan of Care

Nursing care is directed toward enabling the child and the parent to

1. Verbalize an understanding of the ramifications of hernias and hydroceles and the recommended treatment.
2. Demonstrate the ability to reduce an inguinal hernia.
3. Distinguish bowel irritability related to the hernia from the signs and symptoms of gastroenteritis.
4. Provide comfort measures to relieve the minor discomfort of a hernia.
5. State the signs and symptoms of bowel incarceration and when to seek prompt medical attention.

### Intervention

When counseling the child with an inguinal hernia or hydrocele and the parents, the nurse first determines their understanding of the condition as described by their physician or from common knowledge. Because of the prevalence of inguinal hernias in the general population, parents are often well versed in the cause of the problem and the surgical management. Often, the father or a close male relative will have undergone a herniorrhaphy as an adult. Rather than this common experience having a reassuring effect, the father may respond with a great degree of anxiety. Reassure the parents that contrary to the experience in adults, surgical correction of hernias and hydroceles in the very young child is a simple procedure with minimal postoperative discomfort.

Use visual aids to illustrate the defect, showing them how bowel or omentum may slip through the muscle wall defect and how the hernia is reduced. Be sure to mention that intestinal involvement may affect an infant's normal bowel pattern and possibly cause mild discomfort.

Surgery is often delayed until the infant approaches 1 year of age, when the defect is quite large, or until the infant weighs more than 10 lb. Consequently, there may be a prolonged period when the parents need to manage this problem at home. Explain that infants and children with hernias or hydroceles may experience episodic bouts of discomfort. During times of fussiness, ask the parents to correlate the increased irritability with more pronounced signs of the hernia or hydrocele, bowel straining, or strenuous physical activity. Discomfort may be managed by soothing the child with a subsequent rest period in a slight Trendelenburg position. Teach the parents how to avoid constipation (e.g., Karo syrup in the formula and gentle rectal stimulation for infants and high-fiber diets for children).

Signs and symptoms of bowel incarceration, such as inguinal or scrotal discoloration, severe persistent crying, abdominal distention, vomiting, and diarrhea, require prompt action by the parents to seek medical attention. Be sure they know how to contact the physician at any time or where to obtain emergency care.

Before the surgical correction, provide parents with anticipatory teaching of the hospital experience, including location of the incision, projected length of stay, postoperative fluid management, and comfort measures such as rocking the infant or child and use of analgesics. Most herniorrhaphies and hydrocelectomies are ambulatory procedures, unless the infant was premature or required home monitoring for apnea bradycardia, bleeding disorder, significant heart disease, or sudden infant death syndrome; these infants require a 1- or 2-day stay with postoperative monitoring. When a child has pronounced scrotal edema preoperatively, explain to the parents that this fluid will persist in the scrotal sac and take several weeks to be completely reabsorbed. Discharge instructions are minimal and focus on wound precautions dictated by the incisional covering material used and on activity restrictions for several days.

### Patient Outcomes

1. The child and the parents verbalize an awareness of the signs and symptoms,

cause, and treatment of hernias and hydroceles.

2. The parents are able to reduce the hernia successfully.
3. The parents are able to report differences between bowel irritation related to a hernia and the signs and symptoms of gastroenteritis.
4. The parents are able to comfort their child when the hernia or hydrocele causes irritability.
5. The parents seek prompt medical attention if the bowel becomes incarcerated.

# CRYPTORCHIDISM

## Perspective on Disease Entity

**Etiology.** Normally, the testes descend from the abdomen into the scrotum during the seventh to ninth months of gestation. This descent is aided by the gubernaculum, a tract of tissue containing smooth muscle attached to the lower pole of the testes, and assisted by endogenous androgens. The upper segment of the processus vaginalis usually atrophies and closes, and the lower portion forms the tunica vaginalis of the testes. When one or both testes fail to descend through the inguinal canal, cryptorchidism occurs. The failure of this descent may occur at any point along the normal pathway.

Cryptorchidism may be unilateral or bilateral. The classification of cryptorchidism is based on the testicle's location and ability to be palpated, being divided into the following categories: retractile testis, ectopic testis, undescended testis, monorchism, and anorchism. A retractile testis has completely descended, yet it retreats into the groin owing to a hyperactive cremasteric reflex. Clinical presentation of the retractile testis is demonstrated as a testicle that may be palpated at any level along the tract of descent into the scrotum. Most commonly, it is palpated at the inguinal ring; gentle coaxing may draw the testicle into the sac without tension. Most retractile testes require no surgical intervention and are consistently descended by puberty. The ectopic testis is a palpable mass found outside the external inguinal ring, most commonly in the superficial inguinal pouch. Other locations include the perineal, penile, transverse scrotal, femoral, or abdominal regions. The truly cryptorchid testis is nonpalpable because of its position along the inguinal canal or within the abdomen and therefore can-

not be manipulated into the scrotum. Intra-abdominal surgical exploration for the nonpalpable testis fails to detect a gonad in one of five procedures.

Theories attempting to explain abnormal testicular descent include inadequate hormonal stimulation, ineffective traction by the gubernaculum, abnormal epididymal development, or insufficient abdominal pressure. Abnormalities of hormone function and disorders of testosterone production and androgen utilization have also been associated with cryptorchidism.

Cryptorchidism represents one of the most common structural defects among males, occurring in 3% or 4% of full-term male births and 30% to 33% of premature male infants. Generally, the incidence of cryptorchidism is inversely dependent on gestational age and birth weight. Continuation of testicular descent occurs spontaneously during the first few months of life, until only 0.7% to 0.8% of boys remain cryptorchid after 1 year of age.

There appears to be a familial tendency toward cryptorchidism, with an incidence of 2% to 10% among male offspring (Ellis, 1990). A definitive pattern of inheritance has not been identified at this point, however.

**Pathophysiology.** Abnormal development of the testicle is thought to occur early in the presence of cryptorchidism. The undescended testis is often smaller, softer, and more ovoid compared with a normal gonad. The epididymis may be malpositioned or poorly attached to the testis; in 90% of the patients, there is also a patent processus vaginalis. Histologic changes in the undescended testicle are usually not evident until the child is older than 2 years of age, when a decreased spermatogenic count and tissue fibrosis are noted (Ellis, 1990). These changes are believed to be a result of prolonged exposure to higher ambient temperatures within the various extrascrotal locations. The degree of histologic change seems to correlate with the position of the testis—less pronounced changes are found as the testis lies distal to the abdomen. Deterioration of the testis may also occur secondary to other causes, such as a congenital malformation of the spermatic duct, primary hormonal understimulation resulting in germ cell atrophy, or anomalies of the peritoneum or inguinal canal (Kogan, 1992).

Fertility has been found to be diminished in the cryptorchid testis owing to decreased spermatogenesis, which can occur even after early orchiopexy (Kogan, 1992). Spermatozoan counts of the nondescended testis decrease proportionately with increasing age after the boy's second year of life. Endocrine function, which controls the development of secondary sexual characteristics, is usually unaffected by cryptorchidism. However, the patient with cryptorchidism is at increased risk for later development of a testicular malignancy, even in the contralateral testis (Kogan, 1992). Cryptorchidism is 35 times more likely to have been found in men with testicular tumors than in the general male population. Additionally, the risk factor for the abdominally placed undescended testis is six times greater than the inguinal undescended testis (Martin, 1982). Hernias are associated with the cryptorchid testis, and testicular torsion occurs more commonly in the undescended testis.

**Medical-Surgical Management.** Cryptorchidism is one of the most common urologic defects among male children. The goals of management, whether using a medical or a surgical approach, are to preserve testicular function, avoid damage from excess body heat, reduce the likelihood of torsion, enable the performance of testicular self-examination to detect malignancy, and allow for a normal scrotal appearance.

The initial approach to cryptorchidism is often watchful waiting, because spontaneous descent may occur during the child's first 12 months of life. Further treatment may be necessary to correct a patent processus vaginalis, if present.

Human chorionic gonadotropin (hCG), the pituitary hormone that stimulates testosterone production, has been used to correct cryptorchidism with reported success in some instances (Kogan, 1992). Treatment protocols vary among practitioners but generally include a biweekly or triweekly series of injections given over a 2- to 5-week time span. Side effects of hCG include increased scrotal pigmentation, penile growth, and growth of pubic hair; these manifestations are reversible after cessation of injections. Recently, the use of intranasal gonadotrophic-releasing hormone to provide local testicular stimulation and induce passage of the gonad into the scrotum has produced marginal results (Rajfer et al., 1986). Currently, the most useful application of hCG therapy is to increase testicular and vasal vasculature before surgical exploration of the nonpalpable testis (Gandhi, 1993). The treatment of choice for cryptorchidism is surgical orchidopexy, preferably performed in boys between 1 and 10 years of age to decrease the risk of malignancy. A groin incision is made, followed by extraperitoneal dissection of the testis and the spermatic cord. The testicle and spermatic vessels are mobilized and situated in the scrotum. The corresponding inguinal hernia usually is corrected. The testis is then secured by suture through a scrotal incision.

In unusual instances, surgery reveals a complete absence of the organ or a severely atrophic, nonfunctional, or strangulated testis. The necrotic tissue is excised, and a scrotal prosthesis will be implanted during adolescence for cosmetic reasons.

## Approaches to Patient Care

### Assessment

Physical examination is the best way to evaluate cryptorchidism. Begin by inspecting the scrotum for the presence of testicles and degree of scrotal rugae. Next, try to palpate the testis, keeping in mind that the cremasteric reflex produces testicular recoil into the inguinal canal. Several techniques help counteract this reflex. When examining infants, use a gentle milking action, initiated at the superior iliac crest and running down to the scrotum to coax the testicle in place. An effective technique for the older boy is to place him in a cross-legged position, leaning forward slightly, to relax the cremasteric reflex and facilitate testicular palpation. The nurse's hands must be warm to avoid stimulating testicular retraction. A positive diagnosis of cryptorchidism is made if the testis cannot be easily guided into the scrotum.

Throughout the health encounter, the nurse should further evaluate the parents' understanding of testicular function and the importance of treating undescended testes. An adequate opportunity should be provided for parents to express concerns and ask questions. Their understanding of recommended therapies should be ensured.

### Nursing Diagnosis

The nursing diagnoses for the child with cryptorchidism and his parents may include the following:

1. Knowledge deficit related to the cause and treatment of cryptorchidism, including the effects on sexual development and functioning.
2. Potential for noncompliance with pharmacologic protocol related to the frequency of medical visits, patient discomfort, or the occurrence of side effects from hormone administration.

3. Knowledge deficit related to the potential for testicular malignancy and the need to perform regular testicular self-examinations.

### Plan of Care

Nursing care is directed toward enabling the child and the parent to

1. State an understanding of the causes and treatments of cryptorchidism.
2. Portray signs of reassurance concerning sexual development and functioning and the appearance of the genitalia.
3. Maintain compliance with the recommended pharmacologic protocol.
4. Undergo an orchidopexy without complications.
5. Perform, or reinforce the need for, testicular self-evaluation.

### Intervention

Nursing interventions for the child with cryptorchidism first are directed to patient and parent education. Specific health care teaching about this disorder focuses on clarification and reinforcement of information previously supplied by the physician. Areas for discussion include the cause of undescended testicles, treatment options, and potential ramifications on the child's psychosexual functioning and physical development, particularly if the condition is bilateral or if the affected testis is atrophic or absent. In these circumstances, the child and parents may benefit from consultation with an endocrinologist, a psychologist, or a counselor.

If hormonal therapy is attempted, parents should be made aware of the importance of cooperating with the treatment regimen. Mention the potential for side effects from hCG and their transient nature, so that parents will not be deterred from continuing with the injection schedule.

If surgery is planned, provide anticipatory preoperative teaching to reduce anxiety and allay fears postoperatively. Explain to parents that during the immediate postoperative phase, movement may be difficult for the child; however, the pain resolves quickly during the following 1 or 2 days. Forewarn the parents that scrotal ecchymosis and edema are expected as a result of oozing and manipulation of the area.

The nurse who is caring for the child immediately postorchidopexy must be alert to signs and symptoms that indicate surgical complications. Inspect the scrotal wound site frequently for excessive bleeding. Some oozing is normal; reinforce or change the scrotal dressing as needed. Both the abdominal and the scrotal incisions should be checked on a regular basis. Monitor the child's level of discomfort, and administer analgesics as necessary. Because nausea or vomiting may occur after this surgery, ensure adequate fluid intake before discontinuing intravenous fluids.

Discharge instructions are directed to teaching parents the signs and symptoms of wound infection, including fever, redness, increased swelling and drainage from either incision, or discomfort that is progressive in nature. The importance of careful hygiene (e.g., frequent diaper changes) to reduce the risk of this complication should be emphasized. Inform the parent that strenuous activity, such as sports and riding straddle toys, should be avoided for 7 to 10 days, depending on the child's age.

The need for follow-up evaluation, continuing throughout puberty and into childbearing years, should be emphasized. Special attention should be given to the importance of regular testicular self-examination to detect changes that may be indicative of malignancy. In some instances, follow-up fertility evaluation and counseling may need to be pursued, depending on the child's age at the time of surgical correction and the condition of the affected testis.

### Patient Outcomes

1. The child or parents express an understanding of the causes and treatments of cryptorchidism by asking questions pertinent to health teaching.
2. The child or parents do not demonstrate signs of anxiety, such as restlessness, irritability, inability to listen, and inappropriate verbalization or behavior.
3. The child receives the recommended hormonal therapy as planned.
4. The child exhibits no postoperative complications, such as bleeding, infection, and wound separation.
5. The parents are able to repeat the postoperative instructions in their own words.
6. The child or parents are able to describe the procedure for testicular self-examination.
7. The child and parents are alert to resources that address concerns regarding sexual development and functioning.

# TORSION OF THE TESTICLE

## Perspective on Disease Entity

**Etiology.** Torsion, or twisting, of the testis is a urologic condition that affects males usually between birth and young adulthood. The incidence is 1:160 males; two thirds occur in early puberty, and 6 of 127 occur in the neonatal period (James, 1953). The three forms of torsion are

1. Intravaginal torsion—a twisting of the testis within the tunica vaginalis.
2. Extravaginal torsion—a strangulation of the spermatic cord at the external inguinal ring.
3. Torsion of the appendix testis—a twisting of one of the four testicular appendages.

Extravaginal torsion is most often found among newborn males, although it may occur in utero. Intravaginal torsion or torsion of the appendix testis typically presents among young adolescents.

The cause of testicular torsion is poorly understood, but elevated hormonal levels and anomalous scrotal attachment of its testicular contents (bellclapper deformity) have been suggested as factors. Torsion is most prominent during the perinatal and the peripubertal periods when testosterone levels are high; the exact mechanism that causes torsion to occur is unclear, however. The left testis, which has a longer spermatic cord, becomes coiled twice as often as does the right. Scrotal trauma may precipitate torsion among susceptible males. Worsening scrotal pain after even minor trauma requires close evaluation to detect this complication.

**Pathophysiology.** Torsion of the spermatic cord creates venous congestion and testicular edema, followed by vascular obstruction and eventual tissue necrosis. Twisting may occur intermittently or incompletely, resulting in sporadic testicular ischemia. In some instances, torsion resolves spontaneously. When vascular compromise is unrelieved, however, testicular atrophy ensues. Testicular salvage is more likely if the duration of torsion was less than 6 hours before surgery; however, when longer, the results are poor (Donohue, 1978).

Neonates who are noted to have a unilateral nonpalpable testis require careful examination of the contralateral testis. Although a nonpalpable testis in the neonate may indicate nondescent, another possible cause is in utero extravaginal torsion. The remaining testicle must be checked for anomalous epididymal attachment and horizontal lie (bellclapper deformity), which make it at great risk for torsion.

**Medical-Surgical Management.** Torsion of the testicle is one of the most common pediatric urologic emergencies. Physical examination and a thorough history are paramount to ac-

curately diagnose this condition. If misdiagnosed or not promptly treated, twisting of the vascular pedicle compromises testicular blood flow. Infarction quickly ensues and the testicle is lost. Thus, swift assessment and surgical treatment are warranted to prevent such a complication.

Typically, the hallmark symptom of testicular torsion is scrotal pain, usually sudden in onset. Occasionally, the pain gradually increases in intensity or is intermittent. The pain can occur spontaneously while resting or after an episode of trauma. It is usually localized to the scrotum but may radiate to the abdomen. Nausea and vomiting may be accompanying symptoms. A past history of similar episodes that have resolved without treatment may also be noted. Torsion of an undescended testis also produces abdominal or groin pain. Torsion of the testicular appendage produces similar but less intense symptoms with localized tenderness to the appendiceal attachment.

The most commonly occurring condition whose presentation mimics testicular torsion is epididymo-orchitis. The primary differentiating factor is age, with torsion usually limited to males younger than 20 years of age. Increasing sexual activity among adolescents and the rising prevalence of sexually transmitted diseases in this age group have made accurate diagnosis a greater challenge. In general, genitourinary infections produce fever and urinary symptoms; previous episodes of testicular pain are rare. The cremasteric reflex is generally present during infections or torsion of the appendix testis but is extinguished during torsion. Absence or presence of these physical findings, however, is not completely reliable in making an accurate diagnosis, and further diagnostic studies may be employed.

Arterial flow to the scrotum may be measured by the Doppler stethoscope. Torsion reduces blood flow, whereas circulation is increased during infections; however, this test is associated with a high rate of false-negative results for torsion. Testicular scanning, using technetium 99m, also assesses the blood flow. Results are reliable if obtained early in the disease process and evaluated by an experienced radiologist (Fig. 19–2). Most institutions are not capable of testing after regular office hours, which limits the usefulness of testicular scanning (Leape, 1990). If the diagnosis of testicular torsion is not confidently excluded by physical examination and diagnostic studies, surgical exploration must be performed to ensure the viability of the testis.

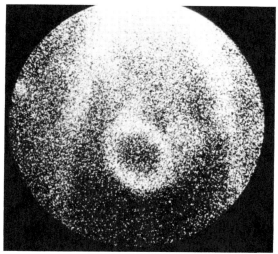

FIGURE 19–2 Nuclear testicular scan demonstrating torsion of the testicle. Note the increased density around the testicle (inflammatory response) and the decreased density in the center (decreased blood flow).

The treatment for testicular torsion is immediate detorsion of the testicle and pexis to the scrotum (Figs. 19–3 and 19–4). If surgery must be delayed, local infiltration of the spermatic cord with lidocaine may permit manual derotation. An open procedure is then scheduled as soon as feasible.

The surgical incision is made through the scrotum to examine the testicle and, if necessary, untwist the cord under direct visualiza-

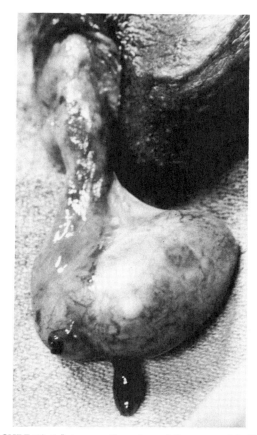

FIGURE 19–4 Intraoperative view of the exposed testicle after detorsion.

tion. A testicle that has become necrotic or infarcted should be removed. Owing to the risk of torsion of the contralateral testicle, that testicle should also be fixed to the scrotum at the time of surgery.

Treatment for the neonate with extravaginal torsion is varied. There is no universal agreement as to the need for inguinal exploration. Orchiectomy is recommended if the organ is totally necrotic (Leape, 1990). Contralateral orchidopexy is essential to prevent damage to the remaining functional testis.

## Approaches to Patient Care

### Assessment

If extravaginal torsion is present, examination of the scrotum in the infant reveals a firm or hard scrotal mass that does not transilluminate and is painless. The scrotal skin may be discolored and edematous. If intravaginal torsion is present, the scrotum may be edematous,

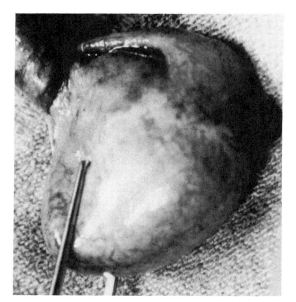

FIGURE 19–3 Intraoperative view of an exposed torsive testicle before detorsion.

painful, warm to the touch, and erythematous. The testicle may appear to be immobilized or fixed and may be higher in the scrotum because of a shortening or twisting of the spermatic cord. An absence of the cremasteric reflex is often noted. The contralateral testis should be examined for a transverse lie. Pain may localize in the abdomen and may be accompanied by nausea and vomiting. Dysuria occurs infrequently.

The nurse should be alert to the possibility of a torsive undescended testicle. Symptoms include pain, tenderness, and a mass in the groin, with a correspondingly empty scrotum.

### Nursing Diagnosis

The nursing diagnoses for the child with torsion of the testicle may include the following:

1. Alteration in comfort: pain related to compromised testicular blood supply.
2. Knowledge deficit related to the need for prompt medical attention.

### Plan of Care

Nursing care is directed toward enabling the child and the parents to

1. Understand that there is no intervention short of seeking medical attention that corrects the underlying condition.

### Intervention

The greatest deterrent to successful management of this medical condition is the child's reluctance to admit his symptoms. Because the pain occurs in a sexually charged area, young boys are embarrassed to describe the pain to adults. They may anticipate reprisal and accusations of the condition being induced through self-manipulation or resulting from sexually arousing fantasies. Modesty or fear that medical intervention may damage their genitalia compels youngsters, especially adolescents, to ignore their symptoms until the pain becomes unbearable.

Likewise, parents hesitate to seek medical attention early for fear of being considered alarmists or in the belief that a few aches and pains are part of growing up. By delaying early treatment, precious hours are lost, and the viability of the testis becomes threatened.

The nurse needs to be aware that testicular torsion is a medical emergency and that any occurrence of scrotal pain necessitates immediate attention. Because of the difficulties in determining an accurate diagnosis, a detailed history is paramount. Gather as much information as possible from the child, parent, school, or babysitter to help determine the likely source of discomfort and probable diagnosis.

When performing the history and physical examination, provide as much privacy as possible. Reduce anxiety by reassuring the child that his pain is a result of a physical abnormality and probably not owing to his own actions, rough play, or physical manipulation of his genitalia. Beyond the onset of puberty, the adolescent should be questioned about his sexual experiences and the presence of symptoms related to sexually transmitted disease. He may be more comfortable divulging this information to a male staff member, if available. The nurse must bear in mind that adolescents are bombarded with sexual messages and macho images, yet often possess a sexual understanding that is incomplete, inaccurate, or a mixture of myth and misconception. Create an atmosphere of professionalism that encourages respect, acceptance, and openness, using opportunities to dispel sexual ignorance.

In the public health setting, the urologic nurse may play a role in the expeditious treatment of this condition by ensuring that parents, school nurses, and the general public are aware of the seriousness related to testicular pain. The nurse may be influential in the discussion of testicular torsion in the school health curriculum, among parent-teacher groups, and in lay literature, such as newspapers, magazines, and health bulletins.

### Patient Outcomes

1. The child and parent seek immediate medical attention.

# HYPOSPADIAS

## Perspective on Disease Entity

**Etiology.** Hypospadias is a relatively common urologic defect that is recognized by the ectopic ventral termination of the urethra, often associated with chordee or ventral curvature of the penis. Classification of hypospadias is dependent on the meatal site (Belman, 1985; Smith, 1990) (Figs. 19–5 to 19–7). The four major classifications include distal, midshaft, penoscrotal, and perineal. They can be further classified as:

Glanular—off-center but still on the glans.
Subglanular—along the distal penile shaft.
Midpenile—along the mid to lower penile shaft.
Penoscrotal—at the base of the penis, but without a bifid scrotum.
Scrotal—centered between scrotal sacs.

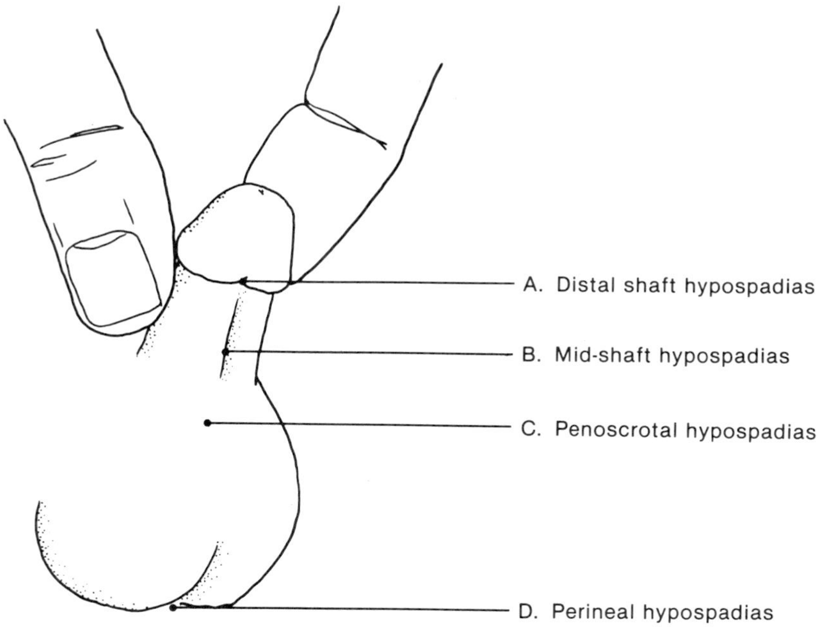

FIGURE 19–5 The type of hypospadias depends on the location of the meatus. (From Sugar, E. C. [1984]. Hypospadias and postoperative nursing care. *AUAA Journal, 5*[2], 9–14. Reprinted by permission.)

A. Distal shaft hypospadias

B. Mid-shaft hypospadias

C. Penoscrotal hypospadias

D. Perineal hypospadias

Perineal—along the perineal bridge and including a bifid scrotum.

Subglanular hypospadias is further classified as coronal (at coronal groove) or distal penile hypospadias.

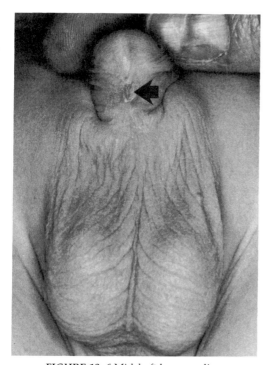

FIGURE 19–6 Midshaft hypospadias.

Chordee, by its curvature effect on the penis, masks the severity of hypospadias; it occurs in approximately 35% of the cases of hypospadias (Belman, 1992). After the surgical correction of chordee, the true, more proximal location of the meatus becomes apparent. Although hypospadias and chordee may occur independently, most defects include varying degrees of both.

Reports of the incidence of hypospadias vary from 2.6 to 8.2 per 1,000 male births. Eighty percent to 85% of the cases of hypospadias are coronal or glanular, 10% to 15% have penile presentations, and 3% to 6% have penoscrotal or perineal presentations (Belman, 1992). There is a possible slight hereditary tendency to develop hypospadias, with a 1.4% risk when the father had hypospadias and a 12% risk among siblings of a hypospadiac child (Angerpointner, 1984; Bauer et al., 1981). Inheritance is theorized to be multifactorial and non–sex linked. There is a slightly greater proportion of whites to blacks who develop hypospadias (Belman, 1985).

Studies have demonstrated an increased risk of inguinal hernias or cryptorchidism associated with hypospadias (Belman, 1992; Dwoskin & Kuhn, 1974; Ross et al, 1959). A higher than expected incidence of ureteral reflux has also been demonstrated (Dwoskin & Kuhn, 1974; Shafir et al., 1982), especially among boys with more severe degrees of hypospadias.

Much research has focused on pinpointing the cause of hypospadias; it is now believed

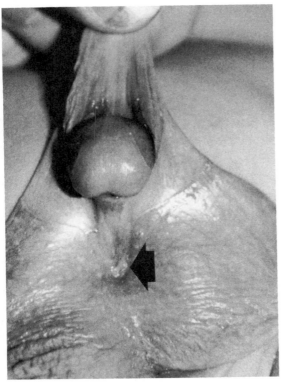

*FIGURE 19-7* Penoscrotal hypospadias.

that genetic, environmental, and hormonal influences all may play a part in the urologic anomaly. As noted earlier, there appears to be a multifactorial mode of transmission for the defect, as well as abnormal chromosomal karyotyping in rare cases (Smith, 1990). Maternal ingestion of progestin during pregnancy may also be a cause of hypospadias (Aarskog, 1979). Hormonal influences center on the possibility of inadequate production or insufficient cellular uptake of testosterone during a critical phase of fetal development, probably between the 6th and 12th weeks of development (Belman, 1985). The result is a failure of the urethral folds to fuse completely, stunting the tubularization of the anterior urethra at some point from the perineum to the glanular level.

**Pathophysiology.** Phallic development begins by the sixth week of gestation when the genital tubercle elongates and is capped by the glans. The medially positioned genital folds, found immediately caudad to the genital tubercle, are stimulated to fuse in a proximal to distal configuration. This newly created tube communicates between the urogenital sinus to the base of the glans. To create the glanular urethra, an epithelial ingrowth is tunneled into the

ventral glans, giving it a splayed appearance. As the groove deepens, the glanular folds fuse to complete the urethral tubularization. Formation of the foreskin is directly dependent on normal urethral development. Completion of the external genitalia is accomplished by 12 to 14 weeks of gestation.

The manifestation of hypospadias depends on the degree of urethrogenesis at the point of arrest. Early interruption of the tubularization produces a bifid scrotum, whereas in later stages, the meatus is found along the ventral penile shaft or glans and the scrotum is fused. Meatus stenosis is common. The ventral foreskin is absent, giving the prepuce a "hooded" appearance. Chordee, or ventral angularization, is caused by fibrosis of the corpus spongiosum, thickening of the tunica albuginea, or constricted ventral tissue (Belman, 1985). There is a general correlation between the degree of hypospadias and the severity of chordee.

Because hypospadias is an anomaly of the anterior urethra, urinary continence is unaffected. Testicular development is normal in most patients, affording adequate spermatogenesis capabilities.

**Medical-Surgical Management.** Surgical intervention for hypospadias is based on evaluation of the degree of pathologic changes present in the child. The genital structures are examined carefully to ascertain the following:

1. The direction of the urinary stream—the ability to void in a physiologically and socially acceptable manner decreases as the degree of hypospadias increases.
2. The compromise to intercourse—the effects of chordee on penile erection may make penetration painful; severe chordee with a shortened penis makes intercourse impossible.
3. The direction of seminal ejaculation—a proximal meatal site adversely affects the potential for fertilization.
4. The amount of physical anomaly—a cosmetic defect of the male genitalia has enormous psychological and sexual consequences (Smith, 1990).

Hypospadias is usually detected at birth. Because the foreskin may be needed as a skin graft to extend the urethra, circumcision is contraindicated. Some urologists recommend the performance of voiding cystourethrogram (VCUG) or renal ultrasonography to screen for coinciding urologic defects, especially in the presence of more proximal hypospadias. However, others will not perform further tests until the first evidence of a urinary tract infection.

**TABLE 19–1. Hypospadias Classifications and Surgical Repair**

| Types of Hypospadias | Meatal Location | Surgical Repair |
|---|---|---|
| Glanular | Off center, on the glans | MAGPI, Duplay, GAP |
| Subglanular | | |
|   Coronal | Coronal juncture | MAGPI, Duplay, GAP |
|   Distal | Distal shaft | Meatal-based flap urethroplasty, Duplay |
| Penile | | |
|   Mid | Midshaft | Ventral penile strip or island flap, Duplay |
|   Proximal | Proximal shaft | Island flap or free graft, Duplay |
| Penoscrotal | Penoscrotal angle | Island flap or free graft |
| Scrotal | Along scrotal raphe | Two-staged |
| Perineal | Perineal bridge | Two-staged |

MAGPI, meatoplasty and glanuloplasty; GAP, glans approximation procedure.

The goals of surgical repair for hypospadias are to

1. Create a penis that is straight during erection.
2. Fashion the meatal placement so that voiding and ejaculation are physiologically normal.
3. Devise a urethra without residual strictures, fistulas, sacculation, or meatal stenosis.
4. Fashion a cosmetically acceptable appearance of the penis.
5. Complete the repair as expeditiously as possible, sparing the child from undue psychological trauma (Smith, 1990).

At least 300 different types of surgical repair of hypospadias are known (Smith, 1990). Individual procedures are often slightly varied adaptations from an established operation, and techniques quickly change or become less popular owing to technologic advances in surgery. Because most urologists have preferential procedures for the various degrees of hypospadias, the reader is advised to become familiar with the corrective repairs most often employed by any particular surgeon.

The intent of surgical intervention is to extend the urethra, preferably to the tip of the glans, recolumnize the splayed glans, correct chordee, and tailor the penis for cosmetic acceptability. Creation of a neourethra is accomplished by techniques based on skin mobilization, pedicle grafts, or free grafts performed as single-, two-, or, rarely, multiple-staged procedures (Dwoskin, 1978). Grafts are fashioned from nonhairy tissue, usually preputial skin or penile or scrotal strips. In complicated multiple reconstructions, graft skin may be obtained from the ileac crest, the inner arm, or behind the ear (Belman, 1985).

Chordee must be alleviated to accurately de-termine the meatal site. After the penile shaft is degloved, the fibrous bands are relaxed using a "feathering" technique. Penile straightening is tested by performing the Gittes "pseudoerection technique," which inflates the shaft with a sterile solution. At that time, with an accurate assessment of the amount of urethral extension needed, the surgeon then chooses the corrective surgery.

Current procedures used most often (Table 19–1) are the meatoplasty and glanuloplasty (MAGPI) or the glans approximation procedure (GAP) (Zaontz, 1989) for distal hypospadias without chordee (Fig. 19–8), or a meatal-based flap urethroplasty for distal hypospadias with chordee (the Mustardé, or the "flip-flap" procedure). A single-staged procedure that uses the ventral tissue mobilization (Thiersch-Duplay) may be chosen to repair distal and midshaft hypospadias. More complex variations of midshaft to penoscrotal hypospadias may be corrected by a transverse island flap urethroplasty or free-graft procedure (Belman, 1992). Some urologists prefer to use a two-staged procedure, such as the Denis Browne, the Byars, and the Bell-Fuqua repair, to achieve satisfactory results. Correction for perineal or scrotal hypospadias demands the expertise of highly skilled urologic specialists who generally achieve best results with a two-staged surgical plan. Details of these procedures are found in comprehensive urologic texts such as *Clinical Pediatric Urology* (Kelalis et al., 1985) and *Pediatric Urology* (Ashcraft, 1990).

Postoperatively, urinary diversion is generally required to allow for adequate healing. Most surgeons use a silicone urethral stent or Foley catheter. A suprapubic tube and a stent that has been tied off are sometimes used in the older continent child. The urethral stent continues to act as a splint for a period after

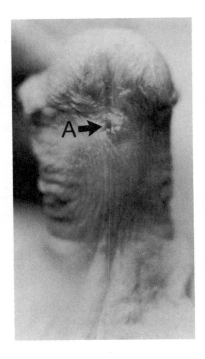

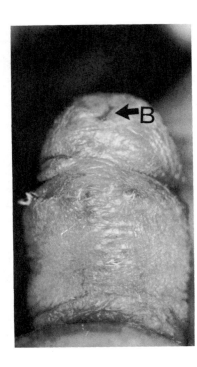

*FIGURE 19–8* Distal hypospadias before surgery *(A)* and after surgery *(B)*.

removal of the feeding tube, as an attempt to reduce the formation of a urethral stricture. Some urologists use the "double-diaper" technique of urinary drainage, whereby the child is diapered, the end of the stent is placed through a hole in this diaper, and a second diaper is applied. This procedure keeps the operative site dry.

Because of the magnitude of postoperative edema and the vascularity of penile tissue, a compression dressing is advocated. Some surgeons also insist on bed rest or activity only by wheelchair or cart for the first few days after surgery.

Timing of the surgery is extremely important because of parental concerns and the child's psychosexual development. Feelings of guilt and anger are aroused when a child is born with hypospadias, and some parents, especially fathers, have difficulty expressing acceptance of their child. Blaming themselves for producing a less-than-perfect boy, coupled with feeling diminished self-esteem and fearfulness for the child's future sexual abilities, many fathers distance themselves from their son or expect the boy to overachieve as a compensation for his "altered sexuality." Therefore, it is important from a perspective of bonding to correct the defect as early as is technically feasible. The urologist must also weigh the psychological effects of surgical intrusion on the male genitalia during critical

phases of personality development and consider the child's limitations in managing the prescribed postoperative regimen. The recommended age for repair of hypospadias, therefore, varies among individual practitioners and even among individual patients. It is believed that all corrective procedures should be completed before the child enters school, at the average age of 6 to 18 months (Belman, 1986).

Postoperative complications include meatal stenosis, urethrocutaneous fistula, urethral stricture, and urethral diverticulum (Belman, 1986). Residual chordee is a serious complication that signals the need for reoperative intervention, with the risk of compromising the neourethra (Belman, 1985). Development of postoperative complications may result from tissue friability, infection, or scarring at the anastomosis site. Scrupulous adherence to the intraoperative as well as postoperative regimen is important to enhance the surgical success rate.

## Approaches to Patient Care

### Assessment

The presence of hypospadias is detected during inspection of the penis, when the meatus is noted to be ventrally ectopic. Chordee may be present with or without hypospadias; likewise, not all cases of hypospadias include chordee.

The prepuce is hooded because of the absence of ventral tissue, and the glans is flattened or splayed. The meatus is often concealed, especially in more pronounced hypospadias. To determine the meatal location and patency, the examiner should take hold of the glans and simultaneously retract the ventral shaft skin. The meatus becomes readily apparent.

Attention should likewise be given to the external genitalia for evidence of cryptorchidism or inguinal hernia. The parents should be questioned about the urinary stream, frequency of voiding, continence, dribbling, urinary infections, and family history of renal disease to detect underlying uropathology. Palpate the abdomen for bladder distention and the flanks for kidney enlargement.

Because treatment of hypospadias consists of surgical repair, it is important to assess the child's and parents' understanding of, and readiness for, the operation. The parents' knowledge of postoperative care activities, as well as their willingness to participate in the child's care during hospitalization and following discharge, should also be ascertained.

### Nursing Diagnosis
The nursing diagnoses for the child and the parent of a child with hypospadias may include the following:

1. Parent and child anxiety related to the diagnosis of hypospadias, the options for treatment, and the implications for long-term follow-up.
2. Knowledge deficit related to immediate postoperative and posthospital care.
3. Potential for impaired tissue integrity related to urethral and penile edema and compromised circulation to the neourethra.
4. Alteration in urinary elimination related to the need for urinary diversion.
5. Potential for urinary tract infection related to urinary diversion.
6. Pain related to bladder spasms.
7. Impaired physical mobility related to the effects of surgical correction of the penis.

### Plan of Care
Nursing care is directed toward enabling the child and the parent to

1. Verbalize an understanding of the hypospadias anomaly and surgical correction.
2. Participate in postoperative and posthospital care.
3. Experience adequate urethral and penile healing.
4. Maintain adequate, sterile urine output.

5. Obtain relief from bladder spasms.
6. Adjust to altered mobility.
7. Develop a positive self-concept and sexual identity.

### Intervention
It is important for the parents to meet with the urologist as soon as the diagnosis of hypospadias is made, so they may be given immediate reassurance and the treatment plan may be discussed. A full explanation of the defect should be provided, including visual aids to portray the penis before and after correction. Emphasis should be placed on the fact that the penis is not "malformed" but is "incompletely formed." The goal of surgery is to finish the formation of the penis. The surgeon needs to candidly inquire about prenatal or familial risk factors to provide counseling about future family planning. To encourage parental acceptance and bonding, highlight the fact that development of hypospadias is probably a result of factors outside the parent's control. In all likelihood, there is nothing the parents could have done to prevent their son from developing the defect.

Nursing encounters with the parents and child focus on validation of the family's understanding of the disorder and corrective procedure. Clarify any misconceptions about the causes of hypospadias or the effects on other body systems. Observe the parent-child interaction, being alert to clues of poor parental acceptance, such as poor growth, lack of attachment, use of negative terms toward the child, and inappropriate expectations. Watch for overprotective or distancing behaviors. Because it is recognized that gender identity begins quite early in infancy, observe for signs that may signal the potential or actual emergence of a negative sexual self-concept within the boy.

Once the specific surgical procedure has been determined, the nurse then focuses attention on anticipatory guidance for the hospitalization. The preoperative orientation should be based on the developmental needs and skills of the child. Parents must be aware of the child's postoperative condition and restrictions so they may become emotionally prepared and mobilize supportive resources in anticipation of the child's home convalescence. Use of photographs, a video presentation, and an anatomically correct doll, coupled with a preoperative hospital tour, make the hospitalization a less stressful event.

Timing of the surgical correction is based on three considerations: the degree of hypospadias, the chosen procedure, and the child's age. Because of psychosexual, emotional, and developmental influences that have an impact on the child's hospital adjustment, surgery is completed before the start of school. The nurse should offer interventions to ease the child's postoperative course that corollate with his developmental skill level and emotional stage (see Chap. 17 for suggestions on techniques that encourage positive adjustment after urologic surgery).

The length of hospitalization required after hypospadias surgery varies, although technical advances have encouraged more urologists to favor same-day procedures or one overnight stay before discharge. The current era of condensed hospitalization mandates detailed postoperative teaching, because the parents assume responsibility for skilled care of the wound and urinary diversion, plus observation and management of complications.

*Care of the Urinary Diversion.* Urine must be shunted from the bladder to maintain a dry surgical site and prevent increased voiding pressures against the fragile urethral anastomosis. Numerous types of urinary diversion have been advocated, including suprapubic cystotomy, perineal urethrotomy, Foley or feeding tube catheterization, and use of a penile stent. Currently, most urologists prefer a silicone Foley catheter or urethral stent, which has the added advantage of becoming a splint for the healing neourethra. Principles of catheterization that must be addressed are (1) the assurance of adequate urine flow, (2) the prevention of urinary tract infection, and (3) proper tube anchoring (when a Foley catheter is used). To maintain the free flow of urine, the child should be offered a liberal supply of fluids, including milk, water, juices, milk shakes, frozen fruit bars, soups, or ice cream. Observe the urine for the presence of mucous shreds or hematuria that may be a precursor of obstruction. Instructions and supplies for catheter irrigation should be provided to the parents if the child will have a Foley catheter at home.

The hospitalized child with a catheter requires scrupulous technique to prevent infection, including continuous tube patency, no separation of drainage tubing, and proper handling of the collecting bag. An antibiotic is administered prophylactically (Sugar, 1988), and vitamin C may be added to acidify the urine. Urethral drainage may be connected to a collection bag; be sure it is lower than the child's body, whether in bed or a wheelchair. If a leg

bag is used, it must be emptied often to avoid backup pressure (Fig. 19–9).

It is extremely important that the Foley catheter be positioned and anchored properly. The tube or catheter must be secured to the abdomen and again to the upper thigh to reduce movement along the anastomosis site, to prevent downward pressure on the penile incision and avoid premature removal (Fig. 19–10). Before the child is discharged with a catheter, parents should demonstrate their ability to perform the taping properly.

As with any bladder drainage, the child may experience bladder spasms. During these bladder contractions, urine may drip from the penis or become blood tinged, and coinciding bowel movements may precipitate bladder spasms. Spasms are stimulated by tube movement, physical activity, or a full rectum; therefore, their frequency may be reduced by adherence to proper tube taping, reduced physical activity, and regular, soft bowel movements. Bowel cleansing done preoperatively may delay spasms or reduce their frequency. Use of an anticholinergic, such as oxybutynin chloride, after surgery is effective in managing this problem.

Minor hypospadias repairs, such as the

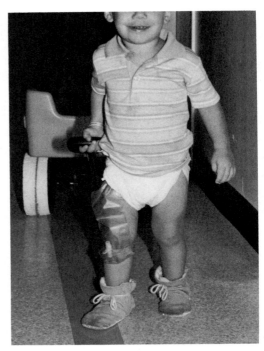

*FIGURE 19–9* Child with Foley catheter connected to a leg bag postoperatively. (From Sugar, E. C. [1984]. Hypospadias and postoperative nursing care. *AUAA Journal,* 5[2], 9–14. Reprinted by permission.)

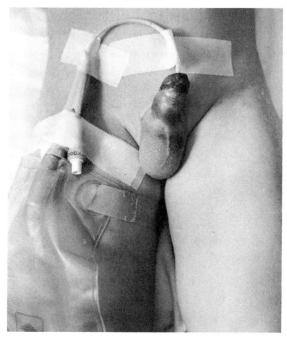

FIGURE 19–10 Proper taping of the Foley catheter to the thigh and abdomen after hypospadias surgery. (From Sugar, E. C. [1984]. Hypospadias and postoperative nursing care. *AUAA Journal, 5*[2], 9–14. Reprinted by permission.)

MAGPI procedure, use a urethral stent that protrudes slightly from the meatus. The stent is secured by two sutures to the glans and may be encircled with a small bead of silicone to prevent retraction. Minimal home care is required, except for frequent diaper changes and avoidance of irritating clothing. Showers or sponge baths are recommended until removal of the compression dressing; thereafter, 5- to 10-minute baths twice daily are encouraged. The sutures dissolve in approximately 7 days, at which time the boy expels the stent while voiding, or it is removed on the 10th postoperative day (Fig. 19–11).

*Incisional Care.* To ensure postoperative comfort, a caudal block may be administered by an anesthesiologist after the completion of the operation. This will afford greater comfort for several hours during the immediate postoperative period.

The penis is extremely vascular, and the surgical bed seeps for some time after surgery, causing pronounced penile edema. To control the swelling, a compression dressing is applied circumferentially to the penis by the surgeon immediately after completing the surgery and is left untouched for 4 to 7 days (see Fig. 19–

11). The exposed glans becomes ecchymotic and edematous during the first 1 or 2 days postoperatively, then slowly returns to normal size and color. Residual penile edema may last for several weeks after the procedure.

Wound healing is encouraged by good dietary intake and reduced physical activity. Some urologists restrict ambulation for several days postoperatively, only allowing the child to be held by his parents or moved by a wheelchair or cart. Ingenious use of diversional activities helps the child cope with immobility, for example, coloring, fingerpainting, storybooks, arts and crafts, videos, and leg exercises that do not require walking (see Chap. 17 for additional suggestions). The dressing should be kept dry until the penile incision has healed (approximately 4 to 7 days, depending on the surgeon's preference). To ease its removal, a 15- to 30-minute tub soaking may be ordered to loosen the dressing (Fig. 19–12).

The nurse should be alert for signs and symptoms that indicate possible complications. These include marked decrease or absence of urine output, voiding around the catheter despite irrigation, inadvertent tube removal, penile bleeding, clots in the urine, unrelenting bladder spasms, penile odor or discharge, nausea, vomiting, fever, chills, or pain. After early discharge, parents should be instructed never to reinsert the catheter if it falls out and to

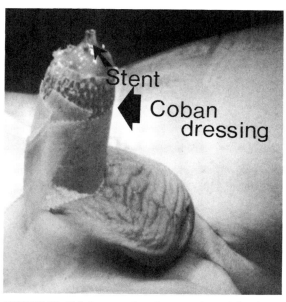

FIGURE 19–11 Intraoperative close-up view of the dressing and urethral stent immediately after hypospadias surgery.

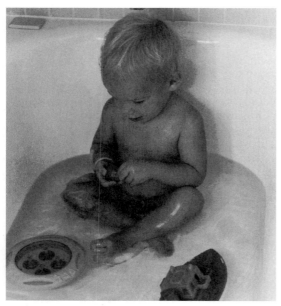

*FIGURE 19–12* Child with a Foley catheter and leg bag soaking the penile dressing 4 days after hypospadias surgery to ease removal of the dressing. (From Sugar, E. C. [1984]. Hypospadias and postoperative nursing care. *AUAA Journal, 5*[2], 9–14. Reprinted by permission.)

immediately contact the urologist if problems arise.

At the conclusion of the first postoperative week, wound healing should be well established, and the urine drainage apparatus is removed. The mild dysuria of initial voiding may be relieved with acetaminophen. The preoperative level of bladder control returns readily. To promote continued wound healing, parents are instructed to restrict baths to 5 to 10 minutes, twice a day, to change soiled or wet diapers often, and to apply an antimicrobial ointment to the incision line for the next week (Fig. 19–13). Strenuous play, such as riding straddle toys and playing contact sports, must be avoided for another 2 or 3 weeks. Incisional erythema, drainage, or marked edema must be reported to the urologist.

Successful reconstruction of hypospadias is a testament to the continuous evolution of surgical and technical expertise that minimizes tissue handling, vascular compromise, and trauma at the urethral anastomosis site. There exists, however, the potential for surgical complications, most commonly meatal stenosis, urethrocutaneous fistula, and urethral stricture, which may become apparent as long as several years after surgery. When detected early, these problems may be managed with minor surgical

intervention. Long-standing presence of these conditions may gradually undermine the urethral integrity. Parents should be advised to periodically observe their son's voiding, looking for a pinpoint or intermittent stream, hesitancy, urgency, dysuria, or ventral leakage. As the boy matures, his surgical history should be explained, with the expectation that he will assume responsibility to monitor his functional voiding ability.

The birth of a son with hypospadias confronts the parents with two issues of deep concern: how the child and family will cope with the surgical experience and whether the child's psychosexual maturation will be adversely affected. The former issue has become increasingly less dramatic for both parents and children because surgical repair is accomplished at a younger age with a briefer hospitalization period. The infant or toddler's memories of discomfort and separation from parents quickly fade, and disruption of the family routine is minimized. As the child approaches an age of genital awareness, the surgical reconstruction has normalized his penis. Parental acceptance of their son's defect is enhanced when steps toward correction are taken early.

If surgery must be delayed until the child is preschool aged, it is beneficial to have the surgery performed at an institution where his psy-

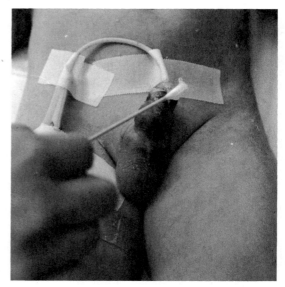

*FIGURE 19–13* Application of an antimicrobial ointment to the incision after hypospadias surgery and after the dressing has been removed. (From Sugar, E. C. [1984]. Hypospadias and postoperative nursing care. *AUAA Journal, 5*[2], 9–14. Reprinted by permission.)

chosocial needs are recognized and addressed. The movement to humanize hospitalization for children, characterized by comprehensive pre-operative preparation, liberal parental involvement, and developmentally focused activities that promote coping skills, has significantly negated the untoward psychological effects previously associated with hospital stays (Bright & Gavin, 1985; Vernon et al., 1966; Visintainer & Wolfer, 1975).

Parental concern for their son's psychosexual development and future sexual maturity is well founded, particularly with greater degrees of hypospadias and chordee. Because of the integral role the external genitalia assume in male sexual identity and the development of intimate relationships, parents fear that the genital defect will have a devastating impact on their child. The nurse needs to provide parents with thorough explanations of the surgery and expected results, along with support and counseling to allay their fears. Reassure them of the high success rate for a penile reconstruction whereby physical appearance, urinary function, and sexual performance will be adequate, given the technical advances of modern urologic surgery. Offer first-hand insights into coping with hypospadias by connecting the family with former patients. At each health encounter, the nurse should be sensitive to signs indicating poor self-esteem or negative adjustment of either the child or his parents, such as regressive behavior, undue aggressive tendencies, personality extremes, or chronic feelings of failure and worthlessness. Professional counseling should be suggested when problems become apparent.

**Patient Outcomes**

1. The parent and child are able to describe the hypospadias defect and the chosen repair.
2. The penile incision heals without incident.
3. The child's preoperative level of bladder control returns after surgery.
4. The child's urine output is adequate for his age and intake.
5. The child does not acquire a urinary tract infection.
6. The child verbalizes relief from bladder spasms.
7. The child pursues appropriate outlets to compensate for changes in his mobility.
8. The parents verbalize or demonstrate the expected care after discharge.
9. The child and parents express positive feelings about the child's male identity and emerging sexuality.

# URETHRAL OBSTRUCTIVE DISORDERS

Anomalous urethral structures almost exclusively affect males and include malformations such as valves, strictures, and diverticula. Because these defects all contribute to varying degrees of outflow obstruction, the child is at risk for urinary tract infection, increased intravesical pressure, and renal damage.

The most common obstructive disorders of the urethra are posterior and anterior urethral valves, urethral strictures, and urethral diverticula. Because the embryologic nature and the significance of each disorder are unique, they are presented individually. Nursing care of the child is dictated by the medical-surgical approach chosen to manage the child's condition and, therefore, is discussed within a treatment context.

## Perspective on Disease Entity

### POSTERIOR URETHRAL VALVES

**Etiology.** The phenomenon of posterior urethral valves has been recognized only recently as a congenital urologic entity. Incidental autopsy findings reported the presence of membranous leaflets in the posterior urethra of adult male cadavers in the early 1800s; however, detection of posterior urethral valves by endoscopic examination in a patient occurred more than 100 years later. In 1919, Young and his cohorts published the classic paper that defined a broad spectrum of morbidity in posterior urethral valves.

Posterior urethral valves are positioned between the verumontanum and the bladder neck. There are several types of valves, endoscopically resembling either a sail or a diaphragm and blocking the inner lumen substantially. Although the cause of posterior urethral valves is unclear, several theories have been promoted. Stephens (1963) has implicated errors in the embryologic evolution of the urethra and defective attachment of the wolffian ducts into the urethra, abnormal locations of the original orifices in the cloaca, and their abnormal migration. Other investigators have proposed that the lesion is a persistent remnant of the urogenital membrane or represents hypertrophy of the urethrovaginal folds (King, 1985).

No genetic predisposition to develop posterior urethral valves has been found; neither is there an association with genetically determined multisystemic syndromes. Pathologic effects from posterior urethral valves are confined to the urinary tract. Incidence of posterior urethral valves is estimated as 1:5000 to 8000 males births (King, 1985).

The broad spectrum of manifested effects in the urinary tract accounts for the wide variation in the age at which the diagnosis of posterior urethral valves is established. More severe urologic disturbances, such as oliguria and retention, obstructive uropathy, and frank renal failure, are detected during the early neonatal period. Hydronephrosis may be discovered with ultrasonography prenatally, which may lead to this diagnosis on further investigation. Milder involvement may delay diagnosis until late adolescence or even adulthood, when the discovery of posterior urethral valves emerges during an evaluation of enuresis or hypertension. Like many congenital urologic disorders, posterior urethral valves is an insidious disease. Without prior sensations of normal voiding, the child assumes that straining, hesitancy, and incomplete bladder emptying are universal experiences. Especially among first-time parents, the presence of wet diapers is adequate assurance of their son's voiding ability. At times, diagnosis of posterior urethral valves is a serendipitous hunch made in combination with observations of voiding, plus noting of prolonged delays in voiding (as long as 14–16 hours), vague complaints of abdominal fullness, stomachaches, poor appetite, and pubic distention. Posterior urethral valves may also be found during ultrasonography for another medical condition.

**Pathophysiology.** Posterior urethral valves are composed of transitional epithelium, initially thickwalled, that thins and balloons from the pressure of an obstructed urinary stream. The valves arise from a site at or immediately distal to the verumontanum, and they terminate close to the junction of the membranous and bulbous urethral segments. The prostatic urethra proximal to the valves elongates and expands, whereas the vesical urethra becomes thickened, trabeculated, and prone to diverticula (Fig. 19–14). Effects on the bladder neck cause hypertrophy; in some children, however, the bladder neck becomes noncompliant and incontinence develops.

Further effects on the urinary tract depend on the location of the valves and the degree of blockage, but they follow a predictable sequence of retrograde systemic involvement (Fig. 19–15). Reflux, a common coincident de-

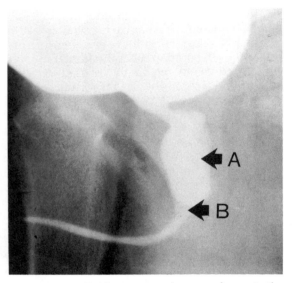

**FIGURE 19–14** Voiding cystourethrogram demonstrating dilatation of the proximal urethra *(A)* and the location of the posterior urethral valves *(B)*.

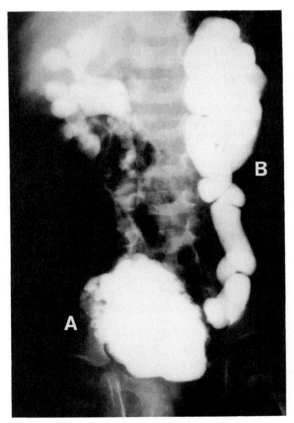

**FIGURE 19–15** Cystogram of a child with posterior urethral valves demonstrating bilateral hydronephrosis, bladder trabeculation *(A)*, and left vesicoureteral reflux *(B)*.

fect, is potentiated by bladder trabeculation and obstruction. The high intravesical pressures induce paraureteral diverticula and functional reflux. Hydronephrosis and mega-ureters are common sequelae, with varying degrees of renal insufficiency. Severe intrauterine valvular obstruction generates the classic triad of renal dysgenesis, oligohydramnios, and pulmonary hypoplasia, often culminating in stillbirth or neonatal death.

**Medical-Surgical Management.** The widespread use of prenatal ultrasonography has made the early diagnosis and treatment of an obstructed urinary tract more possible. At the current level of medical skill, the value of prenatal detection is to alert the health care team to a high-risk neonate, requiring immediate surgical intervention. Intrauterine therapy to relieve urinary obstruction poses many risks for both mother and infant, and even when successful, fails to reverse the devastating effects on the kidneys and lungs.

The infant with severe urinary occlusion develops signs of renal failure within the first few weeks of life, such as abdominal ascites, failure to thrive, acidosis, azotemia, hypertension, vomiting, and diarrhea. Fever and urinary tract infection may progress to gram-negative sepsis. Flank and bladder masses may be palpable. Immediate attention is directed at correcting the metabolic imbalance and eradicating infection. Bladder drainage requires the insertion of a No. 5 feeding tube. Postobstructive diuresis is closely monitored for needed fluid and electrolyte replacement.

Urologic workup then proceeds, including urinalysis, renal ultrasonography, and VCUG (see Fig. 19–14). Excretory urograms are not performed because the neonate's inability to concentrate the contrast material compromises a diagnostic renal image. The typical VCUG findings of bladder trabeculation and cellules, enlarged capacity, elongated and dilated posterior urethra, plus a postvoid urine residue, are hallmarks of posterior urethral valves.

Treatment is based on the degree of obstructive uropathy but most commonly incorporates temporary diversion by loop cutaneous ureterostomy or pyelostomy or by cutaneous vesicostomy. Some urologists prefer percutaneous nephrostomy or pyelostomy drainage, particularly if the infant is mildly ill and recovers quickly and if diversion is anticipated to last only a few weeks or months.

The surgical procedure to disintegrate the valves is known as valve ablation. Fiberoptic resectoscopes are used to fulgurate the valve leaflets. Insertion of the resectoscope is through the urethral meatus or, if trauma to a narrowed inner lumen is a concern, through a perineal urethrotomy or percutaneous cystotomy. Great care must be taken to avoid urethral dilatation, because overmanipulation may cause rebound stricture formation. Valve ablation is delayed for 6 to 12 months after the urinary diversion to allow for growth of the child and resolution of urethral irritation prompted by high-pressure voidings.

Attention to the associated uropathology also is delayed for several months until the organic structures are more amenable to surgical intervention. Ureteral replantation, with tapering if necessary, and vesical diverticulectomy are undertaken before undiversion. Residual incontinence may be problematic, requiring reconstructive treatment for the bladder neck. (For more detailed descriptions of urinary diversion and replantation, see Chap. 20. Bladder neck surgery is discussed in Chap. 21.)

In the older boy with less severe posterior urethral valves, the disease may surface after a urinary tract infection or with failure to achieve complete bladder control by conventional therapy. Primary treatment is valve ablation with cystoscopy. Postfulguration, a Foley catheter may be inserted for several hours to assist hemostatis. A course of antibiotics is often recommended. Success of the valve ablation is assessed with follow-up VCUG study, because a repeat resection may be necessary to completely obliterate the redundant tissue.

## ANTERIOR URETHRAL VALVES

**Etiology.** Another type of urethral obstruction is anterior urethral valves, a rare anomaly that affects only males. The incidence is estimated at 1:40,000 births (King, 1985). These valves may be located anywhere along the anterior urethra, from the bulbous segment to the distal portion.

Anterior urethral valves are often, but not always, associated with a proximal diverticulum; however, there is always antecedent urethral distention. Whether this represents two distinct entities or the variance of a single presentation is unclear. Anterior urethral valves are believed to be the result of defective embryonic development. Williams and Retik (1969) postulated that the anomaly is produced by outgrowths at the attachment site of the periurethral glands. Another theory is that the valves may be the arrested beginnings of a duplicate urethra (Burstein & Firlet, 1985).

**Pathophysiology.** Anterior urethral valves appear to be mucosal folds arising from the ventral portion of the inner urethra, assuming a liplike or semicircular shape. As the inner-lumen diameter decreases, typical changes associated with urinary obstruction occur. Initially, changes begin with proximal urethral distention, followed by a definite diverticular structure. Increased outflow resistance affects the bladder, stimulating trabulation, cellules, and distention. Ureteral reflux may now occur. The most severe degree of blockage produces the obstructive uropathy seen in grades IV and V reflux.

**Medical-Surgical Management.** Obstructed urinary stream, hematuria, and ventral penile swelling are signs that may alert the practitioner to this disorder. Dribbling after voiding may occur as a large diverticulum drains. Marked obstruction leads to a poor growth pattern, gradual hydronephrosis, acidosis, azotemia, and possibly urosepsis. A carefully performed VCUG study is necessary to make the definitive diagnosis (Fig. 19–16). Further diagnostic studies, such as intravenous pyelography and renal scan, may be ordered, depending on the extent of renal involvement.

Renal failure, if present, must be treated initially. Surgical treatment of the valves is by endoscopic resection. A diverticulum with a distinct rim of demarcation requires open resection and urethroplasty, followed by a period of urinary diversion, similar to that for a hypospadias repair (Burstein & Firlet, 1985).

## URETHRAL DIVERTICULUM AMONG MALES

**Etiology.** Male urethral diverticula are saclike weaknesses located along the ventral urethra. The cause of this rare congenital anomaly is unknown but may be the result of deficient development of the corpus spongiosum, which fails to provide support to the urethra. Another possible theory is that the urethral groove columnizes incorrectly, encasing an epithelial cyst or diverticulum (Burstein & Firlit, 1985). Although these diverticula are not a sequela to distal obstruction, they disturb the urinary stream because of turbulence and poor drainage.

**Pathophysiology.** Two distinct diverticular entities are the saccular ("wide-mouth") diverticulum and the globular ("small-mouth") diverticulum. The diverticula are similarly lined

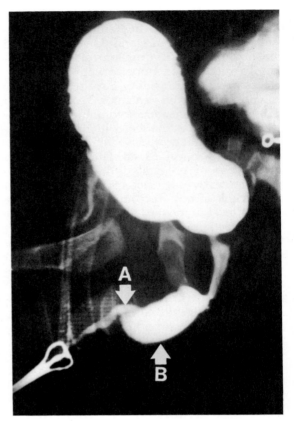

*FIGURE 19–16* Voiding cystourethrogram demonstrating anterior urethral valves *(A)* and an associated urethral diverticulum *(B)*.

with epithelial cells and encapsulated in a fibrous sheath. Their urethral attachment differs in location and configuration. The globular diverticulum is positioned ventrally along the proximal urethra, with a tiny orifice communicating to the body of the diverticulum by a peduncle. The saccular diverticulum has no true neck but rather is a rimmed opening located along the ventral bulbous to midpendulous urethra. The distal circumference of the rim may gradually become undermined and develop a flaplike appendage, which acts as a valvular obstruction. The potential for retrograde obstruction and upper tract deterioration is present, but these complications rarely occur (Burstein & Firlit, 1985).

**Medical-Surgical Management.** Urethral diverticula may be noted as palpable penile bulges that emerge during micturition. Compression on the penis may prompt further urinary dribbling. Some boys experience diminished flow, dysuria, frequency, or hematuria. Urinary stasis within the globular diverticulum may be a source of infection or lithiasis.

Visualization of the diverticulum with VCUG study confirms the diagnosis and demonstrates the obstructive effects of the saccular rim. Surgical correction involves open excision and urethral reapproximation, using a Foley catheter as a splint. Some instances of small saccular diverticula with mobile distal rims may respond satisfactorily to simple avulsion or fulguration of the valvular tissue.

## URETHRAL STRICTURES

**Etiology.** Among males, anterior urethral strictures may be congenital or acquired as a consequence of medical intervention, trauma, or inflammation. Embryologic considerations in congenital strictures suggest that they may be the result of an incomplete anastomosis between the prostatic and distal urethral segments. A soft, membranous "diaphragm" remains at this juncture (Gibbons et al., 1979).

Iatrogenic strictures may develop as an aftermath of urethral manipulation. The most frequently implicated procedures are urethroplasty, fulguration of posterior urethral valves, and prolonged indwelling catheterization. The bulbous urethra is vulnerable to straddle injury, pelvic fracture, and perineal trauma.

Within the older male pediatric population, urethral strictures may be the sequelae to gonococcal infections or nonspecific urethritis. The bulbous urethra, with its numerous mucus-secreting glands, is particularly susceptible to the inflammatory effects of infection.

Congenital urethral strictures are also present in females. Labeled as *distal urethral stenosis* or *Lyon's ring*, the stricture is a band of fibrous tissue that encircles the urethra immediately proximal to the external meatus (Lyon & Smith, 1963). The cause of distal urethral stenosis appears to be the persistence of the cloacal membrane.

**Pathophysiology.** Congenital strictures in males are composed of nonfibrous tissue remnants from the urogenital portion of the cloacal membrane (Burstein & Firlit, 1985). The irritation or inflammation that produces acquired strictures creates histologic tissue changes, fibrosis, or cellular compaction. The proximal urethral segment elongates and dilates, and bladder neck incompetence may develop. Vesical changes, such as hypertrophy, trabeculation, and reduced compliance, may also result.

Distal urethral stenosis obstructs urine flow, creating turbulence throughout the length of the girl's urethra. The bladder neck gives the urethra a "spinning-top" appearance, whereas the bladder hypertrophies in response to the outflow obstruction. It has been postulated that the whirlpool flow of urine carries pathogens from the external meatus into the bladder neck, increasing the risk of bacterial colonization (Kedar, 1968).

**Medical-Surgical Management.** The symptoms of urethral strictures relate to a disrupted urinary stream, incontinence, or urinary tract infection. Typical complaints include dysuria, hesitancy, frequency, diminished stream, and symptoms of cystitis. Relapsing enuresis or failure of conservative measures to provide urinary control may suggest the presence of a stricture or distal urethral stenosis. Prior history of penile or perineal trauma, such as toilet seat and bicycle injuries, should be explored to aid in diagnosis. Visual inspection of the external meatus, especially among young girls, is inconclusive in demonstrating distal urethral stenosis. However, distinctive findings on VCUG study confirm the diagnosis.

For soft urethral strictures, cystoscopic dilatation is indicated. Fibrous strictures and distal urethral stenosis may respond to resectoscopic splaying during cystoscopy (Farrar et al., 1973; Mahony & Laferte, 1974; Vermillion et al, 1971). More complex strictures are best treated with urethroplasty, either end-to-end anastomosis or one of many procedures advocated to correct hypospadias.

## Approaches to Patient Care

Obstructive anomalies of the urethra include a broad range of pathophysiologic changes and target organ involvement. Urinary tract consequences range from minor bladder dysfunction (incontinence, urgency, or small residual volumes) to severe obstructive uropathology, possibly culminating in death from renal-pulmonary failure.

Medical management for the child is dictated by not only correction of the organic anomaly but also the alleviation of the systemic effects. Therapeutic intervention often assumes a "symptom approach" (a generic protocol of treatment determined by the degree of disease) to target organs rather than the underlying defect. Consequently, medical therapy for the various urethral obstructive disorders may be identical to treatment of vesical or upper urinary tract obstruction, including replantation, vesical diverticulectomy, or urinary diversion.

The nursing approach is dictated more by the particular surgical intervention chosen to alleviate the child's symptoms than by the specific diagnosis. The nursing goals, diagnoses, and implementations mimic those of other urinary obstructive disorders or urethral anomalies. Therefore, the reader is directed to other parts of this text for a complete description of the nursing care of a child with the following disorders:

Vesicoureteral reflux—see Chapter 20
Hydronephrosis and obstructive uropathy—see Chapter 20
Bladder neck decompensation—see Chapter 21
Continence disorder—see Chapter 22
Urethral anomaly requiring urethroplasty—see the section on hypospadias in this chapter

## CONCLUSION

Surgical correction of disorders of the external genitalia in children must be handled delicately by the health care professional. Understanding the disease entities, performing a thorough assessment, and providing appropriate treatment and compassionate nursing care to meet the physical and psychological needs of the child are paramount to the child's healthy recovery and his or her future growth and development. If the anxiety of the parent and the child becomes excessive, the guilt, embarrassment, and misunderstanding may leave permanent effects on the child's personality development. A supportive environment, reassurance, comfort, and adequate explanations allow the child and the family greater capacity for understanding and coping with the illness and treatment. Awareness of the possible reactions that children with disorders of the external genitalia may demonstrate is absolutely essential in planning the care of such children. The collaborative efforts of the health team and the family benefit the child's emotional development and assist in coping with the stresses of treating children with disorders of the external genitalia.

## REFERENCES

Aarskog, D. (1979). Maternal progestins as a possible cause of hypospadias. *New England Journal of Medicine, 300*(2), 75–78.

Angerpointner, T. (1984). Hypospadias: Genetics, epidemiology and other aetiological influences. *Zeitschrift Fur Kinderchirurgie, 39*(2), 112–118.

Ashcraft, K. W. (1990). *Pediatric Urology.* Philadelphia: W. B. Saunders.

Bainbridge, D. R., Whitaker, R. H., & Shepheard, B. G. F. (1971). Balanitis xerotica obliterans and urinary obstruction. *British Journal of Urology, 43*, 487.

Bauer, S., Retik, A., & Colodny, A. (1981). Genetic aspects of hypospadias. *Urologic Clinics of North America, 8*(3), 559–564.

Belman, A. (1985). Urethra. In P. P. Kelalis, L. R. King, & A. B. Belman (Eds.), *Clinical pediatric urology* (2nd ed., pp. 751–792). Philadelphia: W. B. Saunders.

Belman, B. (1986). Hypospadias. In K. Welch, et al. (Eds.), *Pediatric surgery* (4th ed., pp. 1286–1302). Chicago: Year Book Medical Publishers.

Belman, B. (1992). Hypospadias and other urethral abnormalities. In P. P. Kelalis, L. R. King, & A. B. Belman (Eds.), *Clinical pediatric urology* (3rd ed., pp. 619–663). Philadelphia: W. B. Saunders.

Boyce, W. (1983). Care of the foreskin. *Pediatrics in Review, 5*:1, 26–30.

Bright, C., & Gavin, K. (1985). *Post-hospital adjustment following urologic surgery.* Research presented in Meeting of the American Urologic Association Allied. Atlanta, May 1985.

Burstein, J., & Firlit, C. (1985). Anterior urethra. In P. P. Kelalis, L. R. King, & A. B. Belman (Eds.), *Clinical pediatric urology* (2nd ed., pp. 558–581). Philadelphia: W. B. Saunders.

Davenport, C., & Romberg, R. (1984). Hospital survey of circumcision rates in the United States. *Birth, 11*(4), 247–250.

Donohue, R., & Utley, W. (1978). Torsion of the spermatic cord. *Urology, 11*(1), 33–36.

Dwoskin, J. Y. (1978). Hypospadias. *Urologic Clinics of North America, 5*(1), 95–105.

Dwoskin, J. Y., & Kuhn, J. (1974). Herniograms and hypospadias. *Urology, 4*, 458–460.

Ellis, D. (1990). Undescended testes: Cryptorchidism. In K. Ashcraft (Ed.), *Pediatric urology* (pp. 415–427). Philadelphia: W. B. Saunders.

Ephgrave, K., & Chang, J. (1983). Pediatric circumcision revisited. *Texas Medicine, 79*, 62–65.

Farrar, D., Green, N., & Ashken, M. (1973). An evaluation of otis urethrotomy in female patients with recurrent urinary tract infections. *British Journal of Urology, 45*, 610–615.

Gandhi, K., & Maizels, M. (1993). Management of the undescended testis. *Comprehensive Therapy, 19*(1), 3–7.

Gardner, D. (1983). The fate of the foreskin: A study of circumcision. *British Medical Journal, 2*, 1433–1437.

Gearhart, J. P., & Callan, N. A. (1986). Complications of newborn circumcision. *Contemporary OB/GYN, 27*, 57–68.

Gibbons, M., Koontz, W., & Smith, J. (1979). Urethral strictures in boys. *Journal of Urology, 121*, 220.

Ginsburg, C., & McCracken, G. (1982). Urinary tract infections in young infants. *Pediatrics, 69*, 409.

Holve, R., Bromberger, P., Groveman, H., Klauber, M., Dixon, S., & Snyder, J. (1983). Regional anesthesia during newborn circumcision. *Clinical Pediatrics, 22*, 813–818.

James, T. (1953). Torsion of the spermatic cord in the first year of life. *British Journal of Urology, 25*, 56.

Kaplan, G. (1977). Circumcision: An overview. *Current Problems in Pediatrics, 73*, 3.

Kaplan, G. (1983). Complications of circumcision. *Urologic Clinics of North America, 10*, 543–549.

Kedar, S. (1968). The urethra in the female child. *British Journal of Urology, 40*, 441–444.

Kelalis, P., King, L., & Belman, A. (1985). Clinical pediatric urology (2nd ed.). Philadelphia: W. B. Saunders.

King, L. (1985). Posterior urethra. In P. P. Kelalis, L. R. King, & A. B. Belman (Eds.), *Clinical pediatric urology* (2nd ed., pp. 527–558). Philadelphia: W. B. Saunders.

Kirya, C., & Werthman, M. (1978). Neonatal circumcision

and penile dorsal block: A painless procedure. *Journal of Pediatrics, 96*, 998–1000.

Klauber, G., & Sant, G. (1985). Disorders of the male external genitalia. In P. P. Kelalis, L. R. King, & A. B. Belman (Eds.), *Clinical pediatric urology* (2nd ed., pp. 825–863). Philadelphia: W. B. Saunders.

Kogan, S. (1992). Cryptorchidism. In P. P. Kelalis, L. R. King, & A. B. Belman (Eds.), *Clinical pediatric urology* (3rd ed., pp. 1050–1083). Philadelphia: W. B. Saunders.

Leape, L. (1990). Testicular torsion. In K. Ashcraft (Ed.), *Pediatric urology* (pp. 429–436). Philadelphia: W. B. Saunders.

Lyon, R., & Smith, D. (1963). Distal urethral stenosis. *Journal of Urology, 45*, 610–615.

Mahony, D., & Laferte, R. (1974). Studies of enuresis: VII. Results of distal internal urethrotomy in girls with juvenile urinary incontinence. *Urology, 4*(2), 162–172.

Marchette, L., Main, R., Redick, E., Bagy, C., & Leatherleand, J. (1991). Pain reduction interventions during neonatal circumcision. *Nursing Research, 40*(4), 241–244.

Martin, D. (1982). Malignancy in the cryptorchid testis. *Urologic Clinics of North America, 9*(3), 371–376.

Mudge, D., & Younger, J. (1989). The effects of topical lidocaine on infant response to circumcision. *Journal of Nurse-Midwifery, 34*(6), 335–340.

Peevy, K., Speed, F., & Hoff, C. (1986). Epidemiology of inguinal hernia in preterm neonates. *Pediatrics, 77*(2), 246.

Persky, L., & deKernion, J. (1986). Carcinoma of the penis. *CA, 36*, 258–273.

Rajfer J., Handelsman, D. J., Swerdloff, R. S., Hurwitz, R., Kaplan, H., Vandergast, T., & Ehrlich, R. M. (1986). Hormonal therapy of cryptorchidism: A randomized, double-blind study comparing human chorionic gonadotropin and gonadotropin-releasing hormone. *New England Journal of Medicine, 314*(8), 466–470.

Rawlings, D., Miller, P., & Engel, R. (1980). The effect of circumcision on transcutaneous $PO_2$ in term infants. *American Journal of Diseases in Children, 134*, 676–678.

Ross, J., Farmer, A., & Lindsay, W. (1959). Hypospadias: A review of 230 cases. *Plastic Reconstructive Surgery, 24*, 357–368.

Shafir, R., Hortz, M., Bocchis, H., Tam, H., Aladjam, M., & Jonas P. (1982). Vesico-ureteral reflux in boys with hypospadias. *Urology, 20*(1), 29–30.

Schiff, D. (1989). *AAP member alert.* Elk Grove Village, IL: American Academy of Pediatrics.

Scorer, C. G., & Farrington, G. H. (1971). *Congenital deformities of the testis and epididymis.* New York: Appleton-Century-Crofts.

Smith, E. (1990). Hypospadias. In K. Ashcraft (Ed.), *Pediatric urology* (pp. 353–395). Philadelphia: W. B. Saunders.

Stang, H., Gunner, M., Svellsman, L., Condon, L., & Kestenbaum, R. (1988). Local anesthesia for neonatal circumcision. *Journal of the American Medical Association, 259*, 1507–1509.

Stephens, F. (1963). *Congenital malformations of the rectum, anus, and genitourinary tract* (pp. 219–245). Edinburgh: E&S Livingstone.

Sugar, E. (1984). Hypospadias and postoperative nursing care. *AUAA Journal, 5*(2), 9–14.

Sugar, E., & Firlit, C. (1988). Urinary prophylaxis and postoperative care of children after hypospadias repair. *Urology, 32*(5), 418–420.

Tree-Tarkarn, T., Parayavaraporn, S., & Lutakyamenee, J. (1987). Topical analgesia for relief of post-circumcision pain. *Anesthesiology, 67*, 395–399.

Vermillion, C. Halvestadt, D., & Leadbetter, G. (1971). Internal urethrotomy and recurrent urinary tract in female children: II. Long-term results in the management of infection. *Journal of Urology, 106*, 154–157.

Vernon, D., Schulman, J., & Foley, J. (1966). Changes in children's behavior after hospitalization. *American Journal of Diseases in Children, 111*, 581–593.

Visintainer, M., & Wolfer, J. (1975). Psychological preparation for surgical pediatric patients: The effect on children's and parents' stress responses and adjustment. *Pediatrics, 56*, 187–202.

Williams, D., & Retik, A. (1969). Congenital valves and diverticula of the anterior urethra. *British Journal of Urology, 41*, 228.

Wiswell, T., Engenauer, R., Cornish, J., & Hankins, C. (1987). Declining frequency of circumcision: Implications for changes in the absolute incidence and male to female ratio of urinary tract infections in early infancy. *Pediatrics, 79*(3), 338–343.

Young, H., Frontz, W., & Baldwin, J. (1919). Congenital obstruction of the posterior urethra. *Journal of Urology, 3*, 289–292.

Zaontz, M. (1989). GAP (glans approximation procedure) for glanular/coronal hypospadias. *Journal of Urology, 141*, 359–361.

# CHAPTER 20

# Congenital Anomalies That Affect the Kidney, Ureter, and Bladder

■

*Barbara Montagnino, Valre W. Welch,*
*and Christine Hoyler-Grant*

## OVERVIEW

Congenital anomalies that affect the kidney, ureter, and bladder involve a wide spectrum of defects. Abnormalities of the renal unit range from complete absence of the organ to structural malformation or ectopia. Defects of the ureter include obstruction, duplication, and termination anomalies. The classic triad of flaccid abdominal musculature, vesical anomalies, and genital defects comprise the complex disorder known as prune belly syndrome. Physiologic effects from these anomalies vary greatly; in some cases, their detection is merely a serendipitous radiologic finding, whereas in others, the defect is incompatible with life.

Current advances in medical technology, in particular the prenatal detection of urinary tract anomalies, afford the nurse an earlier opportunity to meet with parents and plan for the anticipated needs of their child. The goals of early nursing intervention are, therefore, to offer teaching and support to parents and to enhance their decision-making skills concerning the health care needs for their child who will be born with a defective urinary tract.

This chapter familiarizes the nurse with the various congenital abnormalities that may occur in the upper or lower urinary tract, followed by discussions to help the nurse appreciate the clinical significance of each disorder, the medical-surgical approach to disease management, and the plan for nursing care, which incorporates the needs of the child and family.

## BEHAVIORAL OBJECTIVES

After studying this chapter, the reader should be able to

1. Discuss the role of prenatal testing in diagnosing congenital upper urinary tract disorders.

2. Identify diagnostic criteria or physiologic signs that suggest anomalies that affect the upper or lower urinary tract in children.

3. Implement a plan of nursing care for the child undergoing corrective intervention to treat a congenital urologic condition of the kidney or upper urinary tract, incorporating patient and family needs.

4. Create strategies for child-parent education that anticipate immediate and long-term health care requirements and promote home management of a congenital urologic disorder.

## KEY WORDS

**Ectopic ureter**—an abnormal termination of the distal ureter outside the bladder trigone; the ureter may empty into the urethra, vagina, or rectum, but rarely into the cervix or ureters, seminal vesicles, vas deferens, or epididymis.

**Hypoplastic kidney**—a renal unit with reduced numbers of nephrons or cells.

**Multicystic kidney**—unilateral renal dysplasia characterized by numerous cysts, ranging from microscopic to massive in size, which are destructive to functional units of the kidney.

**Nephrectomy**—the surgical removal of the kidney.

**Polycystic kidney**—a hereditary renal disorder, usually occurring bilaterally, highlighted by pockets of cystic development within the nephron.

**Potter's facies**—the characteristic appearance of infants with renal agenesis, consisting of flattened face,

blunted nose, prominent fold and skin crease beneath each eye, hypertelorism, prominent depression between the lower lip and chin, and low-set ears.

**Renal agenesis**—the complete absence of kidney; may be unilateral or bilateral.

**Renal aplasia**—a severe form of dysplasia, characterized by a scant cluster of nonfunctional tissue.

**Renal atrophy**—the involution of a normal kidney as a reaction to infection or ischemia.

**Renal dysplasia**—kidneys that contain primitive structures; these structures may be localized to focal areas or to a specific segment, or they may infiltrate the total organ.

**Renal ectopia**—the failure of the mature kidney to reach its normal location.

**Renal ultrasound**—a noninvasive study using sound waves to examine the anatomy of the upper urinary tract.

**Urachus**—a fibrous cord that extends from the dome of the bladder to the umbilicus.

**Ureterocele**—a saclike engorgement of the terminal segment of ureter, resulting from stenosis of the ureteral meatus (the terminal ureter is sandwiched within the layers of the bladder muscle).

**Ureteroneocystostomy (ureteral reimplantation)**—surgical transplantation of the ureter to a different site in the bladder.

**Ureterovesical junction (UVJ)**—the point at which the ureter inserts into the bladder muscle; normally, the terminal segment is sandwiched within layers of vesical musculature.

**Vesicoureteral reflux**—the regurgitation of urine from the bladder into the ureter due to an incompetent valve mechanism at the ureterovesical junction.

**Voiding cystourethrogram (VCUG)**—the radiographic study of the bladder, in which contrast material is instilled into the bladder and the lower urinary tract is visualized during voiding.

## DISORDERS OF THE KIDNEY

Abnormal renal development is termed *renal dysgenesis;* this label is applied to a broad spectrum of clinically defined disease states identifiable by microscopically incomplete or pathologic renal structures. Dysgenetic entities are grouped by results of histologic examination, disease states, and genetic influence to overcome the confusion caused by morphologic similarities among the various renal conditions.

*Renal dysplasia* applies to kidneys that contain primitive structures. Clinical expression of dysplasia is not uniform; in fact, by gross appearance these kidneys may look normal or be obviously malformed, range in size from subnormal to massive, and contain large cysts, microcysts, or no cysts. Dysplasia may be limited to focal areas of the renal unit or a kidney segment, or it may affect the total organ. The most extreme form of dysplasia is *aplasia*, characterized by a "nubbin" of nonfunctional renal mass.

*Renal hypoplasia* signifies a renal unit with reduced numbers of nephrons or cells. Although renal dysplasia always includes renal hypoplasia (hence the more accurate label *hypodysplasia*), the opposite is not true. In renal hypoplasia, nephrons function normally and are anatomically mature.

The congenital absence of kidney tissue is *renal agenesis. Renal atrophy* represents a normally developed kidney that undergoes involution secondary to insult by infection or ischemia.

Among the pediatric population, renal dysplasia is categorized as either renal hypodysplasia or renal cystic disease. Two clinically distinct presentations of renal cystic disease are differentiated by inheritance: genetic transmission causes autosomal recessive polycystic kidney disease, whereas multicystic dysplasia of the kidney has no genetic predetermination.

### Unilateral or Bilateral Renal Agenesis

#### PERSPECTIVE ON DISEASE ENTITY

**Etiology.** Renal agenesis is a result of the failure of the ureteral bud to develop from the wolffian duct, leading to absence of the kidney and its corresponding ureter. This happens at about the 24th to 26th day of gestation. Renal agenesis, a rare anomaly, has a familial predisposition (Kohn & Borns, 1973; Rizza & Downing, 1971; Winter et al., 1968). Reports of unilateral renal agenesis disclose an incidence that ranges from 1:450 to 1:1800 live births. However, these statistics may be misleadingly low, because the anomaly can remain undetected unless discovered during the evaluation of other congenital anomalies (such as skeletal, cardiovascular, gastrointestinal, and genital defects) (Fig. 20–1).

Bilateral renal agenesis, a condition incompatible with life, has a less frequent incidence. Estimates place its occurrence at 1:4800 births

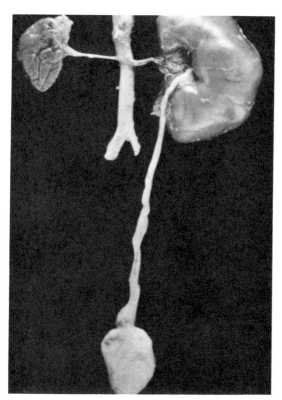

FIGURE 20–1 Unilateral renal agenesis. (From Kelalis, P., King, L. R., & Belman, A. B. [Eds.] [1985]. *Clinical pediatric urology* [p. 645]. Philadelphia: W. B. Saunders. Reprinted by permission.)

often bowed with club feet. Potter's syndrome appears to be triggered by oligohydramnios, which results from the intrauterine nonproduction of urine. The effects of bilateral renal agenesis are devastating; nearly 40% of infants are stillborn. Of the remaining live births, most succumb within 48 hours owing to respiratory insufficiency secondary to pulmonary hypoplasia, another feature of Potter's syndrome. Those infants who survive this period die within days or weeks, depending on the rate at which renal failure progresses.

Unilateral renal agenesis occurs more often in males; corresponding urologic defects may include ipsilateral absence of the vas deferens, testicular hypoplasia or anorchism, or possibly hypospadias. Females with unilateral agenesis may likewise be diagnosed because of associated defects to their external reproductive organs, such as vaginal absence or aplasia. Other genital anomalies may include unicornuate or bicornuate uteri, hypoplastic ovaries or tubes, and uterine hypoplasia. Genital anomalies are present in females four times more frequently than in males, at a rate of 44% compared with 12%, respectively (Thompson & Lynn, 1966).

Hypertrophy of the solitary kidney compensates to maintain adequate renal function; how-

(Potter, 1965). Males are affected more frequently, with a male to female ratio of 3:1.

A familial tendency exists for both unilateral and bilateral renal agenesis, although the route of genetic transmission and rate of occurrences are unknown. Of all children found to have unilateral renal agenesis, 40% are diagnosed by 1 year of age and another 35% before their fifth birthday.

**Pathophysiology.** The kidneys are completely absent in the child with bilateral renal agenesis. Ureters are either wholly or partially absent, and the bladder is dysplastic. Renal umbilical vessels likewise are totally absent. Children with bilateral renal agenesis also develop Potter's syndrome, easily identifiable by the characteristic "Potter's facies" (Fig. 20–2). Facial features include increased width between the eyes; flattening and broadening of the nose; large, low-set ears; and an unusually prominent fold arising from the inner canthus. The infant's appearance resembles that of premature aging, with excessive dry and loose skin. The hands are spadelike, and the legs are

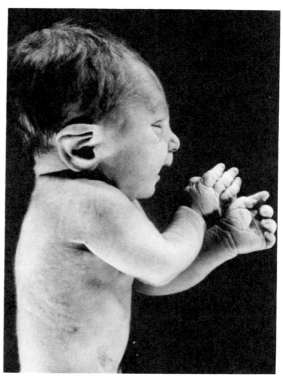

FIGURE 20–2 Potter's facies.

ever, this kidney is at increased risk to develop pathologic changes, particularly ectopia and malrotation. This risk is specific to the congenitally solitary kidney, not to the unilateral kidney, which is acquired as a result of nephrectomy.

Unilateral renal agenesis may be detected during evaluative studies for congenital syndromes such as Turner's, Klippel-Feil, or fetal alcohol syndromes, or in children with numerous vertebral or long bone defects, cardiovascular malformations, gastrointestinal abnormalities, or "dysmorphogenesis" (a collective spectrum of defects involving all three systems). Belman and King (1972) reported a high association of renal agenesis with imperforate anus or scoliosis. Radiologic clues that suggest renal agenesis may be found on a flat-plate examination of the abdomen. Radionuclide studies or ultrasonography confirm the absence of the renal unit. Incomplete development of the trigone, an incidental finding during cystoscopy, would suggest ipsilateral renal agenesis.

**Medical-Surgical Management.** For the infant born with bilateral renal agenesis, medical care is supportive. In the absence of adequate renal function, the life expectancy of the anephric child is only a few days or weeks. Many of these children die from complications of pulmonary hypoplasia rather than from renal failure.

When unilateral renal agenesis is diagnosed, attention is then focused on evaluating the anatomy, function, and position of the solitary kidney. Radiologic studies, such as an excretory urogram (intravenous pyelogram [IVP]) and voiding cystourethrogram (VCUG), radionuclide imaging, and hematologic determinations of renal function are obtained at the time of diagnosis and at periodic intervals during the child's growth years. Compromising conditions that exist in the remaining kidney may require corresponding surgical intervention to preserve renal function.

Children born with a solitary kidney can anticipate a normal lifespan and may engage in all activities, with the exception of contact sports that pose a potential risk of trauma.

A significant increase in the use of prenatal ultrasonography to assess urologic functioning allows early detection and close surveillance of the fetus with renal agenesis, with diagnosis possible as early as 20 weeks of gestation (Gonzales, 1985). Accuracy of prenatal ultrasound varies from 60% to 85% (Smith et al., 1987; Turncock & Shawis, 1984). Prenatal diagnosis affords the urologist an opportunity to counsel parents who are faced with the impending birth of a child with a defective urinary tract. Plans may then be made to deliver the baby in a facility that provides specialized neonatal care.

## APPROACHES TO PATIENT CARE

### Assessment

Renal agenesis is frequently discovered by prenatal ultrasonography. Unilateral renal agenesis is suspected when a solitary, enlarged kidney is detected. Bilateral renal agenesis is demonstrated by ultrasound findings, which include the absence of renal outlines, oligohydramnios, a negative furosemide challenge test administered to the expectant mother, and nonfilling of the fetal urinary bladder (Campbell, 1973).

At birth, the newborn with bilateral renal agenesis presents with signs of severe renal failure and respiratory decompensation. The baby is of low birth weight, is anuric, and has Potter's facies. The skin is excessively dry, and the chest is bell-shaped. Abdominal palpation fails to reveal kidneys. Respiratory maintenance is necessary immediately, along with constant monitoring of all vital functions.

Unilateral renal agenesis, conversely, may not be readily apparent by assessment techniques. A careful abdominal examination may disclose an absence of renal tissue or contralateral renal enlargement. In males, the homolateral epididymis may be absent; in females, the external vaginal opening may be absent, septate, or hypoplastic (Bryan et al., 1949).

Without these presenting signs, unilateral renal agenesis may defy detection unless the child correspondingly exhibits other anomalies that have a high association to the kidney disorder. The nurse should therefore assess the urologic function of all children with multiple congenital malformations or skeletal, cardiovascular, or gastrointestinal deformities. Because renal tissue is difficult to palpate in children beyond the infancy stage, the abdominal examination may not be an effective technique in discerning a solitary kidney.

## Bilateral Renal Agenesis

### Nursing Diagnosis

The nursing diagnoses for the child with bilateral renal agenesis may include the following:

1. Potential altered parenting/bonding related to the birth of a child with a life-threatening urologic defect.
2. Anticipatory grieving related to the potential loss of a child as a result of a life-threatening urologic defect.

### Plan of Care
Nursing care is directed toward enabling the child or parent to

1. Demonstrate increased attachment and bonding behaviors.
2. Verbalize positive feelings regarding the child.
3. Initiate an active role in the child's care.
4. Express and manage grief.

### Intervention
The birth of an infant with bilateral renal agenesis requires that parents receive support from the heath care team, which may include some or all of the following members: neonatologist, urologist, radiologist, nephrologist, pulmonary specialist, nurse, social worker, clergy, and geneticist; all of whom need to be sensitive to the needs of parents whose child has a life-threatening disease.

Parents anticipate the delivery of a healthy infant. When faced with the reality of having a newborn with a birth defect and a life-threatening problem, they may react negatively. The nurse must be able to accept the parents' feelings and assist the family members in dealing with their feelings of sadness, anger, denial, blaming, and fear of the unknown. The parents should be encouraged to bond with the newborn (i.e., hold the infant, have skin-to-skin contact, and focus on the infant's positive characteristics). The nurse should be alert to the parents' behavior when interacting with the infant. Some parents may distance themselves from the child by infrequent visits or calls to the nursery, lack of interest in the care of the child, or a reluctance to name the child or speak about the child as part of the family unit. Although recognizing that some people may choose not to share their feelings, convey to the family that you are available if they desire to do so later. By being a positive role model (i.e., holding the newborn, pointing out positive features), the nurse can assist the parent in accepting the child. Provide parents with information from the American Kidney Foundation or other organizations devoted to renal disease. Additionally, grief support groups, such as "Compassionate Friends," can help parents cope with the loss of their child.

### Patient Outcomes
Evidence of parental acceptance of the baby can be described in a variety of ways. Ideally, parents verbally accept the infant as an individual by talking to their child, providing care, and seeking eye contact. They are able to express concerns candidly, revealing information as they feel comfortable doing so. Acceptance of assistance from outside agencies, such as parent support groups, also suggests that the family is coping with the child's poor prognosis.

## Unilateral Renal Agenesis

### Nursing Diagnosis
Nursing diagnoses for the child with unilateral renal agenesis may include the following:

1. Potential for body image disturbance related to discovery of missing renal unit.
2. Knowledge deficit related to the functional ability of the remaining kidney as well as the durability and integrity of entire urinary tract.
3. Ineffective individual coping related to restriction of physical activity.

### Plan of Care
Nursing care is directed toward enabling the child and parent to

1. Accept his or her altered body image.
2. Pursue regular urologic evaluation of the remaining kidney and urinary tract.
3. Choose appropriate physical activities.

### Intervention
The discovery of unilateral renal agenesis often comes as a shock to the child and family, especially when there are no other apparent urologic anomalies. For the child whose renal defect is an incidental finding elicited during the evaluation of other organic malformations, the involvement of another body system may be overwhelming. When providing care for this child and his or her family, the nurse needs to let them express their fears and anger, while providing education about the durability of the urinary tract. Emphasize the rejuvenation and compensatory nature of kidney tissue, plus the fact that, in nonstress circumstances, adequate renal function can be maintained with less than 50% of the kidney tissue. Conversely, because renal disease may be present without symptoms, it is important to emphasize the need for urologic evaluation of the remaining urinary tract. Be sure to point out any positive struc-

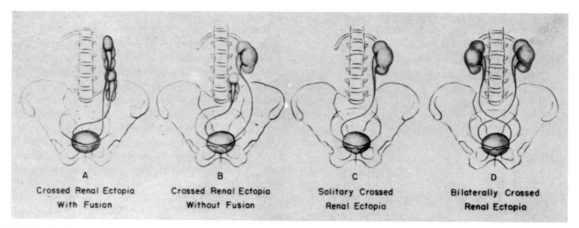

*FIGURE 20–3* Four types of crossed ectopia. (From Walsh, P. C., Retik, A. B., Stamey, T. A., & Vaughan, E. D. Jr. [Eds.] [1992]. *Campbell's urology.* [Vol. 2, 6th ed., p. 1371]. Philadelphia: W. B. Saunders. Reprinted by permission.)

tural findings. Discuss coping techniques, and acknowledge appropriate coping behaviors.

Contact sports represent an unnecessary risk of trauma to the solitary kidney. Many school districts prohibit such children from participating in school-sponsored organized contact sports. The nurse can provide the child and parents with alternative activities and interests, such as swimming, tennis, golf, and biking. Physical education teachers can work with the nurse to plan adaptive physical education programs that incorporate the activity restrictions.

**Patient Outcomes**

1. The child verbalizes positive feelings about self.
2. The child or parents seek and follow medical advice regarding care of the solitary kidney.
3. The child chooses activities that do not pose a risk to the solitary kidney and that are personally satisfying.

## Renal Ectopia or Renal Fusion

### PERSPECTIVES ON DISEASE ENTITY

**Etiology.** The progression of kidney formation is embryologically unique, because the organs follow a caudad-cephalad direction of development. Between the fourth and eighth week of fetal life, the mesodermal renal tissue ascends upward from the nephrogenic cord to its permanent position beside L2 and rotates 90 degrees on its lateral axis. Blood circulation is supplied by vessels present along the path of ascent. This process is extremely complex and depends on numerous factors; the risk of

anomalous development or placement as a consequence is high.

*Renal ectopia* is a term applied to a kidney that is not located in the usual flank position. Most often, the organ is found in the bony pelvis (pelvic or sacral kidney), with a correspondingly short ureter. Renal ectopy is further defined as *simple ectopy,* in which the kidney is on the same side as its ureteral attachment site, or *crossed ectopy,* in which the kidney is contralateral to the ureter's insertion site. McDonald and McClellan (1957) classified crossed ectopia as crossed ectopia with fusion, crossed ectopia without fusion, solitary crossed ectopia, and bilateral crossed ectopia (Fig. 20–3).

The incidence of renal ectopia is 1:500 to 1:1100 births, with a higher occurrence in postmortem studies. Boys are affected more often than girls. Most commonly, it is the left kidney that is ectopic. A crossed kidney is far more likely to be fused than separated.

When two or more kidneys are joined, the resultant kidney unit is termed *renal fusion.* Most commonly occurring is the horseshoe kidney (Fig. 20–4), which is composed of two distinct renal masses lying vertically along the midline and connected at their lower pole by an isthmus. This abnormality occurs during the fourth to sixth fetal week. Other variations include crossed fused ectopia (unilateral fused kidney) or pelvic fused kidney. An extremely rare form of crossed fused ectopia includes joined renal units that are attached to a solitary ureter. Varying degrees of malrotation are present in all fused kidneys, compromising the blood supply in some cases.

The incidence of renal fusion is uncertain, because this defect may be asymptomatic.

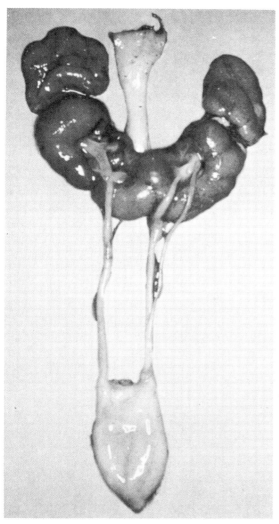

*FIGURE 20–4* Horseshoe kidney. (From Walsh, P. C., Retik, A. B., Stamey, T. A., & Vaughan, E. D., Jr. [Eds.]. [1992]. *Campbell's urology* [Vol. 2, 6th ed., p. 1377]. Philadelphia: W. B. Saunders. Reprinted by permission.)

Horseshoe-type fusion occurs most often, affecting anywhere from 1:600 to 1:1800 births, usually males. When horseshoe kidneys are discovered at birth, it is generally during the workup for other life-threatening defects. These infants may succumb from the related systemic defects; rarely is death a result of renal factors.

Causes of ectopy and fusion are uncertain and perhaps multifactorial. Possible explanations include pressure from abnormally placed umbilical arteries (Wilmer, 1938) to malalignment and abnormal rotation of the fetus's caudad structures (Cook & Stephens, 1977). Genetics certainly exert an influence, as evidenced by

a familial incidence (Greenberg & Nelsen, 1971; Hildreth & Cass, 1978). Ectopy may be an outgrowth of an abnormal ureteral bud or metanephros.

Children born with renal ectopia or fusion are likely to have other anomalies. Within the genitourinary system, frequently associated problems are hypospadias or cryptorchidism (Sharp, 1990). The skeletal, gastrointestinal, or cardiovascular systems are often affected, sometimes severely (i.e., imperforate anus, dysplastic vertebrae, and cardiac valvular defects), although defects present in children with horseshoe kidneys tend to be milder. About 60% of children with Turner's syndrome have horseshoe kidneys (Smith, 1982).

**Pathophysiology.** For the child with fused or ectopic kidneys and no other systemic anomalies, the condition is often asymptomatic. Detection occurs by chance during an evaluation for other concerns, probably resulting in significant underreporting of these defects.

Uropathology, when it does occur, is related to the kidney's close proximity to bony structures or to the malrotation that is a component of renal fusion. Ectopy, without the protection and support of ribs and retroperitoneal tissue, leaves the kidney vulnerable to trauma. A minimal blow to the abdomen may be sufficient to create hematuria or renal hematoma, particularly if the child has horseshoe kidneys. By reducing the benefit of gravity on urine flow to the bladder, the ectopic kidney may encourage stasis, with eventual hydronephrosis, infection, or stone formation. Ureteropelvic junction (UPJ) obstruction is common among fused kidneys and may be the source of presenting symptomatology.

**Medical-Surgical Management.** Treatment for the child with renal ectopy or renal fusion is planned to relieve symptoms that evolve from the degree of underlying pathologic changes. Because these conditions vary greatly in anatomic development and, therefore, in risk for disease, an astute uroradiologic evaluation is mandated. Findings must be carefully evaluated to ensure an accurate assessment of urinary tract structures and function.

Urinary tract infections resulting from urostasis are treated with organism-specific antibiotics. Management of kidney stones may include surgical intervention or extracorporeal shockwave lithotripsy if the child is a candidate for the procedure. Hydronephrosis from UPJ obstruction can be relieved by pyeloplasty. Renal trauma is monitored by computed tomography (CT) scans or other radiologic procedures. Activities are restricted until the kidney heals. The child whose kidney is vulnerable to trauma should avoid contact sports or use of equipment such as some gymnastic apparatus and trampolines.

## APPROACHES TO PATIENT CARE

### Assessment

Typically, there is no symptomatology of the child with renal ectopia or fusion (barring other systemic defects). Certainly, children with a family history of uropathology or "solitary kidney" should be observed closely for urinary tract infections, abdominal mass, or chronic low abdominal or even pelvic pain. Minor incidents of blunt abdominal trauma that produce hematuria or prolonged pain may alert the nurse to the possibility of fusion or ectopy. Sharp, colicky abdominal or pelvic pain in conjunction with hematuria may signal renal stones.

### Nursing Diagnosis

The nursing diagnoses for the child with renal ectopia or fusion may include the following:

1. Knowledge deficit related to
   a. Potential for infection.
   b. Potential formation of renal calculus.
   c. Risk of renal trauma.
2. Ineffective individual coping related to activity restriction.

### Plan of Care

Nursing care is directed toward enabling the child and parent to

1. Maintain a sterile urinary tract.
2. Promote adequate urinary output to reduce the potential for calculus formation.
3. Reduce the risk of renal trauma.
4. Detect abnormal coping responses and develop appropriate coping skills.

### Intervention

To prevent urinary stasis in a malrotated or ectopic kidney, adequate fluid intake is necessary. In the infant, 2 to 3 oz of fluid per pound of body weight per day should be ensured. A 1-year-old child requires 1000 mL/day with an additional 100 mL added for each year of life up to age 10 years. Offer the child a variety of fluids, with the exception of caffeine-containing products, because these may irritate the bladder.

Signs of potential complications, such as urinary tract infection and calculus, should be taught to the family, with instructions to seek immediate medical attention at their onset. Because of the silent nature of chronic uropathology, the nurse should emphasize the need for periodic evaluation to detect any insidious changes that occur from growth or maturation.

Recommendations for activity restrictions need to be clearly explained and defined to both parents and the child, yet be presented in a way that does not make the child feel abnormal or inferior. Coordinating an adaptive physical education program with the gym teacher or school nurse affords the urology nurse an opportunity to advocate for the child's inclusion in age-appropriate but non-risky gym activities. Parents should be encouraged to offer a variety of allowable activities without emphasizing the sports that cannot be performed. Many of these activities are well suited for adult participation; a greater degree of family unity and involvement may be a positive result.

### Patient Outcomes

1. The child does not develop urinary tract infection, as evidenced by normal urine culture and absence of symptomatology.
2. The child does not develop renal calculus, as evidenced by absence of pain and associated symptoms.
3. The child avoids activities that may result in abdominal trauma and hematuria.
4. The child and parents verbalize an understanding of the need for ongoing urologic evaluation.
5. The child becomes involved in permitted activities, verbalizes positive self-esteem, and interacts appropriately with peers.

# Renal Hypoplasia (Oligomeganephronia)

## PERSPECTIVE ON DISEASE ENTITY

**Etiology.** Congenital hypoplasia indicates a small kidney that is devoid of dysplastic or embryologic structures, although more accurately it is a small kidney composed of a reduced population of nephrons and calices. Hypoplasia may occur sporadically or totally within one or both kidneys and is often associated with reflux. However, reflux nephropathy (renal changes associated with reflux) may be an acquired condition that results from pyelonephritis and, therefore, may not be diagnostic of renal hypoplasia. Radiologic studies of the small kidney may be equivocal for diagnosis of hypoplasia; identification of insufficient numbers of calices often is the only distinguishing feature between true hypoplasia and secondary atrophy or hypodysplasia.

Oligomeganephronia is a specific form of renal hypoplasia, first described in 1962 (Habib et al.; Royer et al.), which presents shortly after birth. Oligomeganephronia does not appear to demonstrate a genetic transmission, but a 3:1 male predominance has been noted. Low birth weight (<2500 g) and maternal age older than 35 years are common factors among 30% of affected infants (Royer et al., 1962). The cause of the renal disease is unknown.

**Pathophysiology.** In most instances, hypoplasia is bilateral but unevenly distributed between kidneys. On examination, the kidney surface is granular, the cortex and medulla are indistinct, and the usual eight renal segments are reduced. Early histologic examination reveals a reduction in nephrons and glomeruli with marked increase of proximal tubular length and glomerular volume, followed later in the disease by interstitial fibrosis and atrophic uriniferous structures. As the disease progresses, the grossly enlarged glomeruli undergo functional deterioration, eventually resembling structures seen with glomerulonephritis.

Urologic function is disturbed early in the disease, with creatinine clearance at 10 to 50 mL/min/1.73 m$^2$ and urine concentration reduced to a maximum specific gravity of 1.007 to 1.012. Proteinuria is an early finding, and electrolyte imbalances and acidosis become evident; progressive renal failure ensues.

**Medical-Surgical Management.** Typically, the infant is originally seen for failure to thrive, vomiting, dehydration, polyuria, extreme thirst, unexplained fever, and diarrhea. Creatinine, blood urea nitrogen (BUN), and electrolyte levels are elevated. Diagnostic studies, such as an excretory urogram and sonogram, reveal very small kidneys without malformed calices (Scheinman & Abelson, 1970). The definitive diagnosis is made by microscopic examination following renal biopsy.

Treatment is focused on correcting acidosis and electrolyte imbalance, maintaining adequate calcium-phosphorus metabolism, and reducing protein intake to 1.5 g/kg/day. A period of stable azotemia may last until adolescence, when renal function deteriorates rapidly. Dialysis maintains the child until transplant is performed. Prognosis for transplant is favorable, because the child's remaining urinary tract is normal; family members can be suitable donors because oligomeganephronia is nonfamilial.

## APPROACHES TO PATIENT CARE

### Assessment

On examination, the nurse observes an infant who has a history of low birth weight, intense thirst, and polyuria. The infant has the appearance of failure to thrive, accentuated by persistent vomiting and diarrhea. Urine concentration is low, and moderate proteinuria is common. Hematologically, serum electrolyte levels are elevated, along with renal function studies (i.e., BUN and creatinine). To further focus the evaluation of failure to thrive, the family should be questioned regarding the presence of urologic disease for the preceding three generations.

Once the diagnosis of renal hypoplasia is made, the nurse should evaluate the parents' understanding of the disease and long-term consequences. Decisions for treatment are based on degree of renal failure and the child's body size and health status. Because dialysis may be an ongoing option until the child is a suitable candidate for transplant, the ability of the family to cope with the management of a child on dialysis should be ascertained.

### Nursing Diagnosis

The nursing diagnoses for the child and parent with oligomeganephronia may include the following:

1. Altered physical growth related to the effects of renal disease and abnormal protein metabolism.
2. Knowledge deficit related to disease process, treatment options, follow-up care, and home management.
3. Altered family processes related to the effects of the child's chronic renal disease on family life.
4. Body image disturbance related to delayed physical growth, inadequate renal function, and perception of the body as imperfect.

### Plan of Care

Nursing care is directed toward enabling the child and parent to

1. Provide meals that supply adequate nutritional requirements while also complying with dietary restrictions.
2. Recognize need for ongoing medical intervention.
3. Make informed decisions regarding the long-term health management.
4. Cope with the stressors related to a chronically ill child and the altered family interactions.
5. Develop a sense of positive self-worth with

the abilities and skills to accomplish and be accepted by peers.

### Intervention

During the initial hospitalization phase, the child's health care is managed by the pediatrician or neonatologist and urologist, with additional support services provided by the dietitian and social worker. The nurse creates an environment of concern and support through the efforts of health care planning, education of the disease process, and clarification of the medical management. Parents are understandably fearful for the child's prognosis; therefore, providing anticipatory guidance for home management and long-term follow-up can buoy the parents' feelings of adequacy. Allow them an opportunity to grieve for the birth of a child with a chronic and progressively debilitating deficit, and emphasize the normalcy of feeling guilty, overwhelmed, and angry. If possible, contact with support groups for families with chronically ill children can help parents develop skills to cope with their feelings and enhance the development of their child.

For the older child, continued dietary management is necessary to ensure that the child's intake is adequate for growth needs yet maintains the protein restriction guidelines. Incorporating the child's food preferences as much as possible encourages compliance. Emphasize the need for increased fluids, especially during hot weather or if the child is very active. Encourage the child to pursue hobbies, sports, or other activities, praising his or her efforts.

As the child approaches end-stage renal disease, both parents and child need honest explanations of the treatment options. The child should be included in the management and decision making of the disease process. Referral to a support group for the child with renal failure can be extremely beneficial. At this phase, the urology nurse becomes the liaison between the family and the nephrology team members who manage the dialysis. Patient teaching is directed at the complexities of dialysis, renal transplantation, and further follow-up after surgery.

### Patient Outcomes

1. The child's metabolic status is maintained as close to normal as possible through dietary management and increased fluid intake.
2. The parents and child participate in the decision-making process for issues surrounding health management and plan of treatment.
3. The child receives continued health care as recommended.

4. The parents express positive feelings about the child, demonstrate confidence in their skills to support the child, and respond to the needs of the total family unit.
5. The child interacts appropriately with peers and expresses positive feelings about self.

## Autosomal Recessive Polycystic Kidney Disease

### PERSPECTIVE ON DISEASE ENTITY

**Etiology.** Of the two variations of genetically predetermined renal cystic disorders present in the pediatric population, autosomal recessive polycystic kidney disease (ARPKD) is more prevalent. To develop ARPKD, the child must inherit the defective gene from both parents; only the homozygote is symptomatic. The incidence of ARPKD is approximately 1:6000 to 1:14,000 births, with males affected twice as often as females (Sharp, 1990).

Kidney involvement manifests as renal tubule dilatation and is bilateral and concomitant with congenital hepatic fibrosis. It is certain that all children with ARPKD have associated liver involvement; whether congenital hepatic fibrosis is axiomatic with ARPKD is unknown. The degree of involvement between the liver and the kidney is inversely proportional and has a direct effect on the onset of disease and the child's prognosis. Nearly complete renal involvement is evidenced in the neonatal period as oligohydramnios, high flank masses, and severe respiratory distress (Potter's syndrome); periportal fibrosis, however, is minimal. These infants succumb within 6 weeks. At the opposite extreme, when fewer than 10% of the renal tubules are dilated, the age of diagnosis may be as late as mid-childhood; the symptomatology is generally related to the consequences of marked hepatic fibrosis, such as portal hypertension and esophageal varices.

Children whose renal dysfunction is moderate (25–60% renal involvement) may exhibit a slower progression of renal failure, allowing them to survive to an age at which renal transplantation becomes a treatment option. In the past, ARPKD was called *infantile polycystic kidney disease,* referring to the fact that the disease always presents in childhood, usually infancy. Likewise, autosomal dominant polycystic kidney disease (ADPKD) was generally known as *adult polycystic kidney disease* owing to its usual occurrence in patients older than 30 years of age. Using the terms ''infantile'' and ''adult'' may be confusing, because ARPKD is not limited to infancy and ADPKD may actually appear in childhood; therefore, their use is discouraged (for more information on ADPKD, refer to a nephrology text).

**Pathophysiology.** On gross examination, the enlarged organ has a typical reniform shape, and normal fetal lobulation is present. A cross-section examination of the kidney reveals a radial configuration of small subcapsular cysts, representing dilated fusiform collecting ducts. The tubules originate in the medulla and extend to the subcapsular zone. Pathologic changes beyond the collecting ducts are usually not evident, because the proximal nephron, renal pelvis, ureter, and renal pedicle are spared. Studies by Zerres, Volpel, and Weib (1984) suggest that the underlying pathogenesis is related to hyperplasia of the cells that line the collecting ducts.

**Medical-Surgical Management.** Prenatal detection of ARPKD currently is not possible, because fetal ultrasonography is not sensitive enough to demonstrate the cysts, and there are no genetic markers indicative of the disease. Diagnosis of ARPKD begins with an abdominal and renal ultrasound, the recommended course for all infants born with abdominal masses. Massively enlarged kidneys with increased and uniform medullary echogenicity (Sanders, 1979) are found, along with small medullary cysts. The intravenous urogram exhibits the characteristic image of "sun-ray" streaks that radiate outward toward the cortex (Ashcraft, 1990).

Renal insufficiency is evidenced hematologically by a decreased glomerular filtration rate, renal plasma flow, reduced concentration ability, anemia, and acidosis. Serum creatinine levels, normal at birth, begin to increase shortly after birth.

To determine genetic inheritance, a thorough investigation of the family's medical history must be obtained. The presence of kidney disease in the previous three generations should be explored to differentiate dominant from regressive inheritance, so that parents can be presented with potential risks for disease in future progeny. A liver biopsy, which may demonstrate periportal fibrosis, may be necessary to accurately diagnose ARPKD.

Medical management is dependent on the age of diagnosis and the degree of organic involvement. Because of overwhelming pulmonary hypoplasia, newborns usually succumb to respiratory failure soon after birth. For the child with less severe kidney involvement, sup-

portive management of renal and hepatic failure, hypertension, and congestive heart failure may delay the course of progression, allowing the option of dialysis and transplantation. The effects of marked liver disease in the older child may require venous shunting to correct venous hypertension and gastric transection with reanastomosis to manage esophageal varices.

## APPROACHES TO PATIENT CARE

### Assessment

The infant born with ARPKD may have renal masses large enough to obstruct vaginal delivery. Flank tenderness may be present. Oligohydramnios may be noted and, at birth, respiratory distress may be marked. The classic features of Potter's facies are ominous markers of pulmonary hypoplasia. Death may occur as a result of a rapid progression of uremia and respiratory failure.

Renal or hepatic enlargement in the older infant or child with ARPKD may be elicited during abdominal palpation. As liver involvement increases, abdominal ascites and spider varicosities may be noted. Growth retardation and signs of anemia may be evident. Hematuria and urinary tract infection are commonly found.

Urinalysis shows proteinuria and low specific gravity. Microscopically, increased numbers of red and white blood cells are seen.

When assessing the patient and family, the nurse should evaluate their capacity to participate in the dialysis program. Economic, cultural, and psychosocial strengths and weaknesses should be identified in preparation for the impending progression of disease. If the child is in a terminal phase of disease, the nurse can begin to prepare the child or the family for the child's death.

### Nursing Diagnosis

The nursing diagnoses for the child with ARPKD may include the following:

1. Potential for fluid volume deficit related to an inability to concentrate urine.
2. Altered nutrition related to impaired absorption of nutrients due to renal failure.
3. Knowledge deficit related to disease progression, genetic transmission, and treatment options.
4. Altered parent-infant bonding and anticipatory grief related to the birth of a child with a terminal illness.
5. Ineffective family coping: compromised by

the effects of a child's chronic, life-threatening disease.

**Plan of Care**

Nursing care is directed at enabling the child and parent to

1. Maintain a normal fluid and electrolyte balance.
2. Achieve optimal growth through adequate dietary management.
3. Accept the child's diagnosis and manage his or her health care needs to achieve the child's potential for wellness.
4. Make informed decisions regarding family planning.
5. Develop a nurturing relationship with the chronically ill infant.
6. Express grief over the anticipated or actual loss of the child.
7. Establish self-esteem and positive family patterns of interaction.

**Intervention**

The birth of an infant with such a grim prognosis is shattering to the parents. Unprepared because of a seemingly normal pregnancy, the parents may recoil from any form of emotional attachment and become overwhelmed with guilt, anger, bewilderment, and grief. If the infant survives the immediate neonatal period, the parents are faced with the responsibility of caring for their terminally ill infant. The nurse can assist the family by encouraging them to verbalize their fears and frustrations, by validating their responses as normal, and by enlisting the aid of hospital and community social service resources. A parent support group can be extremely helpful, both before and after the child's death.

Parents need detailed discharge instructions to prepare them for the progression of symptoms. Providing parents with a system to contact the nurse as problems arise allays many of their anxieties, making the prospect of home care more manageable. Remind the parents that respite time, for themselves as individuals and as a couple, helps place family stressors in a more objective context and relieve tension.

Dietary management for the infant or child with ARPKD is geared toward providing calories for growth without overloading the deficient kidneys. Fluid intake should be carefully increased, especially in warm weather, when salt supplements may also be required. Acidosis can be controlled by the addition of sodium bicarbonate solutions. Protein intake may need to be adjusted, depending on BUN and serum creatinine levels, along with the degree of proteinuria. Enlist the aid of the hospital nutritionist to develop menus that are nutritionally sound yet incorporate the child's preferences.

Parents of children with ARPKD require genetic counseling to explore the potential for disease recurrence in future offspring, especially because no prenatal markers currently exist. Reiterating to parents that, owing to the recessive inheritance of the disorder, they both contributed genes responsible for ARPKD helps them cease blaming solely themselves or the other parent for the child's condition.

As infants with ARPKD survive into their childhood years, they become candidates for dialysis and, ultimately, renal transplantation. Peritoneal dialysis is usually the treatment of choice for end-stage renal disease, because it can be performed at home, is less disruptive to the family's lifestyle, and does not require venous access (the reader is referred to a pediatric nephrology text for an in-depth discussion of peritoneal dialysis). The child and family should be told that, at this point, the course of the disease is variable and that progression is not always immediate. Prolonged survival does occur, even with marked renal impairment (Vathibhagdee & Singleton, 1973). Encourage the child to remain as actively involved with peers as possible, offering praise for accomplishments. The nurse may need to work in partnership with the school setting to help provide a program that reflects the child's needs and restrictions. As with any child, the chronically ill child should have regular household chores and be given guidelines for acceptable behavior.

**Patient Outcomes**

1. The child grows and develops within established parameters.
2. The child remains adequately hydrated.
3. The parents are able to develop meal plans that supply adequate nutrients yet reflect the child's metabolic status.
4. The parents express positive feelings and demonstrate supportive actions toward their child.
5. Parents are compliant with follow-up care and make health care decisions with a stated understanding of the disease and treatment options.
6. The child expresses feelings of worthiness and pride in accomplishments.
7. The parents and family use positive coping mechanisms to deal with the death of the child.

# Multicystic Dysplasia of the Kidney

## PERSPECTIVE ON DISEASE ENTITY

**Etiology.** Multicystic dysplasia of the kidney is broadly applied to a severely dysplastic, cyst-filled renal structure originating from a nongenetic cause. Renal expression of multicystic dysplasia varies greatly; the disease may be bilateral or unilateral, kidney size may range from slightly below normal to massive, and the cysts may vary from microscopic to readily apparent on gross examination. The presence of cysts can range from focal or segmental involvement to permeation of the total organ. The only common factors linking the multiple clinical manifestations are the lack of typical lobar development and abnormal caliceal drainage.

Multicystic dysplasia of the kidney has a high degree of clinical significance, representing the most common finding in infants with palpable abdominal mass. Sixty percent of the patients are diagnosed within the first year of life. It is also the most prevalent cystic disorder in the pediatric population (DeKlerk et al., 1977; Longino & Martin, 1958). The disorder is found equally or slightly more commonly among males than females and generally is unilateral, most often affecting the left kidney. The contralateral urinary system must be carefully evaluated, because there is a 20% to 30% risk of pathologic changes (Glassberg & Filmer, 1992), usually evidenced as UPJ obstruction, reflux, ureterovesical junction (UVJ) obstruction, ureteral ectopy, or urethral obstruction. Bilateral multicystic dysplasia is a fatal disease. Unilateral multicystic dysplasia is not life-threatening and is often diagnosed incidentally during the process of evaluation for other diseases; the severity of symptomatology depends on the status of the opposite renal structures. There appears to be no familial inheritance in the transmission of the disorder.

Associated systemic anomalies occur frequently in conjunction with dysplasia. Congenital defects of the gastrointestinal system, especially esophageal atresia, and anomalies of the cardiovascular, skeletal, and neural systems all signal the need for a thorough urologic workup.

Although the cause of multicystic dysplasia is unknown, several theories have been proposed. A documented concurrence of ureteral ectopy with multicystic dysplasia suggests the possibility that an abnormal interaction between the ureteral bud and the metanephric blastema may be a cause. Ureteral obstruction occurring early in fetal development has also been implicated as a precipitating factor, with the resultant hydronephrosis evolving into extreme dysplasia. Intrarenal reflux is known to be present in some affected kidneys; however, its role is currently unclear. Animal research has uncovered a link between mesenchymal insult and the development of multicystic dysplasia (Sharp, 1990). Because the disease encompasses a wide array of anatomic findings, all these factors may, individually or interrelatedly, induce the formation of multicystic dysplasia.

**Pathophysiology.** The multicystic dysplastic kidney, on gross inspection, has the appearance of "a bunch of grapes" (Fig. 20–5). It is a coarsely lobulated mass that may occupy almost an entire hemiabdomen and cross the midline. There is no obvious renal pelvis or parenchymal tissue, and glomeruli are usually sparse and immature. The cysts are separated by stroma tissue and primitive ducts and usually have no communicating structures. The ipsilateral ureter is generally atretic in part or totally.

**Medical-Surgical Management.** The widespread practice of fetal ultrasonography has resulted in better prenatal detection of renal obstruction or enlargement, with UPJ obstruction creating hydronephrosis and multicystic dysplasia being the most likely causes. After birth, the sonogram should be repeated to differentiate between cyst-filled and solid mass kidneys. A typical finding that suggests multicystic dysplasia is the presence of nonmedial, noncommunicating cysts; multiple cysts; absence of renal parenchyma; and a nondilated renal pelvis. A technetium 99m dimercaptosuccinic acid (DMSA) renal scan fails to show function. If the diagnosis still is equivocal, CT scan may be useful, particularly in cases of renal or ureteral ectopy. A final diagnostic tool, not often employed, is cystoscopy and retrograde studies. Endoscopic findings include an atretic ureter and possibly an absent or ectopic ipsilateral ureteral orifice.

Because of the high risk of pathologic changes in the opposite kidney, it is recommended that a sonogram, excretory urogram, and VCUG be performed to evaluate the contralateral system (Greene et al., 1971; Pathak & Williams, 1964). Hematologic studies of the child with unilateral multicystic dysplasia should be within the normal range; any abnormal findings are suggestive of associated anomaly in the opposite kidney.

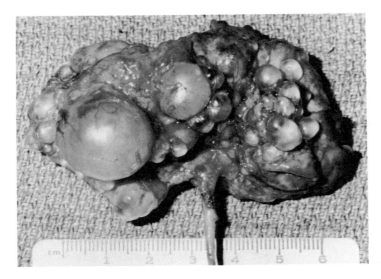

*FIGURE 20–5* Multicystic kidney.

Once the diagnosis of multicystic dysplasia is established, the urologist has the option of choosing medical or surgical management to treat the disease. Evidence to support both views can be presented; therefore, either approach is justified.

Previously, it was recommended that surgical exploration be performed to discern malignant tissue; however, modern imaging techniques have made this view obsolete. In fact, clinical reports have uncovered only six cases of concomitant malignancy (Sharp, 1990). Some clinicians have advised surgical exploration to positively differentiate between multicystic dysplasia and hydronephrosis, choosing to correct the UPJ obstruction if hydronephrosis is found. However, current assumptions are that when the renal scan elicits minimal or complete nonfunction, the hydronephrotic renal unit has little potential for functional return, making correction pointless (Glassberg & Filmer, 1992). Hypertension has been cited as a long-term sequela of multicystic dysplasia that could be abated by surgical intervention; again, clinical reports have failed to substantiate this finding, except in rare cases (Glassberg & Filmer, 1992).

Urologists who favor surgical treatment for dysplasia claim that the oppressing mass of such an enlarged organ can impinge on a child's normal activities as a result of frequently accompanying pain; there is also a predisposing risk of urinary tract infection. Given the relatively minor anesthetic risk and the savings recovered from the dispensation of medical monitoring and follow-up, removal of the dysplastic kidney may be in the child's best interest.

Nephrectomy is accomplished through a small flank incision, followed by decompression of the major cysts. The kidney is then detached from the obliterated ureter, the blood supply is ligated, and the organ is removed. Nylon suture is used to close the wound, and a polyfilm or Penrose drain, if used, is left in place from 4 to 7 days. The hospital stay is short; sutures are removed after 7 days.

## APPROACHES TO PATIENT CARE

### Assessment

The infant born with bilateral multicystic dysplasia demonstrates evidence of severe renal obstructive disease (i.e., Potter's facies, respiratory distress, and ensuing renal failure). Death usually occurs quickly. In rare cases when the infant has had some renal capacity, medical attention was sought because of the child's failure to thrive, acidosis, polyuria, polydipsia, and urosepsis.

Unilateral multicystic dysplasia not discovered by prenatal ultrasonography is most commonly detected by palpation of an abdominal mass. In cases when the renal unit is normally sized, the diagnosis is made serendipitously during an evaluation for contralateral kidney disease or associated congenital anomalies. Symptoms of renal obstruction, such as flank fullness, hematuria, and urinary tract infection, signal the need for a complete urologic evaluation to determine the status of both kidneys.

### Nursing Diagnosis

The nursing diagnoses for the child with bilateral multicystic dysplasia may include the following:

1. Anticipatory grieving related to the birth of

a child with a disorder incompatible with life.

The nursing diagnoses for the child with unilateral multicystic dysplasia may include the following:

*Prenephrectomy*
1. Pain related to pressure from an abdominal mass.
2. Potential for urinary tract infection related to inadequate urine drainage.
3. Knowledge deficit related to
   a. Need for follow-up care of the medically managed multicystic kidney.
   b. Possible uropathology of the contralateral kidney.
4. Potential for injury to remaining functional kidney related to participation in highly physical activities.

*Postnephrectomy*
1. Pain following nephrectomy.
2. Fluid volume deficit, actual or potential, related to surgical removal of kidney.
3. Potential for infection related to
   a. Disruption of skin integrity.
   b. Discharge from surgical drain.
4. Fear related to hospitalization experience, or threat to the child's health status as a result of nephrectomy.

**Plan of Care**
The nursing care is directed toward enabling the child or parent to

1. Express grief over the infant's impending death and cope with the overwhelming experience.
2. Recognize the need to evaluate the functional urinary system.
3. Receive ongoing medical surveillance of the urinary tract if the multicystic dysplastic kidney is not removed.
4. Choose appropriate physical activities that pose a minimal risk of harm to the functional kidney.
5. Remain comfortable after surgery.
6. Maintain or restore adequate fluid volume during the postoperative phase.
7. Experience proper incisional healing.
8. Develop strategies to cope effectively with surgery and hospitalization.

**Intervention**
Bilateral multicystic dysplasia is a life-threatening condition that quickly progresses to renal failure. The infant ultimately dies, leaving the parents with an unfulfilled promise of their child's life potential. The ensuing grief can be devastating, consuming everyday activities and disrupting personal relationships. If the infant survives long enough to be discharged, the parents' response may vacillate between detachment and compulsive overattentiveness. The nurse should assess the parents for signs of inappropriate coping, such as neglect of self-care or care for other children; anger or hypercriticism directed toward the doctor, hospital, or each other; extreme change in personal habits; decision-making inability; and denial of sorrow. If the parents are willing to acknowledge their feelings, provide a comfortable emotional climate for them to express their grief and then plan time to listen to them. Validate their appropriate grieving responses as normal experiences to extreme stress. Contact the hospital chaplain for spiritual intervention, and also inform the family of local support groups.

Unilateral multicystic dysplasia is generally a benign condition when considered by itself. The disorder is often silent; in fact, detection of the anomaly is frequently serendipitous during the evaluation of other systemic defects. Unless the kidney is massive and encumbers respiratory action, even newborns with a palpable dysplastic kidney and no other gross defects are asymptomatic, having the appearance of perfectly formed infants. This dichotomy—a seemingly healthy child who possesses a completely dysfunctional organ in a major body system—may arouse feelings of disbelief, anxiety, or doubt in the parents.

The nurse who is caring for the child with unilateral multicystic dysplasia needs to bear the following considerations in mind:

1. Shock at the child's diagnosis may have blocked the parents' ability to comprehend the urologist's explanation and teaching.
2. Even though the renal disease may have a minimal effect on the child's health, parents feel overwhelmed when a child with systemic malformations is additionally diagnosed with multicystic dysplasia.
3. Denial of the problem and generalized hostility are coping mechanisms used by both the child and parents.
4. When approaching the child and parents at the initial contact, the nurse should first assess their knowledge of the disorder; then using this information as a base, supplement or reiterate the urologist's teaching. Use anatomic drawings to illustrate the normal urinary tract, then show the results of evaluative studies to demonstrate the urinary tract defect. It is necessary to advise parents of the potential for uropathology to the contra-

lateral renal system; temper this recommendation with the reassurance that most congenital urologic anomalies are amenable to surgical intervention. Emphasize the rejuvenative capacity of the kidney, especially among infants, after reconstructive surgery.

Interacting effectively with a family that is hostile or in a state of denial is difficult, but the nurse should keep in mind that these responses are actually a façade to mask their deeper emotions of fear, guilt, or sorrow, especially if the child has a spectrum of organic defects. Linking this family with others who have experienced similar circumstances can be very helpful. Also allow the child or parents an opportunity to ventilate their feelings in a nonjudgmental atmosphere.

When surgery is contemplated for a child, parents often express fear at the child's ability to cope with the experience physically and emotionally. Neonates, particularly, are believed to be "too fragile" to withstand surgery. The nurse should counsel the parents on how to make the hospital and surgical experience a positive one for the child, incorporating principles based on the child's developmental age. Preoperative preparation is essential. Many pediatric institutions provide preadmission orientation programs; this may allay most of the parents' fears. Hospital policies that encourage care by parents and open visitation play an important role in reducing the anxieties surrounding surgery.

The care of the child who undergoes a nephrectomy involves monitoring fluid balance, providing comfort measures, and assessing wound healing. Intravenous feedings restore fluid volume until the child can retain clear to full liquids, usually within 24 hours. Diet is advanced as tolerated.

Analgesia is induced through the use of meperidine hydrochloride (Demerol), 1 to 1.5 mg/kg, intramuscularly or orally every 4 hours as needed. After 24 to 48 hours, milder analgesics such as acetaminophen may be employed. Parents of infants and young children are encouraged to cuddle them, but they may hesitate for fear of causing pain. The nurse should direct the parents in the proper handling of their child to avoid discomfort.

The incision should be inspected regularly to determine the extent of healing and to assess for infection. Discharge is expected from the drain, and soiled dressings should be changed daily. On the fourth to seventh postoperative day, the drain is removed, and the drain site is covered with a light bandage for another 24

hours. Tub baths are allowed after complete wound healing.

If surgery is not the treatment recommended by the urologist, parents need to be aware of the need for periodic medical surveillance to monitor the child's urinary status. Teach the signs and symptoms of urinary tract infection, along with techniques to reduce the child's risk, such as a high fluid intake, hygienic measures, and frequent voiding. Hematuria, frequent intestinal upsets, or abdominal distention and pain should always be reported to the urologist. A yearly blood pressure measurement after age 5 years is also suggested.

Because the multicystic dysplastic kidney is a nonfunctional renal unit, the child with this condition should be considered as if he or she has a solitary kidney. It is prudent for the child to avoid contact sports or activities with an increased risk of damage to the remaining functional kidney. In many school systems, team sports are prohibited for the child with only one of a paired organ. The nurse may advise parents of appropriate physical activities and also collaborate with the physical education teacher for an adaptive gym program.

**Patient Outcomes**

1. The family expresses feelings related to grief.
2. The family uses appropriate coping mechanisms to deal with grief.
3. The child undergoes urologic evaluation of the contralateral system.
4. The family of the child who undergoes nephrectomy receives preparation for the surgery and hospital experience, and the child responds to the experience in an age-appropriate, positive manner.
5. The child has a comfortable postoperative period.
6. Adequate hydration is maintained, as evidenced by adequate voiding (1 mL/kg/h) and good skin turgor.
7. Wound healing occurs without dehiscence or infection.
8. The parents comply with ongoing medical surveillance and report signs of potential complication.
9. The child acquires hobbies and pursues activities that preserve the functional kidney yet still provide an outlet for creative expression and stimulate physical development.

## DISORDERS OF THE URETER

Ureteral defects encompass a grouping of various organ anomalies that are distinguished by etiology, pathophysiologic changes, and symptomatology. Medical-surgical management is diversified but is always governed by the location and degree of actual or functional obstruction and the extent of end-organ disease. Consequently, the treatment of the child with a specific congenital ureteral anomaly lacks uniformity or consistency; instead, treatment is individually tailored to the circumstances of each child's disease. Table 20–1 shows the terminology proposed as standard nomenclature for the disorders by the American Academy of Pediatrics.

The nursing plan of care for the child is consequently fashioned as a response to perceived needs arising from alterations in normal urinary function or as supportive care after surgical intervention. The nursing approach, therefore, is not focused on the child's anatomic defect but rather is driven by the specific medical-surgical management techniques selected.

The material presented in this section deviates from the previous format to reflect this altered perspective. First, the specific ureteral anomaly is explained and the potential treat-

---

**TABLE 20–1. Nomenclature of Duplex Systems, Ectopic Ureters, and Ureteroceles**

The following is a synopsis of the report of the Committee on Terminology, Nomenclature and Classification of the Urology Section of the American Academy of Pediatrics. It is an attempt to standardize the terminology used for duplex system, ectopic ureters, and ureteroceles and obviate the ever-present confusion in the use of these terms.

| | |
|---|---|
| Duplex system | An upper-tract unit in which the kidney has two pelves and is associated with either a single ureter, bifid ureter, or two ureters emptying separately into the bladder; includes both complete and incomplete duplicated systems. |
| Duplex kidney | A kidney in which two pelves are present. |
| Bifid system | Incomplete duplication; bifid pelvis means two pelves that join at the ureteropelvic junction; bifid ureter signifies two ureters that join before emptying into the bladder. |
| Upper-pole kidney (UPK) | Refers to that segment of a duplex kidney that is drained by the superior (upper-pole) pelvis. |
| Upper-pole ureter (UPU) | The ureter that drains the superior pole of a duplex kidney. |
| Upper-pole (ureteric) orifice (UPO) | The ureteric orifice that is associated with the ureter that drains the superior pole of a duplex kidney. |
| Lower-pole kidney (LPK) | Refers to that segment of a duplex kidney that is drained by the inferior (lower-pole) pelvis. |
| Lower-pole ureter (LPU) | The ureter that drains the inferior pole of a duplex kidney. |
| Lower-pole (ureteric) orifice (LPO) | The ureteric orifice that is associated with the ureter that drains the inferior pole of a duplex kidney. |
| Ectopic ureter | A ureter that drains to a site located outside the bladder (that is, bladder neck or beyond). It may be used to identify a ureter that is associated with a duplicated system or a single system. |
| Lateral ectopia | Site of orifice is lateral to A or normal position (B, C, D, D1, D2). C represents severe lateral ectopia, and B lies midway between A and C. D, D1, and D2 represent, respectively, orifices located at the mouth of a hiatal diverticulum, just inside the diverticulum, and well inside the diverticulum. |
| Caudal or medial ectopia | Site of orifice is at the proximal lip of the bladder neck (F) or beyond (G and H). In the male, G represents the urethra and H, the genital tract (vas deferens, seminal vesicle, and so on). In the female, G1 represents the proximal half of the urethra, G2, the distal half of the urethra and urethrovaginal bridge, and H, the vagina, Gartner's duct, and hymen. Orifices located on the trigone but caudal or medial to the A position are not regarded as ectopic and are designated by the letter E. |
| Intravesical ureterocele | When the ureterocele and its orifice are located entirely within the bladder. It usually is associated with a single system, but may be associated with the upper-pole ureter of a completely duplicated system and, in extremely rare circumstances, with the lower-pole ureter. |
| Ectopic ureterocele | When some portion of the ureterocele is located at the bladder neck or in the urethra. The orifice may not be clinically apparent or may be located in the bladder, at the bladder neck, or in the urethra. |

Stephens (1971; *Australian and New Zealand Journal of Surgery, 40,* 239) has avoided the customarily used adjective for ureteroceles and instead has defined them anatomically as follows: stenotic, sphincteric, sphincterostenotic, caeco-, blind, and nonobstructive. When appropriate, these terms can be employed to further describe either the intravesical or ectopic ureterocele.

---

From Caldamone, A. A. (1985). Duplication anomalies of the upper tract in infants and children. *Urologic Clinics of North America, 12*(1), 77. Reprinted by permission.

ment modalities are described. Following this is a global approach to patient care of all children with ureteral defects, further categorized by the nursing management of the child after specific surgical interventions.

## Perspective on Disease Entity

### ECTOPIC URETER

**Etiology.** An ectopic ureter occurs when there is abnormal development of the ureteric bud on the wolffian duct. Normally, the ureteric orifice is in the bladder. With the ectopic ureter, the ureteric bud remains with the wolffian duct for a longer period, and the orifice is carried closer to the vesical neck and develops in some area arising from the wolffian duct or urogenital sinus (i.e., vesical neck, prostatic urethra, seminal vesical, vas deferens, or ejaculatory duct in males, or the vesical neck, urethra, or vestibule in females) (Caldamone, 1985; Kelalis, 1985a; Williams, 1982). Ectopic ureteral orifices have also been found in Gartner's ducts, in cysts, or within urethral diverticula in young girls (Kelalis, 1985a). Structures deriving from the müllerian duct, such as the uterus, cervix, and vagina, are also possible sites for ectopic orifices. Remnants of the distal wolffian duct have been found in the walls of the vagina and broad ligament in a significant number of women. These anomalous locations provide an embryologic explanation for the association between ectopic ureters and the uterus or vagina.

Extravesical ectopic ureters are frequently present in association with a duplex renal–ureteral system; it is usually the upper renal segment that drains into an ectopic ureter. The child with unilateral ectopy is likely also to have developed contralateral duplication and should be evaluated for coinciding ectopia, which occurs infrequently (Kelalis, 1985a). Females have a sixfold higher incidence of ectopic ureters than males.

**Pathophysiology**

*Ectopic Ureter in the Female.* The most common extravesical location for an ectopic orifice in females is in the urethra or vestibule; therefore, the presenting manifestations are usually recurrent urinary tract infections and dribbling incontinence without maturation in the neurologically normal female. Vaginal abnormalities may also be present (Williams, 1982).

When the ectopic orifice is located distal to the bladder neck or in the vagina, cervix, or uterus, the girl who is toilet trained and has a normal voiding pattern also complains of constant dampness or dribbling (Churchill et al., 1987). Occasionally, the child with incontinence wets only when in an upright position. This leakage is due to the pooling effect in a dilated ureter when the child is recumbent.

Some females experience a vaginal discharge, but this is an inconsistent finding. Many cases of ectopic ureters in females are not diagnosed until adulthood, after either childbirth or pelvic musculature relaxation. Ureteral ectopy, in unusual cases, is diagnosed during the neonatal period, when a palpable abdominal mass is actually a massively dilated ectopic ureter (Caldamone, 1985; Kelalis, 1985a).

*Ectopic Ureter in the Male.* A single ectopic ureter that drains a dysplastic or ectopic kidney and terminates at the bladder neck or posterior urethra, the seminal vesicles, the ejaculatory duct, or the vas deferens is the most common presentation in the male. Urinary infection is a more common manifestation than is incontinence, because the ectopic ureter is always proximal to the external sphincter. Epididymitis in the prepubertal male should suggest ectopic ureter.

*Bilateral Single Ectopia.* Bilateral single ectopia is a rare congenital defect that affects females six times more often, and with greater severity, than males. The spectrum of pathologic changes is broad and involves the total urinary tract. Both kidneys are severely abnormal and drain into extravesical ectopic ureters, which open into the urethra. The trigone is undifferentiated, the bladder neck incompetent and, because of ureteral diversion, bladder capacity is limited. A short, patulous urethra is a common finding among girls.

The child with bilateral single ectopia has a history of total incontinence dating back to infancy. Urinary tract infection often compounds the problem. On physical examination, the patulous urethra is observed to have a constant dribble of urine. Development of systemic manifestations suggestive of renal failure is related to the degree of kidney involvement.

**Medical-Surgical Management.** The initial diagnostic evaluation of the child with ureteral ectopy begins with a VCUG and an excretory urogram. Depending on the terminal location of the ureter, signs of obstruction or reflux may be present. The bladder outline may appear irregular, and capacity may be limited owing to the exteriorized urine flow. Varying degrees of renal function may be visualized, affecting the kidney completely or in segments. Further renal studies, such as ultrasonography and a delayed renal scan, may be useful in the presence of renal damage.

Direct visualization with cystourethroscopy and vaginal examination may help in the diagnosis and the location of the ectopic ureteral meatus. An abnormal trigone and the absence of a ureteral meatus, noted during cystoscopy, may suggest ureteral ectopy; these signs are also seen with ureteral agenesis.

Final diagnosis may require the use of dyes such as indigo blue or indigo carmine, administered intravenously or instilled into the bladder, to distinguish clear urine flow from colored urine drainage.

To conserve renal function, surgical intervention is often pursued. If the renal scan shows reasonable function, then replantation of the ectopic ureter is advised. For children with duplication, this conservative approach may entail splicing the ectopic ureter into the normal ureter and discarding the abnormal distal segment (ipsilateral ureteroureterostomy). In some cases, however, function is poor and nephroureterectomy is advocated. With duplication, the surgeon must take care to avoid damaging or compromising the blood supply to the normal ureter and the lower-pole kidney (Williams, 1982).

Treatment of bilateral single ectopic ureters is a challenging problem, requiring reimplantation of the ureter, as well as reconstruction of the bladder neck and, frequently, augmentation cystoplasty (see Chaps. 21 and 22). Many times, unfortunately, the kidneys have sustained scarring and damage from reflux or severe hydronephrosis, and their management must include surveillance and therapy by a pediatric nephrologist.

## URETERAL AGENESIS

**Etiology.** The presence of an incomplete or absent ureter occurs when the ureteric bud does not form. In this situation, the ipsilateral hemitrigone is absent and the kidney does not develop, because differentiation of the metanephros is dependent on contact with a ureter.

**Pathophysiology.** There can be several variations of incomplete ureter, ranging from total absence of the ureter, including the renal pelvis, to the presence of a narrow, thin-walled tube, or a solid, threadlike structure. The ureter may narrow and end several centimeters from the kidney. Occasionally, the ureter may be discontinuous, with normal segments proximally and distally. Usually, severe renal dysplasia accompanies this degree of ureteral anomaly (Johnston, 1982).

It is uncertain whether the ureteric abnormality is responsible for the renal dysplasia; such a hypothesis seems likely. It is also assumed that with abnormal sections or gaps in the ureter, the ureter developed normally but was then subjected to some period of ischemia or other untoward effect. Bilateral ureteric absence with associated renal agenesis is incompatible with life.

**Medical-Surgical Management.** In cases of partial or total ureteral agenesis with a functional renal system on the contralateral side, no treatment is necessary. However, a VCUG should be performed to determine if reflux occurs into the incomplete ureteral stump. A stump that becomes dilated owing to reflux may become a cause of infection and should be excised (Williams, 1982).

## URETEROCELE

**Etiology.** A ureterocele is a congenital cystiform dilatation of the terminal ureter. It may be classified as either simple or ectopic and may involve a single or duplicated system.

Simple (orthotopic) ureteroceles are entirely intravesical in both position and drainage. The ballooning occurs as a result of stenosis of the ureteric orifice. These ureteroceles are usually restricted to the trigonal area because of their appropriate location between the muscular layers. The enlargement is often symmetric (Johnston, 1982).

Simple ureteroceles affect either side with equal incidences and are often bilateral. The size of the ureterocele depends on the intravesical length of the ureter and the size of the ureteral orifice. Females are affected seven times more frequently than males (Williams, 1982).

If the stenosis of the ureteral orifice is severe, the cystiform dilatation persists, whereas with lesser degrees of stenosis, the ureterocele remains small and simply fills and empties with each bolus of urine. Large ureteroceles may be palpable on abdominal examination. There is some debate as to whether simple ureteroceles are congenital or acquired, because they are rarely detected among children.

The ectopic ureterocele arises from an ectopic ureter in a duplicated system. More often, it affects the draining of the upper pole of the affected kidney. The ureterocele may protrude into the bladder neck and obstruct the bladder outlet. In females, prolapse of the ureterocele can present with a fleshy projection from the external meatus, either acutely with voiding or chronically. In boys, the prolapse can obstruct the membranous urethra. Depending on the dilatation of the ectopic ureteral orifice, reflux can occur. Incontinence may result, usually from cystitis but occasionally from the position of the ectopic orifice. The incidence of ectopic ureteroceles is six times greater among females than males and affects either ureter with equal frequency. The condition is unilateral in more than 90% of the cases (Royle & Goodwin, 1971). Single-system ectopic ureteroceles, which are more prevalent among males, often occur in conjunction with cardiac or genital defects (Johnson & Perlmutter, 1980).

**Pathophysiology.** The development of a ureterocele occurs in the embryo when there is a disruption in the normal development of the distal portion of the ureter. According to some authors, the presence of a ureterocele can be attributed to changes in the caudal end plate prior to tubularization and its connection with the wolffian ducts.

An ectopic ureterocele most frequently opens in the upper urethra close to the bladder neck. The ureter proximal to the ureterocele is usually dilated, and the musculature of the long submucosal segment may be defective. The ectopic orifice may or may not be stenotic. In some instances, it is large enough to result in reflux.

Ectopic ureteroceles obstructing the upper pole of a duplicated system are classified in relation to the site of obstruction: stenotic, for the obstructed ureteral orifice that terminates intravesically; sphincteric, for the ureter that tunnels through the internal sphincter, creating obstruction; or sphincterostenotic, for the combined features of both.

**Medical-Surgical Management.** The child with a ureterocele most often presents with a severe urinary tract infection, which can quickly progress to sepsis in infants. Kidney obstruction may also be marked; renal failure or failure to thrive is a potential sequela. Bladder outlet obstruction, although uncommon, may result from a pendulous or prolapsed ureterocele.

The initial management of the child with a ureterocele consists of treating the urinary tract infection with appropriate antibiotics, as determined by a urine culture and sensitivity. When the ureterocele has caused upper tract obstruction, resolution of infection may not be achieved without drainage procedures, including catheterization or, possibly, placement of a nephrostomy tube. Sepsis, renal failure, and failure to thrive require medical management and metabolic adjustment after drainage has been accomplished (Kelalis, 1985b).

Once the infection has been adequately treated, a VCUG and an excretory urogram are obtained. The excretory urogram usually demonstrates a bladder that has a nonopaque filling defect due to little or no contrast material in the ureterocele. The size of the ureterocele may vary from only a few centimeters to occupying almost the entire bladder, and it fluctuates with the filling of the bladder. The defect is usually smooth, but if the ureterocele is very edematous or has ruptured, it is irregular. The ureterocele is usually in contact with the bladder floor and located to one side or the other of midline; occasionally, it may be positioned at the bladder neck. Also, there is the typical cobra-head dilatation surrounded by a ring of contrast (Williams & Johnston, 1982). The lesion has been confused at times with gas in the rectum, a stone, a tumor, or a blood clot (Kelalis, 1985b).

A VCUG should be performed whenever a ureterocele is diagnosed to determine if reflux is present. Once the diagnosis is made, renal ultrasonography and radionuclide scanning provide more information prior to surgical intervention. Cystoscopy provides the definitive diagnosis.

Surgical management is the preferred treatment. When planning the type of surgical intervention for ureterocele, factors to be considered include the amount of damage or dysplasia of the upper renal segment associated with the defective ureter, the degree of reflux present in the ureterocele and in the ureter itself, as well as the obstruction of the bladder outlet by the ureterocele (Kelalis, 1985b). A current protocol recommends excision of the ureterocele and ureteral reimplantation. The procedure of transurethral unroofing, or incision of the ureterocele, has been less favored, because it often results in reflux and the need for a second surgery (Caldamone, 1985).

Some infants with ureterocele have ureteral duplication and intact renal function in both segments of the kidney. In these cases, ureteropyelostomy with partial ureterectomy of the distal segment is the treatment of choice. If the renal portion draining into the ureterocele functions poorly, a heminephrectomy with subtotal excision of the accompanying ureter could be performed. The excision of the ureterocele and ureteroureterostomy with antirefluxing reimplantation is yet another choice for surgical correction.

When the infant is very sick or a poor surgical risk for a lengthy procedure, cutaneous ureterostomy or a percutaneous nephrostomy is an excellent temporary procedure to decompress the system, allowing the infant the opportunity to stabilize. Surgical correction is then rescheduled electively.

The procedure of reimplantation is frequently complicated by a ureter that requires tapering and placement into a trabeculated, thick-walled bladder, which also needs a bladder base reconstruction. Under these circumstances, the technique of collapsing the ureterocele may still be chosen as a preliminary measure to allow the bladder to recover. At a later date, the ureterocele would be excised and reimplantation would be performed.

## URETERAL DUPLICATION

**Etiology.** Ureteral duplication can exist in several forms. Complete ureteral duplication occurs when two ureteral buds arise from one wolffian duct. The orifice of the ureter draining the upper segment is usually positioned medially and inferiorly to the orifice for the lower segment. The anatomic position of these orifices accounts for the greater likelihood that the upper ureter segment will be stenotic or ectopic and the lower segment ureter will develop reflux (Kelalis, 1985a).

Incomplete ureteral duplication occurs when two ureters drain a single kidney but unite and enter the bladder as a single ureter. This embryologic event occurs owing to early branching of a single ureteral bud. The partially duplicated ureter that bifurcates extravesically is described as a Y-type ureter, whereas a V-type ureter splits within the intramural lumen.

A blind-ending duplication occurs when one of the branches of the bifid ureteral bud fails to evolve into metanephria tissue as a result of arrested development. This blind-ending ureter does not connect to any portion of the kidney (Churchill et al., 1987).

Ureteral duplication is the most common urinary tract anomaly, observed in 2% to 4% of the clinical population (Hartman & Hodson, 1969; Nation, 1944; Nordmark, 1948). It occurs twice as frequently in females as males. Unilateral duplication is approximately six times more prevalent than bilateral duplication (Kelalis, 1985a).

There is a familial tendency toward duplication, with a 12% incidence among parents and siblings.

**Pathophysiology.** Renal hypoplasia and renal dysplasia can be seen with uncomplicated ureteral duplication, but in most cases the renal parenchyma is normal (Caldamone, 1985). The patient with incomplete ureteral duplication may experience ureteroureteral reflux from one segment into the other. This yo-yo phenomenon is responsible for urinary tract infections and abdominal or flank pain (Kelalis, 1985a).

Vesicoureteral reflux, which occurs with complete duplication, commonly originates from the superiorly placed ureteral orifice, whereas the inferior orifice is more likely to be obstructed. Children with ureteral duplication are prone to an increased incidence of acute and chronic urinary tract infections. Certainly, severe reflux with recurrent or persistent urinary tract infection may lead to renal damage.

**Medical-Surgical Management.** The management of ureteral duplication depends on the symptomatology and range of urologic problems consequent to the duplication. For the child with a symptomatic urinary tract infection, medical management with appropriate antimicrobial therapy is the initial treatment. This may be the only treatment indicated, with routine follow-up. For the child with chronic or persistent urinary tract infection secondary to vesicoureteral reflux or obstruction, careful attention must be paid to the thorough performance and precise interpretation of diagnostic studies such as excretory urogram, furosemide augmented excretory urogram, VCUG, or cineradiogram.

There are many surgical options, depending on the anatomy involved. The urologist determines the feasibility of performing pyeloureterostomy, heminephrectomy and ureterectomy, or replantation of both ureters into the bladder. The degree of renal scarring often determines the optimal procedure (Williams, 1982).

## MEGAURETER

**Etiology.** *Megaureter* describes a ureter that is markedly dilated and has decreased peristalsis. It occurs more often in boys, with a male to female ratio of 1.5:1 to 5:1; in 25% of the cases, both ureters are involved. Unilateral megaureter involves the left ureter four times more often than the right (King, 1985). The causes of megaureter are varied and include vesicoureteral reflux, UVJ, abnormal development of ureteral musculature, or high urine flow from poor renal concentrating ability. The neonatal ureter, conversely, may dilate tremendously yet not lose any peristaltic capability because of its structural anatomy and elasticity. The diversity of causes of megaureter has prompted an International Classification (Fig. 20–6) to help organize and delineate diagnosis and management based on etiology and concomitant symptomatology (King, 1985). For the purposes of this discussion, only primary obstructed megaureter and nonrefluxing, nonobstructed megaureter are described. Refluxing megaureter is discussed in the section in this chapter on vesicoureteral reflux.

*Primary Obstructed Megaureter.* In this condition, the juxtovesicular ureteral segment is markedly dilated, stenotic, or poorly innervated. As urine drainage is impeded, the ureter dilates and peristaltic activity becomes further diminished, causing obstruction at the UVJ or just above it. It occurs more frequently in males than females and, if unilateral, the left ureter is more likely to be affected than the right. In these cases, there is no evidence of bladder outlet obstruction or vesical dysfunction. The condition usually presents during the first year of life with symptoms of urinary tract infection, including fever, abdominal pain, and flank pain. Hematuria may be present, perhaps because of damage to mucosal vessels secondary to the marked dilatation (Johnston, 1982).

The distal ureter is always abnormal and markedly dilated, requiring reconstruction. Prenatal ultrasonography has aided in making the diagnosis of obstructed megaureter possible before a urinary tract infection or symptoms develop.

*Nonobstructed, Nonrefluxing Megaureter.* The cause of this condition is unknown. Without evidence of stenosis, there is no obstruction at the UVJ; the ureter nonetheless is markedly dilated, beginning just above the bladder.

There is no reflux present or any bladder anomaly, leading to a suspicion of either innate hypoplasia of the ureteral musculature or abnormally low intra-abdominal pressure.

In the child with secondary nonobstructive, nonrefluxing megaureter, the cause of the dilated upper tract is usually urinary tract infection, diabetes insipidus, or another metabolic cause. Dilatation of the lower ureter is most prominent, but the entire ureter or, occasionally, only the mid-portion may be affected (King, 1985).

**Pathophysiology**

*Primary Obstructed Megaureter.* This type of megaureter can be present in a form ranging from mild to severe. The ureter can be dilated at the distal or pelvic segment, with tapering to a relatively normal caliber. The kidney can demonstrate some cortical atrophy or show marked renal atrophy with caliceal clubbing and parenchymal thinning. The nondilated portion of the ureter is unable to transmit the peristaltic wave through the dilated distal segment and, therefore, is functionally obstructed. Cussen (1971) found that congenitally dilated ureters structurally demonstrate muscle hypertrophy and hyperplasia. This pathologic finding does not appear to exist with refluxing megaureters or megaureters associated with prune belly (Eagle-Barrett) syndrome (Hanna, 1988).

*Nonobstructed, Nonrefluxing Megaureter.* The congenitally nonobstructed megaureter is often associated with megacalicosis (caliceal dilatation without obstruction). Detailed studies are essential to prove that obstruction is not present. The upper urinary tracts in children with nonobstructive, nonrefluxing megaureter appear quite functional, and the megacalicosis

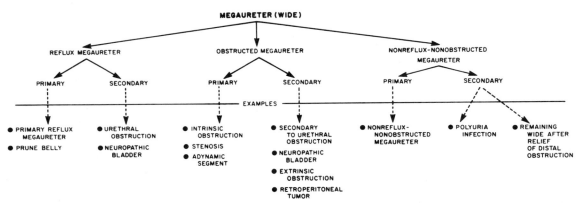

*FIGURE 20–6* Classification of megaureter. (From Hanna, M. K. [1988]. *Urologic surgery in neonates and young infants* [p. 161]. Philadelphia: W. B. Saunders. Reprinted by permission.)

gradually resolves with growth and increasing age.

**Medical-Surgical Management.** Most children with megaureter present with a urinary tract infection, hematuria, abdominal or flank pain, or a palpable flank mass. Renal ultrasonography, VCUG, and excretory urogram should be ordered once the infection is treated. These studies demonstrate the dilated ureter without evidence of reflux or intravesical obstruction. A furosemide renal scan is performed to induce diuresis as a means to determine renal function and to ascertain the degree of obstruction; however, there is great variance in the interpretation of this study. Children with nonobstructed, nonrefluxing megaureter usually drain all contrast material within 1 to 2 hours, indicating that surgical intervention is unnecessary. The condition tends to improve with age or remain stable as the ureter becomes progressively less dilated. These patients are monitored for urinary tract infections and with routine ultrasonography evaluation.

The child with obstructed megaureter usually presents with a urinary tract infection, abdominal or flank pain and, occasionally, hematuria. The excretory urogram highlights a ureter that is markedly dilated and tortuous until immediately proximal to the UVJ, where it abruptly tapers to an extremely narrow segment. Decreased ureteral peristalsis delays emptying of the ureter. Such findings are best seen when the bladder is empty (Aaronson & Cremin, 1984). Occasionally, the renal concentration impairment that occurs prevents adequate demonstration of the defect, and a retrograde pyelogram is necessary.

The surgical management, following resolution of the urinary tract infection, depends partially on the degree of function of the ureter and the kidney. Prompt correction of the obstructed megaureter is paramount, especially in the infant, to increase the potential for renal preservation (Hanna, 1988). Decompression of the kidney by placement of a nephrostomy tube may be the initial intervention, followed by re-evaluation of the upper urinary tract. Temporary diversion with a loop cutaneous ureterostomy is also another useful procedure for the infant with severe ureterectasis. A stoma is created in the ureter, close to the UPJ, and then is sutured to the skin. Urine flows unobstructed into a diaper that is wrapped in waistband fashion around the infant. Ureteral reconstruction occurs later, as indicated by radiologic monitoring.

If function is present, ureteral reimplantation with tapering and excision of the affected ureteral segment is the preferred surgical procedure. Care should be taken to preserve the ureteric blood supply and prevent any angulation of the ureter. A nonfunctional kidney and ureteral unit require nephroureterectomy.

Antibiotics are prescribed postimplant for 10 to 14 days and prophylactically for 3 months, followed by an excretory urogram and a VCUG to ascertain surgical success.

## URETERAL STRICTURE

**Etiology.** Congenital strictures of the ureter were once believed to be a rare occurrence. A major study by Cussen (1971) detected an incidence of mid-ureteral strictures of 30% among all ureteral obstructions.

Allen (1970, 1973) described strictures in the region of the pelvic brim as the ureter crosses the common iliac vessel. These strictures are believed to result from compression by the vessels during fetal life (King, 1985). Studies by Beck suggest that the ureter may develop normally in these cases but then is subjected to an ischemic episode (Johnston, 1982). It seems unreasonable to suspect that an abnormality of the ureteric bud would cause a stricture, because the renal parenchyma is usually normal. When the ureteric bud is abnormal, development of the kidney from metanephric tissue is usually grossly abnormal.

**Pathophysiology.** Ureteral strictures cause compensatory hyperplasia and hypertrophy in the preceding ureteral segment. Depending on the severity, the stenosis causes varying degrees of hydronephrosis. Chronic hydronephrosis may be asymptomatic, whereas stress conditions such as high fluid intake may result in intermittent renal colic.

**Medical-Surgical Management.** Management of ureteral stricture depends on the degree of functional renal impairment and hydronephrosis. If hydronephrosis is extreme, having caused extensive renal scarring and damage, nephrectomy is the treatment of choice. When renal function is preserved, a ureteroureterostomy is performed. The cut ends are anastomosed after excision of the strictured segment. A wide anastomosis, modified by spatulation to expedite matching discrepant calibers, is imperative. Recovery of normal ureteral function is usually seen by the fourth postoperative week.

# URETEROPELVIC JUNCTION OBSTRUCTION

**Etiology.** Obstruction of the UPJ is a condition that culminates in hydronephrosis. The cause is not uniform but rather may be traced to intrinsic or extrinsic causes. In its most common presentation, the musculature of the UPJ is replaced with inelastic collagen that creates an aperistaltic segment (Allen, 1970; Snyder et al., 1980). Another plausible theory of intrinsic etiology postulates that there is an arrest of ureteral development as it proceeds from the solid phase to recanalization (Ruano-Gil et al., 1975).

Extrinsic factors that produce UPJ obstruction include adhesions, kinks, or bands that wrap circumferentially around the ureter. Aberrant fetal blood vessels also may compress the ureter early in embryologic development (Allen, 1970). A high ureteral insertion at the renal pelvis, with subsequent angulation at the UPJ, may be a predisposing factor that leads to obstruction or may be an aftermath of the condition (Mann, 1990).

The left side is affected more frequently than the right side. UPJ obstruction predominates among males, especially in infancy, and they are usually more severely affected than females. Over half of the children with UPJ obstruction are diagnosed by the time they are 5 years old, and 25% are diagnosed before the age of 1 year. Evidence of dysplasia can be seen in the more severe cases of UPJ obstruction. Multicystic, dysplastic kidney with ureteral atresia is the most severe associated anomaly. UPJ may also be associated with other urinary tract abnormalities, including hypospadias, malrotation, duplex kidneys, agenesis, renal ectopia, stones, and undescended testes. Contralateral UPJ obstruction may be present in as many as 25% of cases (Snyder et al., 1980).

Symptoms of UPJ obstruction are often intermittent. When stressed with increased urine production, the pelvis is unable to drain urine adequately through the partial obstruction. The obstruction then causes dilatation of the pelvis and increasing hydronephrosis and pain, often accompanied by nausea and vomiting. These symptoms often suggest a gastrointestinal disorder, but the diagnosis of UPJ obstruction is usually made after the intestinal tract has been excluded through appropriate studies.

Urinary tract infection, pyelonephritis, or cystitis may also be the presenting event, occurring more frequently in females. Occasionally, reflux is present and demonstrated on a VCUG. Hematuria, particularly after minor trauma, appears to be one of the most common presenting signs in children aged 4 to 12 years. This is believed to be caused by intrapelvic pressure changes or acute obstruction, which could cause rupture of a dilated vessel (King, 1985). In the child younger than 1 year of age, the presence of an abdominal mass often calls attention to the problem. Of all abdominal masses in infants, one half are from renal origin; 40% of these cases of kidney enlargement occur from UPJ obstruction. The appreciation of this diagnosis has been markedly increased with the use of antenatal ultrasonography. Children with disorders that would have been undetected until they presented with symptoms of infection or a mass are now detected antenatally, and appropriate therapy initiated in the neonatal period conserves renal tissue and allows for functional restoration (Snyder et al., 1980).

**Pathophysiology.** The child with UPJ obstruction demonstrates a dilated ureter, renal pelvis, and calices. Peristaltic activity from the renal pelvis to the ureter is disrupted, and contractility may be weakened as well as prolonged. The rhythmic progression of peristalsis becomes uncoordinated and counteractive. Renal impairment varies according to the severity of hydronephrosis and is a consequence of destruction to the renal tubules and glomeruli (Mann, 1990).

**Medical-Surgical Management.** The medical management is based on an appropriate diagnosis. The most important diagnostic test is the excretory urogram, which differentiates between UPJ and UVJ obstruction. In neonates with immature concentrating ability, the excretory urogram is not reliable; therefore, renal ultrasonography and renal scanning are the initial evaluative studies. With the increased use of prenatal ultrasonography, many cases of hydronephrosis are diagnosed antenatally.

A furosemide-augmented excretory urogram or renal scan gives a clear picture of the degree of obstruction if renal function is adequate to preserve concentrating ability. The major diagnostic problem with UPJ obstruction is that symptoms tend to be related to variability in urine flow rates. A diuretic administered at the time of the excretory urogram or scan may be required to increase the urine production and precipitate the pain and hydronephrosis. A VCUG is also performed to rule out the presence of vesicoureteral reflux. Occasionally, a retrograde ureterogram at the time of surgical intervention is necessary to confirm the obstruction when conventional testing fails to outline the ureter completely.

In the neonate with marked hydronephrosis, after definitive diagnosis is made, placement of a percutaneous nephrostomy is sometimes performed. This measure decompresses the kidney, gives time to evaluate renal function, and makes surgical correction less traumatic. Nephrostomy drainage allows time to determine if the kidney is salvageable. Temporary nephrostomy is also used to allow time for a small neonate to reach a more optimal weight and maturity for anesthesia. In some instances, when renal function is so diminished that it is not recoverable, nephrectomy is performed.

In most cases, a dismembered pyeloplasty is performed. In this procedure, the surgeon excises the obstructed segment and anastomoses the ureter to the renal pelvis. Improvement in the excretory urogram study is generally demonstrated within 6 months. Placement of a ureteral stent to carry urine to an external drainage collector helps eliminate the problem of postoperative obstruction due to edema. Stents are removed at the surgeon's discretion, either several days or several weeks later. Internal drainage with a double-J stent, which allows urine to bypass the anastomosis site, is another option.

A urethral catheter may be inserted for 3 to 4 days to provide bladder decompression. An incisional Penrose drain is left in place and removed when incisional drainage ceases. Administration of antibiotics intraoperatively and postoperatively is routine.

## VESICOURETERAL REFLUX

**Etiology.** Primary vesicoureteral reflux is believed to be caused by anomalous development of the ureterovesical tunnel. It becomes evident by the fifth fetal month, when urine production initiates. The reason for the defect in normal development is unknown but is associated with a deficiency of the longitudinal muscle of the submucosal ureter (Levitt, 1981).

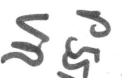

ary reflux is the result of another
rary tract, such
blad-
e. The
stigat-

reflux
urinary
anomalies
own. However, evaluation of the urinary tract following urinary tract infec-

tion has demonstrated vesicoureteral reflux in 25% to 50% of this pediatric population (Smellie & Normand, 1966; Walker et al., 1977). Age seems to be a factor in the incidence of reflux, because the percentage of children with the anomaly decreases progressively throughout childhood. There is a 10:1 ratio between white and black females, both positive for urinary tract infection, who have associated vesicoureteral reflux (Askari & Belman, 1982).

Siblings of children with vesicoureteral reflux are at increased risk for the disease; reflux is often unaccompanied by urinary tract infection or voiding disorder. Vesicoureteral reflux may affect as many as 45% of this population, with both sexes affected equally (Abbeele et al., 1987; Dwoskin, 1976; Jenkins & Noe, 1982; Screening for reflux, 1978). Although the exact mechanism of genetic transmission is unclear, it is postulated to be by polygenic or multifactorial inheritance (Screening for reflux, 1978).

**Pathophysiology.** The definition of vesicoureteral reflux is the abnormal backflow of urine from the bladder into the ureter or into the ureter and the kidney. The normal valve mechanism of the ureter depends on the oblique entry of the ureter into the fixed posterolateral portion of the floor of the bladder, an adequate intramural ureteral length in proportion to its diameter, and an adequate amount of support by the detrusor muscle for both the intramural and submucosal ureters. These factors together prevent reflux by producing a passive valve mechanism. In the patient with vesicoureteral reflux, the ureteral orifice is laterally displaced to a more direct intravesical entry angle, the submucosal ureter is foreshortened, and the valve mechanism does not function properly because of the decrease in the ratio (normally, 4:1 or 5:1) between the submucosal length and ureteral diameter (Anderson & Smey, 1985).

The major concern with vesicoureteral reflux is the potential for renal scarring and damage. Most scarring seems to occur in children between birth and 5 years of age; often, it relates to the process of intrarenal reflux, defined as the extension of vesicoureteral reflux into the collecting tubules and nephrons, which theoretically allows urinary bacteria to gain access to the renal parenchyma and begin the process of renal scarring. The scarring usually takes place in the polar areas of the kidney, where the papillae are either flat or concave, as opposed to convex. These papillae are refluxing and allow urine to enter the renal parenchyma. The result is a permanent alteration in the pa-

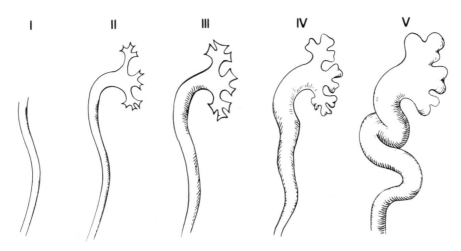

## GRADES OF REFLUX

*FIGURE 20–7* Grades of reflux—international study. (From Anderson, G. F., & Smey, P. [1985]. Current concepts in the management of common urologic problems in infants and children. *Pediatric Clinics of North America, 32*[5], 1145. Reprinted by permission.)

renchyma (fibrosis and scarring), and the morphology of the papillae is eventually changed, no longer allowing intrarenal reflux (Anderson & Smey, 1985; Levitt, 1981). Some researchers are questioning the role of bacteriuria in the formation of renal scars, having observed patients who incurred renal damage but have no history of urinary tract infection (Keenin, 1987). On initial evaluation for vesicoureteral reflux, 30% to 60% already show evidence of renal scarring. As the age of onset for urinary tract infection increases, the associated finding of vesicoureteral reflux decreases, suggesting that children gradually outgrow the condition (Levitt, 1981). Kidneys subjected to vesicoureteral reflux are smaller than normal kidneys not experiencing vesicoureteral reflux but there is still controversy over whether there is an increased or accelerated rate of growth in the affected kidney once the condition is eliminated. It has also been noted by some researchers that somatic growth in prepubertal children increases once vesicoureteral reflux is eliminated (Levitt, 1981). Research by Wettlaufer (1989) demonstrated a significant increase in height and weight postreplant that was directly proportional to the degree of reflux.

Another potential consequence of vesicoureteral reflux is the development of hypertension. The exact incidence of hypertension associated with renal scarring from vesicoureteral reflux in children is currently not available. A certain number of patients who manifest renal scarring associated with vesicoureteral reflux have ele-

vated renin levels and eventually develop hypertension. Some ultimately progress to end-stage renal disease (Holland, 1979; Smellie & Normand, 1979). This sequence is not predictable, because the degree of scarring is not directly correlated with outcome. Long-term follow-up of patients with a history of vesicoureteral reflux and renal scarring is therefore essential (Levitt, 1981).

**Medical-Surgical Management.** The management of the patient with vesicoureteral reflux is dictated in most instances by the grade of reflux present. The International Study Classification (Fig. 20–7) developed the definitions of gradation. These gradings are based solely on VCUG results. An excretory urogram is employed to assess the anatomy of the upper tracts, whereas the renal scan (DMSA) or glucoheptonate cortical scan can provide evidence of renal scarring and indicate renal function. Appropriate treatment is guided by the radiologic findings.

A cystoscopy is often useful, enabling the urologist to determine the diameter and position of the ureteral orifices by direct visualization.

Medical management for grade I or II reflux consists of vigilant monitoring for urinary tract infection and continuous, low-dose prophylactic antibiotics. Such management is continued until the vesicoureteral reflux has resolved as documented by two negative VCUGs 1 year apart. The child must be kept on continuous antibiotic prophylaxis. The encouragement of frequent voiding, good perineal hygiene, and prevention of constipation are also recommended.

Serial urine cultures monitor the maintenance of urine sterility. The medical approach is based on the fact that vesicoureteral reflux tends to improve or resolve with time. Resolution can occur in children with dilated or non-dilated ureters. Studies indicate that spontaneous resolution most often occurs in the first months or years of treatment, up to puberty, after which it is unlikely that the child will outgrow reflux. Because vesicoureteral reflux may hamper continence, parents should be discouraged from unduly pressuring the young child to be dry until the reflux resolves.

The debate of medical versus surgical treatment involves reflux grades III through V. Surgical correction of vesicoureteral reflux has a very high rate of success—usually higher than 98% in the hands of the experienced pediatric urologist. The technique of ureteral replantation is a definitive treatment for reflux. The exact procedure is based on the individual case and surgeon's preference; the degree of ureteral dilatation, the location of ureteral orifices, and the presence of voiding abnormalities all may affect the choice of technique. The techniques currently employed are either the Politano-Leadbetter intravesical approach or the transtrigonal technique of Cohen. Both techniques are quite effective (Bellinger, 1985).

A controversial issue related to vesicoureteral reflux is the management in newly diagnosed cases among adolescents or young adults. It has been shown that adults with renal scarring often had vesicoureteral reflux in childhood. There is also a definite connection between adults with renal scarring and renal insufficiency and hypertension. Surgical correction in these adult patients decreased the incidence of pyelonephritis but not the overall progression of the disease process. There are also studies to document that pregnant women with vesicoureteral reflux are more likely to have problems with pyelonephritis and bacteriuria (Bellinger, 1985) and have premature births. Consequently, reimplantation is recommended if conservative treatment fails to resolve reflux by puberty (King, 1985).

The last issue concerns the familial tendency of vesicoureteral reflux and the screening of asymptomatic siblings of patients found to have the condition. Numerous studies have shown the incidence in asymptomatic or symptomatic siblings of patients with vesicoureteral reflux to be from 8% to 45%. This is in sharp contrast to the general population, in which the incidence is approximately 1%. For all of the reasons previously discussed, screening of siblings seems to be prudent (Abbeele et al., 1987; Dwoskin, 1976; Jenkins & Noe, 1982; Screening for reflux, 1978).

## URETEROVESICAL JUNCTION OBSTRUCTION

UVJ obstruction is usually related to the condition known as primary obstructive megaureter, previously discussed in this chapter. In addition to primary obstructive megaureter, other causes of UVJ obstruction include strictures, diverticula, ureteroceles, calculi, or polyps. The reader is referred to other sections of this chapter, along with Chapters 4 and 6, for further discussion on the pathophysiology and management of these and other related conditions.

## Approaches to Patient Care

The nursing care of patients with a congenital anomaly of the ureter is similar, regardless of the specific anomaly. The symptomatology is similar, as are the problems and health care needs. Therefore, this section addresses the overall strategy for nursing care.

### Assessment

The initial history may begin with a diagnosis of hydronephrosis or ureteral tortuosity recognized on antenatal ultrasonography. An incomplete ureter may precipitate hydronephrosis in the ipsilateral kidney or compensatory hydronephrosis in the contralateral kidney. The child with bilateral incomplete ureters associated with renal agenesis will not survive. It is possible to identify or suspect the presence of a ureterocele, duplicated ureter, megaureter, incomplete ureter, or UPJ or UVJ obstruction by prenatal ultrasonography. The technique of the ultrasonographer, as well as the experience and expertise of the obstetrician or maternal–fetal medicine physician and pediatric urologist, increases the recognition of these problems. In most instances, there is consultation with a pediatric urologist to determine the most likely diagnosis based on the ultrasound findings. This review allows the urologist to meet with the prospective parents to discuss the urologic findings and provide them with an understanding of what the proposed plan of care will be once the infant is born. The consultation also permits the medical and nursing staff members (the clinical nurse specialist in many institutions) to prepare for the child having this urologic problem and to ensure appropriate studies while the patient is in the neonatal nursery. The early detection and subsequent intervention of hydronephrosis interrupt the potential progression of renal damage and help reduce the risk of urinary tract infection.

A high percentage of children present initially with a urinary tract infection. The child has a wide range of symptoms, depending on age of onset, the virulence of the bacteria, and the presence of intrarenal reflux. The physical examination may disclose abdominal or costovertebral tenderness; cloudy, foul-smelling urine; and fever higher than 38.5°C. The urinalysis shows bacteriuria, leukocytosis, possibly hematuria, and mild proteinuria, and possibly tests positive for nitrate. A urine culture is obtained for microorganism identification and sensitivity as determined by the usual spectrum of antibiotics. (For specific details regarding the nursing assessment of a child with urinary tract infection, see Chapter 18.)

In many instances, gross ureteral defects in young infants are detected by prenatal ultrasonography or during palpation for a flank mass. The degree of hydronephrosis or ureteral tortuosity determines if a mass can be felt. The likelihood of palpating an abdominal mass in an infant older than 6 months of age is minimal because of increased deposits of subcutaneous fat and the muscular development of the abdomen and retroperitoneum.

The older infant or young child with a ureteral disorder may have a history of delayed growth or even failure to thrive. Height and especially weight measurements are consistently below the appropriate range for age. Parents report that the child is colicky, lethargic, irritable, and "sickly." Indeed, the child may have experienced frequent colds, fevers, or respiratory infections and appears to succumb to each new bout of virus or flu. The underlying cause for the child's fragile health is most likely an undiagnosed urinary tract infection.

Another frequent symptom of ureteral anomalies that compromise renal urine flow is sudden or intermittent, sharp flank pain, often accompanied by nausea and vomiting. On examination, the child demonstrates abdominal tenderness. Gastrointestinal causes are initially suspected, and the child is treated for gastroenteritis. Occasionally, appendicitis is diagnosed, and the appendix is removed only to have an attack recur. The persistence of the symptomatology, or the discovery that the ingestion of large volumes of fluid can precipitate the pain, leads the investigator to suspect hydronephrosis from UPJ obstruction, megaureter, or ureteral stenosis. These children sometimes present with episodes of hematuria unrelated to specific trauma.

When assessing a child for the possibility of a ureteral disorder, inquire about the child's voiding pattern. A history of urgency, frequency, dysfunctional voiding, or dribbling incontinence (constant dampness in spite of regular voidings) is a clue to ureteral ectopia or ureteral duplication with an ectopic ureter distal to the bladder neck. Urinary obstruction may be a manifestation of a prolapsed ureterocele, which acts as a ball valve to obstruct the bladder neck. Occasionally, the prolapse may be seen as a bubble of smooth pink tissue protruding from a girl's urethra.

Inquiry should be made about symptoms of acute epididymitis in young boys or about vaginal infections or chronic vaginal discharge in young girls. On rare occasions, these symptoms are the result of ectopic ureters that terminate in the genital organs.

### Nursing Diagnosis

The nursing diagnoses for the patient and family with a congenital anomaly of the ureter may include the following:

1. Ineffective family coping related to the birth of an infant with a congenital anomaly.
2. Potential for infection related to urinary stasis, instrumentation of the urinary tract, or placement of urinary drainage devices.
3. Pain related to
   a. Symptoms of urinary tract infection or hydronephrosis.
   b. Surgical intervention or accompanying bladder spasms.
4. Urinary incontinence related to inflammation, irritation, or infection of the urinary tract or possible anomalous placement of the ureter.
5. Knowledge deficit related to a specific ureteral anomaly, treatment modalities, postoperative care, or long-term management.
6. Patient/family anxiety related to the need for diagnostic evaluation, hospitalization, or surgical intervention.
7. Potential impairment of skin integrity related to urine incontinence or wound drainage.

### Plan of Care

The nursing care is directed toward enabling the patient or parents to

1. Understand the nature of the ureteral defect,

its evaluation and management, and how the condition impacts the child's future care needs.

2. Acquire knowledge of prescribed diagnostic procedures, including proper preparation, how tests are performed, and postprocedural instructions.

3. Understand the importance of completing the prescribed antibiotic course as an initial therapy for the child with a ureteral defect.

4. Recognize the signs and symptoms of urinary tract infection.

5. Remain free of postoperative infection.

6. Remain free of pain postoperatively, thereby providing for adequate rest and daytime activity.

7. Maintain the patency of urinary drainage tubes and resume normal voiding patterns after tube removal.

8. Prevent skin breakdown, redness, or excoriation from urine incontinence or wound drainage.

### Interventions

The nursing care of a patient with a congenital anomaly of the ureter begins as soon as the family or patient is aware of the problem, even prenatally when the diagnosis is made by sonography. The parents have been anticipating a perfectly normal infant and are shocked to receive news that something is wrong. They are usually seen by the pediatric urologist or their obstetrician, who counsels them on the ramifications of the ultrasound findings. The clinical nurse specialist or pediatric urology nurse can become involved at that time to answer the parents' questions or reiterate and reinforce the information provided by the physician. As concerns arise later, the parents may need to contact the nurse for further information or support.

Once the infant is born, nursing intervention takes a more active role in the care of patient and family. Assessing what family support system is available (e.g., grandparents, friends, or siblings) to help the family cope with the situation is important. The birth of an infant with an abdominal mass that was not detected prenatally by ultrasonography is always a shock and source of dismay for the family. Providing the parents and immediate family with an explanation of the diagnostic testing and helping reinforce or interpret explanations given by the physician are essential. When a child has been born with bilateral incomplete ureters associated with bilateral renal agenesis, it probably will not survive. Nursing care is then directed toward providing grief counseling for parents and family members.

The nurse caring for the baby with hydronephrosis and suspected ureteral defect needs to monitor accurately the infant's intake and urine output. If a urethral catheter has been inserted, meticulous meatal care, especially after stooling, is needed to reduce the risk of development of a urinary tract infection.

After an evaluation of renal function, the neonate may undergo placement of a percutaneous nephrostomy tube into the renal pelvis, under the guidance of fluoroscopy, to decompress the kidney. The nephrostomy tube siphons off the retained urine and allows for constant urine flow that bypasses the obstruction. As renal parenchymal tissue heals, kidney function often improves; subsequent function studies are obtained to evaluate kidney response to this treatment.

The nephrostomy tube is carefully coiled around its insertion site and covered with a transparent occlusive dressing, then connected to a sterile closed system for gravity drainage. Immediately postplacement, strict monitoring of urine output from the tube is essential. The nephrostomy tubes must be handled carefully, because they are prone to kinking and obstruction. Once a crease is created in the tubing, it must be splinted to prevent disruption of urine flow. Hematuria is common but usually is transient. Other complications, such as infection and bleeding from actual placement of the tube, are rare.

The family needs to be prepared for the insertion of the nephrostomy tube and then be provided with instructions for home care. The drainage system should remain closed and sterile. Gentle handling to prevent kinking or dislodgement, good hand-washing technique, and an adequate drainage bag reduce the risk of infection. Arranging follow-up with a home health agency to provide nursing care at home to assess the nephrostomy tube, answer questions the parents might have once they are caring for the infant at home, and assessment of adequate urine output is reassuring to both family and physician.

The child who presents with a urinary tract infection or a history of recurrent urinary tract infections needs a different type of intervention. Once the definitive diagnosis of urinary tract infection has been made (based on the results of a urine culture with sensitivities), the patient or family needs to be instructed on proper antibiotic therapy. The nurse should review the dose, dosage schedule, and possible side effects of the medication and emphasize the need for adequate fluid intake. Reinforce the importance of maintaining the prescribed duration of antibiotic therapy. Any diagnostic studies ordered postinfection should be explained to the patient and the parents.

If the child is hospitalized for pyelonephritis, vital signs should be monitored until the child is afebrile. Observe the child closely for signs of gram-negative shock, such as hyperventilation, hyperthermia, vomiting, diarrhea, chills, and warm, dry skin. Assurance of adequate urine output (at least 1 mL/kg/h) depends on increased oral intake or is accomplished by intravenous fluid therapy. Parenteral antibiotics are ordered and should be carefully administered at the prescribed times to maintain adequate blood levels.

On discharge, the family should be given detailed instructions about the medication administration. Stress the importance of completing the prescribed therapy. Scheduling a return visit to the physician's office or clinic for a follow-up urine culture or diagnostic studies should be arranged at the time of discharge (see Chap. 18 for other interventions pertaining to the care of a child with a urinary tract infection).

Once the diagnostic studies are completed and a diagnosis has been determined, surgical intervention may be required. The patient and family receive an explanation of the diagnosis and proposed surgical procedure from the physician. Initially, the nurse discusses the operation and hospitalization with the parents to determine their level of understanding of what they have been told. They often need some reinforcement or further explanation. Early-morning admission for most surgical procedures has had a great impact on nurses' ability to perform preoperative teaching. In instances when the clinical nurse specialist or a nurse from the day surgery department or the physician's office has been unable to spend some time with the patient and family to provide the necessary preoperative teaching, the nurse needs to provide all of the teaching postoperatively.

The child who undergoes pyeloplasty to correct a UPJ obstruction returns from the operating room with intravenous fluid, an anterior flank incision with a Penrose drain in place, subcuticular sutures, and either an occlusive dressing or sterile gauze covering the incision. The child may have a Foley (urethral) catheter inserted. Generally, a ureteral stent connected to a closed drainage is in place. Careful record-

ing of urine output, oral and intravenous intake, plus incisional drainage measurements should be maintained.

The Foley catheter at times requires irrigation with normal saline solution if flow is inadequate and the catheter appears obstructed. Meticulous stent or catheter care during each shift is essential. The child is started on oral fluids once completely awake postanesthesia and is advanced as tolerated. Turning or positioning and coughing and deep breathing (using incentive spirometry with preschool and school-age children) to prevent pulmonary complications are encouraged. The children are allowed to ambulate when medically feasible.

The Foley catheter is removed by the third postoperative day, and the ureteral stent is withdrawn by the sixth day, following a tubogram to ensure patency at the anastomosis site. Proper administration of analgesics, such as morphine sulfate, meperidine, acetaminophen (with or without codeine), as well as antispasmodics, such as opium and belladonna suppositories or oxybutynin chloride, for treatment of bladder spasms is essential to keep the child as comfortable as possible postoperatively. The use of distraction techniques, favorite toys, and security objects (blankets, pacifiers) for the younger child also helps reduce the anxiety associated with hospitalization and separation from the family. Encouraging the family to have one parent stay with the child as much of the time as possible, including overnight, also helps reduce the child's fear and anxiety related to hospitalization and surgery.

If there is not a large increase in drainage from the Penrose drain after removal of the Foley catheter or ureteral stent, the Penrose drain is removed and the child is ready for discharge. The child is continued on oral antibiotics at home for approximately 7 days and on prophylactic or suppressive doses for several weeks postoperatively. A follow-up excretory urogram is scheduled approximately 3 to 6 months later.

*Ureteral Reimplant.* The nursing interventions for the child having either unilateral or bilateral ureteral replantation to correct primary vesicoureteral reflux or megaureter with reflux or UVJ obstruction begin with a careful explanation to the family and patient of the procedure as described by the physician. Most children are admitted to the hospital on the day of surgery, having had their preoperative laboratory work done as an outpatient.

Postoperatively, urine is diverted from the bladder either by a urethral catheter or a suprapubic tube that exits through the dome of the bladder and out a puncture site approximately 2 to 4 cm above the incision. Ureteral stents may be inserted to ensure adequate drainage when postoperative edema may hinder urine flow. All drainage tubes are connected to a closed collection system. The Pfannenstiel incision includes a superficial, and possibly a deep, Penrose drain (if no suprapubic tube has been used).

Urine output initially should be monitored every 1 or 2 hours, then decreased to every 4 to 8 hours as the child heals. Vital signs are assessed at least every 4 hours, once stable, after the child leaves the postanesthesia care unit. The incision is covered with a transparent occlusive dressing, then with sterile gauze bandages. It should be checked every 4 hours for signs of drainage, redness, swelling, or increased tenderness, and the dressings changed as needed. Serosanguineous drainage is expected from Penrose drains, but a sudden marked increase should be reported to the physician. Usually, the drainage subsides in 24 to 48 hours postoperatively.

The superficial drain is removed as drainage slows, and the deep drain or ureteral stents are removed on the fourth postoperative day, unless ureteral tapering has been performed. Removal of the stent may be delayed until imaging studies confirm healing and patency. The patient is initially treated with analgesics, such as morphine sulfate or meperidine. The need for this usually subsides after 24 to 48 hours postoperatively. Acetaminophen, with or without codeine, is also prescribed once the child is taking oral fluids well. Oxybutynin chloride orally and belladonna and opium suppositories are helpful in treating bladder spasms. Oxybutynin chloride, 2.5 to 5 mg twice or three times a day, is prescribed and adjusted as needed on an individual basis, whereas belladonna and opium (B & O) suppositories (one half or one) are administered every 4 to 6 hours. Proper documentation of pain relief following administration of medication helps ensure adequate medication dosage.

Intravenous antibiotics, usually a second- or third-generation cephalosporin, are ordered postoperatively; the child is switched to an oral cephalosporin when the intravenous form is discontinued.

The child is encouraged to sit in a chair as soon as possible to hasten recovery and decrease the risk of pulmonary complications. Demonstrate to the parents how to use nonpharmacologic comfort measures to ensure a smoother postoperative period. Encourage parents to bring the child's favorite toys or cuddlies from home. They serve as a diversion while the child waits for relief from the analgesic, as well as provide familiarity and entertainment.

The urethral catheter or suprapubic tube is usually removed between 4 and 6 days postoperatively if there do not appear to be any clots present. Initially, the urine appears very bloody but clears over the next few days. Bladder spasms may be accompanied by urine discharge. Encourage a large fluid intake to help clear the urine. Stress to parents and the child that maintaining a high fluid intake reduces the risk of future urinary tract infection (Colbert & Lilien Thal, 1988; Cross, 1976).

The scheduling of a renal scan to check on adequate blood flow to the kidneys postoperatively is sometimes done before the patient is discharged. This test is not for the purpose of determining the elimination of reflux, because postoperative edema produces some degree of obstruction and does not allow a good evaluation of the status of the reflux. Some degree of obstruction secondary to edema always remains. The follow-up VCUG is scheduled between 3 and 6 months postoperatively, depending on the degree of ureteral reconstruction that was necessary.

Teaching the family the names, dosages, and duration of antibiotic therapy is part of the discharge process. Patients are discharged on therapeutic doses of antibiotics for approximately 5 to 7 days and then are continued on the prophylactic dose until the follow-up radiologic studies confirm the cessation of reflux. Patients are seen for follow-up between 1 and 2 weeks postoperatively.

Parents need to be instructed that their child may return to school and is able to bathe or, preferably, shower once they get home (the suprapubic site usually closes sufficiently within 24 hours of removal). Activity basically returns to normal, except for excessive rough play or contact sports, within a week after the return home.

***Ureterostomy.*** The infant with massive ureterectasis sometimes is treated surgically with cutaneous ureterostomy (or ureterostomies). This procedure of implanting the ureter or ureters into an opening on the abdominal wall is performed to divert the urine temporarily (Walker, 1988). At times, one ureter is anastomosed to the other ureter and then brought out through the abdominal wall to the skin in a single stoma (transureteroureterostomy). A third technique is a loop cutaneous ureterostomy. The ureter immediately adjacent to the UPJ is dissected and opened to the flank. The diversion allows the hydronephrosis associated with the obstruction to subside, then the urologist re-evaluates the renal function in several months.

Postoperatively, the child needs careful observation and accurate measurement of intake and output every 1 or 2 hours, progressing to every 4 hours. The urine is initially blood tinged but clears rapidly within a day or two. The infant only requires a diaper and petroleum jelly gauze dressing over the stoma postoperatively. The nurse should check the color of the stoma every 4 hours and observe for any drainage or evidence of infection. Any marked edema, prolapse, stenosis, or skin breakdown should be reported to the physician. Vital signs should be monitored every 4 hours for the first 48 hours postoperatively, then routinely. Intravenous fluids are ordered until the patient is able to tolerate oral feeding. Analgesics should be administered as needed. Intravenous morphine is ordered immediately postoperatively, and then acetaminophen, with or without codeine, should be sufficient to manage pain control. The infant can be held by the parent immediately after the surgery is completed. Diet is initiated with clear fluids and advanced as tolerated to age-appropriate feedings.

Home care following cutaneous ureterostomy entails keeping the area clean, monitoring urine output, and detecting signs of urinary tract infection (i.e., fever, foul-smelling urine, and dysuria). The skin can be washed with mild soap and water and carefully dried. Water-soluble salves can be used to provide skin protection. Frequent diaper changes are necessary. If only one ureter has been implanted into the abdominal wall, the child will still urinate, and the parents should monitor this output as well. The patient is administered parenteral, then oral, antibiotics while in the hospital and is discharged on antibiotics for at least 5 to 7 more days in a therapeutic dose. If there was any evidence of reflux, prophylactic doses of antibiotics will be maintained until the reflux resolves or is surgically corrected. Involvement of a home health agency is frequently beneficial; the caregivers provide reassurance and ongoing assessment of the child for a short time after discharge. Follow-up is usually scheduled 1 or 2 weeks postoperatively. Further radiographic studies are scheduled 3 to 6 months later to re-evaluate renal and ureteric function.

**Patient Outcomes**

1. The family or patient verbalizes an understanding of ureteral anomaly, proposed plan of treatment, and long-term management.
2. The patient exhibits no signs or symptoms of urinary tract infection.
3. The patient verbalizes or expresses a decrease in pain by facial expression, body position, or attitude.
4. An adequate urine output is maintained at approximately 1 to 3 mL/h.
5. The patient shows no signs of postoperative complications (e.g., wound infection, pneumonia).
6. Catheters (ureteral or urethral) remain patent for their duration.
7. The patient's voiding pattern normalizes after surgical correction or catheter removal.
8. The patient shows no signs of skin breakdown, redness, or excoriation and patient or family can provide appropriate stoma care.
9. The family verbalizes an understanding of the prescribed postoperative medications and follow-up instructions.
10. The child or family demonstrates an ability to cope with the urologic disorder while in the hospital, as well as after discharge.

# PRUNE BELLY SYNDROME (EAGLE-BARRETT SYNDROME)

## Perspective on Disease Entity

**Etiology.** *Prune belly syndrome* is the most common term for congenital absence, deficiency, or hypoplasia of the abdominal musculature. It is a condition characterized by a large hypotonic bladder, dilated and tortuous ureters, and bilateral cryptorchidism. The syndrome occurs almost exclusively in males. Its occurrence is about 1:35,000 births (Kratochwil, 1986).

The cause of prune belly syndrome is unknown; however, several theories have been suggested. Some researchers believe that the abdominal wall defect and intra-abdominal cryptorchidism are secondary to distention of the urinary tract. Because of its predominance in males, an obstruction at the level of the posterior urethra might cause this distention. From an embryologic viewpoint, it is theorized that a primary mesodermal error may result in the prune belly defect. It may also be caused by a complex chromosomal mutation (Riccardi & Grumm, 1977), possibly with a sex-linked inheritance.

**Pathophysiology.** Most children with prune belly syndrome have similar appearances (Fig. 20–8). The wrinkled abdominal wall in the infant tends to take on a pot-bellied appearance in early childhood. Bilateral cryptorchidism is evident. The testes are intra-abdominal, and orchiopexy is technically more challenging owing to the shortened spermatic vessels. Various orthopedic anomalies that are also associated in conjunction with prune belly syndrome are thought to be a direct result of fetal compression from oligohydramnios. These conditions range from a dimple in the outer aspect of the knee to the absence of the lower portion of the leg. Clubfoot and congenital hip dislocation are also seen. Intestinal defects include malrotation, imperforate anus, and Hirschsprung's disease. Chronic constipation is often a problem. Approximately 10% of the infants with prune belly syndrome have cardiac anomalies such as ventricular septal defect, atrial septal defect, or tetralogy of Fallot (Adebonojo, 1973).

In the more severely affected infants, pulmonary hypoplasia is a major complication and may be fatal. Those children that survive are more prone to pneumonia because they lack accessory respiratory muscle action that enables them to cough effectively.

The kidneys may be normal, although renal dysplasia and hydronephrosis are typically associated with this syndrome. Renal deterioration is usually caused by infection rather than obstruction; therefore, hydronephrotic kidneys have relatively good function. The child's long-term prognosis is determined by the degree of dysplasia, which is exacerbated by urethral stenosis, megalourethra, or imperforate anus (Potter, 1972).

The prune belly bladder is large and thick walled. Vesicoureteral reflux is often present. Patent urachus may be present in some patients (Fig. 20–9).

**Medical-Surgical Management.** Fetal ultrasonography has made the presumptive diagnosis of prune belly syndrome possible. The earliest diagnosis was reported by Fremond and Babut (1986) in a 15-week-gestation fetus. However, no effective prenatal intervention has yet been identified. At birth, these children may have impaired renal function. The serum creatinine and blood urea nitrogen (BUN) levels may be elevated. Radiographic evaluation shows hydronephrosis and vesicoureteral reflux. Because of stasis of urine in the dilated system and inadequate detrusor contraction, urinary tract infections are a chronic problem.

Children with prune belly syndrome face multiple reconstructive procedures. Temporary urinary diversion may be necessary early in life. Often, the already-patent urachus is surgically opened even wider to allow temporary urinary diversion. Cutaneous vesicostomy is most often the procedure advocated. Vesicostomy is a surgical procedure in which the bladder is opened on the abdominal wall just below the umbilicus. The bladder mucosa is sutured to the abdomen, creating a stoma from which

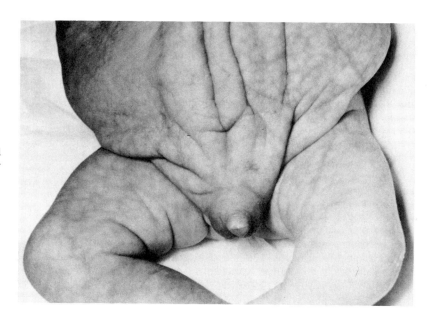

*FIGURE 20–8* Wrinkled abdominal wall of child with prune belly syndrome.

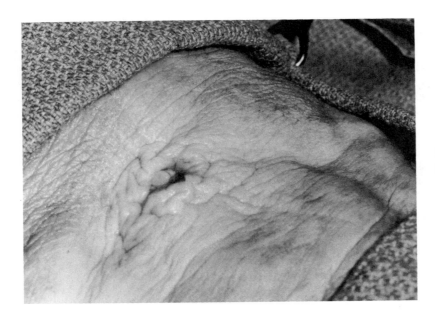

*FIGURE 20–9* Patent urachus in patient with prune belly syndrome.

urine drains freely. High-loop cutaneous ureterostomies may be required in patients having urosepsis or progressive renal deterioration. This surgical procedure is a form of temporary diversion in which the ureters are brought out onto the flank, creating a stoma to drain the upper portion of the urinary tract unimpeded. Urinary tract reconstruction after either procedure can be readily performed later.

As the child progresses beyond infancy, more extensive reconstructive procedures may be performed. The ultimate aims of any urologic intervention are to relieve urinary stasis, which predisposes the child to bacteriuria, and to conserve renal function.

The bladder of a child with prune belly syndrome typically is large, thickened, and humped at the dome. To eliminate urine stasis within this pseudodiverticulum, a reduction cystoplasty may be performed. A ureteral reimplantation treats reflux, a condition that may cause renal deterioration from urine regurgitation into the calices. The ureter is replanted into a more stable area of the bladder base to create a one-way, passive valve mechanism. Lifetime surveillance of these patients is necessary, because renal function may deteriorate over time.

Adults with prune belly syndrome are infertile. However, the testicles appear to have good androgenic function and, therefore, orchiopexy is part of the treatment of this syndrome. In recent years, abdominal wall plication has been performed to improve the appearance of these boys. Because this aspect of the defect seems to improve with age, many parents provide their children with a corset for external support rather than go through another surgical procedure.

## Approaches to Patient Care

### Assessment

The oligohydramnios of prune belly syndrome may be detected by prenatal ultrasonography or at delivery. The most obvious manifestation of the syndrome is the loose, wrinkled skin over the abdomen and torso. Bilateral cryptorchidism is also evident. A patent urachus draining urine can be seen. Other anomalies associated with prune belly syndrome that the nurse may observe are lower limb anomalies and clubfoot. The appearance of the infant may shock the parents and impair the bonding process. Support should be given to them.

Chronic upper respiratory infection or pneumonia may occur because the infant has inadequate muscular support of the diaphragm. As the child grows and is in a more upright position, these problems decrease.

Constipation can result from the lack of muscular support to the lower abdomen. The child is unable to push during bowel movements and may not empty the rectum completely; fecal retention may be noted during abdominal palpation.

Skin integrity may deteriorate from the constant drainage of urine through the patent urachus. The nurse may observe redness, excoriation, rash, or actual breakdown.

### Nursing Diagnosis

The nursing diagnoses for the patient with prune belly syndrome and the family may include the following:

1. Ineffective family coping related to the birth of a child with congenital anomalies.
2. Urinary retention or infrequent voiding related to ineffective voiding mechanisms.
3. Ineffective breathing patterns related to a decrease of respiratory effort.
4. Constipation related to lack of abdominal musculature and decreased peristalsis.
5. Actual or potential impaired skin integrity related to a patent urachus or temporary urinary diversion.
6. Body image disturbance related to flaccid abdominal musculature, testicular nondescent, and externalized urinary discharge.
7. Altered sexuality patterns related to failure to ejaculate or inability to produce viable sperm.

### Plan of Care

Nursing care is directed toward enabling the child or parents to

1. Understand the etiology, treatment options, and long-term management of prune belly syndrome.
2. Demonstrate increased attachment behavior.
3. Achieve regular and complete bladder emptying.
4. Achieve maximum pulmonary function.
5. Maintain skin integrity.
6. Prevent constipation.
7. Develop a positive body image.
8. Acquire a satisfying pattern of sexual functioning.

### Intervention

With the birth of an infant with a birth defect as obvious as prune belly syndrome, many parents react with fear, disgust, and shame. The nurse can intervene at this time by accepting the parents' feelings, providing simple explanations of the birth defect and pointing out positive aspects of the baby that the parent can expect, such as normal intellect, ability to ambulate, and surgical correction of the abdominal skin deformity. Encourage the parents to hold and touch the infant. Assist the parent as a role model by talking to and cuddling the infant.

Urinary tract infections need prompt medical attention. The parents should be taught to watch for signs of infection, such as listlessness, poor appetite, fever, and urine with a foul odor. Older children may also complain of dysuria and back pain. Medical intervention is necessary in the event of a urinary tract infection.

Management of urine drainage at the vesicostomy or ureterostomy site is best accomplished by diapering around the abdomen of infants or by using a disposable, gel-filled pad over the stoma, held in place with a diaper or abdominal binder in the older child. External appliances may be used on the ureterostomy stomas in some cases, but usually this is not necessary, because the urinary tract is often reconstructed before the child reaches an age when diapers are no longer acceptable.

The nursing care of the child who undergoes a reduction cystoplasty and ureteral replantation for prune belly syndrome is similar to the care needed by children having surgery for other ureteral defects (refer to the previous sections of this chapter for further information). Despite successful ureteral intervention, the child may still not empty the bladder completely. If this is the case, older children may be taught to void on a timed schedule and use double-voiding technique. After urinating, they should wait a few minutes and attempt to urinate again. Credé maneuvers (applying gentle pressure to the lower abdomen) may also help to empty the bladder. If this fails and the child continues to carry high residual volumes, thereby causing frequent urinary tract infection, clean intermittent catheterization may then be started.

The parents are taught signs of impending respiratory infection such as fever, congestion, and increased respirations. Frequent changes in the infant's position help drain the lungs. Pulmonary therapy (humidification, nasal suction, and chest clapping) during an acute episode may be required to prevent the progression of an upper respiratory infection to pneumonia. The parents should contact the pediatrician at the first indication of a respiratory problem.

Bowel irregularity, particularly constipation, may be a problem for children with prune belly syndrome. Measures taken to prevent constipation in infants include increased fluid intake, addition of fruits to the diet as tolerated, a stool softener such as docusate sodium taken daily, and glycerin suppositories used as needed. Enemas may be given as a last resort. Older children have fewer problems with constipation, because they are generally more active. Dietary changes, such as additional fluids, bulk, and roughage, may improve the situation. Also, establishing a regular time for elimination helps these children regulate bowel function.

In the infant and young child, skin care is a problem owing to constant contact with urine. Instruct the parents to use a perineal wash and waterproof, protective skin barrier and to inspect the skin daily for evidence of breakdown redness, excoriation, and rash. Skin breakdown that is intractable to home care requires medical attention. Superinfection may require a 3-day course of nystatin cream applied to the affected area two or three times daily. Diaper rashes are treated with nonprescription preparations. Disposable, gel-filled pads are used over the stoma site if a disposable diaper is inadequate in collecting the urine. The pads are held in place with a diaper or abdominal binder.

As the child with prune belly syndrome becomes more aware of his unusual appearance, he may develop feelings of shame or embarrassment. The school years can be a major source of stress as the child is exposed to common bathroom facilities, physical education classes, and group dressing and shower areas. The nurse works closely with the family and school personnel to monitor the child's adjustment pattern, his emotional response, and peer relationships in this stage in his development. Further assistance from the school psychologist, the school nurse, a clinical psychologist, or a social worker may ease the difficulties that arise during this time.

Sexual maturation ushers in a new realm of development problems. During adolescence, the teen is preoccupied with issues, fantasies, and activities that affirm his ability to be sexually capable and competent. Not only is he aware of the emerging secondary sex characteristics, but the adolescent recognizes the role of sex and intimacy in the quest for satisfying adult relationships. Sexual inadequacies, either imaginary or real, may be devastating to the adolescent's passage through these years and to the development of a positive feeling of self-worth. The nurse, using a background of developmental theory, can detect clues that suggest poor peer relationships and social adjustments. The adolescent and his family may be directed to a psychoendocrinologist, clinical psychologist, or sex therapist for help during this phase of development.

### Patient Outcomes

1. The parents become attached to the infant, as evidenced by seeking eye contact, talking to the infant, and providing sensory stimulation.
2. The parents effectively manage the special problems related to elimination, respiratory function, and skin integrity.
3. The child maintains optimal respiratory function, as evidenced by normal temperature and normal respiratory rate and pattern.
4. The child has regular bowel movements.
5. The child has good bladder function, as evidenced by sterile urine and urinary continence.
6. The child has good skin integrity.
7. The child and parents express a positive body image.
8. The child forms satisfying peer relationships.
9. The child expresses a positive sexual image.

## REFERENCES

Aaronson, I., & Cremin, B. (1984). *Clinical pediatric uroradiology* (pp. 203–205). London: Churchill Livingstone.

Abbeele, A., Treves, T., Lebowitz, R., Bauer, S., Davis, R., Retik, A., & Colodny, A. (1987). Vesicoureteral reflux in asymptomatic siblings of patients with known reflux: Radionuclide cystography. *Pediatrics, 79*(1), 147–153.

Adebonojo, F. O. (1973). Dysplasia of the abdominal musculature with multiple congenital anomalies: Prune belly or triad syndrome. *Journal of the National Medical Association, 65,* 327.

Allen, T. D. (1970). Congenital ureteral strictures. *Journal of Urology, 104,* 196.

Allen, T. D. (1973). Ureteral strictures. In Lutzeyer & Melchior (Eds.) *Urodynamics: Upper and lower urinary tract,* (pp. 137–147). Berlin: Springer-Verlag.

Anderson, W., & Smey, P. (1985). Current conception in the management of common urologic problems in infants and children. *Pediatric Clinics of North America, 32*(5), 1133–1149.

Ashcraft, K. W. (1990). *Pediatric urology.* Philadelphia: W. B. Saunders.

Askari, A., & Belman, A. B. (1982). Vesicoureteral reflux in black girls. *Journal of Urology, 127,* 747.

Bellinger, M. (1985). The management of vesicoureteral reflux. *Urologic Clinics of North America, 12*(1), 23–29.

Belman, A. B., & King, L. R. (1972). Urinary abnormalities associated with imperforate anus. *Journal of Urology, 108,* 823–824.

Bryan, A. L., Nigro, J. A., & Counseller, V. S. (1949). One hundred cases of congenital absence of the vagina. *Surgery, Gynecology and Obstetrics, 88,* 79–86.

Caldamone, A. (1985). Duplication anomalies of the upper tract in infants and children. *Urologic Clinics of North America, 12*(1), 75–91.

Campbell, C. (1973). Ultrasound detection of fetal abnormality [abstract]. In A. G. Motulsky (Ed.), *International Congress Series* No. 297, Fourth International Conference on Birth Defects.

Churchill, B., Abara, E., & McLorie, G. (1987). Ureteral duplication, ectopy and ureteroceles. *Pediatric Clinics of North America, 34*(5), 1273–1289.

Colbert, P., & Lilien Thal, M. (1988). Nursing management of the child with vesicoureteral reflux. *AUAA Journal, 8*(4), 15–20.

Cook, W. A., & Stephens, F. D. (1977). Fused kidneys: Morphologic study and theory of embryogenesis. In D. Bergsman & J. Duckett (Eds.), *Urinary systems—Malfor-*

mations in children (pp. 327–340). New York: Allen R. Liss.

Cross, P. (1976). Ureteral reimplantation: Nursing care of the child. *American Journal of Nursing, 76*(11), 1800–1803.

Cussen, L. J. (1971). The morphology of congenital dilation of the ureter: Intrinsic ureteral lesions. *Australian and New Zealand Journal of Surgery, 41,* 185.

DeKlerk, D. P., Marshall, F. F., & Jeffs, R. D. (1977). Multicystic dysplastic kidney. *Journal of Urology, 118,* 306–308.

Dwoskin, J. Y. (1976). Sibling uropathy. *Journal of Urology, 115,* 726.

Fremond, B., & Babut, J. (1986). Obstructive uropathies diagnosed in utero: The postnatal outcome—A study of 43 cases. *Progress in Pediatric Surgery, 19,* 160–177.

Glassberg, K. I., & Filmer, R. B. (1992). Renal dysplasia, renal hypoplasia and cystic disease of the kidney. In P. D. Kelalis, L. R. King, & A. B. Belman (Eds.), *Clinical pediatric urology* (3rd ed., pp. 1121–1184). Philadelphia: W. B. Saunders.

Gonzales, E. T. (1985). Urologic considerations in the newborn. *Urologic Clinics of North America, 12*(1), 43–51.

Greenberg, L. W., & Nelson, C. E. (1971). Crossed fused ectopia of the kidneys in twins. *American Journal of Diseases of Children, 122,* 175–176.

Greene, L. F., Feinzaig, W., & Dahlin, D. C. (1971). Multicystic dysplasia of the kidney: With special reference to the contralateral kidney. *Journal of Urology, 105,* 482–487.

Habib, R., Courticuissi, V., & Mathieu, H. (1962). Congenital bilateral hypoplasia, oligonephronia. *Journal d'Urologie et de Nephrologie* (Paris), *68,* 139.

Hanna, M. (1988). Megaureter. In L. King (Ed.), *Urologic surgery in neonates and young infants* (pp. 160–204). Philadelphia: W. B. Saunders.

Hartman, G. W., & Hodson, C. J. (1969). The duplex kidney and related abnormalities. *Clinical Radiology, 20,* 387.

Hildreth, T. A., & Cass, A. S. (1978). Cross renal ectopia with familial occurrence. *Urology, 12,* 59–60.

Holland, N. (1979). Reflux nephropathy and hypertension. In J. Hodson & P. Kincaid-Smith (Eds.), *Reflux nephropathy.* New York: Masson.

Jenkins, G. R., & Noe, H. N. (1982). Familial vesicoureteral reflux: A prospective study. *Journal of Urology, 128,* 774.

Johnson, D. K., & Perlmutter, A. D. (1980). Single system ectopic ureteroceles with anomalies of the heart, testis and vas deferans. *Journal of Urology, 123,* 81.

Johnston, J. H. (1982). Upper urinary tract obstruction. In D. Innes Williams & J. H. Johnston (Eds.), *Pediatric Urology* (2nd ed., pp. 189–213). London: Butterworth Scientific.

Keenin, C. (1987). *Detection, prevention and management of urinary tract infections* (4th ed.). Philadelphia: Lea & Febiger.

Kelalis, P. (1985a). Renal pelvis and ureter. In P. Kelalis, L. King, & A. B. Belman (Eds.), *Clinical pediatric urology* (2nd ed., pp. 672–725). Philadelphia: W. B. Saunders.

Kelalis, P. (1985b). Surgical correction of vesicoureteral reflux. In P. Kelalis, L. King, & A. B. Belman (Eds.), *Clinical pediatric urology* (2nd ed., pp. 381–417). Philadelphia: W. B. Saunders.

King, L. (1985). Ureter and ureterovesical junction. In P. Kelalis, L. King, & A. B. Belman (Eds.), *Clinical pediatric urology* (2nd ed., pp. 486–512). Philadelphia: W. B. Saunders.

Kohn, G., & Borns, P. F. (1973). The association of bilateral and unilateral renal aplasia in the same family. *Journal of Pediatrics, 83,* 54–97.

Kratochwil, A. (1986). Prenatal diagnosis of fetal malformations by ultrasonography. *Progress in Pediatric Surgery, 19,* 143–157.

Levitt, S. (1981). Medical versus surgical treatment of primary vesicoureteral reflux—Special article—Report of the International Reflux Study Committee. *Pediatrics, 67*(3), 392–400.

Longino, L. A., & Martin, L. W. (1958). Abdominal masses in the newborn infant. *Pediatrics, 21,* 596–604.

Mann, C. M. (1990). Ureteropelvic junction obstruction. In K. W. Ashcraft (Ed.), *Pediatric urology.* Philadelphia: W. B. Saunders.

McDonald, J. H., & McClellan, D. S. (1957). Crossed renal ectopia. *American Journal of Surgery, 93,* 995–1002.

Nation, E. F. (1944). Duplication of the kidney and ureter: A statistical study of 230 new cases. *Journal of Urology, 51,* 456.

Nordmark, B. (1948). Double formations of the pelves of the kidneys and ureters: Embryology occurrence and clinical significance. *Acta Radiologica, 30,* 267.

Pathak, I. G., & Williams, D. I. (1964). Multicystic and dysplastic kidneys. *British Journal of Urology, 36,* 318–331.

Potter, E. L. (1965). Bilateral absence of ureters and kidneys: A report of 50 cases. *Obstetrics and Gynecology, 25,* 3–12.

Potter, E. L. (1972). Abnormal development of the kidney. In E. L. Potter (Ed.), *Normal and abnormal development of the kidney* (pp. 3–305). Chicago: Year Book Medical Publishers.

Ransley, P. G. (1982). Vesicoureteral reflux. In D. I. Williams & J. H. Johnston (Eds.), *Pediatric urology* (2nd ed., pp. 151–165). London: Butterworth Scientific.

Riccardi, V. M., & Grumm, C. M. (1977). The prune-belly anomaly: Heterogeneity and superficial X-linkage mimicry. *Journal of Medical Genetics, 14,* 266–270.

Rizza, J. M., & Downing, S. E. (1971). Bilateral renal agenesis in two female siblings. *American Journal of Diseases of Children, 121,* 60–63.

Royer, P., Habib, R., & Mathieu, H., & Courtecuisse V. (1962). Congenital bilateral renal hyperplasia with reduction of the number and hypertrophy of the nephrons in children. *Annales de Pediatrie* (Paris), *9,* 133–146.

Royle, M. G., & Goodwin, W. E. (1971). The management of ureteroceles. *Journal of Urology, 106,* 42.

Ruano-Gil, D., Coca-Payerus, A., & Tejedo-Maten, A. (1975). Obstruction and normal recanalization of the ureter in the human embryo: Its relation to congenital ureteric obstruction. *European Urology, 1,* 287.

Sanders, R. C. (1979). Renal cystic disease. In M. I. Resnick & R. C. Sanders (Eds.), *Ultrasound in urology* (pp. 97–121). Baltimore: Williams & Wilkins.

Scheinman, J. I., & Abelson, H. T. (1970). Bilateral renal hypoplasia with oligonephronia. *Journal of Pediatrics, 76,* 369.

Screening for reflux [Editorial]. (1978). *Lancet, 2,* 23.

Sharp, R. J. (1990). Developmental anomalies of the kidney. In K. W. Ashcraft (Ed.), *Pediatric urology.* Philadelphia: W. B. Saunders.

Smellie, J. M., & Normand, C. S. (1979). Reflux nephropathy in childhood. In J. Hodson & P. Kincaid-Smith (Eds.), *Reflux nephrology.* New York: Masson.

Smellie, J. M., & Normand, C. S. (1966). The clinical features and significance of urinary infection in childhood. *Proceedings of the Royal Society of London, 59,* 415.

Smith, D. W. (1982). XO syndrome (Turner's syndrome). In M. Markowitz (Ed.), *Recognizable patterns of human malformation—Genetic, embryologic and clinical aspects* (pp. 72–75). Philadelphia: W. B. Saunders.

Smith, D., Egginton, J., & Brookfield, D. (1987). Detection of abnormality of fetal urinary tract as a predictor of renal tract disease. *British Medical Journal, 294,* 27–28.

Snyder, H. M., Lebowitz, R., Colodny, A., Bauer, S., & Retik, A. (1980). Ureteropelvic junction obstruction in children. *Urologic Clinics of North America, 7*(2), 273–290.

Thompson, D. P., & Lynn, H. B. (1966). Genital anomalies associated with solitary kidney. *Mayo Clinic Proceedings, 41,* 538.

Turncock, R., & Shawis, R. (1984). Management of fetal urinary tract anomalies detected by prenatal ultrasonography. *Archives of Disease in Childhood, 59,* 962–965.

Vathibhagdee, A., & Singleton, E. (1973). Infantile polycystic disease of the kidney. *American Journal of Diseases of Children, 125,* 167–170.

Walker, R. D. (1988). Who needs temporary diversion? In L. King (Ed.), *Urologic surgery in neonates and young infants* (pp. 226–238). Philadelphia: W. B. Saunders.

Walker, R. D., Duckett, J., & Bartone, F. (1977). Screening schoolchildren for urologic disease. *Pediatrics, 60,* 239.

Wettlaufer, J. (1989) Growth following ureteral reimplantation. Paper read at the American Urological Association Allied Conference, Dallas, Texas, May, 1989.

Williams, D. I. (1982). Ureteric duplications and ectopia. In D. I. Williams, & J. H. Johnston (Eds.), *Pediatric urology* (2nd ed., pp. 167–187). London: Butterworth Scientific.

Williams, D. I., & Johnston, J. H. (Eds.) (1982). *Pediatric urology* (2nd ed.). London: Butterworth Scientific.

Wilmer, H. A. (1938). Unilateral fused kidney: A report of five cases and a review of the literature. *Journal of Urology, 40,* 551–571.

Winter, J. S., Kohn, G., Mellman, W. J., & Wagner, S. (1968). A familial syndrome of renal, genital and middle ear anomalies. *Journal of Pediatrics, 72,* 88–93.

Zerres, K., Volpel, M. C., & Weib, H. (1984). Cystic kidneys: Genetics, pathologic anatomy, clinical picture and prenatal diagnosis. *Human Genetics, 68,* 104–135.

CHAPTER 21

# Bladder Exstrophy and Epispadias

■

*Vicki Bowers, Kathleen F. Hannigan, and Karen L. Kushner*

## OVERVIEW

Classic and cloacal bladder exstrophy and epispadias are disfiguring congenital anomalies that threaten not only the health of the kidneys but also a child's body image, self-esteem, and future social adaptation.

This chapter describes the embryologic alterations resulting in these congenital defects and the anatomic variations present at birth. Emphasis is placed on the importance of early neonatal assessment, staged surgical reconstruction, and continuous follow-up. Methods to obtain functional closure of the bladder are examined; advances in these techniques provide for improved renal preservation, a more pleasing genital appearance and, most importantly, a greater opportunity for achieving urinary continence.

The chapter progresses according to the recommended sequence of surgical procedures. Its focus is the specialized nursing care required for each stage of repair. The developmental needs of the child and parent-child coping are incorporated throughout.

## BEHAVIORAL OBJECTIVES

After studying this chapter, the reader should be able to

1. Summarize the structural defects and corrective surgical procedures associated with classic bladder exstrophy.

2. Generate a plan of care for the bladder exstrophy newborn and his or her family to promote parent-infant bonding.

3. Interpret the system used to provide urinary drainage for the child following any of the reconstructive surgeries and predict potential causes of obstruction for that system.

4. Contrast nursing techniques that help maintain the infant versus the toddler sufficiently immobile while in traction following primary bladder closure.

5. Summarize the methods by which nurses and family members may positively influence the initial voiding experience following bladder neck reconstruction.

## KEY WORDS

**Bladder dehiscence**—rupture of the abdominal incision following the surgical closure of bladder exstrophy, allowing the bladder to move out of the pelvic ring.

**Bladder neck plasty**—a surgical procedure to reconstruct the bladder neck by creating a new urethra (neourethra) to provide for continence.

**Bladder outlet resistance**—the amount of opposing pressure exerted against the bladder by the internal sphincter; must be low enough pressure to allow for complete emptying of the bladder during voiding; must be high enough pressure to maintain continence between voidings; may be surgically increased, as in the tightening of the urethra to achieve continence.

**Bryant's traction**—a type of skin traction used to immobilize both lower extremities to allow for healing of the reapproximated pelvis following bladder exstrophy closure; elevates the lower extremities to a vertical position with the child supine; the trunk and lower extremities form a right angle; used primarily with newborns or very young infants.

**Bryant's traction, modified**—the pelvis is immobilized in the same manner as in Bryant's traction; however, the knees are flexed to prevent damage to arterial circulation; used in older infants and children.

**Classic exstrophy**—a congenital defect of the bladder and lower abdominal wall exposing an open, protruding bladder and urethra through the defect in the anterior wall of the abdomen.

**Cloacal exstrophy**—a severe variation of bladder exstrophy in which the normal separation of the intestinal tract from the urinary tract is interrupted, resulting in a fused bladder and intestine.

**Diastasis of the pelvis**—the nonunion of the pubic bones at the anterior midline (symphysis pubis).

**Dorsal chordee**—an upward curvature of the pelvis.

**Epispadias**—an opening at any point along the dorsal shaft of the penis, exposing the urethra; the internal sphincter mechanism is intact, and continence is maintained.

**Epispadias, complete**—an opening along the entire shaft of the penis, exposing the urethra; the internal exstrophy sphincter is cleft and rendered incompetent, resulting in continuous incontinence; associated with bladder exstrophy.

**Marshall-Marchetti bladder neck suspension**—the surgical suspension of the bladder neck to the symphysis pubic bone to create an increased urethrovesical angle, providing increased outlet resistance for achieving urinary continence; an anti-incontinence procedure.

**Mitrofanoff procedure**—a surgical procedure to reconstruct a catheterizable urinary stoma using bowel tissue, most frequently the appendix. An antireflux connection between the bladder and bowel segments provides for continence between inte mittent catheterization.

**Neourethra**—the surgical reconstruction of the urethra using urethral mucosa to form a new urethra.

**Pelvic osteotomy**—the bilateral incision of bone wedges from the innominate bone of the pelvis, allowing for anterior closure of the symphysis pubic bones to form a more normal pelvic ring, thus correcting the diastasis of the pelvis present in bladder exstrophy.

**Young-Dees-Leadbetter bladder neck plasty**—a surgical procedure to promote urinary continence by tightening the bladder neck. The procedure involves re-implantation of the ureters higher on the bladder wall to allow excision of a midline strip of trigone muscle to form a neourethra. The neourethra is supported by trigone muscle wrapped in a double-breasted fashion.

**Young's urethroplasty, modified**—a surgical procedure to correct the epispadias defect. A dorsal strip of penile skin is tubularized to form a neourethra. Triangular areas on either side of the strip of skin are reapproximated to form the glans.

---

## PERSPECTIVE ON DISEASE ENTITY

### Etiology

The exstrophy–epispadias complex is a group of serious congenital defects of the lower genitourinary tract and musculoskeletal structures of the pelvis. There are several variations of the complex, ranging in severity. They are all closely related and result from an interruption in the early embryonic development of the caudal end of the embryo.

The cause of exstrophy–epispadias complex is unknown. The incidence of bladder exstrophy is approximately 3.3:100,000 live births and occurs twice as often in males as in females (Gearhart & Jeffs, 1992; Lancaster, 1987). The risk of recurrence of bladder exstrophy in any given family is approximately 1:100. There does not appear to be a direct inheritance pattern. From a study involving 225 offspring of exstrophy–epispadias complex parents, the risk of bladder exstrophy appearing in offspring was determined to be approximately 1:70 live births (Shapiro et al., 1984).

### Pathophysiology

Normal embryonic development of the urinary tract involves a precise sequence of steps. Early in gestational life, the bladder and the distal intestine emerge principally from the cloaca, a blind oval chamber appearing in the caudal end of the embryo. The anterior wall of the cloaca is formed by the cloacal membrane, a temporary structure that gradually diminishes in size as surrounding structures develop. The bladder is not fully separated from the intestinal tract until the embryo is at least 6 weeks old. The complete migration of mesodermal cells toward the midline is essential for this important division of the cloaca into the intestinal tract and the bladder (Fig. 21–1), and later for the formation and closure of the anterior walls of the bladder, genitalia, and abdomen (Muecke, 1986).

When the migration of mesodermal cells is interrupted, the prominent cloacal membrane persists and acts as a wedge, preventing the completion of essential developmental steps (Muecke, 1986). Eventually, the cloacal membrane weakens and ruptures, resulting in an exposed lower urinary tract and abdominal wall (Fig. 21–2). In effect, the closing mechanism is never completed.

The variations of the exstrophy–epispadias complex have in common some degree of persistent cloacal membrane responsible for interrupting embryonic development. The timing is most important. The earlier the interruption in gestational life, the more severe the defect, because less time is available for the normal developmental process. The later the interruption in gestational life, the less severe the defect, because more time is available for normal development.

The following are the four variations of the exstrophy–epispadias complex, classified according to severity.

**Cloacal Exstrophy.** Cloacal exstrophy is the

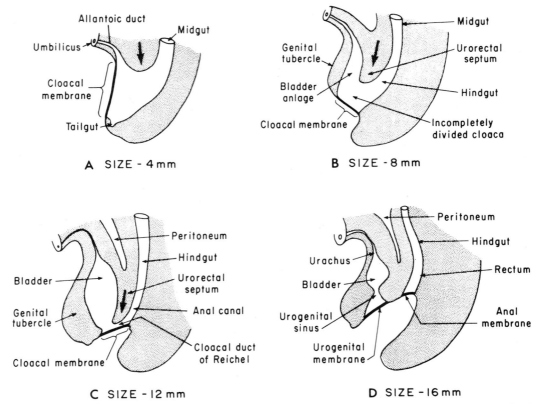

**A** SIZE - 4 mm

**B** SIZE - 8 mm

**C** SIZE - 12 mm

**D** SIZE - 16 mm

_FIGURE 21–1_ Developmental changes of the cloaca and cloacal membrane in the normal embryo. _Arrows_ show the division of the intestinal tract from the bladder. (From Walsh, P. C., Retik, A. B., Stamey, T. A., & Vaughan, E. D., Jr. [1992]. _Campbell's urology_ [Vol. 2, 6th ed., p. 1774]. Philadelphia: W. B. Saunders. Reprinted by permission.)

most severe and rarest form of the exstrophy complex. The incidence is approximately 1:400,000 live births (Gearhart & Jeffs, 1992). This form of the exstrophy defect occurs early in gestational life (fourth to sixth week). The prominent cloacal membrane ruptures before there is time for complete division of the bladder from the intestinal tract. The result is that the cloaca itself exstrophies. Intestinal mucosa is present in the center of the exposed bladder. In addition, the ureteral orifices are always incompetent, with resulting bilateral reflux; the internal urethral sphincter is cleft, resulting in complete incontinence (Gearhart & Jeffs, 1992).

**Classic Exstrophy.** Classic exstrophy is a less severe form of the exstrophy complex, which has a higher incidence of approximately 1:40,000 live births. The male to female ratio is estimated to be 3:1 (Gearhart & Jeffs, 1992). This defect occurs when the cloacal membrane ruptures 1 or 2 weeks later (sixth to eighth week). More time is available for the complete separation of the intestinal tract from the urinary bladder. However, the lower anterior wall

of the bladder and abdomen do not completely close, because the cloacal membrane persists for a longer time than normal before rupturing. The bladder is then exposed through the defect in the abdominal wall. Within the bladder itself, the ureteral orifices are always incompetent, resulting in bilateral vesicoureteral reflux; the internal urethral sphincter is cleft, resulting again in complete incontinence (Gearhart & Jeffs, 1992).

**Complete Epispadias.** Complete epispadias is an opening along the entire dorsal shaft of the penis. In females, the anterior wall of the urethra remains open, but the defect is hidden within the surrounding pelvic structures. The internal urethral sphincter is cleft and rendered incompetent, resulting in complete incontinence. This defect is always associated with both cloacal and classic exstrophy. It is, however, important to note that complete epispadias may occur alone, without the presence of an exstrophied bladder. The embryologic basis for complete epispadias without bladder exstrophy may be traced to a late rupture of the

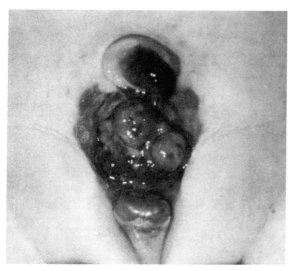

FIGURE 21–2 Exstrophy of the bladder. (Courtesy of Dr. John Gearhart, Baltimore, MD.)

cloacal membrane that had already diminished in size (after 8 weeks). More time has been available for closure of the bladder and abdominal wall (Gearhart & Jeffs, 1992).

**Epispadias.** Epispadias is the least serious defect in the exstrophy–epispadias complex. It is an opening at any point below the internal sphincter along the dorsal shaft of the penis. Embryologically, the exposed urethra is caused by a persistent remnant of the cloacal membrane that ruptures late in gestational development (eighth week or later). This defect differs from complete epispadias in that the internal urethral sphincter remains intact and continence is maintained (Gearhart & Jeffs, 1992).

For both cloacal and classic exstrophy, the defect includes significant alteration in the lower musculoskeletal structures. The persisting cloacal membrane prevents the complete closure of not only the bladder and the abdominal wall but also the anterior pelvic ring. This results in an outward rotation of the hips, a diastasis or widening of the pelvis at the symphysis pubis, and a separation of the musculature of the pelvic floor essential for support of the bladder (Fig. 21–3). These musculoskeletal defects are present in all exstrophy patients, but to a greater degree in those with cloacal exstrophy (Muecke, 1986).

## Medical-Surgical Management

Previously, ureterosigmoidostomy and ileal conduit urinary diversion were the methods of choice for urinary drainage of exstrophy patients, because of the complexity of the exstrophy defects and surgical failures at attempts to achieve functional bladder repair. During the past 20 years, significant surgical progress has contributed to the success of diversion. A multistaged approach to reconstruction is now recommended, after careful individualized assessment of the defects by the surgical team.

Primary goals for the surgical management of bladder exstrophy are (1) to secure the primary bladder, abdominal wall, and pelvic ring closure; (2) to achieve a functional bladder, capable of maintaining continence and renal preservation; and (3) to reconstruct a functional and cosmetically acceptable penis in the male and external genitalia in the female. These goals may be achieved through the following surgerical procedures: (1) primary bladder closure, with or without pelvic osteotomies; (2) epispadias repair; and (3) bladder neck reconstruction and ureteral reimplantation.

The sequence for these surgical procedures after the first stage of primary bladder closure is variable and highly individualized. Ongoing assessment of the upper and lower urinary tracts helps evaluate the success of the previous surgical procedures and determine the prospective surgical plan (Gearhart & Jeffs, 1992).

The overall surgical outcome depends on the surgical technique, the quality of nursing care, and the development of a positive parent-child relationship.

## APPROACHES TO PATIENT CARE

### Presentation of Bladder Exstrophy at Birth— Preoperative Care

**Assessment**

An extensive health history should be obtained as soon as possible to plan for the needs of the family of the child born with bladder exstrophy. The interviewer should obtain the mother's prenatal history and a record of the events at birth. The child's history should include any medical and surgical procedures that have been previously performed. The parents' knowledge base regarding bladder exstrophy should also be established to prepare an individualized teaching plan. This is especially important when the teaching plan must be revised to accommodate the needs of the toddler

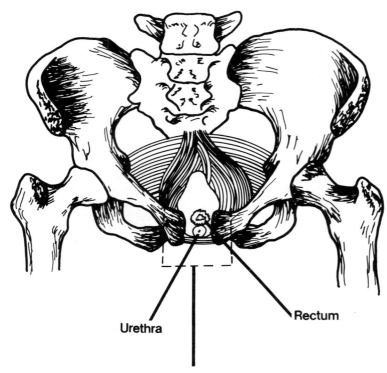

*FIGURE 21–3* Diastasis of the pelvis and separation of the pelvic musculature. (Courtesy of Linda Wheatley Mateer, Doraville, GA.)

Urethra

Rectum

## Diastasis of the symphysis pubis

when the initial attempt to reapproximate the pelvis and close the bladder have failed as a result of the nonunion of the symphysis pubis or bladder dehiscence.

Most parents are willing to discuss the events that occurred after the birth of their child. They may describe how their feelings of joy and anticipation quickly turned to fear and uncertainty. These feelings may have been intensified if the obstetrician and obstetric nursing staff were unfamiliar with the exstrophy defect and were unable to give the parents the necessary information and support they so desperately needed.

Some parents may disclose misconceptions about the cause of the exstrophy defect. Through feelings of guilt, the parents may attribute the cause of the defect to problems that occurred during pregnancy, such as prolonged nausea, excessive weight gain, and a physical injury sustained by the mother. Left uncorrected, these misconceptions may foster feelings of an inability to care for the child or may alter the couple's decision to have more children.

The family background, available support systems, and usual methods of coping should be determined. Because of the lengthy hospital-ization usually required, the care of siblings, employment problems, and financial concerns must be discussed. Identification of available support systems is especially important when a child has been admitted to a medical institution far from home, and close family and friends are not nearby. A description of how the parents have coped with stressful events or a family crisis in the past gives an indication of their needs during this crisis. However, coping methods of the past are not necessarily effective in all situations, and alternate methods of assisting the family may be required.

Children presenting with bladder exstrophy are usually healthy, full-term infants with the anomalies confined to the lower pelvic area. Early surgical management, during the first 72 hours of life, is highly recommended following a complete neonatal assessment. Special emphasis is placed on the cardiopulmonary status of these neonates and their subsequent ability to withstand the stress of surgery. If circumstances are less than favorable at birth, surgery may be deferred until the child's condition improves or until the child can be transported to a medical center with specialized pediatric urology services (Gearhart & Jeffs, 1992).

For the neonate, the potential for successful

reconstructive surgery is assessed as soon as possible following birth. The upper urinary tracts, bladder, and genitalia must be examined to ensure normal kidney function and drainage, a reasonably sized bladder, and genitalia that have potential function following reconstructive surgery (Gearhart & Jeffs, 1992).

*Renal Assessment.* Kidney function may be assessed by ultrasonography or nuclear renal scanning immediately following the birth or by an intravenous pyelogram after the first 24 to 48 hours of life. These diagnostic tests disclose the presence of a major kidney malformation or hydronephrosis.

*Bladder Assessment.* The severity of the bladder defect, bladder size, and bladder contractility are essential parameters to consider in the selection of patients for functional bladder reconstructive surgery.

At birth, the bladder mucosa is smooth, thin, and reddened in appearance. It is also extremely sensitive and easily denuded. It is essential that bladder mucosa trauma be prevented by ensuring that special nursing care measures are instituted before primary bladder closure is performed.

Exstrophied bladders vary in size, although most are quite small. An exstrophied bladder with an estimated capacity of only 5 mL is acceptable for functional repair (Gearhart & Jeffs, 1992). The estimation of bladder size may be made by attempting to close the bladder around a Malecot urethral catheter or by indenting the bladder with a gloved finger. An acceptable capacity may also be demonstrated by observing a bladder bulge when the infant cries (Chisholm, 1962). Despite the size and the limited capacity of an exstrophied bladder, the tissue has the potential to increase in size once primary closure and epispadias repair are completed.

In some instances, there is an absence of contractility because of a small, fibrotic bladder "patch." Unfortunately, children with this variation may not be candidates for the multistaged functional bladder reconstruction and may require urinary diversion.

*Genitalia Assessment.* Males born with bladder exstrophy have a very short penis that has an unnatural upward curvature (dorsal chordee). A wide separation of the symphysis pubis contributes to the shortening of the penis. The length and angle of the urethral groove in the male is assessed to determine if penile lengthening and release of chordee are necessary at the time of primary bladder closure (Muecke, 1986).

Females born with bladder exstrophy often present with a bifid clitoris and nonfused labia. These defects, however, may be surgically corrected during a subsequent surgical procedure to produce cosmetically acceptable genitalia (Muecke, 1986).

Females born with epispadias alone are sometimes not readily diagnosed because the defect is hidden within the pelvic structures. The nurse needs to be alert to the possibility of this defect when a female child presents with a history of an inability to be toilet trained, dribbling incontinence, or leakage of urine between voidings. This defect may be corrected in one reconstructive surgical procedure (Muecke, 1986).

Commonly associated with bladder exstrophy are bilateral undescended testes and inguinal hernias. These conditions may be surgically corrected during the first stage of exstrophy surgery.

*Musculoskeletal Assessment.* The degree of pelvic separation varies in exstrophy patients, with cloacal exstrophy presenting with the widest defect. Computed tomography (CT) scans of the pelvis are obtained to determine the degree of separation and to identify the full extent of the defect (Muecke, 1986).

**Nursing Diagnosis**

The nursing diagnoses for the child born with bladder exstrophy and his or her family may include the following:

1. Ineffective family coping related to the birth of a child with a congenital anomaly.
2. Impaired skin integrity related to the exposed bladder mucosa.
3. Actual or potential altered parenting related to impairment or interrupted parent-infant attachment.

**Plan of Care**

Nursing care is directed toward enabling the child or parent to

1. Verbalize an understanding of the diagnosis and treatment plan for bladder exstrophy.
2. Express feelings associated with the birth of a child with a congenital defect.
3. Prevent damage of the bladder mucosa, ureteral orifices, and surrounding skin.
4. Participate in care activities to facilitate bonding.

**Intervention**

As with any congenital anomaly, the family of the exstrophy newborn experiences a multitude of emotions, including shock, disbelief, anger, fear, and guilt. These emotions make it difficult to process the information needed to make decisions regarding the child's care and treatment plan. The parents of the child with exstrophy must be helped to comprehend their child's defect and its implications as well as assisted to appreciate the positive features of their child. Encourage the parents to examine and discuss the infant's resemblances to family members, hair color, and size and proportion of the eyes, nose, and mouth. These observations are a natural part of the parent-child bonding process.

Providing the parents with information about bladder exstrophy helps reduce the fear associated with the unknown. The time for and extent of the explanation required depends on the previous assessment of the parents' level of understanding and present coping ability. Clarifying misconceptions about the child's defect, the child's care, and the possible outcomes following surgical intervention gives a foundation for making informed decisions and helps the parents answer questions from family and friends.

Assist in the preparation of extended family members before their first visit with the child. A grandparent's refusal to look at or to hold the infant may be devastating to the parents and may contribute to feelings of failure. Education of family members and friends helps them understand the birth defect and therefore adapt more easily.

Encourage the family to use the coping methods and support systems with which they are familiar. Arrange for other families of children with bladder exstrophy to talk with them so that similar feelings and experiences may be acknowledged and discussed. Helpful information regarding care techniques may also be solicited. Suggest other resources that provide information and support, such as the clergy, social services, parent support groups, and birth defect foundations.

The care of the exposed bladder and surrounding skin is essential to prevent infection and denuding of the bladder mucosa. Should these conditions occur and be left untreated, the bladder's contractility may be affected, decreasing the child's potential for achieving optimal bladder function and control.

Neonates with bladder exstrophy should not have a clamp applied to the umbilical cord in the delivery room, because of the close proximity of the exposed bladder and the umbilical cord—the umbilical clamp may scrape or lacerate the bladder tissue. Instead, the umbilical cord should be tied off with strong suture material.

To prevent infection of the tissue, the area must be kept as clean as possible. Preventing contamination of the area by the child's stool may be achieved by placing a large piece of plastic wrap, such as Saran Wrap, over the exposed bladder tissue. The plastic wrap should be changed with each soiled diaper. The plastic wrap also functions as a protective layer between the bladder tissue and the diaper, preventing denuding of the bladder epithelium (Radebaugh, 1986).

Frequent warm water rinses help prevent ammonia burn and excoriation of the sensitive bladder surface and surrounding skin. The area may be lightly dried using a blow dryer at the lowest temperature setting with the dryer held at least 12 inches away from the infant. Ointments, powders, and corn starch must not be used, because damage to the bladder tissue may occur when attempts are made to clean the bladder surface of these products. In addition, the ureteral orifices can become obstructed and impede the flow of urine from the kidneys. Baby powders and corn starch are also considered too abrasive and may promote bacterial growth.

Constrictive clothing also must be avoided. The infant can be placed on its abdomen if the plastic wrap is in place and the diaper loosely applied.

The parents of a child born with bladder exstrophy need a lot of support and reassurance in their ability to care for the newborn child. Fear of hurting the infant, along with their feelings of disappointment and guilt, may hinder the bonding process. Depending on the health of the child, it may be several hours before they are able to see the child for the first time. If the infant has no problems other than the exstrophied bladder, the parents should be encouraged to hold, examine, and care for the child. If the mother wishes to breast-feed the infant, she should be allowed to do so as soon as possible. Demonstration of bladder care as previously described helps reassure the mother that the bladder surface is protected while she is holding and feeding her infant.

Observe the parent-child interactions and reinforce attachment and child care behaviors. It is important to remember that during the first 2 to 3 days after the birth of a child, many women exhibit a "taking-in" phase, in which their activity is largely passive; at this time, the new mother prefers the nursing staff to attend to her needs as well as care for her infant. This "taking-in" phase should not be confused with signs of delayed bonding or rejection of the infant. As the mother's physical strength returns and her discomfort lessens, her interest in caring for herself and the child will improve (Pilliteri, 1981).

### Patient Outcomes

1. Parents and family members verbalize their feelings related to the perceived loss of a "normal" infant.
2. Parents and family identify their strengths and weaknesses and use their support systems effectively.
3. Parents ask appropriate questions about the care and treatment plan for their child.
4. The exposed bladder mucosa remains smooth, moist, and reddened.
5. The bladder mucosa remains clear, without signs of infection or scar tissue formation.
6. The skin surrounding the bladder is not excoriated or does not exhibit signs of breakdown.
7. Urine flows freely from the ureteral orifices.
8. The parents exhibit appropriate attachment behaviors, such as cuddling, touching, and talking about their infant.
9. The parents participate in the daily care activities of the child.
10. The parents verbalize positive feelings about their ability to care for their child.

# Primary Bladder Closure with Osteotomies— Postoperative Care

To achieve primary bladder and abdominal wall closure, it is essential for the widened symphysis pubis to be reapproximated to reduce tension on the abdominal wall. Infants with bladder exstrophy seen within the first 48 hours of life have an advantage in that the pelvis is still malleable and closure of the pelvic ring can be accomplished manually. If, however, the pelvis is not malleable and there is an unduly wide diastasis, surgical osteotomies are preferred to aid in the reapproximation of the pelvis.

Posterior iliac osteotomies are used in the initial closure of the pelvic ring. The procedure involves bilateral vertical surgical incisions into the innominate bone of the pelvis to allow the two sides of the pelvis to hinge and close anteriorly (Gearhart & Jeffs, 1992). The reapproximation of the pelvis creates a pelvic ring, essential for successful bladder function. Pelvic ring closure allows not only midline approximation

of the abdominal wall structures but also the surrounding levator ani and puborectalis muscles to lend support to the bladder outlet (Fig. 21–4A). Providing muscular support aids in resisting urine flow, essential in achieving urinary continence (Gearhart & Jeffs, 1992).

Occasionally, repeat pelvic osteotomies are necessary if approximation of the symphysis pubis is not attained. Anterior pelvic osteotomy, as opposed to posterior osteotomy, is a new approach that may be used. There are several advantages of the anterior pelvic ring closure. Intraoperatively, it takes less time to perform an anterior osteotomy, and it is not necessary to turn the child, which is required with a posterior osteotomy. Increased mobility of the pubis and less blood loss are other advantages. The disadvantages to this approach include the necessity of pin placement to secure the pelvis in place while healing takes place. Several instances of temporary femoral nerve dysfunction have also occurred (Fig. 21–4B).

Once the pelvic osteotomies are completed, the bladder and bladder neck are then indented and closed anteriorly. The bladder is placed within the pelvic ring, forming a more normal anatomic relation with the vertical axis of the bladder. This procedure is an additional aid in achieving the future goal of urinary continence.

To complete the primary closure, the pelvic ring is firmly fixed by placing horizontal mattress sutures at the midline fibrocartilage of the symphysis pubis.

At the time of primary bladder closure, penile lengthening of a very short penis may be undertaken. Because separation of the symphysis pubis is an important factor that results in shortening of the penis, lengthening may be accomplished after reapproximation of the pelvis by advancing the split corpora cavernosa into a penile shaft (Fig. 21–5). Also, release of dorsal chordee at this time may reduce the number of stages of later genital reconstruction (Jeffs & Lepor, 1986).

### Assessment

Immediately after primary bladder closure, the bladder is drained by a suprapubic Malecot urethral catheter for 4 weeks. Ureteral stents are used to provide ureteral drainage during the first two postoperative weeks, when edema of the bladder mucosa could obstruct the ureters. To avoid necrosis of the urethra, a urethral stent is not used. The suprapubic catheter and the ureteral stents emerge from the umbilical area through midline sutures (Fig. 21–6). The frequent assessment of the appearance and

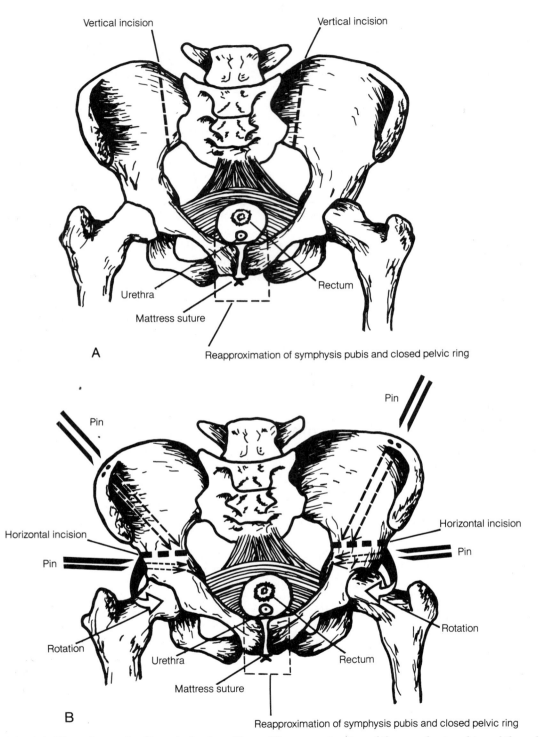

**FIGURE 21–4** *A,* Bilateral posterior iliac osteotomies with resulting approximation of the symphysis pubis and the pelvic musculature. *B,* Bilateral anterior innominate osteotomies with pin placement and rotation. (*A* and *B* courtesy of Linda Wheatley Mateer, Doraville, GA.)

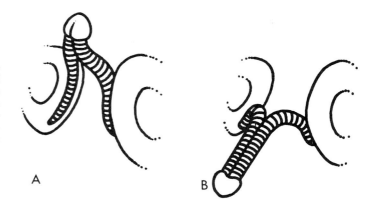

*FIGURE 21–5 A, B,* Penile lengthening accomplished by reapproximation of the pelvis and advancement of the split corpora cavernosa into a penile shaft. (From Walsh, P. C., Retik, A. B., Stamey, T. A., & Vaughan, E. D., Jr. [1992]. *Campbell's urology* [Vol. 2, 6th ed., p. 1796]. Philadelphia: W. B. Saunders. Reprinted by permission.)

A

B

quantity of urine draining from the suprapubic catheter and ureteral stents remains a priority nursing care concern throughout the hospitalization. The abdominal and osteotomy incisions and suprapubic catheter sites must be closely observed for evidence of healing and signs of infection.

Postoperatively, newborns and young infants are placed in Bryant's traction for approximately 4 weeks to allow for healing of the reapproximated pelvis (Gearhart & Jeffs, 1992). This type of skin traction elevates the lower extremities to a vertical position, with the child

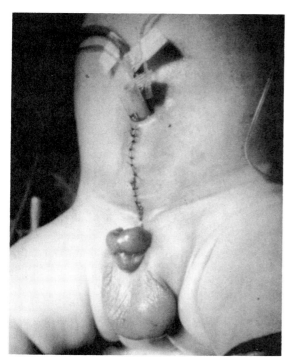

*FIGURE 21–6* Postoperative primary bladder closure. (Courtesy of Dr. Robert Jeffs, Baltimore, MD.)

supine. The trunk and lower extremities form a right angle. The traction mechanism is held in place by elastic bandages wrapped around the legs (Fig. 21–7A). Older children are immobilized in modified Bryant's traction or by interfragmentary pins and an external fixation device with light Buck's traction (Fig. 21–7 B and C) (Gearhart & Jeffs, 1992).

The child's alignment while in traction needs to be monitored, especially as the child's level of activity increases. Early detection of altered neurocirculation to the lower extremities helps prevent unnecessary discomfort and potential injury.

Other methods to achieve immobilization of the legs and pelvis include the application of a hip spica cast or elastic bandages wrapped about the hips and legs. However, the greatest success for achieving normal bladder continence is obtained when an external fixation is used (Sponsellor et al., 1991).

Pain management encompasses an assessment of all of the potential problems a child having bladder exstrophy may develop. Through a process of elimination, the source of a child's discomfort may be determined. For example, a crying, flailing infant should be approached with the following questions in mind: Is the discomfort related to an impeded urine flow? Are there signs of inadequate circulation to the lower extremities, causing discomfort? Is there a source of skin breakdown, causing irritation and pruritus, or a wound showing signs of infection? Is the child demonstrating pain related to incisional pain or bladder spasms? Is the pain medication sufficient? Is there a need for warmth and comfort that cuddling and music might provide? Or is the infant in need of stimulation and human interaction? Hunger, constipation, or other gastrointestinal ailments must also be considered when an infant is crying. Once comfort measures are instituted,

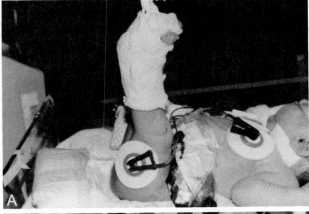

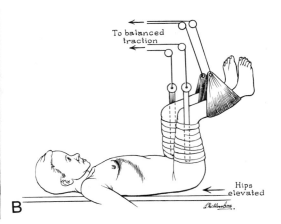

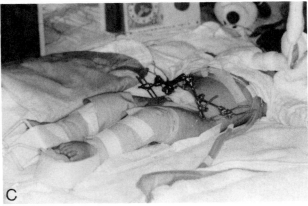

*FIGURE 21–7* *A,* Bryant's traction. *B,* Modified Bryant's traction. *C,* Pins and external fixation with light Buck's traction. (*B* from Walsh, P. C., Retik, A. B., Stamey, T. A., & Vaughan, E. D., Jr. [1992]. *Campbell's urology* [Vol. 2, 6th ed., p. 1790]. Philadelphia: W. B. Saunders. Reprinted by permission.)

their effectiveness must be ascertained and appropriate changes made.

The nurse must also be constantly aware of how the family and child are coping with the hospitalization. Their knowledge base and level of coping ultimately affect how teaching and support are provided. A complete developmental history and ongoing assessment of the child's reaction to the many changes in the hospital determine the appropriate stimulation needed.

### Nursing Diagnosis

The nursing diagnoses formulated from the postoperative assessment of the child and family following primary bladder closure may include the following:

1. Altered pattern of urinary elimination related to the placement of multiple urinary drainage tubes.
2. Impaired physical mobility related to the use of Bryant's traction or pins with external fixation device, potential wound dehiscence, and potential catheter displacement.
3. Pain related to the effects of surgical incisions and presence of urinary drainage catheters.
4. Impaired tissue integrity related to altered circulation induced by traction.
5. Actual or potential impaired skin integrity related to immobility, wound healing and potential infection, or skin traction.
6. Actual or potential altered parenting related to impaired parent-infant attachment.
7. Ineffective family coping related to the child's lengthy postoperative hospitalization.
8. Alteration in sensory perception related to deprivation as a result of immobility.
9. Knowledge deficit related to home care.
10. Potential for infection related to placement and maintenance of interfragmentary pins.

### Plan of Care

Nursing care is directed toward enabling the child or parent to

1. Maintain a urinary output of at least 1 mL/kg/h.
2. Remain immobilized to facilitate wound healing and prevent bladder dehiscence.

3. Be sufficiently free from discomfort so as to participate in normal daily activities and obtain adequate rest.
4. Have adequate circulation to the lower extremities while in traction.
5. Heal without infection and have skin remain intact, without breakdown.
6. Interact effectively, providing for parent-infant attachment.
7. Verbalize an understanding of the postoperative treatment plan.
8. Express feelings related to the environmental changes in the hospital.
9. Obtain age-appropriate stimulation necessary for normal growth and development.
10. Demonstrate an understanding of discharge plans and home care.

### Intervention

*Urinary Elimination.* Understanding the probable causes of an inadequate urine output provides the basis for the nursing interventions initiated. After surgery, hydration is one of the most likely causes of decreased urine output. Close monitoring of the child's intake and output measurements is essential. An output of less than 1 mL/kg/h and a specific gravity higher than 1.015 may indicate a need for an increase in fluid intake, and intravenous and oral fluids should be adjusted accordingly.

Patency of the urinary drainage system is essential to ensure adequate kidney drainage. Urine flow through the suprapubic catheter or ureteral stents may be obstructed by an internal source, such as mucus, tissue, or blood clots. Providing for adequate hydration (as described) helps dilute the blood and tissue drainage and maintain urine flow.

External sources that may cause an obstruction in urine flow include the kinking or twisting of the drainage tubing and inaccurate placement of drainage bags. The suprapubic catheter and ureteral stents should be taped securely to the abdomen, and the extra tubing should be coiled and loosely fastened to the bed. Suspension of the drainage bags at the level of the mattress permits free flow of urine by gravity without significant change in the bladder pressure, which is important in the management of bladder spasms (see Pain in this section). Older infants and children may also require hand and ankle restraints to prevent dislodging of the drainage tubes.

The normal healing process also affects the amount and color of urine drainage from the suprapubic catheter and ureteral stents. Stents are placed in the ureters to allow urine to drain from the kidney pelvis when bladder and ure-

teral swelling would otherwise prevent normal flow. When this postoperative swelling subsides, urine from the kidneys may drain around the stents into the bladder, where the suprapubic catheter then provides for drainage. Therefore, the ureteral stents may be expected to drain most of the urine initially, whereas the suprapubic catheter drains small amounts of blood. Consequently, after several days the amount of suprapubic catheter drainage should increase and stent drainage decrease as swelling subsides. Any significant decrease in urine output from the stent without a relative increase in output from the suprapubic catheter may indicate a possible stent obstruction. If no external obstruction is found, and if hydration is sufficient, irrigation of the affected stent may be required. Increased patient discomfort and elevation in vital signs usually accompany any impediment to urine flow from the kidney. A catheter that has been successfully irrigated begins to drain urine, signifying removal of the internal blockage. Shreds of mucus, tissue, or blood may be visible in the urine. The child's discomfort should also subside.

Changes in urine color also follow a pattern as healing progresses. The urine should gradually change in color from bright red to tealike, and eventually, after 7 to 10 days, to the amber yellow characteristic of urine. Reappearance of blood in previously clear yellow urine may indicate a bladder spasm. Persistence of blood in the urine is abnormal, and the physician should be notified.

*Mobility.* Proper positioning of the child following primary bladder closure is imperative in preventing bladder dehiscence and in achieving optimal bladder function. To maintain the bladder within the reapproximated pelvis and to allow for adequate healing, the child is placed in Bryant's traction or immobilized with external fixation, depending on the age and size of the child. Routine adjustment of the Bryant's traction is not the responsibility of the nurse. However, any alteration in the position of the child's legs caused by displacement of the weights, rope pulleys, or elastic bandages should be brought to the physician's attention so that appropriate adjustments may be made. The weights should hang freely from the pulley ropes, and objects should not be suspended from the overhanging bars or ropes.

Maintaining proper body alignment, especially as it relates to the hips and legs, is of concern when diapers and bed linens are changed and as the child's activity increases. Trochanter or towel rolls may be placed along both sides of the hips and against the buttocks to help maintain the correct position. During bathing and diaper changes, both legs should be lifted simultaneously by pulling upward on the traction ropes to prevent undue stress on the pelvic band.

Once movement of the traction bed is allowed, usually 1 week after surgery, care must be taken not to disrupt the traction or jostle the child unnecessarily during transport.

Antispasmodics and narcotic analgesics are usually prescribed around the clock during the initial postoperative period to facilitate immobilization of the child.

**Pain.** As described previously, management of the child's discomfort and activity is necessary in attaining the most successful outcome possible following a bladder exstrophy closure. Determining the cause of the child's discomfort is essential in providing appropriate nursing interventions. The abdominal and pelvic incisions and bladder spasms are the primary sources of pain. Incisional pain may be expressed by irritability, restlessness, or verbal complaints, depending on the child's age and development. Bladder spasms occur as the bladder contracts in response to a clot passing through a catheter or because the catheters are irritating the swollen and sensitive bladder wall. Discomfort caused by spasms may be differentiated by a rapid onset and termination of the child's response. The older child may clutch the perineum or arch the back. A sleeping child may abruptly wake crying and soon fall back to sleep once the spasm subsides. A small amount of blood may also be forced through the open urethra or drainage tube, causing the urine to become blood tinged for a short time following a spasm. The frequency of spasms differs among children, as does their ability to tolerate the spasms. The potential for bladder spasms remains as long as there are catheters present in the bladder.

Maintaining a constant flow of urine through the suprapubic catheter and ureteral stents helps prevent bladder spasms as blood and tissue are more easily passed from the bladder. Therefore, a greater intake of fluids must be encouraged.

The amount of pressure exerted on the bladder as urine flows into the drainage bag has been identified as a contributing factor in bladder spasms. By placing the drainage bags at the level of the mattress, the gradient at which the urine must flow from the bladder to the drainage bag is decreased. As a result, the pressure exerted on the bladder is reduced and a potential source of spasms is minimized.

Medications available to control the discomfort of bladder spasms include anticholinergics, antispasmodics, and narcotic analgesics. These medications are administered on a continuous schedule to obtain the best possible pain relief. Continuous administration of anesthetics by way of a caudal catheter is the best possible method of pain management postoperatively. Whatever type of pain medication is prescribed, it is important to anticipate pain before it becomes severe and to closely monitor the child so that an accurate assessment of the pain relief is made.

Once the initial postoperative pain has lessened and pain medications are needed less frequently, the child becomes more active and requires more diversional activities to help him or her cope with discomfort. Encourage parents to cuddle and talk to their children. Intrauterine sound tapes and soft music are often comforting to the newborn. Provide pacifiers, and support mothers in their decision to breastfeed. The infant should be placed in traction in a regular-sized bed, rather than a crib, so that the mother may lie next to her child and breastfeed without interfering with the traction. Older children may be diverted with games and crafts and may participate in activities with other children.

*Tissue Integrity.* The potential for impaired neurocirculation to the lower extremities is present while the child is immobilized in Bryant's traction. Constrictive elastic bandages or leg slings often contribute to this problem. Signs of neurocirculation impediment include edematous feet, cyanotic nail beds, sluggish capillary refill, and weak or absent pedal or posterior tibial pulses. Should these symptoms occur, minor adjustments in the sling or elastic bandages without disruption of the traction alignment may be made. The physician should be notified if neurocirculation does not improve.

*Skin Integrity.* Prolonged bed rest in traction signifies the need for scrupulous skin care. Routine skin care with special attention to the back and buttocks is necessary to prevent a young child's sensitive skin from breaking down. Daily bathing, frequent application of lotions, and the use of egg-crate mattresses or sheepskin pads may be effective in preventing pressure areas and decubitus formation. Alternate methods of securing urinary tubes and abdominal dressings may be needed because of the frequent skin irritation resulting from the use of adhesive tapes. Using a Montgomery strap dressing or wrapping the torso with gauze may be useful.

Wound care involves the routine cleansing of the surgical sites (and pins) and assessment of healing. The suprapubic catheter and ureteral stent sites are cleansed with hydrogen peroxide and covered with a sterile dressing twice daily and as needed. The abdominal incision is usually closed with sutures and requires the same routine cleansing and dressing changes.

If a Penrose drain is in place, the surrounding skin also requires cleansing with hydrogen peroxide. Once the Penrose drain is removed and the abdominal incision has healed, 1 or 2 weeks later, the sutures are removed and the area is left open to air.

Often, a small amount of blood or urine leaks from the open urethra during a bladder spasm. This drainage may collect at the distal end of the incision and cause skin irritation and breakdown. Gently wick the area dry with a sterile gauze and cleanse it with hydrogen peroxide. Blowing warm air over the area with a blow dryer is also effective in keeping the area dry.

The osteotomy incisions on the lower abdominal wall are usually covered with clear Op-Site and gauze dressings and do not require routine changing. Once the gauze dressings are removed, the clear Op-Site dressing allows for assessment of wound healing. If pins with external fixation are used, then daily pin care with hydrogen peroxide is needed. An increase in drainage around the pins may be suggestive of an infectious process; therefore, immediate wound cultures should be done.

All the wound sites described have the potential to become infected. Erythema, swelling, or purulent drainage at the wound sites should be noted. Unusual discomfort and an elevated temperature are also significant, and the physician should be notified.

Once the child is taken out of skin traction and the elastic bandages are removed from the legs, areas of skin breakdown may be expected. Prepare the parents for this unavoidable complication to help alleviate undue concern when they initially view the red, excoriated skin. Depending on the severity of the breakdown, the areas are usually treated like minor burns and appropriate creams or dressings are applied. The affected areas of the legs usually heal quickly.

*Parenting.* The significance of the initial bonding that occurs between an infant and his or her parents has been verified in research studies (Bowlby, 1969). It has also been shown that this process may be hindered when a child is born with a serious defect and must be hospitalized to undergo surgery (Brazelton, 1986). After the initial surgical repair, the infant is immobilized in traction, further inhibiting the normal process of parent-infant attachment. Facilitating this bonding is an ongoing challenge.

Encourage rooming-in as available, and support breast-feeding mothers, as previously described. Using the nurse as a role model, parents can be shown that talking and cuddling can still take place while the child is in traction. Encourage their efforts in providing age-appropriate stimulation and diversion. Allow the parents to participate in the daily care activities as much as possible.

*Coping.* To facilitate the family's ability to cope with the stressful recovery period and lengthy hospital stay after bladder closure, nursing measures used preoperatively should be continued. Interventions particular to the postoperative child and family include soliciting the family's active participation in the care management problems. For example, bladder spasms are often difficult to control, despite medical and nursing interventions. The ability to help relieve the child's discomfort is a source of stress for the parents. Suggest the family assist by increasing the child's oral fluids and by keeping a record of intake. Also, a cool or warm cloth may be placed on the perineal area for comfort, and the parents may change this cloth as needed.

The parents may become so closely involved in their child's care that objectivity is obscured and fatigue interferes with their ability to cope. Living-in has many positive effects on a child's hospitalization, but parents need to be encouraged to take time for themselves away from the bedside. Suggest that another family member stay with the child awhile. A break from the hospital routine provides the parents with time to regroup and better manage the stresses that accompany the care of their child.

*Sensory Perception.* When a child is immobilized in traction, sensory deprivation is a potential problem. An understanding of the child's developmental needs and a cooperative effort on the part of the nurses, family, and child life staff may provide the child with age-appropriate stimulation.

The infant needs to acquire a sense of trust and to feel secure. Facilitating parent-infant bonding by encouraging verbal and tactile stimulation from the parents helps meet this need. Mirrors, mobiles, and brightly colored objects arouse the visual interest of an infant. Music boxes, cassette tapes, and intrauterine sound tapes are also soothing.

Toddlers tend to feel a loss of control as a result of the environmental changes within the hospital. As a result, the child may exhibit regressive behaviors. Reassure parents that these behaviors are temporary, and provide suggestions for promoting the child's independence. Despite the physical restrictions placed on the child, some daily routines may be continued. While the child is closely supervised, his or her hands may be freed to allow for self-feeding and self-care activities. Craft activities and games that promote free expression and release of energy should be offered. Painting, doll play, musical instruments, and punching bags may help the child express feelings and gain some control over his or her environment at an age when autonomy is important. Meeting the child's need for stimulation while limiting his or her activity to promote healing is the ultimate goal (Fig. 21–8).

*Knowledge Deficit.* Preparation for discharge should be ongoing throughout the child's hospitalization. Any parental misconceptions about the child's care following bladder closure and about plans for future surgical repair should be corrected.

Home care includes a daily assessment of the surgical sites for signs of infection. By the time the child is discharged, the pelvic osteotomy and abdominal incisions have usually healed completely. However, pin sites require long-term care, so parents should continue daily cleansing of the area. The suprapubic catheter site may leak a small amount of urine for 24 to 48 hours after removal of the catheter. Until this area has completely healed, the parents should cleanse the site twice daily with hydrogen peroxide, as was the hospital routine. Bandages are not necessary, unless active drainage persists.

The parents should contact their physician should a wound site exhibit any signs of infection, as previously described (see Skin Integrity in this section).

Soliciting the parents' assistance in wound care while still in the hospital should give them the confidence to proceed on their own at home. Provide encouragement and constructive suggestions, and discuss any concerns or misconceptions they may have about wound care and assessment.

To help prevent future urinary tract infections, the parents should encourage their child to drink plenty of fluids. Bubble baths should be avoided, and parents should be taught to cleanse the perineum from front to back. Symptoms of urinary tract infection should also be reinforced in the teaching plan.

Prophylactic antibiotic therapy continues at home. Prescriptions and directions pertaining to drug administration should be conveyed to the family.

Providing numerous opportunities for discussion and questions throughout the hospitalization makes the transition to home much smoother as parents become secure in their knowledge and their capabilities.

**Patient Outcomes**
1. Urine output is more than 1 mL/kg/h.
2. Urine specific gravity is lower than 1.015.
3. The child remains in traction in good body alignment, with the hips and legs at a 90-degree angle.
4. Pelvic x-ray film confirms the presence of calcification at the symphysis pubis.
5. Bladder dehiscence has not occurred.

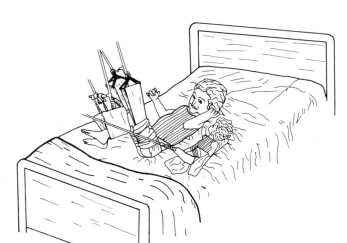

*FIGURE 21–8* Environmental stimulation and medical play are provided while the child is restricted to bed rest. (Courtesy of Linda Wheatley Mateer, Doraville, GA.)

6. The child participates in play activities, demonstrates a good appetite, and sleeps well at naptime and at night.
7. Pedal and posterior tibial pulses are strong and easily palpated.
8. Toe nail beds are pink, with a rapid capillary refill.
9. The child is able to move his or her toes without complaint of tingling, numbness, or pain.
10. Wound approximation is evident without erythema, edema, or purulent drainage.
11. The back and buttocks are pink, without areas of discoloration.
12. The leg wounds present after removal of the skin traction are free of infection and gradually heal as regeneration of skin layers occurs.
13. The parents actively engage in conversation with the child, maintaining good eye contact.
14. The parents attempt to soothe the child when the child is agitated or crying.
15. The child responds to the parents' comforting by becoming less agitated and more playful or by improving his or her appetite.
16. The parents verbalize an understanding of the postoperative plan of care following primary bladder closure.
17. The parents express their feelings related to the stress of a lengthy recovery period in the hospital.
18. The family identifies and effectively uses available support systems.
19. The child continues to perform age-appropriate behaviors and skills previously demonstrated.
20. The parents confirm prior to discharge an accurate understanding of the wound care, medications, personal care, activity restrictions, infection identification, and the importance of follow-up appointments.
21. The parents accurately perform wound care prior to discharge, including daily care to pins and fixation (if used).
22. On subsequent contacts made with the family after discharge, it is noted that wound edges are approximated without signs of infection.
23. On subsequent contacts after discharge, the parents verbalize that they were adequately prepared to care for their child at home.

## Interim Medical-Surgical Management

Following bladder closure, the bladder and pelvis are restored to a more normal anatomic position. The bladder neck and sphincter mechanism are nonfunctioning, and continuous urinary incontinence is expected. A freely draining bladder at low pressure is essential to protect the kidneys from the inevitable bilateral reflux of urine until ureteral replantation may be performed. In addition, epispadias is still present and will be corrected at a later stage.

In summary, the major goal following primary bladder closure is to convert the bladder exstrophy to a closed bladder with complete epispadias and continuous incontinence for preservation of renal function.

During the "incontinent interval," from birth to approximately 3 years of age, continuous monitoring is required to ensure that the urinary tract remains free of infection and that urinary drainage is unimpeded. Between 2 and 3 years of age, assessment of bladder capacity by cystogram is recommended. A bladder capacity of 60 mL or more is necessary before bladder neck reconstruction is performed (Gearhart & Jeffs, 1992).

The sequence of surgical procedures following primary bladder closure is determined by ongoing assessment of the following four criteria: (1) ureteral reflux, (2) urinary tract infections, (3) hydronephrosis, and (4) bladder capacity.

By the age of 2 years, epispadias repair is performed if recovery from the first stage of correction has progressed well. The epispadias repair adds some resistance to urine flow, causing the bladder wall to enlarge and, it is hoped, stimulate bladder growth. Once the capacity of 60 mL is achieved, the child may then undergo bladder neck reconstruction. Bilateral ureteral reimplantation always accompanies bladder neck reconstruction, because the bladder shape and position within the pelvis change. Subsequently, ureters must be reimplanted to sites higher on the bladder wall (Gearhart & Jeffs, 1992).

If attempts to increase the bladder capacity to 60 mL are unsuccessful, the bladder may not have the potential to attain normal bladder function and continence, and alternate procedures may be considered. These procedures are discussed in the section on persistent incontinence at the end of this chapter.

The sequence of surgical procedures just discussed is highly individualized, depending on the child's success following each stage and the surgeon's preference (Fig. 21–9).

## Epispadias Repair

Reconstruction of the male genitalia to a more acceptable appearance is a delicate repair

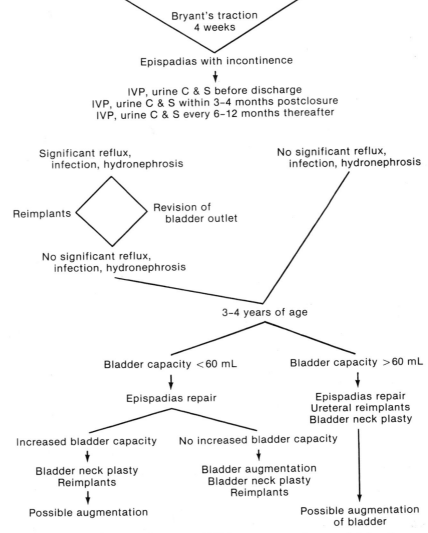

*FIGURE 21–9* Bladder exstrophy surgical sequence. IVP, intravenous pyelogram; C & S, culture and sensitivity.

because of the intricate plastic surgery involved, as well as the significance it has on the developing self-esteem of the school-aged and adolescent male. This repair usually involves penile lengthening, release of dorsal chordee, and one or more urethroplasties to obtain the desired cosmetic results.

The epispadias defect is corrected by performing a modified Young urethroplasty or Cantwell-Ransley procedure. During the primary bladder closure, the utmost care is taken by the surgeon to preserve the limited penile skin necessary for the intricate epispadias re-

pair procedure. Preoperative administration of testosterone also usually is required to increase the size of the unusually small penis. The dosage is usually 2 mg/kg at 5 weeks and again at 2 weeks prior to surgery (Gearhart & Jeffs, 1987).

During the urethroplasty, the surgeon selects a dorsal strip of penile skin to be rolled into a urethral tube (tubularization) to form a neourethra (Fig. 21–10 *A*). Triangular areas on either side of the dorsal strip of skin are denuded of mucosa and are then reapproximated to form the glans. The urethral strip is closed in a linear

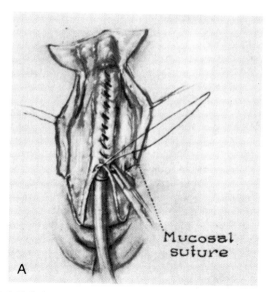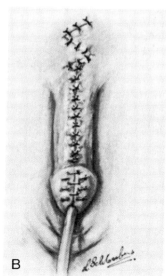

*FIGURE 21–10 A,* Tubularization to form a neourethra. (*A* and *B* from Walsh, P. C., Retik, A. B., Stamey, T. A., & Vaughan, E. D., Jr. [Eds.]. [1992]. *Campbell's urology* [6th ed., p. 1797]. Philadelphia: W. B. Saunders. Reprinted by permission.)

fashion over an indwelling feeding tube, which serves as a stent (Fig. 21–10 *B*). The penis is then wrapped in a dressing such as Op-Site, and a prosthetic foam dressing is applied to protect the surgical site. When there is insufficient penile skin available for construction of the neourethra, a ventral prepuce graft or full-thickness graft from the thigh serves as an additional source (Hendron, 1979; Jeffs & Lepor, 1986).

Urethral fistulas are an infrequent complication following an epispadias repair. Many fistulas heal over time if kept dry and free from the pressure of the passage of urine. Closure of the fistula may occur during the postoperative period, because urine is diverted by an indwelling catheter. Other fistulas may require a minor surgical intervention later.

Female reconstruction of the external genitalia and urethra presents a less complicated situation. Reapproximation of the bifid clitoris and mons pubis usually provides satisfactory cosmetic results in one stage (Dees, 1949).

### Assessment

As with any surgical patient, the general preoperative and postoperative assessment data are included in the overall patient assessment to formulate the patient-specific nursing diagnoses and plan of care.

Following epispadias repair, the urine is drained from the bladder by a suprapubic catheter or a urethral stent for approximately 10 to 14 days. Assessment should include urine output measurements and catheter patency. (Information regarding the assessment of the urinary drainage system is presented in the section on primary bladder closure.) Male patients who have a suprapubic catheter also have a urethral stent, a thin tube used to maintain the tubularized shape and patency of the neourethra. The stent is not intended to act as a urinary drain. The distal end of the stent extends beyond the urethral meatus. Female patients are usually managed with a suprapubic catheter to minimize potential damage to the urethra. Female patients do not usually require placement of a urethral stent.

The prosthetic foam dressing stabilizes the penis in an upright position, allowing for proper healing of the incisions and protection of the surgical site. The dressing is made of a flexible material that expands with the expected postoperative swelling, but which is firm enough to maintain proper positioning of the penis. The dressing remains in place for approximately 10 days (Fig. 21–11).

Most of the penile incisions are covered by the foam dressing. However, assessment of the exposed meatal surface for signs of infection or decreased circulation due to penile swelling should also be noted. Penile enlargement due to preoperative administration of testosterone

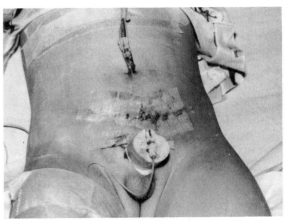

*FIGURE 21–11* Postoperative epispadias repair and bladder neck reconstruction. The foam dressing and urethral stent are for support, and the suprapubic catheter is for urinary drainage.

should not be confused with unusual postoperative edema. The suprapubic catheter site and abdominal incisions should also be assessed for signs of infection and proper healing.

The back, buttocks, shoulders, elbows, and heels are primary sites for pressure ulcer formation because of the long period of bed rest required. Thorough skin assessments should be made several times each day.

The two primary sources of discomfort are incisional pain and bladder spasms. Comfort assessment is discussed in depth earlier in this chapter, in the section on primary bladder closure.

An accurate assessment of the child's mastery of age-appropriate developmental tasks is necessary to plan for his or her psychological needs. The child being considered for an epispadias repair is usually 2 or 3 years of age. At this age, the child should be developing self-esteem and a sense of autonomy. Mastery of bladder control is one of the major milestones contributing to the positive feelings related to such accomplishments. Following epispadias repair, the child is still incontinent because of the incompetent bladder neck, and a sense of shame and doubt may develop. In addition, society places a great deal of importance on the accomplishment of this task, adding to the pressure and guilt felt by the parents and, ultimately, the child.

Changes in environment due to hospitalization may result in the loss of previously demonstrated developmental skills and other regressive behaviors. Ongoing assessment of

these behaviors determines how nursing may facilitate the child's ability to cope.

**Nursing Diagnosis**

The nursing diagnoses for the child and family after epispadias may include the following:

1. Altered pattern of urinary elimination related to the placement of urinary drainage tubes.
2. Actual or potential impaired skin integrity related to immobility and wound healing.
3. Impaired physical mobility related to the potential for wound dehiscence and catheter displacement.
4. Pain related to the effects of surgical incision and the presence of urinary drainage catheters.
5. Ineffective family coping related to lengthy postoperative hospitalization.
6. Knowledge deficit related to home care.

**Plan of Care**

Nursing care is directed toward enabling the child or parent to

1. Maintain a urine output of 1 mL/kg/hr.
2. Heal without wound infection and without skin breakdown.
3. Remain sufficiently immobilized to allow wounds to heal and to ensure correct catheter placement.
4. Be sufficiently free from discomfort to allow participation in normal daily activities and obtain adequate rest.
5. Demonstrate appropriate coping behaviors.
6. Verbalize an understanding of the postoperative treatment plan.
7. Express feelings related to the environmental changes in the hospital.
8. Demonstrate an understanding of discharge plans and home care.

**Intervention**

*Urinary Elimination.* The various methods of urinary drainage have been described earlier in the chapter. Urinary drainage system management includes the same nursing care considerations discussed in the section on primary bladder closure.

When a suprapubic catheter is used with a urethral stent, the urethral stent is not intended to act as a urinary drain. However, bloody drainage or urine may be present in the stent and may ooze from the top of the stent during a bladder spasm or when the child is too active. If this occurs, the meatus should be carefully cleansed with hydrogen peroxide and dried.

A few days after surgery, the physician may elect to shorten the drainage tubing and allow the urine to be collected by a technique that has been called the *double-diaper system.* A round hole large enough to accommodate the penile dressing is cut out of the first diaper. The diaper is placed on the child so that the penile dressing protrudes through the hole. A second diaper is placed on the child, with the drainage tube tucked between the two diapers. This allows the urine to flow out of the tube with decreased gravitational pull, which has been associated with causing bladder spasms. At the same time, the drainage tube is kept away from possible contamination by stool. Another advantage to using this system is that there is less tubing to get tangled or accidentally pulled, decreasing the possibility of accidental tube displacement or removal (Fig. 21–12).

*Skin Integrity.* Suprapubic catheter site care has been described in the section on primary bladder closure in this chapter. The urethral meatus should be cleansed routinely with hydrogen peroxide and gently dried with cotton-tipped applicators. Petroleum jelly (Vaseline) may be applied to the meatus after cleansing to keep the meatal tissues soft and supple.

Because the child is to remain resting in bed

in a supine position for 7 to 10 days, prevention of skin breakdown is imperative. Skin care management necessary for the child restricted to bed has been discussed in the section on primary bladder closure.

*Mobility.* Maintaining a toddler on strict bed rest presents a challenge to nurses, child life teachers, and parents. Wrist restraints may be removed for play activities while the child is being supervised. Bed cradles may also be used to allow the child to participate in games and other table activities. Care must be taken to ensure that the bed cradle is not resting against the urinary drainage tubing or penile dressing. Stretchers, reclining wheelchairs, and wagons may be used to transport the child to play and family visitation areas as the physician permits. Additional diversional activities outside the patient room may be helpful in reducing boredom and restlessness.

*Pain.* Management of incisional pain and bladder spasms has been discussed previously in the section on primary bladder closure.

*Coping.* Methods to facilitate the toddler's need for autonomy can be found in the section on primary bladder closure. Parents often have

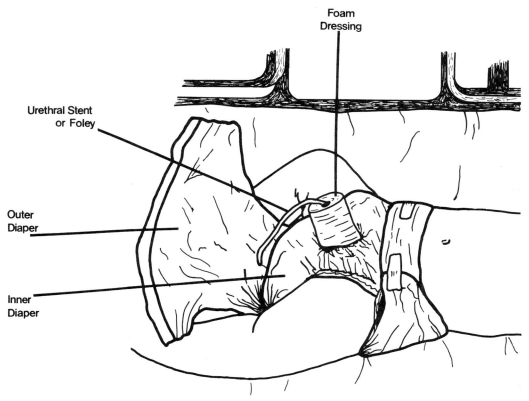

*FIGURE 21–12* Double-diaper system. (Courtesy of Linda Wheatley Mateer, Doraville, GA.)

difficulty coping with social pressures related to their child's inability to gain urinary continence when other parents of toddlers are boasting accomplishment of potty training. Encourage verbalization of these feelings, and arrange for other parents of exstrophy children to discuss such social pressures. Decreasing the parents' anxiety concerning the achievement of bladder training at this time helps reduce the pressure the parents may exert on the child. The child is more likely to gain a positive self-esteem if the parents demonstrate a positive attitude toward their child and his or her abilities.

*Knowledge Deficit.* Home care of the surgical incisions, assessment for infection, and prophylactic antibiotic therapy have been described in the section on primary bladder closure.

### Patient Outcomes

1. Urine output is more than 1 mL/kg/h.
2. Urine specific gravity is lower than 1.015.
3. Wound healing is evident without erythema, edema, or purulent drainage.
4. The skin is without areas of breakdown.
5. Urethral fistula does not occur.
6. The suprapubic catheter remains in correct position.
7. The child participates in play activities, demonstrates a good appetite, and sleeps well at night and during naps.
8. The child demonstrates or verbalizes relief of discomfort.
9. The parents and child verbalize an understanding of the post-operative plan of care and goals.
10. The parents express feelings related to the stress of hospitalization.
11. The family identifies and effectively uses available support systems.
12. Prior to discharge, the parents confirm an accurate understanding of wound care, signs of infection, personal care, activity restrictions, medication administration, and the importance of follow-up appointments.
13. The parents accurately perform wound care prior to discharge.
14. In subsequent contacts made with the family after discharge, it is noted that wound edges are approximated without signs of infection.
15. In subsequent contacts after discharge, the parents verbalize that they were adequately prepared to care for their child at home.

## Bladder Neck Reconstruction

Bladder neck reconstruction is essential to promote continence in the patient with exstrophy. A bladder capacity of 60 mL or more under anesthesia is required before this procedure can be attempted. The surgical goal is to reconstruct the bladder neck so that it is tight enough to achieve continence but not too tight to cause complete urinary retention. Several factors aid in this endeavor: (1) initial firm closure of the pelvic ring during primary bladder closure, (2) bladder neck reconstruction with intraoperative profilometry to measure closure pressure, and (3) bladder neck suspension to provide additional outlet resistance by increasing the urethrovesical angle.

A Young-Dees-Leadbetter bladder neck plasty begins with a transverse incision that is extended vertically to expose the small bladder. Bilateral ureteral reflux is corrected by a transtrigonal reimplantation of the ureters to a site higher on the bladder wall. When bilateral reimplantations have already been completed at an earlier date, it is often necessary for this procedure to be repeated. If the ureteral orifices are low, they must be moved to a higher position on the bladder wall, well away from the bladder neck, to allow for the reconstructive procedure.

During a bladder neck plasty, the surgeon selects a midline strip of muscle from the trigone area of the bladder to be rolled into a urethral tube (tubularization) to form a neourethra (Fig. 21–13*A*). The neourethra is reinforced with adjacent trigonal muscle, wrapped in a double-breasted fashion to give it firm support. It is then anastomosed to the distal end of the urethra (Fig. 21–13*B*). Note in both diagrams that the ureters have been reimplanted higher on the bladder wall.

During the surgery, intraoperative profilometry determines the closure pressure. The goal is for the neourethra to resist a pressure of at least 60 cm $H_2O$ without leaking through the repairs (Gearhart et al., 1986). If necessary, adjustments may be made before closure of the bladder.

A bladder neck plasty is usually supplemented with a Marshall-Marchetti type of bladder neck suspension (Marshall et al., 1949). This helps reduce incontinence by increasing the urethro-vesical angle and outlet resistance. The suspension is fixed by suturing the bladder to the suprapubic structures (Fig. 21–14). Outlet resistance is then measured by intraoperative profilometry (Gearhart et al., 1986).

### Assessment

The bladder neck plasty and bladder neck suspension may be the final reconstructive surgery for the child born with bladder exstrophy. It is an exciting time for the child and family,

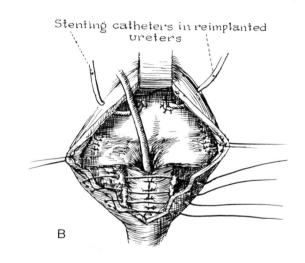

FIGURE 21–13 A, Bladder neck reconstruction. A midline strip of urethral mucosa is rolled into a urethral tube. B, Trigone muscle flaps are wrapped around the urethra to give firm support to the urethra and bladder neck. (A and B from Walsh, P. C., Retik, A. B., Stamey, T. A., & Vaughan, E. D., Jr. [1992]. *Campbell's urology* [Vol. 2, 6th ed., p. 1800–1801]. Philadelphia: W. B. Saunders. Reprinted by permission.)

because an end to hospitalization is anticipated. There are also heightened expectations as to the prospective voiding capabilities of the child after surgery. The contemplation of these events, along with the impending 3- to 4-week hospital stay, certainly can cause a great deal of stress.

The family's history should include a description of past surgeries and hospitalizations and any problems the child or family may have encountered. Any nursing interventions that proved especially helpful should be noted, as well as those that were less useful. The child's perception of previous hospitalizations should also be determined, and any misconceptions should be clarified. The nurse should be aware of any significant family dynamics that may affect the family's coping ability and should identify support systems that are available.

In preparation for this final surgery, enthu-

siastic parents may have told their child that diapers will no longer be needed when they leave the hospital. The child and the family are setting themselves up for disappointment, because urinary continence usually occurs over time and is not necessarily achieved before discharge from the hospital. Correcting any such misconceptions and preparing the family for the possible short- and long-term outcomes after bladder neck reconstruction helps them cope with the postoperative course and necessary follow-up bladder training.

The postoperative physical examination following a bladder neck reconstruction includes the routine assessment of the child's cardiopulmonary status and gastrointestinal motility.

On examination, the child has a lower abdominal "Steri-stripped" incision with a subcutaneous running suture. A suprapubic catheter and two ureteral stents drain the bladder

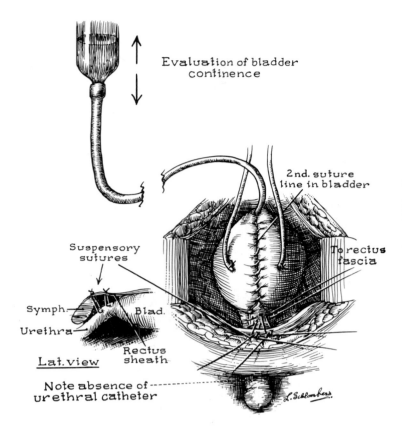

Evaluation of bladder
continence

2nd. suture
line in bladder

Suspensory
sutures

To rectus
fascia

Symph.                          Blad.

Urethra

Rectus
sheath

Lat. view

Note absence of
urethral catheter

*FIGURE 21–14* Suspension of the bladder by securing the bladder neck to the suprapubic structures. (Adapted from Walsh, P. C., Retik, A. B., Stamey, T. A., & Vaughan, E. B., Jr. [1992]. *Campbell's urology* [Vol. 2, 6th ed., p. 1801]. Philadelphia: W. B. Saunders. Reprinted by permission.).

and reimplanted ureters, respectively, and exit the body through a small opening several centimeters above the suture line at the midline. A wound drain may also be present. The ureteral stents are removed 1 or 2 weeks after surgery, once bladder and ureteral swelling has diminished and urine drains freely from the kidneys into the bladder (see Urinary Elimination in the section on primary bladder closure). The suprapubic catheter diverts urine away from the bladder neck and urethra for a full 3 weeks to prevent undue pressure on the reconstructed bladder neck. The child remains on strict bed rest for approximately 1 week and progresses to a reclining wheelchair if the physician allows, depending on the child's activity level. Three weeks following bladder neck reconstruction, adequate healing of the bladder is evaluated and the drainage of the upper urinary tracts is determined by an intravenous pyelogram. If healing is adequate and kidney and ureteral drainage are efficient, bladder training begins with the intermittent clamping of the suprapubic catheter.

Further nursing assessment considerations coincide with those described in the section on epispadias repair.

**Nursing Diagnosis**

The nursing diagnoses for the child undergoing bladder neck reconstruction and his or her family may include the following:

1. Altered pattern of urinary elimination related to
   a. Placement of urinary drainage tubes.
   b. The child's initial voiding experience secondary to the continence procedure (bladder neck reconstruction).
2. Actual or potential impaired skin integrity related to immobility and wound healing.
3. Impaired physical mobility related to potential wound dehiscence and catheter displacement.
4. Pain related to the effects of the surgical incisions and the presence of urinary drainage catheters.
5. Ineffective family coping related to a lengthy postoperative hospitalization.
6. Knowledge deficit related to home care.

**Plan of Care**

Nursing care is directed toward enabling the child or parent to

1. Maintain a urine output of 1 mL/kg/h.
2. Heal without wound infection and without skin breakdown.

3. Remain sufficiently immobilized to allow wounds to heal and to ensure correct catheter placement.
4. Be sufficiently free from discomfort to allow participation in normal daily activities and adequate rest.
5. Demonstrate age-appropriate coping behaviors.
6. Verbalize an understanding of the postoperative treatment plan.
7. Express feelings related to environmental changes in the hospital.
8. Void with minimal discomfort and efficient bladder emptying.
9. Demonstrate an understanding of discharge plans and home care.

### Intervention

*Urinary Elimination.* The nursing care considerations related to urinary elimination are the same as those described in the sections on primary bladder closure and epispadias repair.

*Skin Integrity.* The nursing care considerations related to skin integrity are the same as those described in the section on epispadias repair.

*Mobility.* The nursing care considerations related to mobility are the same as those described in the section on epispadias repair.

*Comfort.* The nursing care considerations related to comfort are the same as those described in the section on primary bladder closure.

*Coping.* The child and family require much support and encouragement because of the heightened stress surrounding the bladder neck reconstruction and impending bladder training. The sensation of a full bladder and subsequent contractions are new experiences for the child. The control he or she initially develops over his or her bladder may be influenced by a positive, supportive family and nursing staff. Providing the family with accurate information regarding potential complications and their implications may assist in dealing with these often temporary difficulties. For example, a better understanding of how a bladder increases in size over time as it begins to fill with urine and stretch reassures a parent whose child is voiding every 5 to 10 minutes at first. Frequent dribbling or difficult voiding due to persistent swelling or an impassable urethra or bladder neck are other conditions that require physiologic explanations and care alternatives, should they persist. During this sensitive time, the child may assume guilt for not achieving his or her parents' or medical caregivers' expectations. Reassure the child that he or she is not to blame for any setbacks. Provide encouragement and age-appropriate explanations. Additional support may be necessary, depending on the emotional development of the child. (See the section on coping following epispadias repair for further measures to assist the child and his or her family with coping.)

*Urinary Elimination Related to Initial Voiding.* The physician specifies how the clamping regimen will proceed. Anticholinergic medications, such as oxybutynin chloride, must be discontinued at least 12 hours before the child's initial attempt to void, so that bladder contractions are not inhibited. The length of time the clamp should remain in place and the indications for notifying the physician should be clearly established.

Once the clamp is applied to the suprapubic catheter, it is usually left in place no longer than 1 or 2 hours. If the child complains of discomfort before this time, he or she is encouraged to void. Any urine voided is measured, and the residual urine left in the bladder is drained through the suprapubic catheter by removing the clamp. Accurate recording of the amount of urine voided and the amount of residual urine is imperative in assessing the child's ability to effectively empty his or her bladder. Parents may be encouraged to assist with the recording of urine output at the bedside.

During the initial phase of the clamping process, the residual urine tends to be much greater than the amount voided. Within a couple of days, these numbers should reverse, with the residual urine decreasing to less than 20 mL.

The force of the urine stream and the child's discomfort during the initiation and cessation of the stream are also important details to note. Any dribbling between voids should also be documented, as well as the occurrence of any stress incontinence.

It is not unusual for the child to be unable to pass urine the first few times he or she attempts to void. Persistent swelling of the bladder neck and urethra may prevent urine flow. Old blood or tissue debris may also obstruct the urethra. If the child is uncomfortable and is unable to void, the bladder should be emptied through the suprapubic catheter. If the child continues to be unable to pass urine, the physician may establish urethral patency by catheterizing the child. The catheter also helps dilate the bladder neck and urethra. The child may be sedated or undergo anesthesia for the catheterization procedure, depending on the child's ability to co-operate. A difficult catheterization may contribute to the child's experiencing physical and emotional trauma and should be avoided.

A cystoscopy may also be performed to assess the bladder neck and urethra if the child's inability to void persists. The physician may opt to use a urethral Foley catheter for dilation over time to allow bladder neck swelling to subside completely. These children may be sent home and then return after several days to resume the clamping regimen.

Some children may experience the effects of a hypersensitive bladder and express the need to void every few minutes. In addition, the small bladder contracts in response to small amounts of urine. Gradually, as the bladder adapts and begins to fill with urine, the volumes of urine causing contractions should increase. This is the first time the bladder has ever acted to store and expel urine. The child is also experiencing the sensation of a full bladder for the first time. The newness of these sensations, along with the related fear, anxiety, and discomfort, may certainly be overwhelming for the child. Being sensitive to the child and lending nonjudgmental support and encouragement help him or her cope better during this stressful time. Allowing uninterrupted sleep at night and eating at mealtimes by placing the suprapubic catheter to straight drainage gives the child and parents a much needed break from the clamping routine and provides the child with adequate periods of rest.

*Knowledge Deficit.* Home care of the surgical incisions, assessment for infections, and prophylactic antibiotic therapy have been described previously in the section on primary bladder closure. The parents should notify the physician immediately if the child has unusual pain, difficulty voiding, or urinary retention.

The parents should understand that during the next few months there will be gradual changes in their child's voiding pattern. Evaluating the child's progress involves the assessment of two parameters: the frequency of incontinent episodes and the average daytime dry interval. The frequency of incontinent episodes may be monitored by keeping a chart of how often the child is wet. The average daytime dry interval may be documented by noting the length of time between incontinent episodes and by calculating the average time interval.

A 3-hour dry interval is usually achieved by 1 year after bladder neck reconstruction. To be socially acceptable, the child should experience no incontinent episodes within that period. Children who do not achieve a dry interval of at least 1 hour within 1 year after bladder neck reconstruction seldom achieve a sufficient continence mechanism (Gearhart & Jeffs, 1992).

Staying dry through the night may be accomplished after the child has achieved good daytime control and is aroused from sleep by the sensation of bladder fullness. This state may take an additional year after bladder neck reconstruction to be achieved (Jeffs, 1987).

Parents may also need guidance in dealing with the problems of frequent voiding and episodes of incontinence when the child participates in a day care center or attends school. A few brands of incontinence pads or briefs are available in pediatric sizes. Some types are easy enough for the child to use with little or no assistance. A second set of clothing should be available at the day care center or school in the event of an incontinent episode. Bladder exstrophy support groups and other service organizations may be helpful in providing additional information and support.

It is important that the parents discuss their child's special needs with the teachers and school administrators, so that the physical inability to remain dry is clearly understood. Feelings of shame, doubt, and isolation may be prevented by a teacher's sensitive manner of dealing with the frequent personal care needs of the child.

**Patient Outcomes**
1. Urine output is more than 1 mL/kg/h.
2. Urine specific gravity is lower than 1.015.
3. Wound healing is evident without erythema, edema, or purulent drainage.
4. The skin is without areas of breakdown.
5. The suprapubic catheter and ureteral stents remain in correct position.
6. The child participates in play activities, demonstrates a good appetite, and sleeps well at night and during naps.
7. The child verbalizes relief of discomfort.
8. The parents verbalize an understanding of the postoperative plan of care after bladder neck reconstruction.
9. The parents express their feelings related to the stress of a lengthy recovery period in the hospital.
10. The family identifies and effectively uses available support systems.
11. The child expresses minimal discomfort when voiding.
12. The child has a postvoid residual of less than 20 mL of urine prior to discharge.
13. Prior to discharge, the parents confirm an

accurate understanding of wound care, signs of infection, activity restrictions, medication administration, and the importance of follow-up appointments.

14. The parents accurately perform wound care prior to discharge.

15. On subsequent contacts made with the family after discharge, it is noted that wound edges are approximated without signs of infection.

16. On subsequent contacts after discharge, the family members verbalize that they have been adequately prepared to care for their child at home.

## Persistent Incontinence

There are several alternatives for patients who have less than a 1-hour daytime dry interval or who have marked stress incontinence 2 years after bladder neck reconstruction. A repeat bladder neck repair with Marshall-Marchetti suspension or collagen injections may be considered for these patients. In the future, collagen injection into the bladder neck may provide support and increased outlet resistance to urine flow. The surgery is relatively simple and involves a shorter hospital stay and recovery period than does repeat bladder neck reconstruction.

Occasionally, persistent outlet resistance with incomplete bladder emptying results, and long-term intermittent catheterization is necessary. The advantage to this is that the patient may achieve total continence between catheterizations. Children with bladder outlet dysfunction may learn to perform self-catheterization as early as their preschool years with the assistance of specially developed patient teaching techniques (Hannigan, 1982; Hannigan & Elder, 1988).

If the bladder remains small and contracted, it is often useful to augment the size of the bladder with a bowel segment (augmentation cystoplasty). This has been successful in increasing the capacity of the bladder and lengthening the dry interval. However, most patients who undergo augmentation need to perform intermittent catheterizations (Gearhart & Jeffs, 1988).

Anti-incontinence devices to achieve continence in exstrophy patients are somewhat risky in young children because of the complication of eroding into a urethra that has become poorly vascularized after earlier surgeries (Gearhart & Jeffs, 1988; Hanna, 1981).

More recently, the Mitrofanoff procedure has been selected for some patients with persistent incontinence. In this procedure, the urethra may be closed and the appendix is tunneled into the bladder to serve as a passage directly into the bladder. The distal end of the appendix is tunneled submucosally to maintain continence between catheterizations. To increase bladder capacity, bladder augmentation is also included (Gearhart & Jeffs, 1988). This surgery is a definite improvement over the more radical urinary diversions used in the past, because the urinary bladder remains intact and external appliances are not necessary.

## Social Adjustment

An adolescent needs to be accepted by his or her peers and identify with a certain group. A positive self-image is a prerequisite for this stage, and a socially acceptable appearance is of great concern, especially because intimacy with others is likely to occur. Feelings of inferiority and insecurity are heightened if social continence has not been achieved. The cosmetic appearance of a short, stubby penis may be somewhat improved by undergoing a penile lengthening procedure (Johnston, 1974). However, the scars of the multiple surgical repairs may alter pubic hair distribution and make the altered penile appearance more noticeable. The adolescent's ability to cope with his or her perceived imperfection may affect how he or she deals with intimate relationships with the opposite sex. Reluctance to engage in intimate relationships may lead to isolation and depression.

Fortunately, most patients with exstrophy have overcome the potential for social maladjustment, as determined by a study of 64 bladder exstrophy patients by Woodhouse et al. (1983). In addition, the libido and sexual function of patients with exstrophy have been evaluated as being very high (Woodhouse et al., 1983).

The ability to reproduce offspring is much higher in females than in males. Damage of the prostatic portion of the urethra during primary bladder closure may contribute to retrograde ejaculation and low sperm counts in male patients with exstrophy. Vaginal deliveries in females with functionally closed bladders may cause injury to the urinary sphincter. To avoid this trauma, cesarean sections are usually performed (Gearhart & Jeffs, 1992).

## SUMMARY

Advancements in the medical and nursing management of the patient with bladder exstrophy have contributed to the attainment of improved outcomes for bladder function and emotional adjustment. Nurses must recognize their influential roles as skilled caregivers, resources of knowledge, and providers of emotional support in the overall management of the child with bladder exstrophy and his or her family. The opportunity to provide care for these patients is both challenging and gratifying.

## *REFERENCES*

Bowlby, J. (1969). *Attachment and loss: Separation* (Vol. 2). New York: Basic Books.

Brazelton, T. B. (1986). *On becoming a family: The growth of attachment.* New York: Dell Publishing.

Chisholm, T. C. (1962). *Pediatric surgery* [vol. 2, p. 933]. Chicago: Year Book Medical Publishers.

Dees, J. E. (1949). Congenital epispadias with incontinence. *Journal of Urology, 62,* 513.

Gearhart, J. P., & Jeffs, R. D. (1987). The use of parenteral testosterone therapy in genital reconstructive surgery. *Journal of Urology, 138,* 1077–1078.

Gearhart, J. P., & Jeffs, R. D. (1988). Augmentation cystoplasty in the failed exstrophy reconstruction. *Journal of Urology, 139,* 790–793.

Gearhart, J. P., & Jeffs, R. D. (1992). Exstrophy of the bladder, epispadias, and other bladder anomalies. In P. C. Walsh, A. B. Retik, T. A. Stamey, & E. D. Vaughn (Eds.), *Campbell's urology* (6th ed., Vol. 2, pp. 1772–1821). Philadelphia: W. B. Saunders.

Gearhart, J. P., Williams, K. A., & Jeffs, R. D. (1986). Intraoperative urethral pressure profilometry as an adjunct to bladder neck reconstruction. *Journal of Urology, 136*(5), 1055–1056.

Hanna, M. K. (1981). Artificial urinary sphincter for incontinent children. *Urology, 18,* 370.

Hannigan, K. F. (1982). Self-catheterization: An alternative to surgical diversion. *Infection Control and Urological Care, 7*(2), 5–8.

Hannigan, K. F., & Elder, J. (1988). Teaching intermittent catheterization to children. *Urologic Clinics of North America, 15*(4), 653–660.

Hendron, W. H. (1979). Penile lengthening after previous repair of epispadias. *Journal of Urology, 12,* 527.

Jeffs, R. D. (1987). Exstrophy, epispadias, and cloacal and urogenital sinus abnormalities. *Pediatric Clinics of North America, 34*(5), 1233–1254.

Jeffs, R. D., & Lepor, H. (1986). Management of the exstrophy-epispadias complex and urachal anomalies. In P. C. Walsh, R. F. Gittes, A. D. Perlmutter, & T. A. Stamey (Eds.), *Campbell's urology* (5th ed., Vol. 3.) Philadelphia: W. B. Saunders.

Johnston, J. H. (1974). Lengthening of the congenital or acquired short penis. *British Journal of Urology, 46* 685.

Lancaster, P. A. L. (1987). Epidemiology of bladder exstrophy: A communication from the international clearing house for birth defects monitoring systems. *Teratology, 36,* 221.

Marshall, V. S., Marchetti, A. A., & Krantz, K. E. (1949). The correction of stress incontinence by single vesicourethral suspension. *Surgery, Gynecology and Obstetrics, 88,* 509.

Muecke, E. (1986). Exstrophy, epispadias, and other anomalies of the bladder. In P. C. Walsh, R. F. Gittes, A. D. Perlmutter, & T. A. Stamey (Eds.), *Campbell's urology* (5th ed., Vol. 2, pp. 1856–1867). Philadelphia: W. B. Saunders.

Pilliteri, A. (1981). *Maternal–newborn nursing: Care of the growing family* (2nd ed., pp. 367–380). Boston: Little, Brown.

Radebaugh, L. (1986). Nursing care of the infant with bladder exstrophy. *American Urological Association Allied Journal, 7*(2), 11–15.

Shapiro, E., Lepor, H., & Jeffs, R. D. (1984). The inheritance of classical bladder exstrophy. *Journal of Urology, 132,* 308–310.

Sponsellor, P. D., Gearhart, J. P., & Jeffs, R. D. (1991). Anterior innominate osteotomies for failure or late closure of bladder exstrophy. *Journal of Urology, 146*(1), 137–140.

Woodhouse, C. R., Ransley, P. C., & Williams, D. I. (1983). The exstrophy patient in adult life. *British Journal of Urology, 55,* 632.

# CHAPTER 22

# Pediatric Voiding Disorders

■

*Catherine-Ann Lawrence\**

## OVERVIEW

Pediatric voiding disorders may be divided into those that are associated with intact neurologic innervation of the bladder and those associated with impaired neurologic innervation of the bladder. There are also several congenital structural defects that alter voiding patterns in the newborn period.

Based on the physical assessment of the newborn, the nurse often makes observations that may indicate a potential voiding disorder. Assessment cues and the development of urinary control are discussed as the basis for understanding altered physiologic states.

Most children brought to the urologist for evaluation of voiding disorders have negative findings on neurologic examination. These children may have enuresis or urge incontinence associated with a urinary tract infection and are often treated nonsurgically. Therefore, this chapter discusses the management of those children with intact innervation of the bladder experiencing an alteration in urinary elimination.

*The author acknowledges the enhancement of this chapter by the contribution of Karen A. Karlowicz, M.S.N., C.U.R.N., Editor, of the section "Urodynamics in Children."

Children born with specific congenital defects are categorized as having an alteration in the neurologic innervation of the bladder. Presented in the chapter are the medical and nursing management of the child with myelodysplasia, sacral agenesis, and spinal dysraphism. These children require a more extensive workup, a combination of intervention techniques, and long-term follow-up.

## BEHAVIORAL OBJECTIVES

After studying this chapter, the reader should be able to

1. Recognize findings in a newborn physical examination that may indicate a potential voiding disorder.
2. Define the term *neurogenic bladder*.
3. Differentiate between voiding disorders associated with a neurogenic bladder and those associated with a nonneurogenic bladder.
4. Apply at least one management technique used to treat enuresis.
5. Write the components of a teaching plan for clean intermittent catheterization.

## KEY WORDS

**Enuresis**—the involuntary diurnal or nocturnal loss of urine.

**Encopresis**—the involuntary loss of feces.

**Hyperreflexia**—uninhibited detrusor activity.

**Hypotonic**—a diminution or loss of muscular tone.

**Incontinence**—the involuntary loss of urine, semen, or feces through loss of sphincter control or cerebral or spinal lesions.

**Intermittent catheterization**—the periodic emptying of the urinary bladder with a catheter.

**Meningocele**—a type of spina bifida cystica with protrusion of the meninges through unfused vertebral arches.

**Myelomeningocele**—a type of spina bifida cystica with protrusion of the spinal cord and its membranes through unfused vertebral arches.

**Myelodysplasia**—a defect that occurs during the formation of the spinal cord.

**Neurogenic bladder**—a bladder dysfunction resulting from a lesion of the central nervous system or the spinal cord.

**Nonneurogenic bladder**—an idiopathic voiding dysfunction, usually associated with encopresis without evidence of a neurologic deficit.

**Posterior urethral valves**—congenital urethral folds in the posterior urethra that cause an obstruction to the outflow of urine.

**Retention**—the inability to expel body waste.

**Sacral agenesis**—a congenital anomaly that involves the absence of part or all of two or more sacral vertebrae.

**Spina bifida cystica**—includes two groups of disorders: meningocele and myelomeningocele.

**Spina bifida occulta**—an occult or hidden defect of the spinal vertebrae. External manifestations may include a tuft of hair at the base of the spine, hemangioma, hyperpigmentation, or lipoma.

**Spinal dysraphism**—a term applied to a group of structural abnormalities of the caudal end of the spinal cord and vertebral column; includes lipoma, dermoid cyst or sinus, aberrant sacral roots, fibrous traction on the conus medullaris, or a tight filum terminale.

# VOIDING DISORDERS IN THE NEWBORN

## Perspective on Disease Entity

### ETIOLOGY

Voiding disorders in the newborn may range from a delay in the onset of the first voiding in a child with an intact urinary system to an obstruction in the flow of urine, such as with posterior urethral valves, or to anuria in the child born without kidneys. If an infant is born without kidneys (a condition termed *renal agenesis*), no urine is produced. The most likely cause of a delay in spontaneous voiding in an otherwise healthy neonate is inadequate perfusion of functioning kidneys (Moore & Galvez, 1972). Inadequate kidney perfusion is most commonly caused by dehydration.

A delay in the first voiding may also be caused by an obstructive lesion within the urethra. One of the most common obstructive lesions in the urethra is posterior urethral valves. Posterior urethral valves are primarily a lesion of the male urethra, and their obstructive cause is unknown (Glassberg, 1985).

### PATHOPHYSIOLOGY

**Delay in First Voiding.** In a study of 500 full-term infants, Sherry and Kramer (1955) found that, within 12 hours after birth, two thirds of all neonates have passed urine. By the first 24 hours, at least 92% of all neonates have passed urine and, by 48 hours, 99% have passed urine. Failure to pass urine within the first 48 hours after birth may be a normal, individual physiologic variation or the first sign of renal disease (Moore & Galvez, 1972). The presence of an obstruction may alter the caliber of the urinary stream, as well as delay the first voiding in any infant with an intact urinary system.

**Posterior Urethral Valves.** The congenital defect of posterior urethral valves may cause either a partial or complete obstruction of the urethra. Urethral valves consist of transitional epithelial tissue that forms folds within the walls of the urethra. When posterior urethral valves partially obstruct the urethra, the characteristics of the urinary stream are altered. If posterior urethral valves completely occlude the urethra, urine flow is obstructed. In utero, obstruction to the free flow of urine may be associated with damage to the parenchyma of the developing kidney. The developing kidney

is damaged by increased pressure within the bladder, ureters, and kidney as a result of the blockage of the free flow of urine through the urethra. Posterior urethral valves offer no resistance to the retrograde passage of a catheter but balloon out during voiding, thereby obstructing the flow of urine through the urethra and increasing pressure within the bladder (Gauthier et al., 1982). Because the obstruction with posterior urethral valves ranges from partial to complete, kidney damage is variable and depends on the extent of urethral obstruction. It is essential that the diagnosis of posterior urethral valves is arrived at early in the workup of the child.

**Tight Foreskin.** Although rare, a male infant may be born with an extremely tight foreskin that restricts the flow of urine.

**Renal Agenesis.** Fetal development follows an organized pattern, called *differentiation*. Three layers of fetal tissue—mesoderm, ectoderm, and endoderm—are the primary structures from which all other tissues and organ systems are formed. Cells arise from these layers and, in an organized pattern, differentiate or change to become various predetermined structures in the body. During the fourth to sixth week of fetal life, the urogenital tract develops. A disruption in the normal developmental pattern in this period may cause failure in the development of the ureteral bud. The ureteral bud differentiates into the renal pelvis, the calices, and a portion of the renal pelvis. If these structures fail to develop, the kidneys will be absent. The absence of kidneys is referred to as *congenital renal agenesis*. The failure of the kidneys to develop is usually associated with other anomalies. Because the kidneys are required for the production of urine, an infant born with renal agenesis is anuric. (See Table 22–1 for a list of congenital anomalies commonly associated with urinary tract malformations.)

### MEDICAL-SURGICAL MANAGEMENT

Prenatal ultrasonography has been used to diagnose disorders of the urinary tract, allowing for early intervention in obstructive uropathy (Gonzalez, 1985). Ultrasonography may alert the health team to the delivery of a potentially compromised infant. The presence of both a nephrologist and a urologist, working in consultation with the pediatrician, is required for the management of an infant born with anatomic changes suggestive of an obstructive lesion of the urinary tract. When intrauterine surgical intervention for urinary tract obstruction is to be attempted, cooperation and coordination with the obstetrician are also required.

**Delay in First Voiding.** If dehydration is the cause of the delay of the first voiding, the infant should void after adequate hydration. Following hydration, a nephrourologic assessment is done if a newborn fails to pass urine within 72 hours of birth. The assessment focuses on determining if the kidneys, ureters, bladder, and urethra are present and if there is an obstruction in the flow of urine at any point between the kidney and the urethral meatus. In the rare instance in which the newborn does not urinate within 72 hours, the physician considers the diagnoses of bilateral renal agenesis, urinary tract obstruction, or renovascular accident (Edelmann, 1978). Radiographic and serum chemistry studies are used to assist in diagnosing the cause of a delay in voiding.

An obstructive lesion is not demonstrated by ultrasonography; however, this diagnostic test assists in evaluating nephrourologic impairment as a result of obstruction. The following information may be obtained: the size of the kidney, the thickness of the parenchyma of the kidney, the severity of the dilatation of the calices and renal pelvis as a result of hydronephrosis, enlargement of the bladder, and thickening of the bladder wall. The voiding cystourethrogram (VCUG) is the primary method of diagnosing posterior urethral valves. Endoscopy may be used to confirm the radiologic findings obtained from the VCUG (Cendron & Melin, 1987).

**Posterior Urethral Valves.** Obliteration of posterior urethral valves is almost always possible with current technology (Cendron & Melin, 1987). The size of the urethra is calibrated, and the appropriate size of cystoscope or rectoscope is passed. The valves are visualized and fulgurated or incised. If the size of the urethra is small, such as in a premature infant, the passage of a cystoscope may be contraindicated. Instrumentation of a small urethra may

cause urethral stricture (Glassberg, 1985). If the urethra is small, a temporary cutaneous vesicostomy is done. A vesicostomy allows urine to drain until the infant is mature enough for surgical obliteration. Most infants, however, are suffering the consequences of obstruction when diagnosed with posterior urethral valves and may not be candidates for surgical intervention until they are stabilized. The treatment of urinary tract obstruction must address the cause of the obstruction, as well as any physiologic deviations caused by the obstruction, such as dehydration, electrolyte imbalance, decreased renal function, and acidosis.

In addition to the surgical creation of a vesicostomy, temporary measures to establish urinary drainage while the infant is medically stabilized include the insertion of an indwelling urethral catheter or percutaneous nephrostomies.

*Vesicostomy.* A vesicostomy is one of the simplest forms of temporary diversion. The procedure is done in the operating room, under anesthesia. An incision is made in the lower abdomen, so that the dome of the bladder is exposed. The bladder is opened and the edges of the opening are sutured to the fascia and skin.

*Indwelling Urethral Catheter.* The passage of a urethral catheter initiates decompression and drainage of the obstructed system. The French size and type of catheter used depends on the preference of the urologist and the size of the child. For example, a 5 Fr plastic feeding tube may be used in a premature infant, and an 8 Fr feeding tube may be used in a newborn.

*Percutaneous Nephrostomies.* The percutaneous insertion of a drainage tube directly into the kidneys may be completed using sedation and local anesthesia. The dilated system is visualized using fluoroscopy or sonography. An 18-gauge needle with a guide wire is passed percutaneously. The needle is removed and the opening is widened by dilators. The appropriate size tube is then inserted. The type of tube differs with the preference of the urologist; however, most use a Malecot tube.

**Tight Foreskin.** If the foreskin is abnormally tight, circumcision is the recommended surgical procedure. In cultures in which the foreskin may have ethnic importance, the foreskin may be retained and rendered functional by means of a minor surgical procedure.

**Renal Agenesis.** If a newborn is suspected to have renal agenesis, the physician will order emergency ultrasonography to confirm the diagnosis. Unfortunately, the child with this condition rarely lives longer than 6 to 12 hours after birth, even with aggressive intervention with life-support measures. In most instances, parents are counseled concerning the condition and are recommended to have life-support systems removed. Comfort measures are employed until the child's eventual death.

# Approaches to Patient Care

### Assessment

A maternal or family history of nephrourologic impairment is an important piece of information in the prediction of neonatal voiding abnormalities. If the infant's mother received prenatal care, determine if the mother was evaluated by ultrasonography and if oligohydramnios was detected. Oligohydramnios is a maternal-fetal condition in which there is a scant amount of amniotic fluid. Because the fetus swallows and excretes fluids in utero, a diminished amount of fluid is usually the result of obstruction in the urinary tract or failure of the kidneys to develop.

The nurse in the delivery suite may be the first to observe the initial spontaneous voiding of the infant. The time of the first voiding, as well as the quality of the stream, if observed, should be noted in the appropriate section of the hospital record and reported to the nurse receiving the infant in the nursery area. Lattimer, Uson, and Melicow (1962) suggest that not only should nurses record the time of the first void but, in male infants, they should also note the characteristics of the urinary stream. Deviations include observing a stream that is not large and forceful, a stream that is like a spray, an intermittent stream, or the lack of a stream, such as with dribbling. Observation of the urinary stream in males should also include noting if the foreskin balloons during voiding, a sign of an extremely tight foreskin. Abnormalities in the timing and quality of micturition are often indications for referral for urologic investigation; however, the force and caliber of the urinary stream are more important parameters than timing (Gonzalez, 1985).

Some nursery units keep the infant in the nursery until the first voiding and the first water feeding. If the infant is rooming-in with his or her mother, the nurse monitors the infant and instructs the parents to notify the nursery nurse when the infant voids.

If the kidneys have failed to develop, as in renal agenesis, infants often have a typical facies, which consists of flattening of the nose,

recession of the chin, and abnormal ears (Lattimer et al., 1962). Abnormalities of the form and position, usually described as "low set," of the external ear may indicate renal anomalies, and microcephaly (small head) is sometimes associated with posterior urethral valves. A tuft of hair and dimpling over the lower spine suggest the presence of spinal defects. The most common defect associated with the presence of a tuft of hair is spina bifida occulta. Sacral agenesis is suspected when there is absence of a normal buttock cleft (Gauthier et al., 1982). Spina bifida and sacral agenesis are discussed in the section on neurogenic bladder.

In an infant who has not voided since birth, palpation of the abdomen with the finding of a full bladder may indicate an outlet obstruction, such as posterior urethral valves, or neurogenic bladder. Despite the abdominal position of the bladder, it is not easily palpable in the newborn. Therefore, a distended, tense bladder is abnormal (Gonzalez, 1985). The presence of a distended bladder helps differentiate obstruction to flow versus the absence of urine formation (Moore & Galvez, 1972). If the infant has an abdominal mass, the physician must perform diagnostic radiologic studies to eliminate hydronephrosis, cystic kidneys, and tumor. Obvious congenital defects, such as prune belly syndrome and exstrophy of the urinary bladder, demand immediate urologic assessment and appropriate management. Infants born with the congenital anomaly of agenesis of the kidneys either die in utero or do not survive long after birth.

Table 22–2 contains a list of nursing observations appropriate for use in the delivery room and newborn nursery. This list may be reformulated into an observation and recording checklist. It is understood that the nurse

---

**TABLE 22–2. Assessment of Voiding in Newborns**

1. Observe infant for facial deviations associated with nephrourologic impairment, including
   a. Form and position of the ears.
   b. Flattened nose.
   c. Recession of the chin.
   d. Small head.
2. Observe infant for lower back deviations associated with an occult spinal defect, including
   a. Absence of buttocks cleft.
   b. Dimpling over the lower spine.
   c. Tuft of hair at the base of the spine.
3. Document the time of the first passage of urine.
4. Observe the urinary stream for force, including
   a. Continuous or intermittent stream.
   b. Dribbling.
   c. Spray.

takes into account the effects of the passage of the infant's head through the birth canal or the temporary effects of the use of forceps to assist the delivery before noting the observations in items 1 and 2 to be deviations.

**Nursing Diagnosis**

The nursing diagnosis for the child with a delay in voiding in the newborn period may include the following:

1. Altered pattern of urinary elimination—delay in the onset of first voiding related to (select cause)
   a. Dehydration.
   b. Agenesis of the kidney.
   c. Posterior urethral valves.
   d. Tight foreskin.
   e. Congenital abnormality.
   f. Unknown at present.

**Plan of Care**

Nursing care is directed toward enabling the child or parent to approximate physiologic urinary drainage according to the method selected by the physician.

**Intervention**

If the infant is born with an obstruction in the urethra, such as posterior urethral valves, nursing management is related to the method of intervention selected by the physician and may include any of the following.

*Vesicostomy.* The most important aspect of nursing management of the child with a vesicostomy is attention to skin care. A vesicostomy drains urine from the bladder through an opening in the skin. Therefore, urine is continuously draining on the skin of the abdomen. A thin layer of petroleum jelly applied to a wide area of skin around the vesicostomy opening forms a protective barrier against skin rash. If the application is too thick, the jelly may occlude the vesicostomy opening and prevent the free flow of urine. The child is then diapered as usual, monitored for urinary output, and changed frequently. If the physician wants an approximation of the amount of urine voided, the diaper may be weighed (Table 22–3).

*Indwelling Catheter.* Caring for an indwelling catheter in an infant is similar to managing a catheter in an older child or adult. Most important, however, is to ascertain that the drainage bag is secured at a level that promotes adequate urinary flow from the bladder. A drainage bag and tubing placed too far below the level of the child's bed mattress actually prevents urine from freely flowing from the bladder to the drainage bag. For other guidelines, follow the procedure outlined in your hospital nursing procedure manual pertaining to the care of indwelling urinary catheters. Most procedures include instructions for cleaning the perineum, inserting the catheter under aseptic technique, checking the catheter and drainage tubing for kinks, noting the quantity and quality of the urinary drainage, and collecting a specimen for a culture and sensitivity examination of the urine. Usually a culture and sensitivity test is done (1) if the infant has a fever, (2) a sepsis workup is ordered, (3) the urine is cloudy, (4) before removing the catheter, and (5) 24 hours after removing the catheter.

*Ureterostomy.* The ureter is brought out to the skin level when the physician surgically creates a ureterostomy. A ureterostomy may be performed for some of the following reasons: (1) when the simpler procedure of a vesicostomy will not adequately drain an obstructed, tortuous ureter; (2) in an acutely ill child, anesthesia and surgical times are shorter for the ureterostomy procedure compared with a conduit procedure; and (3) entering the peritoneum should be avoided.

As with a vesicostomy, urine drains directly on the skin. It is possible to apply a pediatric-sized drainage appliance over the ureterostomy to collect the urine and protect the skin. Consult an enterostomal therapy nurse to assist with the management of this infant. The professional nurse who is specially trained in enterostomal management may assist in making an assessment of the stoma and surrounding skin, and in selecting appropriate products to protect the skin from drainage, the correct size and the best pouch to collect the urine, and in methods of removing and reapplying the pouch.

*Nephrostomy.* The physician may create an opening from the skin directly into the kidney to decompress a hydronephrotic kidney. A

**TABLE 22–3. Weighing of Diapers**

1. Place a dry diaper, the same size and brand that the infant is wearing, on a balanced scale.
2. Record the weight of the dry diaper.
3. Weigh the child's wet diaper.
4. Subtract the weight obtained in step 2 (the weight of the dry diaper) from the weight obtained in step 3 (the weight of the wet diaper).
5. Using the equation: 1 g = 1 mL, you can obtain an approximate output amount for the infant. For example, if the weight obtained in step 4 is 46 g, the infant voided approximately 46 mL of urine.

stent or catheter may or may not be inserted into the kidney. As with a ureterostomy, skin care is important. If a stent or catheter is in place, it is connected to a drainage bag. Most often, a stent or catheter is not in place and an appliance is used. Pediatric-sized collecting devices are available, and an enterostomal therapy nurse may assist with the management of this infant.

### Patient Outcomes

1. The urinary system is intact and the infant is urinating at regular intervals.
2. The urinary system is draining with the assistance of (select a method)
   a. Vesicostomy.
   b. Indwelling catheter.
   c. Ureterostomy.
   d. Nephrostomy.
3. The skin surrounding the ostomy (vesicostomy, ureterostomy, or nephrostomy) is intact and free of irritation.
4. The indwelling catheter is patent and free of kinks.
5. The infant is free of urinary tract infection.

# VOIDING DISORDERS AND THE NONNEUROGENIC BLADDER

## Enuresis

### PERSPECTIVE ON DISEASE ENTITY

**Etiology.** Enuresis is defined as the inappropriate or involuntary voiding of urine in a child who has reached an age at which bladder control is expected (Meadow, 1978). In children who do not have psychological, developmental, or physiologic problems, bladder control is achieved sometime between the first and fifth year of age. According to a study of 738 children, 91% of girls and 79% of boys were able to verbalize the need to void by the age of 30 months (Roberts & Schoellkopf, 1951). Therefore, if a child has failed to achieve bladder control by age 5 years, he or she is considered enuretic. The reason some children fail to achieve complete bladder control at the age when most of their peers have completed this developmental task is unknown (Gauthier et al., 1982).

There are two types of enuresis: primary and secondary. The term *primary enuresis* is used if a child has never achieved consistent urinary control. The term *secondary enuresis* is used if the child had a period of urinary control prior to the onset of enuresis. Bed wetting, or noctur-

nal enuresis, is the most common form. In a study of 859 children from birth to 12 years of age, primary nocturnal enuresis was associated with a low birth weight, being a middle child or a withdrawn female, or having a neurologic impairment (Oppel et al., 1968). Nocturnal enuresis is generally regarded as being present in 15% to 20% of 5-year-old children (Perlmutter, 1985). Approximately 10% of children with nocturnal enuresis also have some diurnal or daytime enuresis (Meadow, 1978).

Enuresis is a symptom, not a disease, and many hypotheses have been proposed to describe its cause. Maturational age, sleep disorder, genetic factors, and failure to concentrate urine are most commonly associated with primary enuresis. Secondary enuresis is most commonly associated with urinary tract infections, organic disease, and severe psychological stress. If any of these conditions exist, a thorough evaluation of the urinary tract is completed and treatment of the underlying cause is initiated.

### Pathophysiology: Primary Enuresis

*Maturational Lag.* Primary enuresis is known to resolve with increasing age. Most likely, this is related to a delay in the functional maturation of the central nervous system, termed *maturational lag*. The exact nature of the developmental delay is unknown; however, it may result from slow myelinization of the neural pathways that are involved in inhibiting bladder contraction (Ruble, 1981). In diurnal enuresis, the symptoms are thought to result from the persistence of a neonatal type of bladder caused by delayed neuronal maturation (Pillen et al., 1985).

*Sleep Disorder.* There is controversy as to whether nocturnal enuresis is a sleep disorder. Parents of enuretic children often report that the child is a deep sleeper. However, when enuretic children were compared with a control group of nonenuretic children, no statistically significant differences in the sleep patterns of enuretic and nonenuretic children of the same age were found (Kales et al., 1977).

*Genetic Factors.* Enuresis is commonly found to be a familial disorder. When taking a history of the family with an enuretic child, one often finds that one or both of the parents were bed wetters.

*Failure to Concentrate Urine.* A loss of urine-concentrating ability is one of the earliest changes in renal function as a result of primary renal disease. Loss of concentrating ability results in an increased volume of urine, which may be more than the bladder is able to hold;

therefore, the child leaks urine. The child may be referred to the urologist for management of enuresis, but on diagnostic evaluation, primary renal disease is diagnosed (Perlmutter, 1985).

**Pathophysiology: Secondary Enuresis.** Secondary enuresis is often associated with organic disease, urinary tract infection, and psychological stress. Organic disease associated with enuresis is any pathophysiologic alteration that causes polyuria, such as diabetes mellitus and insipidus. However, the involuntary loss of urine in either of these diseases is a result of an increased volume of urine. The child may not be able to hold the large volume of urine produced and therefore may experience urgency and the involuntary loss of urine. A child with a urinary tract infection may also involuntarily lose urine, but this is as a result of bladder mucosa irritability, urgency, and frequency.

Enuresis associated with psychological stress may have various causes. One of the most common is separation from the parents during the stress of hospitalization, in a situation in which parent rooming-in is not allowed. Others include stress within the family, such as the addition or loss of a family member, and environmental change, such as moving to a new area.

**Medical-Surgical Management: Primary Enuresis.** The management of enuresis includes behavioral modification techniques, such as conditioning or the use of an alarm system that alerts the child when the underpants are damp, medications, and psychotherapy when indicated. Behavioral modification is the most common form of management, followed by the use of medication.

*Behavioral Modification.* Behavioral modification using the technique of conditioning is an attempt to establish a physiologic response to bladder fullness. An enuresis alarm is often used to establish this response. The alarm consists of a sensor or electrode that clips onto the child's underpants. The sensor is connected to an alarm that is worn on the wrist like a watch. When the sensor detects moisture in the child's underpants, the alarm is activated.

Initially, the child awakens after an almost complete emptying of the bladder. After several weeks of nightly use of the alarm, the child awakens more quickly, until eventually the child awakens to the sensation of a full bladder rather than the alarm. An adjunct component of this management technique includes rewarding the child for acceptable behaviors, such as having a dry night. Parents are instructed to keep a calendar or chart and place a sticker or star on each day that the child remained dry. After 2 or 3 dry days or nights, the child receives a reward that is agreed on by both parent and child (Pillen et al., 1985).

*Pharmacotherapy.* If medication is the method of choice, the physician may initially prescribe imipramine (Tofranil) for the child. This drug acts on the bladder neck, causing local constriction, and relaxes the detrusor muscle. The usual dose is 1 to 2 mg/kg of body weight, given 1 hour before bedtime. Another medication often prescribed for the enuretic child is oxybutynin chloride (Ditropan). This drug may be beneficial for the child suspected of having bladder irritability or uninhibited contractions. The usual dosage for the child older than 5 years of age is 5 mg twice a day.

Occasionally, a combination of pharmacologic agents is used to treat enuresis in the hope that some degree of improvement may be achieved. This approach often proves beneficial in children whose symptoms persist despite the use of imipramine or oxybutynin chloride. Although diazepam (Valium) and phenoxybenzamine (Dibenzyline) are drugs that are still used when combination pharmacotherapy is indicated, most physicians now use desmopressin (DDAVP). Desmopressin is a synthetic form of vasopressin, which has as one of its effects that of an antidiuretic. Desmopressin is given in a spray intranasally at bedtime. The mechanism of action of this drug is in the production of a small volume of concentrated urine. It has been found effective in stopping or considerably decreasing bed wetting (Gauthier et al., 1982).

**Medical-Surgical Management: Secondary Enuresis.** Secondary enuresis, often associated with urinary tract infection, psychosocial disturbances, or organic disease, is managed by diagnosing and treating the underlying cause. If the cause of secondary enuresis is a urinary tract infection, antibiotic therapy and a urologic evaluation are completed. If the cause of enuresis is an organic disease, such as diabetes mellitus or insipidus, the child is referred for medical management. Psychosocial disturbance or problems of family stress are managed by referral to a psychotherapist or family counselor to diagnose and treat the underlying problem.

## APPROACHES TO PATIENT CARE

### Assessment
The role of the nurse in caring for the child with enuresis includes obtaining an extensive

history, assisting with or performing a physical examination that includes a neurologic evaluation, and formulating a teaching plan based on the method of treatment.

Questions asked in taking the history of a child who presents with enuresis are extensive and should be designed to collect information about some of the following: age of attaining urinary control, length of time the child maintained urinary control, average duration of dry intervals, and events surrounding the loss of control (e.g., urgency, unaware of loss of urine, participation in strenuous physical activity, and giggling). Also, does the child squat or cross his or her legs to suppress voiding? Does the loss of urine occur at any particular place (home, school, at play, while visiting a parent who does not live with the child) or any particular time of day? What is the frequency of nocturnal enuresis (e.g., every night, two to three times per week, or other)? Is there any particular stress in the child's life (e.g., socioeconomic, emotional, family problems, death of a family member, birth of a sibling, problems in school, hyperactivity)? Because familial incidences of enuresis have been found, it is not unusual to also elicit a history of enuresis in parents of enuretic children. Finally, determine what methods the parents have employed to manage their child's enuresis. What has worked for them, if anything?

A psychosocial assessment is done to uncover any particular stressors in the child's life that might contribute to the enuresis. Determine the composition of the family—who are the people the child lives with, and what is their relationship to the child? Has there been a change in the family composition as a result of a particular event, such as birth, marriage, divorce, illness, or death? Has the family recently moved? Has the child changed schools? Has there been an illness or death of a playmate? Is the child under any stress known to, or suspected by, the parent or guardian?

Following a complete history, a physical examination is completed. The examination, which should include a neurologic workup, is usually found to be negative. This is often the case if the child has primary enuresis. If the history leads to the diagnosis of secondary enuresis, the nurse assists the physician in determining the underlying cause by assessing the child for a causative systemic disease, such as diabetes mellitus or insipidus. A urinalysis and urine culture should be obtained. If a urinary tract infection is found, prompt treatment is essential. Once the infection is cleared, the nurse may be involved in preparing the child for further urologic assessment, such as an intravenous pyelogram (IVP), VCUG, or urodynamic testing.

During the physical examination, be sure to inspect the child's skin (particularly the lower abdomen, perineum, and inner thighs) for any signs of irritation. Are there areas of redness or rash? Are there open sores? At this point in the examination, it is appropriate and important to inquire about hygiene practices. Find out how frequently the child bathes and what type of soap is used. Are any powders or ointments used on the irritated areas of the skin? How often is the clothing changed?

The child with enuresis is almost certain to have an odor problem. What measures have been taken to control the odor? Has the odor problem interfered with the child's willingness to interact with others, and to what extent?

**Nursing Diagnosis**

The nursing diagnoses for the child with enuresis may include the following:

1. Alteration in the pattern of urinary elimination related to (select appropriate etiology)
   a. Primary enuresis.
   b. Secondary enuresis.
2. Knowledge deficit related to (select appropriate cause)
   a. The appropriate age for achieving urinary control.
   b. The causes of enuresis.
   c. Treatment or management options, including the use of bed-wetting alarms, medications, counseling, special protective bed linens or undergarments, dietary and fluid modifications, and voiding schedules.
3. Potential impaired skin integrity related to recurrent episodes of enuresis and prolonged contact to wet linens or clothing.
4. Self-esteem disturbance related to the embarrassment, shame, or guilt experienced as a result of enuresis.
5. Self-care deficit: inability to control body odors caused by enuresis as a result of ineffectual personal hygiene practices.

**Plan of Care**

Nursing care is directed toward enabling the child or parent to

1. Establish or regain urinary control by decreasing or eliminating episodes of enuresis.
2. Cooperate in an agreed-on management plan.
3. Protect the skin from rashes, redness, or excoriation.

4. Verbalize positive statements about self as enuretic episodes decrease.
5. Improve personal hygiene to diminish body odor.

### Intervention

Nursing intervention is based on the diagnosis and management plan selected by the urologist. If the use of an alarm or conditioning is the method of choice, the nurse should provide the family with information on where to purchase the device. An enuresis alarm is easily obtained in a pharmacy or surgical supply house. Depending on the supplier, the alarm may be available for rental. Instructions on the use of the alarm should be given to the child as well as the parents and should include an explanation and demonstration about inserting batteries, attaching the sensor clips to the child's underpants, and attaching the alarm to the wrist (it is worn like a watch) or shoulder (Fig. 22–1). Spend extra time with the child explaining how the device works. Demonstrate on the child or on a doll how the sensor responds to moisture on the underpants with an audible tone. This rehearsal provides the child with information, prepares the child for the use of the alarm, and allows the child some control in the treatment plan. The parents are instructed to set up a chart or use a calendar to record dry nights (Fig. 22–2). A sticker or star is placed on the chart to indicate a dry night. The parent and child agree on how many consecutive dry nights merit an award. Usually the chart is not started until after the first few nights to give the child time to accommodate to the device.

Sometimes enuresis may be resolved without using an alarm. Simple strategies that do not require an expenditure for a special device should be considered and explained to the child and parents. Such strategies might include the implementation of a voiding schedule that requires urinating before going to bed; the use of night lights in the bedroom and bathroom for a child who is afraid of the dark; a reduction in the child's fluid intake 2 or 3 hours before bedtime; a modification in the child's diet that would restrict the intake of milk products, carbonated beverages, caffeinated drinks, chocolate, and salty snacks; as well as an incentive plan that rewards for dry intervals during the day and dry nights (Esperanca & Gerrard, 1969).

Regardless of the management alternative selected, the nurse should be certain to explain to the child and parents that feelings of embarrassment, shame, or guilt are not unusual. To combat such feelings, the children need to understand that there are other children their age who have the same bladder control problem. Moreover, they need to know that they will very likely overcome the problem as they mature and as they incorporate specific management strategies into their lifestyle. Such information is also appreciated by parents, who may have feelings of inadequacy and frustration over their inability to resolve the child's urine control problem.

If the physician prescribes medication for the treatment of enuresis, the nurse must make certain that the parents understand how the drug works, as well as the dosage schedule. Carefully review all possible reactions and side effects with the parents because, in many instances, indications for the use of some pharmacologic agents in the pediatric population have not been clearly defined.

The condition of the child's skin, particularly the lower abdomen, perineum, and inner thigh area, is always a concern when enuresis has been a long-standing problem. Irritation, rashes, and breakdown occur if these vulnerable areas are not carefully cleansed and thoroughly dried at least twice daily and between each change of undergarments (Jeter, 1990). In some instances, the nurse may want to recom-

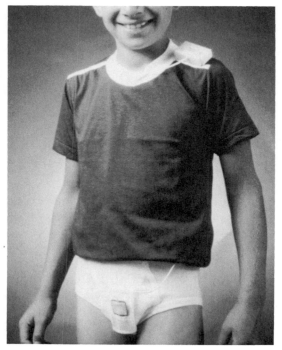

**FIGURE 22–1** Child wearing the Palco Wet-Stop enuretic device. (Courtesy of Palco Labs, Santa Cruz, CA.)

Name _____

Date commenced _____

*Remember: Always go to the toilet before going to bed. In the morning stick on a blue star for a dry night. For the third dry night in a row stick on a GOLD star.*

| | 1st Week | 2nd Week | 3rd Week |
|---|---|---|---|
| Monday | ☆ | ☆ | ☆ |
| Tuesday | ☆ | ☆ | ☆ |
| Wednesday | ☆ | ☆ | ☆ |
| Thursday | ☆ | ☆ | ☆ |
| Friday | ☆ | ☆ | ☆ |
| Saturday | ☆ | ☆ | ☆ |
| Sunday | ☆ | ☆ | ☆ |
| | 4th Week | 5th Week | 6th Week |
| Monday | ☆ | ☆ | ☆ |
| Tuesday | ☆ | ☆ | ☆ |
| Wednesday | ☆ | ☆ | ☆ |
| Thursday | ☆ | ☆ | ☆ |
| Friday | ☆ | ☆ | ☆ |
| Saturday | ☆ | ☆ | ☆ |
| Sunday | ☆ | ☆ | ☆ |

*FIGURE 22–2* Continency star chart. (From Jeter, K. F., Faller, N., & Norton, C. [1990]. *Nursing for continence* [p. 100]. Philadelphia: W. B. Saunders. Reprinted by permission.)

mend the use of skin care products. Depending on the severity of the irritation, a cleanser and moisturizing cream may be used along with a barrier cream. This three-step regimen promotes healing of damaged skin while protecting the integrity of surrounding areas that are unaffected. Parents should be instructed to avoid the use of powders, which can cause additional irritation to the skin.

Controlling odor is an issue that must be addressed when a child experiences frequent and repeated episodes of wetting. This is especially important when day care or schooling may be affected by the child's inability to control his or her bladder. Regular bathing and meticulous skin care are essential to prevent odors. In addition, clothing should be changed immediately after an episode of involuntary voiding and rinsed in a solution of white vinegar and water to eliminate the odor of urine. Rinsing should be followed by a thorough washing with laundry soap.

Enuresis related to a stressful event in the child's life may require referral to a therapist or appropriate social service agency. Sometimes, the child may be enrolled in a program designed just for enuretic children. Such programs are usually coordinated by a nurse specialist and combine counseling techniques with behavior modification and instruction in self-care. The decision to refer a child for psychological counseling or special training programs needs to be considered on an individual basis.

Finally, if a urinary tract infection is detected, the nurse should instruct the family in the appropriate administration of medication. As with any medication used to treat an infection, the parents are instructed to complete the entire course of medication, usually 10 days, and return on a specified date for follow-up urine culture. Medication instruction includes name of the drug, dose, how often to administer, common side effects, what to do if side effects are suspected, and telephone numbers to call in case of questions. It is also helpful to practice pouring out the correct dose of medications with parents.

**Patient Outcomes**

1. The parents are able to express their feelings and concerns about the proposed management plan, as well as about the child's expected progress toward resolving the enuresis.
2. The child and parents have incorporated specific management strategies into the child's daily routine.
3. The child and parents verbalize an understanding of the use of a bed-wetting alarm.
4. The child verbalizes positive statements about himself or herself, as well as progress with the prescribed management plan.
5. The child's skin remains free of rashes, redness, or excoriation.
6. The child and parents incorporate specific strategies for controlling odors associated with repeated episodes of involuntary wetting.
7. The child is continent of urine both day and night.

# VOIDING DISORDERS AND THE NEUROGENIC BLADDER

For the bladder to accomplish its physiologic functions of storing and emptying urine, the neurologic pathways leading to and from the bladder must be intact. Children born with specific congenital defects fall into the category of pediatric voiding disorder caused by an alteration in the neurologic innervation of the bladder.

Unlike children with a pediatric voiding disorder associated with an intact neurologic innervation of the bladder, children with an alteration in the neurologic innervation to the bladder require a more extensive workup, often require surgical intervention and, in almost all cases, require long-term follow-up care. Children in this category include those with myelodysplasia, which includes spina bifida occulta and spina bifida cystica (meningocele and myelomeningocele), sacral agenesis, and spinal dysraphism.

## Myelodysplasia

### PERSPECTIVE ON DISEASE ENTITY

**Etiology.** Myelodysplasia is a neural tube defect, or an abnormality in the development of the spinal column. The exact cause of myelodysplasia is unknown; however, combined factors of heredity and environment are suspect. One factor that has been studied is the use of vitamins by pregnant women. Differences have been found in neural tube defect risk between women who used multivitamins in the 3 months before conception, including the first trimester, and women who did not report multivitamin use. The authors do caution that the differences may not be totally attributed to vitamin use but may be the result of a combination of factors, including adequate nutrition and a healthy lifestyle (Mulinare et al., 1988). In another study, Mills and associates (1989) found no significant difference in the rate of vitamin use between mothers of infants with neural tube defects and mothers in two control groups; one control group consisted of mothers of normal infants and a second control group consisted of mothers of infants who had defects other than one involving the neural tube or who were stillborn. One fact is known: the rates of occurrence and recurrence of neural tube defects is higher in the United Kingdom than in the United States (Rhoads & Mills, 1986).

**Pathophysiology.** Myelodysplasia includes a group of related disorders that occur during the third to fourth week of gestation and represents a failure of the midline neural plate to close as it forms the neural tube. In other words, as the spinal column and vertebral arches are developing and forming a tube shape, the closure of the tube is incomplete. As a result of this incomplete closure, the fetus may have spina bifida occulta or spina bifida cystica.

Spina bifida occulta is a defect of the spinal vertebrae in which the posterior vertebral arches have failed to fuse. It is called "occulta" because the defect is hidden; that is, the meninges are not exposed at the skin surface. External skin manifestations that are cues to the presence of an occult spinal defect may be detected on physical examination. These skin manifestations, found at the base of the spine, may be any of the following: a small hemangioma, a dimple in the skin, a pilonidal sinus tract, or a tuft of hair.

Spina bifida cystica is characterized by an external sac protruding over a bony defect in the spine. The two most common types of spina bifida cystica are meningocele and myelomeningocele.

Meningocele is a herniation of meninges and spinal fluid through the bony defect. The spinal cord is not involved. The meningocele is usually located in the lumbosacral or sacral area of the lower spine and looks like a soft, cystic mass covered with a membrane or epithelial tissue (Smith, 1985). The location of the spina bifida cystica may be in the thoracic, lumbar, lumbosacral, or sacral area of the spine. The defect of hydrocephalus is often associated with myelodysplasia. Hydrocephalus may be present at birth or may develop within the first year of life.

Myelomeningocele (also called *meningomyelocele*) is a herniation of cord segments, neural tissue, and spinal fluid through the bony defect. Myelomeningocele is the single most common cause of neuropathic bladder dysfunction in children (Bauer, 1984).

From a urologic perspective, the function of the urinary bladder to store and completely empty urine is altered in the newborn with spina bifida cystica. The newborn may have either of two types of bladder problems. One type is retention with overflow. In other words, the newborn retains urine in the bladder as a result of increased sphincter activity and leaks urine but does not completely empty the bladder. If the newborn is catheterized after an observed leak of urine, a residual urine volume of more than 10 mL is usually obtained. Once a newborn with a high urine residual volume is identified, it is important to further investigate for the presence of upper tract dilatation. This can be done by ultrasonography of the kidneys and bladder. Decompression of the dilated system may be obtained by intermittent catheterization or by a temporary vesicostomy. If this type of bladder function alteration is not identified and treated promptly, the bladder

walls may thicken, bladder diverticula may form, upper tracts may become dilated as a result of vesicoureteral reflux, and frequent urinary tract infections may occur.

The other type of bladder function alteration is total urinary incontinence. This occurs as a result of a complete absence of tone in the external urethral sphincter or because of a hyperreflexic bladder. These newborns are constantly wet but are less likely to suffer frequent urinary tract infections and upper urinary tract dilatation. When catheterized, these newborns have low or negative urinary residual volume.

**Medical-Surgical Management.** Urologic management of the child with myelodysplasia begins at birth or as soon as the defect has been detected. If surgery is performed to close the spine, postoperative monitoring of the infant's urinary tract function is critical (Table 22–4).

Children with a neurogenic bladder often require a combination of medical and surgical interventions for them to approximate or even achieve urinary continence. Surgical methods used include vesicostomy, augmentation cystoplasty, artificial urinary sphincter, and urinary diversion. Nonsurgical methods used to manage the neurogenic bladder include pharmacotherapeutics and clean intermittent catheterization.

**Surgical Management**

*Vesicostomy.* A vesicostomy, or surgical opening from the skin level directly into the urinary bladder, is most often used in new-

**TABLE 22–4. Urologic Management After Surgical Repair of Spina Bifida Cystica**

1. Blood urea nitrogen and creatinine levels, urinalysis, urine culture study.
2. Because all infants develop some degree of urinary retention after surgery as a result of spinal shock, intermittent catheterization should be done three or four times a day in the first few postoperative days. If that has to be nursed in the prone position, a self-retaining catheter may be necessary.
3. VCUG and ultrasonography; IVP if ultrasonography is abnormal.
4. Urodynamic studies within 6 weeks after closure of the spinal defect to determine the leak-point pressure.
5. VCUG and ultrasonography at 6 months of age and renal ultrasonography every 6 months thereafter for patients who have high leak-point pressures. Annual ultrasonography for patients with low leak-point pressures.

IVP, intravenous pyelogram; VCUG; voiding cystourethrogram.

Adapted from the protocol of Bhagwant Gill, MD, Associate Clinical Professor of Urology, Albert Einstein College of Medicine and J. D. Weiler Hospital, Bronx, NY; with permission.

borns who are in a state of retention or who do not completely empty their bladders. This procedure is usually a temporary measure to allow for the unobstructed flow of urine while the spinal defect is stabilized and repaired surgically. A vesicostomy may also be used in selected infants to provide a temporary urinary outlet for an obstructed urinary system or for reflux when an infant is not stable enough to undergo antireflux surgery (Bellman & King, 1973). The procedure is relatively simple to perform and is completely reversible. (A description of the surgical technique is found in the section on voiding disorders in the newborn in this chapter.)

*Augmentation Cystoplasty.* Older children with neurogenic bladder may require a procedure called *augmentation cystoplasty*, a surgical procedure designed to overcome the failure of the bladder to function as an adequate urinary reservoir (Decter et al., 1987). Depending on the preference of the urologist, a segment of the ileum, cecum, or sigmoid colon may be used. The selected bowel segment, which is freed up and removed, is implanted into the bladder, thus increasing the capacity to store urine. Augmentation cystoplasty has been used more recently in children as an alternative to urinary diversion and as an adjunct in procedures designed to eliminate an existing urinary diversion (King et al., 1987).

*Urinary Diversion.* Historically, most children with neurogenic bladder secondary to myelomeningocele were managed by a surgical technique that diverted the ureters away from the bladder. Known as a conduit or urinary diversion, the procedure involved dissecting the ureters away from the bladder and inserting them into a segment of bowel that had been freed up from the ileum or sigmoid colon and fashioned into a pouch. The open end of the pouch was then brought out to skin level to create a stoma. The primary reason for this procedure was to preserve renal function. The surgery left the child with a draining stoma on the abdomen that required the use of an appliance to collect the urine. Recent advances in both surgical and nonsurgical management of the neurogenic bladder have led to the reconstruction of the urinary tract or undiversion. Augmentation cystoplasty and clean intermittent catheterization have caused the slow decline in the use of urinary diversion. There remains a small population of patients who may benefit from diversion. Included in this group are severely ill infants with urinary tract obstruction or sepsis and patients institutionalized with se-

vere neurologic impairment (Mitchell & Rink, 1985).

In the past it was considered state of the art to remove the urinary bladder at the same time that the urinary diversion was created. Although extensive reconstructive surgery is required, these patients may also be undiverted. An artificial bladder may be created using a segment of bowel, and continence may be achieved with the use of clean intermittent catheterization. Mitchell and Rink (1985) describe the use of the cecum and the ileocecal valves in an undiversion procedure involving a patient whose bladder had been removed as a result of bladder exstrophy.

*Artificial Urinary Sphincter.* The artificial urinary sphincter (AUS) was first used for patients with neurogenic bladder dysfunction in 1972 (Scott et al., 1974). The surgical procedure involves implanting an inflatable occlusive cuff around the urethra. After several device modifications, the components of the AUS in current use include the occlusive cuff, a pressure-regulating balloon, and a control–pump assembly to deflate the cuff (Fig. 22–3). The components constitute a closed system filled with sterile fluid. The control–pump mechanism is implanted in the scrotum of males (Fig. 22–4) and in the labia of females (Fig. 22–5). When the pump is activated by manually locating the

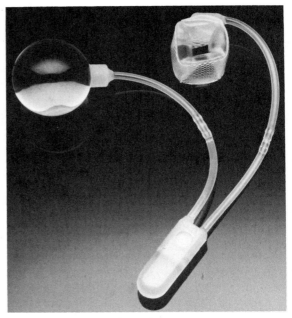

*FIGURE 22–3* AMS Sphincter 800 urinary prosthesis. (Courtesy of American Medical Systems, Inc., Minnetonka, MN.)

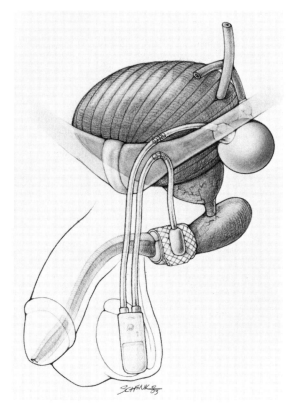

FIGURE 22–4 AMS 800 prosthesis implanted in the male. (Courtesy of American Medical Systems, Inc., Minnetonka, MN. Medical illustration by Michael Schenk.)

pump in the subcutaneous tissue and squeezing it, fluid drains from the cuff. The cuff is now relaxed around the urethra and the patient voids. The fluid cycles within the closed system and returns to the cuff, thereby occluding the urethra and providing continence. Success with this device depends on patient-family selection. It is imperative to choose compliant families who understand the workings of the AUS, the importance of maintaining a schedule of bladder emptying, and the need for frequent follow-up. Satisfactory continence using the AUS has been reported (Churchill et al., 1987; Light et al., 1983).

### Nonsurgical Management

*Pharmacotherapeutics.* Advances in the understanding of the neurology and neuropharmacology of the urinary tract have led to a better understanding of the different types of drugs that affect the physiologic activity of the bladder. Table 22–5 presents a list of drugs commonly used in the management of the child with neurogenic bladder.

*Clean Intermittent Catheterization.* Inter-

mittent bladder catheterization, performed using sterile technique, was first used by Guttman and Frankel (1966) in patients with spinal trauma. Clean intermittent catheterization was first used by Lapides in 1971. Since then, the procedure has gained wide popularity in the management of neurogenic bladder in both adults and children. The major benefits include the protection of the upper urinary tracts and improved urinary control (Crooks & Enrile, 1983). For many patients, the stigma of incontinence and social isolation resolves as patients are freed from urinary leakage, odor, and wearing of incontinence pads.

## APPROACHES TO PATIENT CARE

### Assessment

*Spina Bifida Occulta.* On admission to the newborn nursery, the infant's temperature is stabilized and routine care follows. One component of routine care completed by the nurse is a bath. This activity gives the nurse an excellent opportunity to assess the newborn for any deviations from the norm. The diagnosis of spina bifida occulta is sometimes made in the neonatal period through observation of any of the external skin cues. The nurse assesses the lower spine for the presence of a hemangioma, a dimple in the skin, or a tuft of hair. Often, the diagnosis of spina bifida occulta is not made in the neonatal period but later in life. A

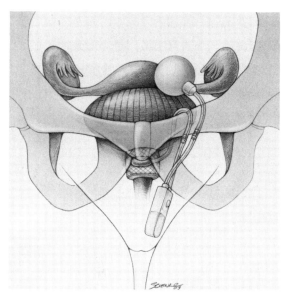

FIGURE 22–5 AMS 800 prosthesis implanted in the female. (Courtesy of American Medical Systems, Inc., Minnetonka, MN. Medical illustration by Michael Schenk.)

TABLE 22–5. Drugs Commonly Used
in the Management of Children
With Neurogenic Bladder

| TRADE NAME | GENERIC NAME |
| --- | --- |
| Bentyl | Dicyclomine |
| Dibenzyline | Phenoxybenzamine |
| Ditropan | Oxybutynin chloride |
| Ornade | Phenylpropanolamide |
| Sudafed | Pseudoephedrine |
| Tofranil | Imipramine |
| Urecholine | Bethanechol chloride |
| Urispas | Flavoxate |
| Valium | Diazepam |

toddler or older child may be referred to the urologist for assessment of frequent urinary tract infections, enuresis, or other urinary tract symptoms. During the physical examination and diagnostic workup, radiologic studies may demonstrate the vertebral arch defect.

*Spina Bifida Cystica.* The child born with spina bifida cystica is easily diagnosed at birth because of the obvious deformity at the base of the spine. Close examination may determine that there is also a leak of spinal fluid from the defect. Hydrocephalus is sometimes present at birth in children with spina bifida cystica, or it may develop later. Newborns with spina bifida cystica require rapid assessment and intervention by all members of the health care team. At this time, the physiologic stability of the child, the spinal level of the lesion, and the status of the urinary bladder are determined. This information helps the team assess the child's ability to undergo surgical closure of the spinal defect and predict the future ability and disability of the infant in terms of ambulation, bowel control, and bladder control. The information also assists the team as they discuss the prognosis of the child with the parents.

The nurse's role in the assessment of the newborn includes the following:

1. Daily measurement of head circumference.
2. Determining the neurologic status of the lower extremities by observing leg movement as well as applying a stimulus to elicit a response (e.g., stroking feet).
3. Assessing anal sphincter tone, usually by perineal pin prick.
4. Palpating the abdomen for bladder distention.
5. Observing the urinary stream.
6. Checking the amount of residual urine, either by Credé's maneuver (if physician permits) or catheterization.
7. Examining the urine for signs of infection.

8. Noting the frequency and amount of stooling in a 24-hour period.
9. Noting the average urinary output in 24-hour period; for newborns, this can be accomplished by weighing diapers (see Table 22–3).
10. Questioning parents to determine if there was prenatal detection of the defect.
11. Soliciting comments from parents concerning their perceptions and understanding of the problem.

If it is a preschool or school-aged child presenting with spina bifida cystica, the nurse should seek answers to the following questions:

What is the child's daily voiding pattern?
Has the child had repeated fevers? Are fevers related to infection in the urine, or is the cause unknown?
Were there problems or difficulty with toilet training?
Does the child have a problem with enuresis or encopresis?
What type medical management has been previously employed?
Have the parents complied with medical follow-up? Where? How often?

**Nursing Diagnosis**
The nursing diagnoses for the patient with myelodysplasia may include the following:

1. Altered pattern of urinary elimination related to (select cause)
   a. Retention of urine.
   b. Incontinence of urine.
   c. Surgical creation of vesicostomy.
   d. Construction of urinary diversion.
   e. Implantation of AUS.
   f. Use of clean intermittent catheterization for bladder emptying.
2. Potential for urinary tract infection related to (select cause)
   a. Incomplete bladder emptying and stasis of urine.
   b. Noncompliance with clean intermittent catheterization regimen.
   c. Noncompliance with AUS bladder-emptying protocol.
   d. Inadequate perineal hygiene.
3. Compromised, ineffective family coping related to (select cause)
   a. Birth of a child with a spinal defect.
   b. Prediction of child's ability and disability in terms of ambulation, bowel control, and bladder control.

c. Knowledge deficit concerning recommended medical or surgical therapies.
4. Potential for noncompliance related to (select cause)
   a. Difficulty or inability to adhere to prescribed therapeutic regimen (e.g., clean intermittent catheterization or use of AUS) because of age, dexterity, or mobility.
   b. Inability or failure to participate in long-term medical follow-up.
   c. Knowledge deficit concerning the benefits of the prescribed treatments.

**Plan of Care**
Nursing care is directed toward enabling the child or parents to

1. Approach the level of continence consistent with medical-surgical intervention.
2. Learn management techniques to approximate or to achieve urinary continence (select technique to be taught)
   a. Care of a vesicostomy.
   b. Clean intermittent catheterization.
   c. Care of a urinary diversion.
   d. Use of the AUS.
   e. Use of medications.
3. Prevent urinary tract infection by recognizing early signs and symptoms and seeking evaluation and treatment promptly.
4. Comply with recommended therapies and medical follow-up.
5. Verbalize perceptions, feelings, and concerns about the child's condition and prognosis.

**Intervention**
*Newborn.* Intensive nursing intervention is required in the first few hours of life when the child is born with spina bifida cystica. Temperature regulation and rapid assessment of the newborn must be done simultaneously. This is best accomplished if the child is placed in a radiant warmer or an Isolette. Protection of the cystic mass or sac is vital, especially if the sac is ruptured and leaking spinal fluid. The sac should be covered with sterile, saline-soaked dressings, followed by the application of a plastic film cover such as a Vi-Drape dressing. This reduces the possibility of contamination of the sac with urine and stool. Other nursing activities include assisting with the stabilization of the newborn by monitoring cardiovascular, respiratory, neurologic, and fluid balance parameters.

Parental support is essential as the newborn is undergoing assessment and diagnostic tests.

Allowing the parents to express their feelings and mourn over the birth of a less-than-perfect infant is a difficult task. Often, the nurse assigned to care for the infant is unable to sit with the parents and offer support because the primary concern is stabilization of the newborn. In this case, another nurse or member of the psychosocial support team (clergy, social worker, psychiatric nurse specialist, member of the bereavement team) should be available to meet with the parents. The decision to close the defect is usually made within the first few hours of life. If the hospital where the child was born does not have a neonatal intensive care unit and the range of medical specialists needed to manage the child, transfer of the patient to another facility may occur. This situation is an added stressor for the parents that signals the need for ongoing support.

*Postoperative Care.* Postoperative management includes monitoring the temperature, pulse, respirations, and blood pressure every 15 minutes until the infant is stable. Once the vital parameters are stable, they may be assessed every 30 minutes and advanced to hourly, depending on the infant's condition. The dressing over the closure of the defect must be kept free of contamination from urine and stool. In the operating room, a sterile dressing is applied to the wound, followed by an occlusive plastic film. If the dressing becomes contaminated with urine or feces, the surgeon should be notified immediately and the wound should be redressed. Fluid balance is assessed every 15 to 30 minutes. Because spinal shock is common after surgery, most infants are in some degree of urinary retention. The urologist most often orders the infant to be catheterized every 3 or 4 hours. The catheterization may be accomplished with the use of a feeding tube. Pediatric feeding tubes, usually used for orogastric feeding, may be obtained in 5 and 8 Fr sizes. Consult the urologist to select the appropriate-sized tube for the infant. Feeding tubes are safe to use as urinary catheters because they have an atraumatic rounded tip. A suction catheter should not be used to catheterize the bladder, because the tip is usually open and blunt cut. To reduce the risk of hospital-acquired, or nosocomial, infection, some hospitals require that clean intermittent catheterization be performed using sterile technique when done by hospital staff. Follow the policy and procedure established by the hospital infectious control staff. If there is a difference between hospital and home clean intermittent catheterization procedures, explain the rationale clearly to the parents. At this time, the nurse may be able to assess the parents' readiness to learn the components of catheterization if they are required to do the procedure at home.

If the infant was found to be in retention with upper urinary tract dilatation, and clean intermittent catheterization or an indwelling tube is contraindicated, a vesicostomy may have been performed. In this instance, the peristomal skin is protected from the urinary drainage with a thin layer of petroleum jelly. A thin layer of petroleum jelly is usually sufficient to protect the skin and not occlude the vesicostomy opening. Output from the vesicostomy is monitored, and a decrease in output is reported to the urologist. If accurate output measurement is ordered, a small, pediatric-sized drainage pouch may be applied to the stoma or the diaper-weighing method in Table 22–3 may be used.

During the recovery process, the parents are prepared for managing the infant at home. Often, medical and nursing team members are focused on ill baby care, such as care of the wound and bladder management, and they neglect or skim over routine infant care. Feeding, bathing, safety, skin care, handling, and dressing need to be reviewed with the parents.

Wound care is often just a simple dressing held in place with paper tape. The parents are instructed to change the dressing daily and report any change in the appearance of the wound, such as drainage, redness, and an opening in the suture line.

If the child has a vesicostomy, demonstrate the use of a thin layer of petroleum jelly on the peristomal skin to prevent a rash from developing. Teach the parents to contact the urologist if the infant has a fever, if there is decreased urine output from the stoma, or if the urine is milky or has an odor.

If the child will require intermittent catheterization, the parents are given the following information: the name and the size of the catheter, the supplies needed for catheterization (lubricant and cleansing agent), and where the supplies may be obtained. The following components of the catheterization procedure are taught to the parents: preparation of supplies; positioning the infant in a safe position on a bed or table; the location of the urinary meatus; cleansing the meatus; lubricating and inserting the catheter; holding the catheter in place until the flow of urine stops; pinching the catheter before withdrawing it from the urethra (to prevent back spillage of urine from the catheter into the bladder); noting the color, odor, and clarity of the urine; measuring the output if requested to do so by the urologist; cleaning the used catheter with soap and water, rinsing well; and storing the catheter in a clean plastic sandwich bag when the catheter is dry.

The method of teaching may be a demonstration on an anatomic model or anatomically correct doll, followed by observation of the nurse catheterizing the infant, or observation of the nurse followed by the parent doing the next catheterization under the supervision of the nurse. The most effective method is to use a model or doll, because this is nonthreatening and less anxiety producing and allows the parents to ask questions and master the technique before catheterizing their infant. It is most helpful to provide parents with a written instruction sheet so that they may review the catheterization procedure at home whenever necessary. The instruction sheet should also contain symptoms to be reported to the urologist, such as bleeding from the urethra, difficulty passing the catheter, inability to obtain urine when the catheter is inserted (which may indicate the presence of a false urethral passage), milky urine, mucous shreds in the urine, or an odor to the urine. The information sheet should also contain the telephone numbers of the urologist, the hospital, and the place where supplies may be ordered.

Additional support may be provided for the parents by making referrals to community agencies. The public health or visiting nurse may reinforce the catheterization instructions (send a copy of the instructions with the referral request), monitor wound healing, and teach infant care. The local Spina Bifida Association may be a source of information, support groups, and counseling for parents.

*Older Child.* The older child with spina bifida cystica may be a candidate for the AUS. Children selected for this procedure must be competent in self-care, have manual dexterity, and be compliant with medical management. Some urologists require that the child be assessed by a child psychologist before surgery to ensure that the child fully understands the importance of his or her full participation in the care and his or her ability to comply with the component steps to activate the AUS. The components of the activation procedure are locating the bulb (found in the scrotal sac for males and the labia majora for females); pressing the bulb to release the cuff pressure, thus allowing urine to flow; noting the color, odor, and clarity of the urine; and measuring the output if requested to do so by the urologist. The child and parent are also given a list of symptoms to report to the urologist. The list includes fever, pain in the area of implantation of the AUS (lower abdomen, labia, or scrotum), redness over the area of implantation, difficulty locating the bulb, inability to obtain urine after pressing the bulb, leakage of urine, blood in the urine, and urine that is cloudy or has an odor.

The older child who is referred to the pediatric urologist for voiding dysfunction may be found to have spina bifida occulta. Various diagnostic tests are used to confirm the diagnosis. Tests may include serum chemistry for blood urea nitrogen and creatinine levels; a routine urinalysis and urine for culture; a complete physical examination, including a neurologic assessment; IVP or VCUG and ultrasonography, depending on the urologist's choice; and urodynamic studies.

The nurse plays an important role in ensuring that the child is adequately prepared for all tests and procedures. For example, if the child is unable to see the room where urodynamics is performed, a photo book may be used to orient the child to the equipment in the room. The child should also have an opportunity to "dry run" the procedure by seeing the procedure performed on a doll or reviewing a picture book. Letting the child know in advance what he or she will see, hear, and feel allows the child to master the event in a nonthreatening way. Children who have been given these opportunities to rehearse what will happen to them are often more cooperative during tests and procedures.

Possible urologic management of the child may include pharmacotherapeutics alone or in conjunction with clean, intermittent catheterization. If medication is used, the parents must be instructed in the drug's action, side effects, dose, and route and the hours to administer the drug, the length of time the child will be on the drug, and any blood or urine tests that need to be done because the child is receiving the drug. (Refer to Table 22–5 for a list of drugs that affect the bladder.)

Regardless of the prescribed management plan, the parents and child must be made to realize that long-term medical and nursing follow-up are required. Keeping appointments, undergoing diagnostic procedures, adjusting medications, and modifying management regimens may at times be inconvenient, but nonetheless are necessary to ensure optimal function of the urinary tract, as well as the child's general well-being.

*Teaching Children to Perform Clean Intermittent Catheterization.* Clean intermittent catheterization is a popular therapy frequently recommended for the child with bladder dysfunction associated with myelodysplasia. It is a safe and effective procedure that has improved and simplified the long-term care of children with neurologically impaired bladders (Hannigan & Elder, 1988).

The optimal age for beginning instruction on clean intermittent catheterization is 4 or 5 years, although some 3-year-old children may also be capable and ready to learn the procedure. The child's ability to master the technique depends on his or her age, manual dexterity, and mental capability, as well as interest and willingness to learn (Fig. 22–6). For the child who must learn to do clean intermittent catheterization, an early introduction to the procedure offers the opportunity to achieve independence. Early instruction of clean intermittent catheterization also helps the child with myelodysplasia develop a positive body image and improve his or her self-esteem.

Children are initially taught the procedure of clean intermittent catheterization using anatomically correct dolls for simulation. Once the child has become proficient with doll catheterization and is able to verbally state the steps of the procedure, he or she may then be advanced to self-catheterization.

Initially, girls may be taught to catheterize themselves using a mirror affixed to the toilet seat, which permits visualization of the urethral meatus. When the child becomes comfortable with the procedure and is able to locate the urethral meatus by touch, use of the mirror may be eliminated. An 8 or 10 Fr, 6-inch, polyvinyl catheter is often recommended for use in young girls.

Boys may be taught to do the procedure in either the sitting or standing position, depending on their mobility. A size 8 to 12 Fr catheter is recommended. Although boys are readily able to visualize the urethral meatus, they are reluctant to insert the catheter all the way into the bladder. Therefore, they should be taught (and encouraged) to continue passing the catheter until urine begins to flow from it; this is their cue that the catheter is in the bladder. A water-soluble lubricant may be used to facilitate the passage of the catheter through the male urethra.

Other aspects of clean intermittent catheterization that must be stressed to the child to avoid problems and complications, include the following:

Code:
P: Parent
C: Child
I: Instructed
D: Demonstrated

Patient:

| | Clinic Appointments | | | | | |
|---|---|---|---|---|---|---|
| 1. Readiness for Self-Catheterization Lessons (Assessed during doll cath.) | 1 | 2 | 3 | 4 | 5 | 6 |
| Emotional readiness | | | | | | |
|   Accepting behaviors | | | | | | |
|   Anxious behaviors | | | | | | |
|   Distressed behaviors | | | | | | |
|   Spontaneous performance | | | | | | |
|   Inhibited performance | | | | | | |
| Attention span | | | | | | |
|   Short (5 min) | | | | | | |
|   Long (15–20 min) | | | | | | |
|   Attentive behaviors | | | | | | |
|   Distractable behaviors | | | | | | |
| Comprehension | | | | | | |
|   States simple explanation | | | | | | |
|   Describes procedure | | | | | | |
|   Follows directions | | | | | | |
| Manual dexterity | | | | | | |
|   Imitates behaviors with ease | | | | | | |
|   Imitates behaviors awkwardly | | | | | | |
|   Fine-motor precision | | | | | | |
| 2. Self-Catheterization Performance | | | | | | |
|   Washes hands | | | | | | |
|   Gathers equipment | | | | | | |
|   Positions self | | | | | | |
|   Positions and adjusts mirror | | | | | | |
|   Separates labia/straightens penis | | | | | | |
|   Identifies urethral meatus | | | | | | |
|   Inserts catheter | | | | | | |
|   Withdraws catheter | | | | | | |
|   Washes catheter | | | | | | |
|   Replaces equipment | | | | | | |
| Total Procedure | | | | | | |

*FIGURE 22–6* Self-catheterization flow sheet. (From Hannigan, K., & Elder, J. S. [1988]. Teaching catheterization to children. *Urologic Clinics of North America, 15*[4], 653–660. Reprinted by permission.)

1. Careful hand washing with soap and water before and after the procedure; for convenience in public facilities, prepackaged wet towelettes may be used.
2. Cleansing catheters with soap and water after each use, followed by storage in a clean, dry container (such as a plastic sandwich bag).
3. Holding the catheter in the bladder until urine stops draining.
4. Removing the catheter slowly, observing for the restart of the flow. If this occurs, stop

withdrawing the catheter, and hold the catheter in place until the flow stops. Continue to slowly remove the catheter. Pinch the catheter before it is withdrawn to prevent urine backflow.

5. Compliance with the total procedure and with the established catheterization schedule.

The goal of catheterization is the facilitation of complete bladder emptying with achievement of a dry interval of 3 or 4 hours. However, the child may need to begin by performing the procedure more often and then gradually extending the time between catheterizations to reach that goal. Factors that may indicate to the nurse the frequency for catheterization include the child's age, the type and amount of fluid intake, the bladder capacity, and the type of voiding disorder.

If a school-aged child must perform clean intermittent catheterization, the urologic nurse should provide the child's teachers and school nurse with information about the program. In some instances, it may be helpful to visit the school and offer instruction to school personnel about the technique. Their thorough understanding of the child's needs ensures that the child is permitted the time, privacy, and assistance necessary to comply with the self-catheterization schedule.

**Patient Outcomes**

1. The parents of newborns with spina bifida cystica are able to verbalize their feelings in a supportive environment with a caring staff member.
2. The parent or guardian demonstrates appropriate skin care for the child with a vesicostomy.
3. The child with a vesicostomy is free of peristomal skin rash.
4. The child and parent or guardian demonstrate the application of an appliance for the child with a urinary stoma.
5. The parent or guardian is able to state the following, if drug therapy is used to assist in attaining urinary continence:
   a. The name of the drug.
   b. The action of the drug.
   c. The side effects of the drug.
   d. The dose, route, and hours to administer the drug.
   e. How long the child will take the drug.
   f. Any blood or urine tests that need to be performed while the child is taking the drug.
6. The child and parent or guardian demonstrate the appropriate technique for clean,

intermittent catheterization, including the following:
   a. Preparation of supplies.
   b. Cleansing the urinary meatus.
   c. Lubricating and inserting the catheter.
   d. Pinching the catheter before removal.
   e. Noting the color, odor, and clarity of the urine, and measuring the output if requested to do so by the urologist.
   f. How to obtain supplies.
   g. When to come for follow-up urine culture and sensitivity, blood, or radiology tests.
   h. Symptoms to report to the urologist (e.g., fever, nausea and vomiting, urethral bleeding, difficult catheterization, and cloudy or foul-smelling urine).
7. The child and parent or guardian demonstrate the appropriate technique in emptying the urinary bladder with the aid of the AUS, including the following:
   a. Locating the bulb.
   b. Pressing the bulb to allow urine to flow.
   c. Noting the color, odor, and clarity of the urine, and measuring the output if requested to do so by the urologist.
   d. Symptoms to report to the urologist (e.g., pain, urinary leak, inability to palpate or locate the bulb, blood in the urine, and signs of urinary tract infection).

# Sacral Agenesis and Spinal Dysraphism

## PERSPECTIVE ON DISEASE ENTITY

**Etiology.** As with myelodysplasia, the cause of sacral agenesis and spinal dysraphism is unknown. However, 1% of mothers who have diabetes mellitus have newborns with sacral agenesis.

**Pathophysiology.** *Agenesis* means lack or failure of development. Sacral agenesis is a rare congenital anomaly that involves the absence of part or all of two or more sacral vertebrae and is associated with lower urinary tract dysfunction and orthopedic deformities (Guzman et al., 1983). Vesicoureteral dysfunction may be absent, minimal, or severe, depending on the extent of damage to the nerves supplying the bladder.

The term *spinal dysraphism* is applied to a group of structural abnormalities of the caudal end of the spinal cord and vertebral column. The following anomalies are included in this group: lipoma, dermoid cyst or sinus, aberrant sacral roots, fibrous traction on the clonus med-ullaris, or a tight filum terminale (Mandell et al., 1980).

**Medical-Surgical Management.** Children suspected of having sacral agenesis have the diagnosis confirmed through anteroposterior and lateral x-ray films of the lower spine (Bauer, 1984). Other diagnostic studies may include an IVP, a VCUG, and urodynamic procedures. The child who has a presumptive diagnosis of spinal dysraphism has the diagnosis confirmed by myelogram, computed tomography scan, magnetic resonance imaging, or surgical exploration.

Management of the child with a neurogenic bladder secondary to sacral agenesis or spinal dysraphism is dependent on urodynamic findings. Urodynamic evaluation that includes electromyography of the external urethral sphincter assists in determining the extent and type of the neurologic defect (Mandell et al., 1980). Based on these findings, the urologist may choose a drug or combination of drugs to control uninhibited bladder contractions or to augment voluntary bladder contractions when the child fails to empty the bladder completely. Clean intermittent catheterization may be used in conjunction with drug therapy, or it may be the only therapy (Guzman et al., 1983).

Surgical management of the primary diagnosis of spinal dysraphism involves a laminectomy with release of compression or tethering of the spinal cord. This procedure helps prevent continuing damage to the nerves as the child grows (Anderson, 1975).

## APPROACHES TO PATIENT CARE

### Assessment

Nursing management of the child with bladder dysfunction secondary to spinal dysraphism or sacral agenesis is centered on the resolution of parent-child knowledge deficits concerning tests and procedures, the diagnosis and the child's progress, alteration in bladder functioning secondary to the diagnosis, and treatment methods to restore or approximate physiologic bladder functioning. This goal is accomplished by an assessment of the current level of parent-child understanding and a resolution of questions before the formulation of a care plan appropriate to the age and developmental level of the child.

During the interview portion of the nursing assessment, an inquiry should be made as to any history of maternal diabetes. Although the incidence is low, there appears to be a relation between diabetic mothers and children with sacral agenesis. Additionally, the parent (or child) should be asked to describe the child's voiding habits, voiding schedule, and characteristics of the urinary stream. If possible, a urine specimen should be obtained so that it may be examined for signs of infection.

The part of a complete newborn physical examination that may be performed by the nurse includes an examination of the spine for defects. The diagnosis of sacral agenesis may be overlooked during the newborn examination as the lower spine is palpated. A clue to the presence of sacral agenesis is the absence of a gluteal or buttocks cleft, widely spaced buttocks dimples, absence of the sacrum on palpation, and flattened buttocks (Guzman et al., 1983). If not diagnosed in the newborn period, the child may be referred to the urologist because of enuresis or encopresis.

Spinal dysraphism is often not diagnosed at birth but is suspected when the child is brought to the urologist for an assessment of voiding dysfunction. An infant may be referred to the urologist because of abnormal voiding patterns or frequent urinary tract infections. The toilet-trained child or older child may be referred for an assessment of incontinence or infection.

In a study of eight children diagnosed with spinal dysraphism, Mandell and associates (1980) found some of the following on physical examination: a neurologic or orthopedic abnormality involving the lower extremities, scoliosis, ankle deformity, leg-length discrepancy, diminished ankle-jerk reflexes, weakness of the lower extremities, and poor anal tone. Therefore, during the physical examination of a child suspected of having spinal dysraphism, the nurse should include an assessment of the lower extremities, including size, length, and symmetry; a visual inspection and palpation of the lumbosacral area; and an assessment of anal tone and the response to eliciting the sacral, bulbocavernous, and anocutaneous reflexes (Mandell et al., 1980).

### Nursing Diagnosis

The nursing diagnoses for the patient with sacral agenesis or the patient with spinal dysraphism may include the following:

1. Alteration in the pattern of urinary elimination related to (select cause)
   a. The failure to store urine.
   b. The failure to empty urine.
2. Knowledge deficit related to (select all that apply)

a. The diagnosis of sacral agenesis or spinal dysraphism (including its cause and the child's prognosis).

b. Diagnostic tests and procedures.

c. Treatment options, including the administration of medications and method of clean intermittent catheterization.

3. Impaired mobility related to neurologic or orthopedic abnormalities involving the lower extremities.

4. Potential for infection related to an alteration in urinary elimination.

**Plan of Care**

Nursing care is directed toward enabling the patient to

1. Approach or reach a physiologic control of urination consistent with the urologist's plan of management.

2. Develop an understanding of the diagnosis of sacral agenesis or sacral dysraphism.

3. Cope with tests and procedures.

4. Comply with instructions for drug use.

5. Comply with the components of the clean intermittent catheterization procedure.

6. Prevent urinary tract infection.

**Intervention.** The management plan of the urologist often includes the use of medications or clean intermittent catheterization. Therefore, nursing intervention is directed toward preparing the family to comply with the selected plan. Specific nursing actions that may be employed are similar to those described for the child with myelodysplasia. (Refer to the previous section for a complete description of appropriate nursing interventions.)

**Patient Outcomes**

1. The parents verbalize an understanding of their child's condition.

2. Parents are sufficiently prepared for tests and procedures that their child will experience as demonstrated by their ability to support and assist their child to cope.

3. The child is prepared for procedures to the extent that he or she is cooperative.

4. The parent or child demonstrates awareness of the medication regime, including knowledge of

a. The name of the drug.

b. The appropriate dose.

c. The method of administration.

d. The route of administration.

e. The frequency of administration.

f. The common side effects of the drug and the action to be taken if a side effect occurs.

g. The duration of drug use and if follow-up serum or urine studies are needed.

5. The parent or child demonstrates proficiency with the components of clean intermittent catheterization, including

a. Hand washing before performing the procedure.

b. Appropriate cleansing of the perineum.

c. Lubrication of the catheter.

d. Insertion of the catheter.

e. Collection of urine (measure quantity if requested by physician).

f. Pinch catheter before slowly removing (to prevent the urine remaining in the tube from flowing back into the bladder as the catheter is withdrawn).

g. Method of cleaning and storing equipment.

6. The child is continent.

7. The child exhibits no signs or symptoms of a urinary tract infection.

## URODYNAMICS IN CHILDREN

Urodynamic studies should be performed to accurately and completely evaluate voiding problems in pediatric patients. However, performing such studies on a child is challenging and sometimes complicated. Often, techniques must be modified to ensure completion of the study with reliable and reproducible measurements.

The difficulties encountered during urodynamic assessment are generally attributed to a child's short attention span, low tolerance for discomfort, fear of having an invasive test, difficulty following commands during testing, difficulty communicating sensations, and inability to remain still during the procedures (Abrahams et al., 1983; Bauer, 1984, 1991). In addition, the size of the child's urethra may make catheterization with more than one catheter difficult, thereby preventing an adequate recording and measurement of bladder pressure.

Every child with a voiding disorder does not require a urodynamic evaluation. The decision to proceed with urodynamic testing depends on information obtained during the health history and physical examination. Data from laboratory and radiologic studies, as well as the age and sex of the child, also are determining factors. In general, a child is referred for urodynamic evaluation if he or she is suspected of having a voiding disorder as a result of congenital or anatomic abnormality, a neurologic

**TABLE 22–6. Clinical Indications for Pediatric Urodynamics**

| CATEGORY | DISEASE OR DISORDER |
|---|---|
| Congenital or anatomic abnormalities | Posterior urethral valves |
| | Bladder exstrophy |
| | Epispadias |
| | Urethral stricture |
| | Prune belly syndrome |
| Neurologic disorders | Myelodysplasia |
| | Spinal dysraphism |
| | Sacral agenesis |
| | Traumatic myelitis |
| | Central nervous system malignancy (primary or metastatic) |
| | Meningitis |
| Functional conditions | Enuresis |
| | Encopresis |
| | Diurnal frequency/urgency syndrome |
| | Recurrent urinary tract infections |
| | Nonneurogenic bladder |

disorder, or a functional condition (Table 22–6).

The primary objective of a urodynamic evaluation is to reproduce the natural act of voiding to study those symptoms or conditions that contribute to a child's inability to appropriately store or eliminate urine. A variety of urodynamic procedures and techniques are available to accomplish this purpose, and all may be performed on children. However, each child referred for urodynamic testing does not require every procedure available. A good rule to follow when faced with a child needing urodynamic testing is to consider the child's specific problem, then select and perform those procedures that provide the needed information with the least amount of invasiveness. In every instance, consultation with the referring physician is advised so that the child is appropriately studied and the necessary information is obtained.

When working with children, procedure techniques often require modification to ensure that usable and reproducible results are obtained. The extent to which a urodynamicist should modify each procedure technique depends on the age of the child, the child's ability and willingness to cooperate with the testing, the type of information to be obtained by the testing, and the pediatric urologist's preferences. Alternative investigational techniques that may be used when performing urodynamic testing on a child include some of the following:

1. A single-lumen catheter with $CO_2$ infusion offers quick screening for uninhibited bladder contractions, especially when voiding studies are not needed. However, water cystometry offers a more physiologic result and is less irritating. The use of water or $CO_2$ depends on the preference of the physician.

2. Abdominal wall electromyelography, accomplished with surface electrodes applied to the skin, is a simple way to monitor abdominal muscle involvement during voiding, especially when a balloon catheter inserted in the rectum is deemed undesirable or uncomfortable by the child (although perineal electrodes and small rectal probes are used successfully on children in some centers).

3. Surface electrodes applied to the perineum offer a noninvasive alternative for monitoring pelvic floor activity. This type of monitoring does not discriminate pelvic floor activity from other nearby muscle groups but does allow the examiner to determine if pelvic floor activity is appropriately coordinated with urine storage and bladder emptying. The trick to obtaining a good recording is to apply the electrode on an area of skin that has been thoroughly cleaned with an abrasive skin cleanser; this reduces resistance and artifacts and helps the electrodes adhere better. Throughout the study, it is important to monitor any movement by the child and note it on the printout; movement artifact must be clearly identified so that an accurate interpretation of the data may be completed.

4. When voiding studies are needed, investigate the feasibility of having a suprapubic catheter inserted for measuring bladder pressure. A suprapubic catheter may easily be inserted at the same time the child is anesthetized for cystoscopy. If necessary, bladder filling can also be accomplished through the same tube. Although placement of a suprapubic tube is not a routine practice, it may represent the only viable alternative for completion of a urodynamic evaluation in some children.

5. Keep in mind that a child's bladder capacity is smaller than an adult's. Therefore, the filling rate during cystometry should be adjusted accordingly. For most children, slow-fill cystometry is desirable (up to 10 mL/min).

6. For the 4- or 5-year-old toilet-trained child, flow rate measurement is the easiest to obtain and may be the only testing with which

the child is willing to cooperate. If measurement of residual urine is needed at the same time, consider using ultrasonography for a noninvasive means of making this determination. The availability and sophistication of portable ultrasound units make this an option (Fig. 22–7).

7. If the child is scheduled to have a cystogram or VCUG, consider scheduling the urodynamic testing at the same time that either of these tests are done. Extra catheterizations may be eliminated, and the examiner may collect additional valuable information from the fluoroscopic imaging.

Soliciting a child's cooperation during urodynamic testing requires that the examiner be persuasive and creative. To get the child to endure the entire testing procedure, the nurse may employ one of the following strategies:

1. Explaining the procedure before beginning urodynamic testing is often beneficial. However, offering an explanation too far in advance may frighten the child to the point of wanting to refuse testing. Descriptions of urodynamic procedures sound much worse than the actual testing. Therefore, consider each individual child's ability to compre-

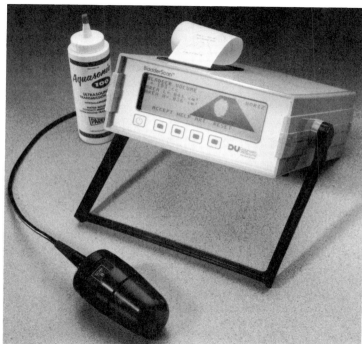

*FIGURE 22–7* BladderScan BVI 2500 and printout showing how residual urine is graphically depicted. (Courtesy of Diagnostic Ultrasound Corporation, Kirkland, WA.)

hend preprocedural teaching before offering the information. If possible, permitting the child to see the room, demonstrating the equipment, and explaining the procedure may help allay fears and allow the child to be more cooperative.

2. Some physicians prefer that children be medicated before urodynamic testing to reduce discomfort and enhance cooperation. Meperidine, 1 mg/kg, administered intramuscularly, may be used (Bauer, 1984, 1991). However, analgesics, narcotics, and smooth muscle relaxants alter bladder sensations and contractility, which may cause the study results to be inconclusive.

3. Storybooks are a good diversion for young children during urodynamic testing. Depending on the age of the child, he or she may look at the books with or without a parent, or a parent or health professional may read aloud.

4. Encourage the child who is apprehensive about having urodynamic testing to bring a doll or stuffed animal along. Having a familiar comforting object is often a great consolation to children.

5. Children are curious about complicated technical equipment. They want to know how it works and what it sounds like. Therefore, if the child shows interest in the mechanical aspects of urodynamic testing, let him or her "help" in some way with the testing. Also involve the child in creating the study results by showing what you are seeing and how he or she can affect the results.

6. The reinforcement of urodynamic testing as a positive experience is especially important for those children who may require repeated studies. Therefore, when the testing is completed, offer a treat or reward, and praise the child's braveness so that he or she may be able to associate the urodynamic test with a caring examiner.

## REFERENCES

Abrahams, P., Feneley, R., & Torrens, M. (1983). *Urodynamics.* New York: Springer-Verlag.

Anderson, F. M. (1975). Occult spinal dysraphism: A series of 73 cases. *Pediatrics, 55*(6), 826–835.

Bauer, S. B. (1991). The urodynamic evaluation of children. In R. J. Krane & M. B. Siroky (Eds.), *Clinical neuro-urology* (2nd ed.; pp. 299–316). Boston: Little, Brown.

Bauer, S. B. (1984). Urodynamics in children: Indications and methods. In D. M. Barrett & A. J. Wein (Eds.), *Controversies in neuro-urology.* New York: Churchill Livingstone.

Belman, A. B., & King, L. R. (1973). Vesicostomy: Useful means of reversible urinary diversion in selected infants. *Urology, 1*(3), 208–213.

Cendron, J., & Melin, Y. (1987). Congenital obstructive lesions of the male urethra. In A. B. Retik & J. Cukier (Eds.), *Pediatric urology* (pp. 452–468). Baltimore: Williams & Wilkins.

Churchill, B. M., Gilmour, R. F., Khoury, A. E., & McLorie, G. A. (1987). Biological response of bladders rendered continent by insertion of artificial sphincter. *Journal of Urology, 138*(4 Pt 2), 1116–1119.

Crooks, K. K., & Enrile, B. G. (1983). Comparison of the ileal conduit and clean intermittent catheterization for myelomeningocele. *Pediatrics, 72*(2), 203–206.

Decter, R. M., Bauer, S. B., Mandell, J., Colodny, A. H., & Retik, A. B. (1987). Small bowel augmentation in children with neurogenic bladder: An initial report of urodynamic findings. *Journal of Urology, 138*(4 Pt 2), 1014–1016.

Edelmann, C. M., Jr. (1978). *Pediatric kidney disease* (Vols. 1 and 2). Boston: Little, Brown.

Esperanca, M., & Gerrard, J. W. (1969). Nocturnal enuresis: Comparison of the effects of imipramine and dietary restriction on bladder capacity. *Canadian Medical Association Journal, 101,* 721–724.

Gauthier, J. A., Edelman, C. M., & Barnett, H. L. (1982). *Nephrology and urology for the pediatrician.* Boston: Little, Brown.

Gill, B. (1988). [Personal communication].

Glassberg, K. I. (1985). Current issues regarding posterior urethral valves. *Urologic Clinics of North America, 12*(1), 175–185.

Gonzalez, E. T. (1985). Urologic considerations in the newborn. *Urologic Clinics of North America, 12*(1), 43–51.

Gutmann, L., & Frankel, H. (1966). The value of intermittent catheterization in the early management of traumatic paraplegia and tetraplegia. *Paraplegia, 4*(1), 63–83.

Guzman, L., Bauer, S. B., Hallett, M., Khoshbin, S., Colodny, A. H., & Retik, A. B. (1983). Evaluation and management of children with sacral agenesis. *Urology, 22*(5), 506–510.

Hannigan, K., & Elder, J. S. (1988). Teaching catheterization to children. *Urologic Clinics of North America, 15*(4), 653–660.

James, J. A. (1968). *Renal disease in childhood.* St. Louis: C. V. Mosby.

Jeter, K. (1990). The use of incontinence products. In K. Jeter, N. Faller, & C. Norton (Eds.), *Nursing for continence* (pp. 209–222). Philadelphia: W. B. Saunders.

Kales, A., Kales, J. D., Jacobson, A., Humphrey, F. J., & Soldatos, C. R. (1977). Effects of imipramine on enuretic frequency and sleep stages. *Pediatrics, 60*(4), 431–436.

King, L. R., Webster, G. D., & Bertram, R. A. (1987). Experiences with bladder reconstruction in children. *Journal of Urology, 138*(4 Pt 2), 1002–1006.

Lapides, J. (1971). Clean intermittent self-catheterization in the treatment of urinary tract disease. *Transactions of the American Association of Genito-Urinary Surgeons, 63,* 92–95.

Lattimer, J. K., Uson, A. C., & Melicow, M. M. (1962). Urologic emergencies in newborn infants. *Pediatrics, 29*(2), 310–323.

Light, J. K., Hawila, M., & Scott, F. B. (1983). Treatment of urinary incontinence in children: The artificial sphincter versus other methods. *Journal of Urology, 130*(3), 518–521.

Mandell, J., Bauer, S. B., Hallett, M., Khoshbin, S., Dyro, F. M., Colodny, A. H., & Retik, A. B. (1980). Occult spinal dysraphism: A rare but detectable cause of voiding dysfunction. *Urologic Clinics of North America, 7*(2), 349–356.

Meadow, S. R. (1978). Enuresis. In C. M. Edelmann Jr. (Ed.), *Pediatric kidney disease* (Vols. 1 and 2; pp. 1176–1181). Boston: Little, Brown.

Mills, J. L., Rhoads, G. G., Simpson, J. L., Cunningham, G. C., Conley, M. E., Lassman, M. R., Walden, M. E., Depp, O. R., & Hoffman, H. J. (1989). The absence of a relationship between the preconceptional use of vitamins and neural tube defects. *New England Journal of Medicine, 321*(7), 430–435.

Mitchell, M. E., & Rink, R. C. (1985). Urinary diversion and undiversion. *Urologic Clinics of North America, 12*(1), 111–122.

Moore, E. S., & Galvez, M. B. (1972). Delayed micturition in the newborn period. *Pediatrics, 80*(5), 867–873.

Mulinare, J., Cordero, J. F., Erickson, J. D., & Berry, R. J. (1988). Periconceptional use of multivitamins and the occurrence of neural tube defects. *Journal of the American Medical Association, 260*(21), 3141–3145.

Oppel, W. C., Harper, P. A., & Rider, R. V. (1968). The age of attaining bladder control. *Pediatrics, 42*(4), 614–626.

Perlmutter, A. D. (1985). Enuresis. In P. P. Kelalis, L. R. King, & A. B. Belman (Eds.), *Clinical pediatric urology* (2nd ed.; pp. 311–325). Philadelphia: W. B. Saunders.

Pillen, T., Kroeger, R. M., Mardis, H., & Kammandel, H. (1985). Voiding disorders in children. *Physician Assistant, 9*(4), 30–32, 61–62.

Rhoads, G. G., & Mills, J. L. (1986). Can vitamin supplements prevent neural tube defects? *Clinical Obstetrics and Gynecology, 29,* 569–579.

Roberts, K. E., & Schoellkopf, J. A. (1951). Eating, sleeping, and elimination practices of a group of two- and one-half year-old children. *American Journal of Diseases of Children, 82*(2), 121–152.

Roy, C. C., Silverman, A., & Cozzetto, F. J. (1975). *Pediatric clinical gastroenterology* (2nd ed.). St. Louis: C. V. Mosby.

Ruble, J. A. (1981). Childhood nocturnal enuresis. *MCN: American Journal of Maternal Child Nursing, 1*(6), 26–31.

Scott, F. B., Bradley, W. E., & Timm, G. W. (1974). Treatment of urinary incontinence by an implantable prosthetic urinary sphincter. *Journal of Urology, 112,* 75–80.

Sherry, S. N., & Kramer, I. (1955). The time of passage of first urine by the newborn infant. *Journal of Pediatrics, 46*(2), 158–159.

Smith, P. (1985). Innervation and mobility: Implications of altered neurological and neuromuscular function. In S. R. Mott, N. F. Fazekas, & S. R. James (Eds.), *Nursing care of children and families: A holistic approach* (pp. 1544–1548). Menlo Park, CA: Addison-Wesley.

# CHAPTER 23

# Problems of Sexual Differentiation and Development

■

*Kathleen A. Thompson*

## OVERVIEW

At birth, the sex assignment of an infant is usually a simple task, based on a quick examination of the external genitalia. However, when an infant is born with ambiguous genitalia, this assignment is often approached with considerable confusion on the part of the medical personnel and shame or guilt on the part of the parents. These children present a challenge to pediatricians, surgeons, urologists, geneticists, and endocrinologists, as well as to the support staffs of nursing, social services, and psychiatry. This chapter explores the complex problems of ambiguous genitalia, including the medical, psychosexual, and social implications of the diagnosis and treatment.

## BEHAVIORAL OBJECTIVES

After studying this chapter, the reader should be able to

1. Identify five determinants of the sex of an individual and discuss their relevance in the sex assignment of an infant with ambiguous genitalia.

2. Differentiate between the five major classifications of anomalous sexual development.

3. Recognize the importance of obtaining an accurate family and prenatal history and conducting a thorough physical examination of an infant with ambiguous genitalia.

4. Formulate a teaching plan for the parents of an infant with ambiguous genitalia.

## KEY WORDS

**Adrenocorticotropic hormone (ACTH)—** a hormone produced by the pituitary gland that stimulates the cortex of the adrenal gland to secrete its hormones.

**Androgen—**any substance that stimulates male characteristics. Although the key androgen, testosterone, is manufactured daily by the testes, it is also produced in small amounts by the adrenal glands in both sexes and by the ovaries in females.

**Arrhenoblastoma—**an ovarian tumor composed of masculine sex cells, which produce male sex characteristics.

**Bifid scrotum—**the condition in which the scrotum is divided into two lobes by a median cleft.

**Clitoromegaly—**enlargement of the clitoris, the erectile body in the female.

**Dysgenesis—**a defective development or malformation.

**Endoscopy—**the inspection of cavities with the use of an endoscope.

**Feminization—**the development of female secondary sex characteristics and external genitalia.

**Gender identity—**the unified and persistent experience of oneself as male or female. Gender identity is not determined by chromosomes, gonads, or prenatal hormones but by rearing.

**Genotype—**the total genetic constitution of an individual.

**Glucocorticoid—**a substance that increases gluconeogenesis, (e.g., cortisol or hydrocortisone).

**Gynecomastia—**abnormally large mammary glands.

**Hirsutism—**an excessive growth of hair, or the presence of hair in unusual places.

**Hypospadias—**a developmental anomaly in which the urethra opens onto the underside of the penis or on the perineum.

**Karyotype—**the chromosomal constitution of the cell nucleus.

**Luteoma—**an ovarian tumor containing lutein cells.

**Mineralocorticoid—**any hormone of the adrenal cortex that affects the electrolyte composition of the extracellular fluid.

**Mosaicism—**when cells in an individual are derived from the same zygote but have a different chromosomal constitution.

**Müllerian ducts—**paired embryonic ducts that develop into the vagina, uterus, and uterine tubes in the female. They usually become obliterated during normal male development. Appendices testes are the normal müllerian remnants in the male.

**Müllerian regression factor (or müllerian inhibition factor)—**a substance produced by the fetal Sertoli's cells and secreted by the fetal testes to cause a regression of the müllerian ducts in the male.

**Orchidectomy (also orchiectomy, orchectomy)—**surgical removal of one or both testes.

**Phenotype—**the external physical expression of an individual as male or female.

**Pseudohermaphrodite—**an individual in whom the gonads are of one sex but the external physical expression is to some degree contradictory. A female pseudohermaphrodite is an individual who is genetically female and has female gonads, but is partially masculinized. A male pseudohermaphrodite is an individual who is genetically male and has male gonads, but is incompletely masculinized.

**Streak gonads—**an underdeveloped ovary or testicle. In most cases, endocrine-producing cells do not occur in streak gonads.

**Testicular feminization—**an individual who is genotypically male but phenotypically female.

**True hermaphrodite—**a person who possesses both ovarian and testicular tissue.

**Urogenital sinus—**the common receptacle of the genital and urinary ducts. In the embryo, the wolffian ducts and bladder empty into the urogenital sinus, which opens into the cloaca.

**Vaginoplasty—**the plastic repair or creation of a vagina.

**Virilization (or masculinization)—**the development of male secondary sex characteristics and genitalia.

# PERSPECTIVE ON AMBIGUOUS GENITALIA

## Etiology and Contributing Factors

The most common causes of anomalous sexual development include chromosomal anomalies; excessive androgen production in the genetic female, causing virilization of the external genitalia; and defective androgen production or action in the genetic male, causing feminization of the external genitalia. Infants are affected at the rate of 1:1000 live births, making genital ambiguity relatively common (Parks, 1977).

## Pathophysiology

### SEXUAL DIFFERENTIATION

A thorough understanding of normal sexual differentiation is important for understanding the various classifications of anomalous sexual development. (For a review of normal embryologic development, see Chap. 1.) Normal sexual differentiation includes three phases: differentiation of the gonads, development of the internal ducts, and differentiation of the external genitalia. During the third to the fifth weeks of gestation, an indifferent gonad is formed. Prior to the onset of sexual differentiation, two sets of primordial ducts, the wolffian and the müllerian, are present in both the male and the female fetus. The chromosomes direct the future differentiation of the gonad into either an ovary or a testis.

The testis differentiates much earlier in gestation than does the ovary. The fetal testis secretes two hormones: müllerian regression factor, which causes regression of the müllerian ducts, and testosterone, which stimulates development of the internal wolffian duct structures. The wolffian duct structures give rise to the vas deferens, seminal vesicles, and epididymis. In the female fetus, because of the lack of a testis, müllerian regression factor is not produced, and the müllerian ducts give rise to the fallopian tubes, the uterus, and the upper vagina. Also, because of the lack of testosterone stimulation in the normal female, the wolffian ducts regress.

Before differentiation of the external genitalia at 8 to 15 weeks, the genitalia of both sexes are identical and consist of the genital tubercle (the precursor of the clitoris in the female and the glans penis in the male), the inner labio-urethral folds (the precursor of the urethra and the ventral shaft of the penis in the male and the labia minora in the female), and the outer labioscrotal swellings (the precursor of the scrotum in the male and the labia majora in the female) (Glassberg, 1987).

In the male fetus, for testosterone to produce the final differentiation of the external genitalia, it must be converted to dihydrotestosterone by the 5-alpha-reductase enzymes. In the female fetus, it is the absence of androgens that causes the development of the external genitalia. In summary, early testicular function is required for regression of the müllerian structures, growth of the wolffian ducts, and the differentiation and growth of the external genitalia in the male. Female genital development, however, does not depend on ovarian function but on the absence of androgenic stimulation (Parks, 1977).

### CLASSIFICATION OF ANOMALOUS SEXUAL DEVELOPMENT

The classification of anomalous sexual development as discussed in the following sections is summarized in Table 23–1.

## Female Pseudohermaphrodism

Female pseudohermaphrodism occurs when a genetic female (46,XX) is exposed in utero to endogenous or exogenous androgens, causing virilization of the external genitalia. Endogenous androgenization is most commonly caused by congenital adrenal hyperplasia (CAH), also referred to as *adrenogenital syndrome*. CAH accounts for 60% of all cases of anomalous sexual development and occurs in 1:40,000 female births (Donahoe & Crawford, 1986). CAH is an inherited (autosomal recessive) enzymatic block in the synthesis of cortisol. By attempting to compensate for the lowered cortisol levels, adrenocorticotropic hormone (ACTH) stimulates the adrenal gland to secrete an excessive amount of androgens (Walsh et al., 1978). The two most common enzyme defects that cause CAH are a 21-hydroxylase deficiency, which may be associated with an excessive salt loss, and an 11-hydroxylase deficiency, which may cause hypertension. CAH with an excessive salt loss is usually evidenced at 7 to 10 days of age by weight loss, vomiting, and cardiovascular collapse. Of all the conditions that may cause ambiguous genitalia, only CAH is potentially life threatening

(Donahoe & Hendren, 1984). An unusual endogenous cause of female pseudohermaphrodism is a virilizing tumor of the maternal ovary, either an arrhenoblastoma or a luteoma.

Exogenous androgen exposure caused by maternal drug ingestion was a significant cause of female pseudohermaphrodism in the past, when progestational steroids were used in managing threatened abortion (Canty, 1977). A few reports note drug-induced virilization in infants of women who continued to use oral contraceptives after conception occurred (Parks, 1977).

Excessive androgens cause virilization of the female fetus. The degree of virilization of the urogenital sinus and the external genitalia depends on the gestational age of the fetus and the amount and strength of the androgen present (Glassberg, 1987). The phenotype varies from a mild clitoromegaly to a penis-like phallus with a vagina that opens very proximally into the urogenital sinus (Fig. 23–1*A* and *B*).

Individuals with female pseudohermaphrodism are fertile females and are therefore always raised as female. Surgical correction consists of clitoral reduction and vaginoplasty. Individuals with the salt-losing type of CAH require close medical management for cortisol and mineral replacements.

## Male Pseudohermaphrodism

*Male pseudohermaphrodism* is the term used to describe genetic males who usually have a normal 46,XY karyotype but who have incomplete masculinization of either internal or external genital structures (Donahoe et al., 1977). The multiple and complex causes in male pseudohermaphrodism reflect the complicated biosynthetic and hormonal processes required for the initiation of normal development of the male external genitalia (*Atlas of pediatric physical diagnosis*, 1987). Although the cause is known in only about 50% of individuals given the diagnosis of male pseudohermaphrodism, inheritable single gene disorders characterize the group (Eil et al., 1984). There are five known causes of male pseudohermaphrodism: a decreased amount of müllerian regression factor, inadequate androgen production, androgen insensitivity, 5-alpha-reductase deficiency, and dysgenetic testes.

Male pseudohermaphrodism due to a decreased amount of müllerian regression factor is rare. Although these individuals have both müllerian and wolffian internal ducts, they are in most cases, with the exception of cryptor-

chidism, normal appearing males. The diagnosis is usually established when a herniorrhaphy is performed to correct a symptomatic hernia and the hernia is found to contain a uterus. This condition has also been referred to as *hernia uteri inguinalis* (Allen, 1976). These individuals are raised as males.

Inadequate androgen production in male pseudohermaphrodism is the result of a deficiency in one of five enzymes required to synthesize testosterone from cholesterol. These individuals are phenotypic females but may have palpable inguinal testes. After orchidectomy is performed in infancy, these individuals are raised as females, with estrogen therapy initiated at puberty.

Male pseudohermaphrodism may also be caused by an unresponsiveness of the external genitalia to androgens because of an absence of androgen-binding protein in the cells; the condition occurs in a complete and an incomplete form. A complete androgen insensitivity is an X-linked recessive trait that causes the genetically normal male fetus (46,XY) to passively develop as a female and is commonly referred to as *testicular feminization syndrome.* Because these individuals are normal-appearing phenotypic females, the diagnosis is usually made during adolescence, when amenorrhea is noted. Because of the presence of müllerian regression factor from the normal testes, there are no female internal structures. Occasionally, the diagnosis is made in infancy when a testis is found during a hernia repair. These individuals all remain in the female role. Because the incidence of gonadoblastoma increases from approximately 4% before puberty to more than 30% by 50 years of age, it is generally recommended that the testes be removed as soon as possible and the patient be given appropriate hormonal replacement in puberty (Manuel et al., 1976). Some surgeons, however, recommend leaving the testes until after puberty, because testosterone cannot cause virilization, and normal breast enlargement occurs as a result of the conversion of the testosterone to estradiol (Donahoe et al., 1977).

The incomplete form of androgen receptor malfunction or insensitivity produces a broad spectrum of ambiguous genitalia. The sex assignment is variable and based on the degree of virilization. If the diagnosis is made in infancy, the individual is usually given a female assignment, because it is uncertain what degree of virilization will take place at puberty. Griffin and Wilson (1992) have described this incomplete androgen insensitivity as familial in-

## TABLE 23–1. Classification of Anomalous Sexual Development

| | BARR BODIES | CHROMO-SOMES | GONADS | INTERNAL DUCTS | EXTERNAL GENITALIA | PUBERTY | SEX ASSIGN-MENT | FERTILITY | TREATMENT |
|---|---|---|---|---|---|---|---|---|---|
| **Female Pseudohermaphrodism** | | | | | | | | | |
| Endogenous androgenization | Chromatin + | 46,XX | Ovaries | Female | Variably virilized | Amenorrhea with virilization without treatment | Female | Normal fertile female | Medical: steroid and salt replacement as needed. Surgical: clitoral reduction + vaginoplasty |
| Exogenous androgenization | Chromatin + | 46,XX | Ovaries | Female | Variably virilized | Normal | Female | Normal fertile female | Surgical: clitoral reduction + vaginoplasty |
| **Male Pseudohermaphrodism** | | | | | | | | | |
| A decreased amount of müllerian regression factor | Chromatin − | 46,XY | Testes | Müllerian & wolffian | Phenotypic male except for cryptorchidism in most cases | Normal | All are reared as male | None | Surgical: removal of the uterus. The testes are preserved |
| Inadequate androgen production | Chromatin − | 46,XY | Testes palpable in the inguinal canal | Wolffian | Phenotypic female | Infantile if left untreated | Female | None | Surgical: orchidectomy in infancy. Medical: estrogen therapy at puberty |
| Androgen insensitivity Incomplete | Chromatin − | 46,XY | Testes | Wolffian | Variable | Variable; may respond imperfectly to testosterone in adolescence | Variable, based on the degree of masculinization | None | Male assignment: surgical repair of the hypospadias and bifid scrotum. Female assignment: clitoral recession, labioscrotal reduction, gonadectomy in infancy, vaginal reconstruction in late adolescence |
| Complete (testicular feminization) | Chromatin − | 46,XY | Testes; 80% have inguinal hernias | Wolffian | Phenotypic female, but only the lower ⅓ of a vagina is present | Feminization; no menses | Female | None | Surgical: bilateral orchidectomy and herniorrhaphy as needed. In some cases, small doses of exogenous estrogen may be needed |
| 5-Alpha-reductase deficiency | Chromatin − | 46,XY | Testes | Wolffian | Phenotypic female, except that testes are found in the groin | Full virilization | Variable | None | Female assignment. Surgical: orchidectomy and vaginoplasty. Medical: estrogen therapy at puberty |
| **Dysgenetic testes** | | | | | | | | | |
| Due to both deficient androgen production and müllerian regression factor | Chromatin − | 46,XY | Testes | Wolffian & müllerian | Ambiguous | Virilization | Variable | None | Surgical: removal of gonads due to potential for malignancy |
| Due to deficient androgen production only (Klinefelter's syndrome) | Most chromatin + | Most commonly 47,XXY | Testes | Wolffian | Phenotypic male | Partial virilization | Usually male, because the diagnosis is usually not made until puberty | None | Testosterone treatment in puberty (age 11 or 12 yr) |

| Condition | Chromatin | Karyotype | Gonads | Internal Ducts | External Genitalia | Pubertal Development | Fertility | Gender of Rearing | Treatment |
|---|---|---|---|---|---|---|---|---|---|
| **True Hermaphrodism** | 80% chromatin + | ≥80% 46,XX, remainder 46,XY or 46,XX/46,XY | Testis + ovary, ovary + ovotestis, testis + ovotestis + ovotestis | Vas on side of testis + uterus + fallopian tube on side of ovary or ovotestis | Ambiguous, but 80% favor the male with varying degrees of hypospadias; cryptorchidism is common | Unpredictable; 80% have gynecomastia, 50% menstruate | Possible but unlikely | 75% are reared as female; if patient presents in newborn period with small phallus, a female assignment should be made | Female assignment: testicular tissue and wolffian structures are removed, scrotum is reduced, clitoris is recessed, and vagina is exteriorized; ovarian tissue is preserved. Male assignment: ovarian and müllerian structures are removed; hypospadias is repaired, and testicular prosthesis is inserted as needed |
| **Mixed Gonadal Dysgenesis** | Chromatin – | Almost all are mosaics, usually 45,XO/46,XY | Most commonly a dysgenetic testis on one side and a streak ovary on the other | Variable, retained müllerian structures and occasionally a vas is found | Varies from a normal-appearing female with clitoromegaly to a normal-appearing male with or without hypospadias | Partial virilization sometimes complete | None | Variable; if patient presents early, usual decision is to rear as female, even if phallus is of an adequate size | Female assignment: clitoral recession, vaginoplasty and labioscrotal reduction; estrogen and progesterone replacement at puberty. Male assignment: hypospadias repair and removal of the streak gonads and any müllerian duct derivatives; all gonads should be removed by age 30 yr. If needed, androgen replacement is initiated in adolescence and mastectomy is done if needed |
| **Pure Gonadal Dysgenesis (Turner's Syndrome)** | 50% chromatin – | 45,XO, 45,XO/46,XX or 45,XO/46,XY | Bilateral streaks | Immature müllerian | Phenotypic female | No pubertal development | None | Female | Estrogen therapy at puberty |

Data from Allen, 1986; *Atlas of pediatric physical diagnosis*, 1987; Donahoe & Crawford, 1986; Griffin & Wilson, 1992; Hendren & Crawford, 1972; Parks, 1977.

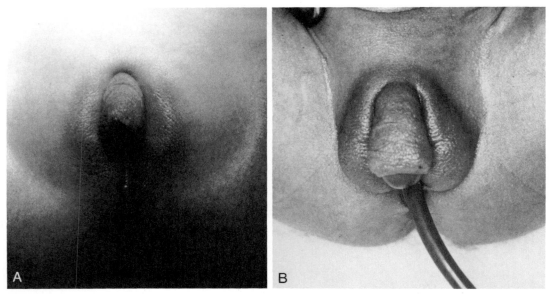

**FIGURE 23–1** The external genitalia of two patients with congenital adrenal hyperplasia, depicting the variation in external masculinization that may occur, ranging from *(A)* simple clitoral hypertrophy to *(B)* severe clitoral hypertrophy with marked labioscrotal development. (*A* and *B* courtesy of James Mandell, MD, Boston, MA.)

complete male pseudohermaphrodism type 1. These individuals have also been labeled anatomically into syndromes, including Lubs', Reifenstein's, and Gilbert-Dreyfus syndromes (Allen, 1976).

Another cause of male pseudohermaphrodism is a 5-alpha-reductase deficiency, which causes the defective metabolism of testosterone to dihydrotestosterone and leads to an inadequate masculinization of the external genitalia. This condition is also referred to as *pseudovaginal perineal-scrotal hypospadias*. Although the 5-alpha-reductase deficiency has been found to be an autosomal recessive trait, studies by Pinto et al. (1977) suggest that maternal ingestion of hydantoins causes an inhibition of 5-alpha-reductase in male fetuses. These individuals are phenotypic females but have testes found in the groin. The sex assignment is female, and orchidectomy, vaginoplasty, and estrogen therapy are undertaken at puberty.

The final cause of male pseudohermaphrodism is dysgenetic testes resulting from a deficiency in either androgen production alone or both androgen production and müllerian regression factor. The deficiency in androgen production alone is referred to as *seminiferous tubule dysgenesis* or *Klinefelter's syndrome*, and it affects 1:400 newborn males (*Atlas of pediatric physical diagnosis*, 1987). The most common karyotype is XXY, but other chromosomal patterns have been described, varying from XXXY

to XXXXYY, as well as some mosaics, varying from XX/XXY to XO/XY/XXY.

Klinefelter's syndrome is usually not obvious until puberty, when the onset of spermatogenesis is blocked by the presence of the two X chromosomes, causing the germ cells to die and the seminiferous tubules to become scarred. This results in a reduction in the size of the testicles (*Atlas of pediatric physical diagnosis*, 1987). Although testosterone levels are usually about half the normal level, they may vary and cause a range of virilization. As puberty progresses, gynecomastia occurs in 40% of individuals with Klinefelter's syndrome. Once gynecomastia occurs, it can only be corrected surgically. Testosterone treatment, beginning by age 11 or 12 years if virilization has not begun, prevents gynecomastia from occurring (*Atlas of pediatric physical diagnosis*, 1987). The physical manifestations include relatively narrow shoulders, female distribution of pubic hair, a small to normal-sized penis, and a small scrotum because of the small size of the testicles. Males with more than two X chromosomes are usually mentally retarded. The average intelligence quotient in individuals with Klinefelter's syndrome is 87 (*Atlas of pediatric physical diagnosis*, 1987).

## True Hermaphrodism

True hermaphrodism is one of the rarest forms of sexual ambiguity—only 400 cases have been reported in the literature (Berkovitz et al., 1982). Although the cause is unknown, the most likely hypothesis is that translocation of a fragment of the short arm of Y chromosome to X chromosome occurs (Glassberg, 1987). The most common karyotype is 46,XX, with the remainder being either 46,XY or a mosaic including 46,XX/46,XY, 46,XY/47,XXY, or 45,XO/46,XY (Van Niekerk, 1981). Although 80% of true hermaphrodites are chromatin positive, the H-Y antigen is manifested despite the XX karyotype. It is presumed that the gene bearing the fragment of the short arm of Y chromosome is present somewhere, resulting in the expression of the H-Y antigen and in testicular differentiation and male development.

Both well-developed ovarian and testicular tissue is present with the ovotestis, a gonad with both ovarian and testicular tissue combined, being the most commonly found gonad. Other gonadal possibilities include a testis on one side and an ovary on the other, a testis or ovary on one side and an ovotestis on the other, or ovotestes bilaterally. The internal ducts include a uterus and a fallopian tube on the side of the ovary or ovotestis and a vas on the side of the testis. The external genitalia may vary from those of a phenotypic male with the urinary meatus on the glans to a phenotypic female with mild clitoromegaly.

Puberty is unpredictable. Eighty percent of individuals with true hermaphrodism have gynecomastia, and 50% menstruate. Although fertility is possible, it is not common (Walsh et al., 1979). The incidence of tumor formation in true hermaphrodism is 6.2%, which is low when compared with that of mixed gonadal dysgenesis (Van Niekerk, 1981).

If the individual presents in the newborn period with a small phallus, the female sex should be assigned. Treatment involves removal of all testicular tissue, excision of the wolffian structures, and reduction of the scrotum. The clitoris is recessed and the vagina exteriorized; all ovarian tissue is preserved. If the phallus is of an adequate size and the individual is committed to the male role, the individual should remain in the male role. Ovarian and müllerian structures should be removed and the hypospadias should be repaired.

## Mixed Gonadal Dysgenesis

The pathophysiology in mixed gonadal dysgenesis remains unknown. Masculinization and müllerian duct inhibition in utero are in-

complete. The external genitalia varies from a phenotypic female with clitoromegaly to a male with or without hypospadias. Almost all individuals with mixed gonadal dysgenesis are mosaics chromosomally, with 45,XO/46,XY being the most common (Walsh et al., 1979). The key to remember in establishing this diagnosis is that there is asymmetry both internally and externally. It is most common to find a dysgenetic testis on one side and a streak ovary on the other (Donahoe et al., 1979). Other possibilities include a unilateral gonadal agenesis or tumor, bilateral streak gonads with rudimentary tubular elements, or a gonad on one side and a gonadal tumor on the other. The gonads exhibit increased fibrosis, with sparse follicles or tubules, and are prone to neoplastic formation. Twenty-five percent of the individuals reared as males develop testicular tumors, with gonadoblastomas being the most common type (Walsh et al., 1979).

## Pure Gonadal Dysgenesis

Turner's syndrome is one of the three most common chromosomal abnormalities found in early spontaneous abortions; only 2% of the affected fetuses are ever born. It is estimated that Turner's syndrome is found in 1:700 newborns (*Atlas of pediatric physical diagnosis*, 1987). Physical features include short stature, unusual faces, webbing of the neck, low posterior hairline, epicanthal folds, prominent ears, small mandible, high-arched palate, broad chest with widely spaced nipples, pigmented nevi, and hyperconvex fingernails. It is common to find associated cardiac anomalies, particularly coarctation of the aorta, as well as several renal anomalies, including rotation of the kidney, horseshoe kidney, duplication of the renal pelvis and ureter, and hydronephrosis secondary to ureteropelvic obstruction.

At birth, the external genitalia appear to be those of a normal female. The gonads, however, are bilateral streaks, the internal ducts are immature müllerian structures, and the karyotype is either 45,XO, 45,XO/46,XX, or 45,XO/46,XY. The second sex chromosome is missing or abnormal in some or all of the cells. Pubertal development is infantile, and there is primary amenorrhea, sparse pubic and axillary hair, underdeveloped breasts, short stature, and sterility (*Atlas of pediatric physical diagnosis,* 1987). The uterus remains infantile, and the ovaries consist of only strands of connective tissue. Mental development is usually normal.

# Medical-Surgical Management

## GENDER ASSIGNMENT

The medical management of the child with ambiguous genitalia must be carefully approached, because if incorrectly handled, a lifetime of unhappiness for both the parents and the child may follow. The exact nature of the defect must be determined quickly and accurately so that a definite plan of care may be presented to the parents before the infant's discharge to allow them to rear the child in a socially acceptable role (Donahoe & Crawford, 1986). Although gender assignment should be treated as a "social emergency," an arbitrary or erroneous sex assignment must be avoided (Canty, 1977).

The normal determination of the sexual differentiation of an individual is based on the following physical findings: the appearance of the external genitalia, the internal ductal differentiation, and the gonads, as well as the social and psychosexual aspects of gender identity, gender role, and sexual orientation. In the individual born with ambiguous genitalia, however, the determination of gender assignment must be based on the existing anatomy and not the genetic sex. Although it is possible to surgically construct functional female genitalia for satisfying sexual performance and normal sociosexual development, it is not currently possible to reconstruct a satisfactory phallus (Weber, 1978). The sex assignment should be consistent with adequate phenotypic appearance and function after surgical reconstruction.

Money (1968) noted that gender is a learned role that is firmly entrenched by the age of 18 to 24 months. Therefore, the sex of a child cannot be changed beyond the age of 18 months without anticipating severe psychological problems throughout life (Griffen & Wilson, 1992). However, an infant may be reared as either male or female, regardless of the genetic sex. If an individual born with ambiguous genitalia is treated as a male, that individual generally assumes a male gender role, despite having ovaries. Likewise, if an individual is reared as a female during development, even though the internal sex organs and chromosomal patterns are those of a male, the individual usually develops a female gender role. Sex rearing consistent with the assigned sex is the most significant factor in both cognitive and personality development (Money, 1968).

## DIFFERENTIAL DIAGNOSIS

The initial evaluation for gender assignment should take place as soon as possible, ideally within the first 24 hours of life. A preliminary diagnosis may be established with 90% accuracy using the following two criteria: a buccal smear for chromatin mass (see the section on assessment) and the symmetry or asymmetry of the gonads (Donahoe & Crawford, 1986). Symmetry refers to the position of the gonads in relation to each other, either above or below the external inguinal ring. For example, asymmetry occurs if one gonad has differentiated as a testis and the other one as an ovary.

Figure 23–2 depicts the diagnostic modalities that may be used to differentiate between the major classifications of intersex abnormalities and arrive at a diagnosis. The diagnostic studies are described in further detail in the section on assessment.

## SURGICAL INTERVENTION

It is generally recommended that surgery be performed early in the child's life to prevent a subconscious rejection of the child by the parents and to promote a positive body image and self-esteem in the child (Donahoe & Hendren, 1984). The surgical treatment of an individual with ambiguous genitalia initially involves the removal of inappropriate gonads and ductal structures. These gonads are usually removed early in life, often at the time of the laparotomy, to avoid inappropriate hormonal changes during and after puberty, to avoid the risk of tumor formation, and because the individual is usually infertile. However, the ovaries of female pseudohermaphrodites are never removed, because the individuals have the potential for normal fertility. Likewise, true hermaphrodites should not have the gonad appropriate to the assigned sex removed.

### Female Sex Assignment

The reconstructive procedures in the infant given a female sex assignment may include clitoral recession, vaginoplasty, and labioscrotal reduction (Donahoe & Crawford, 1986). Although timing of the clitoroplasty is optional, surgery in the newborn period helps alleviate parental distress caused by observing a large phallus every time they change their daughter's diaper. The timing of the vaginoplasty and labioscrotal reduction depends on the point of entry of the vagina into the urogenital

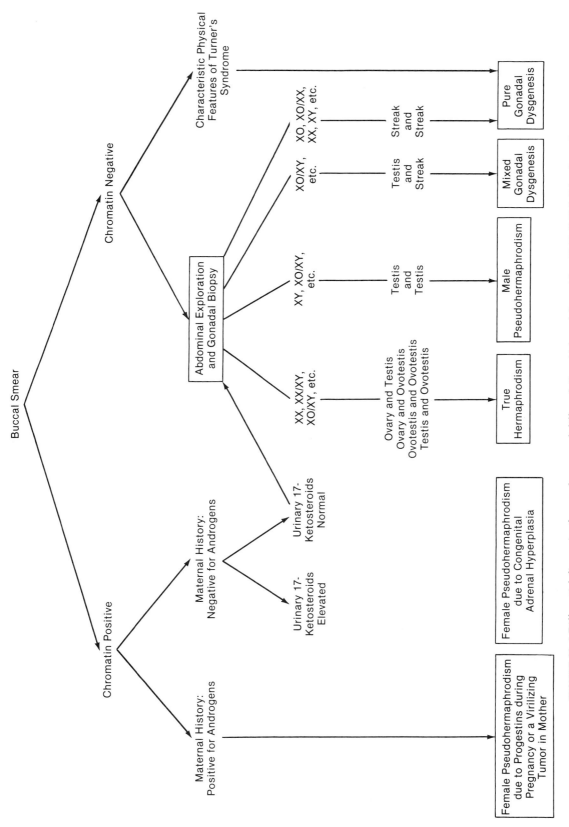

*FIGURE 23–2* Differential diagnosis of anomalous sexual differentiation. (Adapted from Allen, T. D. [1976]. Disorders of sexual differentiation. *Urology,* 7 [4 Suppl], 1–32. Reprinted by permission.)

sinus. Surgical repair may be completed by 6 months of age, unless the vagina enters the urogenital sinus at a high level, in which case the vaginoplasty is delayed until the child is approximately 2 years of age.

In the past, an enlarged clitoris was reduced by simple amputation at the level of the pubic symphysis. With more awareness of satisfactory sexual functioning, the goal of surgery now is not only cosmetic reduction in phallic size but preservation of erectile function and sensation of the glans clitoris.

Depending on the size of the clitoris, surgical options include either recession and relocation of the entire organ beneath the symphysis, or partial corporectomy and reanastomosis. This preserves erectile function and, by dissection of the neurovascular bundles, the sensation to the glans is preserved (Weber, 1978). Figure 23–3 contains a description of the surgical procedure. The phallic skin and the foreskin may be used in the formation of labia minora (Marburger, 1975). Research by Sotiropoulous et al., (1976) revealed satisfactory coitus by most individuals followed into the sexually active years.

The goal of the next reconstructive procedure, the vaginoplasty, is to provide an adequate opening of the vagina onto the perineum.

The decision as to the type of vaginoplasty depends on whether the vagina enters the urogenital sinus proximally (higher) or distally (lower) in relation to the external sphincter. In mild cases, in which the vagina sits under the skin of the perineum, a simple incision is used to exteriorize the vagina. In most cases, when the vagina enters the urogenital sinus distal to the external sphincter, the surgical procedure involves raising an inverted V- or U-shaped perineal flap and swinging it back into the floor of the vagina (Glassberg, 1987). This procedure, called a *flap vaginoplasty*, is often performed in the newborn period, usually between 3 and 6 months of age (Fig. 23–4*A* and *B*).

In rare cases, the vagina enters the urogenital sinus in a high position near the bladder neck. In these cases, Hendren and Crawford (1969) recommend a vaginal pull-through operation to avoid damaging the urinary sphincter mechanism, which could make the child incontinent. The procedure involves raising several flaps and separating the vagina from the urethra, which is then sutured. The vagina is mobilized, and the orifice, which is often narrow, is opened in four quadrants, advanced, and sutured. Because the surgical procedure is technically difficult to perform during infancy, Hendren and Crawford (1969) recommend

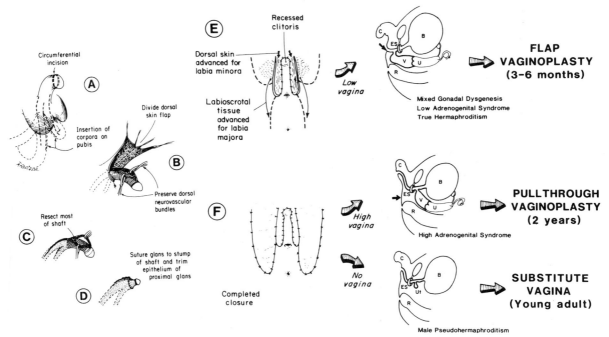

*FIGURE 23–3* Clitoral recession surgical procedure, followed by vaginoplasty, or surgical creation of a substitute vagina, as indicated by the individual patient's anatomic structure. (From Donahoe P. K., & Hendren, W. H. III. [1984]. Perineal reconstruction in ambiguous-genitalia infants raised as females. *Annals of Surgery, 200,* 363. Reprinted by permission.)

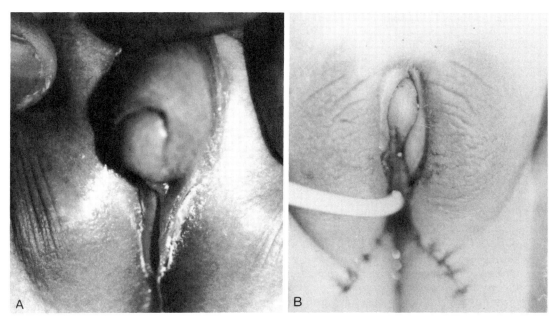

*FIGURE 23–4 A*, Preoperative view of a genetic female with clitoral hypertrophy, diagnosed with congenital adrenal hyperplasia. *B*, Patient with congenital adrenal hyperplasia, shown after reduction clitoroplasty and flap vaginoplasty. (Courtesy of James Mandell, MD, Boston, MA.)

postponing surgery until the child is at least 2 years of age. For psychological reasons, however, the reduction clitoroplasty is still performed in the newborn period.

Stenosis is a common postoperative complication of vaginoplasty and may be prevented by dilatations. Approximately 1 or 2 weeks after surgery, dilatations are begun using the appropriate-caliber Hegar sound or dilator. Parents are instructed to perform the procedure, which involves generous lubrication of the dilator, followed by gentle insertion of the sound or dilator into the vagina as far as it will go, and then removing it. Dilatations are initially done daily and then with decreasing frequency over the next few months, until healing is complete and the perineal tissues are soft and supple (Hendren & Crawford, 1972).

If no vagina is found, clitoral and labioscrotal reductions are performed in infancy, and vaginal replacement is planned for late adolescence. If an introitus is present, dilatations over a 6- to 12-month period may be recommended before surgery in adolescence to enlarge and deepen the introitus. Occasionally, dilatations alone may provide an adequate vagina (Donahoe & Crawford, 1986).

The sigmoid colon has been used in the creation of a vagina. A vagina may also be constructed from split-thickness skin grafts sewn over a plastic vaginal mold and tunneled up into the perineum in a space dissected between the bladder and the rectum (Hendren & Crawford, 1972). Again, stenosis is the most common long-term postoperative complication and may be prevented by dilatations. The dilatations help keep the introitus supple until the individual engages in sexual intercourse regularly, which then serves as a natural dilator.

## Male Sex Assignment

Surgical intervention in the infant given a male sex assignment usually begins with the repair of the hypospadias anomaly. Hypospadias repair in these individuals may be challenging to the surgeon, because the meatal opening is often perineoscrotal; marked chordee is often present, and the phallus is usually small (Donahoe & Crawford, 1986). Some individuals may need endocrine stimulation preoperatively to cause penile growth. The choice of a one- or multistage repair depends on the surgeon and the amount of available skin. Hypospadias repair is not discussed further here, because the repair is the same as that for any male infant with severe hypospadias (see Chapter 19).

Other possible surgical procedures in an infant given a male sex assignment may include the insertion of a testicular prosthesis as needed for cosmetic reasons; mastectomy in males developing gynecomastia as puberty approaches; and, if a uterus is present, a hysterectomy, which is often recommended to avoid uterine bleeding and any possible tumor development.

## MEDICAL MANAGEMENT

Individuals with female pseudohermaphrodism due to congenital adrenal hyperplasia need close endocrine follow-up. Those individuals who are salt losers require treatment with both glucocorticoids (e.g., cortisol) and mineralocorticoids. Villee (1982) recommends a cortisol dose of approximately 15 mg/m² per 24 h with careful monitoring, because too large a dosage depresses bone growth and too small a dosage allows an increased production of androgen and an accelerated bone maturation with an eventual overall short stature. Villee (1982) further recommends a dose of 0.1 mg of fludrocortisone acetate (Florinef) daily for salt retention. Medical management includes close follow-up of linear growth, bone age, urine 17-ketosteroids, and serum 17-hydroxy-progesterone. The cortisone dose is adjusted so that bone growth and maturation are achieved. Nonsalt losers are usually treated with glucocorticoids alone. In puberty, longer-acting glucocorticoids such as prednisone may be used (Villee, 1982).

Some individuals who are given a female gender assignment may require hormonal therapy (Fig. 23–5). Synthetic estrogen therapy is initiated between the ages of 13 and 15 years on a cyclical basis to promote breast development and menses. One regimen that may be prescribed is ethinyl estradiol 0.02 mg on days 1 through 21 and medroxyprogesterone 5 mg on days 15 to 21 of a 28-day cycle (Parks, 1977).

If it has been determined that hormones are required at puberty in an individual given a male sex assignment, injectable, sustained-release preparations are more effective than oral agents, which have the potential side effect of being carcinogenic. Parks (1977) recommends testosterone cypionate or enanthate in a dosage of 100 to 400 mg per month.

## APPROACHES TO PATIENT CARE

### Assessment

The evaluation of the newborn with ambiguous genitalia (Table 23–2) should begin with a detailed history. Because many of the intersex disorders are familial, the family history should include not only any similarly affected individuals but also any other type of abnormal sexual development. Genital abnormalities, including hypospadias, cryptorchidism, any unexplained deaths of young infants during the first few weeks of life, or any history of placental insufficiency should be explored. The existence of any infertile family members, such as maternal aunts with amenorrhea, sterility, or inguinal hernia with a "prolapsed ovary" should be included, as well as any inappropriate changes noted at puberty (e.g., hirsutism

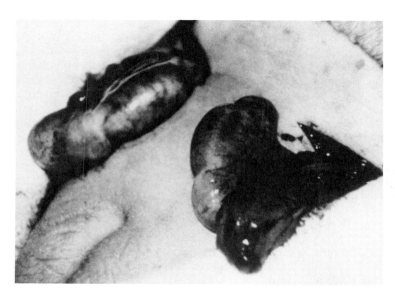

FIGURE 23–5 A phenotypic female infant found to have bilateral testes during surgical repair of bilateral inguinal hernias. The diagnosis of complete testicular feminization was given to this genetic male, who will have bilateral orchidectomies and remain in the female role. Hormonal treatment will begin at puberty. (Courtesy of James Mandell, MD, Boston, MA.)

**TABLE 23–2. Initial Evaluation of the Infant With Ambiguous Genitalia**

**Immediate**
  Detailed history
  Physical examination
  Buccal smear for Barr body studies
  Serum for Y fluorescence studies; karyotyping; sodium, potassium, glucose, gonadatropins (follicle-stimulating and luteinizing hormones) and steroid analyses (including testosterone, cortisol, and 17-alpha-hydroxyprogesterone)
  Urine for creatine and 17-ketosteroids
**Possible Additional Studies**
  Sonography, genitography, or endoscopy
  Laparotomy, gonadal biopsy, and genital skin biopsy

in a phenotypic female). Histories for any of the infant's siblings should include growth and development, menstrual history, and any hypertension, salt craving, or vasomotor collapse (see the section on female pseudohermaphrodism).

A pregnancy history of the mother of the infant with ambiguous genitalia should include the forms of contraception used before or during pregnancy, as well as any maternal illnesses or drug ingestion, including alcohol, phenytoin (Dilantin), or androgenic or progestational substances. Dates and length of exposure also should be noted. Any history of virilization of the mother during her pregnancy is important in the diagnosis of an infant with ambiguous genitalia.

The physical examination of the newborn with ambiguous genitalia should begin with an assessment of symmetry (Donahoe & Crawford, 1986). If one gonad is above and the other gonad is below the inguinal ring, the gonadal asymmetry is usually the result of structural defects. If both gonads are either above or below the inguinal canal, the gonadal symmetry is usually the result of hormonal influences. Next, assess the scrotum for symmetry. Note if one hemiscrotum is much larger than the other one and if the scrotum is bifid and positioned normally; also determine the degree of labioscrotal fusion (Donahoe & Crawford, 1986).

Next, the number of perineal orifices should be noted. Finding only one perineal opening does not rule out the possibility that a vagina is present. A single opening may represent the opening to a urogenital sinus that divides into a urethra anteriorly and a vagina posteriorly (Glassberg, 1988). The position of the urethral meatus and any chordee, if present, should also be noted.

The size of the phallus should be ascertained

by measuring the length along the dorsum, from the pubic symphysis to the tip of the stretched glans. The average phallic size of a full-term infant is 3.5 ± 0.4 cm (Flateau et al., 1975). The average phallic diameter in a full-term infant is between 1 and 1.5 cm. Length and width measurements less than 2 × 0.9 cm are a cause for concern. Length and width measurements less than 1.5 × 0.7 cm are a cause for alarm (Donahoe & Crawford, 1986).

A rectal examination should be done to determine if a cervix is present. The uterus in the newborn is usually palpable, because it is relatively large as a result of the intrauterine stimulation by estrogen (Donahoe & Hendren, 1984). Also, any increased pigmentation of the areolar or labioscrotal folds should be noted, as well as any associated congenital anomalies.

Immediately after the history and physical examination, diagnostic studies should be obtained. Those studies that yield the most rapid results should be completed first. The most common diagnostic studies are described in detail in the following paragraphs.

*Buccal Smear.* Useful information concerning the number of X or Y chromosomes may be obtained from stained smears of buccal mucosa cells, which are easily collected by rubbing a swab over the interior lining of the infant's cheek. In normal females, one of the two chromosomes is condensed during interphase to form the sex chromatin, or Barr, body, which is located on the inner surface of the nuclear membrane. Genetic females typically have more than 20% Barr body–positive cells, whereas genetic males have fewer than 1% to 2% (Walsh et al., 1979). Results are usually available within 24 hours.

*Y Fluorescence.* Although buccal mucosal cells may be used, leukocytes are easier to work with. A variety of fluorescent DNA-binding dyes have been used; the most effective is quinacrine mustard. The stained cells are then examined by a fluorescent microscopic technique; the distal half of the long arm of Y chromosome exhibits a bright spot of fluorescence. Present evidence indicates that it is the nonstaining short arm of Y chromosome that determines maleness. Fifty percent of leukocytes from a normal male exhibit the bright spot of fluorescence when examined under ultraviolet light. The results of this test are available within 24 hours.

*Karyotyping.* Determination of the total number and types of sex chromosomes should be performed routinely on all individuals with ambiguous genitalia. A normal female has two

X chromosomes, and a normal male has one X and one Y. Cytogenetic studies offer the most precise differentiation of the disorders of gonadogenesis. Abnormalities such as aneuploidy (the incorrect number of chromosomes due to the failure of two chromosomes to separate subsequent to metaphase in meiosis or mitosis, so that one daughter cell has both and the other neither of the chromosomes), deletion, breakage and rearrangement, and structural abnormalities such as translocation may be detected. Eighty percent of true hermaphrodites have a 46,XX karyotype, and the mosaic karyotype 45,X/46,XY is found in most individuals with mixed gonadal dysgenesis. The process of obtaining the karyotype involves fixing the cells in the metaphase and placing them in a hypotonic solution. The nuclear chromosomes are then stained, photographed, enlarged, and mapped. Although the chromosomal studies are highly informative, they are generally not available for several weeks, during which time the gender assignment is often made.

*Urine 17-Ketosteroids.* The purpose of the test is to aid in the diagnosis of CAH and to monitor cortisol therapy in the treatment of the disorder. Steroids and steroid metabolites, characterized by a ketone group on carbon 17 in the steroid nucleus (17-ketosteroid [17-KS]) originate primarily in the adrenal glands. The testes produce one third of 17-KSs in males, and the ovaries produce a minimal amount of 17-KSs in females. Although not all 17-KSs are androgens, they cause androgenic effects. Excessive secretion of 17-KSs in a female fetus may cause virilization (Quigley, 1981).

*X-ray Films.* Radiologic examination of the genitourinary tract is performed to delineate the exact anatomic structures. Conventional cystourethrography may not be accurate for determining the presence or absence of a vagina within the single perineal opening. Hendren and Crawford (1969) recommend the use of a flush genitogram, which is performed by placing a blunt-tipped syringe of dye in the single perineal opening. The dye-flushed retrograde better discloses the presence of a vaginal cavity branching off the common urogenital sinus.

*Sonography.* Sonography may be performed readily on the first day of life and is helpful in determining the presence of a cervix and a uterus.

*Endoscopy.* The perineal opening in all patients should be examined endoscopically in the neonatal period. In combination with radiologic studies, the internal and external genital anatomy may be ascertained, and reconstruction may be planned.

*Exploratory Laparotomy.* An exploratory laparotomy is a diagnostic procedure used for the inspection and biopsy and, occasionally, removal of gonadal tissue. The biopsy involves a wedge excision of a segment extending the full length of the gonad to avoid missing an ovotestis. Laparotomy of the newborn is undertaken only if the gonadal biopsy findings will influence the sex of rearing (Donahoe et al., 1977). For example, laparotomy is not required in infants with female pseudohermaphrodism caused by CAH, because their internal anatomic structure is always that of a normal female (Hendren & Crawford, 1972).

*Genital Skin Biopsy.* A biopsy of the genital skin is often obtained at the same time as the laparotomy and is used to assess alpha-reductase and androgen-receptor activity (Glassberg, 1988).

*Human Chorionic Gonadotropin Stimulation.* One way that human chorionic gonadotropin (HCG) may be used is by giving 3000 $IU/m^2$ of HCG once a day for 5 days and obtaining steroid levels on the sixth day (Glassberg, 1988). If there is an increase in testosterone levels following the administration of HCG, an enzyme block in testosterone synthesis may be ruled out. An increase in specific steroid precursors in conjunction with decreased testosterone or dihydrotestosterone levels suggests the specific enzyme deficiency (Glassberg, 1988).

Many parents of children born with ambiguous genitalia are devastated at having created a child with a birth defect, and they feel embarrassed by the freakish nature of the anomaly. A psychosocial assessment of these families should be undertaken by the nurse as early as possible, so that appropriate support may be provided.

The assessment should begin with the anxiety levels of the parents, which are often high because of a lack of understanding of how the defect occurred, as well as how it is diagnosed and treated. It is important to ascertain what prior knowledge, if any, the parents had of individuals born with anomalous sexual development. A question such as "Before your child's birth, had you ever heard the term ambiguous genitalia or hermaphrodite?" may elicit some information (see the discussion on family history earlier in this section). Next, the parents' current understanding of their child's problem should be explored. Much misinformation may be passed on by well-meaning but misinformed obstetricians, delivery room nurses, and pediatricians. It is also important to learn what the parents have retained from all that they have heard during the often overwhelming first few hours or days since their child's birth. In many instances, parents may focus only on the fact that their child's sexual organs are improperly formed. Although one may expect them to be concerned about immediate treatment options, most often their concern is related to their child's growth and development and eventual ability to participate in normal sexual activity with genitalia that appear normal to others. Another major concern is the ability of their child to reproduce offspring. Therefore, an open-ended question such as, "What have you been told about your child's condition?" may help to establish what parents have learned, as well as what other concerns or questions they have.

An assessment of the parents' coping abilities and support system is essential. Inquire about prior stressful life events, including who and what helped them cope. Explore who they have notified of their child's birth and which individuals they believe will be most helpful to them in dealing with this crisis.

Finally, and most important, the psychosocial assessment of the parents of these children, like the parents of any child born with a birth anomaly, should include an assessment of the bonding between the parents and the child. Cues to observe include the following: does the parent hold the child, does he or she make eye contact while feeding or changing the child, do the parents speak lovingly or protectively of the child, or do they seem detached or uninterested, is either parent overly concerned that a particular sex be assigned? It is important that the nurse assess and acknowledge that the process of grieving the loss of a normal healthy child has begun. It is often the first time that these families are given the opportunity to express how devastated and how angry they feel, which facilitates the grieving process and acceptance of their child's condition.

### Nursing Diagnosis

The nursing diagnoses for the parent of a child born with anomalous sexual development may include the following:

1. Anxiety related to the delay in determining the sex assignment of the infant.
2. Knowledge deficit related to the cause and treatment of the intersex anomaly.
3. Ineffective family coping related to the birth of a child with a congenital anomaly.

4. Anticipatory grieving related to the probable infertility of the child.

### Plan of Care

Nursing care is directed toward enabling the parents to

1. Assess their own abilities to cope with the process of sex assignment.
2. Verbalize an understanding of their infant's birth anomaly and the diagnostic tests and medical or surgical interventions required to treat the anomaly.
3. Express their feelings concerning parenting a child with a birth anomaly.
4. Use appropriate support services.
5. Express their fears and loss, as well as verbalize concerns regarding the future infertility of the child.

### Intervention

The family of a child born with ambiguous genitalia needs a tremendous amount of emotional support, beginning the first few minutes after the child's birth, when they learn that there is a problem with their infant, until 3 or 4 days later, when a gender assignment has been made and the future plan of care is discussed. This is an extremely difficult time for the family, because the first question asked concerning the birth is the sex of the child. Advise the family to consider delaying the announcement of the birth beyond the immediate family until a gender assignment has been made.

Reinforce to the parents that the gender assignment must be delayed until the preliminary test results are completed. Explain, in advance, exactly what diagnostic studies will be done and why (see section on assessment). The parents must understand that there is a logical process for establishing the diagnosis and treatment plans. Giving parents an estimate of the time required to establish the diagnosis and gender assignment (i.e., it takes approximately 4 days for the test results to be completed and then reviewed by the appropriate specialist or team of specialists) helps allay their anxiety during this uncertain time.

The child with ambiguous genitalia represents an enormous medical challenge, as well as an emotional and educational one. The primary goal of the nursing staff is to provide support to the parents and to help them understand their child's birth anomaly and how it happened. A good way to describe this birth anomaly to the parents is to explain that their infant's sex organs are incompletely formed or that their infant has a birth defect of unfinished genitalia. It might be helpful also to discuss normal dimorphic reproductive system development by using diagrams that depict the internal müllerian and wolffian ductal systems and the development of the genital tubercle. The parents need to understand that all people, both male and female, start out anatomically identical and that these identical parts undergo changes over time because of the influence of hormones. The genital tubercle, for example, in the presence of the male hormone testosterone enlarges to become a penis in the male. In the female, because of an absence of the male hormone, the genital tubercle shrinks in size to become the clitoris. Reiterate that males and females are more alike anatomically than most people realize. It is also important for the parents to recognize that pubertal development is largely dependent on the sex hormones, which may be substituted medically in most instances. Moreover, it is important to reinforce that sex rearing consistent with the assigned sex is the most significant factor in both cognitive and personality development.

Frequent contact with a few key medical personnel is helpful in assisting the parents to cope at this extremely difficult time. Nurses, as 24-hour caretakers, are in an ideal position to provide consistent support to the family of a child with ambiguous genitalia. Primary nursing enables the parents to deal with a limited number of caretakers and to become comfortable asking questions and verbalizing needs, fears, and concerns.

An important nursing function is to assist the parents in identifying a support system within their circle of family and friends and then to encourage communication with these individuals. In collaboration with the primary care physician, the nurse may coordinate the additional support services of social workers and psychologists. Some large medical centers may have an interdisciplinary team of specialists who are involved in the treatment of individuals with intersex disorders; the team typically includes endocrinologists, urologists, and geneticists. It is imperative that members of the of nursing, psychology, and social services also be part of this team to provide coordinated care to these families.

Many parents find it extremely helpful to communicate with other parents of children born with ambiguous genitalia. It is reassuring to parents to know that their child is not the only one born with such a defect and that medical personnel are able to provide treatment for the problem. Although providing statistical data on the prevalence of a particular disorder is helpful, talking with or actually meeting another family who has been through a similar experience may be extremely reassuring. Parents are often amazed to see how well adjusted the child with an intersex disorder is in the assigned gender role. A common remark is how feminine looking a genetic male, given a female sex assignment, can be.

Parents should be offered reassurance that the plan of care established for their child will be carefully monitored and that the appropriate follow-up services will be arranged before their infant's discharge from the hospital. The need for close follow-up care by the various specialists of the interdisciplinary team should be reinforced to the parents as recommended. Close endocrine follow-up is imperative for infants with CAH and includes pharmacologic management of possible electrolyte imbalance and steroid therapy. The endocrinologist also may assist the family in dealing with the possible future issues of lack of menstruation, the need for hormone replacement beginning in puberty, and infertility.

Finally, it is important to reinforce to the parents that, following surgical reconstruction, their child will have a "near normal" appearance to the genitalia and, with the exception of infertility, may lead a normal life. The issue of infertility should be approached positively using a statement such as, "your child will need to achieve parenthood through adoption." This approach does not prohibit the issue of parenthood but rather provides an alternative to achieve that goal. Parents also may find consolation in knowing that the incidence of infertility among the general population is quite high. Refer to Table 23–1 to determine which diagnoses involve infertility.

**Patient Outcomes**

1. Parents define, in basic terms, the rationale for the diagnostic studies their child must undergo.
2. Parents define, in basic terms, the cause of their child's birth anomaly.
3. Parents express acceptance of their child's sex assignment.
4. Parents ask appropriate questions concerning the treatment plan for their child.
5. Parents verbalize their feelings of loss related to the birth of a child with a genital anomaly.
6. Parents verbalize their feelings of loss related to the future infertility of their child.
7. Parents identify their coping strengths and use the appropriate support services.

# REFERENCES

Allen, T. D. (1976). Disorders of sexual differentiation. *Urology, 7*(4 Suppl), 1–32.

*Atlas of pediatric physical diagnosis.* (1987). New York: Gower.

Berkovitz, G. D., Rock, J. A., Urban, M. D., & Migeon, C. J. (1982). True hermaphrodism. *Johns Hopkins Medical Journal, 6,* 290–297.

Canty, T. G. (1977). The child with ambiguous genitalia: A neonatal surgical emergency. *Annals of Surgery, 186*(3), 272–281.

Donahoe, P. K., & Crawford, J. D. (1986). Ambiguous genitalia in the newborn. In K. J. Welch, J. G. Randolph, M. M. Ravitch, J. A. O'Neill, & M. I. Rowe (Eds.), *Pediatric surgery* (pp. 1363–1381). Chicago: Year Book Medical.

Donahoe, P. K., Crawford, J. D., & Hendren, W. H. (1977). Management of neonates and children with male pseudohermaphroditism. *Journal of Pediatric Surgery, 12*(6), 1045–1056.

Donahoe, P. K., Crawford, J. D., & Hendren, W. H. (1979). Mixed gonadal dysgenesis, pathogenesis, and management. *Journal of Pediatric Surgery, 14*(3), 287–299.

Donahoe, P. K., & Hendren, W. H. (1984). Perineal reconstruction in ambiguous genitalia infants raised as females. *Annals of Surgery, 200*(3), 363–372.

Eil, C., Crawford, J. D., Donahoe, P. K., Johnsonbaugh, R. E., & Loriaux, D. L. (1984). Fibroblast androgen receptors in patients with genitourinary anomalies. *Journal of Andrology, 5*(5), 313–320.

Flateau, E., Josefsberg, Z., & Reiner, S. H. (1975). Penile size of the newborn male infant. *Journal of Pediatrics, 87,* 663.

Glassberg, K. I. (1987). Intersex disorders: Classification and management. In A. B. Retik & J. Cukier (Eds.), *Pediatric urology* (pp. 330–351). Baltimore: Williams & Wilkins.

Glassberg, K. I. (1988). Ambiguous genitalia. In D. Evans & L. Glass (Eds.), *Perinatal medicine* (p 437). New York: Harper & Row.

Griffin, J. E. & Wilson, J. D. (1992). Disorders of sexual differentiation. In P. C. Walsh, A. B. Retik, T. A. Stamey, & E. D. Vaughan, Jr. (Eds.), *Campbell's urology* (6th ed., pp. 1509–1532). Philadelphia: W. B. Saunders.

Hendren, W. H., & Crawford, J. D. (1969). Adrenogenital syndrome: The anatomy of the anomaly and its repair—Some new concepts. *Journal of Pediatric Surgery, 4,* 49–59.

Hendren, W. H., & Crawford, J. D. (1972). The child with ambiguous genitalia. *Current Problems in Surgery, 11,* 4–64.

Manuel, M., Katayama, K. P., & Jones, H. W. (1976). The age of occurrence of gonadal tumors in intersex patients with a Y chromosome. *American Journal of Obstetrical Gynecology, 124,* 293.

Marburger, H. (1975). *Hunterian lecture.* London: Royal College of Surgeons.

Money, J. (1968). *Sex errors of the body: Dilemmas, education and counseling.* Baltimore: John Hopkins Press.

Parks, J. S. (1977). Endocrine disorders of childhood. *Hospital Practice, 12,* 93–108.

Pinto, W., Gardner, L. I., & Rosenbaum, D. (1977). Abnormal genitalia are presenting signs of two male infants with hydantoin embryopathy syndrome. *American Journal of Diseases in Children, 62,* 170.

Quigley, E. J. (1981) *Diagnostics.* Springhouse, PA: Intermed Communications.

Sotiropoulos, A., Morishima, A., Homsy, Y., & Lattimer, J. K. (1976). Long-term assessment of genital reconstruction in female pseudohermaphrodites. *Journal of Urology, 115,* 599–601.

Van Niekerk, W. A. (1981). True hermaphrodism. In N. Josso (Ed.), *The intersex child* (pp. 80–99). Basel: S. Karger.

Villee, D. B. (1982). Management of congenital adrenal hyperplasia. *Dialogues in Pediatric Urology, 5*(6), 2–4.

Walsh, P. C. (1978). The differential diagnosis of ambiguous genitalia in the newborn. *Urologic Clinics of North America, 5*(1), 213–221.

Walsh, P. C., Hensle, T., & Wigger, H. G. (1979). Ambiguous genitalia in a child. *Urology, 14*(4), 405–409.

Weber, C. H. (1978). A management approach to the newborn with ambiguous genitalia. *Weekly Urology Update, 19*(1), 3–7.

# CHAPTER 24

# Pediatric Urologic Oncology

■

*Julie Wettlaufer and Judith Atkinson-Tighe*

Wilms' Tumor—Nephroblastoma
Neuroblastoma
Rhabdomyosarcoma

## OVERVIEW

The diagnosis of a malignant tumor no longer heralds inevitable death. Improved chemotherapeutic drug combinations, radiotherapy, and surgical techniques provide many children with a cure and others with a longer life expectancy. Understandably, the diagnosis of ``cancer'' causes a state of shock and helplessness, psychological disarray, and crisis within the family. To add to this confusion, the child is often transferred to a large medical center that is unfamiliar and many miles from home, increasing the family's anxiety and emotional stress.

The initial diagnostic interview with the physician usually confirms the parents' deepest suspicions. Initially they may be unable to hear or understand the implications of the disease process and the proposed treatments. The honest and empathetic support of the pediatric urology nurse is key to the parents' attitude toward their child's illness and, in turn, their child's attitude toward his or her own illness. A trusting relationship and an expressed sense of hope that everything possible will be done without giving unrealistic expectations will help the family adapt to their new situation. Most importantly, the nurse should encourage the family to reach out for support from the health care team, other parents, and community resources.

This chapter provides the reader with a comprehensive review of malignant tumors affecting the genitourinary tract in the pediatric population. The tumors to be discussed are the three most common: Wilms' tumor, neuroblastoma, and rhabdomyosarcoma.

## BEHAVIORAL OBJECTIVES

After studying this chapter, the reader should be able to

1. Contrast the different clinical presentations of malignant tumors affecting the pediatric urinary tract.

2. Identify common areas of metastases of malignant tumors affecting the pediatric urinary tract.

3. Cite factors that contribute to survival of children with tumors of the urinary tract.

4. Explain the importance of comfort and relaxation techniques for children undergoing painful and invasive procedures and treatments.

5. Identify nursing measures to preserve the normality of childhood and to lessen the effect of oncologic therapy.

## KEY WORDS

**Nephroblastoma**—synonymous with Wilms' tumor. A tumor arising from the renal parenchyma.

**Beckwith-Wiedemann syndrome**—infant giant syndrome or viseromegaly.

**Hemihypertrophy**—an overgrowth of one side of the body, a condition that may coexist with Wilms' tumor.

**Aniridia**—a sporadic, nonfamiliar absence of the iris of the eye, a condition that may coexist with Wilms' tumor.

**Hamartomas**—the presence of hemangiomas, multiple nevi, and café au lait spots.

**Neuroblastoma**—a tumor of the neural crest that can arise in the sympathetic ganglia anywhere from the neck to the pelvis, particularly in the adrenal medulla.

**Malignant malaise**—symptoms of abdominal pain and distention, failure to thrive, fatigue, pyrexia, and anemia.

**Rhabdomyosarcoma**—a soft tissue sarcoma that arises from the primitive mesenchyme.

## PERSPECTIVE ON DISEASE ENTITY

### Wilms' Tumor— Nephroblastoma

In 1899, a German surgeon known as Max Wilms first correctly described the kidney tumor that bears his name. Sometimes referred to as renal embryoma or nephroblastoma of the kidney, Wilms' tumor was initially treated by surgical excision and the survival rate was 10%. Improvements in surgery and pediatric anesthesia, the addition of radiation and chemotherapy, along with the formation of the National Wilms' Tumor Study Committee has increased the survival rate to 90%. Wilms' tumor was the first childhood cancer in which combining surgery, radiation therapy, and chemotherapy attained significant cure rates. Today Wilms' tumor is considered one of the most responsive of all childhood cancers.

### ETIOLOGY

The etiology of Wilms' tumor is unknown; most cases occur sporadically. Recent studies have shown several chromosomal anomalies, including 11p, trisomy 8, trisomy 18, and XX/XY mosaicism, to be associated with Wilm's tumor. Analysis of cytogenetic abnormalities in Wilms' tumor indicates that deletion or rearrangements involving the short arm of chromosome 11 may occur in 30% to 40% of cases (Slater et al., 1985). These relationships suggest the existence of a Wilms' tumor suppressive gene that resides in the 11p band. On rare occasions Wilms' tumor may be inherited by autosomal dominant transmission. It has been suggested that all bilateral Wilms' and 1% or less of unilateral tumors are inherited.

Wilms' tumor is the most common tumor of the urinary tract in children. The incidence of Wilm's tumor is remarkably constant worldwide. It affects males and females equally and does not appear to be related to race, climate, or environment. In the United States, there are approximately 500 new cases of Wilms' tumor reported each year. In approximately 75% of cases, the diagnosis is made between 1 and 5 years of age. Of all patients with Wilms' tumor, 90% are seen before age 7 years, with the peak incidence between ages 3 and 4 years. Only 1% of cases of Wilms' tumors are diagnosed in patients older then 10 years of age.

Approximately 15% of children with Wilms' tumor have other congenital abnormalities, suggesting an intrauterine event (Miller et al., 1964). The most commonly associated anomalies are as follows:

1. Genitourinary—found in 4.4% of Wilms' tumor cases. These include renal hypoplasia, duplications, cystic disease, hypospadias, cryptorchidism, and pseudohermaphroditism.
2. Hamartomas—presence of hemangiomas, multiple nevi, and cafe-au-lait spots. A 30-fold increase in the incidence of neurofibromatosis is found in patients with Wilms' tumor (Stay & Vawter, 1977).
3. Hemihypertrophy—characterized by an asymmetry of the body; found in 2.9% of cases of Wilms' tumor. This asymmetry may be partial, involving one limb, or complete, involving one half of the body. Careful history and/or observation will diagnose hemihypertrophy.
4. Beckwith–Wiedemann syndrome—Approximately 1 in 10 children with this syndrome develops a neoplasm. Visceromegaly involving the adrenal cortex, kidney, liver, pancreas, and gonads characterizes this syndrome. Omphalocele, hemihypertrophy, microcephaly, mental retardation, and macroglossia may also be found. Many cases of hemihypertrophy may represent incomplete forms of the Beckwith–Wiedemann syndrome.
5. Aniridia—absence of the iris of the eye. There are two forms of aniridia, sporadic and familial. When the sporadic form is associated with chromosomal 11p deletion there is a 33% risk of developing Wilms' tumor. In the first National Wilms' Tumor Study, aniridia was present in 1 in 70 pa-

tients with Wilms' tumor (the rate in the general population is 1 in 50,000).

## PATHOPHYSIOLOGY

Wilms' tumor is thought to originate from an abnormal growth of metanephric blastoma (the embryologic tissue that develops into functional renal tubules and glomeruli). The tumor may occur in any part of the kidney and is usually encapsulated; necrosis is often found, leading to hemorrhage or cyst formation. The usual large size of the tumor at the time of diagnosis distorts the calyceal anatomy, accounting for the typical radiographic presentation. Uncommonly, the tumor grows into the renal pelvis, where it may lead to hematuria or obstruction. Invasion of the renal vein occurs in 20% of cases. Lymph node metastases are not present in a majority of cases.

Microscopically there appear to be favorable and unfavorable histologic subtypes of tumor cells. Favorable subtypes are associated with a lower mortality rate, while unfavorable subtypes have a higher mortality rate. The unfavorable histologic types make up only 10% of Wilms' tumors, however, and are responsible for 60% of deaths.

Three distinct lesions have been identified as "unfavorable" Wilms' tumor lesions: (1) Anaplasia (diffuse and focal), (2) rhabdoid (ongoing debate exists as to whether this should be considered a Wilms' variant), and (3) clear cell sarcoma of the kidney.

Two associated tumors merit discussion in this section, although they are not "true" Wilms' tumors, as they are considered favorable subvariants. The first is congenital mesoblastic nephroma. Often found in children less then 1 year of age, congenital mesoblastic nephroma is a benign, infiltrating, aggressive tumor of the kidney. The second is nephroblastomatosis, which is said to be a precursor of Wilms' tumor. Nephroblastomatosis is abnormal persistence of embryonal renal tissue that is immature. The tumor itself is nonmalignant, yet it is considered "premalignant."

## MEDICAL-SURGICAL MANAGEMENT

### Diagnosis

The most prominent feature of Wilms' tumor is a fast-growing abdominal mass, which is present in 75% of children with disease. Many tumors are discovered by the primary care pro-

TABLE 24–1. Differential Diagnosis of Flank Masses in Children

| DIAGNOSIS | PROMINENT FEATURES | ORIGIN | AGE AT ONSET |
|---|---|---|---|
| Wilms' tumor | Large mass, not crossing the midline<br>Child appears healthy<br>If metastasis, usually to lungs | Renal | 2–5 years |
| Neuroblastoma | Large, firm, irregular mass that often crosses the midline<br>Displaced kidney noted on x-ray<br>Child with generalized malaise, weight loss, pyrexia; appears sick | Adrenal or sympathetic chain | Neonate, infant, or child |
| Mesoblastic nephroma | Benign hamartomas<br>Determined by postoperative pathology | Renal | Neonate or infant |
| Hydronephrosis | Cystic kidney disease, obstruction, posterior urethral valves or reflux | Renal | Neonate |
| Fecal mass | Transient masses, history of abnormal bowel function, child may appear septic in severe cases, abdominal pain, impaction detected on physical examination or x-ray, may be functional or structural etiology | Bowel | Infant or child |
| Renal tumor, non-Wilms' | Sarcoma of kidney<br>Hypernephroma<br>Renal cell carcinoma<br>All above have poor prognosis and frequently have metastasized by the time of detection | Renal | Varies with tumor |

vider during a routine physical assessment. The child's parents may notice an enlarging abdomen or waistline, which prompts a visit to the family's health care provider. In older children, complaints of abdominal pain or hematuria may be noted.

The physical exam will reveal a flank mass that is smooth, firm, and nontender. Most often, the tumor is unilateral and does not extend across the midline; however, in some instances of Wilms' tumor this is not the case. Increase in blood pressure may be caused by compression of the vascular supply to the renal parenchyma and the production of renin in as many as 60% of children. Other than these findings, most children presenting with Wilms' tumor are in remarkably good health.

The child with Wilms' tumor is best cared for by a multidisciplinary subspecialty team. Diagnosis may include the following baseline studies:

1. Complete blood count and coagulation studies to rule out anemia, which could be secondary to intratumor hemorrhage.
2. Liver and renal function tests to determine the patient's metabolic status.
3. Twenty-four hour urine collection for catecholamine levels to rule out neuroblastoma.
4. Abdominal ultrasound to determine extent of the tumor.
5. Chest x-ray to detect pulmonary metastasis (pulmonary computed tomography [CT], bone scan, and a skeletal survey are recommended when metastasis is present).
6. Computed tomography to establish intrarenal origin of the tumor and to assess the extent of the tumor and lymph node involvement.
7. Magnetic Resonance Imaging (MRI) is used in many tumor centers in place of CT since it does not require ionizing radiation.

Prior to beginning cardiotoxic chemotherapy (anthracyclines), the following tests may also be performed:

1. M-mode electrocardiogram.
2. MUltiple Gaited Acquisition scan (MUGA)—continuous image of the heart cycle using labeled or flagged red blood cells.

Since other renal tumors have similar features to Wilms' tumor, it is necessary to investigate the differential diagnosis so that prompt and accurate treatment can begin (Table 24–1).

**Tumor Staging.** The National Wilms' Tumor Study (NWTS) is a cooperative group that formed to collect and evaluate treatment regimens. Initially the NWTS was used only in the United States, but it is now accepted internationally, thus unifying the knowledge and treatment of children with Wilms' tumor. The NWTS classification particularly emphasizes nodal involvement and tumor spillage. One problem that emerged from NWTS-I and NWTS-II was that adequate discrimination between groups II and III (presently called stages II and III) was lacking. When the NWTS-III was completed, the *grouping system* was modified to the present *staging system* (D'Angio et al., 1989). All patients with positive lymph nodes were assigned to stage III. Better discrimination between stages II and III promises to be useful in treatment and overall survival rate (Table 24–2).

Tumor staging is assigned postoperatively since it is based on (1) tumor and node findings as detected during the surgery and (2) the success of tumor excision. The purpose of staging, therefore, is to determine the prognosis and to identify appropriate treatment regimens for chemotherapy and radiation. Also, the presence of Wilms' tumor in the contralateral kidney may only be detected by surgical exploration. Bilateral disease will have profound ramifications on the treatment protocol.

## Treatment

**Surgery.** The classic surgical intervention for Wilms' tumor is nephrectomy. This is per-

formed once the diagnosis has been made and preliminary investigations have determined that the tumor is operable. If the upper pole of the kidney is involved, the adrenal gland is also excised. A generous thoracoabdominal incision is necessary to have adequate access to the tumor and to minimize potential rupture. During the surgery the anterior and posterior surfaces of the contralateral kidney are scrupulously inspected for evidence of tumor, as over 30% of bilateral tumors are diagnosed intraoperatively (Blute et al., 1987). If any abnormalities are noted, they are biopsied along with routine lymph node samplings to provide more accurate staging results. Radical lymph node dissection has not resulted in any significant increase in survival and is therefore not routinely performed.

**Radiation.** Since Wilms' tumor is a radiosensitive cancer, the response to this treatment modality is quite good. If radiation is indicated, it should begin within 5 days after surgery. Dosage and area of radiation are determined by staging and the child's age. Under current NWTS-IV guidelines, radiation is not given to patients with stage I or II disease. The goal is to narrowly focus the radiation at the diseased tissue and to avoid normal tissue, the remaining kidney, and sensitive organs, such as the ovaries, bone growth centers, joints, and muscle. Radiation is known to be toxic to the heart, lungs, and liver, and may cause asymmetric growth. Secondary tumors have developed as late as 15 years postnephrectomy, making long-term follow-up necessary (Jaffe et al., 1980).

**Chemotherapy.** Wilms' tumor was the first pediatric solid neoplasm to be successfully treated by chemotherapy following the addition of actinomycin D to the treatment protocol. Within two decades vincristine, actinomycin, cyclophosphamide (Cytoxan), and Adriamycin have become primary chemotherapeutic agents in the treatment of Wilms' tumor.

Chemotherapy is initiated once staging has been done. The schedule and length of time for treatment is carefully laid out by the NWTS-IV protocol. Dosages for infants are halved to reduce toxicity (Table 24–3). As with many forms of chemotherapy, nutritional support may be required to promote growth of the child.

## Long-Term Follow-Up and Future Considerations

The excellent survival of patients with Wilms' tumor has lead to recent studies to

**TABLE 24–2. Current Staging of Wilms' Tumor**

| STAGE | DESCRIPTION |
|-------|-------------|
| I | Tumor limited to kidney, completely excised, capsular surface intact; no tumor rupture; no residual tumor apparent beyond margins of resection |
| II | Tumor extends beyond kidney but is completely excised. Regional extension of tumor; vessel infiltration; tumor biopsied or local spillage of tumor confined to the flank. No residual tumor apparent at or beyond margins of excision |
| III | Residual nonhematogenous tumor confined to the abdomen. Lymph node involvement of hilus, periaortic chains, or beyond; diffuse peritoneal contamination by tumor spillage or peritoneal implants of tumor; tumor extends beyond surgical margins either microscopically or macroscopically; tumor not completely removable because of local infiltration into vital structures |
| IV | Deposits beyond stage III, i.e., lung, liver, bone, brain |
| V | Bilateral renal involvement at diagnosis |

Adapted from D'Angio, G. J., Breslow, N., Beckwith, J. B., et al. (1989). Treatment of Wilms' tumor: Results of the Third National Wilms' Tumor Study. *Cancer, 64*(2), 349–360. Reprinted with permission.

TABLE 24–3. National Wilms' Tumor Study IV: Procedures and Study Design at a Glance

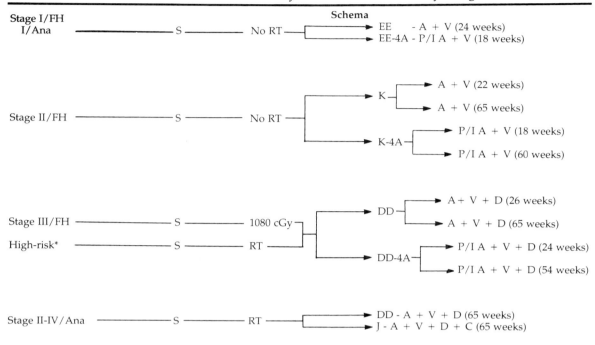

### PROCEDURES

1. All patients should have an excretory urogram or opacified CT scan of the abdomen for accurate placement of radiation therapy portals.
2. The initial randomization to standard or pulsed, intensive chemotherapy *need not await final determination of stage or histology* because the initial randomization is the same for virtually all patients.† Randomization is to take place within 72 hours of nephrectomy, *which will be considered day zero,* but not later than 5 calendar days thereafter. If a patient must be randomized during the weekend or on a holiday to remain eligible, the Data and Statistical Center (DSC) should be called ahead of time and special arrangements will be made.

---

*High risk = clear cell sarcoma of kidney (CCSK) (all stages) and stage IV/FH. CCSK patients receive RT (1080 cGy) and stage IV/FH patients receive RT (1080 cGy) if the primary tumor would qualify as stage III were there no metastases.
†Re-randomization will be offered should the tumor qualify later as stage II–V/Ana.
S, surgery; A, actinomycin D; D, doxorubicin (Adriamycin); V, vincristine; C, cyclophosphamide; Ana, anaplastic tumors; P/I, pulsed, intensive; FH, favorable histology; RT, radiation therapy.
From Snyder, H. M., D'Angio, G. J., Evans, A. E., & Raney, R. B. (1992). Pediatric oncology. In P. C. Walsh, A. B. Retik, T. A. Stamey, & E. D. Vaughan, Jr. (Eds.), *Campbell's urology* (6th ed., p. 1982). Philadelphia: W. B. Saunders. Reprinted by permission.

track their offspring. These studies have shown a correlation between abdominal radiation and delivering a stillborn or low birthweight infant. There is no evidence to date that the offspring is any more likely to develop Wilms' tumor (Li et al., 1987).

NWTS-IV is currently in progress to further refine and improve the treatment protocols. Its objectives are to reduce toxicity complications and to preserve renal function. Efforts to improve outcomes for children with anaplastic and rhabdoid tumors are being studied, while genetic, familial, and etiologic markers indicating risk of disease are being sought.

## Neuroblastoma

### ETIOLOGY

Neuroblastoma is a tumor derived from neural crest tissue that ordinarily would develop into the adrenal medulla and the sympathetic ganglion. The cause for the transformation of normal ganglion cells into malignant neuroblastoma, as for most other cancers, is unknown. There appears to be a mediated immunologic response, as some children produce antibodies to the tumor, while others block their regulatory cytotoxic lymphocytes. There may also be genetic influences (Pui and Crist, 1991).

There are three types of tumors derived from this neural crest tissue: (1) ganglioneuroma (benign), (2) ganglioneuroblastoma (mixed tissue-benign and malignant), and (3) neuroblastoma (malignant). There may be a link between neuroblastoma and other neural-crest derived disorders, such as neurofibromatosis, pheochromocytoma, tuberous sclerosis, Hirschsprung's disease, and heterochromia of the iris.

Neuroblastoma is the most common malignant tumor in infants. It accounts for 50% of all neonatal malignancies. Approximately 50% of patients with neuroblastoma are diagnosed by age 2 years, and more than 75% are diagnosed by the fourth year of life. Neuroblastoma is slightly more common in white children than in black children and slightly more common in boys.

The tumor is peculiar among neoplasms in its ability to spontaneously regress in the very young. While performing autopsies for deaths due to other reasons, Beckwith and Perrin (1963) made the incidental finding of microscopic clusters of neuroblastoma cells in the adrenal glands in a number of infants under 3 months of age. Autopsies on older infants failed to show any neuroblastoma clusters. These findings indicate that the incidence of the disease is some 40 times less than expected because of this spontaneous regression.

## PATHOPHYSIOLOGY

Neuroblastomas are highly malignant and spread early in the disease course. Metastasis is unrelated to the size of the primary neoplasm. On gross examination, the mass appears solid, vascular, purplish in color, and encased in a pseudocapsule; however, the capsule often fails to contain the tumor from local tissue infiltration. Histologically, the neuroblastoma consists of small, spherical, undifferentiated cells containing catecholamines. These cells are arranged in a rosette configuration, emerge during the seventh gestational week, and are quite evident as nests or clusters in the adrenal gland by the 20th week. At this point, many of these tumorous clusters arrest their development, becoming what is termed *neuroblastoma in situ*. Other clusters will develop into one of the three types of tumors previously described (ganglioneuroma, ganglioneuroblastoma, or neuroblastoma). There is no known histologic pattern or biochemical environmental influence that affects the tumor's maturation, and attempts to artificially induce tumor development have been unsuccessful.

## MEDICAL-SURGICAL MANAGEMENT

### Diagnosis

In its early stage, neuroblastoma is usually a silent tumor. Metastatic dissemination of the tumor often occurs early. Up to 70% of patients have metastatic disease at the time of diagnosis (Gross et al., 1959). "Raccoon eyes" or "panda eyes" caused by periorbital swelling and ecchymosis strongly suggest metastatic neuroblastoma. Young infants may present with abdominal enlargement due to metastasis to the liver, and skin nodules resembling subcutaneous purple grapes may be present.

Children presenting with this tumor usually appear ill. They present with "malignant malaise": unexplained weight loss, complaints of abdominal pain, "bone pain," abdominal distention, pyrexia, pallor, and fatigue. These symptoms may be due, in part, to anemia, from bone marrow invasion or hemorrhage within the tumor. Other symptoms may relate to catecholamine excretion from the tumor and include sweating, hypertension, headaches, palpitations, and skin flushing.

Neuroblastoma, ganglioneuroma, and ganglioneuroblastoma can form anywhere along the sympathetic chain from the head to the pelvis. Their presentation and differential diagnosis will vary with the site of tumor origin. More than 50% of neuroblastomas originate in the abdomen (66% of these arise from the adrenal gland). The breakdown of the primary tumor site is as follows: head 2%, neck 5%, chest 13%, abdomen 55%, pelvis 4%, other 9%, and unknown 12%. By virtue of this breakdown, the most common presenting feature is an abdominal mass that is irregular, firm, nontender, fixed, and often extends beyond the midline.

The clinical investigation for the child suspected of harboring a neuroblastoma must be detailed and thorough, due to the likelihood of metastasis. Recommended studies include:

1. Hematologic and biochemical tests—complete blood count (CBC) with sedimentation rate, coagulation studies, liver and renal function studies, ferritin, and neuron-specific enolase.
2. Urinalysis and urinary catecholamine assay for the two major metabolites of catecholamine production: vanillylmandelic acid (VMA) and homovanillic acid (HVA). These

## TABLE 24–4. Neuroblastoma Staging

| STAGE | CRITERIA | TREATMENT | 2-YR SURVIVAL |
|---|---|---|---|
| 0 | Neuroblastoma in situ | Spontaneous resolution | 95–100% |
| I | Tumors confined to organs or structures of origin | Primary tumor excision | 90% |
| II | Tumors with regional infiltration not crossing midline; may have ipsilateral lymph node involvement | If resectable, primary tumor excision; if not resectable, chemotherapy possibly followed by surgery | 80% |
| III | Tumors extend in continuity beyond midline; contralateral regional lymph nodes also involved | Chemotherapy regimen: single or combination use of: Cyclosphosphamide Doxorubicin Cisplatin Etoposide (VP 16) Vincristine | 37% |
| IV | Distant metastasis—bone, bone marrow, brain, skin, liver, lung, soft tissue, distant lymph nodes | Bone marrow transplant protocol: Lethal dose chemotherapy and total body irradiation, bone marrow transplant Experimental: Targeted radiation using MIBG Chemotherapy alone | 10% |
| IV-S | Stage I or II criteria, plus remote spread to bone, liver, or skin (primarily in children <1 yr) | Spontaneous regression, observe for respiratory compromise—use of low level radiation or chemotherapy | 80% |

Data from Snyder, H. M., D'Angio, G. J., Evans, A. E., & Raney, R. B. (1992). Pediatric oncology. In P. C. Walsh, A. B. Retik, T. A. Stamey, & E. D. Vaughan, Jr. (Eds.), *Campbell's urology* (6th ed., pp. 1967–1986). Philadelphia: W. B. Saunders. Reprinted by permission.

markers can be detected with 24-hour urine collection or spot test.
3. Radiologic studies—computed tomography (CT) or magnetic resonance imaging (MRI) of primary site, bone scan, skeletal survey, and, depending on the primary and metastatic sites, chest film; abdominal CT and ultrasound; CT of head, orbit, and chest; liver scan and intravenous pyelogram (IVP).
4. [131]I-Meta-Iodobenzylguanidine (MIBG)—competes with norepinephrine and is taken up by adrenergic secretory vesicles in neuroblastoma, thus permitting imaging of the primary and metastatic sites.
5. Bone marrow aspirate and biopsy—very important because the bone marrow is a common site of metastasis, and a typical pattern in bone marrow and elevated urine catecholamine may obviate the need for an open biopsy of the tumor.

**Tumor Staging.** Neuroblastomas are best managed by a multimodal approach, which may combine surgery, chemotherapy, and radiation. The specific protocol is guided by the stage assignment determined by the initial exploratory procedure, lymph node involvement, and disease dissemination. Evan's system of neuroblastoma staging is the most commonly used tool to set treatment protocols (Evans et al., 1971). Table 24–4 outlines staging criteria, treatments, and 2-year survival rates.

Evans' classification continues to be the most widely used neuroblastoma classification today because of its clinical applicability. A variation of this schema has been adopted for international use (Brodeur et al., 1988). Factors other than those listed in Table 24–4 also seem to be prognostic factors of survival. Cure equals survival for 2 years with no evidence of disease. The four major indices are age, stage of disease, serum ferritin level, and the Shimada index. Using these four prognostic indices, it is possible to divide patients with neuroblastoma into two groups: those with favorable tumors and those with unfavorable tumors. In those with favorable tumors, therapy can be limited; in those with unfavorable tumors, it must be more aggressive (Silber et al., 1991).

1. Age
   a. Children under 1 year of age have a 74% survival rate.
   b. Children 12 to 23 months of age have a 26% survival rate.
   c. Children over 2 years of age have a 12% survival rate.

d. Children who present with the disease when they are over 6 years of age have a 25% survival rate (Evans, 1980; Sather et al., 1981).
2. Stage—see Table 24–4.
3. Serum ferritin level
   a. Neuroblastoma excretes elevated levels of this serum protein
   b. The higher the ferritin level, the worse the patient's survival rate (Hann et al., 1979).
   c. In 40% to 50% of stage III or IV disease, the serum ferritin level is elevated.
   d. Stage III
      (1) Nonelevated serum ferritin survival rate is 76%.
      (2) Elevated serum ferritin survival rate is 23%.
   e. Stage IV
      (1) Nonelevated serum ferritin survival rate is 27%.
      (2) Elevated serum ferritin survival rate is 3%.
4. Shimada Index
   a. A histologic index that is important in the prognosis of low-stage disease (I, II, and IV-S).
   b. For disseminated disease (stage III and IV), ferritin level alone appears to be the most important prognostic variable (Shimada et al., 1984).

Recent research has shown two prognostic molecular studies of the neuroblastoma tumor cells:
(1) If the N-*myc* oncogene is increased in the neuroblastoma, the prognosis is poor.
(2) If the DNA index is greater than 1, the prognosis is favorable (the average DNA index is 1).

## Treatment

The management of neuroblastoma remains a clinical challenge. It continues to be a very frustrating pediatric malignancy to treat. Results of diverse treatment protocols using single or combination therapies have been inconclusive, with the long-term prognosis remaining unchanged over the last two decades.

### Surgery

*Treatment of Favorable Disease.* In the treatment of well-localized favorable disease, simple surgical removal of the primary tumor is the major mode of treatment. Complete removal is accomplished in stage I or II disease,

yet is more difficult once the tumor crosses the midline.

*Treatment of Unfavorable Disease.* Other than tumor biopsy, there is little the surgeon is able to do. Operations to "debulk" the tumor do not improve the survival rate and may worsen the outcome (Sitarz et al., 1983).

A second role for surgery is to stage the tumor. It should be determined if the tumor infiltrates beyond the midline or involves the contralateral lymph nodes. Lymph node biopsy is only a staging maneuver, and there is no evidence that radical dissection is of any value in treating neuroblastoma. Second-look surgery in and of itself does not improve the overall survival rate; however, it may be useful as part of an aggressive chemotherapy and total body radiotherapy that is part of a bone marrow transplant program.

### Radiation

*Treatment of Favorable Disease.* Neuroblastoma is a radiosensitive tumor. Little treatment other than surgical removal of the tumor is needed, since the prognosis is not improved with the advent of radiation.

*Treatment of Unfavorable Disease.* This is used for palliation of painful or unsightly metastases only. More aggressive radiation therapy in stage IV disease appears to have little to contribute to overall survival.

### Chemotherapy

*Treatment of Favorable Disease.* No evidence indicates that chemotherapy improves the survival in stage I or II disease. Little treatment other than surgical removal is needed.

*Treatment of Unfavorable Disease.* Neuroblastoma is a chemotherapy-responsive tumor. Most major medical centers have chemotherapy drug programs; however, no clear advantage has been shown for any particular combination of agents.

## Long-Term Follow-up and Future Considerations

In general, survival for 2 years with no evidence of disease is equivalent to a cure. Bone marrow transplantation can be followed at times by a rather late disease relapse. Two new therapeutic approaches include targeted radiation therapy with labeled metaiodobenzylguanidine, a substance that is taken up by the neuroblastoma, making it tumor specific. The second new therapeutic approach involves total body irradiation and lethal chemotherapy, followed by bone marrow transplant. These two treatments may be beneficial for patients with unfavorable disease or those children who relapse.

Immunotherapy seems to be a potential future treatment for neuroblastoma. It has been demonstrated that lymphocytes from children with neuroblastoma are capable of specific inhibition of neuroblastoma cells. Although not proven successful to date, there are early data on the use of interferon, interleukin-2, and cytotoxic and radiation-conjugated antibodies in the treatment of neuroblastoma (Bernstein, 1982; Hellstrom and Hellstrom, 1972; Sawada et al., 1981).

# Rhabdomyosarcoma

Soft tissue sarcomas are the fifth most common solid tumors in childhood after central nervous system tumors, lymphomas, neuroblastomas, and Wilms' tumor. Of all sarcomas, rhabdomyosarcoma accounts for about half, making it the most common soft tissue sarcoma.

## ETIOLOGY

Rhabdomyosarcoma has been associated with neurofibromatosis, fetal alcohol syndrome, and specific types of basal cell nevus syndromes. There appears to be a familial link with other sarcomas. Family members of children with rhabdomyosarcoma have a high frequency of carcinoma of the breast, brain, and lung. In the United States, the incidence of rhabdomyosarcoma is approximately 4.4 per million white children and 1.3 per million black children per year. The ratio of males to females is 1.4:1. Two age peaks occur, the first between 2 and 6 years (most tumors in this age group occur in the head and neck or genitourinary tract—prostate, bladder, and vagina) and the second between 15 and 19 years (most tumors in this age group occur in the extremities or the male genitourinary tract, particularly testicular or paratesticular tissue). Seventy percent of cases occur before the age of 10 years (Pui and Crist, 1991).

As many as 20% of rhabdomyosarcomas originate in the pelvis or genitourinary tract. The vast majority of these tumors are of the embryonal histopathologic type, making them "favorable" tumors with good treatment outlooks. The morbidity and mortality are most dependent on the stage of the tumor at the time of diagnosis. Genitourinary rhabdomyosarcoma can be divided into subgroups according to the anatomic location of the primary tumor: (1) paratesticular, (2) bladder and bladder-prostate, and (3) gynecologic.

## PATHOPHYSIOLOGY

Rhabdomyosarcoma is described as a tumor of striated muscle, arising from primitive or undifferentiated mesenchyme, the portion of mesoderm that produces connective tissue and striated muscle. These tumors can originate anywhere in the body, and the most common site is the head and neck. Since the urogenital tract and lymphatic system evolve from embryonal mesenchyme, the genitourinary (GU) system is also a common site, accounting for approximately 20% of all rhabdomyosarcomas (Maurer et al., 1988).

On gross examination, there are no remarkable features common to rhabdomyosarcoma (with the exception of sarcoma botryoides). The mass is nodular, firm, and appears to be well contained. Microscopic examination, however, reveals extensive local infiltration, tissue hemorrhage, and necrosis. Cellular composition of the tumor is predominantly the rhabdomyoblast, a large cell with an immature, irregular nucleus and acidophilic cytoplasm. The variety of microscopic forms that rhabdomyosarcoma can take reflects the wide range of mesenchymal differentiation seen in this tumor. Mierau and Favara (1980) have suggested that all childhood rhabdomyosarcomas are basically embryonal tumors, which only vary in the degree to which they have differentiated. The microscopic/pathologic evaluation of the tumor is critical in staging and treatment, and can be a very complex process (Table 24–5).

Rhabdomyosarcomas spread by local extension, via the lymphatic system to regional lymph nodes or by the hematologic route to the lungs, liver, bone marrow, bones, and occasionally the brain. The incidence of lymphatic spread correlates with the preponderance of lymph nodes at the primary site. For example, lymph node metastases are relatively common in the genitourinary subgroup (15–20%) and are particularly common in the paratesticular subgroup (40%).

## MEDICAL-SURGICAL MANAGEMENT

### Diagnosis

The child with a genitourinary rhabdomyosarcoma is most often diagnosed following the

### TABLE 24–5. Histologic Grouping for Rhabdomyosarcoma

| TYPE | DESCRIPTION | LOCATION | PROPORTION OF PEDIATRIC CASES |
|---|---|---|---|
| Embryonal (favorable) | Large, acidophilic myoblasts, round and spindle cells, cross-striations in cytoplasm | Head, neck, GU tract | 50–60% |
| Sarcoma botryoides | Subtype of embryonal—this is a favorable tumor that has a characteristic appearance that can be identified easily on gross examination—polypoid, looks like a "bunch of grapes" | Forms in any hollow structure—vagina, uterus, bladder, nasopharynx, or middle ear | 5% of all rhabdo's are this type |
| Alveolar (unfavorable) | Pseudoalveolar appearance, common in adolescents and young adults | Extremities, perineum, metastasis to lymph nodes | 20% |
| Pleomorphic | Racket-shaped to large, round cells with large or multiple nuclei. Rare in children | Extremities or trunk | 1% |
| Undifferentiated (unfavorable) | Primitive, small, round cells may resemble Ewing's sarcoma. Three subtypes of undifferentiated tumors 1. Anaplastic 2. Monomorphous round cell 3. Mixed | Soft tissue | 10–20% |

GU, genitourinary; rhabdo's, rhabdomyosarcomas.

detection of a palpable mass. Pelvic tumors may be quite large before the child experiences symptoms necessitating medical attention. Common symptoms include bowel-related complaints, such as constipation, frequent liquid stools, or any other general changes in bowel habits. Children with large tumors in the abdomen frequently complain of bladder changes, including hematuria, dribbling, leaking, incontinence, frequency, infection, or retention. The tumor can cause obstruction in any area of the abdomen as the size of the tumor increases and puts pressure on surrounding organs. Scrotal pain or a foul vaginal discharge may be present with genital/gynecologic tumors. Sarcoma botryoides may prolapse within the vagina or urethra. Lymphadenopathy, especially in the groin, is common.

Sites of tumor metastasis include the regional lymphatics, lung, liver, bone and marrow, and brain. The disease is often widespread, mandating a meticulous workup to detect all sites and to properly stage the disease. Components of the diagnostic evaluation may include:

1. Complete blood count
2. Liver and renal function studies
3. Skeletal survey and bone scan
4. Chest x-ray
5. CT or MRI of brain, abdomen, and pelvis
6. Analysis of cerebrospinal fluid
7. Abdominal ultrasound
8. Evaluation of upper and lower urinary tract voiding ceptourethrogram (VCUG)
9. Gallium scan to detect involved lymph nodes
10. Cystoscopy and vaginoscopy

Actual diagnosis of rhabdomyosarcoma requires a tissue biopsy, either by endoscopy or laporatomy. The open procedure also allows for scrutiny and sampling of lymph nodes, which is necessary for accurate tumor staging.

**Tumor Staging.** The Intergroup Rhabdomyosarcoma Study (IRS) reported a staging system that is widely accepted, although many large oncologic centers have developed their own adaptation (Table 24–6).

## Treatment

Rhabdomyosarcomas of the bladder and prostate are difficult to manage and are rarely cured by one method of treatment alone. Unlike Wilms' tumor, they are not encapsulated and infiltrate submucosally despite appearing well-differentiated intraoperatively. By the time of diagnosis, approximately 20% of these tumors have spread to the lymphatics through

**TABLE 24–6. Staging and Outcome of Rhabdomyosarcoma**

| STAGE | CRITERIA | PROPORTION OF PATIENTS | 8-YEAR SURVIVAL |
|---|---|---|---|
| I | Localized disease, completely resected (no regional node involvement, confined to muscle or organ of origin, contiguous involvement with infiltration outside the muscle or organ of origin, as through fascial plane). | 15% | 74% |
| II | Grossly resected tumor with microscopic residual disease; no evidence of gross residual tumor; no evidence of regional node involvement. Regional disease, completely resected (regional nodes involved or extension of tumor into an adjacent organ); all tumor completely resected with no microscopic residual tumor. Regional disease with involved nodes; grossly resected, but with evidence of microscopic residual disease. | 25% | 65% |
| III | Incomplete resection or biopsy with gross residual disease. | 41% | 40% |
| IV | Distant metastatic disease present at diagnosis (lung, liver, bones, bone marrow, brain, lymph nodes). | 19% | 15% |

Adapted from Maurer, H. M., Behangady, M., Gehan, E. A., et al. (1988). The Intergroup Rhabdomyosarcoma Study I: A final report. *Cancer, 61*, 209–220. Reprinted by permission.

the blood stream. Treatment is most successfully coordinated by a multidisciplinary team composed of pediatric subspecialists, that is, a pediatric surgeon, radiotherapist, and oncologist.

With the ongoing efforts of the Intergroup Rhabdomyosarcoma Study, it has become obvious that collaborative findings obtained from closely monitored follow-up groups are far more promising than single protocols based on the limited experience of individual practitioners. IRS-IV is open at the present time and is utilizing a modified staging system and more intense treatment protocols based on the evaluation of the tumor site and histology. Table 24–7 summarizes the IRS-IV staging and treatment guidelines.

## Special Considerations

Radiation to the pelvis causes considerable untoward effects, especially for the child. It can cause growth disturbances in the pelvic skeletal structure as well as colonic, rectal, and ovarian complications. The morbidity of radiation and the extent of surgery are major considerations in the care of each child with rhabdomyosarcoma. Many centers begin treatment regimens for patients with pelvic tumors with chemotherapy to shrink the primary tumor and allow for limited surgery. Radiation therapy is not needed if the tumor can be resected with clean surgical margins.

# APPROACHES TO PATIENT CARE

### Assessment

A health assessment and history should be obtained as it is necessary to develop a plan to meet the needs of the child and family. The interviewer should be sensitive to the family's fears and sense of uncertainty with regard to forthcoming tests, treatments, and surgeries. Although the survival rate for urologic malignancies has improved, it does not lessen the dread and anxiety around "cancer, chemotherapy, and radiation." There is also undeniable shock, helplessness, and psychological disarray caused by this crisis. The family is often disoriented by the unfamiliarity of the hospital surroundings. It is also important to provide reassurance to the parents with regard to the lack of emergency behaviors among the medical and nursing staff. It is difficult for parents to comprehend that their child's condition and chance of survival does not warrant emergency intervention.

The accurate assessment of immediate symptoms is necessary to relieve any discomfort for the child. Urinary retention, dysuria, or overflow incontinence; pain on defecation; constipation, or a slight bulging under the perineum can indicate spread to other structures. Sufficient and appropriate analgesia needs to be administered to relieve any pain the child is having. The most effective way to provide pediatric analgesia is oral or continual patient-controlled analgesia or epidural analgesia. All steps are taken to avoid injections.

The initial interview may not provide the nursing staff with an understanding of the family dynamics and needs. The development of a firm and trusting relationship with a primary nurse will provide the parents with an avenue to disclose any feelings of guilt, apprehension, and lack of trust.

The nursing staff should encourage the parents to take breaks away from their child and to be aware of their own physical and emotional well-being. This is often a challenge because the parents feel vulnerable and very needed by their child, with their only comfort and sense of worth coming from this perceived need.

## PRETREATMENT OR PREOPERATIVE PHASE

### Nursing Diagnosis

Nursing diagnosis for the child or parent of a child with a genitourinary malignancy may include the following:

1. Alteration in parenting abilities and patterns related to the diagnosis of their child's illness.
2. Ineffective family coping: compromised related to
   a. Change in environment
   b. Regime of chemotherapy or radiation treatments and inadequate knowledge/understanding of possible side effects.
3. Alteration of body image due to enlarging abdominal mass.

4. Alteration in body function related to encroachment of the tumor on vital structures.
5. Alteration of comfort related to pain from the presence of the tumor.

### Plan of Care

Nursing care is directed toward enabling the patient or parent to

1. Encourage parents/patient to express anxieties and concerns related to their child's/own disease.
2. Discourage indiscriminate palpation of abdominal mass to prevent rupture.
3. Encourage parental discussion of fears related to a change in environment.
4. Provide consistent and accurate information to the parents/patient of disease process, proposed surgical intervention, and chemotherapy treatments and eventual cure.
5. Be sufficiently pain-free to obtain adequate rest and comfort.
6. Have sufficient fluids and total parenteral nutrition to allow for improvement in general condition and to provide adequate hydration and nutritional requirements.
7. Have relief of secondary symptoms associated with the progression of the tumor.
8. Maintain adequate urine flow via insertion of indwelling catheter to relieve urinary obstruction from tumor encroachment.
9. Remain free of urinary tract infection following insertion of Foley catheter.
10. Verbalize an understanding of the medical and surgical management, plan of care, disease process, and prognosis of the neoplasm.

**TABLE 24–7. Intergroup Rhabdomyosarcoma Study Staging and Treatment Guidelines**

| STAGE | CRITERIA | CHEMOTHERAPY | RADIATION |
|---|---|---|---|
| I | All favorable sites, Mo, primary tumor Ta or Tb with no lymph node involvement | Randomized: Vincristine, actinomycin, and cyclophosphamide | No |
| | | OR | |
| II | All favorable sites, Mo, primary tumor Ta, N1 | Vincristine, actinomycin, and ifosfamide | Yes |
| | | OR | |
| III | All unfavorable sites, primary tumor Tb, regional nodes N1 with Mo | Vincristine, actinomycin, and etoposide | Yes |
| IV | All metastatic disease (M1) | May add doxorubicin, cisplatin, dacarbazine, or cyclophosphamide | Not recommended |

Mo, no metastasis; M1, metastasis present; Ta, tumor <5 cm in diameter; Tb, tumor >5 cm in diameter; No, lymph nodes benign; N1, lymph nodes clinically involved.
Data from Maurer, H. M., Beltangady, M., Gehan, E. A., et al. (1988). The Intergroup Rhabdomyosarcoma Study I: A final report. *Cancer, 61,* 209–220. Reprinted by permission.

## Interventions

The medical staff will provide much information on treatment, prognosis, and surgical procedures. It is vital, though, for the primary nurse to be present during these discussions and to become well-acquainted with the options and results of treatments as well as cure rates. This ensures that the nursing staff will provide accurate and consistent information to the parents and the patient.

Initially, parents will be overwhelmed by the amount and content of the information, and may require frequent repetitions and reassurances. They may also be inclined to hang on to the positive prognosis, rather than comprehend the lengthy treatments and surgical interventions. The nurse should reinforce the individual nature of their child's treatment program and reassure parents that a child can sustain an active, healthy life with one functioning kidney or with a urostomy (or other body changes). It is quite common for parents to seek solace from other families and friends during this difficult time, but this often results, unfortunately, in muddled ideas and misinterpretation of health teaching and information. The nurse must be prepared to answer their questions, to clarify teaching, and to provide support.

A child who is being investigated for a tumor requires much support and detailed explanation of the extensive invasive and noninvasive tests required to confirm the diagnosis. It is important to develop a trusting relationship with the child. Honesty is always the best policy. Children have startling abilities if they have trust in their health care team and are provided with accurate information about forthcoming events. It is important not to minimize the pain to be experienced by the child, as this destroys the trust and increases anxiety for the unknown ahead. Testing and surgery should be explained in a simple, concise way, not too far in advance of the impending event.

There are a variety of support mechanisms to assist the child through invasive and painful procedures. They allow the child to have some control over the situation as well as to relax. The preschool child (2–5 years) finds it difficult to concentrate for long periods, so the methods and tools selected for relaxation must appeal to the level of development and cognitive skills. The use of a puppet can be helpful for communicating fears and anxieties. The child is enthralled by the puppet. The operator only needs to suggest a scene or emotion similar to the child's own or potential experience to be rewarded by the response. One soon forgets one's awkwardness in puppeteering.

Play therapy is also used to alleviate stress. Dolls or stuffed toys can be used as recipients of painful procedures and treatments, with minimal equipment. Toys representative of hospital settings can also be helpful. This allows children to recreate a fearful or traumatic scene in their own way. Often the physician or nurse becomes the unsuspecting patient, receiving no treatment to pleasant treatment from the child.

The school-age child requires different aids. The emotional development of a child of this age allows a greater understanding and awareness of the mind and body than with younger children. Relaxation and concentration on a loved pet or object can be used. The therapeutic tools should be selected according to the child's age, maturity, and individual likes. For example, using a windmill to blow to encourage deep-relaxing breathing and blowing bubbles are satisfying and distracting activities. A wand with moving sparkles is hypnotic and soothing. Serene pictures or popular children's characters on the ceiling above a treatment table can also be useful distractors.

The preadolescent and adolescent can use relaxation tapes; either music or specially prepared visual imagery tapes are readily available for use in this age group. Some patients are not helped by the above methods. Hypnosis, biofeedback, and pain specialists are available and have proved to be very successful.

When incontinence is present, measures must be taken to provide frequent cleansing and good hygiene. The use of diapers should be negotiated with older children and adolescents, who see this as a threat to their self-esteem. Relief of constipation may be obtained by dietary modifications if the child is not suffering severe side effects from chemotherapy or from oral medications.

The young child's fear of strangers and the adolescent's fixation on body image and independence are common hurdles to overcome in providing care. A sensitive and compassionate approach to the patient that allows validation of feelings, maintains modesty, and offers choices, when feasible, will help gain cooperation. Nurses must nevertheless act as the patient's advocate in preventing unnecessary manual palpation of any abdominal tumor. Palpation may precipitate rupture and subsequent secondary malignancies. The risk of frequent manual examination, usually by a stranger, is more likely to occur in large teaching centers.

## POSTOPERATIVE PHASE

### Nursing Diagnosis

Nursing diagnosis for the postoperative patient and family may include the following:

1. Pain related to surgery.
2. Impaired physical mobility related to the presence and risk of displacement of drainage/support systems, including a nasogastric tube, urinary catheter, and any other external tubes (oxygen, intravenous (IV), central venous pressure, chest).
3. Body image disturbance related to the presence of a surgical incision.
4. Altered protection related to the effects of presurgical chemotherapy and the surgical insult.
5. Activity intolerance related to the effect of the surgical intervention.
6. Anxiety related to the surgery and technical support equipment.

### Plan of Care

Nursing care is directed toward enabling the patient or family to

1. Be sufficiently pain-free to promote easy mobility, rest, and coping.
2. Resume activities of daily living when the condition permits.
3. Maintain adequate urinary output (1 mL/kg/hr).
4. Maintain patency of all connecting tubes (catheter, IV, nasogastric tube).
5. Maintain accurate and regular recording of vital signs.
6. Maintain a clean, adequately dressed surgical incision.
7. Encourage deep breathing and coughing.
8. Verbalize anxieties of interventions, medications, and diagnosis.
9. Express realistic expectations and understanding of the disease process and prognosis.
10. Participate in direct care.
11. Obtain age-appropriate stimulation for normal growth and development in accordance with the child's physical condition.

### Intervention

Postoperative vital signs should be monitored and recorded every 2 to 4 hours depending on the patient's condition and hospital protocol. The nasogastric tube, if present, should be checked for proper placement. In the initial postoperative period, more than one type of urinary drainage device may be needed. The patency of these tubes as well as the volume and appearance of urinary drainage should be closely monitored. The intravenous/central venous access site needs to be assessed and cared for per institutional practice standards. Observe closely for signs of dehydration (poor skin turgor, sticky mucous membranes, general malaise, and decreasing urinary output).

Analgesia should be given as ordered to keep the child pain-free. The child's response to analgesics should be recorded. The child should be encouraged to move in bed and ambulate on the second postoperative day. Children are usually good monitors of their own capabilities. If they are pain-free and feel well, they can be coaxed by a wheelchair ride or a visit to the playroom or gift shop. If a child refuses to ambulate, the nurse should consider other factors of underlying physical problems requiring medical intervention (i.e., constipation, secondary surgical complications). Incisional care includes cleansing and dressing as well as keeping the surrounding skin as dry as possible to prevent breakdown. An assessment of the wound for signs of infection or dehiscence should be performed on each shift as necessary.

The primary nurse should be certain that the information on the individual patient's disease process and treatment is an accurate reflection of discussions with the surgeon and the oncologist. Although it is important to reassure the family of a successful outcome following the surgical intervention, support is needed to assist them in being realistic about the months of treatment ahead. If possible, arrange for them to meet with the urologic oncology nurse who will be providing outpatient care services. Both the child and parents need to be aware of the side effects of chemotherapy and the possible nausea and vomiting, despite antiemetic agents. There is also the risk of infections, herpetic mouth lesions, and pyrexia due to the drug-induced low white blood cell count.

The loss of hair, including eyebrows and eyelashes, and its emotional impact, depend on the child's age and social activities. Naturally, those of school age are likely to find hair loss far more disturbing than a younger child. The entire body surface should be assessed daily and meticulous hygiene should be adhered to. A sheepskin, air mattresses, or Clinitron beds can be used for the adolescent patient, who may be more susceptible to pressure areas and skin breakdown.

Prior to discharge the parents should be taught to care for the central line and any other unfamiliar body alterations (e.g., urostomy bags). Mouth care is very important for those children requiring chemotherapy. The patient or parents should be instructed to provide the following regular regime twice daily:

Brush teeth and rinse with a mouthwash before and after meals.

Apply petroleum jelly to lips regularly.

Visually check for signs of stomatitis, and if ulcers are found notify the health care professional. A bland diet may be necessary for comfortable eating. Topical anesthetics are available in a viscous compound and may be applied to the ulcers with a cotton-tipped swab. Antifungal agents may be required if *Candida* develops.

### Patient Outcomes

1. The child's pain control is maintained consistently.
2. The child's nutrition is monitored and fluid intake maintained with daily weights and blood work.
3. Peripheral/central lines are correctly monitored to maintain asepsis.
4. The child's urine output is at least 1 mL/kg/hr with a specific gravity below 1.015.
5. Nasogastric tube has remained in the correct position for adequate drainage of stomach fluids.
6. Oral care has been maintained and stomatitis prevented.
7. Skin integrity has been maintained.
8. Wound infection, dehiscence, or delayed healing has not occurred.
9. Frightening procedures are lessened by the use of relaxation or distraction techniques.
10. The parents actively participate with direct care, restoring confidence in their parenting abilities and providing comfort to their child.
11. Parents demonstrate care of central access device prior to discharge.
12. The child responds to parental/nursing encouragement and becomes more cooperative with necessary interventions.
13. The child is able to participate in age-appropriate activities.
14. Parents demonstrate an understanding of treatments, medications, and outpatient appointments prior to discharge.
15. Parents are aware of home care services available to them in their community.

## REFERENCES

Beckwith, J. B., & Perrin, E. V. (1963). In situ neuroblastoma: A contribution to the natural history of neural crest tumors. *American Journal of Pathology, 43,* 1089–1104.

Bernstein, I. D. (1982). Prospects for immunotherapy of neuroblastoma. In A. E. Evans (Ed.), *Advances in neuroblastoma research* (p. 243). New York: Raven Press.

Blute, M. L., Kelalis, P. P., Offord, K. P., Breslow, N., Beckwith, J. B., & D'Angio, G. J. (1987). Bilateral Wilms' tumor. *Journal of Urology, 138,* 968–973.

Brodeur, G. M., Seeger, R. C., Barrett, A., et al. (1988). International criteria for diagnosis, staging and response to treatment in patients with neuroblastoma. *Journal of Clinical Oncology, 6,* 1874–1881.

D'Angio, G. J., Breslow, N., Beckwith, J. B., et al. (1989). Treatment of Wilms' tumor: Results of the Third National Wilms' Tumor Study. *Cancer, 64*(2), 349–360.

Evans, A. E. (1980). Staging and treatment of neuroblastoma. *Cancer, 65,* 1799.

Evans, A. E., D'Angio, G. J., & Randolph, J. (1971). A proposed staging for children with neuroblastoma. *Cancer, 27,* 374.

Gross, R. E., Farber, S., & Martin, L. W. (1959). Neuroblastoma sympatheticum: A study and report of 217 cases. *Pediatrics, 23,* 1179.

Hann, H. L., Levy, H. M., Evans, A. E., & Drysdale, J. W. (1979). Serum ferritin and neuroblastoma (abstract 509). *Proceedings of the American Association Cancer Research Society for Clinical Oncology, 20,* 126.

Hellstrom, K. E., & Hellstrom, I. (1972). Immunity to neuroblastoma and melanomas. *Annual Review of Medicine 23,* 19.

Jaffe, N., McNeese, M., Kayfield, J. K., & Riseborough, E. J. (1980). Childhood urologic cancer therapy, related sequelae and their impact on management. *Cancer, 45,* 1815–1820.

Li, F. P., Williams, W. R., Gimbrere, K., Flamant, F., Green, D. M., & Meadows, A. T. (1988). Heritable fraction of unilateral Wilms' tumor. *Pediatrics, 81*(1), 147–149.

Maurer, H. M., Beltangady, M., & Gehan, E. A., et al. (1988). The Intergroup Rhabdomyosarcoma Study I: A final report. *Cancer, 61,* 209–220.

Mierau, G. W., & Favara, B. E. (1980). Rhabdomyosarcoma in children: Ultrastructural study of 31 cases. *Cancer, 46,* 2035.

Miller, R. W., Fraumeni, J. R., Jr., & Manning, M. D. (1964). Association of Wilms' tumor with aniridia, hemihypertrophy and other congenital malformations. *New England Journal of Medicine, 270,* 922.

Pui, C. H., & Crist, W. M. (1991). Pediatric solid tumors. In A. I. Holleb, D. J. Fink, & G. P. Murphy (Eds.), *American Cancer Society textbook of clinical oncology* (pp. 464–472). Atlanta, GA: American Cancer Society.

Sather, H., Siegel, S., Finkelstein, J., Klemperer, M., Sitarz, A., & Hammond, D. (1981). The relationship of age at diagnosis to outcome for children with metastatic neuroblastoma [abstract]. *Proceedings of the American Society of Clinical Oncology, 22,* 409.

Sawada, T., Takamatsu, T., Tanaka, T., Mino, M., Fujita, K., Kusunoki, T., Arizono, N., Fukuda, M., & Kishida, T. (1981). Effects of intralesional interferon on neuroblastoma: Changes in histology and DNA content distribution of tumor masses. *Cancer, 48,* 2143.

Shimada, H., Chatten, J., Newton, W. A., Sachs, N., Hamoudi, A. B., Chiba, T., Marsden, H. B., & Misugi, K. (1984). Histopathologic prognostic factors in neuroblastic tumors. *Journal of the National Cancer Institute, 73,* 405–416.

Silber, J. H., Evans, A. E., & Fridman, M. (1991). Models to predict outcome from childhood neuroblastoma: The role of serum ferritin and tumor histology. *Cancer Research, 51,* 1426–1433.

Sitarz, A., Finklestein, J., Grosfeld, S., Leikin, S., McCreadie, S., Klemperer, M., Bernstein, I., Sather, H., & Hammond, D. (1983). An evaluation of the role of surgery in disseminated neuroblastoma: A report from the Children's Cancer Study Group. *Journal of Pediatric Surgery, 18,* 147.

Slater, R. M., de Kraker, J., Voute, P. A., & Delemarre, J. F. (1985). A cytogenic study of Wilms' tumor. Cancer genetics. *Cytogenetics, 14,* 95–109.

Snyder, H. M., D'Angio, G. J., Evans, A. E., & Raney, R. B. (1992). Pediatric oncology. In P. C. Walsh, A. B. Retik, T. A. Stamey, & E. D. Vaughan, Jr. (Eds.), *Campbell's urology* (6th ed., pp. 1987–2002). Philadelphia: W. B. Saunders.

Stay, E. J., & Vawter, G. (1977). The relationship between nephroblastoma and neurofibromatosis. *Cancer, 39,* 2550.

Appendix I

# Urologic Instruments

*Nancy C. Brownlee*
*Pamela M. Bilyeu*

## HISTORY OF UROLOGIC INSTRUMENTATION

The historical records of almost all cultures allude to or document the use of instruments in performing surgical procedures. Greece, India, Egypt, and China are among those countries that provide evidence of the first use of instruments for urologic procedures. The most frequent references are to "physicians" who created instruments to remove bladder stones and devised catheters to resolve urinary retention. Of special note is Charaka, an Indian physician of Kaniska, who in the first century A.D. introduced primitive urologic surgery to that country with the use of catheters in patients with urinary retention. In Egyptian medicine, instrumentation is associated with the lithotomist of the day and the various approaches employed for "cutting of the stone."

As the knowledge base grew, examination of the viscera, known as endoscopy, became of interest. In 1806, Phillipp Bozini of Frankfort, Germany, first attempted to see inside the bladder by using a "lichtleiter." The instrument was described as a funnel that was inserted in the urethra and illuminated by a lighted candle. After several attempts by others to develop some type of lighted instrument, Max Nitze, in 1877, produced the first modern cystoscope. This invention brought about the widespread practice of endoscopic examination.

In 1887, Joachin Albarran devised a movable lever (known today as *Albarran's bridge*) to guide catheters and therefore to catheterize a patient. This major technologic advance led to

the development of other devices and techniques used to visualize and manipulate the urinary tract. By the 1950s, technology was advanced enough to have a glass-fiber viewing instrument that improved light transmission to the cystoscopic visual field. Known as *fiberoptics*, the technology is now available in both rigid and flexible endoscopes.

Today, physicians are able to operate on the urinary tract using a variety of sophisticated instruments, in many instances without having an open surgical incision. Among the most common instruments and accessories used by the urologist, and described in this appendix, are the following:

1. Urinary catheters.
2. Instruments used to dilate the urinary tract.
3. Endoscopic instruments to visualize the urinary tract.
4. Equipment designed to biopsy the urinary tract.
5. Devices used in conjunction with endoscopic equipment and designed to manipulate tissue and structures within the urinary tract.
6. Equipment to deliver laser light for tissue destruction.
7. Devices for percutaneous access.
8. Devices for percutaneous ureteral manipulation.
9. Devices for cystoscopic ureteral manipulation.
10. Devices for ureteroscopic manipulation.
11. Ureteral stone extractors.
12. Laser accessories.
13. Stents.

## TABLE I–1. Urologic Instruments Most Commonly Encountered in a Clinical Setting

| NAME | APPEARANCE | PURPOSE/USE | REMARKS |
|---|---|---|---|
| **URINARY CATHETERS** | | | |
| 1. Nélaton red rubber urethral catheter | | One-time, immediate drainage of the bladder; used when indwelling catheter is not needed | Blunt, round-tip straight catheter with one eye |
| 2. Robinson red rubber urethral catheter | | Same as 1. | Round, hollow-tip straight catheter with two eyes |
| 3. Councill red rubber urethral catheter | | Used when passage of a filiform or guide wire is required | Hole at tip |
| 4. Tiemann coudé red rubber urethral catheter | | Used when a catheter must be negotiated through a urethral, prostatic, or bladder neck blockage | Curved, olive-tip catheter with two eyes |

| | Description | Use | Notes |
|---|---|---|---|
| 5. Indwelling Foley urethral catheter | 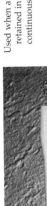 | Used when a catheter must be retained in the bladder for continuous drainage | Various Fr sizes of catheters with 5- or 30-mL balloon |
| 6. Three-way Foley urethral catheter | 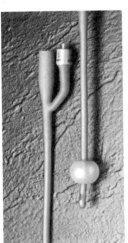 | Used when irrigation of a retention catheter may be needed (e.g., after transurethral resection of the prostate) | Various Fr sizes of catheters with 5- or 30-mL balloon and a third port for irrigation |
| 7. Councill indwelling urethral catheter |  | When insertion of retention catheter must be accomplished with use of filiform or guide wire | Like red rubber catheter, has hole at tip |
| 8. Coudé round-tip Foley urethral catheter | 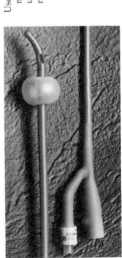 | Used when retention catheter must be passed through urethral, prostatic, or bladder neck blockage | Curved tip |

*Table continued on following page*

**TABLE I–1. Urologic Instruments Most Commonly Encountered in a Clinical Setting** *Continued*

| NAME | APPEARANCE | PURPOSE/USE | REMARKS |
|---|---|---|---|
| 9. Double-balloon Foley urethral catheter | | Used when bladder drainage and pressure on a resected area must be accomplished simultaneously | |
| 10. Malecot catheter | | Sometimes used to drain and irrigate continent reservoirs; for temporary or continuous suprapubic drainage | Self-retaining winged catheter; design may have two or four wings; Stamey type used for suprapubic puncture |
| **INSTRUMENTS USED FOR URETHRAL DILATION** | | | |
| 11. Otis bougie à boule | | Catheterlike device used to dilate urethra; used to calibrate urethral passage | Olive tip; usually available in even sizes from 8–40 Fr |
| 12. Walther sound. *A,* Dilator. *B,* Tapered dilator | | Metal instrument used to dilate female urethra | Tapers toward handle |
| 13. Van Buren sound | | Used to dilate male urethra | Gentle curve in tip |

| 14. Bénique sound | | Same as 13. | Curve in tip is more pronounced than in other sounds |
| 15. LeFort sound | | Often used to dilate severe (usually trauma-induced) urethral strictures in males | Threaded tip for attachment of woven filiform |
| 16. Catheter stylet or guide | | Stiff wire inserted into a channel catheter to make it rigid for easier insertion into the urethra | Another type of guide is the filiform guide wire; has threads at the end to attach filiforms to aid in inserting a Councill catheter |

*Table continued on following page*

**TABLE I–1. Urologic Instruments Most Commonly Encountered in a Clinical Setting** *Continued*

| NAME | APPEARANCE | PURPOSE/USE | REMARKS |
|---|---|---|---|
| 17. Filiforms *(A)* and followers *(B)* | | Used to establish access to the urinary bladder when urethral abnormalities exist or to dilate urethral strictures | Filiform is small and has different-shaped tips; follower attaches to end of filiform once entry to bladder has been established; available in variety of Fr sizes |

**ENDOSCOPIC INSTRUMENTS AND ACCESSORIES**

| | | | |
|---|---|---|---|
| 18. Telescope and lens | | When connected to light cord, lens lights up and magnifies cystoscopic field; different angles give physician the ability to look in all areas | Required for endoscopic procedures. 12° or 30° oblique angle used for viewing urethra and bladder; 70° or 110° lateral angle allows for wide-angle viewing of bladder; 0° angle allows for straight-ahead view of urethra |
| 19. Light cables | | Transmit light from light source to lens | Necessary for endoscopic visualization of urinary tract |

20. Power sources

Electrical device that provides main light source

Same as 19.

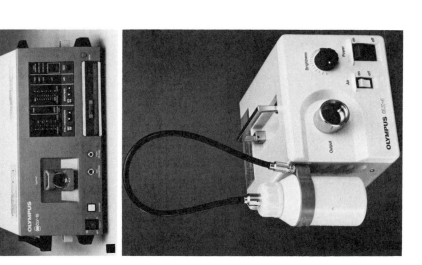

*Table continued on following page*

| NAME | APPEARANCE | PURPOSE/USE | REMARKS |
|---|---|---|---|
| 21. Irrigation sets. *A,* Single. *B,* Dual. | | Tubing that is connected from a bag of solution to the endoscope; used to fill the bladder and wash away debris for better visualization | For cystoscopic procedures, generally only one bag of fluid is used. For prostate surgery, more fluid may be required. The solutions most often used are sterile water and glycerine; normal saline is used for ureteroscopy and continuous bladder irrigation postoperatively |
| 22. Cystourethroscope-urethroscope: sheath (*top*); blind obturator (*middle*); and visual obturator (*bottom*) | | Permits visualization of the lower urinary tract from meatus, through urethra, and into bladder. Rigid cysto-urethroscope that has a sheath made in various sizes and contains ports for irrigation. Through the sheath fits an obturator, which creates a smooth, round nose on the end for safer entrance into the urethra and bladder | Flexible and rigid designs. During cystoscopy, sheaths and obturator are introduced first—all other instruments are then inserted through the sheath or ports. Available in adult and pediatric sizes |
| 23. Lens bridges: straight (*left*); single lumen (*middle*); and double lumen (*right*) | | Most telescope/lens use a bridge to prevent the lens from protruding out the end of the sheath | |
| 24. Albarran's bridge with deflecting mechanism | | Facilitates transurethral catheterization of the ureter, biopsy brushing, and use of biopsy forceps and laser fibers | Fits into a cystoscopic sheath; accommodates a telescope; deflector at distal tip. Bridges also have working ports (e.g., for laser fibers); other type used is Cawood |

25. Stopcock and connecting
    nipple. *A,* Water line adapter
    connecting nipple/Luer-Lok.
    *B,* Water line adapter with
    shut-off valve/Luer-Lok

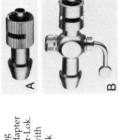
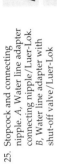

Luer-Lok connectors used to
attach water line or syringes to
cystoscope

26. Rubber tip

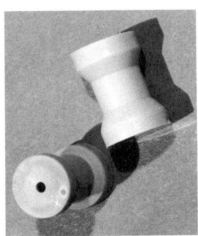

Attaches to metal ports so that
ureteral catheters or guide
wires may be passed through
the cystoscope

Tip has small opening to allow
passage of items such as
catheters and laser fibers but
does not let fluid out

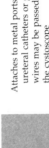

*Table continued on following page*

TABLE I–1. Urologic Instruments Most Commonly Encountered in a Clinical Setting *Continued*

| NAME | APPEARANCE | PURPOSE/USE | REMARKS |
|---|---|---|---|
| 27. Penile clamps. A, Cunningham. B, Baumrucker. C, Zipser | | Used to occlude distal end of penis, usually after instillation of lidocaine jelly before instrumentation | May also be applied for incontinence |
| **EQUIPMENT FOR BIOPSY** 28. Biopsy forceps. A, Closed. B, Open | | Used to obtain tissue specimens from the urethra, bladder, or ureteral orifices | Forceps are passed through the catheter channel of rigid or flexible cystoscope |

29. Cytology brush

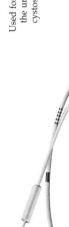

Used for obtaining specimens of the uroepithelium during cystoscopy or ureteroscopy

Available in reusable or disposable form. Brush must be retracted into sheath to have an accurate specimen before it is removed from site

30. Cystoscopic scissors

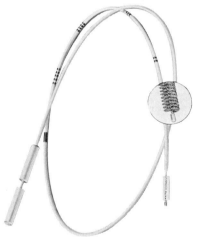

Used for nonelectrical tissue cutting

31. Prostatic biopsy needles and punches. *A,* Tru-Cut biopsy needle. *B,* Buerger prostatic biopsy punch. *C,* Prostatic biopsy aspiration syringe

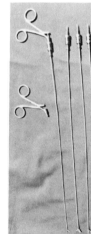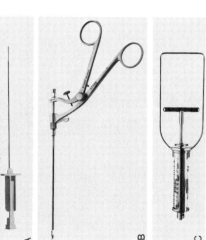

Used to obtain transperineal or transrectal biopsy specimens of the prostate to examine tissue for suspected malignancy

A variety of needles are available. Automatic biopsy systems are used with spring needle for quick and clean split-second sampling

*Table continued on following page*

665

## TABLE I–1. Urologic Instruments Most Commonly Encountered in a Clinical Setting *Continued*

| NAME | APPEARANCE | PURPOSE/USE | REMARKS |
|---|---|---|---|
| **DEVICES USED TO MANIPULATE TISSUE AND STRUCTURES WITHIN THE LOWER URINARY TRACT** | | | |
| 32. *A,* Stone punch. *B,* Lithotrite. *C,* Stone-crushing forceps. *D,* Cystoscopic rongeur | | Used to grasp and crush stones in the bladder | May be introduced through a catheter sheath or passed directly through the urethra |

33. Resectoscope. Working elements: *A*, Iglesias type—passive; *B*, Stern-McCarthy type; *C*, Baumrucker type; *D*, Nesbit type—passive

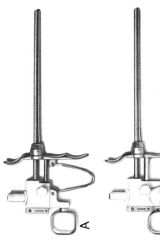

A

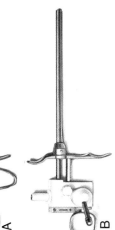

B

C

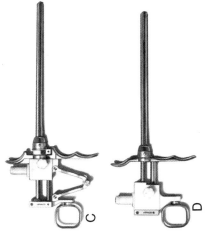

D

A rigid instrument that permits transurethral resection of the prostate and transurethral resection of bladder tumors. If continuous flow, resectoscope is connected by tubing to a pump to allow for emptying of bladder during procedure

Forceps are passed through the catheter channel of rigid or flexible cystoscope. *Iglesias* permits one-handed thumb control, so that prostate may be elevated with free hand. *Stern-McCarthy* is a two-handed element that operates by rack and pinion. *Baumrucker* has spring action that increases stability and reduces fatigue. *Nesbit* works with passive action

34. Electrodes: *A*, Knife; *B*, Roller; *C*, Loop; *D*, Ball; *E*, Loop; *F*, Needle

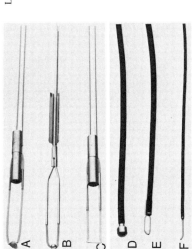

A B C D E F

Loops, blades, or electrodes are attached to the working element for use in combination with items such as lens, catheters, sheaths, and cables during endoscopic procedures. The electrocautery cord is attached to an electrosurgical unit

Specific type selected and used is based on physician preference

*Table continued on following page*

## TABLE I–1. Urologic Instruments Most Commonly Encountered in a Clinical Setting *Continued*

| NAME | APPEARANCE | PURPOSE/USE | REMARKS |
|------|-----------|-------------|---------|
| 35. Urethrotome. *A,* Optical urethrotome. *B,* Urethrotome blades: half-round knife (*upper*); wave-form knife (*middle*); cold knife (*lower*) | | Used to release urethral strictures | Includes lens, sheath, instrument channel, and various styles of cutting knives; blades are connected to electrocautery for ease of cutting |
| 36. Ellik evacuator | | Used to remove clots, tissue, or stones from bladder | Has a bulb and upper and lower bowls; tissue falls into lower bowl, allowing for repeated irrigation and evacuation |

**EQUIPMENT THAT DELIVERS LASER LIGHT FOR TISSUE DESTRUCTION**

37. Lasers—$CO_2$

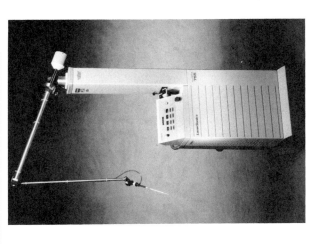

Used in nonendoscopic
procedures for treatment of
external genital lesions, such as
condyloma and carcinoma of
the penis

The $CO_2$ laser uses the $CO_2$
molecule as the active medium.
Its energy is readily absorbed
by water, so most of the energy
from $CO_2$ is absorbed with 0.01
mm of tissue, producing intense
heat and vaporization. Utmost
safety precautions must be
adhered to when using lasers.
Protecting the eyes of the
patient and personnel with
correct eye wear is very
important. Be sure to follow
manufacturer's
recommendations and National
Laser Standards

*Table continued on following page*

## TABLE I-1. Urologic Instruments Most Commonly Encountered in a Clinical Setting *Continued*

| NAME | APPEARANCE | PURPOSE/USE | REMARKS |
|---|---|---|---|
| 38. Lasers—neodymium:yttrium-aluminum-garnet (Nd:YAG) | | Most often used for treatment of bladder tumors | The energy from Nd:YAG is not as easily absorbed by tissue as from $CO_2$ or argon. The Nd:YAG beam is transmitted by optical fibers and passes through water, making it the preferred laser for endoscopic application. The Nd:YAG beam is ideal for treatment of bladder tumors with the use of contact fibers because the laser light may be applied endoscopically to the bladder to cause reproducible full-thickness bladder wall coagulation while maintaining bladder stability and integrity |

**DEVICES FOR PERCUTANEOUS ACCESS**

| NAME | APPEARANCE | PURPOSE/USE | REMARKS |
|---|---|---|---|
| 39. Amplatz renal dilator set | | Used with stiff guide wires for dilation of a percutaneous tract | Sheath permits atraumatic, repetitive in-out passage of scopes and instruments |
| 40. Curved safe T-J guide wire | | Used to establish a percutaneous nephrostomy tract | |
| 41. Renal access catheter | | Used percutaneously to direct a guide wire to a specific site | |
| 42. Amplatz stiff guide wire | | Used with dilators for establishing a percutaneous nephrostomy tract | Fixed core; straight |

43. Lunderquist-Ring torque guide wire

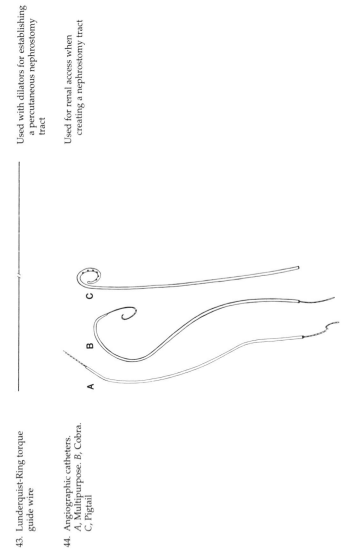

Fixed core with a malleable tip provides rotational control to the distal tip

44. Angiographic catheters. *A*, Multipurpose. *B*, Cobra. *C*, Pigtail

Type used depends on the angle needed

## DEVICES FOR PERCUTANEOUS URETERAL MANIPULATION

45. Ureteropelvic junction occlusion balloon catheter

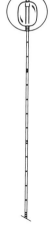

Used to temporarily occlude the ureteropelvic junction to prevent stone fragments from entering the ureter during percutaneous lithotripsy

Contrast medium may also be injected

46. Ultrasonic power source nephroscope and sonotrode

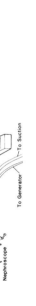

Right-angle nephroscope used for endoscopic examination of renal pelvis. Ultrasonic sonotrode used for fragmenting stones. Sonotrode may be used in the ureter also.

Ultrasonic lithotriptor operated by a foot pedal. Irrigation is used to visualize the collecting system and to assist fragment evacuation.

Table continued on following page

TABLE I–1. Urologic Instruments Most Commonly Encountered in a Clinical Setting *Continued*

| NAME | APPEARANCE | PURPOSE/USE | REMARKS |
|---|---|---|---|
| 47. Percutaneous stone extractor. A, Helical. B, Flat-wire | | Used for stone manipulation in the pelvis under direct vision | The extractor may be introduced percutaneously through any 30-cm cystourethroscope, panendoscope, or endoscope. |
| 48. Malecot nephrostomy catheter | | Used for drainage in the renal pelvis | Also referred to as *mushroom catheter* |
| 49. Smith universal ureteral stent | | Used as a continuous nephroureterostomy stent | |
| 50. Extracorporeal shock wave lithotripsy (ESWL) nephrostomy catheter and stent | | Used to provide nephrostomy or ureteral drainage | |
| 51. Kaye nephrostomy tamponade balloon catheter | | Used for tamponade of nephrostomy tract to control inadvertent hemorrhage | May be used when removing a nephrostomy tube |
| 52. Stamey percutaneous suprapubic catheter | | Used to provide bladder drainage by percutaneous placement of a Malecot (mushroom) catheter. | Softer materials are available with a balloon or a loop for suprapubic placement |

**DEVICES FOR CYSTOSCOPIC URETERAL MANIPULATION**

| NAME | APPEARANCE | PURPOSE/USE | REMARKS |
|---|---|---|---|
| 53. Cohen deflecting guide wire and catheter | | Used to enter displaced ureteral orifice resulting from Cohen transtrigonal ureteral replantation or to negotiate a tortuous or stenotic ureter | Wires may be lubricated to allow for easy passage up the ureter |

| No. | Catheter | Use | Description |
|---|---|---|---|
| 54. | Flexible-tip ureteral catheter | Used for drainage and retrograde pyelogram | Flexible tip allows atraumatic entry of the ureteral orifice and navigation of a tortuous ureter |
| 55. | Whistle-tip ureteral catheter | Used for drainage and retrograde pyelogram | |
| 56. | Round-tip ureteral catheter | Used for drainage and retrograde pyelogram | |
| 57. | Open-end, flexible-tip ureteral catheter | Used for drainage and retrograde pyelogram | The open-end, flexible tip allows for atraumatic placement over a guide wire for negotiation of a looped or stenotic ureter |
| 58. | Spiral-tip ureteral catheter | Used for drainage and retrograde pyelogram | The spiral tip assists in the navigation of a tortuous or partially obstructed ureter |
| 59. | Cone-tip ureteral catheter | Used for retrograde pyelogram | |
| 60. | Rutner universal wedge ureteral catheter. A, Pediatric. B, Adult | Used for retrograde pyelogram | The tip occludes the ureteral orifice and stabilizes the catheter by temporarily wedging in the orifice |

*Table continued on following page*

| NAME | APPEARANCE | PURPOSE/USE | REMARKS |
|---|---|---|---|
| **DEVICES FOR URETEROSCOPIC MANIPULATION** | | | |
| 61. Deflecting guide wire | | Used through flexible or rigid ureteroscope to free or dislodge stones under direct vision | |
| 62. Ureteral dilator set | | Used for dilation of the ureter before ureteroscopy and stone manipulation | Various dilator sizes available |
| 63. Balloon ureteral dilator | | Used for ureteral dilation before ureteral stone manipulation and ureteroscopy | Certain types of balloon catheters may also be used to dilate the musculofascial tract, renal capsule, and parenchyma during percutaneous procedures |
| 64. Inflation gauge | | Used with balloon-dilation catheter to monitor inflation pressure | Uses atmospheres and pounds per square inch |
| 65. Hartley balloon inflation device | | Used for controlled inflation of dilation balloon | Also called a *pressure injector* |
| 66. Rigid ureteropyeloscope with direct and sidearm viewing | | Used to examine ureter and perform procedures through the working channel, such as biopsies, stone basketing, and ultrasonic lithotripsy | A diagnostic ureteroscope is similar to the ureteropyeloscope, except it is shorter and may vary in diameter |

67. Flexible ureteropyeloscope (active)

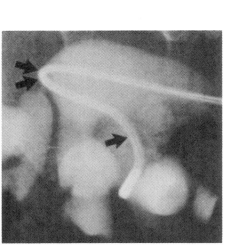

Used for diagnostic and therapeutic procedures involving the renal collecting system

May be referred to as *ureterorenoscope*. An advantage is the manual maneuverability of the distal tip. The deflecting tip allows inspection of virtually all renal calices

68. Flexible ureteroscope (passive)

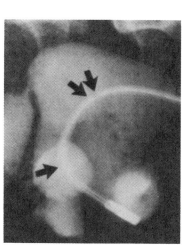

Used for ureteral access with little or no need for dilation. The operator may also perform procedures through the channel

Flexible nephroscopes and cystoscopes are also available

69. Biopsy brush

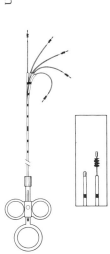

Used to biopsy lesions that cannot be reached in the usual fashion by cup biopsy forceps

*Table continued on following page*

**675**

## TABLE I–1. Urologic Instruments Most Commonly Encountered in a Clinical Setting *Continued*

| NAME | APPEARANCE | PURPOSE/USE | REMARKS |
|------|-----------|-------------|---------|
| 70. Rutner balloon-dilation stone extractor | | Used for ureteral dilation and stone manipulation in the ureter | The balloon assists in the ureteral dilation, and the flexible tip assists in guiding past a stone or up a tortuous ureter |
| 71. Electrohydraulic lithotriptor (EHL) | Electrohydraulic Lithotriptor | Used for fragmenting stones using electrical current. The probe is discharged in a fluid medium to fragment the stone | Irrigation is used for the EHL. May be used in the bladder, ureter, and renal pelvis. Historically, EHL has been used for bladder stones; however, smaller probes (1.9 Fr) are now available for use in the ureter |

### URETERAL STONE EXTRACTORS

| NAME | APPEARANCE | PURPOSE/USE | REMARKS |
|------|-----------|-------------|---------|
| 72. Helical stone extractor. *A,* With filiform. *B* and *C,* 6- and 8-wire helical | A B C | Used for stone manipulation and removal in the urinary tract | May be used with ureteroscope |
| 73. Davis loop stone dislodger | | Used for stone manipulation in the ureter | A monofilament nylon thread passes through angled parts for stone entrapment |

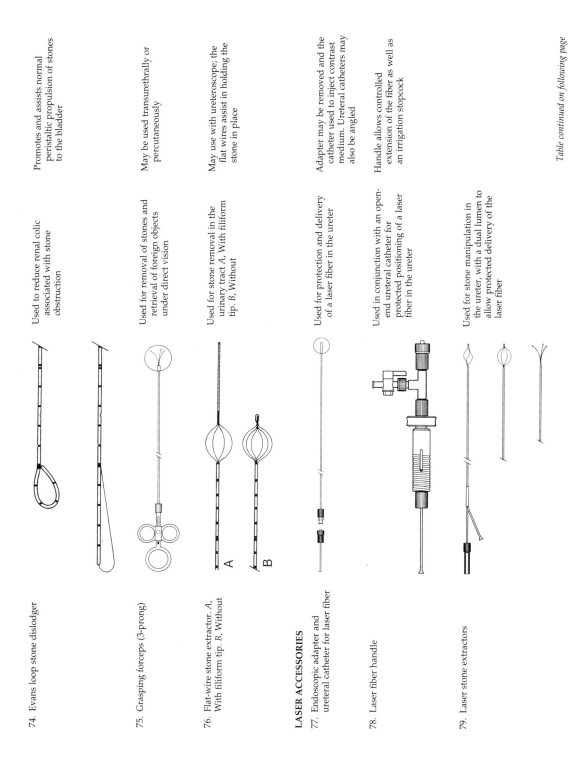

**74.** Evans loop stone dislodger — Used to reduce renal colic associated with stone obstruction — Promotes and assists normal peristaltic propulsion of stones to the bladder

**75.** Grasping forceps (3-prong) — Used for removal of stones and retrieval of foreign objects under direct vision — May be used transurethrally or percutaneously

**76.** Flat-wire stone extractor. *A,* With filiform tip. *B,* Without — Used for stone removal in the urinary tract *A,* With filiform tip. *B,* Without — May use with ureteroscope; the flat wires assist in holding the stone in place

A

B

## LASER ACCESSORIES

**77.** Endoscopic adapter and ureteral catheter for laser fiber — Used for protection and delivery of a laser fiber in the ureter — Adapter may be removed and the catheter used to inject contrast medium. Ureteral catheters may also be angled

**78.** Laser fiber handle — Used in conjunction with an open-end ureteral catheter for protected positioning of a laser fiber in the ureter — Handle allows controlled extension of the fiber as well as an irrigation stopcock

**79.** Laser stone extractors — Used for stone manipulation in the ureter, with a dual lumen to allow protected delivery of the laser fiber

*Table continued on following page*

**677**

**TABLE I–1. Urologic Instruments Most Commonly Encountered in a Clinical Setting** *Continued*

| NAME | APPEARANCE | PURPOSE/USE | REMARKS |
|---|---|---|---|
| **STENTS** | | | |
| 80. Fixed-core straight guide wire | | Used for ureteral stenting and placement of ureteral indwelling stent | |
| 81. Dretler ureteroscopy stent | | Used for postureteroscopy stenting of the ureter | The stent is positioned through the ureteroscope |
| 82. Passive spiral-tip ureteral stent | | Used for temporary stenting of the ureter before, during, and after ESWL | The nylon tether allows removal on an outpatient basis without cystoscopy. The pigtail coil permits retention in the bladder when the spiral tip is located in the renal pelvis |
| 83. Kwart Retro-Inject stent | | Used for retrograde contrast medium injection during ESWL and as internal indwelling ureteral stent after ESWL | |
| 84. Ureteral indwelling double-pigtail stent | | Self-retaining device used for temporary internal drainage from the renal pelvis to the bladder | Stents may be made of different materials, such as polyurethane, soft polyurethane, C-flex, and silicone. Depending on manufacturer may also be referred to as double-J or double-coil stent. |
| 85. Towers peripheral ureteral stent | | Used for temporary internal drainage from the renal pelvis to the bladder | The shape allows peripheral as well as luminal drainage |

Illustration credits are as follows:
Nos. 1–10, 12–17, 27, and 36—Courtesy of Bard Urological Division, C. R. Bard, Inc, Covington, GA.
No. 11—From Walsh, P. C., Gittes, R. F., Perlmutter, A. D., & Stamey, T. A. (Eds.). (1986). *Campbell's urology* (5th ed., p. 521). Philadelphia: W. B. Saunders; with permission.
Nos. 18, 22–26, 31, 32, 34, and 35—Courtesy of Karl Storz, Endoscopy-America, Inc., Culver City, CA.
Nos. 20 and 33—Courtesy of Olympus, Inc., Edina, MN.
No. 21—Courtesy of Baxter Health Care Corporation, Deerfield, IL.
No. 27A and B—From Jeter, K. F., Faller, N., & Norton, C. (1990). *Nursing for continence* (p. 135). Philadelphia: W. B. Saunders; with permission.
No. 27C—Courtesy of Bard Urological and Bard Home Health Division, Murray Hill, NJ.
Nos. 28, 30, 67, and 68—Courtesy of Circon-ACMI, Stamford, CT.
No. 29—Courtesy of Mill-Rose Laboratories, Inc., Mentor, OH.
Nos. 37 and 39—Courtesy of Heraeus Laser-Sonics, Inc., Milpitas, CA.
Nos. 39–43, 45, 47–65, 69, 70, and 72–85—Courtesy of Cook Urological, Spencer, IN.
Nos. 44, 46, 66, and 71—From Clayman, R. V. (1984). *Techniques in endourology.* Chicago: Mosby-Year Book; with permission.

### TABLE I–2. Instruments Required for Operative Procedures

| Procedures | Basic set-up (see Displays) | Bugbee electrodes | Cystourethroscope | Obturator | Bridge | Lens | Water | Glycine | Cautery cord | Resectoscope | Blades or loops | Working element | Ellik | Sachs | Biopsy forceps | Lithotrite rigid | Ultrasound lithotriptor | Electrohydraulic lithotrite | Biopsy needle | Otis urethrotome | Baskets or wires | Balloon and ureteral dilators | Amplatz dilators |
|---|---|---|---|---|---|---|---|---|---|---|---|---|---|---|---|---|---|---|---|---|---|---|---|
| Cystourethroscopy - Flexible | X | | X | | | | X | | | | | | | | | | | | | | | | |
| Adult | X | | X | X | X | X | X | | | | | | | | | | | | | | | | |
| Pediatric | X | | X | X | X | X | X | | | | | | | | | | | | | | | | |
| Metrogram | | | X | X | X | X | X | | | | | | | | | | | | | | | | |
| Prostate biopsy | X | | X | X | X | X | X | | | | | | | | | | | | X | | | | |
| Bladder biopsy | X | X | X | X | X | X | X | | X | X | X | X | X | | X | | | | | | | | |
| Transurethral resection of bladder tumor (TURBT) | X | | X | X | X | X | X | | X | X | X | X | X | | | | | | | | | | |
| Litholapaxy | X | | X | X | X | X | X | | | X | X | X | X | | | X | | | | | | | |
| Direct vision internal urethrotomy (DVIU) | X | | X | X | X | X | X | | X | | X | X | | X | | | | | | X | | | |
| Transuretheral resection of prostate (TURP) | X | | X | X | X | | | X | X | X | X | X | X | | | | | | | | | | |
| Stone manipulation (transurethrally) | X | | X | X | X | X | X | | | | | | | | | | X | X | | | X | X | |
| Percutaneous cystolithotripsy (PCL) | | | | | | X | X | | X | | | | | | | | X | X | | | X | X | X |

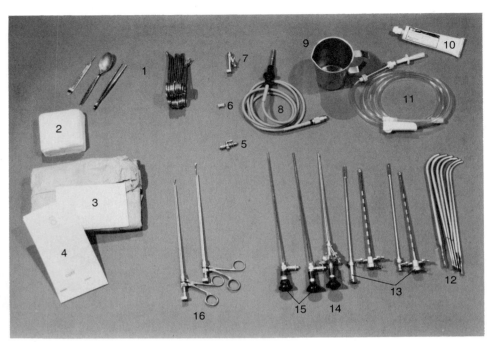

*DISPLAY 1* Basic set-up for cystoscopy. **1.** Vas Set. **2.** Sponges. **3.** Gown. **4.** Gloves. **5.** Fluid Line Adapter. **6.** Rubber Tip. **7.** Bridge. **8.** Light Cable. **9.** Pitcher. **10.** Lubricant. **11.** Fluid Set. **12.** Dilators. **13.** Cystourethroscopes. **14.** Telescope/Bridge. **15.** Telescopes. **16.** Biopsy Forceps. (Courtesy of Pamela Bilyeu.)

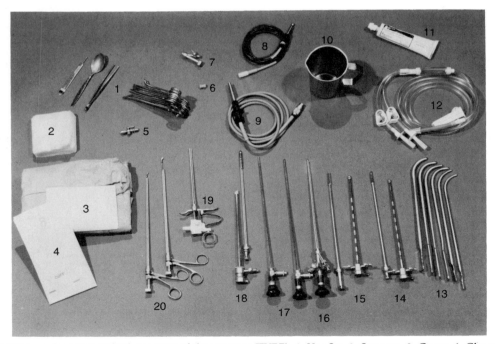

*DISPLAY 2* Set-up for transurethral resection of the prostate (TURP). **1.** Vas Set. **2.** Sponges. **3.** Gown. **4.** Gloves. **5.** Fluid Line Adapter. **6.** Rubber Tip. **7.** Bridge. **8.** Cautery Cord. **9.** Light Cord. **10.** Pitcher. **11.** Lubricant. **12.** Extension Tubing (Y Set). **13.** Dilators. **14.** Cystourethroscope. **15.** Cystourethroscope. **16.** Telescope/Bridge. **17.** Telescope. **18.** Resectoscope. **19.** Iglesias Working Element. **20.** Biopsy Forceps. (Not pictured: loop electrode.) (Courtesy of Pamela Bilyeu.)

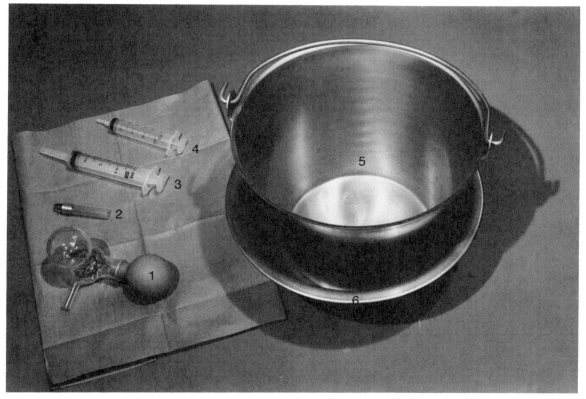

*DISPLAY 3* Additional equipment for transurethral resection of the prostate (TURP). **1.** Ellik Evacuator. **2.** Adapter Between Ellik and Sheath. **3.** Toomey Syringe. **4.** 35-mL Syringe. **5.** Stainless Steel Pail (for irrigation fluid). **6.** Basin. (Courtesy of Pamela Bilyeu.)

## TABLE I–3. Special-Care Instructions for Endoscopic Instruments

1. Handle all instruments with protective gloves.
2. Always follow the manufacturer's recommendations.
3. As soon as the instruments have been used, they should be cleaned of all debris following the manufacturer's recommendations as well as hospital policies and procedures.
4. Instruments should always have all stopcocks opened for cleaning, drying, and soaking purposes.
5. A schedule should be set up so that every stopcock, hinge, joint, and lock is cleaned and lubricated.
6. Handle telescope lenses with care because they are the most expensive part of the instruments. Use distilled water to clean lenses to prevent corrosion.
7. Light cables must be handled with care because they are made of thousands of glass fibers. **Don't** pull, stretch, or coil light cables tightly. Keep light cables clean and scratch free by cleaning with a mild detergent-and-water solution.
8. Sheaths should be cleaned by running water through them as well by using as a soft brush to remove any debris.

Adapted from guidelines prepared by Karl Storz, Endoscopy-America, Inc., Culver City, CA.

## TABLE I–4. Recommendations for Disinfection and Sterilization of Endoscopic Instruments

1. Consult the manufacturer's manuals to identify the recommended sterilization techniques.
2. When disinfection is used, it is recommended that plastic containers be used to help prevent scratches on instruments and eliminate electrolytic corrosion.
3. An EPA-registered hard-surface disinfection solution should be used; avoid solutions containing a surfactant or that have an acidic pH.
4. To prevent damage during disinfection, keep the telescopes separate from the resectoscope sheaths.
5. Make sure that stopcocks are open or disassembled and the obturators have been removed.
6. Rinse the instruments thoroughly (twice in sterile water, in two separate plastic containers with adequate amount of water), because disinfection solutions may cause skin and tissue irritation.
7. Gently moving the instruments in the sterile rinse water helps remove the disinfection solution.
8. After rinsing, transfer the instruments carefully to a sterile table. Dry the instruments thoroughly with sterile sponges.
9. If gas sterilization is to be used to prepare the instruments for procedures, be sure the instruments are disassembled, clean, and dry. Place high-frequency cords and each resectoscope blade in an individual Steri-peel pack.
10. Place individual instruments to be gassed in a large tray on a layer of cloth.
11. *Instruments must be aerated according to the manufacturer's recommendations.*

EPA, Environmental Protection Agency.
Courtesy of Karl Storz, Endoscopy-America, Inc., Culver City, CA.

## TABLE I–5. Methods of Instrument Sterilization and Disinfection*

| INSTRUMENTS | METHODS | | |
|---|---|---|---|
| | Disinfection | Gas Sterilization | Steam Sterilization |
| Bugbee electrodes | Yes | Yes | No |
| Cystourethroscope with obturator | Yes | Yes | Check with manufacturer |
| Bridge | Yes | Yes | Check with manufacturer |
| Lens | Yes | Yes | Check with manufacturer |
| Cautery cords | Yes | Yes | No |
| Resectoscope with obturator | Yes | Yes | Check with manufacturer |
| Blades, loops, and electrodes† | Check with manufacturer | Yes | No |
| Working elements | Yes | Yes | Check with manufacturer |
| Urethrotome | Yes | Yes | Depends on type; check with manufacturer |
| Biopsy forceps—flexible, rigid | Yes | Yes | Check with manufacturer |
| Scissors—flexible, rigid | Yes | Yes | Check with manufacturer |
| Light cables | Yes | Yes | No |

*Rapid, low-temperature sterilization has been recently introduced and may be used for any of the instruments listed. Always follow manufacturer's recommendations.
†Many manufacturers now provide these items in sterile packaging for single use only.
Courtesy of Karl Storz, Endoscopy-America, Inc., Culver City, CA.

# Appendix II

# Imaging Procedures

*Karen A. Karlowicz*
*Nancy J. Reilly*

## TABLE II. Imaging Procedures

| PROCEDURE | DESCRIPTION | PURPOSE AND INDICATIONS | NURSING CARE | COMPLICATIONS |
|---|---|---|---|---|
| KUB (kidneys, ureters, and bladder) | Plain film; visualizes the abdomen and surveys the urinary tract; determines the size, shape, and placement of urologic structures; detects gross structural abnormalities | Often used as an initial diagnostic test for acute flank pain or as a follow-up after treatment of stone disease | Explain procedure, allaying any fears patient may have to x-ray exposure; administer mild laxative the night before procedure, if ordered | None expected |
| Intravenous pyelogram (IVP) or excretory urogram | Contrast material is injected intravenously, either as a bolus or drip infusion; through a series of radiologic films, the contrast material is observed as it passes through the urinary tract; a final film is taken after the patient voids the contrast material | Indications include the identification and evaluation of renal masses, stones, hematuria, hydronephrosis, obstructive uropathy, and congenital anomalies of the urinary tract; renal function may be grossly assessed by the kidney's ability to clear the contrast material; the postvoiding film may indicate the efficiency of bladder emptying; the IVP is rarely used in neonates owing to the risk of volume overload from injection of contrast material, immature proximal tubular reabsorption, and the inability to adequately excrete the contrast material | Patients should be questioned about any known sensitivities to contrast material, iodine, or iodine-containing foods, as well as any allergies to shellfish; steroids may be administered before the procedure to those with known sensitivities to ensure safe completion of the test; a laxative preparation and dietary restrictions are necessary 24 h before the procedure; carefully explain the preparation and procedure; patients with renal failure, labile diabetes or myeloma or those in severely dehydrated states should not undergo an IVP; the IVP is also contraindicated during pregnancy | Hypersensitivity to contrast material may result in pruritus, skin flushing, or difficulty in breathing; a severe anaphylactic reaction may occur in those with an unknown sensitivity to the contrast material; in rare instances, acute renal failure may be precipitated by the use of a contrast material |

*Table continued on following page*

## TABLE II. Imaging Procedures *Continued*

| PROCEDURE | DESCRIPTION | PURPOSE AND INDICATIONS | NURSING CARE | COMPLICATIONS |
|---|---|---|---|---|
| Retrograde pyelogram | A cystoscope is inserted into the urethra under local or regional anesthesia; a ureteral catheter is then passed up into the ureter and contrast material is injected; radiologic films are taken to observe the reverse dispersion of contrast material | Used to visualize the ureters, renal pelvis, and calices when an IVP has failed to adequately highlight these structures; often performed before extracorporeal shock wave lithotripsy in patients with radiolucent stones or as part of a follow-up regimen for patients with urologic cancer who are allergic to intravenous injection of contrast material | Explain procedure and use of anesthesia; ensure dietary restrictions, and administer any ordered medications, including steroid or analgesic, before the procedure; after the procedure, monitor vital signs, measure intake and output amounts, and observe for hematuria and any signs of infection that may result from instrumentation | Possible complications include hematuria, infection, urinary retention, and perforation of the ureter or renal pelvis |
| Antegrade pyelogram | Contrast material is injected percutaneously into the renal pelvis either using a small needle or through a nephrostomy tube; radiologic films are taken as the contrast material travels down the ureter | Performed on patients with ureteral abnormalities that prevent passage of a ureteral catheter or when an IVP is contraindicated after ureteral diversion; it is most commonly performed to evaluate the upper urinary tract after renal surgery for kidney stones when a nephrostomy tube is already in place; often done in conjunction with the Whitaker perfusion test, which measures ureteropelvic pressure to determine the severity of upper urinary tract obstruction | Explain the procedure, and administer any prophylactic steroids or pain medications before it; after the procedure, monitor vital signs, measure intake and output amounts, and observe for signs of infection and hematuria; if procedure was performed with a small needle via percutaneous puncture, the puncture should be dressed and observed for urine drainage or infection | Possible complications include tissue damage as a result of renal puncture, hematuria, infection, and perinephric hematoma |
| Cystogram | Contrast material is injected into the bladder via a transurethral catheter until the bladder is filled; radiologic films of the bladder are then taken, and the contrast material is drained out through the catheter; a final x-ray film is taken after the bladder has been emptied | Evaluates the bladder for gross abnormalities; done after bladder surgery to check for extravasation; used to detect large tumors, bladder diverticula or fistulas, and vesicoureteral reflux; may reveal a voiding disorder; also used to assess bladder injuries as a result of pelvic trauma and in patients with enteritis, diverticulitis, or endometriosis if bladder involvement is suspected; should not be done during pregnancy | If the patient does not have an indwelling catheter, explain that catheterization is required; patients allergic to contrast material may require a steroid preparation; after the procedure, assess the patient for irritative voiding symptoms | Extravasation of contrast material through a small bladder perforation may occur but is usually harmless; systemic absorption of contrast material through the bladder wall is rarely enough to cause a reaction |
| Loopogram | Retrograde injection of contrast material through a stoma and into a pouch or ileal conduit; permits visualization of the anatomic structures of the surgically created urinary diversion | Used to evaluate for ureteroileal obstruction, anastomotic leaks, calculi, abscesses or fistulas, and reflux | Explain that a catheter is inserted into the stoma to permit injection of the contrast material; patients allergic to contrast material may require a steroid preparation; after the procedure, monitor the stoma site for signs of irritation or infection | The risk of systemic absorption of contrast material through bowel used to create the diversion is greater than the risk of absorption through bladder wall |

**TABLE II. Imaging Procedures** *Continued*

| PROCEDURE | DESCRIPTION | PURPOSE AND INDICATIONS | NURSING CARE | COMPLICATIONS |
|---|---|---|---|---|
| Nephrostogram | Contrast material is injected into an existing nephrostomy tube; serial radiologic films are taken as the material passes through the tube and kidney and into the ureter | Used to determine the patency of a nephrostomy tube and the integrity of an obstructed, injured, or repaired ureter | Same as for antegrade pyelogram | Possible complications include hematuria, infection, and irritation as a result of manipulating the nephrostomy tube |
| Voiding cystourethrogram (VCUG) | Through fluoroscopic monitoring, the dynamics of urine storage and bladder emptying are filmed; the study requires that a urethral catheter be inserted and contrast material instilled into the bladder via the catheter; when the patient feels the urge to void and the bladder has been sufficiently filled, the catheter is removed and the patient is asked to void | Used to evaluate the lower urinary tract in patients with voiding dysfunction; commonly employed as a diagnostic aid to establish vesicoureteral reflux, posterior urethral valves, and urethral diverticulum; may be done after urethral surgery to evaluate the integrity of the lower urinary tract and surgical site | Same as for cystogram; contraindicated in patients with suspected urinary tract infection | Same as for cystogram |
| Retrograde urethrogram | Also known as *injecting urethrography*; contrast material is injected retrograde into the urethra to enable visualization of the urinary outlet from the meatus to the bladder neck | Always performed before urethral catheterization if urethral trauma is suspected; used to identify and evaluate abscesses, diverticula, strictures, and other urethral obstructions | Encourage fluids and frequent bladder emptying to relieve irritative voiding symptoms that may persist after the procedure; contraindicated for patients with urinary tract infections or acute urethritis | None expected |
| Vasography | Intraoperative procedure that usually requires a scrotal incision; contrast material is injected into either the vas deferens or the ejaculatory ducts; supine and oblique radiographic films of the pelvis are then taken | Used for evaluation of male infertility if the patient's history, physical examination, and semen analysis suggest obstruction of the ejaculatory ducts or vas deferens | Check scrotal incision site for signs of inflammation | Stricture formation has been suggested as a possible complication but is considered a rare occurrence |
| Cavernosography | Radiologic visualization of the superficial dorsal and deep dorsal veins of the penis; study may require local anesthesia to permit injection of radiopaque contrast medium into the one or both corpora; radiologic films are then taken at specified intervals | Valuable in evaluating impotence, Peyronie's disease, penile trauma, priapism, and metastatic carcinoma of the penis | Explain procedure; check injection site for signs of inflammation or swelling; apply pressure dressing and elevate penis, if necessary | Penile edema with tenderness that may last for hours to a few days; extracorporeal extravasation or development of a hematoma is also possible |

*Table continued on following page*

## TABLE II. Imaging Procedures *Continued*

| PROCEDURE | DESCRIPTION | PURPOSE AND INDICATIONS | NURSING CARE | COMPLICATIONS |
|---|---|---|---|---|
| Lymphangiography | Oily contrast is injected into the lymph system, usually from a site in the foot, to permit visualization of the lymph nodes. Radiologic films are taken during the injection of contrast material, with additional x-ray films required after 24 h for visualization of lymph nodes | Used primarily to detect metastases to the pelvic, inguinal, and retroperitoneal lymph nodes that may occur in advanced stages of cancer of the penis, testes, prostate, and bladder; sometimes used as a diagnostic tool in staging of genitourinary cancers; however, CT scanning and lymph node needle aspiration are considered safer, more important, and more reliable diagnostic tests | Administer prophylactic analgesia before the procedure, if ordered; afterward, observe for signs of shortness of breath, chest pain, fever, or hypotension; also observe injection site for swelling or inflammation, and apply warm compresses; bed rest for 24 h after procedure is usually recommended; elevation of the affected extremity helps reduce edema; contrast material injected may cause skin to be blue tinged and urine and stool to be discolored for as long as 48 h | Infection at the incision or insertion site; pulmonary edema or embolism; chronic edema of legs |
| Angiography (renal arteriogram) | With fluoroscopic monitoring, a catheter is inserted percutaneously at about the L1–L2 interspace or into the femoral artery; contrast material is then injected at a rate of approximately 25 mL/s as x-ray films are taken at serial intervals; an aortogram is often performed as a screening study before renal angiography | Used to evaluate patients who have sustained renal trauma, suspected renal or adrenal masses, hypertension, and acute renal failure; also included in preoperative assessment of renal donors | Carefully explain procedure to the patient; administer analgesia before the procedure, if ordered; after the procedure, monitor vital signs, check injection site for bleeding, swelling, and inflammation, and assess the lower extremities for alteration in neurologic status (e.g., numbness, tingling, and decreased movement) | Renal tissue damage, altered renal function, and altered neurologic function of the lower extremities; at the entrance site of the catheter, localized bleeding may occur; arterial thrombosis, arterial dissection, dislodgement of plaques or thrombi, false aneurysm formation, and arteriovenous fistula formation may also result |
| Computed axial tomography (CT scanning) | Multiple views of a patient are obtained as the x-ray beam is rotated around the body; a computer reconstructs the image and displays it as a digital matrix to provide a cross-sectional view of the body that is seen on x-ray film in varying shades of gray; oral and intravenous contrast material may be administered | Urologic indications include the evaluation of genitourinary and adrenal masses, traumatic injuries to the urinary tract, lymph node involvement in metastatic disease, renovascular disease, nephrolithiasis, and chronic renal infections | Explain procedure; determine if there are any sensitivities to contrast agents; administer preprocedure sedative or steroid if needed or ordered | Radiation exposure is minimal and does not usually pose a threat; any complications that do occur are most often related to the administration of contrast material |

TABLE II. Imaging Procedures *Continued*

| PROCEDURE | DESCRIPTION | PURPOSE AND INDICATIONS | NURSING CARE | COMPLICATIONS |
|---|---|---|---|---|
| Ultrasonography | A transducer is passed over the skin, which has been covered with a conductive gel; internal structures are visualized in real time for the investigator to appreciate three-dimensional organ movement | Multiple urologic indications, including routine screening of kidneys, ureters, bladder, prostate, and testes; instrumental in evaluating clinical problems such as congenital anomalies of the urinary tract, inflammatory conditions and abscesses, calcifications, hydronephrosis, renal failure, renal masses, hematomas, and prostate tumors; useful for assessing arterial and venous blood flow of the penis when evaluating impotency; also used to guide aspiration and biopsy needles, as well as percutaneous injections; there are no contraindications to ultrasonography; the noninvasive nature of ultrasonography makes this an ideal diagnostic procedure for pediatric patients | Explain procedure, and indicate that exposure of the lower abdomen and genitalia may be required for adequate visualization; a bladder ultrasound examination requires a full bladder, and fluids should be encouraged in preparation for the study | None expected |
| Nuclear scans | Requires injection of radioisotopes into the circulatory system; with a special scanning camera, the radioisotopes are then monitored as they move through the vascular network of various organs; some of the more common radioactive tracers used include $^{99m}$Tc-DPTA to assess renal function and for nuclear cystograms, $^{99m}$Tc-DMSA to assess for renal masses, and $^{99m}$Tc bound to methylene diphosphonate for bone scans | Urologic indications for nuclear medicine studies include evaluation of acute and chronic renal failure, renal masses, hydronephrosis, renal blood flow and function before and after renal transplant, as well as evaluation of metastatic bone disease associated with genitourinary carcinoma; the low amount of radiation exposure during nuclear studies makes these diagnostic procedures especially useful in the pediatric population, with nuclear voiding cystograms now state-of-the-art for assessment of vesicoureteral reflux in children | Advise the patient that the radioisotope injection is done at a specified time before the study to achieve concentration of the radioactive tracer in the organ(s) to be evaluated; after the procedure, fluids should be encouraged and intake and output levels monitored; some institutions may require that patients be placed on radiation precaution for at least 24 h after the study | Hypersensitivity reactions to the radioisotopes are rare; nuclear studies are contraindicated during pregnancy |
| Magnetic resonance imaging (MRI) | Scanning procedure that analyzes the magnetic energy in the nuclei of biologic tissue; the resulting image has a brightness that is relative to the number of hydrogen ions in the anatomic site being studied and may be viewed in the coronal, sagittal, or transverse plane | Used to evaluate soft tissue, including the retroperitoneum, abdomen, pelvis, bladder, and prostate | Before the patient enters the MRI area, anything metallic should be removed, including jewelry and clothing with metal fastenings—even purses with credit cards should be left behind; a sedative may need to be administered before the procedure, because claustrophobia in the MRI magnetic tube is often a problem for patients | No known complications; however, MRI is contraindicated in patients with pacemakers, surgical clips, or any metallic foreign body in the eye or elsewhere; MRI scanning is difficult when the patient is grossly obese |

$^{99m}$Tc-DPTA, Technetium 99m diethylene triamine pentaacetic acid; $^{99m}$Tc-DMSA, technetium 99m dimercaptosuccinic acid.

# Appendix III

# Information Resources

*Janice Robinette*
*Karen A. Karlowicz*

This appendix contains a listing of educational and professional resources of interest to the urologic care provider. Included are disease-related organizations, government agencies, professional organizations, and inservice education resources. Although this listing in no way represents a complete compilation of all resources the urologic care provider may access for personal, professional, and clinical development, it does represent the organizations or agencies that offer specific educational-informational programs and publications related to urologic diseases and disorders.

**TABLE III. Urology Care Provider: Professional and Educational Resources**

| FOCUS | ORGANIZATION/RESOURCE | PURPOSE AND DESCRIPTION | SOURCE OR CONTACT |
|---|---|---|---|
| **Disease-Related Organizations** | American Association of Tissue Banks (AATB) | Provides a list of those facilities that practice AATB standards; among lists available are AATB-associated human semen cryobanks in the United States and Canada | Jeanne C. Mowe, Executive Director, 1350 Beverly Rd., Suite 220-A, McLean, VA 22101—(703) 827-9582; FAX: (703) 356-2198 |
| | American Cancer Society, Inc. | National health organization dedicated to eliminating cancer as a major health problem by preventing cancer, saving lives from cancer, and alleviating patient suffering through research, education, and patient services | American Cancer Society, Inc., 1599 Clifton Rd., NE, Atlanta, GA 30329—for information and referral to any state branch of the Society, call 800-ACS-2345 |
| | American Diabetes Association | To improve the well-being of all people with diabetes through information and research to prevent and cure diabetes; referral to local groups | American Diabetes Association, 1660 Duke St., Alexandria, VA 22314—(703) 549-1500 or 800-ADA-DISC |
| | Juvenile Diabetes Foundation International | To support and fund research to find the cause and cure of diabetes and its complications | Juvenile Diabetes Foundation International, 432 Park Ave. South, New York, NY 10016—(212) 889-7575 or 800-JDF-CURE |
| | March of Dimes Birth Defects Foundation | Nonprofit organization dedicated to the promotion of healthy babies and the prevention of prematurity and birth defects | March of Dimes Birth Defects Foundation, 1275 Mamaroneck Ave., White Plains, NY 10605—check telephone directory for the address and phone number of the nearest local chapter |
| | Multiple Sclerosis Society | Dedicated to finding a cause and cure for multiple sclerosis; information and referral organization providing counseling, education, advocacy, and medical equipment assistance; 144 chapters and branches nationwide | Multiple Sclerosis Society, 205 E. 42nd St., New York, NY 10017-5706—(212) 986-3240; Information hotline: 800-624-8236; check telephone directory for address and phone number of the nearest local chapter |
| | Muscular Dystrophy Association (MDA) | Committed to combating 40 neuromuscular diseases through worldwide research, a national network of clinics providing comprehensive medical services, and far-reaching professional and public education | Muscular Dystrophy Association, 3561 East Sunrise Dr., Tucson, AZ 85718—(602) 529-2000; check telephone directory for address and phone number of the nearest local office |

| | | |
|---|---|---|
| National Easter Seal Society | Information and services for disabled children and adults | National Easter Seal Society, 70 Eastlake St., Chicago, IL 60601—(312) 726-6200; check telephone directory for address and phone number of the nearest local chapter |
| National Kidney Cancer Association | Dedicated to providing information to patients and health care providers, encouraging research, and advocating for kidney cancer patients and families | National Kidney Cancer Association, Suite 2100, 320 North Michigan Ave., Chicago, IL 60601—(312) 372-5777 |
| National Kidney Foundation, Inc. | Dedicated to seeking answers to kidney and urinary tract disease through prevention, treatment, and cure; offers professional, patient, and public education materials | National Kidney Foundation, John Davis, Executive Director, 30 East 33rd St, New York, NY 10016—(212) 889-2210; (800) 662-9010 |
| National Rehabilitation Association | Nonprofit organization committed to enhancing the lives of people with disabilities; information and referrals on request | National Rehabilitation Association, 633 S. Washington St., Alexandria, VA 22314—(703) 836-0850 |
| Polycystic Kidney Research Foundation | To promote research into the cause and cure of polycystic kidney disease | Polycystic Kidney Research Foundation, Jean G. Bacon, President and CEO, 922 Walnut St., Kansas City, MO 64106—(816) 421-1869 |
| Spina Bifida Association of America | Offers education and support to families who have a child with spina bifida as well as provides resources to health care providers who care for these patients | Spina Bifida Association of America, 1700 Rockville Pike, STE 250, Rockville, MD 20852-1654—(301) 770-7222; (800) 621-3141 |
| United Network for Organ Sharing | Maintains recipient registry for all patients in the United States who are waiting for donated organs; also maintains a follow-up database on transplants | United Network for Organ Sharing, Gene Pierce, Executive Director, P.O. Box 13770, 1100 Boulders Parkway, STE 500, Richmond, VA 23225—(804) 330-8500 |
| United Ostomy Association, Inc. | Offers educational and product information about ostomies to professionals and the public | United Ostomy Association, Inc., 2001 West Beverly Blvd., Los Angeles, CA 90057—(213) 413-5510 |
| **Government Agencies** Centers for Disease Control and Prevention (CDC) • CDC Recommendations and Treatment Guidelines • Morbidity and Mortality Weekly Report | Statistics, current research findings, and treatment recommendations for STDs and other communicable diseases | Centers for Disease Control, Atlanta, GA 30333—(404) 639-3311 |

*Table continued on following page*

**TABLE III. Urology Care Provider: Professional and Educational Resources** *Continued*

| FOCUS | ORGANIZATION/RESOURCE | PURPOSE AND DESCRIPTION | SOURCE OR CONTACT |
|---|---|---|---|
| | National Cancer Institute (NCI) | Institute within the National Institutes of Health dedicated to the study of cancer | National Cancer Institute, National Institutes of Health, Bethesda, MD 20892—(301) 496-5583 |
| | National Information Center for Handicapped Children and Youth | Provides information regarding educational rights and specialized services | National Information Center for Handicapped Children and Youth, P.O. Box 1492, Washington, DC 20013—(703) 893-6061 |
| | National Institute on Aging (NIA) | Institute within the National Institutes of Health dedicated to the study of aging and needs of the geriatric population | National Institute on Aging, National Institutes of Health, Federal Building, RM 6C12, Bethesda, MD 20892—(301) 496-1752 |
| | National Institute for Diabetes and Digestive and Kidney Diseases (NIDDK) | Institute within the National Institutes of Health dedicated to the study of aging and needs of the geriatric population | National Institute for Diabetes and Digestive and Kidney Diseases, National Institutes of Health, Bethesda, MD 20892—(301) 496-3583 |
| | World Health Organization | Reports on STDs, AIDS, and other communicable diseases; international publications, including statistics and conference proceedings | World Health Organization, Geneva, Switzerland |
| **Professional Organizations** | | | |
| *Multidisciplinary* | Association for the Care of Children's Health (ACCH) | Group of child life specialists, child health nurses, social workers, parents, and others; offers large selection of resources and materials, including parent guides and hospital guidelines | Association for the Care of Children's Health, 3615 Wisconsin Ave., NW, Washington, DC 20016 |
| | Association for Continence Advice—United Kingdom (ACA) | A multidisciplinary group of health care professionals with a special interest in the promotion of continence and the management of incontinence | Association for Continence Advice, c/o Disabled Living Foundation, 380/384 Harrow Rd., London, W9 2HU—(071) 266-3704; FAX: (071) 266-2922 |
| | International Continence Society (ICS) | Group of international health care professionals with clinical and research expertise related to urinary incontinence | International Continence Society, 11 West Graham St., Glasgow G4 9LF, Scotland—(041) 332-6061 |
| *Nursing* | American Association of Spinal Cord Injury Nurses (AASCIN) | Rehabilitation of persons with spinal cord injury; expertise in neurogenic bladder management | American Association of Spinal Cord Injury Nurses, 75-20 Astoria Blvd., Jackson Heights, NY 11370-1178—(718) 803-3782 |

| Organization | Description | Contact |
|---|---|---|
| American Nephrology Nurses' Association (ANNA) | To protect the future of quality care through continuing education, research, standards of clinical practice, quality assurance activities, certification, and interdisciplinary communication and cooperation | American Nephrology Nurses' Association, P.O. Box 56, North Woodbury Rd., Pitman, NJ 08071—(609) 589-2187 |
| American Urologic Association Allied, Inc. (AUAA) | Organization of urologic allied health care professionals dedicated to quality urologic patient care through unity and education | American Urologic Association Allied, Inc., Heather Renehan, Executive Director, 11512 Allecingie Parkway, Richmond, VA 23235—(804)379-1306; FAX: (804) 379-1386 |
| Association of Rehabilitation Nurses (ARN) | Association of nurses who specialize in rehabilitative patient care | Association of Rehabilitation Nurses, 5700 Old Orchard Rd., First Floor; Spokie, IL 60077-1024—(708) 966-3433; FAX: (708) 966-9418 |
| Wound, Ostomy and Continence Nurses Society (WOCN) | Association of nurses who specialize in the prevention of pressure ulcers and the management and rehabilitation of persons with stomas, wounds, and incontinence | Wound, Ostomy and Continence Nurses Society, 2081 Business Center Dr., STE 290, Irvine, CA 92715—(714) 476-0268 |
| International Society of Nurses in Cancer Care | Worldwide organization dedicated to the sharing of knowledge and problems related to oncology nursing care | c/o *Cancer Nursing: an International Journal for Cancer Care*, Lenox Mill Station, P.O. Box 1022, New York, NY 10021 |
| Oncology Nursing Society (ONS) | Sharing knowledge, expertise and problems related to oncology nursing nationwide | Oncology Nursing Society, 1016 Greentree Rd., Pittsburgh, PA 15220-3125—(412) 921-7373 |
| Urology Nurses Interest Group (Canada) | Canadian organization of nurses, formed in 1988, to advance the specialty of urology nursing in order to enhance patient care through a sharing of expertise | Urology Nurses Interest Group (Canada) c/o Kathleen MacMillan, RN, MA, Nursing Administration, Mount Sinai Hospital, RM 342, 600 University Ave., Toronto, Ontario MG5 1X5—or—c/o Debbie Steele, RN, Nursing Manager—Urology Services, Sunnybrook Medical Center, 2075 Bayview Ave., Toronto, Ontario M4N 3M5 |
| ***Urologic Medicine*** | | |
| American Urological Association (AUA) | Professional organization for urologists; publications include the *Journal of Urology* and *AUA Today* (bimonthly newsletter) | G. James Gallagher, Executive Director, 1120 North Charles St., Baltimore, MD 21201—(301) 727-1100 |
| AUA Office of Education | Provides educational programs and services for urologists as well as residents and fellows | Dr. Joseph N. Corriere, Jr., Director of Education, William A. Brubaker, CPA, CAE, Assistant Director, 6750 West Loop South, STE 900, Bellaire, TX 77401—(713) 665-7500 |

*Table continued on following page*

**TABLE III. Urology Care Provider: Professional and Educational Resources** *Continued*

| FOCUS | ORGANIZATION/RESOURCE | PURPOSE AND DESCRIPTION | SOURCE OR CONTACT |
|---|---|---|---|
| | Urodynamics Society | To advance and disseminate scientific knowledge related to the dynamics and bioengineering of the genitourinary system as related to the diagnosis, treatment, and management of voiding dysfunction | Urodynamics Society, Edward J. McGuire, MD, President, 2916 TC/Box 0330, University of Michigan Medical Center, 1500 East Medical Center Dr., Ann Arbor, MI 48109—(313) 936-5775 |
| **Inservice Education Resources** | | | |
| *Cancer: Prostate* | Zoladex | Videotape teaches staff how to inject Zoladex pellet | ICI Pharma, A Division of ICI Americas, Inc., Wilmington, DE 19897 |
| | *Innovations in Urology Nursing* | A quarterly publication with articles written by nurses, for nurses, about prostate cancer | |
| *Child Development* | Case Studies in Human Growth and Development (1986) | 3/4" videocassette—15-minute audiotape: 5-min case studies of newborn, infant, elementary age, and teenage child | Ohio Regional Medical Audio-Visual Consortium, Health Science Communication Center, Case Western Reserve University, Cleveland, OH 44106 |
| | Clinical Advances in the Care of Young Infants—credit: Russel W. Steele, MD (1986) | 3/4" videocassette; color; 48 min | Network of Continuing Medical Education, Roche Laboratories, Nutley, NJ 07110 |
| | A Developmental Approach to Well-Baby Care—credit: Raymond Steuner, MD (1983) | 3/4" videocassette; color; 52 min | |
| | Denver Developmental Materials, Inc. | Programs and tools to screen for developmental delay, including DDST, DASE, and DEST | Denver Developmental Materials, Inc., P.O. Box 6919, Denver, CO 80206-0919—(303) 355-4729 |
| | Kansas Infant Development Screen | An item-based tool to assess for developmental delay | University of Kansas Medical Center, Department of Community Health, 39th Street & Rainbow Blvd., 225 Family Practice Blvd., Kansas City, KS 66103 |
| | Revised Parent Development Questionnaire | Response questionnaire | Benjamin Pasananick, Albany Medical College, Albany, NY 12208 |
| | Techniques of Developmental Assessment: II—credit: Brian Stahler (1976; revised 1981) | 3/4" videocassette 19 min; includes booklet; describes the Denver Developmental Screening Test | Health Sciences Consortium, University of North Carolina at Chapel Hill, Carrboro, NC 27516 |

| | | | |
|---|---|---|---|
| | A Young Child is . . . —credit: Harry Hamp (1983) | ¾" videocassette; 27 min; shows activity of children from 3 months to 4½ yr | Educational Improvement Center, Lawrence Productions, Inc., Mendocino, CA |
| *Clear Intermittent Catheterization (CIC)* | Clear intermittent catheterization—Principles of a successful program (1994). Clinical Education Series. Published by Mentor Urology | Videotape program for health care professionals; discusses indications, contraindications, and the CIC care regimen | Mentor Urology, 5425 Hollister Ave., Santa Barbara, CA 93111—(800) 328-3863 |
| *Cystoscopy* | Outpatient Male Cystoscopy | Videotape shows the use of lidocaine (Xylocaine) jelly with male cystoscopy | Astra Pharmaceuticals, 50 Otis St., Box 4500, West Borough, MA 01581-9981—(800) 225-6333 |
| *Human Embryology* | O'Rahilly, R. (1975). *A Color Atlas of Human Embryology, Part 7—Urogenital System.* | 37 color slides plus booklet | W. B. Saunders Co., Philadelphia, PA 19106 |
| | The Genitourinary System in the Newborn. *Pathology of the newborn* series (Vol. I, number 3, 1986) | Slide series of congenital genitourinary defects often seen in the newborn | Wyeth Laboratories, P.O. Box 8299, Philadelphia, PA 19101 |
| *Incontinence* | Incontinence Assessment and Management: A Self-Study Health Care Program | A self-study continuing education program that is designed to improve skills for making an informed assessment of incontinence problems; 22-page booklet with assessment guide and application for CEU credit | Kimberly-Clark Corp., 2100 Winchester Rd., Neenah, WI 54956—(800) 558-6423 |
| | Working With the Incontinent: A Community Education Kit for Health Care Professionals | Contains slides accompanied by a script, brochures, charts, and evaluations | |
| | Rehabilitating for Continence | Complete inservice training kit for long-term care staffs, includes a monograph for nurses (with assessment forms), handbooks and cue cards for aides, and training guide to help staff developers coordinate training | Beverly Foundation, 70 South Lake, Suite 750, Pasadena, CA 91101—(818) 792-2292 |
| | Diagnosis and Management of Incontinence: A Handbook for Health Care Professionals | Overview of incontinence, including types, causes, neuroanatomy, treatments, and decision tree | Marion-Merrell-Dow, P.O. Box 8480, Kansas City, MO 64114-0480 |
| | Urinary Incontinence | Videotape describing causes, basis of diagnostic studies, and treatments for urinary incontinence | Prospect Associates, Suite 500, Dept. UI-1801, Rockville Pike, Rockville, MD |

*Table continued on following page*

**TABLE III.** Urology Care Provider: Professional and Educational Resources *Continued*

| FOCUS | ORGANIZATION/RESOURCE | PURPOSE AND DESCRIPTION | SOURCE OR CONTACT |
|---|---|---|---|
| *Ostomy* | Types of Ostomies | Describes indications, patient characteristics and management considerations, and recommendations for people with a colostomy, ileostomy, or urostomy | Hollister, Inc., 2000 Hollister Dr., Libertyville, IL 60048 |
| *Ureteroscopy* | Retrograde Stone Manipulation | Videotape demonstrates procedure | Astra Pharmaceuticals, 50 Otis St., Box 4500, West Borough, MA 01581-9981—800-225-6333 |
| | Ureteroscopy | Videotape shows the use of lidocaine (Xylocaine) jelly with ureteroscopy | |
| *Urology: General* | Education Resource Directory | Annotated reference of all abstracts accepted for the "Pearls," Rosetta Stone, and Research Sessions for AUAA's Annual Conference; published in the fall following each Annual Conference | American Urological Association Allied, Inc., 11512 Allecingie Parkway, Richmond, VA 23235—(804) 379-1306 |
| | Patient/Family Educational Resource Directory | A 40-page reference directory of patient education materials, catalogued by topic. $20 members/ $25 nonmembers | |
| | *Urologic Nursing* | Official journal of the AUAA. Contains clinical and scientific articles of interest to urologic nurses; published quarterly by Mosby-Year Book | Mosby-Year Book, 11830 Westline Industrial Dr., St. Louis, MO 63146—(314) 872-8370 |

# Index

Cerebellar ataxia, voiding dysfunction due to, 379t
Cerebellum, in bladder function, 21
Cerebral trauma, voiding dysfunction due to, 379t
Cerebrovascular disease, and impotence, 336
   voiding dysfunction due to, 379t
Cervix, inspection of, 66
Chancroid, 204–205, *205*
   assessment of, 216t
Chemolysis, of stones, 195
Chemotherapy, for penile cancer, 299–300
   for prostate cancer, 278
   intravesical, 244, 249, 249t
Chief complaint, 37
   in children, 445–446
Childhood Depression Assessment Tool, 468, 469t
Children, congenital anomalies in. See *Congenital anomalies.*
   developmental assessment of, 453–454, *460–463*
   developmental tasks of, 470t–480t, *474–477*
   effect of urologic dysfunction on, 466–468
   enuresis in, 599–604, *602, 603*
   evaluation of, 454–456, 456t, *460–463*
   health history for, 445–448, 447t
   malignant tumors in, approaches to patient care for, 649–653
   morbidity in, 441–442
   myelodysplasia in, 604–613, 605t, *606, 607,* 608t, *612*
   neuroblastoma in, 641t, 643–647, 645t
   neurogenic bladder in, 604–605, 605t, *606, 607,* 608t, *612*
   physical examination of, 448–454, 449t–450t, *450–454,* 455t
   rhabdomyosarcoma in, 647–649, 648t–650t
   sacral agenesis and spinal dysraphism in, 613–615
   urinary tract infections in, assessment of, 492–494
      classification of, 490
      defined, 483–484
      etiology of, 485–487
      intervention for, 495–496
      medical-surgical management of, 488–492
      nursing diagnosis for, 494
      pathophysiology of, 487–488
      patient outcomes with, 496–497
      plan of care for, 494–495
      prevalence and incidence of, 485
      recurrent, 487
      risk factors for, 485–486
   urine output in, 459t
   urodynamics in, 615–618, 615t, *617*
   voiding profile for, 446, 447t
   Wilms' tumor in, 639–643, 641t–643t
Chlamydial infection, 202, 216t
Chordee, 312
   and hypospadias, 511
   approaches to patient care for, 319–320
   assessment of, 45, 58, 319
   dorsal, 566, 571
   etiology and pathophysiology of, 318–319
   treatment of, 319, 513
Chyluria, 34
Cigarette smoking, and impotence, 336
Circumcision, 499–502
   and urinary tract infections, 485, 500
Clean intermittent catheterization (CIC), 594
   for myelodysplasia, 607, 610, 611–613, *612*
   for urinary tract infections in children, 491–492
   for voiding disorders, 405–406
   inservice education resources on, 695t
Clean intermittent self-catheterization (CISC). See *Clean intermittent catheterization (CIC).*

Clitoris, anomalies of, 453
   embryology of, 8
Clitoromegaly, 621
Clitoroplasty, 628–630, *630*
Cloaca, 4
   embryology of, 6, 567, *568*
Cloacal exstrophy, 566, 567–568
Clomiphene (Clomid), for infertility, 366
Clotting studies, 82
CMG (cystometrogram), 386–387, *387*
Cohen deflecting guide wire and catheter, 672t
Colic, 34, 43
Collagen injections, 392
Collecting ducts, anatomy of, 10
   embryology of, 6
Colporrhaphy, anterior, 390
Colposuspension, Burch, 390
Combination therapy, defined, 272
Compensation, 108
Computed axial tomography (CT scanning), 686t
Concept formation, 465
Condom catheter, 401
Condylomata acuminata, 209, 312, 325, 327
   assessment of, 216t, 328
Congential adrenal hyperplasia (CAH) 622–623, *626, 632*
Congenital anomalies, autosomal recessive polycystic kidney disease as, 536–538
   ectopic ureter as, 544–545
   etiology of, 442, 443t, 444t
   history of, 48
   impotence due to, 338
   infertility due to, 362, 363
   megaureter as, 547–549, *548*
   multicystic dysplasia of kidney as, 539–542, *540*
   of ureter, approaches to patient care for, 553–558
   organic malformations associated with genitourinary, 442, 444t
   prune belly syndrome as, 558–562, *559, 560*
   renal agenesis as, 528–532, *529*
   renal ectopia or renal fusion as, 532–534, *532, 533*
   renal hypoplasia as, 534–536
   ureteral agenesis as, 545
   ureteral duplication as, 547
   ureteral stricture as, 549
   ureterocele as, 545–547
   ureteropelvic junction obstruction as, 550–551
   ureterovesical junction obstruction as, 553
   urinary tract infections due to, 485
   vesicoureteral reflux as, 551–553, *552*
Conn's syndrome, 222
Consciousness level, 67
Constipation, 484
   and urinary tract infection, 486, 493, 496
Contigen injections, 392
Continence, 20
Continency star chart, 602, *603*
Continent cutaneous urinary diversion, 244, 257–260, *257–260*
   nursing care for, 264–266, 267, 268
Contingency management, 398t
Contralateral, defined, 87, 108
Contusion, 412
   renal, 414, *415*
Conus medullaris, in bladder function, 21
Coping skill, 465
Core-needle biopsy, 277
Corpus cavernosum, 4, 29
   during erection, 341, *343*
Corpus spongiosum, 4, 29